Problem Solving in
PEDIATRIC IMAGING

Problem Solving in
PEDIATRIC IMAGING

Edited by
Sarah Sarvis Milla, MD, FAAP
Chief, Radiology at Children's Hospital Colorado
Vice Chair, Department of Radiology
Professor, Radiology and Pediatrics
University of Colorado School of Medicine
Aurora, CO
USA

Shailee Lala, MD
Clinical Associate Professor
Department of Radiology
NYU Grossman School of Medicinee
New York, NY
USA

LIBRARY OF
CONGRESS
SURPLUS
DUPLICATE

ELSEVIER

Elsevier
1600 John F. Kennedy Blvd.
Ste 1800
Philadelphia, PA 19103-2899

Notice

Practitioners and researchers must always rely on their own experience and knowledge in evaluating
and using any information, methods, compounds or experiments described herein. Because of rapid
advances in the medical sciences, in particular, independent verification of diagnoses and drug dosages
should be made. To the fullest extent of the law, no responsibility is assumed by Elsevier, authors,
editors or contributors for any injury and/or damage to persons or property as a matter of products
liability, negligence or otherwise, or from any use or operation of any methods, products, instructions,
or ideas contained in the material herein.

Library of Congress Control Number: 2021939948

Senior Content Strategist: Melanie Tucker
Content Development Manager: Meghan Andress
Content Development Specialist: Kevin Travers
Publishing Services Manager: Shereen Jameel
Senior Project Manager: Manikandan Chandrasekaran
Cover Design and Design Direction: Bridget Hoette

Printed in India

Last digit is the print number: 9 8 7 6 5 4 3 2 1

Working together
to grow libraries in
developing countries

www.elsevier.com • www.bookaid.org

To my sons, Anderson and Jameson, I hope you will always have curiosity to learn, openness to uncertainty and new experiences, and willingness to share your knowledge and teach others with compassion.

Huge thank you to my partner in this book: Dr. Shailee Lala, who is one of the smartest radiologists I have ever met and an amazing, kind, and caring human being.

Additional and sincere thanks to all the authors of chapters and to Elsevier for their patience and expertise!
*— **Sarah Sarvis Milla***

To
Sarah Milla, for her mentorship
Aditya, Radha, and Akhil, for their patience and love
And Mom, Dad, and Sona, for a lifetime of support.
*— **Shailee Lala***

Contributors

Adina L. Alazraki, MD, FAAP
Associate Professor
Department of Radiology & Imaging Sciences
Department of Pediatrics
Emory University School of Medicine
Children's Healthcare of Atlanta
Atlanta, GA
USA

Michael Baldwin, MD
Attending Physician
Department of Radiology
Connecticut Children's Medical Center
Hartford, CT
USA

Gerald G. Behr, MD
Associate Clinical Member
Memorial Sloan Kettering;
Associate Clinical Professor
Weill Cornell Medical College
New York, NY
USA

Frederic J. Bertino, MD
Senior Clinical Associate
Department of Radiology & Imaging Sciences
Division of Interventional Radiology and Image
    Guided Medicine
Division of Pediatric Radiology
Emory University School of Medicine
Children's Healthcare of Atlanta
Atlanta, GA
USA

Puneet Bhatla, MBBS, MD
Director
Pediatric and Congenital Cardiovascular Imaging in De-
    partment of Pediatrics
Associate Professor
Pediatrics and Radiology
NYU Langone Medical Center
New York, NY
USA

Mark Bittman, MD
Assistant Professor
Department of Radiology
New York Presbyterian – Weill Cornell
New York, NY
USA

Sarah Dantzler Bixby, MD
Associate Professor of Radiology
Radiology
Boston Children's Hospital
Boston, MA
USA

Kiery Braithwaite, MD, FAAP
Associate Professor
Department of Radiology & Imaging Sciences
Department of Pediatrics
Emory University School of Medicine
Children's Healthcare of Atlanta
Atlanta, GA
USA

Dorothy Bulas, MD
Chief, Division of Diagnostic Imaging and Radiology
Childrens National Hospital
Professor of Pediatrics and Radiology
George Washington University
Washington, DC
USA

Michael J. Callahan, MD
Section Chief, Body Imaging
Clinical Director, Computed Tomography
Boston Children's Hospital;
Associate Professor of Radiology
Harvard Medical School
Boston, MA
USA

Jeanne S. Chow, MD
Associate Professor
Harvard Medical School;
Pediatric Radiologist
Boston Children's Hospital
Boston, MA
USA

Neena A. Davisson, MD
Department of Radiology & Imaging Sciences
Division of Interventional Radiology and Image-Guided
    Medicine
Emory University School of Medicine
Atlanta, GA
USA

Nilesh K. Desai, MD
Vice Chief, Quality and Safety
Chief, Division of Neuroradiology
Department of Radiology
Texas Children's Hospital;
Associate Professor of Radiology
Baylor College of Medicine
Houston, TX
USA

Paula Dickson, MD
Department of Radiology & Imaging Sciences
Department of Pediatrics
Emory University School of Medicine
Children's Healthcare of Atlanta
Atlanta, GA
USA

Azam Eghbal, MD
Medical Director
Radiology
Children Hospital of Orange County
Orange, CA
USA

Meryle J. Eklund, MD, FAAP
Associate Professor
Departments of Radiology and Pediatrics
Medical University of South Carolina
Charleston, SC
USA

Thierry A.G.M. Huisman, MD, PD, EDiNR, EDiPNR, FICIS
Professor of Radiology, Pediatrics, Neurosurgery,
    Neurology and OBGYN
Radiologist-in-Chief and Edward B. Singleton Chair of
    Radiology
Texas Children's Hospital and Baylor College of
    Medicine
Houston, TX
USA

Craig Johnson, DO
Division Chief
Interventional Radiology
Nemours Children's Hospital;
Assistant Professor
Radiology
University of Central Florida
Orlando, FL
USA

Matthew M. Jones, MD
Northwest Radiology Network and Peyton Manning
    Children's Hospital at Ascension St. Vincent
Medical Director of Pediatric Radiology
Indianapolis, IN
USA

Amy W. Lai, MD
Pediatric Radiologist
Radiology
John Muir Medical Center
Walnut Creek, CA
USA

Shailee Lala, MD
Clinical Associate Professor
Department of Radiology
NYU Grossman School of Medicine
New York, NY
USA

Sonali Lala, MD
Assistant Professor
Department of Radiology
New York–Presbyterian Columbia University
New York, NY
USA

Jenna Le, MD
Assistant Professor
Department of Radiology, Division of Musculoskeletal
    Radiology
Montefiore Medical Center/Albert Einstein College of
    Medicine
Bronx, NY
USA

Robert D. MacDougall, PhD
Leader, Medical Affairs
Canon Medical Systems USA
Tustin, CA
USA

Alexis B.R. Maddocks, MD
Pediatric Radiology Fellow
Department of Radiology
Children's Hospital of Philadelphia
Philadelphia, PA
USA

Mesha L.D. Martinez, MD
Pediatric Radiology Fellow
Department of Radiology
Children's Hospital of Philadelphia
Philadelphia, PA
USA

William P. McCullough, MD
Pediatric Radiology Fellow
Department of Radiology
Children's Hospital of Philadelphia
Philadelphia, PA
USA

Sarah J. Menashe, MD
Assistant Professor
Department of Radiology
University of Washington School of Medicine
Seattle, WA
USA

Sarah Sarvis Milla, MD, FAAP
Chief, Radiology at Children's Hospital Colorado
Vice Chair, Department of Radiology
Professor, Radiology and Pediatrics
University of Colorado School of Medicine
Aurora, CO
USA

Shreya Mozer, MD
Instructor of Radiology
Pediatric Radiologist
Boston Children's Hospital
Boston, MA
USA

Michael Norred, MD
Medical University of South Carolina
College of Medicine
Charleston, SC
USA

Tina Young Poussaint, MD, FACR
Lionel W. Young Chair in Radiology
Boston Children's Hospital;
Professor of Radiology
Harvard Medical School
Boston, MA
USA

Christian Restrepo, MD
Baylor College of Medicine
Houston, TX
USA

Edward J. Richer, MD
Assistant Professor
Department of Radiology & Imaging Sciences
Department of Pediatrics
Emory University School of Medicine
Children's Healthcare of Atlanta
Atlanta, GA,
USA

Erica L. Riedesel, MD
Assistant Professor
Department of Radiology & Imaging Sciences
Department of Pediatrics
Emory University School of Medicine
Children's Healthcare of Atlanta
Atlanta, GA
USA

Diana P. Rodriguez, MD
Radiologist
Radiology
Nationwide Children's Hospital
Columbus, OH
USA

Bradley S. Rostad, MD
Assistant Professor
Department of Radiology & Imaging Sciences
Department of Pediatrics
Emory University School of Medicine
Children's Healthcare of Atlanta
Atlanta, GA
USA

Sabah Servaes, MD
Associate Professor
Department of Radiology
University of Pennsylvania and The Children's Hospital of
    Philadelphia
Philadelphia, PA
USA

Victoria Michelle Silvera, MD
Associate Professor
Mayo Clinic
Rochester, MN
USA

Naomi Strubel, BS, MD
Assistant Professor
Department of Radiology
New York University School of Medicine
New York, NY
USA

Benjamin Taragin, MD, FACR
Clinical Associate Professor
Department of Radiology
Rutgers University
New Brunswick, NJ
USA;
Associate Professor
Medical School for International Health at Ben Gurion
    University
Israel

Mahesh Thapa, MD, MEd, FAAP
Professor
Department of Radiology
University of Washington School of Medicine
Seattle, WA
USA

Justin T. Tretter, MD
Assistant Professor of Pediatrics
The Heart Institute
Cincinnati Children's Hospital Medical Center
Cincinnati, OH
USA

Smyrna Tuburan, MD
Assistant Professor
Department of Radiology & Imaging Sciences
Department of Pediatrics
Emory University School of Medicine
Children's Healthcare of Atlanta
Atlanta, GA
USA

Jennifer A. Vaughn, MD
Assistant Professor
Department of Radiology, Phoenix Children's Hospital
University of Arizona College of Medicine
Creighton University School of Medicine
Department of Neuroradiology at Barrows Neurological
    Institute
Phoenix, AZ
USA

Matthew Jason Winfeld, MD
Section Chief Pediatric Radiology and OB/GYN imaging
Lancaster General Hospital
Lancaster, PA
USA

Contents

SECTION 1   Chest (Pulmonary/ Cardiac)

1 Imaging the Child With Respiratory Distress 3
Erica L. Riedesel

2 Mediastinal Masses 33
Mark Bittman

3 Approach to Congenital Heart Disease 53
Justin T. Tretter and Puneet Bhatla

SECTION 2   Gastrointestinal

4 Vomiting Infant 81
Naomi Strubel

5 Pediatric Abdominal Pain 98
Adina L. Alazraki and Edward J. Richer

6 Abdominal Masses in Children 127
Benjamin Taragin, Sonali Lala, and Jenna Le

SECTION 3   Genitourinary

7 Scrotal Pain and Swelling 151
Amy W. Lai

8 Imaging Approach to Urinary Tract Dilation 171
Jeanne S. Chow

9 Pelvic Pain 195
Paula Dickson

SECTION 4   MSK

10 Imaging the Limping Child 213
Shreya Mozer and Sarah Dantzler Bixby

11 Skeletal Dysplasias 235
Neena A. Davisson, Adina L. Alazraki, Shailee Lala, and Sarah Sarvis Milla

12 Approach to Pediatric Foot 254
Sarah J. Menashe and Mahesh Thapa

13 Approach to Pediatric Elbow 266
Kiery Braithwaite

14 Imaging Approach to Pediatric Bone Lesions 286
Michael Baldwin

15 Vascular Malformations 313
Frederic J. Bertino

16 Approach to Pediatric Soft Tissue Masses 327
Craig Johnson, Michael Norred, and Christian Restrepo

17 MSK Trauma 346
Azam Eghbal

SECTION 5   General

18 Imaging of the Neonate: Preterm Infant 355
Smyrna Tuburan

19 Imaging of the Neonate: Term Infant 368
Gerald G. Behr

20 Abusive Head and Spinal Trauma 396
Victoria Michelle Silvera

21 Child Abuse (Radiology) 416
Alexis B. R. Maddocks, Mesha L.D. Martinez, William P. McCullough, and Sabah Servaes

22 Dose Optimization and Risk Management in Pediatric CT 429
Robert D. MacDougall, Matthew M. Jones, Shreya Mozer, and Michael J. Callahan

SECTION 6   Fetal

23 Fetal Body MRI 445
Dorothy Bulas and Matthew Jason Winfeld

24 Fetal CNS MRI 472
    Nilesh K. Desai and Sarah Sarvis Milla

SECTION 7 Brain

25 Pediatric Head CT 493
    Jennifer A. Vaughn and Tina Young Poussaint

SECTION 8 Head and Neck

26 Approach to Lateral Neck
    Radiographs 511
    Meryle J. Eklund

27 Pediatric Head and Neck Masses 521
    *Bradley S. Rostad, Adina L. Alazraki, and Erica L.
    Riedesel*

SECTION 9 Spine

28 Imaging of the Pediatric Cervical
    Spine 551
    Diana P. Rodriguez

29 Neonatal Spine Imaging 578
    Thierry A.G.M. Huisman and Sarah Sarvis Milla

30 Imaging of Back Pain 592
    Diana P. Rodriguez

Index 615

Chest (Pulmonary/ Cardiac)

CHAPTER 1
Imaging the Child With Respiratory Distress

Erica L. Riedesel

CHAPTER OUTLINE

Basic Chest Radiograph Interpretation, 3
  "A" for "Airway", 3
  "B" for "Bones", 3
  "C" for "Cardiac" and Mediastinal Structures, 4
  "D" for "Diaphragm", 5
  "E" for "Effusions", 6
  "F" for Lung "Fields", 6
  "G" for "Gastric" Bubble and "Gas" Pattern, 7
  "H" for "Hilum", 7
Differential Diagnosis of Respiratory Distress by Age, 8
  Toddler and Young Child, 8
    Airways, 10

  Reactive Airways Disease/Asthma, 11
  Infection, 12
  Viral Bronchiolitis, 14
  Bacterial Pneumonia, 14
  Aspirated Foreign Body, 19
  Older Child and Adolescent, 20
    Community-Acquired Pneumonia, 20
    Acute Chest Syndrome, 21
    Cystic Fibrosis, 23
    Spontaneous Pneumothorax, 26
Summary, 27

Respiratory distress is one of the most common complaints seen in the pediatric urgent care or emergency department setting. Clinically, respiratory distress is characterized by tachypnea, increased respiratory effort, and poor oxygenation. Radiographs remain the primary imaging modality for evaluation of the pediatric chest because of low cost and easy availability.

A full understanding of normal anatomy on chest radiograph is necessary to recognize important pathology in the setting of respiratory distress. Thus the first portion of this chapter will focus on the normal appearance of fundamental anatomy in children of different ages.

The second portion of this chapter will focus on an organized differential diagnosis of the most common causes of respiratory distress by age, highlighting important diagnostic findings on chest radiographs. Other modalities such as ultrasound, computed tomography (CT), and magnetic resonance imaging (MRI) will be briefly mentioned.

■ Basic Chest Radiograph Interpretation

As with all radiology, approaching the pediatric chest radiograph with a systematic search pattern ensures that important structures are seen and evaluated on each and every study. A common search pattern for chest radiographs is the "ABCDEFGH" checklist. We will use this model to review the fundamentals of pediatric chest radiograph interpretation with a special emphasis on the normal appearance of structures by age.

"A" for "Airway"

A careful evaluation of the trachea should be performed on both frontal and lateral chest radiographs. On the frontal view, normal "shouldering" of the subglottic trachea is seen at the inferior margin of the vocal folds (Fig. 1.1). The intrathoracic trachea is slightly shifted into the right mediastinum in the setting of a normal left aortic arch.

Special attention should be given to the normal appearance of the proximal thoracic trachea in expiration. In the infant and young toddler, the cervical trachea is quite mobile and may buckle at the thoracic inlet on expiration (Fig. 1.2).

"B" for "Bones"

As with adult chest radiographs, evaluation of the bones in the chest can add important information regarding patient position and respiratory effort.

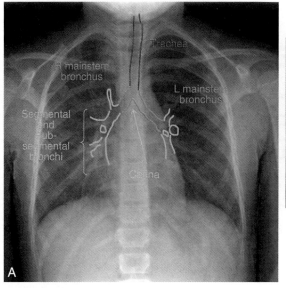

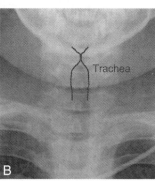

Fig. 1.1 Normal appearance of airway on chest radiograph. (A) Postero-anterior (PA) view of the chest showing the normal thoracic trachea and central airways. (B) Coned down PA view of the chest showing subglottic trachea. Note the normal "shouldering" of the air column. *L,* Left; *R,* right.

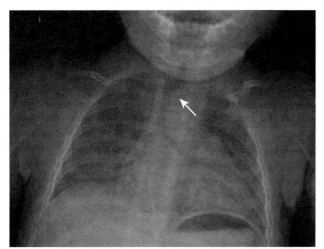

Fig. 1.2 Anteroposterior (AP) view of the chest showing the normal "buckled" appearance of proximal thoracic trachea during expiration, often seen in young children.

In a well-aligned posteroanterior (PA) or anteroposterior (AP) chest radiograph, the spinous processes of the thoracic vertebral bodies should form a vertical line down the center of the thoracic spine, and the medial ends of the clavicles should be equidistant from the center line of the spine.

Lung inflation can be determined by counting the number of posterior ribs (Fig. 1.3). In the newborn, 8 to 9 posterior ribs should be visualized above the associated hemidiaphragm. In toddlers and young children, normal pulmonary inflation is 8 to 10 ribs expansion. In older children and adolescents, normal pulmonary inflation is 10 to 12 ribs expansion. Others use anterior ribs, typically 6 anterior ribs completely above the hemidiaphragm contour.

During this step of chest radiograph evaluation, bones of the thorax should be carefully assessed for fracture. This is especially important in infants and young children because posterior and anterior rib fractures,

scapula fractures, or humeral fractures may be the first and most subtle signs of nonaccidental trauma (Fig. 1.4).

A complete survey of the chest radiograph in children should include evaluation for possible congenital anomalies of the thoracic and upper lumbar spine, ribs, and proximal long bones of the upper extremities (Fig. 1.5). By systematically screening for these abnormalities, an astute radiologist may be the first to suggest underlying genetic syndromes, such as VACTERL (vertebral defects, anal atresia, cardiac defects, tracheoesophageal fistula, renal anomalies, and limb abnormalities).

"C" for "Cardiac" and Mediastinal Structures

Evaluation of the cardiac silhouette should include evaluation of overall cardiac size and gross structure of the heart and mediastinum.

The appearance and appropriate size of the cardiac silhouette on chest radiograph changes with age (Fig. 1.6). Neonates and infants have a more barrel-shaped chest that is equal in transverse and AP dimensions, and the normal cardiac silhouette may take up to 50% (infants) to 60% (neonates) of the transverse thoracic diameter. As children grow, their chest shape changes, and by age 10 to 13 years the normal cardiac silhouette appears similar to that seen in adults, taking up between 30% and 50% of the transverse thoracic diameter.

Gross structures of the heart and great vessels should be evaluated on every pediatric chest radiograph, including the aortic arch, pulmonary artery, and specific cardiac chambers (Fig. 1.7).

Evaluation of aortic arch sidedness is an important exercise in interpretation of pediatric chest radiograph. The normal left-sided aortic arch is a result of normal cardiac looping during embryology. Presence of a right-sided aortic arch may be the first subtle clue of under-

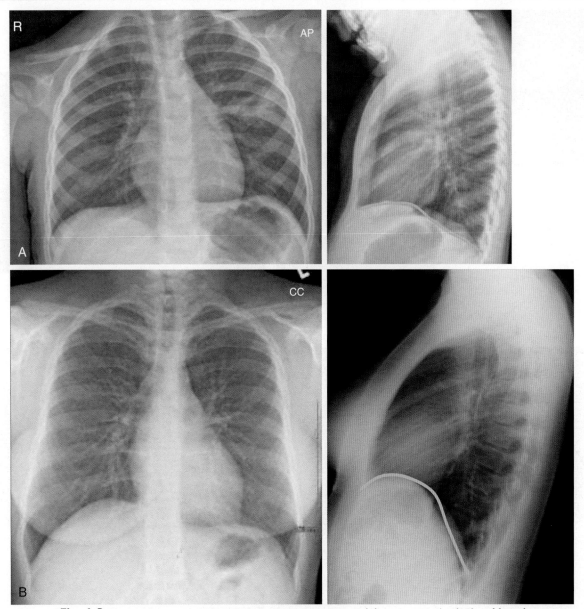

Fig. 1.3 Normal lung expansion and diaphragm contours. (A) Anteroposterior (AP) and lateral views of the chest in a 2-year-old with normal 8 to 10 posterior rib expansion and gentle down-sloping of posterior and lateral diaphragm border. (B) Posteroanterior and lateral view of the chest in a 16-year-old with normal 9 to 12 posterior rib expansion and dome-shaped diaphragm.

lying congenital heart disease. The normal left-sided aortic arch should opacify the left superior mediastinum with gentle rightward shift of the adjacent trachea. In contrast, a right-sided aortic arch will result in gentle leftward shift of the trachea (Fig. 1.8). The descending aorta sidedness may sometimes be confirmed inferiorly toward the level of the diaphragm.

Normal appearance of the mediastinum also varies considerably with age because of variable size of the thymus (see Fig. 1.6). The thymus is most prominent in children younger than 3 years but can occasionally be identified on chest radiographs in children up to age 10 to 12 years. On radiograph, the normal thymus has similar density to the adjacent heart and vascular structures, has soft contours, and does not compress adjacent structures (Fig. 1.9). Full understanding of these imag-

ing features allows the astute radiologist to differentiate normal thymus from mediastinal pathology.

Patients under considerable physiological stress may have decreased thymic size and changes in configuration. Once stress has subsided, the thymus can grow up to 50% of original size, a phenomenon known as "thymic rebound."

"D" for "Diaphragm"

The diaphragm should be evaluated for position, shape, and symmetry. There is minimal variation in appearance of the hemidiaphragms during childhood (see Fig. 1.2).

The right hemidiaphragm is often slightly higher than the left because of mass effect from the underlying liver.

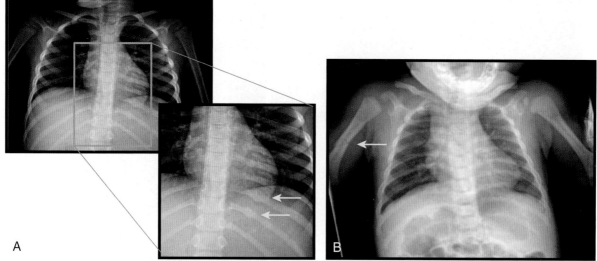

Fig. 1.4 Nonaccidental trauma. (A) Anteroposterior (AP) view of the chest in an infant obtained for respiratory distress that demonstrates multiple posterior rib fractures, highly concerning for nonaccidental trauma. (B) AP view of the chest in a 4-month-old with cough showing a right humeral fracture, concerning for nonaccidental trauma.

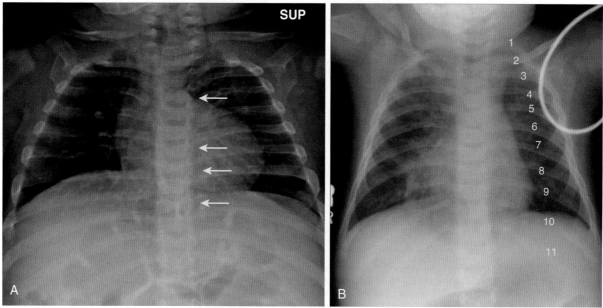

Fig. 1.5 Examples of congenital abnormalities of the skeleton that may be detected on chest radiograph. (A) Anteroposterior (AP) view of the chest in an infant showing multilevel vertebral segmentation anomalies in VACTERL (vertebral defects, anal atresia, cardiac defects, tracheoesophageal fistula, renal anomalies, and limb abnormalities). (B) AP view of the chest in an infant with trisomy 21 showing 11 paired ribs.

Otherwise, the hemidiaphragms should be symmetrical in location and should be able to be outlined easily. Marked asymmetry of diaphragm position should prompt further investigation into underlying pulmonary pathology or diaphragm function (Fig. 1.10). Inability to outline the hemidiaphragm raises concern for adjacent abnormality, such as atelectasis, pneumonia, mass, or pleural effusion.

"E" for "Effusions"

Pleural effusions may be large and obvious or small and subtle. On upright chest radiograph, effusions are seen layering dependently in the costophrenic sulcus. However, many chest radiographs in small children are performed in the supine position, and effusions will layer along the posterior chest in the pleural cavity and may appear as a subtle asymmetrical density (Fig. 1.11).

"F" for Lung "Fields"

A common colloquial term for the pulmonary parenchyma is "lung fields." In chest radiograph evaluation, it is conventional to divide the "lung fields" into three zones: upper, middle, and lower. Lung zones in the right

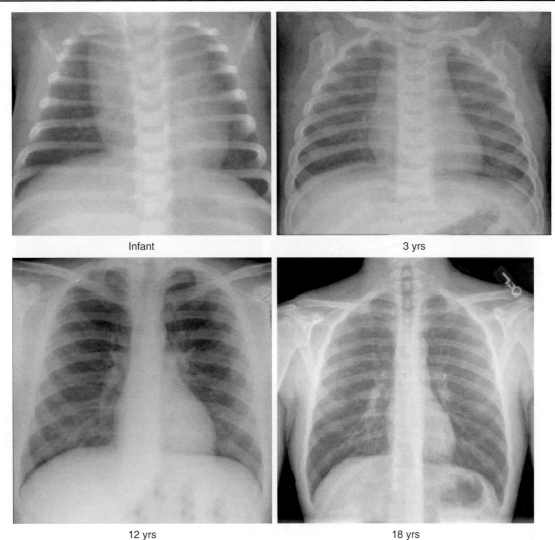

Infant   3 yrs

12 yrs   18 yrs

Fig. 1.6 Changing appearance of the cardiomediastinal silhouette on frontal radiographs of the chest in patients of varying age.

and left chest are compared for uniform aeration and any evidence of asymmetrical opacity. If the lungs appear asymmetrical, it should be determined whether this finding can be explained by asymmetry of normal anatomic structures, technical factors such as rotation, or underlying lung pathology.

The major and minor fissures are not routinely seen against the background normally aerated lung. However, knowledge of the expected position of the pulmonary fissures may assist in defining underlying pulmonary pathology (Fig. 1.12).

Lung markings should be seen to the chest wall. If the visceral pleura is visible, a pneumothorax should be suspected. Again, many chest radiographs in young children are performed in the supine position, and in this position extrapleural gas may move to the anterior or subpulmonic pleural space (Fig. 1.13).

"G" for "Gastric" Bubble and "Gas" Pattern

Gas within the stomach is commonly seen on chest radiograph. In pediatric patients, evaluation of gastric

sidedness is important in conjunction with aortic arch sidedness to detect underlying heterotaxy or situs inversus (Fig. 1.14).

Gas-filled loops of small and large bowel in the upper abdomen are also frequently seen and should be evaluated for size and normal appearance. Free intraabdominal gas can be seen particularly as a subdiaphragmatic lucent crescent on upright chest radiographs.

"H" for "Hilum"

The pulmonary hila, or roots, are complicated structures made up of major bronchi, pulmonary arteries and veins, and hilar lymph nodes. Routine chest radiograph assessment involves evaluation of the hilar structures for normal size, density, and position.

In pediatric patients, careful attention should be made to the relative size of paired bronchovascular structures in the hila. Pulmonary vessels and bronchi should be of similar size on the normal chest radiograph (Fig. 1.15). Difference in size of the pulmonary vessels and bronchi may signal underlying pathology,

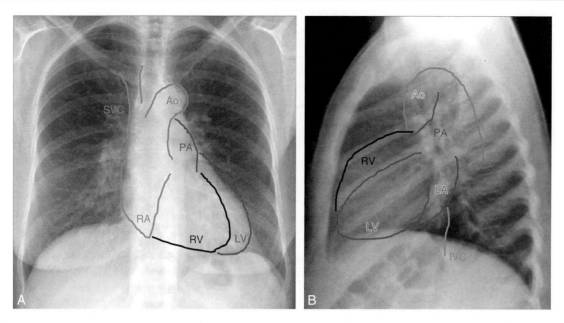

Fig. 1.7 Normal cardiac structures on posteroanterior and lateral radiographs of the chest. *Ao,* Aorta; *IVC,* inferior vena cava; *LA,* left atrium; *LV,* left ventricle; *PA,* pulmonary artery; *RA,* right atrium; *RV,* right ventricle; *SVC,* superior vena cava.

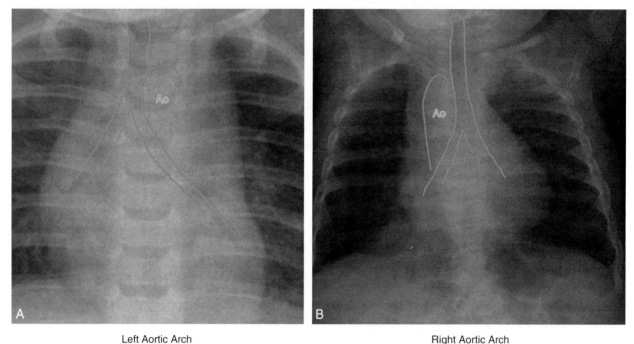

Left Aortic Arch   Right Aortic Arch

Fig. 1.8 Appearance of left and right aortic arch on posteroanterior (PA) views of the chest. (A) Left aortic arch should opacify the left mediastinum with gentle rightward shift of the adjacent trachea. (B) In contrast, a right aortic arch will result in gentle leftward shift of the trachea. *Ao,* Aorta.

such as pulmonary vascular overcirculation or bronchiectasis and air trapping.

■ Differential Diagnosis of Respiratory Distress by Age

The differential diagnosis of respiratory distress is broad and variable by age in the pediatric population. Clini-

cal history and careful physical examination can be extremely helpful in targeting diagnostic evaluation.

Toddler and Young Child

Differential diagnosis of respiratory distress in the toddler and young child includes airways disease, infection, or aspirated foreign body.

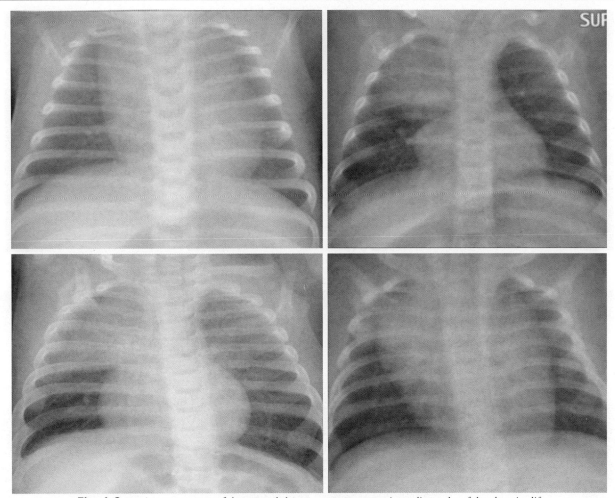

Fig. 1.9 Varying appearance of the normal thymus on anteroposterior radiographs of the chest in different infants. Note its similar density to cardiac structures and its soft, pliable borders that conform to adjacent structures, such as overlying anterior ribs and right minor fissure.

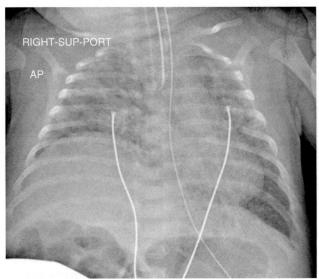

Fig. 1.10 Diaphragmatic paralysis. Anteroposterior (*AP*) view of the chest showing asymmetrical elevation of the right hemidiaphragm in the setting of diaphragm paralysis in pediatric intensive care unit patient.

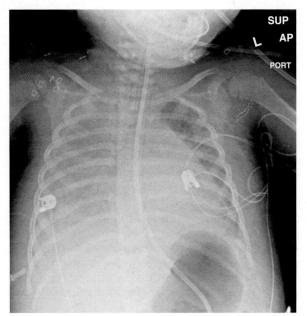

Fig. 1.11 Pleural effusion. Anteroposterior (AP) radiograph of the chest showing asymmetrical hyperdensity of the right chest with obscuration of the right diaphragm plus fluid in the pleural space along the right lateral chest wall, consistent with unilateral layering pleural effusion on a supine chest radiograph.

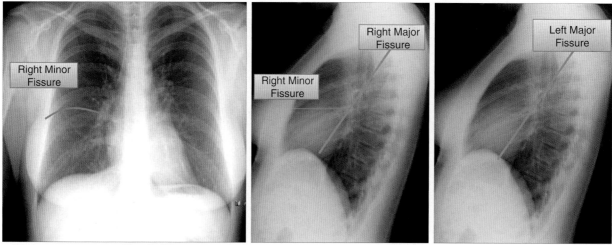

Fig. 1.12 Location of major and minor pulmonary fissures on chest radiograph.

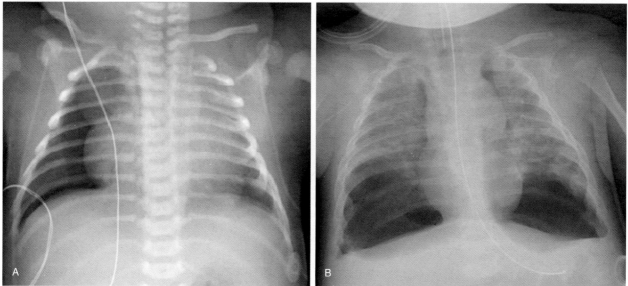

Fig. 1.13 Pneumothoraces on supine radiographs. (A) Anteroposterior (AP) view of the chest showing an anterior pneumothorax in a newborn after positive pressure ventilation during resuscitation. Note subtle increased lucency along right mediastinal and cardiac border. (B) AP view of the chest showing bilateral subpulmonic pneumothoraces in a newborn with meconium aspiration.

Airways

Respiratory distress may occur as the result of an upper or lower airway process. Abnormal breath sounds are frequently associated with respiratory distress in this age group, and the quality of abnormal breath sounds may help target the source of airway pathology.

UPPER AIRWAY OBSTRUCTION

Stertor and stridor are more frequently associated with upper airway obstruction. These clinical findings are best evaluated with radiographs of the soft tissues of the neck (see Chapter 26). Wheezing, grunting, rales, and crackles are more frequently seen in lower airway disease and should prompt imaging evaluation with chest radiograph (Table 1.1).

LOWER AIRWAY STRUCTURAL ABNORMALITY

The main lower airway structural abnormality that may be identified on radiographs is tracheal compression caused by a congenital vascular ring or pulmonary artery sling. Vascular rings occur when there is encircling of the trachea and esophagus by the aortic arch or great vessels. Compression on these structures may cause respiratory distress, abnormal breath sounds, or dysphagia. Findings on chest radiograph are subtle and include identification of a double or right aortic arch impression on the proximal trachea on frontal radiograph or abnormal impression on the posterior trachea on lateral radiograph (Fig. 1.16). Any of these findings should prompt further evaluation with esophagram or cross-sectional imaging with CT or MRI.

Other lower airway structural abnormalities causing respiratory distress, such as tracheobronchomalacia or tracheal or bronchial stenosis, are rarely well seen on radiographs. Occasionally a very narrow trachea can be seen on the lateral radiograph suggesting tracheomalacia. In these patients direct airway visualization with bronchoscopy, dynamic airway imaging with fluoroscopy, or CT is often required for definitive diagnosis.

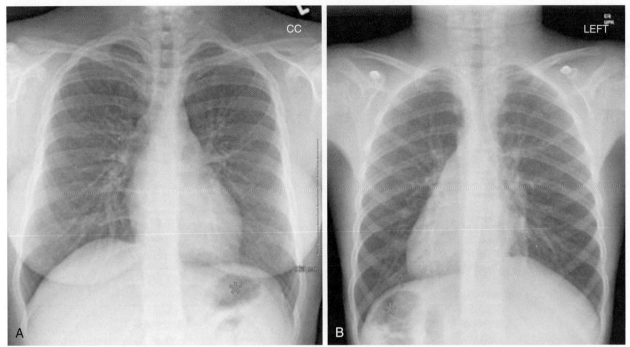

Fig. 1.14 Assessment of abdominal situs. (A) Anteroposterior (AP) view of the chest showing normal thoracic and abdominal situs solitus with left cardiac apex and left gastric bubble (*asterisk*). (B) AP view of the chest showing situs inversus with right cardiac apex and right gastric bubble (*asterisk*).

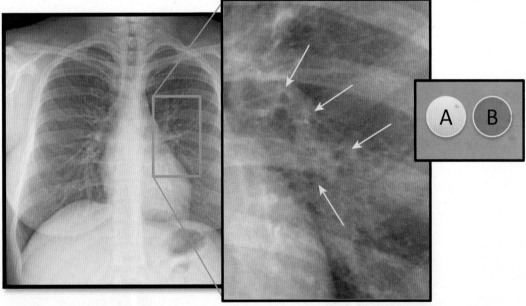

Fig. 1.15 Normal appearance of paired bronchovascular structures in the pulmonary hilum. Vessels (A) will appear as dense rounded structures when seen enface, while bronchi (B) will appear as well demarcated rounded lucencies. Note that normal pulmonary vessels (A) and bronchi (B) are similar in diameter.

Reactive Airways Disease/Asthma

Reactive airways disease, or asthma, is an inflammatory disorder of the lower airways caused by hyperreactivity that is at least partially reversible. Asthma primarily involves the medium and small airways of the lung. Nearly 50% of children with reactive airways disease will have symptoms before the age of 2 years, with approximately 80% of all patients having symptoms by 5 years of age.

Hypersensitivity can be related to a wide variety of factors, including environmental conditions, allergens, exercise, and viral illness. Chronic inflammation results

in hyperplasia of the bronchial wall smooth muscle and increased size of airway mucosal glands. When the airways of patients with asthma are exposed to hypersensitivity triggers, they respond with exaggerated bronchoconstriction and inflammation that results in the classic clinical features of wheezing, cough, and shortness of breath.

The chest radiograph of a young child with asthma in the absence of acute symptoms is often normal. However, in the setting of acute asthma exacerbation the chest radiograph demonstrates pulmonary hyperinflation and findings secondary to airway inflammation, such as bronchial

TABLE 1.1   Abnormal Breath Sounds Frequently Heard in Children With Respiratory Distress May Help Focus Differential Diagnosis and Inform Imaging Evaluation

ABNORMAL BREATH SOUNDS	DEFINITION	CAUSE	IMAGING
Stertor	Sonorous "Snoring" Midpitched Heard loudest near mouth and nose	Nasopharyngeal obstruction	Soft tissue neck x-ray (AP and lateral)
Stridor	High-pitched Associated with respirations Inspiratory—above or at vocal cords Expiratory—lower airway	Laryngeal obstruction	Soft tissue neck x-ray (AP and lateral)
Wheezing	High-pitched Expiratory Heard loudest in chest	Lower airways (small airways) obstruction	Chest x-ray, two views (frontal and lateral)
Crackles/rales	Discontinuous "Rattling" Heard loudest in chest	Lower airways	Chest x-ray, two views (frontal and lateral)

AP, Anteroposterior.

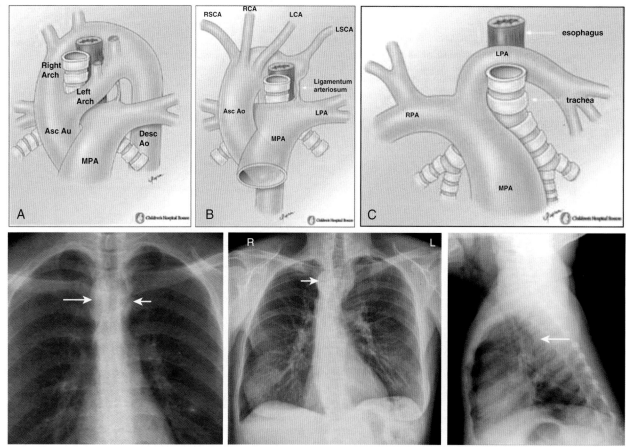

Fig. 1.16 Subtle findings of vascular rings and slings on chest radiograph, including (A) double aortic arch, (B) right arch with aberrant left subclavian artery, and (C) pulmonary artery sling (vessel between trachea and esophagus). *Asc Ao,* Ascending aorta; *Desc Ao,* descedning aorta; *LCA,* left coronary artery; *LPA,* left pulmonary artery; *LSCA,* left subclavian artery; *MPA,* main pulmonary artery; *RCA,* right coronary artery; *RAP,* right pulmonary artery; *RSCA,* right subclavian artery.

wall thickening, ill-defined borders of the airways termed "peribronchial cuffing," and prominence of the central pulmonary interstitium (Fig. 1.17). It should be noted that many of these findings are similar to those seen with viral bronchiolitis, and the two entities cannot be reliably distinguished on chest radiograph without correlation with clinical history and examination findings.

Infection

Respiratory infections are by far the most common underlying cause of respiratory distress in pediatric patients and the most common indication for chest radiograph.

Causes of lower respiratory tract infections in children are often discussed in reference to prevalence by

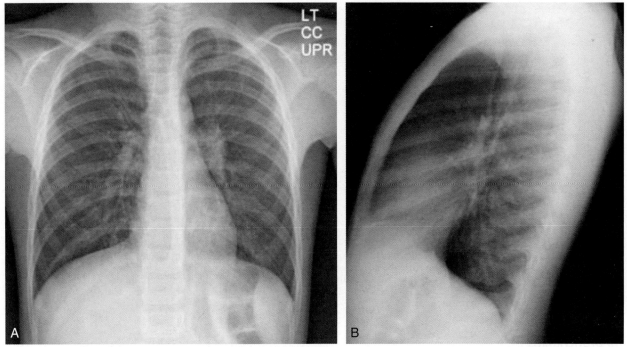

Fig. 1.17 Anteroposterior (AP) (A) and lateral (B) chest radiographs in 7-year-old boy with history of mild persistent asthma presenting with increased "cough and wheeze." Lungs are hyperinflated with flattening of both hemidiaphragms on lateral radiograph. There is also central bronchial wall thickening, peribronchial cuffing, and prominence of the central pulmonary interstitium. These findings are consistent with reactive airways disease/asthma.

TABLE 1.2   Common Pediatric Pulmonary Infectious Pathogens by Age Group

AGE	PATHOGEN	COMMENTS

Neonate	Group B *Streptococcus (GBS)*
	Escherichia coli
	Klebsiella
	Chlamydia trachomatis
		• Vertical transmission
		• Risk factors:
		   • Maternal fever
		   • Prolonged rupture of membranes
		   • (+) Maternal Group B Streptococcus (GBS) status

3 weeks to 3 months	*Chlamydia trachomatis*	• 2–12 weeks of life • Tachypnea, often afebrile
	RSV Parainfluenza	• Viral bronchiolitis often presents with wheezing • May acquire secondary bacterial pneumonia
	Streptococcus pneumoniae	• Most common cause of pediatric bacterial pneumonia
	Bordetella pertussis	• Severe paroxysmal cough • Often afebrile • Secondary bacterial pneumonia as a result of aspiration
3 months to 4 years	RSV Parainfluenza	• Most pneumonia in this age group is viral
	Streptococcus pneumoniae	• Most common cause of pediatric bacterial pneumonia • Associated complications • Parapneumonic effusion/empyema
5 years to adolescence	*Streptococcus pneumoniae*	• Most common cause of pediatric bacterial pneumonia
	Mycoplasma pneumoniae	• Increased incidence in school-age children and adolescents
	Chlamydia pneumoniae	• Similar clinical presentation to *Mycoplasma*

Adapted with permission from Durbin, W. J., & Stille, C. (2008). Pneumonia. *Pediatrics in Review, 29*(5), 147–160. https://doi.org/10.1542/pir.29-5-147
RSV, Respiratory syncytial virus.

age group (Table 1.2). Viral infections are more common than bacterial pneumonia in all age groups. The incidence of community-acquired bacterial pneumonia, most commonly secondary to *Streptococcus pneumoniae*, increases significantly in school-age children, as does the incidence of atypical bacterial infection. However, clinical differentiation between viral and bacterial infection can be extremely difficult in the pediatric population, and imaging can aid clinicians in diagnosis and treatment planning.

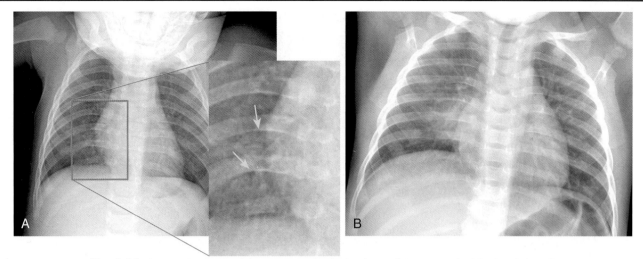

Fig. 1.18 *Viral bronchiolitis.* (A) Anteroposterior (AP) radiograph in 15-month-old girl with "cough and fever" demonstrates bronchial wall thickening and peribronchial cuffing plus prominence of the central pulmonary interstitium, consistent with viral bronchiolitis. (B) AP chest radiograph in the same patient 2 weeks later demonstrates new focal airspace opacity in right middle lobe, consistent with secondary bacterial pneumonia.

Viral Bronchiolitis

By far, the most common cause of respiratory distress in infants and toddlers is viral infection. Viral infection should be suspected in patients with low-grade fever, rhinorrhea, cough, and tachypnea.

In the lower airways, RSV and parainfluenza are the most common viral pathogens; however, rhinovirus, influenza, adenovirus, and human metapneumovirus may also cause viral bronchiolitis.

On chest radiographs, inflammation and edema of the lower airways result in bronchial wall thickening and peribronchial cuffing (Fig. 1.18A). Narrowing of the airways results in air trapping within the lungs, leading to pulmonary hyperinflation. Mucous secretion in the airways may cause lower airway obstruction leading to scattered areas of atelectasis.

Secondary bacterial pneumonia is a common complication of viral bronchiolitis and should be suspected in pediatric patients with a history of viral upper respiratory infection with new-onset fever, worsening cough, or who do not demonstrate expected clinical improvement after diagnosis of viral bronchiolitis. Chest radiographs, frontal and lateral, are suggested to evaluate for new or progressive airspace consolidation (see Fig. 1.18B).

Bacterial Pneumonia

Bacterial pneumonia is often suspected clinically in young children with respiratory distress, cough, and high fever. Tachypnea is the most sensitive and specific clinical finding in pneumonia; however, increased work of breathing and decreased O_2 saturation should also increase clinical concern.

In patients with a classic history and physical examination findings, chest radiography is not required for diagnosis of uncomplicated community-acquired pneumonia. However, symptoms and physical examination findings are sometimes nonspecific, and chest radiograph remains the initial imaging study of choice to confirm diagnosis. Chest radiograph may also identify complications such as pleural effusion, which require hospital management.

Although it is tempting to obtain a single frontal chest radiograph in children, addition of a lateral view significantly increases sensitivity for detection of airspace disease. Thus clinical guidelines from the American Academy of Pediatrics (AAP), Pediatric Infectious Diseases Society of America (IDSA), American College of Radiology (ACR), and Society of Pediatric Radiology (SPR) all recommend two views of the chest, frontal and lateral, as initial radiographic imaging in clinically suspected community-acquired bacterial pneumonia.

Bacterial pneumonia occurs after inhalation of small (0.5–3 μm) infective droplets that travel through the airways and lodge in the pulmonary acini. Infectious debris within the alveoli spread between adjacent acini within each bronchopulmonary segment, resulting in focal airspace opacity and consolidation on chest radiographs. In early bacterial pneumonia, airspace opacities may be small and ill defined. As infection spreads and involves more of the lungs, segmental and lobar airspace opacities may be seen (Fig. 1.19). Localization of infection within the lung can be determined using the "silhouette sign," with density from airspace consolidation resulting in a loss of normal well-defined "silhouette" interface between lucent, normally aerated lung and dense adjacent soft tissues (Figs. 1.20 and 1.21A–B).

In young children, a staphylococcal or pneumococcal pneumonia may appear as a focal, rounded, well-circumscribed opacity (Fig. 1.22). This distinctive appearance is referred to as a "round pneumonia" and is unique to children younger than 8 years. The round shape is thought to be a result of limited spread of bacteria and infectious debris between adjacent pulmonary lobules as a result of immaturity of interalveolar pathways (pores of Kohn) and collateral airways (canals of Lambert). On close inspection, round pneumonia usually will have irregular borders and internal air bronchograms; however, correla-

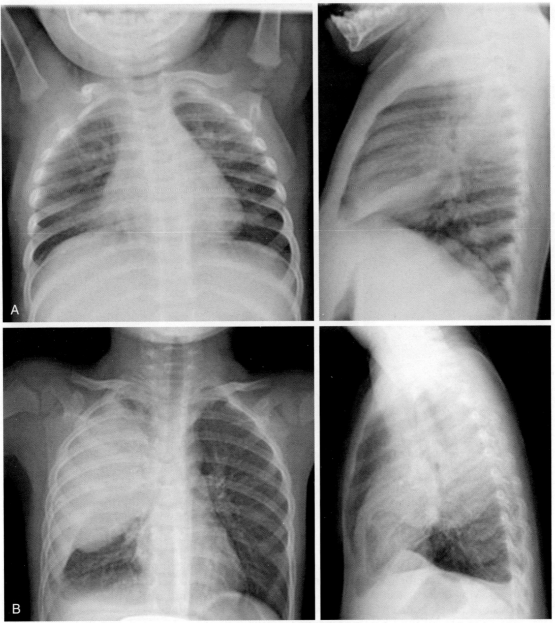

Fig. 1.19 Spectrum of disease seen on chest radiograph in community-acquired bacterial pneumonia (CAP). (A) Early, ill-defined opacity in the right middle lobe. (B) Large, right upper lobar opacity with loculated parapneumonic effusion.

tion with clinical history is imperative because the differential diagnosis of a well-demarcated rounded opacity in the pediatric chest also includes posterior mediastinal or chest wall mass. If the clinical history is not consistent with infection, further imaging with chest CT is suggested. Follow-up radiographs to document resolution also may be obtained. If the opacity does not resolve after appropriate antibiotic therapy, further imaging with chest CT is suggested (Fig. 1.23).

Special mention should be made of pneumonia secondary to *Chlamydia trachomatis* in the young infant. Cervical *C. trachomatis* infection may be transmitted to infants by ascending infection during pregnancy or during passage through the cervix and vagina at the time of delivery. An estimated 30% of infected infants

will acquire *C. trachomatis* pneumonia, which classically presents between 2 and 12 weeks of life with tachypnea and cough in the absence of fever or other signs of illness. The clinical presentation of *C. trachomatis* pneumonia is unique, as are findings on chest radiograph. Chest radiograph findings include pulmonary hyperinflation with patchy interstitial opacities (Fig. 1.24). Lobar consolidation and pleural effusions are typically not seen.

Sterile parapneumonic effusion is a common finding in pediatric community-acquired pneumonia, most frequently seen with *S. pneumoniae*. Clinically, parapneumonic effusion is suspected if there are focally decreased breath sounds at the lung bases or dullness to percussion on physical examination. Chest radiographs can suggest

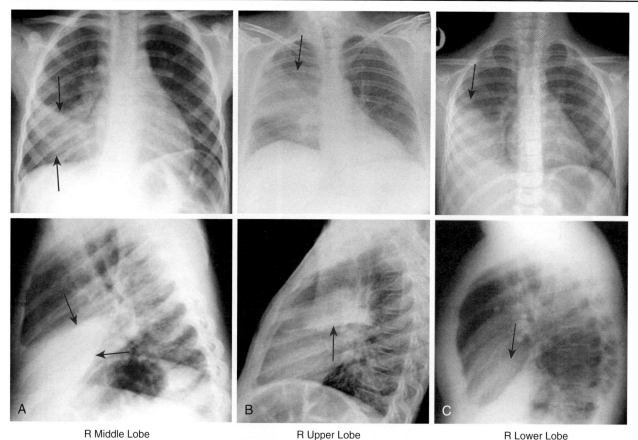

R Middle Lobe   R Upper Lobe   R Lower Lobe

Fig. 1.20 Examples of lobar bacterial pneumonia in the right lung. Localization of infectious process is possible using the "silhouette sign" on chest radiograph. (A) Right middle lobe pneumonia with loss of the right heart border silhouette on frontal view. Note that opacity is bordered superiorly by the right minor fissure and inferiorly by the right major fissure on lateral radiograph. (B) Right upper lobe pneumonia with loss of the lateral chest wall silhouette on frontal view. Opacity is bordered inferiorly by the right minor fissure on lateral radiograph. (C) Right lower lobe pneumonia with loss of the right hemidiaphragm silhouette on frontal view. Opacity is bordered superiorly by the right major fissure on lateral radiograph. *R*, Right.

presence of effusion (Fig. 1.25). A lateral decubitus view or an ultrasound of the chest can help evaluate whether an effusion is free flowing or loculated.

Loculated effusion raises concern for empyema. Empyema occurs when pleural fluid becomes infected and purulent. The most typical organisms responsible for development of an empyema include *S. pneumoniae, Staphylococcus aureus,* and *Hemophilus influenza.* Ultrasound provides complementary information to chest radiography without exposing young children to ionizing radiation, and in well-trained hands it can be a useful tool for the diagnosis of pneumonia complications. Ultrasound can further evaluate quantity and quality of pleural fluid, specifically looking for evidence of complex pleural fluid with internal echogenic debris, internal fibrinous strands and septations, and associated pleural thickening (Fig. 1.26). Ultrasound can also identify an optimal location for chest tube insertion. CT with intravenous (IV) contrast administration may be used for assessment of pleural fluid collections. However, CT is less sensitive than ultrasound for detection of internal fluid septations and pleural thickening, and should be reserved for patients in whom chest ultra-sound is technically challenging. For discussion on radiation reduction, see Chapter 22.

On ultrasound of pneumonia, fluid- and pus-filling alveoli in the lung result in a liver-like or "hepatized" appearance of the lung. Air-filled segmental and subsegmental airways, so-called air bronchograms, can be seen within the consolidated lung as branching linear echogenicities (Fig. 1.27). The adjacent pleural line may appear less echogenic, and normal lung sliding is often decreased or absent.

Major suppurative complications of pneumonia include necrotizing pneumonia and lung abscess. Necrotizing pneumonia occurs secondary to thrombosis of intrapulmonary vessels with subsequent ischemic damage to the lung parenchyma. This, in turn, results in destruction of normal lung architecture and cavity formation, which can result in lung abscess. Clinically, suppurative complications of pneumonia should be suspected in patients who do not respond adequately to appropriate antibiotic therapy. Findings of early necrotizing pneumonia may be better appreciated on ultrasound or CT, which can demonstrate decreased parenchymal blood flow or enhancement (Fig. 1.28).

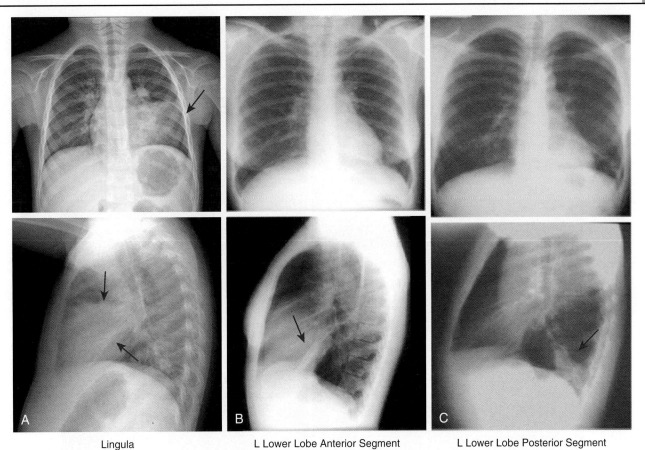

Lingula   L Lower Lobe Anterior Segment   L Lower Lobe Posterior Segment

Fig. 1.21 Examples of lobar and segmental bacterial pneumonia in the left lung. Localization of infectious process is possible using the "silhouette sign" on chest radiograph. (A) Lingular pneumonia with loss of the left heart border silhouette on frontal view. (B) Left lower lobe, anterior segment and (C) left lower lobe, posterior segment pneumonia. Focal airspace opacity is difficult to see on frontal radiograph because of superimposed soft tissue density of the heart. On lateral radiograph, focal airspace opacity is easily seen in left lung base. *L*, Left.

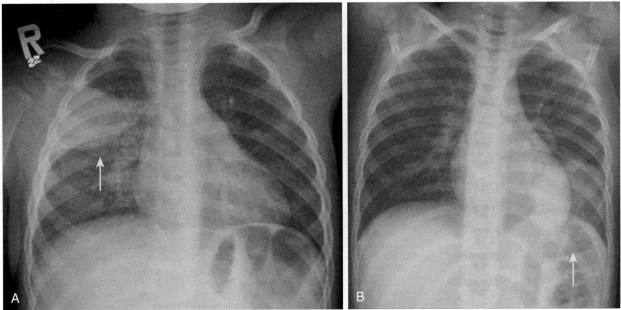

Fig. 1.22 Examples of round pneumonia. (A) Anteroposterior (AP) radiograph of the chest showing a right upper lobe in a 3-year-old with pneumococcal pneumonia. (B) Anteroposterior (AP) radiograph of the chest showing a rounded consolidation in the left lower lobe in a 5-year-old. Focal areas of airspace consolidation cleared on x-ray performed 2 weeks after diagnosis.

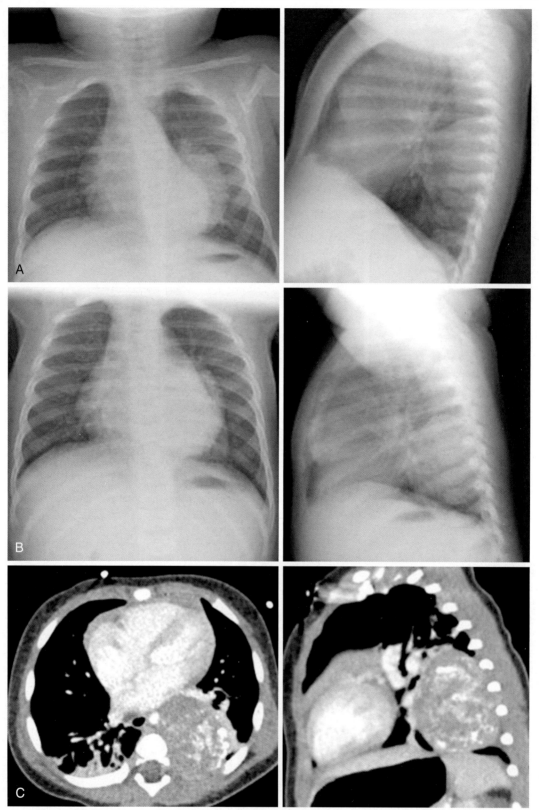

Fig. 1.23 Posterior mediastinal neuroblastoma. (A) 2 view chest radiograph in a 13-month-old child showing a density projecting over the left lower lobe, originally thought to represent round pneumonia. (B) Follow-up chest radiograph 3 weeks later after antibiotics demonstrates no change in size or appearance of focal, round opacity in the left lower lobe. (c) Chest computed tomography (CT) with intravenous contrast demonstrates a round soft tissue mass in the posterior mediastinum with internal calcification and enhancement consistent with neuroblastoma.

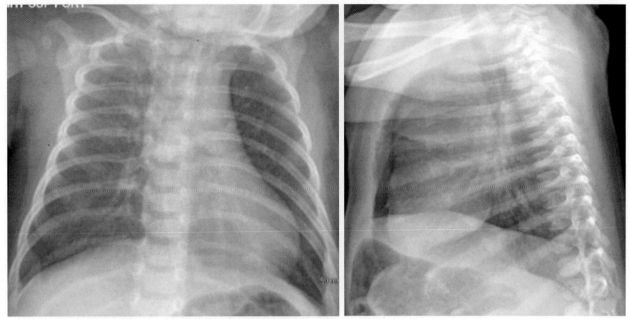

Fig. 1.24 *Chlamydia trachomatis* pneumonia. Anteroposterior (AP) and lateral chest radiograph in 3-week-old infant with "tachypnea" demonstrates pulmonary hyperinflation and subtle pulmonary interstitial opacities. Clinical history and imaging findings are consistent with *C. trachomatis* pneumonia.

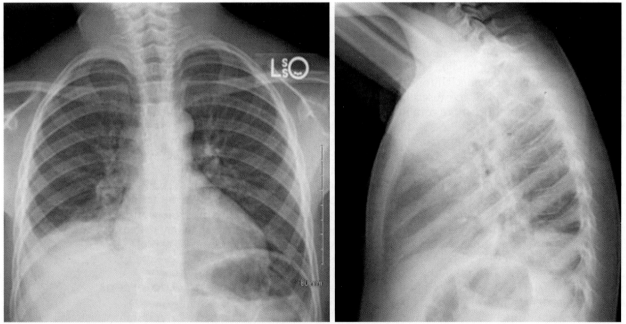

Fig. 1.25 Pneumonia with parapneumonic effusion. Upright posteroanterior (PA) and lateral views of the chest in a 4-year-old boy with right lower lobe pneumonia with parapneumonic effusion in the right costophrenic angle.

Focal, rounded lucencies within areas of consolidated lung on chest radiograph should raise concern for advanced necrotizing pneumonia with pulmonary abscess. Lung abscesses in the lung periphery may be demonstrated on ultrasound as anechoic collections in a background of consolidated lung. CT with IV contrast will demonstrate loss of normal parenchymal architecture and rim-enhancing fluid or air- and fluid-filled abscesses within the lung (Figs. 1.29 and 1.30).

Aspirated Foreign Body

Most foreign body aspirations occur in children younger than 3 years, with a peak incidence between 10 and 24 months. A diagnosis of foreign body aspiration is often missed or delayed because the actual aspiration event is unwitnessed and symptoms are often nonspecific. However, accurate identification of aspirated foreign body is crucial because serious complications, such as airway obstruction or perforation, may occur.

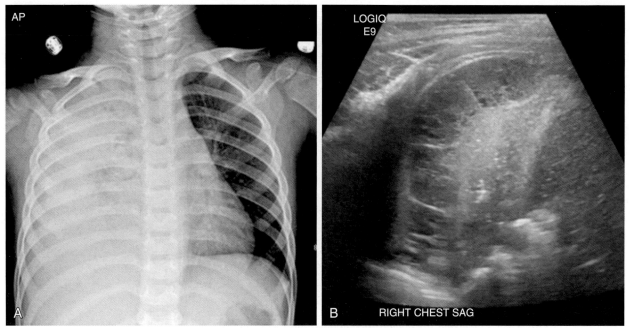

Fig. 1.26 Parapneumonic effusion. (A) Upright anteroposterior (*AP*) chest radiograph in 6-year-old girl with cough and fever showing dense airspace opacity in right lung with increased density along the lateral chest wall concerning for parapneumonic effusion. (B) Grayscale ultrasound of right chest confirms complex pleural fluid collection with internal septations and debris-filled echogenic fluid and pleural thickening consistent with empyema.

Aspiration of nonorganic foreign bodies, such as plastic beads or toy pieces, is actually quite rare. The most commonly aspirated foreign bodies are organic or food objects, such as peanuts. Unfortunately, organic foreign bodies are more likely to cause a localized tissue reaction and tend to produce more complications.

An aspirated foreign body may lodge anywhere within the airways from the upper trachea to the distal bronchioles depending on size. Large foreign bodies tend to lodge in the larynx and are more likely to result in abrupt and severe symptoms of cough, stridor, and difficulty breathing. Smaller foreign bodies in the lower airway are most commonly found in the right mainstem bronchus, which is slightly larger in diameter than the left mainstem bronchus and is more directly aligned with the intrathoracic trachea in upright patients. Symptoms of foreign body in the lower airway include cough and unilateral wheezing on physical examination. Prolonged presence of foreign body, especially organic, may result in chronic and recurrent focal pulmonary infections.

Diagnostic imaging in the setting of suspected aspirated foreign body should include AP and lateral radiograph of the neck and frontal and lateral radiographs of the chest. Radiopaque foreign bodies may be easily seen on these imaging studies and can help to identify location within the airway to guide retrieval, typically by bronchoscopy (Fig. 1.31).

When no radiopaque foreign body is seen, closer evaluation of the chest is needed to identify indirect signs of airway obstruction. When foreign bodies become lodged in the lower airways, they often result in segmental or subsegmental atelectasis from bronchial obstruction (Fig. 1.32).

Alternatively, foreign bodies in the airway may result in focal air trapping through a "ball-valve"-type mechanism. In this setting of incomplete bronchial obstruction, air may pass around and beyond the foreign body in the airway during inspiration as a result of slightly increased diameter of the airways. During expiration, the airway decreases in diameter and air becomes "trapped" distal to the level of airway obstruction, resulting in focal hyperinflation (Fig. 1.33). This can be better demonstrated on expiratory radiographs in patients old enough to cooperate with the technique. In young patients, bilateral decubitus radiographs should be obtained. In this projection, air trapping is evidenced by lack of normal airway collapse because of gravity in the dependent lung (Fig. 1.34).

Older Child and Adolescent

Differential diagnosis of respiratory distress in the older child and adolescent is slightly less broad because many congenital abnormalities have already been diagnosed, and older children are generally able to give more specific details regarding symptoms and clinical history to point toward a specific diagnosis.

Community-Acquired Pneumonia

Infectious disease remains at the top of the list of causes of respiratory distress in this age group. Many of the imaging findings in community-acquired pneumonia in older children are similar to those discussed earlier in this chapter.

Mycoplasma pneumonia is an atypical organism that is a common pathogen responsible for community-

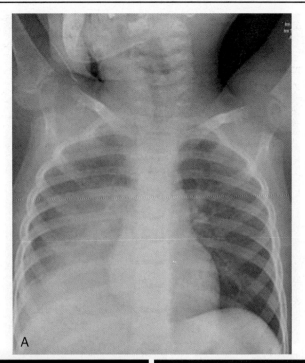

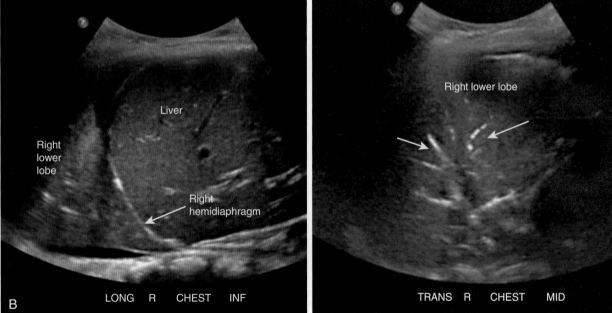

Fig. 1.27 Pneumonia. (A) Anteroposterior (AP) chest radiograph in a 4-year-old with cough and fever shows confluent airspace opacity in the right lung base with obscuration of the right hemidiaphragm concerning for focal pneumonia with possible parapneumonic effusion. (B) Longitudinal and transverse grayscale ultrasound images of the right chest show "hepatized" appearance of the right lower lobe consistent with airspace consolidation with multiple central linear echogenic air bronchograms (→).

acquired pneumonia in children aged 5 to 20 years. Clinical presentation may be more indolent than that of classic community-acquired pneumonia, often presenting with constitutional symptoms such as malaise, headache, and myalgias with low-grade fevers and a dry cough that occurs later in the course of illness.

The appearance of *Mycoplasma* pneumonia on chest radiographs is also different from that seen with classic *S. pneumoniae* or *S. aureus* pneumonia. Findings on chest radiograph include pulmonary hyperinflation and interstitial opacities (Fig. 1.35). In many ways the

radiographic appearance is similar to that seen in the setting of viral bronchiolitis; however, the patient is well beyond the age in which viral bronchiolitis is most commonly seen (>3–5 years).

Acute Chest Syndrome
Acute chest syndrome (ACS) is the leading cause of hospitalization, morbidity, and mortality in pediatric patients with sickle cell disease (HgbSS). Approximately 50% of patients with sickle cell disease will have at least one episode of ACS during childhood.

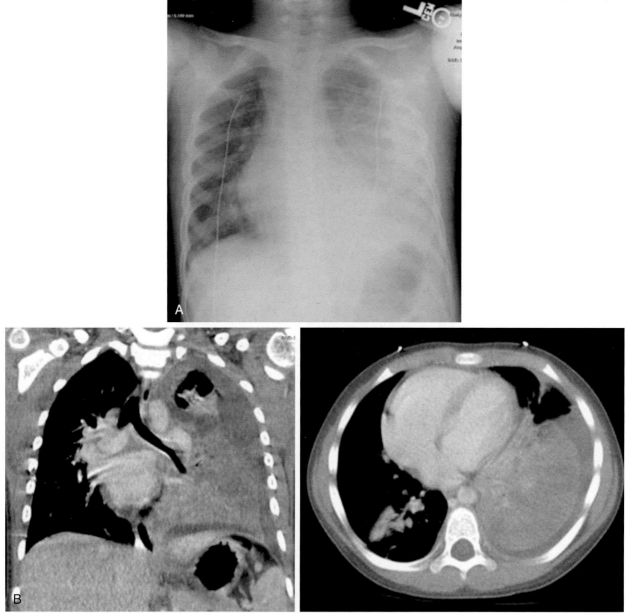

Fig. 1.28 Necrotizing pneumonia. (A) Anteroposterior (AP) radiograph in a 6-year-old with cough and fever showing dense left lower lobe airspace opacity and left pleural effusion. (B) Subsequent chest computed tomography with intravenous contrast demonstrates left lower lobe consolidation with focal regions of decreased contrast enhancement, concerning for early necrotizing pneumonia, and left pleural effusion.

ACS is an acute lung injury syndrome defined as acute respiratory distress associated with fever, chest pain, and signs of pulmonary compromise, such as tachypnea, cough, and dyspnea. The underlying pathophysiology of ACS is complex and likely a result of multiple different processes, such as pulmonary vascular occlusion caused by sickling of red blood cells, fat embolus from bone infarct, or community-acquired bacterial pneumonia.

Diagnostic criteria for ACS include presence of new, focal airspace consolidation on chest radiograph and one of the following clinical findings: chest pain, fever higher than 101.3°F (38.5°C), hypoxemia, and respiratory distress (Fig. 1.36). Pleural effusions also may be seen. Dramatic improvement in airspace opacities on chest radiograph are often seen after treatment, includ-ing antibiotics, IV fluids, pain control, and supplemental oxygen.

Recurrent episodes of ACS and pneumonia may lead to chronic pulmonary disease, seen in approximately 5% of patients with HgbSS. Sickle cell chronic lung disease manifests as interstitial abnormalities on chest radiograph indicative of generalized pulmonary fibrosis and lung scarring, impaired pulmonary function, and pulmonary hypertension. Further imaging with chest CT may demonstrate interlobular septal thickening, dilated secondary pulmonary lobules, traction bronchiectasis, and architectural distortion. Enlargement of the pulmonary vessels may suggest development of pulmonary hypertension, which can be further evaluated with echocardiogram.

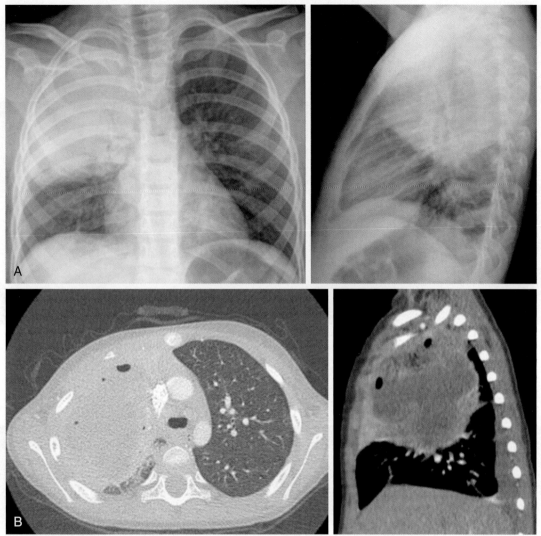

Fig. 1.29 Pneumonia with intrapulmonary abscess. (A) Anteroposterior (AP) and lateral chest radiograph in 3-year-old girl demonstrating dense airspace opacity in right upper lobe. (B) Chest CT with IV contrast demonstrates a fluid-filled collection in the right upper lobe consistent with intrapulmonary abscess.

Cystic Fibrosis

Cystic fibrosis (CF) is an inherited autosomal recessive disorder of exocrine gland function caused by mutations in the *CFTR* gene on chromosome 7q31.2. Mutations lead to abnormal transport of chloride and sodium across epithelial membranes in the lungs, pancreas, liver, and intestine. More than 1000 mutations in the *CFTR* gene have been discovered, and the clinical spectrum of disease is widely variable. Pulmonary involvement ranges from chronic cough and recurrent respiratory infections in older children to chronic pulmonary disease in adolescents and young adults.

In the lungs, thick mucous secretions in the airways result in progressive mucus plugging of the bronchi with superimposed infection. This leads to bronchial wall thickening, mucoid impaction, and diffuse cystic and saccular bronchiectasis. The upper lobes, lingula, and right middle lobe of the lung are the most affected. The natural history of lung disease in CF is one of chronic progression with intermittent episodes of acute wors-

ening of symptoms as a result of inflammation of the large and small airways referred to as acute pulmonary exacerbations.

Diagnosis of CF in the United States is typically made at the time of newborn screening. Patients are followed closely from the time of diagnosis, and advances in preventative and supportive care have resulted in decreased disease complications and significantly prolonged life expectancy and quality of life. Bronchiectasis and small airways disease are important determinants for disease progression, and these pathological findings should be closely monitored.

Chest radiographic findings in CF include pulmonary hyperinflation, bronchial wall thickening, and apical predominant bronchiectasis (Fig. 1.37). Chest CT is superior to chest radiograph for evaluation of the airways and better demonstrates findings of bronchiectasis, bronchial wall thickening, mucus plugging, atelectasis or consolidation, air trapping, and emphysema (Fig. 1.38). Disease severity scoring systems based

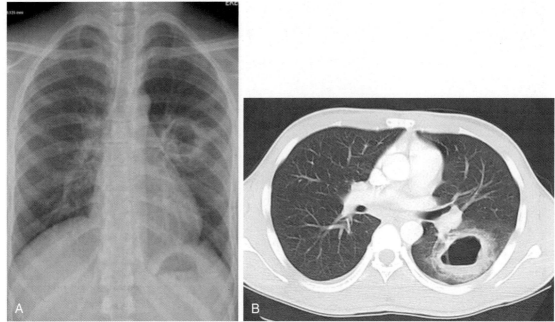

Fig. 1.30 Pneumonia with intrapulmonary abscess. (A) Anteroposterior (AP) chest radiograph in a 16-year-old boy with prolonged history of cough and fever shows well-circumscribed lucency in the left lung with surrounding ill-defined opacity. (B) Chest computed tomography with intravenous contrast demonstrates rim-enhancing pulmonary abscess cavity with small amount of layering internal fluid with surrounding airspace consolidation.

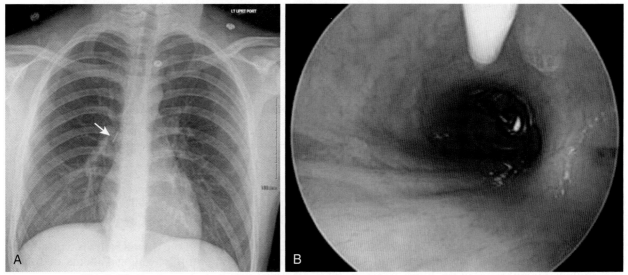

Fig. 1.31 Foreign body aspiration. (A) Anteroposterior (AP) chest radiograph in a 6-year-old showing a linear radiopaque foreign body in expected region of the right bronchus intermedius. (B) Image from bronchoscopy in the same patient confirms the presence of a thumbtack in the airway.

on chest x-ray (e.g., Brasfield score) and chest CT findings (e.g., Brody score, CF-specific CT score, and Perth-Rotterdam Annotated Grid Morphometry Analysis for CF (PRAGMA-CF) score) have been described and can be used to describe lung disease severity.

Routine imaging plays an important role in the care of patients with CF. The Cystic Fibrosis Foundation and American Thoracic Society recommend routine chest imaging beginning at age 1 year. Recommendations include both routine chest radiographs and chest CT in high-risk patients for early detection of disease associated changes.

Acute pulmonary exacerbation presents clinically with increased cough, change in sputum production, and worsening respiratory distress. Incidence of pulmonary exacerbation increases with age and more severe underlying pulmonary disease. These episodes are thought to be an effect of changing airway microbiology caused by

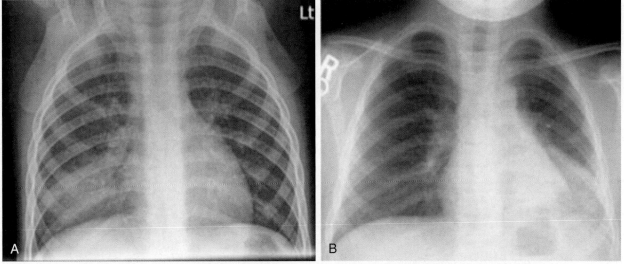

Fig. 1.32 Foreign body aspiration. Anteroposterior (AP) radiographs of the chest in different patients show focal atelectasis caused by non-radiopaque aspirated foreign body in the (A) right middle lobe and (B) left lower lobe bronchus.

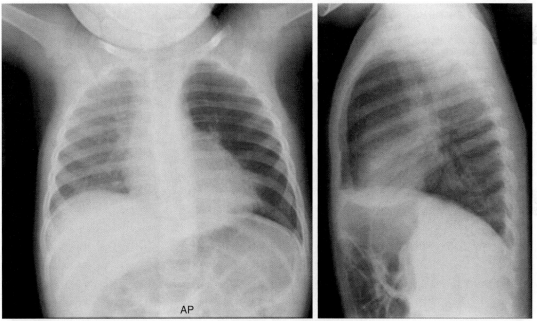

Fig. 1.33 Foreign body aspiration in the left mainstem bronchus. Anteroposterior (AP) and lateral chest radiographs in 2-year-old girl with suspected foreign body aspiration demonstrate asymmetrical hyperinflation of the left lung. Bronchoscopy confirmed cashew nut lodged in left mainstem bronchus.

new viral or bacterial infection or change in colonizing flora on sputum production and airflow obstruction. Diagnosis is predominantly based on clinical symptoms and pulmonary function tests (PFTs). Chest radiograph may demonstrate worsening of bronchial wall thickening and peribronchial cuffing or new regions of focal airspace disease. Chest CT also may be used for further evaluation in patients with worsening symptoms despite appropriate antibiotics and airway clearance. Findings on CT indicative of infection include tree-in-bud opacities, ground-glass opacities, patchy nodular opacities, or

confluent airspace disease (Fig. 1.39). Other acute complications of CF include fungal or mycobacterial infection, allergic bronchopulmonary aspergillosis, pleural effusion, pneumothorax, and secondary pulmonary hypertension.

Angiogenesis and bronchial artery hypertrophy commonly occur in association with chronic airway inflammation in CF. Hemorrhage into the airways may develop from erosions of dilated, thin-walled bronchial vessels after recurrent pulmonary infection. Bronchoscopy and CT angiography are often used to assess and

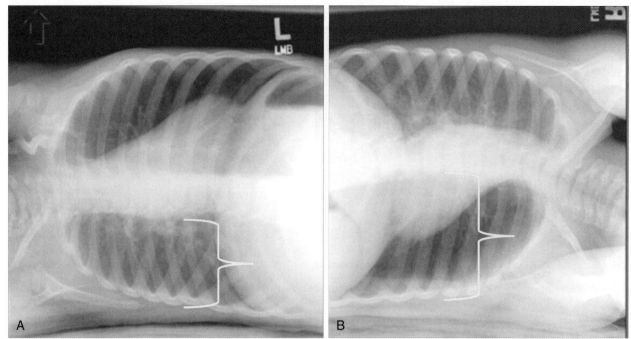

Fig. 1.34 Foreign body aspiration in the left mainstem bronchus. (A) Right lateral decubitus view of the chest shows normal collapse of the dependent right lung. (B) Left lateral decubitus view of the chest shows air trapping in left lung concerning for obstructing foreign body in the left mainstem bronchus. Bronchoscopy confirmed aspirated popcorn kernel in the left mainstem bronchus.

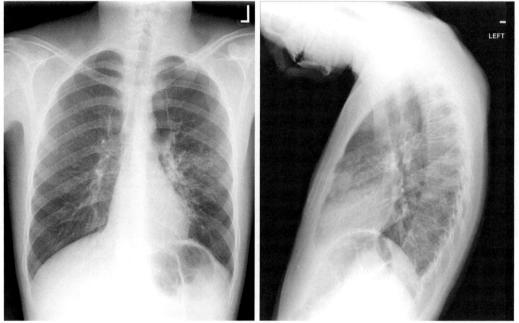

Fig. 1.35 Posteroanterior (PA) and lateral chest radiographs in a 17-year-old boy with "dry cough and fevers" demonstrate reticular and nodular interstitial opacities in the lingula, as can be seen with *Mycoplasma* pneumonia.

localize source of airway bleeding in patients without CF; however, this approach is debated for patients with CF. Approximately 5% of patients with CF may present with massive hemoptysis (expectoration of >300 mL of blood). These patients should have urgent consultation with interventional radiology for consideration of percutaneous endovascular embolization. CT angiograms can be helpful in localization of a dilated bronchial

artery, likely the arterial feeder to active hemorrhage (Fig. 1.40).

Spontaneous Pneumothorax

Primary spontaneous pneumothorax is a relatively rare condition; however, it should be considered in older children with acute respiratory distress. Spontaneous pneumothorax occurs most commonly in tall, thin,

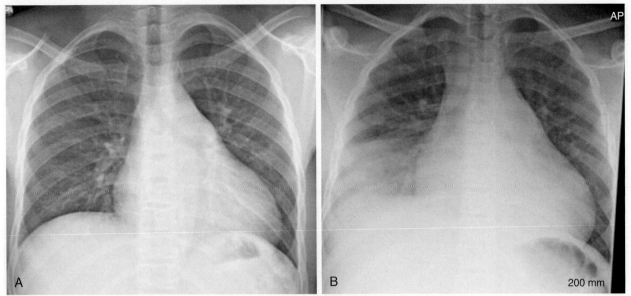

Fig. 1.36 Acute chest syndrome. (A) Baseline Anteroposterior (AP) view of the chest in 12-year-old boy with sickle cell anemia (HgbSS). (B) Chest radiograph obtained 2 days later at time of presentation to the emergency department with chest pain and shortness of breath shows new airspace opacity. Clinical findings and new focal airspace opacity are consistent with diagnosis of acute chest syndrome.

teenage boys and in adolescents with connective tissue disorders, such as Marfan syndrome, or occasionally in patients with asthma.

Spontaneous pneumothorax is generally thought to result from rupture of subpleural blebs in the lung apices. Patients present with acute onset of shortness of breath and local "pleuritic" chest pain that is worse with deep inspiration. On physical examination, primary spontaneous pneumothorax can be associated with unilateral diminished breath sounds and hyperresonance on percussion.

Chest radiograph plays an important role in diagnosis. Unilateral pneumothorax is often easily seen on upright chest radiograph in these older patients (Fig. 1.41A). If there is any ambiguity, then additional expiratory or lateral decubitus radiographs are suggested.

Several methods have been suggested for calculating volume of pneumothorax on chest radiograph. In adults, intervention with chest tube is generally recommended if pneumothorax measures greater than 3 cm from chest wall apex to pleural surface. However, this method has been shown to be unreliable in pediatric patients, and need for pneumothorax management should be dictated by physiological status of the patient. Tension pneumothorax should be suspected if there is depression of the hemidiaphragm, expansion of the intercostal spaces on the side of pneumothorax, or shift of the mediastinum to the contralateral side (Fig. 1.42).

Therapeutic management includes supportive management with rest and supplemental oxygen. Aspiration and chest tube placement may be required for a larger pneumothorax. Surgical management is usually indicated in patients with recurrent ipsilateral pneumothorax, contralateral pneumothorax, or patients with persistent air leak. Chest CT for detection of apical blebs (<2 cm in diameter) and bullae (>2 cm in diameter) may be useful in surgical planning (see Fig. 1.41C). Up to 25% of patients with primary spontaneous pneumothorax will have blebs in the contralateral lung detected on CT. Surgical treatment typically consists of thorascopic bleb resection, pleurodesis, and pleurectomy (see Fig. 1.41C).

■ Summary

Respiratory distress is one of the most common pediatric complaints seen in clinical practice with a broad and variable differential diagnosis. Having a consistent approach to interpreting chest radiographs can assure detection of abnormalities. Knowledge of appropriate pediatric diagnoses and their imaging features, when combined with clinical history and physical examination findings, can direct appropriate diagnosis and treatment.

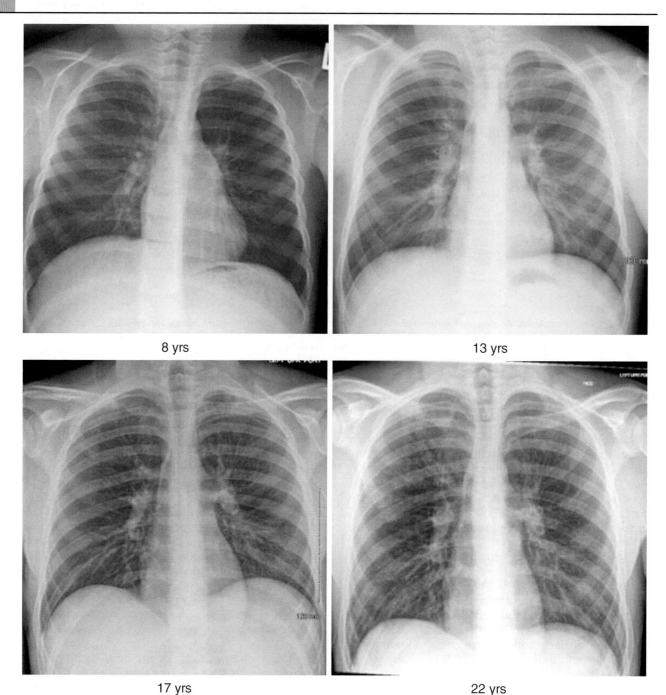

8 yrs   13 yrs

17 yrs   22 yrs

Fig. 1.37 Cystic fibrosis. Anteroposterior (AP) radiographs of chest in same patient with cystic fibrosis over the course of 14 years showing progressive development of apical bronchiectasis, bronchial wall thickening, and pulmonary hyperinflation.

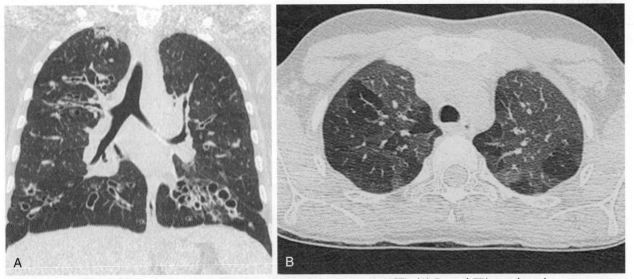

Fig. 1.38 Advanced cystic fibrosis on computed tomography (CT). (A) Coronal CT image through the chest shows extensive bronchiectasis, bronchial wall thickening, and airway mucus plugging. (B) Axial CT images through the chest show mosaic attenuation of lung parenchyma caused by air trapping.

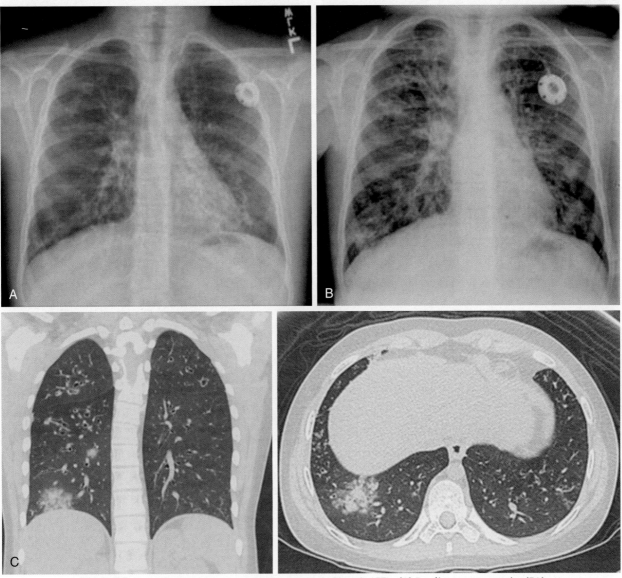

Fig. 1.39 Acute pulmonary exacerbation in cystic fibrosis (CF). (A) Baseline posteroanterior (PA) radiograph of the chest in a patient with history of CF. (B) Posteroanterior chest radiograph in the same patient in the setting of increased cough and sputum production with worsening pulmonary function tests (PFTs) showing increasing bronchial wall thickening, interstitial prominence, and new patchy airspace opacities. (C) Chest CT better demonstrates focal airspace disease consistent with new pulmonary infection superimposed on chronic changes of CF.

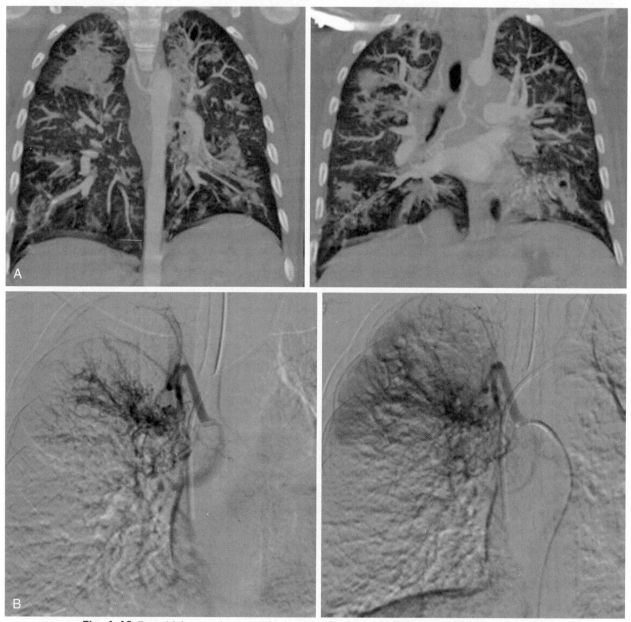

Fig. 1.40 Bronchial artery hypertrophy in cystic fibrosis. (A) Chest computed tomography angiography (CTA) in a patient with cystic fibrosis with massive hemoptysis showing bronchial artery hypertrophy, multiple collateral bronchial arterial vessels, and evidence of alveolar hemorrhage. (B) Bronchial artery angiogram shows contrast "blush" from active bleeding into the alveoli in the right upper lobe.

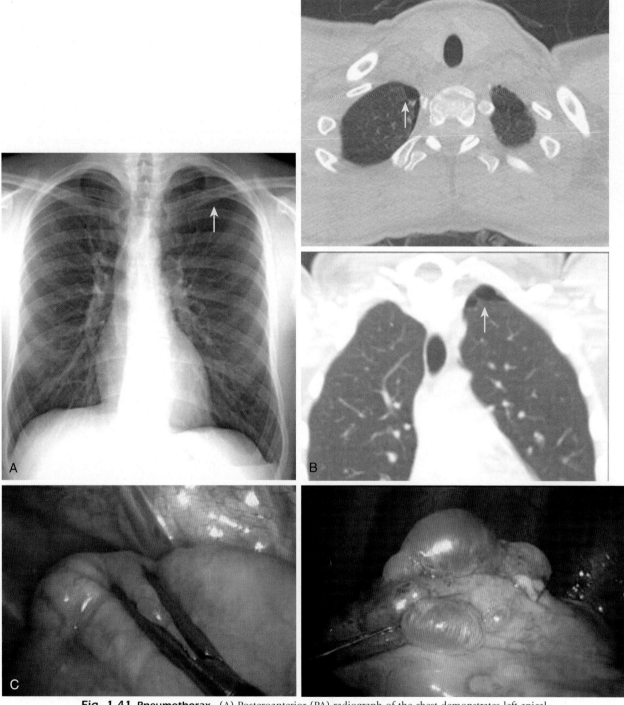

Fig. 1.41 Pneumothorax. (A) Posteroanterior (PA) radiograph of the chest demonstrates left apical pneumothorax in a 16-year-old boy. (B) Chest computed tomography confirms apical pleural blebs bilaterally. (C) Intraoperative photos of right and left lung apex from thorascopic bleb resection.

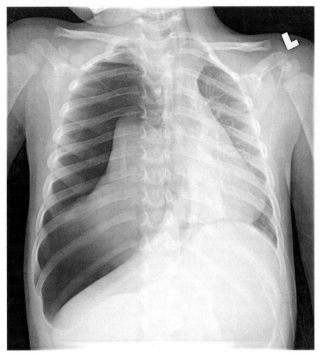

Fig. 1.42 Tension pneumothorax. Anteroposterior (AP) radiograph of the chest showing a right tension pneumothorax with depression of the right hemidiaphragm and shift of mediastinal contents to the left.

Bibliography

Chang, P. T., & Sena, L. (2017). *Chest imaging. The requisites, pediatric radiology* (4th ed.). Elsevier, 1–61.

Cox, M., Soudack, M., Podberesky, D. J., & Epelman, M. (2017). Pediatric chest ultrasound: A practical approach. *Pediatric Radiology, 47,* 1058–1068.

Driscoll, M. C. (2007). Sickle cell disease. *Pediatrics in Review, 28*(7), 259–268.

Durbin, W. J., & Stille, C. (2008). Pneumonia. *Pediatrics in Review, 29*(5), 147–160.

John, S. D., Rmanatha, J., & Swischuk, L. E. (2001). Spectrum of clinical and radiographic findings in pediatric *Mycoplasma* pneumonia. *RadioGraphics, 21,* 121–131.

Laya, B. F., Restrepo, R., & Lee, E. Y. (2017). Practical imaging evaluation of foreign bodies in children: An update. *Radiologic Clinics of North America, 55,* 845–867.

Lonergan, G. J., Cline, D. B., & Abbondanzo, S. L. (2001). From the archives of the AFIP: Sickle cell anemia. *RadioGraphics, 21,* 971–994.

Nasseri, F., & Eftekhari, F. (2010). Clinical and radiologic review of the normal and abnormal thymus: Pearls and pitfalls. *RadioGraphics, 30,* 413–428.

Padlipsky, P. S., & Gausche-Hill, M. (2008). *Respiratory distress and respiratory failure. Pediatric Emergency Medicine.* Saunders Elsevier, 13–27.

Rencken, I., Patton, W. I., & Brasch, R. C. (1998). Airway obstruction in pediatric patients. From croup to BOOP. *Radiologic Clinics of North America, 36,* 175–187.

Schooler, G. S., Davis, J. T., Parente, V. M., & Lee, E. Y. (2017). Children with cough and fever: Up-to-date imaging evaluation and management. *Radiologic Clinics of North America, 55,* 645–655.

St Peter, S. D. (2014). *Acquired lesions of the lung and pleura. Ashcraft's pediatric Surgery.* (6th ed.). Elsevier, 302–314.

White, D. R., Otherson, H. B., & Hebra, A. (2014). *Management of laryngotracheal obstruction in children. Ashcraft's pediatric Surgery.* (6th ed.). Elsevier, 279–301.

CHAPTER 2
Mediastinal Masses

Mark Bittman

CHAPTER OUTLINE

How Do You Differentiate Mediastinal From
   Pulmonary Parenchymal Masses?, 33
How Is the Mediastinum Subdivided?, 33
What Normal Structures Occupy Each Compartment
   of the Mediastinum?, 34
Anterior Mediastinum, 34
   What Is the Normal Appearance of the Thymus on
      Imaging Studies?, 34
   Where Can Ectopic Thymus Implant?, 36
   Thymic Hyperplasia, 37
   Thymic Cyst, 37
   Thymic Epithelial Tumors: Thymoma and Thymic
      Carcinoma, 37
   Thymic and Mediastinal Abscess, 39
   Thymolipoma, 41
   How Can Langerhans Cell Histiocytosis Manifest in
      the Mediastinum?, 41
   Germ Cell Tumors, 41

Lymphoma, 42
   What Subtypes of Lymphoma Most Often Affect the
      Mediastinum?, 42
   How Is Lymphoma Staged?, 42
   What Is the Role of FDG-PET/CT in Lymphoma?, 42
   In Which Compartment Is Lymphoma Most
      Common?, 44
   Lymphatic Malformation, 44
Middle Mediastinum, 47
   Vascular: Rings and Slings, 47
   Foregut Anomalies, 48
Posterior Mediastinum, 49
   What Is the Origin of the Most Common Posterior
      Mediastinal Mass?, 49
   Nerve Sheath Tumors, 49
      What Patient Population Is at Risk for Malignant
         Peripheral Nerve Sheath Tumor?, 49
   Extramedullary Hematopoiesis, 52
Summary, 52

The mediastinum is the most common location for intrathoracic masses in children. Mediastinal masses in pediatric patients are composed of a heterogeneous group of lesions ranging from benign, asymptomatic, and incidentally detected lesions to malignant, symptomatic, and potentially life-threatening masses. Evaluation of the patient with a mediastinal mass often requires a multidisciplinary approach, with imaging playing a critical role in detection, characterization, and monitoring of disease.

■ How Do You Differentiate Mediastinal From Pulmonary Parenchymal Masses?

On radiographs, it is important to differentiate lesions arising from the mediastinum from primary pulmonary parenchymal abnormalities. Mediastinal masses will cause obtuse angles at their interface with aerated lung, whereas intrapulmonary masses will result in acute angles between the mass and adjacent lung. Primary lung lesions may contain air bronchograms, a finding that is not present in mediastinal masses. Masses within the

mediastinum may cause shifting or obliteration of junctional lines and the azygoesophageal recess.

■ How Is the Mediastinum Subdivided?

The mediastinum is a compartment of the thorax located in between the two pleural cavities, posterior to the sternum and anterior to the vertebral column. The superior margin is defined by the thoracic inlet, and the inferior boundary is the diaphragm. The mediastinum is divided into three parts: anterior, middle, and posterior. Because there are no fascial planes anatomically dividing the different sections of the mediastinum, the boundaries of the subdivisions are arbitrarily based on anatomic landmarks delineated on a lateral chest radiograph (Fig. 2.1). Knowledge of the anatomic structures occupying each compartment will help guide a differential diagnosis when evaluating a mediastinal mass (Table 2.1). In addition, the differential can also be narrowed by using the imaging characteristics to suggest tissue type (Table 2.2).

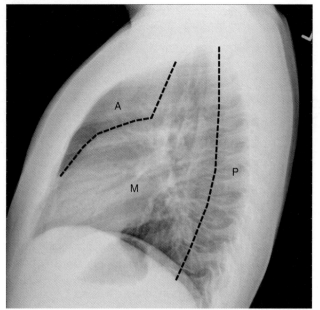

Fig. 2.1 Compartments of the mediastinum. The anterior mediastinum (*A*) is bounded by the sternum anteriorly and the pericardial reflection posteriorly. The middle mediastinum (*M*) is bounded anteriorly by the pericardium and posteriorly by a line drawn 1 cm posterior to the front of the vertebral body. The posterior mediastinum (*P*) is posterior to the line drawn over the vertebral body.

TABLE 2.1   Mediastinal Mass Differential Diagnosis by Location

Anterior mediastinal masses	Normal thymus Thymic hyperplasia Thymoma Thymic carcinoma Thymolipoma Germ cell tumor Lipoma Lymphoma Lymphatic malformation
Middle mediastinal masses	Lymphoma Lymphadenopathy Vascular rings Bronchopulmonary foregut malformation Lymphatic malformation

Posterior mediastinal masses	Sympathetic ganglion tumor
	  Neuroblastoma
	  Ganglioneuroblastoma
	  Ganglioneuroma
	Nerve sheath tumors
	  Schwannoma
	  Neurofibroma
	  Malignant peripheral nerve sheath tumor
	Extramedullary hematopoiesis
	Neurenteric cyst
	Lymphatic malformation

■ What Normal Structures Occupy Each Compartment of the Mediastinum?

The anterior mediastinum, also known as the perivascular space, is the space posterior to the sternum and anterior to the heart and brachiocephalic vessels. Its contents include the thymus, lymph nodes, and fat. The middle

TABLE 2.2   Mediastinal Mass Differential Diagnosis by Tissue Characteristics

LESION CHARACTERISTICS	DIFFERENTIAL DIAGNOSIS
Fat containing	Teratoma Thymolipoma Lipoma
Cystic	Teratoma Thymic cyst Bronchopulmonary foregut malformation Neurenteric cyst Lymphatic malformation
Calcifications	Teratoma Thymoma Thymic carcinoma Neuroblastoma Ganglioneuroblastoma Ganglioneuroma
Homogenous	Lymphoma Neuroblastoma Ganglioneuroma Ganglioneuroblastoma Extramedullary hematopoiesis Schwannoma
Heterogenous	Lymphoma Germ cell tumors Thymoma Thymic carcinoma Neurofibroma Malignant peripheral nerve sheath tumor

mediastinum, or vascular space, is bordered by the pericardial reflections. The contents of the middle mediastinum include the heart, great vessels, trachea, central bronchi, lymph nodes, and fat. The posterior mediastinal compartment, or postvascular space, lies behind the pericardial reflection and extends to the posterior chest wall. The contents include the descending thoracic aorta, esophagus, thoracic duct, azygous and hemiazygous veins, sympathetic nerves, and lymph nodes.

■ Anterior Mediastinum

What Is the Normal Appearance of the Thymus on Imaging Studies?

The thymus is an encapsulated bilobed, soft organ within the anterior mediastinum that functions to produce T cells. The thymus is largest in size at birth, in relation to the patient's body size; however, it is largest in absolute size just before puberty. After puberty, it begins to involute and progressively becomes replaced with fat. On radiographs, it is a prominent soft tissue density in the anterior mediastinum, visible until about 3 years of age. The left lobe is usually larger than the right. On the lateral radiograph, the soft tissue density usually occupies the anterior mediastinum abutting the upper cardiac border. On the frontal projection, it manifests as widening of the mediastinum often with a lobulated margin (wave sign) as a result of indentation from the ribs (Fig. 2.2). Often the right lobe of the thymus has a flat inferior margin at its interface with the minor fissure (sail sign) (Fig. 2.3).

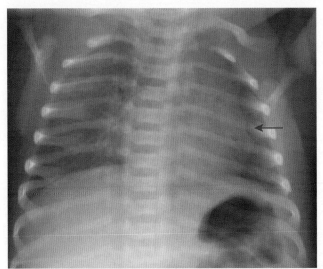

Fig. 2.2 Normal thymus on radiographs. Frontal radiograph of the chest in an infant shows a prominent thymus, a normal finding. The undulating lateral contour of the cardiothymic silhouette is known as the wave sign (*arrow*). Lack of mass effect on the airway is another reassuring finding of a thymus.

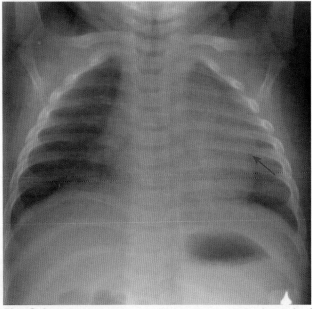

Fig. 2.4 Normal thymus on radiographs. Frontal radiograph of the chest in an infant showing the characteristic notch (*arrow*) at the junction of the left lobe of the thymus and the left heart border.

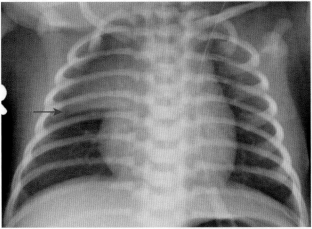

Fig. 2.3 Normal thymus on radiographs. Frontal radiograph of the chest in an infant showing the right lobe of the thymus insinuating into the right minor fissure with a resultant flat inferior margin, known as the sail sign (*arrow*).

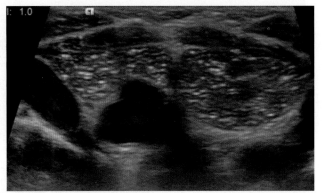

Fig. 2.5 Normal thymus on ultrasound. Thymic tissue has characteristic scattered short linear nonshadowing echogenicities within the tissue.

A characteristic notch may be seen at the junction of the thymus and cardiac silhouette (Fig. 2.4). At fluoroscopy the thymic shadow should widen in expiration and narrow with inspiration because of its pliability. The thymus has a characteristic appearance on ultrasound with short linear echogenic structures corresponding to connective tissue septae (Fig. 2.5). On computed tomography (CT) the thymus occupies the anterior mediastinum and is typically homogenous in attenuation and does not cause mass effect on adjacent structures (Fig. 2.6). On magnetic resonance (MR) imaging (MRI), it is slightly hyperintense on T1-weighted imaging (T1WI) with respect to skeletal muscle and homogeneously mildly hyperintense in signal on T2-weighted imaging (T2WI) (Fig. 2.7). Familiarity of the MR appearance of the thymus is helpful when evaluating for ectopic or aberrant thymus, which should follow thymus signal characteristics on all pulse sequences (Fig. 2.8).

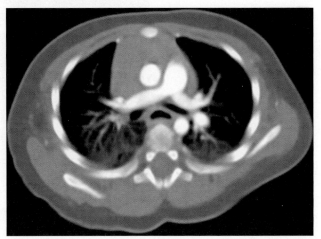

Fig. 2.6 Normal thymus on computed tomography (CT). Axial contrast-enhanced CT of the chest shows a homogeneous soft tissue density in the anterior mediastinum with convex margins compatible with a normal thymus.

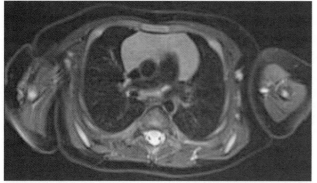

Fig. 2.7 Normal thymus on magnetic resonance imaging.
Axial T2-weighted fat-suppressed image shows a homogeneously
T2 hyperintense structure with convex margins within the anterior
mediastinum, typical of a normal thymus.

Where Can Ectopic Thymus Implant?

Embryologically the thymus is derived from the third
pharyngeal pouch, with minor rudimentary portions
derived from the fourth pharyngeal pouch. Beginning
in the eighth week of gestation, the primordial thymus
descends from the level of the pharynx inferiorly to the
mediastinum along the thymopharyngeal duct, deep to
the thyroid gland and sternocleidomastoid and along
the carotid sheath. During its descent, remnant thymic
tissue may implant along the path of migration, which
may result in a neck or mediastinal mass. In the rare
variant retrocaval thymus, an aberrant portion of the
gland may extend posteriorly between the superior vena
cava and great vessels, mimicking a neurogenic tumor.

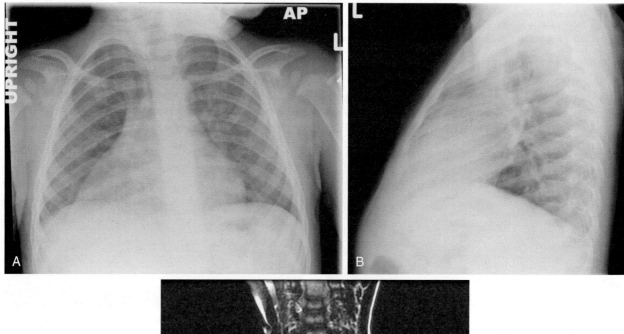

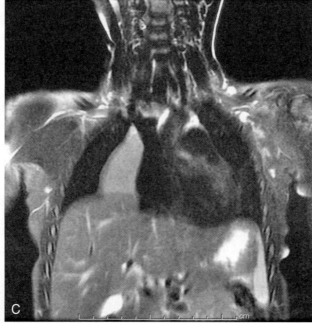

**Fig. 2.8 Aberrant thymus masquerading as a mediastinal mass in a 2-year-old with shortness
of breath.** (A) Anteroposterior and (B) lateral views of the chest show a soft tissue density along the right
anterior inferior heart border. (C) Coronal T2 fat-suppressed magnetic resonance imaging shows that the
density on radiographs represents normal thymus in an aberrant location.

Among reported cases of posterior extension of the thymus, there is a right-sided and male predominance. On cross-sectional imaging, the aberrant thymus should appear identical to the thymus and is usually in continuity with the normally located thymus. Management is typically nonoperative; however, on occasion a large ectopic thymus can cause symptoms as a result of compression of nearby structures prompting surgical resection.

Thymic Hyperplasia

Thymic hyperplasia is a rebound phenomenon seen in patients recovering from thymic atrophy, usually caused by stressors such as chemotherapy, corticosteroids, or radiation therapy. Six months after the cessation of chemotherapy is the average time interval that thymic rebound is observed in pediatric patients. However, it may be seen in just a few weeks if the child was being treated with steroid therapy alone and has been reported as late as 5 years posttreatment. The thymus may rebound to a size even larger than its expected normal size (Fig. 2.9). Differentiating thymic hyperplasia from recurrent neoplasm can be problematic. On cross-sectional imaging, thymic hyperplasia appears as enlargement of the thymus with attenuation at CT and signal intensity at MRI equivalent to that of a normal thymus. In adolescent pediatric patients (>15 years of age), chemical shift MRI can be used to reliably differentiate thymic hyperplasia from neoplasm because of the presence of intracellular lipid in the hyperplastic thymic gland. In thymic hyperplasia, loss of signal on opposed phase images is diagnostic of hyperplasia, a finding not present with neoplasm. In patients younger than 15 years, chemical shift imaging may not be helpful because the physiological process of fatty infiltration of the thymus may not have commenced.

Thymic lymphoid hyperplasia refers to an increase in the number of lymphoid follicles, which is associated with myasthenia gravis and other autoimmune disorders, such as systemic lupus erythematosus, rheumatoid arthritis, scleroderma, and Graves disease. The morphological imaging characteristics of thymic lymphoid hyperplasia and true hyperplasia are indistinguishable; however, lymphoid hyperplasia may be higher in attenuation on CT compared with true hyperplasia.

Thymic Cyst

Thymic cysts are benign cystic lesions arising from the thymus that can be either congenital or acquired. They are typically incidentally identified on cross-sectional imaging performed for unrelated reasons. Although most patients are asymptomatic, there is an association with autoimmune disorders that is reported in up to one-third of patients with intrathymic cysts. Congenital thymic cysts are usually unilocular and contain simple fluid and a thin, imperceptible wall. Acquired thymic cysts, in contrast, may be multilocular and contain complex fluid as a result of hemorrhage or infection. Conditions associated with acquired thymic cysts include Hodgkin lymphoma, thymic tumors, thymic hyperplasia, chest trauma, and HIV infection. On CT, thymic cysts are typically midline, round or oval, well circumscribed, and can be either hypodense or hyperdense on CT depending on the protein content. Calcium and fat attenuation should be absent, distinguishing features from a germ cell tumor (GCT). At MRI, thymic cysts are hyperintense on T2WI, isointense or hypointense to skeletal muscle on T1WI, and thin, peripheral enhancement on postcontrast sequences.

Thymic Epithelial Tumors: Thymoma and Thymic Carcinoma

Thymic epithelial tumors are a group of tumors of epithelial cell origin that arise from the thymus gland and have a variable amount of lymphocytes. In 1999, the World Health Organization (WHO) reclassified thymic epithelial tumors on a continuum as either thymoma (subtypes

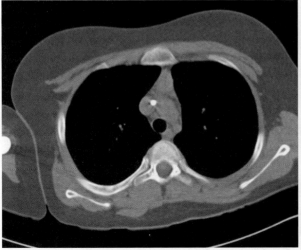 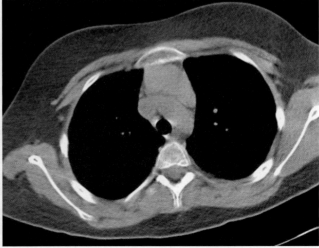

Fig. 2.9 Thirteen-year-old with thymic rebound after chemotherapy for osteosarcoma. Noncontrast chest computed tomography 3 months apart shows interval enlargement of the thymus after cessation of chemotherapy.

A, AB, B1, B2, and B3) or thymic carcinoma (type C), based on their morphological appearance and ratio of lymphocytes to epithelial cells. Thymomas demonstrate no overt atypia of the epithelial cells and retain features specific to the normal thymus. Immature, nonneoplastic lymphocytes are present in variable numbers. Thymomas are the most common type of thymic epithelial tumor, accounting for almost half of all anterior mediastinal masses in the adult patient population. In children, however, they are less common and account for only 1% to 2% of all mediastinal masses. Approximately 40% of patients with thymoma present with a paraneoplastic syndrome, most often myasthenia gravis. Notably, 15% of patients with myasthenia have a thymoma.

Histologically, thymic carcinomas exhibit cellular atypia and no longer demonstrate features specific to a normal thymus. They resemble cytological features of carcinomas of other organs. Thymic carcinomas are usually advanced at the time of diagnosis, have a greater recurrence rate than thymomas, and have a worse 5-year survival. Unlike thymoma, the association of autoimmune disease is uncommon.

Noninvasive type A thymomas have been described as well-defined smooth margins, with a round shape, and tend not to have extracapsular extension. Invasive thymoma, however, does extend beyond the confines of the fibrous capsule with local spread to adjacent structures, such as mediastinal structures and the chest wall. Invasive thymoma may spread to the pleura and often recurs after surgical resection.

Radiographically, thymomas often appear as anterior mediastinal masses with obliteration of the retrosternal clear space on the lateral projection (Fig. 2.10A and B). On frontal radiograph, there is contour abnormality of the mediastinum with a smooth lobulated border. Thin peripheral calcification may be present. Pleural nodu-

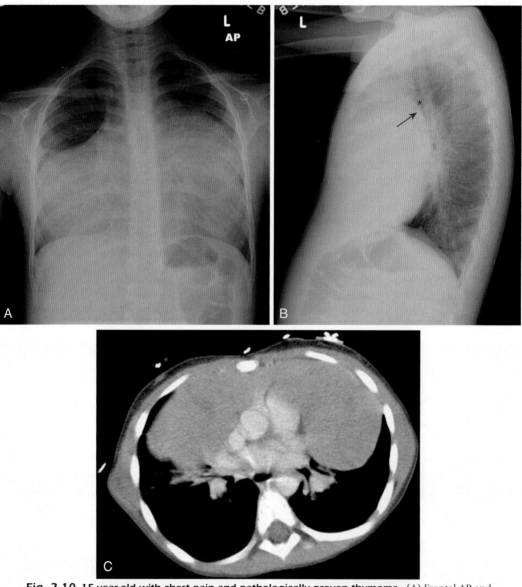

Fig. 2.10 **15-year-old with chest pain and pathologically proven thymoma.** (A) Frontal AP and (B) lateral chest radiographs show a large bilateral anterior mediastinal mass. The mass effect *(arrow)* on the distal trachea *(asterisk)* is best seen on the lateral view. Axial contrast enhanced CT (C) shows a large heterogeneous anterior mediastinal mass.

larity and pleural effusion may indicate invasive disease. Diaphragmatic elevation is suggestive of phrenic nerve involvement.

Among the different subtypes of thymoma, there is significant overlap in the CT imaging findings, making them difficult to distinguish preoperatively (see Fig. 2.10C). The contours are most often smooth or lobulated, round or oval in shape, and the presence of central necrosis is variable and enhancement patterns may be either homogenous or heterogeneous. Invasion of the mediastinal fat, pleural and pericardial effusions, pleural nodularity, and mediastinal lymphadenopathy are more often seen with high-risk thymoma and thymic carcinoma (Fig. 2.11) compared with low-risk thymoma. Great vessel invasion is an imaging feature that is unique to thymic carcinoma, although it is not present in all cases. Thymic carcinomas tend to be larger than thy-

moma at presentation, which is thought to be due to its more aggressive biological behavior or because patients with thymomas seek medical attention sooner from the symptoms caused by the paraneoplastic syndrome.

MR features of thymoma include low-to-intermediate signal on T1WI and hyperintense signal on T2WI with markedly hyperintense signal in areas of necrosis (Fig. 2.12). In contrast with thymic hyperplasia, loss of signal on opposed phase imaging is not present.

Thymic and Mediastinal Abscess

Thymic abscess is a rare cause of fever in a child. Chest radiographs demonstrate an anterior mediastinal mass, and the cross-sectional imaging appearance is similar to abscesses in other locations. A pyogenic thymic abscess

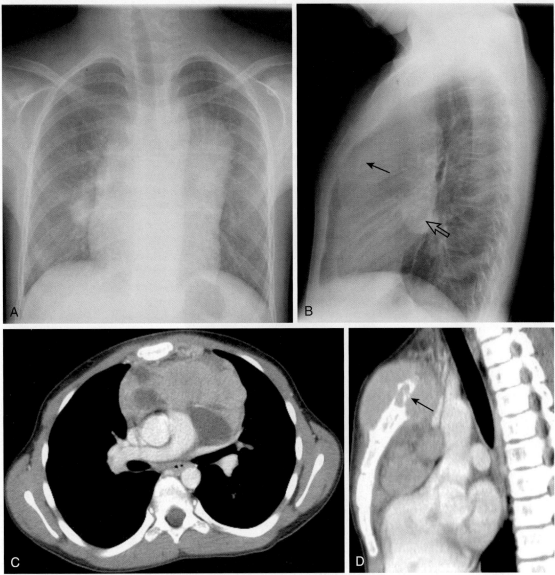

Fig. 2.11 Sixteen-year-old boy with shortness of breath. Frontal (A) and lateral (B) chest radiographs demonstrate a large anterior mediastinal mass with obliteration of the retrosternal clear space (*arrow*). On the lateral view, there is also evidence of a middle mediastinal mass, caused by hilar adenopathy (*open arrow*). Axial (C) and sagittal (D) contrast-enhanced CT image of the chest shows a large, heterogeneously enhancing anterior mediastinal mass with solid and necrotic components. This was a high grade thymoma/thymic carcinoma with invasion of the chest wall and destruction of the sternum (*arrow*).

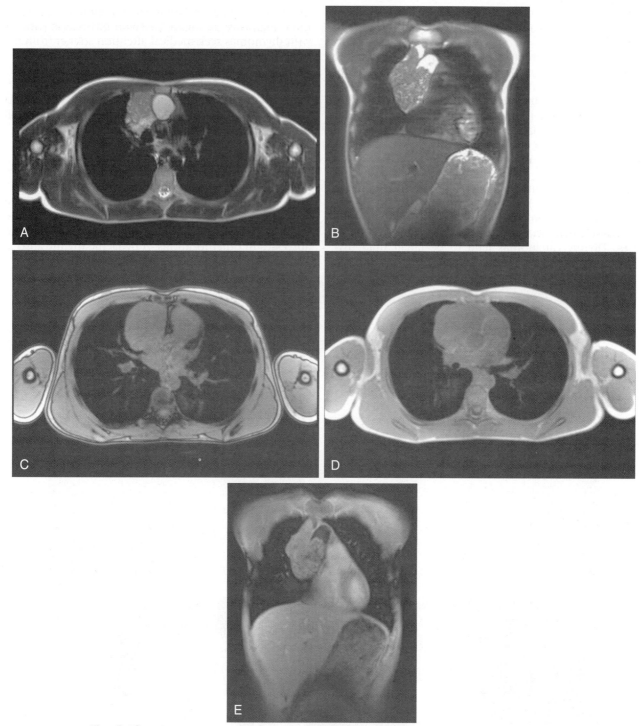

Fig. 2.12 Thymoma in an adolescent patient with myasthenia gravis. Axial (A) and coronal (B) T2-weighted images of the upper chest show a heterogeneous anterior mediastinal mass with a cystic component caused by necrosis or acquired cystic change. Axial (C) and opposed phase (D) images of the mass show no dropout of signal within the mass, a feature that mitigates against thymic hyperplasia. (E) Coronal T1-weighted fat-suppressed postcontrast image shows heterogeneous enhancement of the lesion.

on CT usually presents a multiloculated cystic mass with peripheral enhancement and sometimes with solidly enhancing components. Potential complications include sternal osteomyelitis, which appears as bone destruction with lucency in the adjacent sternum. MRI shows multiloculated collection with peripheral enhancement on postcontrast sequences (Fig. 2.13). Theories of the etiology of a thymic abscess include superinfection of an underlying thymic cyst. Treatment is typically antibiotics and drainage.

Thymolipoma

Thymolipoma is a rare, benign, fat-containing mediastinal mass often located inferiorly within the anterior mediastinum. These lesions are often large at presentation and are usually incidentally detected and asymptomatic. They can occur at any age, with median age of 21 years. When symptomatic, patients present with chest pain, cough, shortness of breath, and arrhythmia as a result of mass effect on adjacent structures. Myasthenia gravis, aplastic anemia, thyrotoxicosis, and Graves disease have been reported in association with thymolipoma.

On chest radiograph a mediastinal mass or widening of the mediastinal silhouette is identified. The margins of the mass are usually smooth, and pulmonary architecture may be seen through the lesion because of the fat content. At CT the lesions are predominantly fat attenuation with some soft tissue elements. There is typically a connection with the thymus that is a helpful finding to differentiate from other fat-containing mediastinal masses. At MR the fat components are hyperintense on both T1WI and T2WI with suppression of signal on fat-suppression sequences. The soft tissue elements are typically intermediate in signal intensity.

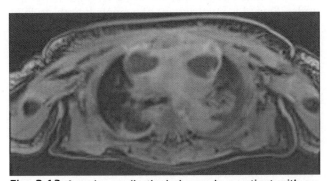

Fig. 2.13 Anterior mediastinal abscess in a patient with purulent pericarditis. Axial T1-weighted postcontrast image demonstrates two peripherally enhancing anterior mediastinal fluid collections compatible with abscesses.

On cross-sectional imaging, these lesions tend to be large, pliable, encapsulated, and do not invade adjacent mediastinal structures.

The treatment of thymolipoma depends on symptoms. Asymptomatic masses can be followed clinically, whereas symptomatic lesions are managed operatively.

The differential diagnosis of a fat-containing mediastinal mass includes lipoma, mediastinal lipomatosis, teratoma, and Morgagni hernia.

How Can Langerhans Cell Histiocytosis Manifest in the Mediastinum?

Thymic involvement in Langerhans cell histiocytosis is uncommon and occurs in the setting of multisystem disease. Concomitant pulmonary involvement is usually present when the thymus is involved. Infiltration of the thymus by histiocytes results in diffuse enlargement and/or heterogeneity on cross-sectional imaging (Fig. 2.14). On radiographs the cardiomediastinal silhouette is enlarged. On CT, calcification and cystic changes have been described. Areas of low attenuation at CT and hyperintense T1 signal on MRI are attributed to a fibroxanthomatous reaction resulting in areas of fatty replacement. These imaging features resolve after favorable response to therapy.

Germ Cell Tumors

GCTs arise within the gonads and extragonadal sites affecting the midline of the body. The anterior mediastinum is the most common extragonadal location, while the pineal region and sacrococcygeum are less commonly affected sites. They are the third most common mediastinal neoplasm after lymphoma and neurogenic tumors, and account for approximately 25% of anterior mediastinal masses in children, with 3% of tumors arising in the posterior mediastinum.

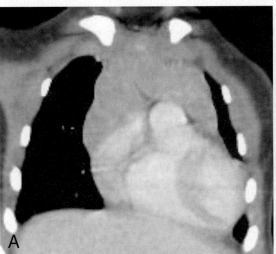
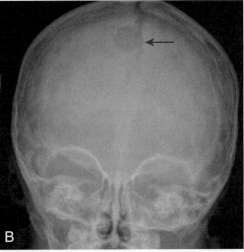
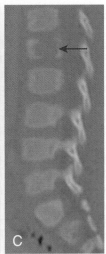

Fig. 2.14 Three-month-old with Langerhans cell histiocytosis (LCH). Coronal computed tomography image of the chest (A) shows heterogeneity and enlargement of the thymus compatible with thymic infiltration. Geographic lucent lesions (*arrows*) in the calvarium (B) and spine (C) are typical of the bony manifestations of LCH.

GCTs can be divided into teratomas (more common), and nonteratomatous GCTs (less common). Nonteratomatous GCTs include seminoma, yolk sac tumor, embryonal carcinoma, choriocarcinoma, and mixed types. Teratomas can be further subdivided into mature, immature, and mixed. Mature teratoma is by far the most common subtype and is almost always benign with a low malignant potential. Immature teratomas have a variable amount of undifferentiated cells and a low malignant potential with the risk for malignancy relative to the proportion of the immature components.

Chest radiographs demonstrate a nonspecific anterior mediastinal mass, often indistinguishable from other mediastinal masses. Calcifications are present in about 25% of cases and may be central or peripheral, a finding that when present on radiography is suggestive of a GCT (Fig. 2.15). The hallmark of teratoma is the presence of fat, fluid, and calcified components on cross-sectional imaging. CT is often the preferred modality and best demonstrates calcifications, as well as the mass's relationship with adjacent structures. The cystic components are low in attenuation, similar to water density, and fat is lower in density with Hounsfield units between –100 and –50 (see Fig. 2.15B). On MRI the fluid components are markedly hyperintense on T2WI, and the fatty elements are bright on both T1WIs and T2WIs with loss of signal on fat-suppressed sequences (see Fig. 2.15C). Fat-fluid levels, when present, are diagnostic of a teratoma. Calcifications are dark on all pulse sequences and show susceptibility artifact on gradient echo sequences. The margins of teratomas are well defined and lobulated, except in rare cases of tumor rupture whereby there is extravasation of internal components into an adjacent site such as lung or the pleural space. Immature teratomas tend to have more solid components than mature teratoma and may invade adjacent mediastinal structures. The treatment of mature teratoma is surgical, whereas immature teratomas require a combination of surgery, radiation, and chemotherapy.

Lymphoma

What Subtypes of Lymphoma Most Often Affect the Mediastinum?

Lymphoma is the third most common childhood tumor in developed countries, accounting for 10% to 15% of all childhood cancers, exceeded in frequency only by leukemia and brain tumors. Lymphoma commonly involves the chest, and involvement can be found in the mediastinum, hilum, parenchyma, chest wall, pleura, and/or pericardium. Non-Hodgkin lymphoma (NHL) accounts for 60% of cases, and Hodgkin disease (HD) accounts for the remaining 40%. The lymphoblastic type of NHL is the most common subtype to involve the anterior mediastinum, seen in 50% of cases (Fig. 2.16). HD, characterized pathologically by the malignant Reed-Sternberg cell, frequently involves the mediastinum, with the nodular sclerosis subtype most commonly involving the anterior mediastinum.

The workup of suspected lymphoma typically begins with a chest radiograph, which can detect an anterior mediastinal mass (Fig. 2.17). Associated findings on chest radiograph include pleural effusions and lung nodules or masses. HD is often associated with bulky hilar lymphadenopathy. At CT the masses are often lobulated and homogeneous. Internal low attenuation represents necrosis or cystic change. The role of cross-sectional imaging is to assess the extent of disease and evaluate for vascular and airway compression, a finding more frequently seen with NHL. Large mediastinal masses often compress venous structures, such as the superior vena cava, brachiocephalic vein, or pulmonary veins. Airway compression is another important complication to evaluate that may influence the ability to safely receive anesthesia. When there is greater than 50% of airway compression, most anesthesiologists would recommend ultrasound-guided biopsy under local anesthesia rather than biopsy under sedation.

How Is Lymphoma Staged?

The purpose of staging lymphoma is to determine a treatment strategy based on risk stratification. In HD the Ann Arbor staging system is used based on the observation that disease spreads along contiguous lymph nodes. Stage I is involvement of a single lymph node or lymphoid structure, stage II involves two or more regions on the same side of the diaphragm, stage III is involvement of lymph node regions on the both sides of the diaphragm, and stage IV is disseminated disease. The modifiers A and B denote whether constitutional symptoms are present, defined as fever, night sweats, and unexplained loss of >10% body weight within 6 months. The St. Jude's Children's Research Hospital has developed a staging system for NHL (Rosolen, et al., 2015).

What Is the Role of FDG-PET/CT in Lymphoma?

Most types of lymphoma are characterized by increased metabolic activity with resultant increased fluorodeoxyglucose (FDG) uptake on positron emission tomography (PET) scans. Although CT offers excellent anatomic information, it lacks information regarding metabolic activity and cannot detect disease within normal-size lymph nodes, both of which can be achieved with PET/CT. Studies have shown that PET/CT can change with stage of disease in 10% to 30% of patients with lymphoma, typically upstaging the disease.

When feasible, PET/CT is obtained before the start of treatment to define the extent of disease. After one to three cycles of chemotherapy, another PET/CT scan is often obtained to evaluate the metabolic changes that take place after induction chemotherapy. These early metabolic changes have been shown to be predictive of final treatment response and progression-free survival. After completion of therapy, many patients have residual mass on diagnostic CT scans. At this time, another PET/CT may be obtained to assess whether the patient achieved a complete metabolic response or partial response to therapy, which will guide treatment strategies (see Fig. 2.17D).

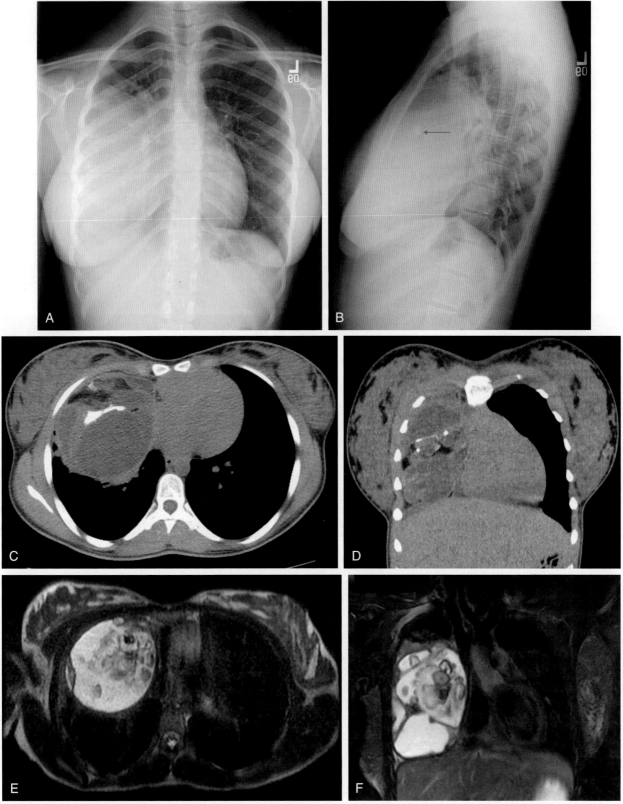

Fig. 2.15 Sixteen-year-old with germ cell tumor. Posteroanterior (PA) (A) and lateral (B) chest radiographs show a large right anterior mediastinal mass with obliteration of the retrosternal clear space on the lateral view. Punctate calcifications are present within the mass (*arrow*), suggestive of germ cell tumor. Noncontrast axial (C) and coronal (D) chest computed tomography images in the same patient show fluid, fat, and calcification, which is diagnostic of a germ cell tumor. Axial (E) and coronal (F) T2-weighted images of the chest demonstrate a heterogeneous mass that is predominantly fluid signal and show hypointense foci that correspond to calcification on the radiographs and computed tomography.

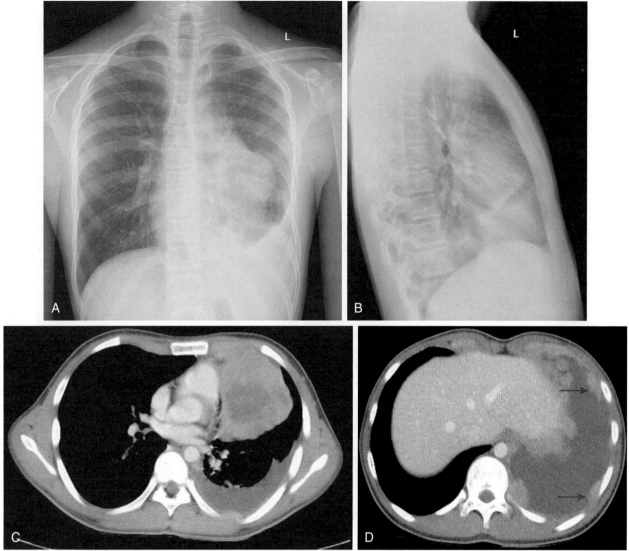

Fig. 2.16 Fourteen-year-old boy with T cell lymphoblastic lymphoma. Posteroanterior (A) and lateral (B) chest radiographs show a left anterior mediastinal mass with an associated left pleural effusion. Axial (C, D) postcontrast computed tomography images demonstrate a heterogeneously enhancing anterior mediastinal mass. There is a left pleural effusion with enhancing pleural nodularity (*arrows*) diagnostic of a malignant effusion.

In Which Compartment Is Lymphoma Most Common?

Lymphoma most often affects the anterior mediastinum, although it can present in any compartment. The middle mediastinum is often concomitantly involved because of associated hilar adenopathy. Rarely, the posterior mediastinum can be involved (Fig. 2.18).

Lymphatic Malformation

Lymphatic malformations (LM) are benign, low-flow lesions composed of dilated lymphatic channels or cysts lined by endothelial cells. LMs are further classified as macrocystic, microcystic, or mixed lesions. They can occur anywhere in the body, with less than 1% localized to the mediastinum. Most mediastinal LMs extend into the mediastinum from adjacent sites, such as the neck or axilla. Although benign, the

clinical course is potentially life threatening depending on the degree of mass effect on the airway and critical vascular structures. On sonography, macrocystic LMs appear as hypoechoic cystic spaces with thin internal septations. MRI is the preferred modality to define the anatomic extent of the malformation and its juxtaposition with other structures, which helps guide in treatment planning. Macrocystic LMs appear as well-defined cysts characterized by hypointense signal on T1WI and markedly hyperintense signal on T2WI. Fluid–fluid levels are common as a result of internal hemorrhage or proteinaceous material, although a feature that is not pathognomonic for LM because they can also be seen in a minority of venous malformations. Hemorrhage within macrocysts is bright on T1WI, dark on T2WI and shows no internal post-contrast enhancement. After gadolinium administration, there is septal and peripheral enhancement, but the cystic spaces do not internally enhance, which is a helpful differentiating feature

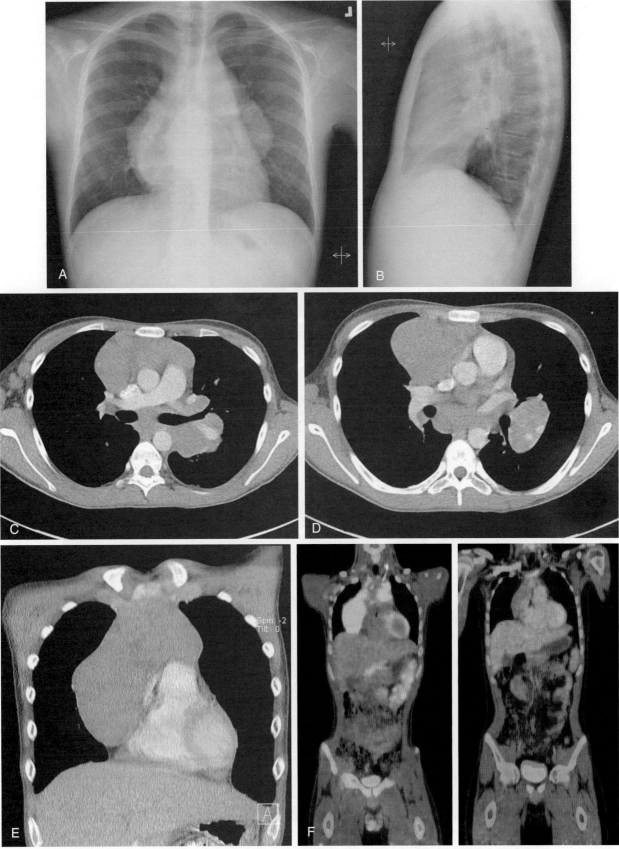

Fig. 2.17 (A) Posteroanterior chest radiograph shows a large anterior mediastinal mass. The lateral (B) view shows obliteration of the retrosternal clear space and middle mediastinal masses compatible with hilar adenopathy. Axial (C & D) and coronal (E) contrast-enhanced computed tomography images of the chest show extensive mediastinal and hilar adenopathy. Coronal FDG-PET image (F) before and after two cycles of chemotherapy show complete metabolic response, a feature of a rapid early responder.

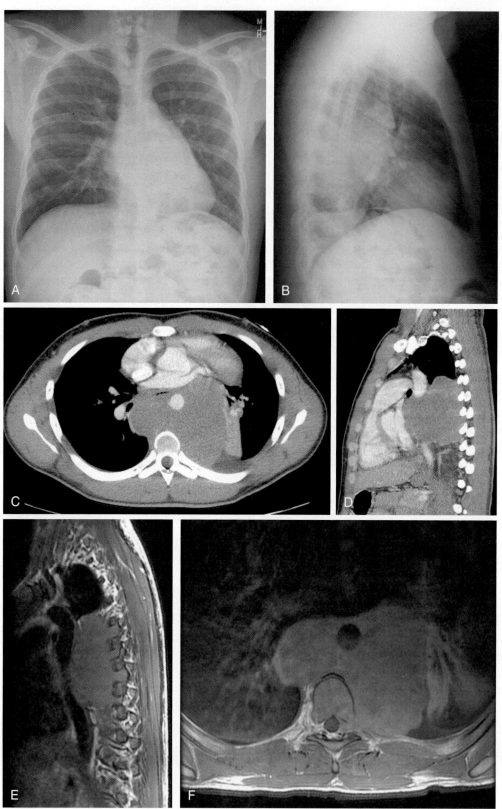

Fig. 2.18 Fourteen-year-old boy with chest pain. Posteroanterior (A) and lateral (B) chest radiographs show a mass involving both the middle and posterior compartments of the mediastinum. Axial (C) and sagittal (D) computed tomography images demonstrate a homogenous mass with encasement of the descending thoracic aorta, which is uplifted away from the spine. Sagittal (E) and axial (F) T1-weighted images of the thoracic spine show neural foraminal invasion.

from VM. Edema and enhancement of the adjacent soft tissue may be present in the setting of an inflamed LM. The cysts in a microcystic LM are usually too small to identify as discrete structures on MRI and usually appear as diffuse areas of low T1 signal and increased signal on T2WI, with mild postcontrast enhancement. Treatment requires a multidisciplinary approach and may be a combination of percutaneous sclerotherapy, surgery, and medical management.

■ Middle Mediastinum

Vascular: Rings and Slings

Aortic arch anomalies may present as middle mediastinal masses. Vascular rings are uncommon anomalies of the aortic arch that result in encircling and compression of the tracheobronchial tree and/or esophagus that may result in respiratory or gastrointestinal symptoms. They account for approximately 1% to 3% of congenital heart disease, with males having a 1.4 to 2 times greater risk than females. Clinical presentation varies from critical airway obstruction in a neonate to an incidental finding in older asymptomatic patients.

Chest radiographs are typically the initial examination performed in symptomatic patients. On the lateral projection, there may be anterior bowing of the trachea and a retrotracheal density secondary to an aberrant subclavian vein or double aortic arch. An abnormal mediastinal contour or widening may be observed on the frontal view. Attention to the tracheal indentation on the frontal view may suggest a right-sided aortic arch (Fig. 2.19A). Unilateral hyperinflation, tracheal narrowing, or a horizontal course of the mainstem bronchi may suggest a pulmonary sling. Cross-sectional imaging (CT or MRI) is necessary to characterize the anomaly

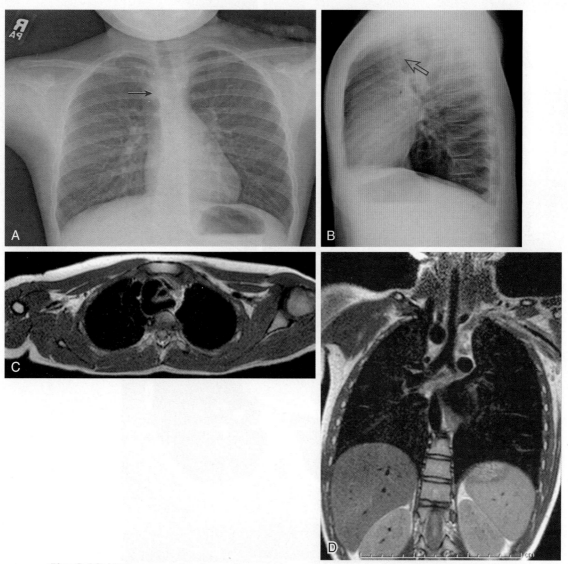

Fig. 2.19 (A) Posteroanterior chest radiograph shows mild widening of the upper mediastinum with indentation on the right aspect of the trachea (*arrow*). (B) On the lateral radiograph, there is mild anterior bowing of the trachea (*open arrow*). Axial (C) and coronal (D) black blood sequences show a right-sided aortic arch with an aberrant left subclavian artery corresponding to the findings on radiographs.

and define its relationship with the aerodigestive tract (see Fig. 2.19B).

Double aortic arch is defined as persistence of the third and fourth aortic arches. More than half of symptomatic arch anomalies are caused by a double aortic arch. The trachea and esophagus are encircled by the aortic arches. Surgical division of a vascular ring is indicated when there are symptoms of airway or esophageal compression.

Foregut Anomalies

Bronchopulmonary foregut anomalies encompass a spectrum of anomalies that includes foregut duplication cysts. Intrathoracic foregut cysts are rare malformations of the embryonic foregut and are composed of three subtypes: bronchogenic, esophageal, and neurenteric. Bronchogenic cysts are thought to result from abnormal lung budding during development and can occur anywhere throughout the tracheobronchial tree, with a predilection for the subcarinal and right paratracheal regions (Fig. 2.20A). Approximately 20% are found intrapulmonary, manifesting as a cyst within lung parenchyma. Bronchogenic cysts are typically well-circumscribed lesions that show water density on CT and are hyperintense on T2WI, hypointense on T1WI, and have thin peripheral enhancement after gadolinium administration. High attenuation within a cyst on CT

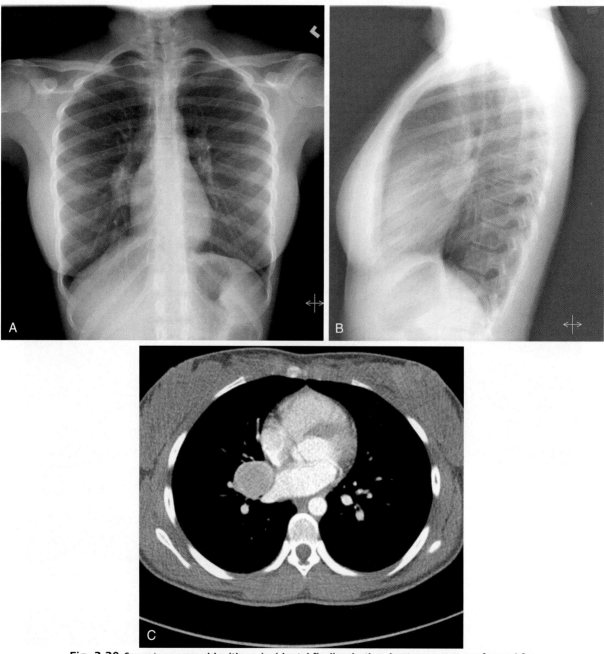

Fig. 2.20 *Seventeen-year-old with an incidental finding in the chest on a scan performed for abdominal pain.* Posteroanterior (A) and lateral (B) chest radiographs show a right hilar, middle mediastinal mass. Axial contrast-enhanced CT of the chest (C) shows a well-circumscribed right hilar mass with soft tissue attenuation (145 Hounsfield units). The high density is likely due to proteinaceous content in this surgically proven bronchogenic cyst.

may be caused by high protein content (see Fig. 2.20C), which is often hyperintense on T1WI. On histological examination the cyst is lined by respiratory epithelium containing smooth muscle, hyaline cartilage, or seromucous glands.

Esophageal duplication cysts result from abnormal development of the posterior division of the foregut. Patients typically present with dysphagia. The upper third of the esophagus is most common, with reports of detached intrapulmonary locations. The histological presence of submucosa or the muscular layer of the gastrointestinal tract provides definitive diagnosis.

Neurenteric cysts are caused by failure of separation of the GI tract from the primitive neural crest during embryonic development. Most neurenteric cysts are located in the posterior mediastinum, often communicate with the spinal canal, and may be associated with congenital vertebral body anomalies.

■ Posterior Mediastinum

What Is the Origin of the Most Common Posterior Mediastinal Mass?

Among all mediastinal masses, about 30% to 40% occur in the posterior mediastinum. The vast majority (approximately 90%) of posterior mediastinal masses are neurogenic in origin, derived from the sympathetic chain located along the vertebral bodies. Neurogenic tumors can be further subdivided into ganglion cell tumors, nerve sheath tumors, and other nervous tissue tumors. Less commonly encountered lesions within the posterior mediastinum include extramedullary hematopoiesis, lipomatosis, vascular malformations, and sarcomas.

Neurogenic masses are on a spectrum of malignancy ranging from the malignant neuroblastoma to the benign ganglioneuroma, with ganglioneuroblastoma having intermediate malignant potential. Neuroblastoma, a malignant tumor of primitive neural crest cells, is most common and typically occurs anywhere along the sympathetic chain. Patients with thoracic neuroblastoma can be asymptomatic, and lesions may be detected incidentally on imaging performed for other complaints. Symptoms are often related to local mass effect of the tumor on nearby structures. For example, tracheal deviation results in stridor, whereas high thoracic and cervical tumors may cause Horner syndrome (ptosis, miosis, anhidrosis) (Fig. 2.21). Neuroforaminal invasion and spinal cord compression may be associated with bowel and bladder dysfunction, extremity weakness, or paraplegia. Patients with metastatic disease typically have constitutional symptoms, including fever, irritability, failure to thrive, and bone pain. Elevated urine catecholamines are highly specific for neuroblastoma; however, sensitivity ranges from 66% to 100%.

Age is an important factor when narrowing a differential diagnosis of a pediatric patient with a posterior mediastinal mass. The median ages of patients with neuroblastoma, ganglioneuroblastoma, and ganglioneuroma are 2, 5.5, and 10 years, respectively. Congenital neuroblastoma may be detected on fetal imaging or imaging performed in the neonatal period.

Chest radiographs show a paraspinal density, which may be associated with rib or vertebral body erosion (Fig. 2.22). Calcifications are common in neuroblastomas, which can be seen in up to 30% of cases on radiographs and 80% of the time on CT, which is more sensitive in the detection of calcifications. CT better delineates the extent of the tumor and assesses for local and distant metastatic disease. Metastases are typically lytic or mixed lytic and sclerotic metaphyseal lesions. Because of the invasive nature of neuroblastoma, it tends to surround and encase blood vessels, and classically extends into the neural foramina. MRI is the modality of choice to evaluate the degree of spinal canal involvement (see Fig. 2.22). On MRI, neuroblastoma is bright on T2WI, hypointense on T1WI, and enhances after gadolinium administration. Bone marrow metastases are well depicted on MRI and are also dark on T1WI and bright on T2WI. Nuclear scintigraphy is used to stage patients with known or suspected neuroblastoma. ^{123}I-MIBG is a catecholamine analogue and localizes in neuroblastoma cells, detecting both the primary lesion and sites of metastatic disease in 90% to 95% of patients (see Fig. 2.21E).

Ganglioneuroma and ganglioneuroblastoma are difficult to distinguish from neuroblastoma on imaging examinations. Ganglioneuromas are benign lesions that typically occur in older patients (Fig. 2.23). Ganglioneuroblastoma, although less aggressive, has malignant potential and is therefore considered to be malignant.

Nerve Sheath Tumors

Nerve sheath tumors are classified as schwannomas or neurofibromas. Schwannomas are encapsulated without nerve fibers coursing through the lesion, whereas neurofibromas are unencapsulated and do have nerve fibers running through the tissue. Imaging characteristics of both types of nerve sheath tumors are similar. They are typically well defined, lobulated soft tissues masses that follow the course of the nerve and may enter the spinal canal via a widened neural foramen creating a dumbbell appearance. On MRI, they are homogeneous on T1WI, and on T2WI show high signal intensity peripherally and central intermediate in signal intensity, giving it a "target" appearance (Fig. 2.24).

What Patient Population Is at Risk for Malignant Peripheral Nerve Sheath Tumor?

Malignant degeneration into malignant peripheral nerve sheath tumors is rare and typically occurs in preexisting neurofibromas in patients with neurofibromatosis type 1. Rapid growth of a preexisting lesion, local invasion, osseous destruction, or associated pleural effusion are signs of malignancy. Imaging features suggesting malignant transformation include significant growth, change in enhancement pattern, and reduced diffusivity on

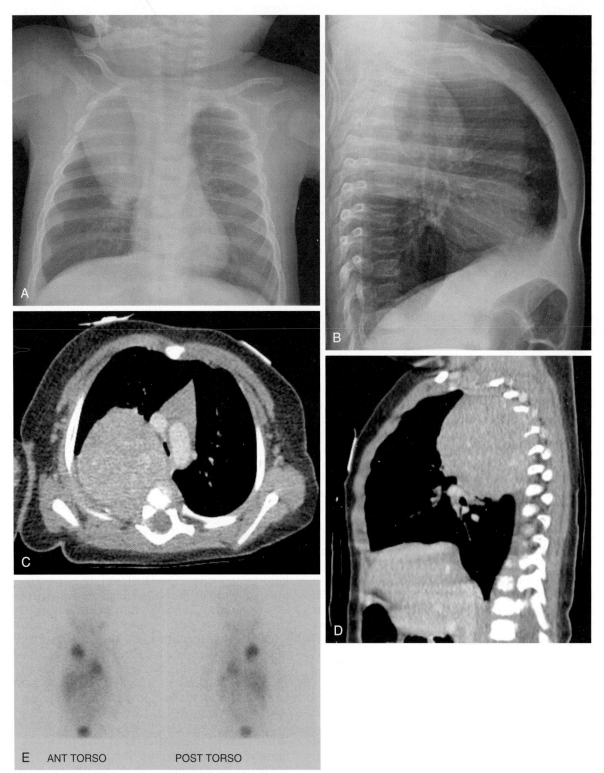

Fig. 2.21 Thoracic neuroblastoma. One-year-old girl with increased work of breathing and Horner syndrome. Frontal (A) and lateral (B) chest radiographs show a large right mediastinal mass that localizes to the posterior mediastinum on the lateral view. Axial (C) and sagittal (D) computed tomography (CT) images demonstrate a heterogeneously enhancing posterior mediastinal mass with marked mass effect on the airway and intraspinal extension. Metaiodobenzylguanidine (MIBG) scan (E) shows increased radiotracer uptake corresponding to the mass seen on radiographs and CT. *ANT*, Anterior; *POST*, posterior.

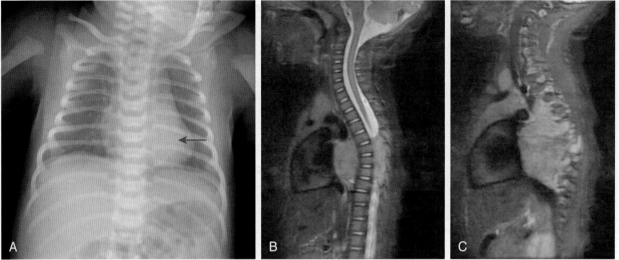

Fig. 2.22 Two-year-old male with lower extremity weakness. (A) Left retrocardiac opacity with splaying of the posterior ribs (*arrow*), a finding inconsistent with pneumonia. Sagittal T1-weighted fat-suppressed postcontrast images of the chest (B, C) performed 3 months later show a large posterior mediastinal mass with neural foraminal invasion and spinal cord compression.

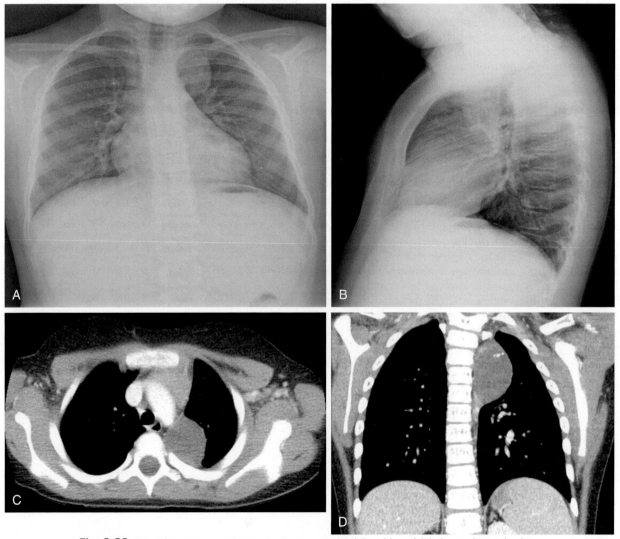

Fig. 2.23 Ten-year-old boy with cough. Posteroanterior (A) and lateral (B) chest radiographs show a left upper posterior mediastinal mass. Axial (C) and coronal (D) contrast-enhanced chest computed tomography images show a well-defined posterior mediastinal hypodense soft tissue mass with a focus of calcification; this mass was pathologically proved to be a ganglioneuroma.

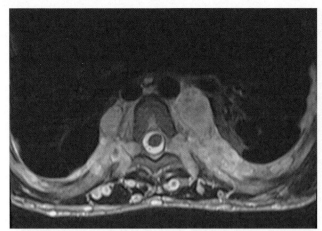

Fig. 2.24 Three-year-old with neurofibromatosis type 1. Axial T2-weighted magnetic resonance imaging of the chest shows bilateral paraspinal masses with intraspinal extension consistent with neurofibromas. The lesions are hyperintense on T2-weighted imaging, some of which have hypointense central zones, giving them a characteristic "target" appearance.

diffusion-weighted imaging. Increased FDG uptake in PET imaging with standard uptake value (SUV), particularly maximum SUV greater than 4, is also concerning for malignant transformation. The treatment for malignant peripheral nerve sheath tumor is surgical excision. Local recurrence is common, and prognosis is poor.

Extramedullary Hematopoiesis

Extramedullary hematopoiesis is defined as formation of hematopoietic tissue in locations other than bone marrow. It is a compensatory process intended to supplement defective hematopoiesis in patients with disorders resulting in chronic anemia. These disorders may be hereditary, as in thalassemia, sickle cell disease, hereditary spherocytosis, and polycythemia vera, or acquired, as in marrow-infiltrating diseases, such as leukemia and lymphoma. The liver, kidney, spleen, lymph nodes, and paraspinal regions are the most common locations. Chest radiographs typically show sharply marginated, bilateral paraspinal masses. Cross-sectional imaging reveals fat or iron content within longstanding lesions and often enhances after contrast administration.

■ Summary

Mediastinal masses in children are composed of a heterogeneous group of masses ranging from benign and incidental to malignant and life threatening. Although the assessment of a pediatric patient with a mediastinal mass requires a multidisciplinary approach, imaging plays a critical role in detection, characterization, and monitoring of disease.

Bibliography

Acker, S. N., Linton, J., Tan, G. M., Garrington, T. P., Bruny, J., Hilden, J. M., et al. (2015). A multidisciplinary approach to the management of anterior mediastinal masses in children. *Journal of Pediatric Surgery, 50*(5), 875–878.

Franco, A., Mody, N. S., & Meza, M. P. (2005). Imaging evaluation of pediatric mediastinal masses. *Radiologic Clinics of North America, 43*(2), 325–353.

Frush, D. P. (2003). Imaging of paediatric mediastinal masses. *Annals Academy of Medicine Singapore, 32*(4), 525–535.

Juanpere, S., Cañete, N., Ortuño, P., Martínez, S., Sanchez, G., & Bernado, L. (2013). A diagnostic approach to the mediastinal masses. *Insights Imaging, 4*(1), 29–52.

Lee, E. Y. (2009). Evaluation of non-vascular mediastinal masses in infants and children: An evidence-based practical approach. *Pediatric Radiology, 39*(Suppl. 2), S184–S190.

Lonergan, G. J., Schwab, C. M., Suarez, E. S., & Carlson, C. L. (2002). Neuroblastoma, ganglioneuroblastoma, and ganglioneuroma: Radiologic-pathologic correlation. *RadioGraphics, 22*(4), 911–934.

Manson, D. E. (2016). Magnetic resonance imaging of the mediastinum, chest wall and pleura in children. *Pediatric Radiology, 46*(6), 902–915.

Merten, D. F. (1992). Diagnostic imaging of mediastinal masses in children. *American Journal of Roentgenology, 158*(4), 825–832.

Meza, M. P., Benson, M., & Slovis, T. L. (1993). Imaging of mediastinal masses in children. *Radiologic Clinics of North America, 31*(3), 583–604.

Ranganath, S. H., Lee, E. Y., Restrepo, R., & Eisenberg, R. L. (2012). Mediastinal masses in children. *American Journal of Roentgenology, 198*(3), W197–W216.

Rosolen, A., Perkins, S. L., Pinkerton, C. R., Guillerman, R. P., Sandlund, J. T., Patte, C., et al. (2015). Revised international pediatric non-Hodgkin lymphoma staging system. *Journal of Clinical Oncology, 33*(18), 2112–2118. https://doi.org/10.1200/JCO.2014.59.7203. 25940716

Takahashi, K., Inaoka, T., Murakami, N., Hirota, H., Iwata, K., Nagasawa, K., et al. (2003). Characterization of the normal and hyperplastic thymus on chemical-shift MR imaging. *American Journal of Roentgenology, 180*(5), 1265–1269.

Thacker, P. G., Mahani, M. G., Heider, A., & Lee, E. Y. (2015). Imaging evaluation of mediastinal masses in children and adults: Practical diagnostic approach based on a new classification system. *Journal of Thoracic Imaging, 30*(4), 247–267.

Yaris, N., Nas, Y., Cobanoglu, U., & Yavuz, M. N. (2006). Thymic carcinoma in children. *Pediatric Blood and Cancer, 47*(2), 224–227.

CHAPTER 3

Approach to Congenital Heart Disease

Justin T. Tretter and Puneet Bhatla

CHAPTER OUTLINE

Segmental Approach to Congenital Heart Disease, 54
Morphological Identification of the Major Cardiac Segments, 54
  Atrial Identification, 55
    Visceroatrial Arrangement or Situs, 55
    Ventricular Identification, 55
    Ventricular Topology or Looping, 57
    Great Arterial Identification, 58
    Great Arterial Arrangement or Situs, 58
  Assessment of the Cardiac Segment Connections, 58
    Atrioventricular Connections, 58
    Ventriculoarterial Connections, 59
    Other Associated Lesions, 59
Septal Defects, 60
  Atrial Septal Defects and Interatrial Communications, 60
    Morphology and Pathophysiology, 60
    Clinical Presentation, 60
    Imaging, 60
    Treatment, 61
  Ventricular Septal Defects, 62
    Morphology and Pathophysiology, 62
    Clinical Presentation, 63
    Imaging, 63
    Treatment, 64
  Atrioventricular Septal Defects, 64
    Morphology and Pathophysiology, 64
    Clinical Presentation, 65
    Imaging, 65
    Treatment, 65
Select Outflow Tract Anomalies, 65
  Transposition of the Great Arteries, 65
    Morphology and Pathophysiology, 67
    Clinical Presentation, 67

    Imaging, 67
    Treatment, 68
  Tetralogy of Fallot, 68
    Morphology and Pathophysiology, 68
    Clinical Presentation, 68
    Imaging, 68
    Treatment, 69
  Double-Outlet Right Ventricle, 69
    Morphology and Pathophysiology, 70
    Clinical Presentation, 70
    Imaging, 70
    Treatment, 70
Select Left Heart Lesions, 71
  Hypoplastic Left Heart Syndrome, 71
    Morphology and Pathophysiology, 71
    Clinical Presentation, 71
    Imaging, 72
    Treatment, 72
  Shone Complex, 72
    Morphology and Pathophysiology, 73
    Clinical Presentation, 73
    Imaging, 73
    Treatment, 73
Aortic Arch Anomalies, 73
  Coarctation of the Aorta and Interrupted Aortic Arch, 73
    Morphology and Pathophysiology, 74
    Clinical Presentation, 74
    Imaging, 74
    Treatment, 74
  Vascular Rings, 75
    Morphology and Pathophysiology, 76
    Clinical Presentation, 76
    Imaging, 76
    Treatment, 76

Congenital heart disease (CHD) can be a challenge for the imagers because it requires a profound knowledge of the morphological and functional characteristics of a broad range of heart defects. Moreover, complex CHD often involves palliative or corrective surgical intervention that can significantly alter the anatomy and blood flow patterns. Therefore complete knowledge of these surgical palliations and repairs is essential to accurately identify associated problems and complications. There has been an increasing use of cardiac magnetic resonance imaging (CMR) and multidetector computed tomography (CT) in the evaluation of these patients. Hence there is an increasing interest among radiologists to understand and learn the various nomenclatures and classifications in place to describe these lesions.

■ Segmental Approach to Congenital Heart Disease

A standardized approach to address the countless variations in complex CHD is necessary to foster understanding of these lesions, along with promoting a common language across disciplines to optimize management of these patients. In 1972, Richard Van Praagh pioneered the segmental approach to CHD. This method involves dividing the heart into three major segments (atria, ventricles, and great arteries) and two interconnecting segments (atrioventricular [AV] junction and conus arteriosus) and then sequentially describing the spatial organization (situs) of each of these three segments using Latin terminology (Van Praagh 1972, 1984). The major groundwork for the segmental approach was laid by Maurice Lev, who coined the morphological method of chamber identification and described the key morphological features of various major segments. Meanwhile an alternate approach was later proposed by Robert Anderson. This involved describing the arrangement of the three major components (atria, ventricular, and arterial components) and emphasizing the two connecting segments (AV and ventriculoarterial connections) using English terminology (Fig. 3.1). The connecting segments can be designated as being either concordant or discordant (Anderson & Shirali, 2009; Shinebourne et al., 1976).

The sequential segmental approach aims to address the following:
1. Perform morphological identification of the three major cardiac segments (atria, ventricles, great arteries).
2. Describe the relationship of the interconnecting segments (AV and ventriculoarterial connections).
3. Describe any associated anomalies involving the valves, atrial and ventricular septum, the great vessels, and the systemic and pulmonary veins.

For example, using Anderson terminology, one would describe the normal heart as having usual atrial arrangement with concordant AV and ventriculoarterial connections and right hand ventricular topology.

The approach taken by Van Praagh uses a three-letter notation within braces to describe the relationships of the three segments, mentioning the connections only if abnormal, with additional notations before or after to describe important associated cardiac anomalies. The spatial relationship of the three main cardiac segments is indicated within the braces: {visceroatrial situs, ventricular situs or looping, great arterial relationship}, with the normal cardiac arrangement stated as {S, D, S}, indicating normal visceroatrial situs solitus, D-looped ventricles, and arterial situs solitus (normally related great arteries). Any ventriculoarterial misalignment, such as transposition of the great arteries (TGA) or double-outlet right ventricle (DORV), may be notated before the braces. Any AV malalignments and associated cardiovascular malformations may be notated after the braces, such as ventricular septal defects (VSDs) or hypoplastic right ventricle (RV). The cardiac position within the chest or position of the cardiac apex may be notated before the braces if abnormal. For instance, dextroposition

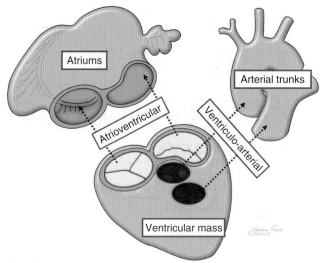

Fig. 3.1 The sequential segmental approach to congenital heart disease involves describing the topological arrangement of the three major cardiac segments (atria, ventricles, and arterial trunks) and describing the two connecting segments (atrioventricular and ventriculoarterial).

refers to the situation when the heart is predominantly positioned within the right hemithorax, and mesoposition when positioned predominantly in the center of the thorax. Dextrocardia refers to the situation where the cardiac apex points rightward, and mesocardia when midline (Anderson & Shirali, 2009; Van Praagh, 1984). Although there are differences to both the Van Praagh and Anderson approaches, there are many similarities to their approaches. Important to this, a recent consensus document of terminology related to the nomenclature of CHD was published by the International Society for Nomenclature of Paediatric and Congenital Heart Disease for the 11th iteration of the *International Classification of Diseases* (ICD-11; refer to this document and to the ICD-11 listing on the World Health Organization website [https://icd.who.int/dev11/f/en] for a detailed listing) (Franklin et al., 2017).

In addition, it is important to recognize that historical cardiac terminology named the attitudinal description with the heart removed from the body and placed on its apex in the Valentine position. This becomes confusing to the cardiac imager who now views the heart as it lies within the body. A review by Mori et al. (2019) describes the detailed normal cardiac anatomy in attitudinally correct fashion as it lies within the body, as revealed by CT three-dimensional reconstructions.

■ Morphological Identification of the Major Cardiac Segments

Recognizing important morphological characteristics of the various cardiac chambers and great arteries is important in classifying the segmental anatomy, because the description of an atrium or ventricle as being "right" or "left" does not refer to its spatial orientation but its morphological identification. Although some of these features are not readily identifiable by current modes of cardiac imaging, with improving technology, most

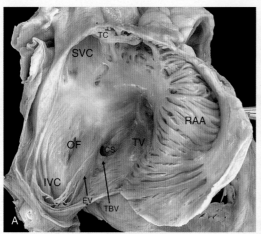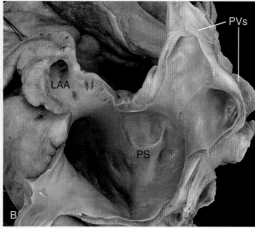

Fig. 3.2 (A) The morphological right atrium is opened, cutting through the terminal crest (*TC*). The broad-based right atrial appendage (*RAA*) is visualized with pectinate muscle extending from within the RAA outside of its confines toward the vestibular of the right atrium near the atrioventricular junction. The superior caval vein (*SVC*) and inferior caval vein (*IVC*) are demonstrated draining into the right atrium. The floor of the oval fossa (*OF*) is surrounding superiorly, posteriorly, and inferiorly by the interatrial infolding or "secondary septum". (B) The morphological left atrium is opened demonstrating the narrow base of the tubular left atrial appendage (*LAA*), with its pectinate muscle contained within the atrial appendage. The pulmonary veins (*PV*) drain into the posterior aspect of the left atrium. The primary atrial septum (*PS*), which forms the floor of the oval fossa on the right side, is visualized. *CS*, Coronary sinus; *EV*, Eustachian valve; *MV*, mitral valve; *TBV*, thebesian valve; *TV*, tricuspid valve. (The specimen images were provided by Diane E. Spicer, Department of Pediatric Cardiology, University of Florida, Gainesville, FL, USA)

of these features can be distinguished. The morphological identification of these chambers and great arteries is then used to assess their respective connections, which help systematically describe the cardiac morphology.

Atrial Identification

The atria are readily distinguished by assessing the inferior vena cava (IVC) and coronary sinus connection, the relation of the primary atrial septum to its "secondary septum," and the atrial appendage morphology, including the extent of pectinate muscle. The right atrium (RA), or systemic venous atrium, receives systemic venous return from the IVC and coronary sinus drainage. Even in the setting of an interrupted IVC, a suprahepatic segment of the IVC tends to drain into the RA, making this a more reliable feature. The RA appendage is broad and triangular shaped, with pectinate muscle extending from the atrial appendage to the vestibule of the RA (Fig. 3.2A). Although the pectinate muscle is difficult to assess by current echocardiographic imaging, it is increasingly detected by CMR and CT imaging.

The left atrium (LA) normally receives all of the pulmonary venous return, although this is highly variable and an unreliable marker for morphological identification. The flap valve of the foramen ovale attaches to the left atrial side of the "secondary septum," the latter of which is technically not a true septum but instead an interatrial infolding that encircles the inferior, posterior, and superior portions of the oval fossa. More reliable is the assessment of the left atrial appendage, which appears long, thin, and "finger-like," with the pectinate muscle contained within the appendage (see Fig. 3.2B).

Visceroatrial Arrangement or Situs

When we assess atrial arrangement or situs, we are assessing the visceral relationship to the respective atrium, or visceroatrial situs. Usual visceral and atrial arrangement or visceroatrial situs solitus {S,-,-} refers to the normal visceral arrangement (right-sided liver, single left-sided spleen, three-lobed right lung with an eparterial bronchus, and two-lobed left lung with a hyparterial bronchus) with a right-sided morphological RA. Mirror image visceroatrial arrangement or visceroatrial situs inversus refers to the mirror image of the normal arrangement described earlier and is denoted as {I,-,-}. The stomach, superior vena cava (SVC), pulmonary venous connections, and cardiac apex position are not reliable markers for determining visceroatrial situs. Visceroatrial situs ambiguous {A,-,-} is used to denote when the atria cannot be morphologically distinguished as right and left, as is commonly the case in heterotaxy syndromes and common atrium (Fig. 3.3). Using Andersonian terminology in a patient with heterotaxy syndrome, one would describe the patient as having right or left atrial appendage isomerism, and the details of the visceral arrangement would be described (Figs. 3.3 and 3.4).

Ventricular Identification

The ventricles are distinguished by assessment of the corresponding AV valve, including valve attachments, the ventricular shape, and the extent and appearance of the muscular trabeculations within the ventricle. By definition, the tricuspid valve (TV) is associated with the morphological RV. The TV is typically trileaflet, composed of the septal, anterosuperior, and inferior leaflets. It contains prominent direct chordal attachments of its septal leaflet to the ventricular septum (referred to as "septophilic") and tends to be more apically positioned

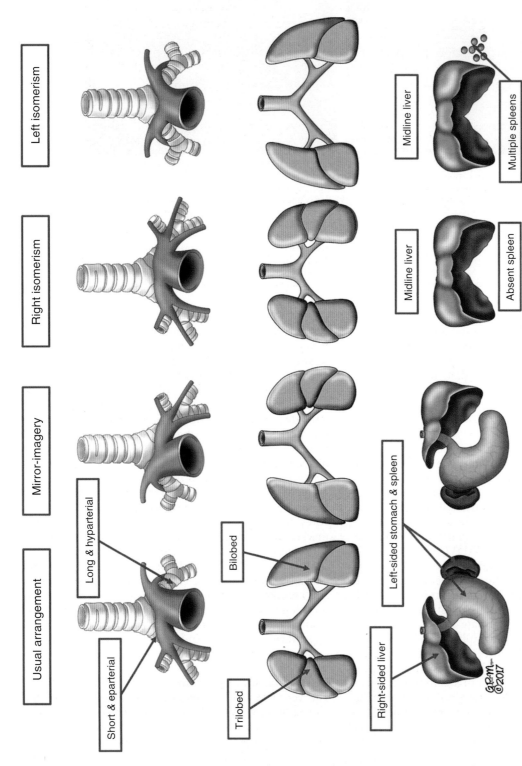

Fig. 3.3 Thoracoabdominal visceral arrangement demonstrated. (Top panel) Morphology of the tracheobronchial tree. In the usual visceral arrangement ("situs solitus"), the right mainstem bronchus is short and eparterial, with the right upper lobe branching over the second branch of the right pulmonary artery, and the left mainstem bronchus is longer and hyparterial, coursing underneath the left pulmonary artery. In mirror image visceral arrangement ("situs inversus," a misnomer as the organs are not switched "upside down"), the bronchial arrangement is the opposite of the usual arrangement, with the right-sided bronchus being longer and hyparterial, and the left-sided bronchus being short and eparterial. In right isomerism, there is bilateral short and eparterial bronchi. In left isomerism, there is bilateral long and hyparterial bronchi. Note that "situs ambiguous" is a poor term, because the visceral anatomy should be described and is never ambiguous. In a usual visceral arrangement the right lung is trilobed and the left lung bilobed. In a mirror image visceral arrangement, this is the opposite. In right isomerism, there are bilateral trilobed lungs. In left isomerism, there are bilateral bilobed lungs. (Lower panel) Morphology of the abdominal organs. In usual visceral arrangement the liver is right sided and the stomach and spleen are left sided. In mirror image visceral arrangement the organs are in the opposite position. In both right and left isomerism, the liver tends to span across the midline. In right isomerism the spleen can be absent, whereas in left isomerism there can be multiple spleens. Alternatively, the spleen may be present but not functional. The splenic anatomy is the least consistent feature of isomeric patients.

relative to the mitral valve (MV). Papillary muscles arise from both the septal and free wall surfaces of the RV. The RV is triangular or pyramidal, and is filled with coarse, heavy trabeculations with a prominent muscular band ("moderator band") coursing from the apical portion of the ventricular septum to the free wall, containing the right bundle branch of the conduction system. In the normal heart, the outlet portion of the RV contains a prominent muscular cone of tissue separating the TV from the pulmonary valve, commonly referred to as the conus or infundibulum. This is highly variable in abnormal cardiac arrangements and cannot be used to identify the RV (Fig. 3.5A).

The left ventricle (LV) is associated with the MV, which is commonly composed of two leaflets, the anterior ("aortic") and posterior ("mural") leaflets. These

two leaflets are attached by chordae to the two free wall papillary muscles, the anterolateral and posteromedial papillary muscles, which when related to the body are in fact positioned superolaterally and inferomedially, respectively. Given the lack of septal attachments of the MV, it is commonly referred to as "septophobic." The MV is more cranially positioned compared with its adjacent AV valve. The LV is prolate ellipsoid or bullet shaped, with fine trabeculations within the apical trabecular component of the ventricle and a smooth septal surface (see Fig. 3.5B). It should be noted that the shape of the ventricle can be an unreliable marker in both pressure- and/or volume-loaded ventricles, which is present in many cardiac defects. In the normal heart, there commonly is no conus or infundibulum present in the LV, resulting in mitral–aortic valve fibrous continuity. Again this is an unreliable marker in CHD.

Ventricular Topology or Looping

In early embryogenesis, the straight heart tube outgrows its containing sac resulting in looping of the tube either to the right (D-dextro-looped) as in normal development, or to the left (L-levo-looped). The "hand rule" is used to determine the topology or looping of any developed heart. The palm of one hand is placed on the ventricular septal surface of the RV with the thumb in the inflow and the fingers in the outflow. This can only be accomplished with one hand. If the right hand is used, then the ventricles are said to have right hand ventricular topology or to be D-looped ventricles {-,D,-}, as seen in normal development. In this arrangement the RV is anterior and to the right of the LV (Fig. 3.6A). If the left hand is used, then the ventricles are said to have left hand ventricular topology or to be L-looped ventricles {-,L,-}. In this arrangement the RV is anterior and to the left of the LV (see Fig. 3.6B). X is used to denote when the ventricular morphology cannot be determined {-,X,-}, or it is referred to as indeterminate.

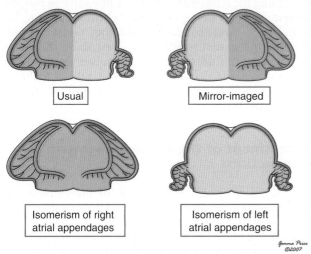

Usual   Mirror-imaged

Isomerism of right atrial appendages   Isomerism of left atrial appendages

Gemma Price
@2007

Fig. 3.4 There are four possible arrangements of the atria using Anderson terminology, as depicted. When using the Van Praagh approach, both of the isomeric arrangements would be described as ambiguous.

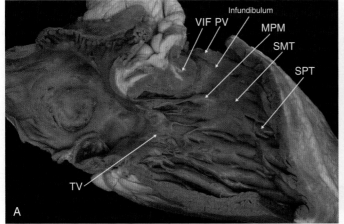

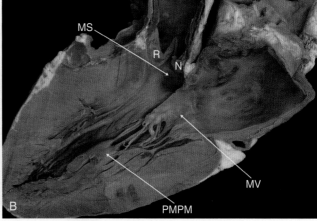

Fig. 3.5 (A) The morphological right ventricle is identified by its triangular or pyramidal shape, prominent septal attachments of the tricuspid valve (*TV*), and heavy apical trabeculations with prominent moderator band (cut in this image near the base of the septomarginal trabeculation [*SMT*]). (B) The morphological left ventricle (LV) is identified by its prolate ellipsoidal or bullet shape, lack of septal attachments of the mitral valve (MV), and fine apical trabeculations. *MPM*, Medial papillary muscle; *MS*, membranous septum; *N*, noncoronary leaflet of the aortic valve; *PMPM*, posteromedial papillary muscle; *PV*, pulmonary valve; *R*, right coronary leaflet of the aortic valve; *SPT*, septoparietal trabeculations; *VIF*, ventricular infundibular fold.(The specimen images were provided by Diane E. Spicer, Department of Pediatric Cardiology University of Florida, Gainesville, FL, USA)

Great Arterial Identification

The artery that gives rise to the branch pulmonary arteries is the pulmonary trunk or main pulmonary artery. The aorta usually gives rise to the coronary arteries, the aortic arch, and its brachiocephalic arteries. A truncus arteriosus, or common arterial trunk, occurs when a common vessel arises from the ventricles and gives rise to the coronary, brachiocephalic, and branch pulmonary arteries. A solitary arterial trunk is defined when there is absence of the intrapericardial pulmonary arteries, and one cannot determine, had they been present, whether the pulmonary trunk and its branches would have originated separately from a ventricle or from a common arterial trunk (Fig. 3.7). As described previously, the conus or infundibulum separates the TV from the pulmonary valve in the normal heart. This is absent in the LV, allowing mitral–aortic valve fibrous continuity. All hearts can have one of the following: bilateral infundibulum (subaortic and subpulmonary), subpulmonary infundibulum (as in the normal heart), subaortic infundibulum only (as usually seen in transposition), or bilaterally absent infundibulum (as can be seen in double-outlet LV). This is highly variable and should be noted on morphological assessment.

Great Arterial Arrangement or Situs

In normally related great arteries (NRGAs) the aorta is aligned with the LV and the pulmonary trunk is aligned with the RV. The subpulmonary infundibulum lifts the pulmonary root superiorly and leftward in relationship to the aortic root, and mitral–aortic valve fibrous continuity is commonly present. In the normal heart (usual atrial arrangement with concordant AV and ventricular arterial connections with NRGAs, or {S,D,S}), the aortic root lies posterior and to the right of the pulmonary root. In I-inversus-NRGAs in a patient with situs inversus of the atria {I,L,I} the aortic root lies posterior and to the left of the pulmonary root. All other great artery relationships are abnormal, with variations in underlying infundibulum. The denotation for abnormal great artery relationships, which is labeled in the third position in the segmental diagnosis, includes L, D, and A, describing the relationship of the aortic valve to the pulmonary valve as being leftward, rightward, or anterior, respectively. Andersonian terminology would simply describe the spatial relationship. Describing this detail is important to fully understand the given morphology. For example, the denotation {-,-,D} could describe an aortic root that is either rightward or rightward and anterior to the pulmonary root.

Assessment of the Cardiac Segment Connections

After identifying the morphology of the three major cardiac segments and their spatial arrangement, the intersegmental connections must be assessed. Further mention of the cardiac chambers in this chapter will reference the morphological identification rather than the spatial arrangement. Normal or concordant connections conclude that the RA is connected to the RV, which is in turn aligned to the pulmonary trunk. Similarly, the LA is connected to the LV, which is aligned to the aorta. Abnormal connections may occur at both the AV connection and the ventriculoarterial connection.

Atrioventricular Connections

In biventricular AV connections, commonly they may be either concordant, in which the RA drains into the

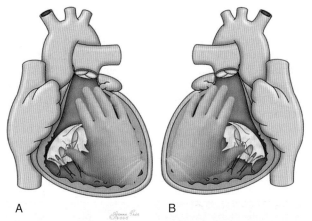

A   B

Fig. 3.6 Looping or topology of the heart is determined by the "hand rule," where the palm of one hand is placed on the ventricular septal surface of the right ventricle with the thumb in the inflow and the fingers in the outflow. The corresponding hand that is able to accomplish this position determines the looping or ventricular topology to be right (A) or left (B).

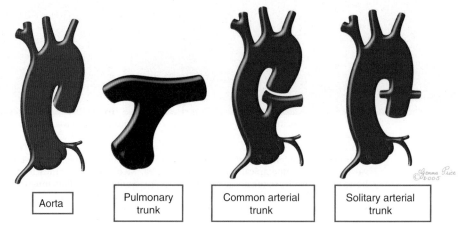

| Aorta | Pulmonary trunk | Common arterial trunk | Solitary arterial trunk |

Fig. 3.7 Morphology of the great arteries is determined by their branching pattern.

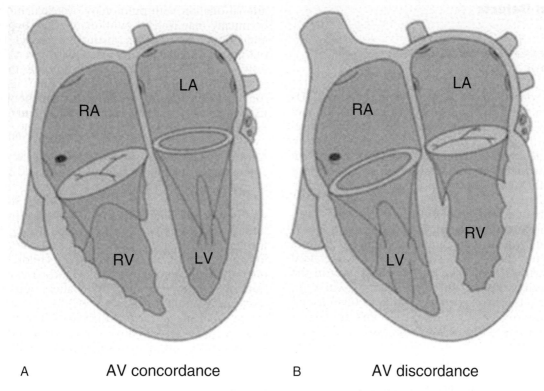

A   AV concordance   B   AV discordance

Fig. 3.8 In biventricular atrioventricular connections, they may be described as either concordant (A) or discordant (B). In the setting of heterotaxy, with isomeric atrial appendages, the atrioventricular connections are considered mixed. *LA,* Left atrium; *LV,* left ventricle; *RA,* right atrium; *RV,* right ventricle.

RV and LA drains into the LV ({S,D,-} or {I,L,-}), or discordant, in which the RA drains into the LV and the LA drains into the RV ({S,L,-} or {I,D,-}) (Fig. 3.8). Less commonly, abnormal AV connections include straddling of the AV valve in which there are chordal attachments crossing over to the opposite ventricle through an interventricular communication, overriding of the AV valve in which the AV valve annulus crosses the interventricular septum lying partially over the opposite ventricle, and a balanced common atrioventricular septal defect (AVSD). Univentricular AV connections can include an atretic AV valve, double inlet LV, or less commonly, RV, and left or right dominant unbalanced common AVSD. In heterotaxy syndrome, whether right or left atrial appendage isomerism, there are mixed AV connections. Any abnormal AV connection should be noted after the braces when describing a lesion using the Van Praagh terminology.

Ventriculoarterial Connections
Normally the pulmonary trunk is aligned with the RV and the aorta with the LV (concordant ventriculoarterial connections), with the presence of subpulmonary infundibulum, and the absence of subaortic infundibulum. The variation in subarterial infundibulum generally determines the relative position of the great arteries, because the presence of the subarterial infundibulum tends to position the respective great artery superiorly and anteriorly. Any other scenario apart from that in NRGAs or anatomically corrected malposition (better

described as concordant ventriculoarterial connections with bilateral subarterial infundibula and parallel arterial trunks) comprises discordant ventriculoarterial connections. In TGA the aorta is aligned with the RV and the pulmonary trunk with the LV. DORV often, but not always, occurs when there are varying degrees of infundibulum under both great arteries, resulting in both great arteries arising from the RV. This is always associated with a VSD to act as an outflow for the LV. Common arterial trunk or truncus arteriosus, and the rare cases of a solitary arterial trunk with absence of intrapericardial pulmonary arteries, were both previously described. When using the Van Praagh approach, any ventriculoarterial connection (the "conotruncal" diagnosis) should be noted before the braces when describing a lesion.

Other Associated Lesions
When using the Van Praagh approach, following the "conotruncal" diagnosis, segmental diagnosis, and any associated AV alignment abnormality, any other associated defect should be listed. These include but are not limited to VSDs, atrial septal defects (ASDs), semilunar valve abnormalities, aortic arch abnormalities, and patent ductus arteriosus (PDA). When using the Anderson approach, applicable lesions are listed sequentially as they relate to the three major segments and two connecting segments, with septal defects often stated last (Allen et al., 2016; Anderson & Shirali, 2009; Van Praagh, 1972; Wernovsky et al., 2019).

■ Septal Defects

Atrial Septal Defects and Interatrial Communications

Interatrial communications makes up to 10% of CHDs in children, with an estimated incidence of 100 per 100,000 live births. The most common of these is a deficiency in the floor of the oval fossa, referred to as an oval fossa defect or secundum ASD. The only other form of a true deficiency in the atrial septum is a deficiency found in the anteroinferior muscular buttress, the so-called vestibular defect (Loomba et al., 2020; Mori et al., 2018). This underappreciated defect is often mistaken for a secundum ASD; however, careful interrogation will demonstrate that it is not found within the confines of the floor of the oval fossa. The remaining interatrial communications are not related to a deficiency in the atrial septum and allow interatrial shunting. These include the sinus venosus defects, which are often found at the mouth of one of the caval veins and are related to a retained venovenous bridge with associated anomalous drainage of a pulmonary vein, and the coronary sinus defect, which is caused by the absence of the walls that usually separate the coronary sinus from the LA. A patent foramen ovale (PFO), which is a normal interatrial communication present in the fetus, remains patent into adulthood in approximately 25% to 30% of healthy adults and is considered a normal variant. The "primum ASD" is not technically an ASD, but instead an AVSD with exclusively atrial-level shunting. In this form of an AVSD the common AV junction is often divided into a right and left AV valve by a tongue of tissue between the superior and inferior bridging leaflets, which is firmly attached to the crest of the ventricular septum. This defect will be discussed in more detail in the Atrioventricular Septal Defects section (Allen et al., 2016; Wernovsky et al., 2019).

Morphology and Pathophysiology

The most common type of ASD, a secundum ASD, results from a deficiency in the primary atrial septum, which normally forms the floor of the oval fossa. The vestibular defect results from a deficiency in the antero-inferior muscular buttress. The sinus venosus defect results from a retained venovenous bridge between the respective systemic and pulmonary veins, allowing indirect communication from the LA to the RA. The coronary sinus defect results from deficiency in the walls that usually separate the coronary sinus from the LA, allowing indirect communication from the LA to the RA. This defect is commonly associated with a persistent left SVC draining into the coronary sinus.

Irrespective of the type of interatrial communication, the degree of left-to-right shunting is determined by the size of the defect and relative compliance of the ventricles. During the first few months of life, RV compliance improves, resulting in increasing right-sided volume overloading. Into adulthood, LV compliance tends to worsen, with further increase in right-sided volume overloading. This left-to-right shunting leads to RA, RV, and pulmonary arterial dilation with pulmonary overcirculation, which eventually may lead to pulmonary artery hypertension and pulmonary vascular obstructive disease. In severe pulmonary vascular obstructive disease, reversal of atrial level shunting, or Eisenmenger syndrome, may occur. It should be noted that smaller secundum ASDs (≤5–8 mm) may become smaller or even close spontaneously in the first few years of life, but thereafter tend to become larger with time (Allen et al., 2016).

Clinical Presentation

The majority of children tolerate this initial left-to-right shunting well and remain asymptomatic into early adulthood, with only up to 5% of patients developing significant pulmonary vascular disease leading to pulmonary hypertension before 20 years of age. However, the incidence may increase fourfold in the third and fourth decades of life. The majority of children with an interatrial communication are diagnosed after evaluation for a murmur or incidentally after evaluation with electrocardiogram, chest x-ray (CXR), or echocardiogram. Adults may present with exercise intolerance, atrial arrhythmias, or paradoxical emboli. If Eisenmenger syndrome develops, patients may present with cyanosis or syncope with exertion.

Imaging

Larger interatrial communications are readily detected in utero with fetal echocardiography; however, small-to-moderate secundum ASDs can be difficult to distinguish in utero from a normal foramen ovale. CXR may be normal during the first decade of life or in smaller interatrial communications. Moderate-to-severe shunting across an interatrial communication can lead to cardiomegaly on CXR as a result of RA and RV enlargement, with prominent main pulmonary artery and increased pulmonary vascular markings extending to the periphery.

Echocardiography is crucial in defining the interatrial communication type, size, degree of shunting, the presence of right chamber dilation, estimation of RV pressure, and any associated defects. Subcostal and high-right parasternal imaging are the primary images used to assess the atrial septum. Transesophageal echocardiogram (TEE) is often used perioperatively to better define the interatrial communication, especially in patients with poor acoustic windows during transthoracic echocardiogram (TTE). TEE additionally plays a crucial role in guiding percutaneous device closure of secundum ASDs. A PFO is differentiated from a small secundum ASD by the overlap of a flap valve on the left side and "secondary septum" or interatrial fold to the right of the interatrial septum, creating a tunneling communication. Intravenous (IV) contrast injection using agitated saline can be used during TTE or TEE imaging to confirm the presence of a PFO or ASD. Real-time three-dimensional echocardiography allows better morphological delineation of the secundum ASD and its surrounding structures, providing helpful information to determine candidacy for percutaneous device closure (Wernovsky et al., 2019).

CMR can be used in patients for whom echocardiography has failed to fully define the interatrial communication

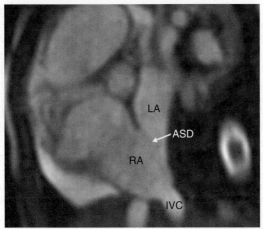

Fig. 3.9 Cardiac magnetic resonance bright-blood short-axis plane image, demonstrating a large secundum atrial septal defect (*ASD*), with dilated right atrium (*RA*). *IVC,* Inferior vena cava; *LA,* left atrium.

(Fig. 3.9) and to better quantify the RV dilation and estimate the left-to-right shunt. To calculate the ASD shunting, the RV stroke volume provides an estimate for Qp (flow to the lungs that includes the shunt at the atrial level), while the LV stroke volume provides an estimate of Qs (systemic flow to the body). The difference in the ventricular stroke volume (RV – LV) in the absence of any valvar regurgitation provides an estimate of shunt volume. CMR phase contrast imaging also can be used to quantify left-to-right shunting by directly estimating Qp (main pulmonary artery flow) as opposed to Qs (ascending aorta flow). It is particularly useful in sinus venosus (Fig. 3.10) and coronary sinus defects, where definition by echocardiogram can be difficult. CT and CMR is often preferred to assure accurate definition of the anomalous pulmonary venous drainage into the SVC or IVC that is commonly associated with sinus venosus defects (Fig. 3.11). In particular, an accurate delineation of anomalous pulmonary veins to the SVC, including the distance from the SVC–RA junction, is critical in surgical decision-making, with the options being direct baffling of the pulmonary veins to LA (pulmonary veins draining in close proximity to SVC–RA junction) as opposed to the Warden procedure (high drainage of pulmonary veins into the cranial SVC), which involves using the caudal SVC as a pulmonary vein baffle and the cranial SVC is surgically connected to the RA appendage. Echocardiography is often adequate when interrogating these structures in the proper imaging planes (Tretter et al., 2017).

Treatment

Closure of an ASD is indicated if there is a large shunt, with Qp (pulmonary flow):Qs (systemic flow) greater than or equal to 1.5 or other evidence of right chamber enlargement. In asymptomatic children with a large shunt, elective closure is often performed between 2 and 5 years of age. In the secundum ASD, closure can be done surgically, or percutaneously with device closure if the rims surrounding the defect are deemed adequate to support a device. Closure is indicated in these scenarios to prevent long-term complications of atrial arrhythmias, paradoxical embolism, pulmonary

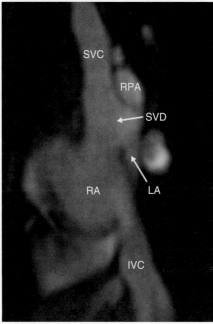

Fig. 3.10 Cardiac magnetic resonance bright-blood sagittal plane image, demonstrating a large superior-type sinus venosus defect (SVD) at the base of the superior vena cava (*SVC*), directly superior to its junction with the right atrium (*RA*), and inferior to the right pulmonary artery (*RPA*), which courses posterior to the SVC. This defect allows an indirect communication between the left atrium (*LA*) and RA. *IVC,* Inferior vena cava.

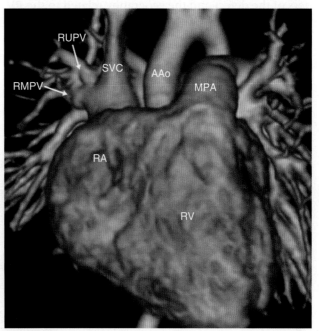

Fig. 3.11 Three-dimensional reconstruction from a cardiac magnetic resonance angiogram dataset in a patient with a superior-type sinus venosus defect, demonstrating associated partial anomalous pulmonary venous drainage of the right upper pulmonary vein (*RUPV*) and right middle pulmonary vein (*RMPV*) into the rightward and posterior aspect of the superior vena cava (*SVC*), just superior to its junction with the right atrium (*RA*). *AAo,* Ascending aorta; *MPA,* main pulmonary artery; *RV,* right ventricle.

hypertension, and severe RV dilation and dysfunction. Surgical closure is the only option for sinus venosus and coronary sinus defects. Anticongestive therapy can be initiated in symptomatic patients until closure is performed. As noted previously, smaller secundum ASDs may close spontaneously or at least get smaller in the first few years of life (Allen et al., 2016; Wernovsky et al., 2019).

Ventricular Septal Defects

VSDs makes up 20% to 30% of CHDs, with an estimated incidence of 5 to 50 per 1000 live births. The spontaneous closure rate of VSDs is approximately 30% (Allen et al., 2016; Wernovsky et al., 2019). Although the VSD is the second most common form of CHD, its description has become confusing and contentious, complicating its understanding. We support the newly proposed ICD-11 terminology, which describes both the borders of the defect (perimembranous, muscular, or doubly committed) and the geography related to the RV aspect of the ventricular septum (inlet, apical trabecular, central, and outlet). Malalignment between the atrial and ventricular septa or of the outlet septum is then additionally described when present. The reader is referred to the International Society for Nomenclature of Paediatric and Congenital Heart Disease consensus document specific to the description of VSDs for more details Lopez et al., 2018).

Morphology and Pathophysiology
Description of the VSD must include both the borders of the defect and the geography related to the RV. It is our preference to begin the description with the borders because this is more objectively defined and relates the margins of the defects to the conduction system. In addition, these three defects account for the three components of septation of the ventricles during development (Tretter et al., 2019). The borders of the defect can be perimembranous, muscular, or doubly committed (Fig. 3.12). Note that a defect that is doubly committed can occasionally extend to

also become perimembranous. The defects can then be subclassified based on their geography related to the RV aspect of the ventricular septum. The RV geography of the defect can be inlet, apical trabecular, central, or outlet. Note that it is erroneous to think of inlet, apical, and outlet components of the septum because a large portion of the inlet of the RV is septated from the outlet of the LV. In addition, a large portion of the outlet of the RV is lifted from the base of the heart by the infundibulum, with its medial wall separating the RV from the pericardial space. It then is important to describe the presence or absence of malalignment of the atrial and ventricular septa, or malalignment of the outlet septum associated with obstruction of either outflow tract.

The perimembranous VSD relates to deficiency in the interventricular portion of the membranous septum and often involves some degree of deficiency of the surrounding muscle. This defect is defined by a fibrous posteroinferior border to the defect. This always involves fibrous continuity between the AV valves and commonly also includes fibrous continuity between the aortic and TV. When small, these defects are located centrally adjacent to the membranous septum. When medium to large, they often extend to open to the inlet and/or outlet of the RV. In the perimembranous inlet VSD, rarely there is malalignment between the atrial and ventricular septa with resulting straddling and override of the TV. This is important to identify when present because the AV node is anomalously displaced posterior and inferiorly. This has historically been mistaken as a "VSD of the canal type"; however, this does not represent an AVSD, and there are separate right and left AV junctions with a bifoliate MV. In the perimembranous outlet VSD, there is often malalignment of the outlet septum either anteriorly or posteriorly, creating some degree of RV or LV outflow tract (LVOT) obstruction, respectively.

The muscular VSD results from incomplete coalescence of the trabeculations resulting in deficiency within the muscular septum. As the name implies, the borders of the muscular VSD are completely muscular. These defects may open to the inlet, apical trabecular, and

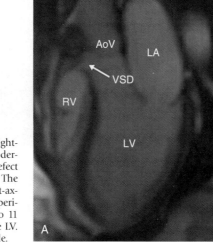
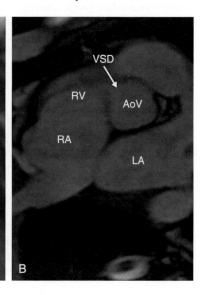

Fig. 3.12 (A) Cardiac magnetic resonance bright-blood three-chamber view demonstrating a moderate-size perimembranous ventricular septal defect (*VSD*) immediately below the aortic valve (*AoV*). The left ventricle (*LV*) appears mildly dilated. (B) Short-axis plane image demonstrating a moderate-size perimembranous VSD, located at approximately 9 to 11 o'clock related to the AoV when viewed from the LV. *LA,* Left atrium; *RA,* right atrium; *RV,* right ventricle.

outlet components of the RV. The muscular inlet defect is important to distinguish from the perimembranous inlet defect, because the conduction system courses anterior and remote to the margins in the former, and posteroinferior and adjacent to the margins in the latter. Therefore just describing it as an "inlet VSD" is insufficient. Likewise it is important to distinguish the muscular outlet defect from the perimembranous outlet defect because the conduction system courses adjacent to the posteroinferior border in the perimembranous form but is protected by the muscular posterocaudal limb of the septomarginal trabeculation along this same border in the muscular form. The muscular outlet VSD also can have malalignment of the outlet septum. Similarly, just calling the defect an "anterior malalignment" or "posterior malalignment VSD" is insufficient, and the borders of the defect must be described. The muscular defects opening to the apical trabecular portion of the RV can be further specified as apical, midventricular, or anterior.

The doubly committed VSD results from failure of development of the proximal outflow cushions and failure of their fusion with the crest of the muscular ventricular septum. Because of the failure of normal formation of the infundibulum and outlet septum, there is fibrous continuity between the aortic and pulmonary valves. This defect can occasionally also extend to become perimembranous when there is deficiency in the posterocaudal limb of the septomarginal trabeculation along the fibrous continuity described earlier for the perimembranous VSD. The relationship to the conduction system can therefore be similar to what was described in the muscular outlet VSD when the borders are only doubly committed, or as described in the perimembranous VSD when the defect additionally extends to become perimembranous. The doubly committed VSD opens to the outlet of the RV by default, and so the geography of the defect can be inferred. Occasionally there is a fibrous remnant of the outlet septum that can be malaligned anteriorly or posteriorly (Wernovsky et al., 2019).

Perimembranous VSDs are the most common, accounting for 80% of VSDs. Doubly committed VSDs, occur in 5% to 7% of VSD, more commonly in those of Asian descent. Both perimembranous and doubly committed VSDs pose risk to the development of aortic valvar regurgitation related to aortic leaflet prolapse through the defect. The perimembranous defect is also associated with risk for development of double-chambered right ventricular outflow tract (RVOT) and LVOT obstruction. Muscular VSDs occur in 5% to 20% of VSDs.

Although much of this section describes the morphology of the defect, outside of the presence of malalignment of the outlet septum, none of these features affect the hemodynamics and clinical presentation. The degree of left-to-right shunting, and hence clinical manifestations, is dependent on the size of the VSD and the relative pulmonary and systemic vascular resistances. The size of the VSD is commonly compared with the aortic valvar diameter (small is <33% aortic valve, moderate is >33% but <50% the aortic valve, and large is >50% the aortic valvar diameter). As the pulmonary vascular resistance decreases over the first few weeks of life, the amount of left-to-right shunting across the defect will increase, and in larger, unrestrictive defects, florid heart failure can ensue within the first few months of life. Pulmonary overcirculation will then lead to increased pulmonary venous return and LA and LV dilation. As pulmonary vascular disease and left atrial hypertension develop, pulmonary vascular resistance increases, leading to a reversal of ventricular level shunting, resulting in Eisenmenger syndrome. Smaller defects restrict flow, preventing equalization of ventricular pressures.

Clinical Presentation

The degree of pulmonary overcirculation dictates the timing and extent of symptoms. Patients with moderate-to-larger VSDs that allow significant shunting leading to pulmonary and subsequently left heart overcirculation can present with symptoms of heart failure within the first few weeks to months of life. These signs and symptoms include failure to thrive, poor feeding, diaphoresis with feeds, tachypnea, tachycardia, and hepatomegaly. The majority of infants are diagnosed after evaluation for a murmur and/or evaluation for signs and symptoms of heart failure. Again, if Eisenmenger syndrome develops, patients may present with cyanosis or syncope with exertion.

Imaging

Larger VSDs are readily detected in utero by fetal echocardiogram. In moderate-to-large VSDs, CXR may show cardiomegaly and a dilated pulmonary trunk with increased pulmonary vascular markings extending peripherally. CXR may also show upward deviation of the left main bronchus secondary to LA dilation.

Echocardiography is important for defining the location and size of the defect, assessing the degree of interventricular shunting and resulting pulmonary artery and left chamber dilation, estimating RV and pulmonary arterial pressures, and defining any associated cardiac defects. TTE often can fully define a VSD; however, TEE is used for intraoperative assessment to clarify anatomic and physiological details and to assess postoperative results.

Cardiac catheterization with angiography has been used not only in quantifying the volume of shunting and determining pulmonary vascular resistance but also in defining multiple smaller VSDs, such as in a "Swiss cheese defect." Similarly, CT and CMR have been used to quantify ventricular size and function and assess shunt volume, along with defining the ventricular septum in the setting of multiple defects (Allen et al., 2016). To calculate VSD shunting, the LV stroke volume provides an estimate for Qp (flow to the lungs returning from the pulmonary veins), while the RV stroke volume provides an estimate of Qs (the systemic flow returning from the systemic veins). The difference in the ventricular stroke volume (LV − RV) in the absence of any valvar regurgitation provides an estimate of shunt volume. CMR phase-contrast imaging also can be used to quantify left-to-right shunting by directly estimating Qp (pulmonary artery flow) as opposed to Qs (ascending aorta flow). Three-dimensional printing from CT or CMR imaging is an emerging technology

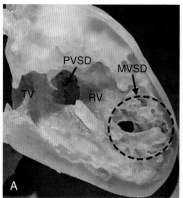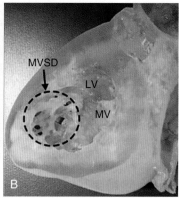

Fig. 3.13 (A) Three-dimensional printed model of the ventricle septum viewed from the right ventricle (*RV*) demonstrating a large perimembranous ventricular septal defect (*PVSD*) and multiple muscular VSDs (*MVSD*) with overlying muscle bundles, trabeculae, and papillary muscle. (B) The multiple MVSDs are seen from the left ventricle (*LV*) side with overlying trabeculae. The PVSD is not demonstrated on the LV view, with the leftward aspect of the LV outflow tract tissue overlying the PVSD and aortic valve. *MV*, Mitral valve; *TV*, tricuspid valve.

that has the potential to better delineate the size and location of the VSDs, as well as define the proximity to adjacent structures, such as the papillary muscles, moderator band, and trabeculations/muscle bundles, which can significantly affect the management approach, especially in surgically remotely accessible muscular VSDs. These models further allow the interventionalist or surgeon to plan and even simulate the procedure before the actual procedure, hence helping to practice personalized medicine (Fig. 3.13) (Bhatla et al., 2017).

Treatment

Surgical closure is indicated in the presence of significant chamber enlargement, greater than half systemic RV systolic pressures, and evidence of progressive aortic valvar regurgitation. A calculated Qp:Qs higher than 2:1 correlates with significant left-sided cardiac dilation and is an indication for surgical closure. Repair is often performed before 12 months of age in those with large defects and evidence of congestive heart failure despite medical management, both to eliminate congestive heart failure and to prevent the development of pulmonary vascular disease. Percutaneous device closure has emerged as an attractive alternative; however, the increased incidence of AV block after device closure has limited its use mostly to muscular VSD. Anticongestive therapy, including diuretics and after-load reducing agents, can be used in those with evidence of heart failure, with the hope of managing symptoms until the defect potentially reduces in size or spontaneously closes, or to promote weight gain before surgery (Allen et al., 2016; Wernovsky et al., 2019).

Atrioventricular Septal Defects

AVSDs makes up 4% to 5% of CHDs, with an estimated incidence of 35 per 100,000 live births. At least 40% of children with Down syndrome have some form of CHD, of which AVSDs are found in 45% (Allen et al., 2016). It is often commonplace to generalize the AVSD into three subtypes: complete AVSD describes common AV valve with both unrestricted atrial and ventricular level shunting; transitional AVSD describes an unrestricted atrial-level shunting, a common AV valve with prominent chordal attachments of the superior bridging leaflet to the crest of the ventricular septum, which results in small, restrictive ventricular level shunting; and incomplete or partial AVSD, which describes exclusively atrial-level shunting with a common AV junction, but with two distinct AV valvar orifices, with a trifoliate left AV valve (Allen et al., 2016; Wernovsky et al., 2019). Due to the conflicting and confusing terminology, as well as the fact that many subtypes do not fit into one of these three general classifications, emphasis has been placed on describing the lesion as it is (Wernovsky et al., 2019).

Morphology and Pathophysiology

Historically the defect has been thought to occur solely from failure of fusion of the endocardial cushions. However, with the advent of episcopic microscopy, we now understand that the deficiency in AV septation is instead related to failure of the mesenchymal cap, which resides on the leading edge of the developing primary septum, to muscularize and fuse with vestibular spine. This then leads to failure of these structures to close the primary atrial foramen and fuse with the endocardial cushions. There are four main features of an AVSD. These include a defect in AV septation, an oval shape of the common AV junction, which leads to the next feature of unwedging of the aortic root (or the "gooseneck" deformity), and the arrangement of the AV valvar leaflets. The common AV valve involves five leaflets: the superior and inferior bridging leaflets, the left mural, the right mural, and the right anterosuperior leaflets. This is true even when there is a tongue of tissue between the bridging leaflets, dividing the common AV junction into two effective AV valvar orifices. The unwedging of the aortic root and resulting elongation of the LVOT result in the increased risk for LVOT obstruction.

It is important to note that we are discussing the AVSD with common AV junction. The "true Gerbode defect" is in fact an AVSD; however, with separate right and left AV junctions. The morphology of the AVSD with common AV junction determining its subtype is then related to three main determinants: the relationship of the AV valve within the AVSD, the size of the AVSD, and the presence or absence of a tongue of tissue between the superior and inferior bridging leaflets. The first two components largely determine the degree of atrial and/or ventricular level shunting. The third component determines whether the common AV junction is guarded by a common AV valve or one that is divided into separate right and left AV valves, both of which will be trifoliate. In the situation where the common AV orifice is divided into two AV valves, the so-called left AV valve "cleft" actually represents the zone of apposition between the leftward aspects of the superior and inferior bridging leaflets. This tongue of tissue also will play a role in determining whether there is ventricular-level shunting depending on its attachments to the crest of the muscular ventricular septum (Wernovsky et al., 2019). In 10% of AVSDs, the AV valve will be maldistributed over the ventricles, resulting in some degree of ventricular hypoplasia. Less commonly, the atrial septum is malaligned to the ventricular septum.

The degree of atrial- and ventricular-level shunting is determined by the respective variables discussed in the earlier Atrial Septal Defects and Ventricular Septal Defects sections. Presentation is dictated by the magnitude of atrial- and ventricular-level shunting, the severity of AV valvar regurgitation, the presence and degree of ventricular hypoplasia, and other associated defects. It should be noted that a patient with AVSD with exclusively atrial-level shunting tends to present earlier than a patient with a secundum ASD.

Clinical Presentation
The presentation is similar to those with an isolated interatrial communication and/or isolated VSD, depending on the degree of atrial- and/or ventricular-level shunting, with earlier presentation and more severe symptoms seen in the setting of a larger combined atrial- and ventricular-level shunting and in those with more significant AV valve regurgitation. In addition to the presentations listed earlier in the sections (Atrial Septal Defects and Interatrial Communications and Ventricular Septal Defects) covering interatrial communications and VSD, infants may be discovered to have an AVSD when an electrocardiogram incidentally reveals a leftward superior axis (Allen et al., 2016; Wernovsky et al., 2019). All children with Down syndrome are generally recommended to have a TTE within the first month of life, which increases the detection rate of associated cardiac defects (McElhinney et al., 2002).

Imaging
Fetal echocardiogram readily detects AVSD in utero, with the presence of the AV valves at the same level being a clue to the diagnosis. Similar to ASD and VSD, CXR may show cardiomegaly and prominent pulmonary vascular markings in the setting of significant shunting. RA enlargement is commonly apparent due to the direction of the left AV valve regurgitation into the RA.

Echocardiography is important for defining the three components of an AVSD, in addition to septal deviation and any degree of AV valvar malposition with associated ventricular hypoplasia and any associated defects. The subcostal en face view is essential for assessing the AV valvar morphology and its relationship to the underlying ventricles (Fig. 3.14). Apical four-chamber imaging is important for defining the ASD and VSD components and the relative ventricular sizes (Fig. 3.15). CT and CMR are rarely used in balanced AVSD but may be more useful in defining abnormal chordal attachments that may interfere with AV septation or in defining AVSD with complex associated anomalies (Fig. 3.16).

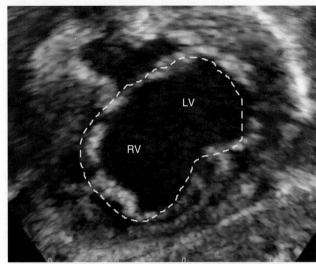

Fig. 3.14 Echocardiographic two-dimensional subcostal atrioventricular valve en face view demonstrates the common atrioventricular valve (*dashed line*) overlying the right ventricle (*RV*) and left ventricle (*LV*) in a patient with a balanced complete atrioventricular septal defect.

Treatment
The goal of surgical repair includes closure of the interatrial and interventricular communications and restoration and preservation of the left AV valvar competence. Patients with a partial AVSD tend to develop symptoms of pulmonary overcirculation earlier than those with a secundum ASD, and repair tends to be at a median age of 2 years. Repair for an AVSD with both unrestricted atrial- and ventricular-level shunting is typically performed between 3 and 6 months of age, before the development of irreversible pulmonary vascular obstructive disease. Palliative surgery with pulmonary artery banding can be performed in younger patients with significant pulmonary overcirculation; however, complete repair involves closure of the AV communications and of the common AV valve. The most common approach is a two-patch repair with closure of the left AV valve "cleft." Deficiency of the left mural leaflet may preclude closure of the left AV valve "cleft". Late reoperation is necessary in 20% of patients, with the most common reasons being significant left AV valvar regurgitation and LVOT obstruction. Similar to ASD and VSD management, anticongestive medication can be used to manage symptoms before surgical repair (Allen et al., 2016; Wernovsky et al., 2019).

■ Select Outflow Tract Anomalies

Transposition of the Great Arteries

TGA accounts for 5% to 7% of CHDs, with an estimated incidence of 30 per 100,000 live births. TGA involves discordant ventriculoarterial connections, with the aorta arising from the morphological RV and the pulmonary trunk arising from the morphological LV. The most common arrangement involves usual atrial arrangement (atrial situs solitus), with concordant AV connections, discordant ventriculoarterial connections, and the aorta positioned anterior and rightward to the pulmonary trunk, described as D-TGA {S,D,D} in Van Praagh termi-nology (Fig. 3.17). There are many other less common variations, including congenitally corrected TGA, which most commonly refers to usual atrial arrangement (atrial situs solitus), discordant AV and ventriculoarterial con-nections, or congenitally corrected TGA {S,L,L} (Fig. 3.18), or its less common form with mirror image atrial arrangement (atrial situs inversus), discordant AV and

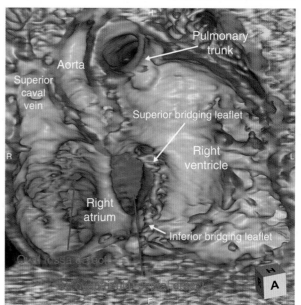

Fig. 3.16 This three-dimensional virtual dissection reconstruction from a computed tomographic dataset with the anterior free walls of the right atrium and right ventricle removed visualize an atrioventric-ular septal defect in a right anterior oblique plane. Although there is a large atrial component to the defect, both the superior and inferi-or bridging leaflets are firmly attached to the crest of the muscular interventricular septum allowing only a small ventricular-level shunt. There is additionally a small oval fossa defect (secundum atrial sep-tal defect) in the center of the oval fossa. While the computed tomo-graphic images were obtained to better assess the mildly hypoplastic aorta in this right ventricular-dominant atrioventricular septal defect, the detail obtained of the intracardiac anatomy is appreciated in great detail.

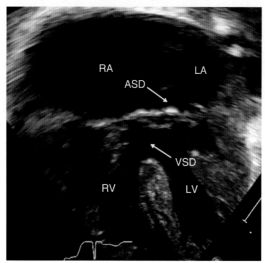

Fig. 3.15 Echocardiographic two-dimensional apical four-chamber image demonstrating the atrial (A) and ventricular (V) components in a patient with a complete atrioventricular septal defect. *ASD*, Atrial septal defect; *LA*, left atrium; *LV*, left ventricle; *RA*, right atrium; *RV*, right ventricle; *VSD*, ventricular septal defect.

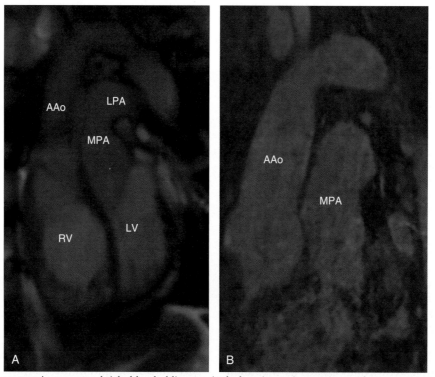

Fig. 3.17 (A) Cardiac magnetic resonance bright-blood oblique sagittal plane image in a patient with D-transposition of the great arteries demonstrating ventriculoarterial discordance, with the left ventricle (*LV*) giving rise to the pulmonary artery and the right ventricle (*RV*) giving rise to the aorta. (B) Oblique sagittal image demonstrating the parallel anterior-posterior relationship of the transposed great arteries as seen in D-transposition of the great arteries. *AAo*, Ascending aorta; *LPA*, left pulmonary artery; *MPA*, main pulmonary artery.

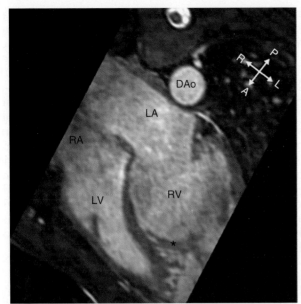

Fig. 3.18 Cardiac magnetic resonance bright-blood axial plane image in a patient with congenitally corrected transposition of the great vessels demonstrating atrioventricular discordance. The right ventricle (*RV*) is heavily trabeculated with a prominent moderator band (*asterisk*). The left ventricle (*LV*) is seen to be smooth walled and bullet shaped. *A,* Anterior; *DAo,* descending aorta; *L,* left; *LA,* left atrium; *P,* posterior; *R,* right; *RA,* right atrium.

ventriculoarterial connections, or congenitally corrected TGA {I,D,D}. Congenitally corrected TGA will not be further discussed (Allen et al., 2016; Wernovsky et al., 2019).

Morphology and Pathophysiology

Although the developmental abnormalities leading to TGA are not fully understood, it is believed to be related to maldevelopment within both the proximal outflow tracts and outflow cushions, with fusion of the outflow cushions in straight rather than their normal spiraling fashion. This results in the subpulmonary component of the proximal outflow tract being transferred to the developing LV, and the subaortic component of the proximal outflow tract to the RV, leading to discordant ventriculoarterial connections.

In TGA, there are two circuits in parallel, with deoxygenated blood entering the right heart and exiting to the systemic arterial system, and oxygenated blood entering the left heart and exiting to the pulmonary arterial system. This inefficient circuit is dependent on various levels of mixing for survival. An interatrial communication is commonly present and supplies effective systemic blood flow shunting left to right in systole. A PDA is also commonly present and supplies effective pulmonary blood flow shunting from the aorta to the pulmonary artery. A VSD is associated with TGA in 40% to 45% of cases, most commonly opening to the outlet of the RV, and provides interventricular mixing dictated by its relative size and other associated anomalies (Wernovsky et al., 2019).

Clinical Presentation

In TGA, clinical manifestations are dictated by the extent of intercirculatory mixing. Minimal intercirculatory mixing leads to early presentation of cyanosis and hypoxemic deterioration. Unrestricted ductal and/or VSD shunting leads to pulmonary overcirculation as the pulmonary vascular resistance decreases with normal transitioning. Reverse differential cyanosis, with upper body cyanosis greater than lower body cyanosis, may be seen early if pulmonary vascular resistance remains elevated causing pulmonary-to-aorta shunting at the PDA. However, this is more commonly seen in the setting of associated aortic arch anomalies, such as coarctation of the aorta (COA) or interrupted aortic arch (IAA).

Imaging

Fetal echocardiogram can miss TGA if only a four-chamber view is used, but visualization of the outflow tracts will show a more parallel arrangement of the transposed great vessels, in contrast with the normal spiraling arrangement. TGA with intact ventricular septum has a characteristic appearance on CXR, with an oval or egg-shaped cardiac silhouette with narrow superior mediastinum, commonly referred to as appearing like an "egg on a string." There may be mild cardiomegaly with increased pulmonary vascular markings. In TGA with VSD, cardiomegaly and increased pulmonary vascular markings tend to be more prominent.

Echocardiogram is crucial not only in identifying the segmental anatomy but also in defining the various levels of mixing, as mentioned earlier, and any other associated anomalies. LVOT obstruction is present in 25% of cases and can be a result of narrowed subpulmonary infundibulum or an outlet VSD (either perimembranous or muscular) with posterior malalignment of the outlet septum. This should be differentiated from dynamic LVOT obstruction caused by bowing of the interventricular septum from the high-pressure RV to the lower-pressure LV, which does not require surgical attention. Coronary artery anatomy is important to define, especially given that the majority of infants with TGA will undergo an arterial switch operation with translocation of the coronary arteries to the neoaorta. The usual pattern found involves the left main coronary artery arising from the left-facing sinus and the right coronary artery arising from the right-facing sinus, which is present in 65% of patients. In about 15% of cases the left circumflex coronary artery arises from the right coronary artery, and a single coronary artery origin occurs in about 8% of cases. If coronary artery anatomy cannot be defined by TTE, angiography during cardiac catheterization is used. Cardiac catheterization with balloon atrial septostomy is commonly performed within the first few days of life in the setting of a restrictive atrial communication not allowing proper mixing. CT or CMR is not commonly used preoperatively but could be used to define coronary anatomy if TTE imaging is inadequate. CMR or CT imaging is particularly helpful in long-term follow-up of adults after TGA repair to assess biventricular size and function, RVOT and branch pulmonary artery obstruction, and proximal coronary artery patency. In addition, CMR can be useful in evaluation of myocardial viability/scarring. CMR also can be valuable in evaluation of the systemic venous baffles and systemic RV size and function in the large adult population who had undergone an atrial switch operation. CT can be used in those with contraindications for CMR, including retrospective gated CT to obtain volumetric and functional information.

Treatment

Immediate postnatal management includes maintaining ductal patency with a prostaglandin infusion until surgical palliation and possible balloon atrial septostomy within the first few days of life, in the setting of a restrictive atrial communication, to allow proper atrial-level mixing before undergoing surgical repair. Historically the atrial switch was commonly performed for TGA as a physiological correction. This, however, keeps the RV as the systemic ventricle and is at risk for venous baffle obstruction or leakage. With improving technology and experience the arterial switch operation became the standard of care in the 1990s and has been used thereafter. The arterial switch is commonly performed within the first few weeks of life. This involves transection of the aorta and pulmonary trunk from their native roots and reattaching to the opposite great arterial root. The pulmonary trunk is placed anterior to the ascending aorta, with its branches laid to course to either side of the ascending aorta (LeCompte maneuver). The coronary arteries are then translocated to the neoaortic root. CMR and CT can be useful in follow-up evaluation of patients after the atrial or arterial switch as described earlier (Allen et al., 2016; Wernovsky et al., 2019).

Tetralogy of Fallot

Tetralogy of Fallot (TOF) is the most common form of cyanotic CHD, with an estimated incidence of 33 per 100,000 live births. With improvement in management of these patients and resulting improved survival, the prevalence of TOF has increased dramatically, with more adults now living with TOF than children. Etienne-Louis Arthur Fallot is credited for defining the four distinct anatomic features present in this cyanotic disease, with subsequent coining of the name "tetralogy of Fallot." The four features recognized include RVOT obstruction, an outlet VSD with anterior malalignment of the outlet septum, hypertrophy of the RV, and rightward deviation with overriding of the aortic root. TOF is now understood to be more of a "monology," with the anterior-cephalad deviation of the outlet septum leading to the development of these four characteristic findings (Allen et al., 2016).

Morphology and Pathophysiology

TOF develops as a result of anterior-cephalad deviation of the outlet septum relative to the malformed septomarginal trabeculation. This insult leads to the outlet VSD with anterior malalignment of the outlet septum; production of subpulmonary muscular stenosis, which includes hypertrophy of the septoparietal trabeculations; and failure of normal incorporation of the aortic outflow tract completely into the morphological LV. The borders of the outlet defect are most commonly perimembranous and less commonly muscular, both with anterior malalignment of the outlet septum. Rarely the defect is doubly committed with anterior malalignment of the fibrous remnant of the outlet septum occasionally extending to also be perimembranous. The importance of distinguishing between the perimembranous, muscular,

and doubly committed outlet defects relates to their relation to the conduction system as highlighted in the Ventricular Septal Defects section (Wernovsky et al., 2019).

The pathophysiology of TOF results in a wide spectrum of presentation depending on the degree of RVOT obstruction. At one end of the spectrum is considered a "pink tet," with mild RVOT obstruction and VSD physiology, resulting in worsening pulmonary overcirculation as normal postnatal transitioning occurs and pulmonary vascular resistance decreases, leading to signs and symptoms of heart failure. At the other end of the spectrum is considered a "blue tet," with severe RVOT obstruction, resulting in right-to-left shunting across the VSD, with deoxygenated blood circulating through the aorta into the systemic circulation, leading to profound cyanosis. The degree of RVOT obstruction thus dictates the pathophysiological consequences.

Clinical Presentation

The clinical presentation is determined by the degree of RVOT obstruction as discussed earlier. Diagnosis of TOF is frequently made after evaluation for the murmur created from RVOT obstruction. Infants with more severe RVOT obstruction and right-to-left shunting across the VSD often present with cyanosis. Those with minimal RVOT obstruction may present with symptoms of heart failure at 4 to 6 weeks of age as a result of pulmonary overcirculation.

Worsening infundibular stenosis and RV hypertrophy may lead to intermittent hypercyanotic episodes or "tet spells," a hallmark of TOF. Tet spells are often provoked by crying and thought to be related to endogenous catecholamine release leading to increased systemic oxygen consumption, acute reduction in systemic vascular resistance, and decreased RV preload. This leads to acute, profound cyanosis and breathlessness, commonly leading to loss of consciousness and, in severe untreated cases, death.

Imaging

With improving fetal echocardiography technology and increasing experience the prenatal diagnosis rate for TOF may be as high as 70% with 90% diagnostic accuracy, with some of the inaccuracy from distinguishing severe RVOT obstruction from pulmonary atresia. Characteristic CXR historically has been described by an upturned apex with a "boot-shaped" appearance secondary to RV hypertrophy, a deficient pulmonary trunk segment, and reduced pulmonary vascularity. More commonly, RV hypertrophy is appreciated by increased proximity of the anterior cardiac border to the sternum on lateral CXR. Right-sided aortic arch can be appreciated on CXR by absence of the usual left-sided aortic knuckle, a bulge to the right of the upper mediastinum, and an impression to the right of the trachea.

Echocardiography is not only important for defining the characteristic features of TOF but also in evaluation of possible associated abnormalities, such as pulmonary atresia, origin of one of the pulmonary arteries from the ascending aorta, absent pulmonary valve leaflets, and associated AVSD. Multilevel RVOT obstruction (from RV to the branch pulmonary arteries) is the hallmark of TOF and must be thoroughly assessed by echocardiography to help determine the necessary repair. TOF leads to clockwise rotation of the aortic root when viewed from the ventricle, best appreciated in parasternal short-axis view, with resulting rotation of the origins of the coronary arteries. Approximately 5% of cases of TOF have anomalous branching patterns of the coronary arteries, most commonly the left anterior descending coronary artery from the right coronary artery. It is important to assess for coronary arteries crossing anteriorly to the subpulmonary infundibulum, such as a prominent conal branch from the right coronary artery, because this may provide difficulties for surgical repair addressing the RVOT obstruction. A right-sided aortic arch with mirror image branching is present in 20% to 25% of patients with TOF, and although it has no clinical significance, it is more commonly associated with 22q11.2 microdeletion, or DiGeorge syndrome. A retroaortic brachiocephalic vein may be present in 5% to 10% of patients with TOF, being more common in those with a right-sided aortic arch.

CT and CMR are rarely used for preoperative assessment, unless to define difficult coronary artery anatomy or other associated vascular anatomy, such as abnormal branch pulmonary artery origins in the setting of pulmonary atresia and associated major aortopulmonary collateral arteries. CMR has, however, become an important component of the postoperative assessment, with serial evaluation of RV volumes, the degree of pulmonary regurgitation, ventricular systolic function, and assessment of differential pulmonary blood flow (Fig. 3.19). Tissue characterization to assess for myocardial viability becomes important in the adolescent and adult patient, with risk for arrhythmia increasing after the second decade of life, especially in patients with significant RV volume overload and RV hypertrophy from residual regurgitation and stenosis, respectively. Criteria for the timing of pulmonary valve replacement (PVR) are partly based on quantification data from CMR, including RV end-diastolic volume, RV and LV ejection fraction, and pulmonary regurgitation fraction (Geva, 2011).

Treatment
A move toward earlier corrective surgery has precluded the need for prolonged medical management in TOF. Medical management may be appropriate when awaiting proper timing for surgical intervention and depends on the degree of RVOT obstruction. Those with mild RVOT obstruction and the development of heart failure may benefit from anticongestive therapy. Oral propranolol, a sympatholytic nonselective beta blocker, is commonly used in those with severe RVOT obstruction, in an attempt to prevent "Tet spells." The acute management of a "Tet spell" involves placing the patient's knees and hips flexed to increase peripheral systemic vascular resistance and giving supplemental oxygen. If there is no improvement, IV colloid or crystalloid fluid can be given to improve cardiac output, IV morphine to relieve pain and anxiety, IV propranolol or esmolol to lower heart rate and improve diastolic filling, and in unremitting cases, an IV systemic vasoconstrictor such as phenylephrine can be given to promote pulmonary blood flow.

Percutaneous palliation with pulmonary valvuloplasty and/or RVOT stent placement may rarely be necessary in

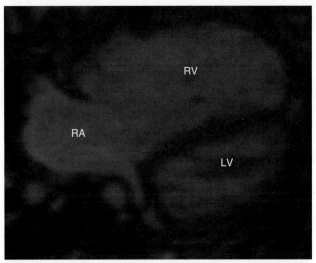

Fig. 3.19 Cardiac magnetic resonance bright-blood axial plane image in a patient with repaired tetralogy of Fallot demonstrating a moderately dilated right ventricle (*RV*) and mildly dilated right atrium (*RA*). *LV,* Left ventricle.

premature or small infants with severe cyanosis who are not yet candidates for full repair. Likewise, surgical palliation with a systemic-to-pulmonary artery shunt, such as a modified Blalock-Taussig-Thomas shunt involving a prosthetic tube graft interposed between the subclavian and branch pulmonary artery, may be used to provide adequate pulmonary blood flow until the patient is an adequate size to undergo successful surgical repair.

An approach toward earlier complete surgical repair, operating between 3 and 12 months of age, has been adapted to not only avoid associated risks with a shunt procedure but also reducing RV hypertrophy and promoting pulmonary arterial growth. Initially surgeons aggressively eliminated RVOT obstruction with liberal use of the transannular patch; however, long-term follow-up showed the detrimental effects of chronic pulmonary regurgitation as a consequence of this strategy. These patients are left with residual lesions, mainly pulmonary regurgitation and, in some cases, both pulmonary stenosis and regurgitation. Long-term follow-up of these patients relies on serial CMR quantification data for RV size and function. Patients with moderate-to-severe pulmonary regurgitation who have RV end-diastolic volumes of greater than 150 mL/m^2 and/or RV or LV systolic dysfunction (RV ejection fraction <47%; LV ejection fraction <55%) are considered high risk and referred for PVR. Options include surgical PVR versus transcatheter PVR, although the latter can be a challenge in patients with a native RVOT with annular dilation. Subsequently a transatrial and transpulmonary approach with valve-sparing technique has been applied in the initial repair whenever possible to avoid the long-term consequences of significant valve incompetence (Allen et al., 2016; Wernovsky et al., 2019).

Double-Outlet Right Ventricle

DORV makes up less than 1% of all CHDs, with an estimated incidence of 6 per 100,000 live births. DORV is defined by both great arteries arising 50% or more from the RV and can broadly be classified into five general categories, with emphasis on the degree of morphological development of the subarterial infundibulum (Allen et al., 2016). Although the presence of bilateral subarterial infundibulum supports the diagnosis, it is not a constant feature, not uncommonly being absent in DORV (Ebadi et al., 2017), and can occasionally be present in the normal heart. The common subtypes relate the great arteries to the VSD: subaortic VSD with pulmonary stenosis or tetralogy type; subpulmonary VSD or transposition type; subaortic VSD with no pulmonary stenosis or VSD type; noncommitted VSD type; and the doubly committed VSD type, with shades of gray between the various types.

Morphology and Pathophysiology

As described earlier, it is the position of the great arteries relative to the VSD and the rotation of the great arteries driven by subarterial infundibular development that generally determine the subtype of DORV (Wernovsky et al., 2019). Underlying infundibular muscle tends to push that respective semilunar valve superiorly and anteriorly, toward the anteriorly positioned RV. In the normal heart, subaortic infundibulum resorbs, creating mitral-to-aortic valve fibrous continuity and leaving the aortic valve positioned inferiorly and posteriorly over the LV. In TOF, there is no subaortic infundibulum with prominent subpulmonary infundibulum, and in TGA, there is no subpulmonary infundibulum with prominent subaortic infundibulum. DORV falls in the middle of this spectrum, with some degree of infundibulum often underlying both semilunar valves, with alignment of both over the RV (Allen et al., 2016). However, as mentioned previously, recent investigations have shown that bilateral infundibulum is not a constant feature in DORV, and the diagnosis of DORV is primarily determined when both great arteries are more than 50% committed to the RV (Ebadi et al., 2017).

The VSD in the noncommitted form is often a muscular VSD opening to the apical trabecular portion of the RV. In all other forms the VSD opens to the outlet. The borders in the outlet VSD can be perimembranous, muscular, or doubly committed, as described in the Ventricular Septal Defects section (Wernovsky et al., 2019).

The diagnosis of DORV in and of itself tells the physician nothing of the hemodynamics and expected clinical presentation. The subtype of DORV determines the pathophysiology. In tetralogy-type DORV, similar to TOF, the degree of pulmonary obstruction determines the degree of cyanosis, with increasing obstruction causing deoxygenated blood entering the RV to preferentially leave through the aorta, leading to profound cyanosis. In transposition-type DORV, the malposed great arteries with subpulmonary VSD allows oxygenated blood from the LV to pass into the pulmonary artery, creating higher pulmonary arterial oxygen saturation relative to the aortic arterial oxygen saturation. VSD-type DORV shares similar pathophysiology to a large VSD, with arterial flow determined by the relative downstream resistances, leading to pulmonary overcirculation and

heart failure. In noncommitted VSD-type DORV, the VSD is not committed to either great artery, and there is complete mixing in the RV, with arterial flow determined by any associated outflow obstruction and the relative downstream resistances. The pathophysiology is less predictable in those with doubly committed defects, and streaming is largely determined by both associated lesions (i.e., outflow tract obstruction) and downstream resistances.

Clinical Presentation

As previously discussed, the morphological variant of DORV determines the clinical presentation. In tetralogy-type DORV, similar to TOF, patients can be diagnosed after evaluation of a murmur, for cyanosis, or can present with a "tet spell." In transposition-type DORV, similar to TGA, patients can present soon after birth with profound cyanosis. In VSD-type DORV and noncommitted VSD-type DORV, patients can be diagnosed after evaluation of a murmur, or present with signs and symptoms of heart failure as the pulmonary vascular resistances falls between 4 and 8 weeks of age.

Imaging

Accurate diagnosis of DORV is possible prenatally with fetal echocardiogram, including assessing the relationship of the great arteries and VSD. CXR findings are similar to that of the CHD for which each morphological variant shares similarities, which have been previously described. Echocardiography can fully define all the anatomic features in most cases of DORV, including the relationship of the great arteries, VSD and AV valves, and associated cardiac anomalies. Defining the presence of AV valve straddling is important when considering biventricular surgical repair, because this may prevent septation. Pulmonary stenosis is present in 50% of patients with DORV and may be valvar or subvalvar. Secundum ASDs are seen in 25% of patients. Coronary artery anomalies occur in 10% of patients and are important to define because they may alter the possibilities for surgical repair. The most common coronary anomaly is the anterior descending coronary artery originating from the right coronary artery. Associated aortic arch anomalies are present in 10% of patients with DORV. Angiography, CT, or CMR may be useful to better define associated complex aortic arch anatomy. In addition, three-dimensional CMR and CT imaging may be helpful for surgical planning, to further define the relationship between the VSD and semilunar valves, and to help define AV valve relationships to the VSD and great arteries when potential baffling pathways need to be better defined (Fig. 3.20). Three-dimensional printing is again emerging as a promising technique that helps print patient-specific heart models that allow us to better understand the complex anatomies in some of these patients and aid in presurgical planning.

Treatment

Potential medical management before surgical repair, timing of surgical repair, and type of surgical repair depend on the morphological variant of DORV, with similarities in management to the CHD in which they share

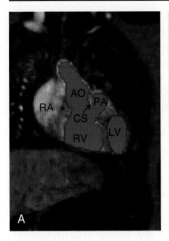
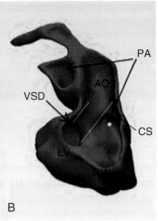
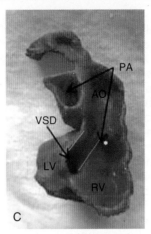

Fig. 3.20 Cardiac magnetic resonance image segmentation (A), virtual three-dimensional representation (B), and three-dimensional printed model (C) in a patient with double-outlet right ventricle demonstrating the subpulmonic region (*asterisk*) inferior to the potential ventricle septal defect (*VSD*)–left ventricle (*LV*)–aorta (*Ao*) pathway (*yellow lines*). CS, Conal septum (outlet septum); *PA*, pulmonary artery; *RA*, right atrium; *RV*, right ventricle.

commonalities. The surgical goal is to restore ventriculoarterial concordance if biventricular repair is possible. In tetralogy-type DORV, surgery is commonly performed between 3 and 12 months of age, with the goal to relieve pulmonary obstruction and to septate the circulations, establishing LV to aortic continuity by baffling the LV to the aorta through the VSD. In transposition-type DORV, surgery is often performed in the neonatal period, commonly performing an arterial switch operation, and baffling the LV to neoaorta through the VSD. In VSD-type DORV, surgical outcomes are excellent in early infancy, and because there is no benefit of deferring surgery once symptoms of pulmonary overcirculation arise, surgery is often performed electively within the first 6 to 12 months of life. This repair often involves baffling the LV to the aorta through the VSD, establishing LV to aortic continuity. Noncommitted VSD-type DORV can present a challenge for surgical repair, because it is often not possible to baffle the remote VSD to the desired great artery, and biventricular repair may not be an option. If significant straddling of an AV valve through the VSD is present, this may also preclude biventricular repair. Single-ventricle palliation is performed in these situations (Allen et al., 2016; Wernovsky et al., 2019).

■ Select Left Heart Lesions

Hypoplastic Left Heart Syndrome

Hypoplastic left heart syndrome (HLHS) makes up only 3% of all CHDs, with an estimated incidence of 36 per 100,000 live births, but it causes approximately 23% of all cardiac deaths within the first week of life. HLHS describes a spectrum of cardiac malformations characterized by variable degrees of an underdeveloped LV and aortic obstruction. The spectrum of HLHS can be broadly classified into the following three categories: aortic stenosis with mitral stenosis, aortic atresia with mitral stenosis, and aortic atresia with mitral atresia.

Morphology and Pathophysiology
The development of HLHS is thought to be a result of either obstructed LVOT or LV inflow. The unifying

theory is that the growth and development of cardiac and vascular structures are dependent on the relative quantity of blood flow during fetal development. One idea is that LVOT obstruction from a hypoplastic ascending aorta and aortic valve leads to underdevelopment of the LV. Others believe that a restrictive foramen ovale, intact atrial septum, or hypoplastic MV leads to reduced preload to the LV, resulting in LV and aortic underdevelopment.

The hypoplastic left heart is commonly unable to fully support systemic blood flow, and the majority of blood is supplied to the branches of the aortic arch and coronary arteries retrograde from the PDA, leading to a variable degree of cyanosis. The hypoplastic aorta and LV cause LA hypertension, leading to left-to-right shunting across the atrial communication. A restrictive atrial communication or intact atrial septum leads to worsening LA hypertension and pulmonary congestion, with resulting "arterialization" of pulmonary veins, dilated pulmonary lymphatic vessels, and hypoplastic pulmonary arteries. Following birth, as the pulmonary vascular resistance falls, worsening pulmonary overcirculation and systemic hypoperfusion ensue. Those with aortic atresia and mitral stenosis subtype have comparatively increased mortality, commonly with coronary fistulous connections to the LV and endocardial fibroelastosis as a result of subendocardial ischemia from suprasystemic LV pressure during development.

Clinical Presentation
The timing of presentation is variable, depending on the ductal patency and the degree of atrial-level shunting, with earlier presentation seen in those with a restrictive atrial septum. Approximately one-quarter of patients with HLHS will present within 24 hours of age, with the majority not developing symptoms until after hospital discharge, after ductal closure, and continued decline of the pulmonary vascular resistance. In the setting of a restrictive atrial septum, LA hypertension leads to pulmonary congestion, possibly presenting with tachypnea and cyanosis. Those with an unrestrictive atrial communication may have a delayed presentation after PDA closure, presenting with feeding difficulties and respiratory distress, rapidly progressing to congestive heart failure and cardiogenic shock from systemic hypoperfusion.

Imaging

HLHS is easily diagnosed by fetal echocardiography, commonly identified during the four-chamber view of the screening obstetric ultrasound. The prenatal challenge is identifying those fetuses with aortic stenosis and a potential for progression to HLHS who would be candidates for fetal aortic valvuloplasty and/or atrial septoplasty. Serial echocardiographic follow-up is necessary in fetuses with aortic stenosis who are at risk for development of HLHS, with serial assessment of the growth of left heart structures and the patterns of blood flow across the foramen ovale and transverse aortic arch. A restrictive foramen ovale or intact atrial septum is a known poor prognostic factor, likely secondary to anatomic changes caused in the lungs.

The CXR in HLHS commonly shows pulmonary overcirculation, with cardiomegaly seen in those with an unrestrictive atrial communication. Echocardiography is used to define the degree of MV, LV, aortic valve, and aortic underdevelopment, along with defining the degree of atrial level and ductal shunting and any associated lesions. The ascending aorta is commonly hypoplastic, with COA present in 80% of patients (Fig. 3.21). Ventriculo-coronary arterial connections should always be assessed for, especially in the aortic atresia with mitral stenosis subtype, as mentioned previously. Assessment of LV size is important when differentiating HLHS from critical aortic stenosis and determining potential candidates for biventricular repair.

Cardiac catheterization with angiography is commonly performed before the second (bidirectional Glenn or Hemi-Fontan) and third (Fontan) stages of palliation, with definition of pulmonary arterial and neoaortic arch anatomy, to determine the presence of venovenous or aortopulmonary collaterals, as well as performing hemodynamic assessment. Some centers instead use CMR and, less commonly, CT to determine the cardiovascular anatomy in select patients. CMR and CT are used to follow up some of these older patients who have undergone Fontan palliation and when the echocardiographic windows are limited.

Treatment

Fetal intervention with aortic balloon valvuloplasty and atrial septoplasty may allow improved fetal growth of left heart structures and ultimately allow biventricular repair in properly selected candidates. However, currently their role has not been established. Immediate postnatal management includes maintaining ductal patency with a prostaglandin infusion until surgical palliation and possible balloon atrial septostomy in the setting of a restrictive atrial communication to decompress the LA.

The most common surgical approach to HLHS is the staged palliation approach, ultimately leading to an in-series single-ventricle circulation. The initial Norwood procedure, or stage 1 palliation, involves creation of an unrestrictive atrial communication, reconstruction of the aortic arch from the RV, separation of the branch pulmonary arteries from the RV, and creation of a restrictive source of pulmonary blood flow from a systemic artery (modified Blalock-Taussig-Thomas shunt) or directly from the RV (Sano modification). This procedure is commonly performed within the first week of life. Stage 2 palliation involves replacing the systemic-to-pulmonary shunt with a superior cavopulmonary anastomosis, either the bidirectional Glenn or hemi-Fontan. This procedure is commonly delayed until at least 6 months of age. Stage 3 palliation, the final stage, involves creating an inferior cavopulmonary anastomosis by connecting the IVC to the pulmonary arteries, with or without a fenestration, referred to as the Fontan procedure. This is generally performed between 18 months and 4 years of age, now creating complete passive flow from the systemic venous return to the pulmonary arteries. Cardiac transplantation can be considered as the primary therapeutic approach in those with previously unsuccessful staged palliation or those who are poor candidates for staged palliation (Allen et al., 2016; Wernovsky et al., 2019).

Shone Complex

Shone complex was first described by John Shone and colleagues in 1963, consisting of four components: a supravalvar mitral ring, parachute MV, subaortic stenosis, and COA (Shone et al., 1963). This complete form is rare, with fewer than 100 patients reported in the literature. An incomplete form with multiple left-sided obstructive lesions is more commonly encountered and can broadly be classified under the Shone spectrum. Left-sided obstructive lesions can include LV inflow

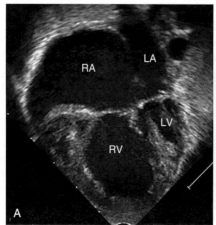
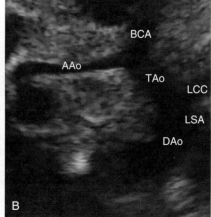

Fig. 3.21 (A) Echocardiographic two-dimensional apical four-chamber image in a newborn with hypoplastic left heart syndrome demonstrating the moderately hypoplastic left atrium (*LA*), mitral valve, and left ventricle (*LV*). (B) Echocardiographic two-dimensional suprasternal sagittal image in the same patient demonstrating a severely hypoplastic ascending aorta (*AAo*), with relatively normal-size transverse aortic arch (*Tao*) and descending aorta (*DAo*). *BCA*, Brachiocephalic artery; *LCC*, left common carotid artery; *LSA*, left subclavian artery; *RA*, right atrium; *RV*, right ventricle.

obstruction, LVOT obstruction, and aortic arch obstruction. Other MV anomalies may include fused MV chordae, arcade MV, single papillary muscle, or MV stenosis. Other LVOT obstructive lesions may include aortic valve stenosis, with or without bicuspid aortic valve, and supravalvar aortic stenosis. Other aortic arch obstructions may include aortic arch hypoplasia or interruption.

Morphology and Pathophysiology

The hemodynamic theory is the dominant theory explaining the development of the Shone spectrum, noting the common association of multiple left-sided obstructive lesions. It states that distal left-sided obstructions, such as COA, develop as a result of hemodynamic disturbances from proximal obstructions causing reduced blood flow through the fetal aortic arch, leading to poor development of the aortic arch.

The involvement and severity of left-sided obstruction determine the degree of compromise to cardiac output. In less severe LVOT and aortic arch obstruction the LV will hypertrophy to improve cardiac output, and the presentation may be delayed. In severe left-sided obstruction, cardiogenic shock may quickly ensue as the ductus arteriosus closes, with no time for LV hypertrophy to develop in an attempt to compensate and improve cardiac output. The long-term prognosis is generally poor, with a perioperative mortality rate of about 25% in those with severe multilevel obstruction, predominantly determined by the extent of MV involvement and associated LV hypoplasia.

Clinical Presentation

Presentation is dictated by the involvement and severity of left-sided obstructive lesions. Severe left-sided obstruction leads to impaired cardiac output and cardiovascular collapse, which tend to rapidly present after ductal closure. Patients with less severe obstruction are mostly detected in childhood either after evaluation of a murmur or for symptoms of congestive heart failure, such as exercise intolerance or dyspnea.

Imaging

Fetal echocardiography commonly will detect the various levels of obstruction seen in Shone spectrum. CXR in those with more severe left-sided obstruction will show cardiomegaly and pulmonary venous congestion. LV hypertrophy may depress the cardiac apex toward the diaphragm and posteriorly toward the IVC. LA enlargement may be apparent with elevation of the left main bronchus.

Echocardiography can accurately assess the multiple levels of left-sided obstruction. Definition of the degree and location of obstruction(s), MV and aortic valve morphology, LV size and functional assessment, and aortic arch anatomy with assessment of associated gradients, along with any other associated defects, will guide management. CT and CMR may be useful in the evaluation of older children with poor acoustic windows or for better delineation of the associated aortic anatomy (Fig. 3.22).

Treatment

The management of patients with Shone complex depends on the severity and levels of obstruction involved.

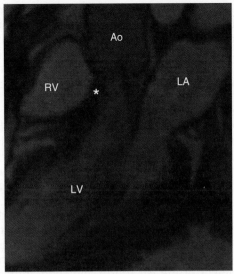

Fig. 3.22 Cardiac magnetic resonance bright-blood three-chamber or left anterior oblique plane image demonstrating a discrete subaortic membrane (*asterisk*) immediately below the aortic valve. Moderate aortic regurgitation is suggested by dephasing artifact. *Ao,* Aorta; *LA,* left atrium; *LV,* left ventricle; *RV,* right ventricle.

In those with severe LVOT and/or aortic arch obstruction, initiation of a prostaglandin infusion immediately after birth may be necessary to maintain ductal patency to sustain adequate systemic perfusion. Anticongestive therapy may also become necessary to counteract manifestations of congestive heart failure before intervention. Percutaneous balloon valvuloplasty may urgently be undertaken to address critical aortic stenosis, or electively in older children to address MV stenosis, aortic valve stenosis, or COA. Stent placement may be considered in adult-size patients with COA. Surgical intervention is often necessary in neonates with severe left-sided obstruction, which may include supramitral valve ring resection, subaortic membrane resection, aortic valve repair or replacement, and aortic arch repair. The timing of any intervention is dictated by the severity of obstruction and the various levels of obstruction involved (Allen et al., 2016; Wernovsky et al., 2019).

■ Aortic Arch Anomalies

Coarctation of the Aorta and Interrupted Aortic Arch

COA makes up 6% to 8% of all CHDs, with an estimated incidence of 36 per 100,000 live births, with about two-thirds of cases presenting soon after birth. COA describes a narrowing of the proximal thoracic aorta or aortic isthmus, and it may involve a discrete or long segment of the aorta. IAA makes up about 1% of all CHDs, with an estimated incidence of 19 per 1 million live births. IAA is commonly associated with a PDA and VSD and is rarely found in isolation. IAA can be classified into three distinct types based on the site of interruption relative to the aortic arch vessels: type A with interruption distal to the origin of the left subclavian artery, type

B with interruption between the left common carotid and left subclavian arteries, and type C with interruption between the right and left common carotid arteries. Type B is the most common, with an incidence rate of 70%, 94% to 100% of which is associated with an outlet VSD with posterior malalignment of the outlet septum.

Morphology and Pathophysiology

The development of the aortic arch and its branches occurs during the sixth to eighth week of human gestation, involving the development of the totipotent arch. The embryological third aortic arches persist as the common carotid arteries, and the left fourth aortic arch forms the thoracic aortic arch and aortic isthmus. The right fourth arch normally involutes leaving a left-sided arch. The embryological sixth aortic arches persist as the proximal branch pulmonary arteries, with the left sixth aortic arch developing distally into the ductus arteriosus. Abnormal development of the left fourth and sixth aortic arches underlies the development of COA, with abnormal development of the left fourth aortic arch underlying development of IAA. Two predominating theories regarding the development of COA include the ductal theory and the hemodynamic theory. The ductal theory notes that COA commonly occurs at the site of ductal insertion and states that COA develops as a result of migration of ductal smooth muscle cells into the periductal aorta, causing constriction and narrowing of the aortic lumen. The hemodynamic theory notes the common association of COA with left-sided obstructive lesions. It states that COA develops as a result of hemodynamic disturbances causing reduced blood flow through the fetal aortic arch, leading to poor development of the aortic isthmus.

The pathophysiology of COA depends on the degree of aortic obstruction and rate of progression, patency of the ductus arteriosus, pulmonary vascular resistance, and any associated cardiac defects. Similarly, hemodynamic consequences of IAA depend on ductal patency, pulmonary vascular resistance, and any associated cardiac defects. As previously stated, about two-thirds of patients with COA present in the neonatal period as a result of severe aortic obstruction in the setting of a closing ductus arteriosus, leading to a rapid decrease in cardiac output. Multiple compensatory mechanisms allow the LV to maintain cardiac output in the setting of aortic obstruction, of which LV hypertrophy is the most important. In severe COA or rapidly progressing COA, which commonly presents in the neonatal period, there is not enough time for LV hypertrophy to develop, and cardiac output is severely compromised.

Clinical Presentation

COA commonly presents as one of three scenarios: an infant in heart failure and shock, a child with a murmur, or a child or adolescent with systolic upper extremity hypertension. Infants with severe aortic obstruction and a closing ductus arteriosus will have reduced LV cardiac output leading to congestive heart failure and cardiogenic shock. Those with less severe aortic obstruction can remain asymptomatic, with the development of significant collateral vessels, and be diagnosed after

evaluation for a murmur or systemic hypertension. IAA presents similarly to severe COA with symptoms of heart failure and cardiovascular collapse as the ductus arteriosus closes.

Imaging

Prenatal diagnosis of both COA and IAA can be challenging, with detailed imaging of the aortic arch, aortic isthmus, and aortic end of the ductus arteriosus crucial in making the diagnosis. The four-chamber view often gives the first clue to COA showing asymmetry of the ventricular sizes, with the RV larger than the LV. This finding is often absent in IAA, because it is associated with a large VSD. The large posterior malaligned VSD is easily seen and should prompt evaluation for IAA.

CXR in severe COA and IAA presenting in infancy commonly shows significant cardiomegaly with increased pulmonary vascular markings and pulmonary congestion. In older children and adolescents the CXR may show a normal heart or mild cardiomegaly with normal vascular markings. A "3 sign" is pathognomonic, with a localized indentation of the aorta at the site of COA. Rib notching may be seen in older patients who have developed prominent intercostal arteries.

Echocardiography is often adequate for assessment of the aorta in infants and young children; however, CMR or CT may be necessary in older children and adults to fully define aortic arch abnormalities. Suprasternal long-axis view allows assessment of the aortic arch, brachiocephalic vessels, aortic isthmus, ductus arteriosus, and proximal thoracic aorta. In COA a "posterior shelf" is often seen protruding from the posterior aspect of the aorta, oriented toward the ductus arteriosus, narrowing the aortic isthmus. Doppler interrogation across the aortic isthmus often shows high-velocity systolic amplitude with continuous antegrade flow throughout diastole, while the descending aorta often shows a blunted systolic upstroke with continuation of flow throughout diastole. In IAA, the arterial duct forms an arch that should not be confused with the aortic arch. The outlet VSD with posterior malalignment of the outlet septum commonly associated with IAA should be evaluated from subcostal, apical, and parasternal views, with assessment of the degree of LVOT obstruction and aortic valve hypoplasia. Both CT and CMR are commonly required in adolescent and adult patients with unrepaired COA because of poor acoustic images (Fig. 3.23). These modalities may also be used to fully define the aorta, brachiocephalic vessels, ductus arteriosus, and collateral arterial circulation in cases where echocardiographic imaging is inadequate (Fig. 3.24). CT and CMR are also necessary for periodic monitoring in patients with repaired COA to monitor for the development of aortic wall injury, such as aortic aneurysms and aortic dissection (Fig. 3.25).

Treatment

Surgical repair is the treatment of choice in neonatal COA, preferentially with resection and end-to-end anastomosis, with PDA ligation if present. A prostaglandin infusion is started immediately after diagnosis to maintain ductal patency in severe COA, and surgery is performed within the first weeks of life. Diuretic therapy may also be necessary before surgical repair. Balloon angioplasty and/or stent implantation are commonly used for recurrent COA or native COA in older children and adults. Surgical repair is the only definitive treatment option for IAA and often is necessary in the immediate neonatal period. Similar to severe COA, a prostaglandin infusion is necessary before surgery to maintain ductal patency, and diuretic therapy may also be needed to address developing congestive heart failure (Allen et al., 2016; Wernovsky et al., 2019).

Vascular Rings

Vascular rings make up only 1% to 3% of all CHDs; however, because many vascular rings do not cause symptoms, the true prevalence is likely underestimated (Allen et al., 2016). A vascular ring is an aortic arch anomaly in which the trachea and esophagus are completely surrounded by vascular structures, which are not necessarily all patent structures. Double aortic arch and right aortic arch with an aberrant left subclavian artery, Kommerell diverticulum, and left ductal ligament are the two most common causes of a vascular ring, together accounting for 90% of cases (Tuo et al., 2009).

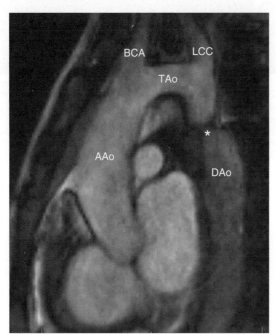

Fig. 3.23 Cardiac magnetic resonance cine image demonstrating a discrete aortic coarctation (*asterisk*). The left subclavian artery is not seen in this image but is directly proximal to the level of the aortic coarctation. *AAo*, Aortic coarctation; *BCA*, brachiocephalic artery; *DAo*, descending aorta; *LCC*, left common carotid artery; *TAo*, transverse aortic arch.

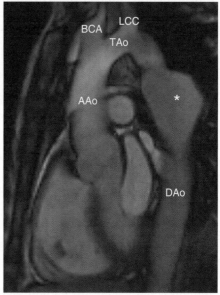

Fig. 3.25 Cardiac magnetic resonance cine image in a patient with a history of aortic coarctation repaired surgically with a Dacron patch, demonstrating a large aneurysm at the site of repair (*asterisk*). *AAo*, Ascending aorta; *BCA*, brachiocephalic artery; *DAo*, descending aorta; *LCC*, left common carotid artery; *TAo*, transverse aortic arch.

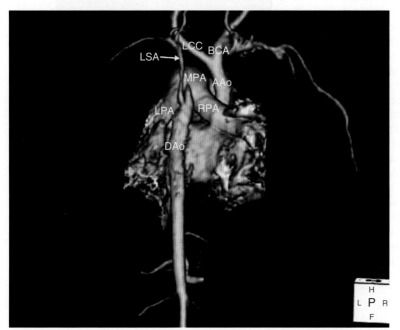

Fig. 3.24 Three-dimensional reconstruction from a cardiac magnetic resonance angiogram dataset from a posterior view in a neonate with an interrupted aortic arch between the left common carotid artery (*LCC*) and the left subclavian artery (*LSA*) (type B). The descending aorta (*DAo*) is supplied from the main pulmonary artery (*MPA*) by a patent ductus arteriosus. *AAo*, Ascending aorta; *BCA*, brachiocephalic artery; *LPA*, left pulmonary artery; *RPA*, right pulmonary artery.

Morphology and Pathophysiology

The development of the aortic arch and its branches occurs during the sixth to eighth week of human gestation, involving the development of the totipotent arch. The embryological third aortic arches persist as the common carotid arteries, and the left fourth aortic arch forms the thoracic aortic arch and aortic isthmus. The right fourth arch normally involutes, leaving a left-sided aortic arch. The embryological sixth aortic arches persist as the proximal branch pulmonary arteries, with the left sixth aortic arch developing distally into the ductus arteriosus. The abnormal persistence or regression of various embryological arches explain the potential for development of various forms of a vascular ring and can be conceptualized by the hypothetical totipotent arch or double-aortic arch model. Vascular rings cause varying degrees of tracheal and esophageal compression, affecting the timing and severity of presentation.

Clinical Presentation

Vascular rings can be asymptomatic or present with symptoms of respiratory distress, stridor, wheezing, dyspnea, chronic cough, recurrent respiratory tract infections, dysphagia, difficulty feeding, recurrent vomiting, failure to thrive, or rarely, present with atypical symptoms such as reflex apnea and cyanosis. These symptoms vary in severity and can present anywhere from infancy to adulthood; however, the majority present during infancy or early childhood.

Imaging

Multiple imaging modalities are commonly used in evaluation of vascular rings, presently with no consensus on the best algorithmic approach. CXR may show tracheal compression but is not diagnostic. Barium esophagram may demonstrate extrinsic compression from a vascular ring, or may reveal other causes for the patient's gastroesophageal symptoms, such as gastroesophageal reflux, aspiration, or tracheoesophageal fistula. Fetal echocardiography is becoming more sensitive in detecting vascular rings in utero in experienced hands. The trachea is fluid filled and, therefore, better imaged in fetal echocardiography. Echocardiography may be sufficient for defining the vascular ring and any associated cardiac defects; however, it poorly visualizes the airway and esophagus, often making further imaging modalities necessary to better define these relationships. CT and CMR angiography are often used to fully define the vascular ring and its relationship to the trachea and esophagus. CMR has the advantage of not exposing the patient to ionizing radiation; however, CT angiogram may be preferred in cases where the airways and lungs must be evaluated together with the vascular anomaly. Atretic vascular segments and the ligamentum arteriosus cannot be visualized by current imaging technologies, but can be suggested by a diverticulum, dimple, or the descending aorta taking an acute turn opposite the side of the aortic arch suggesting a ligamentous connection (Figs. 3.26 and 3.27).

Treatment

Surgical release of the vascular ring is indicated if the patient is symptomatic, or if cardiac surgery is required for other associated cardiac defects. In double aortic arch,

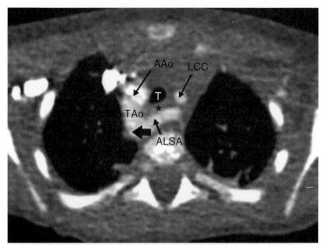

Fig. 3.26 Computed tomography angiogram axial plane image demonstrating a right aortic arch with aberrant left subclavian artery (*ALSA*), diverticulum of Kommerell (*large arrow*), and presumed ductus arteriosus ligament, forming a vascular ring. The rightward aspect of the trachea (*T*) is mildly compressed, and the esophagus (*asterisk*) is completely compressed at this level. *AAo*, Ascending aorta; *LCC*, left common carotid artery; *TAo*, transverse aortic arch.

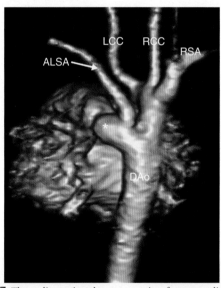

Fig. 3.27 Three-dimensional reconstruction from a cardiac magnetic resonance angiogram dataset from a posterior view in a neonate with a right aortic arch, aberrant left subclavian artery (*ALSA*), diverticulum of Kommerell (*asterisk*), and left ductal ligament, forming a vascular ring. *DAo*, Descending aorta; *LCC*, left common carotid artery; *RCC*, right common carotid artery; *RSA*, right subclavian artery.

the nondominant arch is divided between its last cervical artery and the point where the nondominant arch joins the descending aorta. If a ligamentum or ductus arteriosus forms a border of the vascular ring, it is ligated (Allen et al., 2016; Wernovsky et al., 2019).

Bibliography

Allen, H. D., Driscoll, D. J., Feltes, T. F., & Shaddy, R. E. (Eds.). (2016). *Moss and Adams' heart disease in infants, children, and adolescents* (9th ed.) Lippincott Williams & Wilkins.

Anderson, R. H., & Shirali, G. (2009). Sequential segmental analysis. *Annals of Pediatric Cardiology, 2*, 24–35.

Bhatla, P., Tretter, J. T., Ludomirsky, A., Argilla, M., Latson, L. A., Jr., Chakravarti, S., et al. (2017). Utility and scope of rapid prototyping in patients with complex muscular ventricular septal defects or double-outlet right ventricle: Does it alter management decisions? *Pediatric Cardiology, 38*, 103–114.

Bull, M. J. (2011). Health supervision for children with Down syndrome. *Pediatrics, 128*, 393–406.

Ebadi, A., Spicer, D. E., Backer, C. L., Fricker, F. J., & Anderson, R. H. (2017). Double-outlet right ventricle revisited. *The Journal of Thoracic and Cardiovascular Surgery, 154*, 598–604.

Franklin, R. C. G., Beland, M. J., Colan, S. D., Walters, H. L., Aiello, V. D., Anderson, R. H., et al. (2017). Nomenclature for congenital and paediatric cardiac disease: The International Paediatric and Congenital Cardiac Code (IPCCC) and the Eleventh Iteration of the International Classification of Diseases (ICD-11). *Cardiology in the Young, 27*, 1872–1938.

Geva, T. (2011). Repaired tetralogy of Fallot: The roles of cardiovascular magnetic resonance in evaluating pathophysiology and for pulmonary valve replacement decision support. *Journal of Cardiovascular Magnetic Resonance, 13*, 9.

Loomba, R. S., Tretter, J. T., Mohun, T. J., Anderson, R. H., Kramer, S., & Spicer, D. E. (2020). Identification and morphogenesis of vestibular atrial septal defects. *Journal of Cardiovascular Development and Disease, 10*, 35.

Lopez, L., Houyel, L., Colan, S. D., Walters, H. L., Aiello, V. D., Anderson, R. H., et al. (2018). Classification of ventricular septal defects for the eleventh iteration of the international classification of diseases-striving for consensus: A report from the International society for nomenclature of paediatric and congenital heart disease. *Annals of Thoracic and Cardiovascular Surgery, 106*, 1578–1589.

Mori, S., Tatsuya, N., Tretter, J. T., Spicer, D. E., Hirata, K., & Anderson, R. H. (2018). Demonstration of living anatomy clarifies the morphology of interatrial communications. *Heart, 104*, 2003–2009.

McElhinney, D. B., Straka, M., Goldmuntz, E., & Zackai, E. H. (2002). Correlation between abnormal cardiac physical examination and echocardiographic findings in neonates with Down syndrome. *American Journal of Medical Genetics, 113*, 238–241.

Mori, S., Tretter, J. T., Spicer, D. E., Bolender, D. L., & Anderson, R. H. (2019). What is the real cardiac anatomy? *Clinical Anatomy, 32*, 288–309.

Shinebourne, E. A., Macartney, F. J., & Anderson, R. H. (1976). Sequential chamber localization-logical approach to diagnosis in congenital heart disease. *British Heart Journal, 38*, 327–340.

Shone, J. D., Sellers, R. D., Anderson, R. C., Adams, P., Jr., Lillehei, C. W., & Edwards, J. E. (1963). The developmental complex of "parachute mitral valve," supravalvular ring of left atrium, subaortic stenosis, and coarctation of aorta. *The American Journal of Cardiology, 11*, 714–725.

Tretter, J. T., Chikkabyrappa, S., Spicer, D. E., Backer, C. L., Mosca, R. S., Anderson, R. H., et al. (2017). Understanding the spectrum of sinus venosus interatrial communications. *Cardiology in the Young, 27*, 418–426.

Tretter, J. T., Tran, V. H., Gray, S., Ta, H., Loomba, R. S., O'Connor, W., et al. (2019). Assessing the criteria for definition of perimembranous ventricular septal defects in light of the search for consensus. *Orphanet Journal of Rare Diseases, 14*, 76.

Tuo, G., Volpe, P., Bava, G. L., Bondanza, S., De Robertis, V., Pongiglione, G., et al. (2009). Prenatal diagnosis and outcome of isolated vascular rings. *The American Journal of Cardiology, 103*, 416–419.

Van Praagh, R. (1972). The segmental approach to diagnosis in congenital heart disease. The cardiovascular system. *Birth Defects, 8*, 4–23.

Van Praagh, R. (1984). Diagnosis of complex congenital heart disease: Morphologic-anatomic method and terminology. *CardioVascular and Interventional Radiology, 7*, 115–120.

Wernovsky, G., Anderson, R. H., Kumar, K., Mussatto, K. A., Redington, A. N., Tweddell, J. S., et al. (Eds.). (2019). *Anderson's pediatric cardiology* (4th ed.) Elsevier.

Gastrointestinal

CHAPTER 4
Vomiting Infant
Naomi Strubel

CHAPTER OUTLINE

Bilious Vomiting, 81
  Bilious Vomiting Within the First 2 Days
    After Birth, 81
      Is the Obstruction Proximal or Distal?, 82
      Distal Obstruction, 84
  Bilious Vomiting in Older Infants and Children, 86
Nonbilious Vomiting, 86
  Is the Vomiting Projectile and New in Onset
    (Suspected Pyloric Stenosis)?, 86
  Otherwise Healthy Infant (Suspected Uncomplicated
    Esophogreal Reflux), 88
Imaging Techniques, 89
  Abdominal Radiograph, 89

Upper Gastrointestinal Series, 90
  In the Setting of Bilious Vomiting, 90
  Problems and Pitfalls, 91
  In the Setting of Nonbilious Vomiting, 91
Contrast Enema, 93
Abdominal Ultrasound, 93
To Assess Midgut Malrotation and Volvulus, 94
To Assess Gastroesophageal Reflux, 94
To Assess Pyloric Stenosis, 94
Pitfalls When Assessing the Pylorus With US:, 96
Summary, 96

Vomiting is common in infancy. Parents reporting that their infant is vomiting may be dealing with regurgitation from nonpathological "spitting up" after feeds, which can be normal in newborns and usually resolves over time. Clinicians fear vomiting secondary to obstruction, which can be a life-threatening emergency. Imaging evaluation aids the clinician, in conjunction with the history and physical examination, in distinguishing between these causes. The choice of diagnostic study depends on the suspected etiology of the symptoms, and the appropriate study is performed to diagnose or exclude these potential causes. As discussed throughout this textbook, a systematic approach optimizes imaging evaluation. In the case of the vomiting infant, we always need to ask the age of the infant and if the vomiting is bilious or nonbilious. Only with the answers to these two key questions can the appropriate study be selected. Time of onset of symptoms is also helpful in study selection. Because missing a correctable problem can lead to catastrophic consequences, the most dangerous possible etiologies must be excluded first.

Once the study has been chosen, it must be performed appropriately. We will review optimal techniques for radiographic, fluoroscopic, and ultrasound (US) examinations.

■ Bilious Vomiting

Bilious Vomiting Within the First 2 Days After Birth

Midgut malrotation with volvulus causes vascular compromise of the midgut and, if not promptly surgically corrected, may cause bowel necrosis and death. This is the most dreaded cause of bilious vomiting in infants and, therefore, is the entity that must be first excluded. Bilious vomiting from obstruction of the duodenum by Ladd bands in the setting of midgut malrotation without volvulus may also cause bilious emesis, as can other causes of proximal and distal shiftenterobstruction. Approximately 20% of newborns with bilious emesis have a surgical etiology, typically malrotation, Hirschsprung disease, or atresias. About 10% have a nonsurgical distal obstruction, such as functional immaturity of the colon. However, nearly two-thirds of newborns presenting with bilious vomiting have no obvious cause; this has been called *idiopathic bilious vomiting* and may be secondary to reflux or gastric dysmotility, both commonly seen in otherwise healthy infants.

Is the Obstruction Proximal or Distal?

A radiograph to distinguish between proximal and distal causes of obstruction should be the first study obtained. If the radiograph is normal or nonspecific, malrotation must be excluded. An upper gastrointestinal series (UGI) is usually performed for this purpose. Some prefer an initial attempt at sonographic evaluation of the duodenum and superior mesenteric artery (SMA) and vein (SMV) to assess for midgut malrotation with or without volvulus. If volvulus is detected, surgery can be expedited without need for UGI. If malrotation without volvulus is detected or suspected, urgent confirmatory UGI may be deferred, depending on local surgical preference. If normal location of the duodenal–jejunal junction (DJJ) cannot be demonstrated on UGI series, the patient should be taken for immediate surgical exploration. In addition to midgut malrotation, causes of proximal obstruction that may be discovered at surgery include duodenal stenosis or web, annular pancreas, and preduodenal portal vein.

MIDGUT MALROTATION

During fetal development, the midgut distal to the duodenum herniates into the umbilical coelom and rotates 270 degrees before reentering the abdomen. Subsequent fixation of the various mesenteries to the abdominal wall places the third portion of the duodenum in the retroperitoneum and positions the DJJ in the left upper quadrant and the cecum in the right lower quadrant, with a broad intervening mesentery along which the small bowel runs. Failure of this process can occur at different stages, leading to nonrotation or malrotation of the midgut, without a retroperitoneal duodenum. Depending on the final location of the DJJ and the cecum, the mesentery may therefore

have a narrow attachment at its base. This narrow fan of mesenteric tissue is at risk for rotating around its central axis of the SMA and SMV. Such volvulus may obstruct the SMA and lead to bowel ischemia and even necrosis. In malrotation, the body forms fibrous attachments called *Ladd bands*, possibly in an attempt to fixate the gut. These usually extend from the cecum to the right upper quadrant and may cross the duodenum causing obstruction. The cecum may be located on either the right or left side of the abdomen and is normally located in 20% of malrotations. Imaging to assess malrotation focuses on the location of the duodenum. UGI documents position of the DJJ; on an UGI the normally located DJJ is at the craniocaudal level of the duodenal bulb lateral to the left spinous pedicles (Fig. 4.1). Malrotation may be present without or with obstruction; obstruction may be caused by volvulus or a Ladd band (Figs. 4.2–4.5).

Chronic or intermittent volvulus may present in older infants and children with recurrent abdominal pain and vomiting, failure to thrive, and malabsorption. Internal hernias may also be associated with malrotation and can be difficult to diagnose; patients have symptoms of obstruction. Intestinal malrotation is also present in patients with omphalocele, gastroschisis, congenital diaphragmatic hernia, and heterotaxy syndromes.

DUODENAL ATRESIA, STENOSIS, SHIFTENTERAND WEB

Duodenal stenosis and atresia account for 40% of intestinal atresias. During fetal development the duodenal lumen normally becomes obstructed by rapidly proliferating epithelial cells. If normal luminal recanalization fails, duodenal atresia or stenosis results. Prenatal US

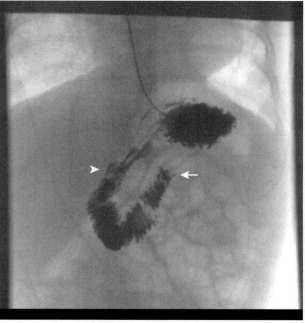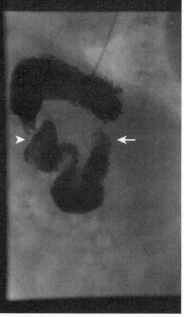

Fig. 4.1 (Left) Normal duodenal–jejunal junction (DJJ): *arrowhead* indicates bulb; *arrow* indicates DJJ. (Right) Lateral view of DJJ at the level of the duodenal bulb.

examinations can be suggestive, but studies performed before gestational age of 20 weeks may not demonstrate the typical findings of polyhydramnios and a "double bubble." The classic appearance on a radiograph in a newborn is a double bubble of air with no distal bowel gas (Fig. 4.6). Complete duodenal atresia can even be missed in full-term, breast-fed infants because these children may not present with classic findings. Breast-fed infants often ingest lower volumes than formula-fed infants in the first days of life, and volume of emesis may be small; difficulties with feeds may initially be attributed to difficulties with breast-feeding rather than obstruction.

A small luminal opening present in an obstructing diaphragm across the duodenum causes a duodenal web. While the web may allow the liquid diet of infants to pass, the partially obstructed proximal duodenum dilates. Radiographically this manifests as a double bubble with distal gas (Fig. 4.7A) and a "wind sock" appearance on contrast studies (Fig. 4.7B). These children often experience feeding difficulties when solid food is introduced to the diet or may have complications after an ingested foreign body.

An *annular pancreas* develops when there is abnormal fusion of the fetal ventral and dorsal pancreatic buds. If the ventral bud does not properly dorsally rotate during duodenal growth, the pancreas may encircle the duodenum when fusing (Fig. 4.8). Patients may present with obstruction in the newborn period or later. Annular pancreas can be associated with malrotation (a more likely cause of obstruction), tracheoesophageal fistula, anal atresia, and cardiac anomalies, often in the setting of trisomy 21 or Cornelia de Lange syndrome.

A *preduodenal location of the portal vein* occurs when there is abnormal involution of the embryological vascular structures that give rise to the portal system. Although by itself this abnormality may cause obstruction, the obstruction is usually due to the entities with which it is associated: midgut malrotation, duodenal web, and annular pancreas, often in heterotaxy syndromes. If detected, its presence should be described to avoid injury during surgery.

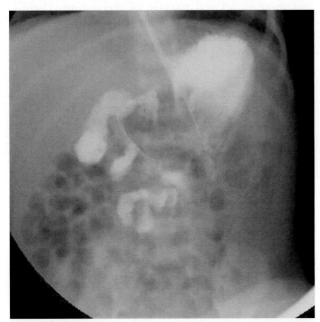

Fig. 4.2 Malrotation without volvulus. Single-contrast upper gastrointestinal series does not show a normally positioned duodenal–jejunal junction. Duodenal loops are located to the right of the spine.

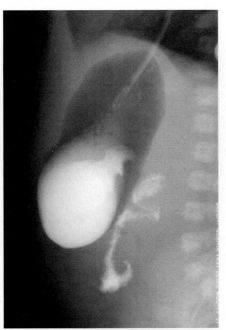

Fig. 4.3 Malrotation with midgut volvulus. "Corkscrew" appearance with proximal small bowel twisting around the axis of the superior mesenteric artery along the mesenteric pedicle.

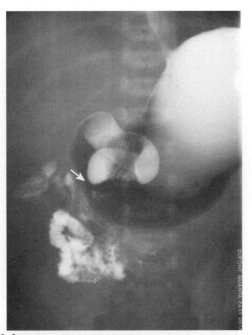

Fig. 4.4 Malrotation with partial proximal obstruction from Ladd bands. Right sided proximal small bowel loops without normal DJJ. Moderate distention of proximal duodenum with abrupt caliber change due to obstruction by Ladd bands (*arrow*).

Distal Obstruction

If the initial radiograph demonstrates distal obstruction with multiple dilated loops of bowel (Fig. 4.9), a contrast enema is indicated to determine the cause. If meconium has already been passed, the differential diagnosis includes Hirschsprung disease, jejunal atresia, and ileal or colonic stenosis; if meconium has not been passed, the differential also includes ileal/colonic atresia, meconium ileus, functional immaturity of the colon, and imperforate anus. Imperforate anus with a fistula may allow passage of minimal meconium, and thus imperforate anus can sometimes be missed without careful physical examination.

JEJUNAL/ILEAL/COLONIC ATRESIA/STENOSIS

Jejunal and ileal atresias comprise half of all intestinal atresias; colonic atresia is less common, accounting for only 9% of atresias. These atresias may be associated with abnormalities in other organ systems. Unlike duodenal atresia, which is caused by a failure of recanalization of the bowel lumen, distal atresias are thought to result from in utero vascular accidents. Multiple foci of bowel atresia may occur in one patient. Proximal small bowel detritus forms meconium; thus in jejunal atresia the infant may pass meconium, whereas with ileal or colonic atresia meconium will not be passed. Radiographs in jejunal atresia typically show dilatation of the stomach, duodenum, and one or a few loops of additional bowel (Fig. 4.10); there may be a "triple-bubble" appearance. In more distal atresias, multiple dilated loops of bowel are more commonly seen (Figs. 4.11 and 4.12). Regardless, further workup is performed with contrast enema to locate the level of the obstruction. The more distal the atresia location, the more "unused" the

colon is, often resulting in a "microcolon" appearance on enema.

FUNCTIONAL IMMATURITY OF THE COLON

Meconium plug and small left colon may represent slightly different presentations of the same entity, caused by functional immaturity of the bowel. These infants are occasionally children of mothers with diabetes, or mothers who received magnesium sulfate, and there is delayed passage of meconium. There is no true obstruction, and the symptoms usually resolve without treatment. If a cast of meconium is seen within the descending colon during contrast enema, it is

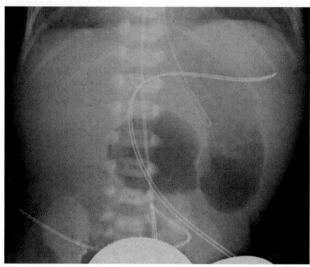

Fig. 4.6 Duodenal atresia. The "double bubble" of duodenal atresia; there is no distal gas.

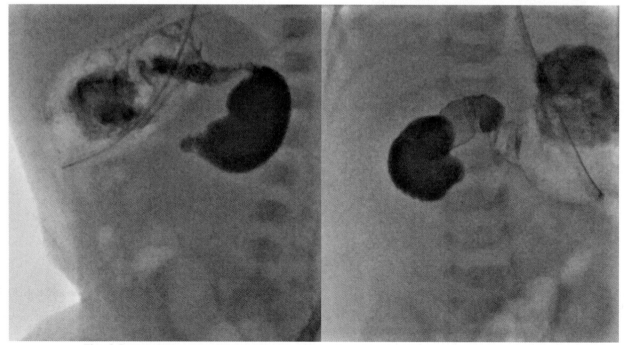

Fig. 4.5 Malrotation with midgut volvulus. Obstruction of proximal duodenum caused by volvulus; note "beaking" at site of obstruction.

termed *meconium plug* (Fig. 4.13); if there is no plug but the descending colon is of decreased caliber compared with more proximal colon, it is termed *small left colon syndrome*. In some cases rectal biopsy is obtained to exclude Hirschsprung disease.

MECONIUM ILEUS

Presenting almost exclusively in infants with cystic fibrosis, meconium ileus is true obstruction of the bowel by dense pellets of meconium. It causes 20% of infantile intestinal obstruction and is the initial presentation in 15% to 20% of patients with cystic fibrosis. Abnormal ion transport caused by the defective Cystic Fibrosis Transmembrane Conductance Regula-

tor (CFTR) chloride channel transporter in this disease yields highly viscous, tenacious meconium that is difficult to pass. This can be seen on radiographs as a bubbly appearance in the bowel loops in the right lower quadrant (Fig. 4.14). Calcifications on initial radiograph suggest meconium peritonitis from intrauterine bowel perforation; meconium spilled in the peritoneal cavity often calcifies and may form a "meconium cyst." Enema with diatrizoate meglumine and diatrizoate sodium solution (Gastrografin, Bracco Diagnostics, 1:5 dilution in water) is suggested when this entity is suspected, because this agent may be therapeutic, assisting in breaking up the meconium for easier clearance.

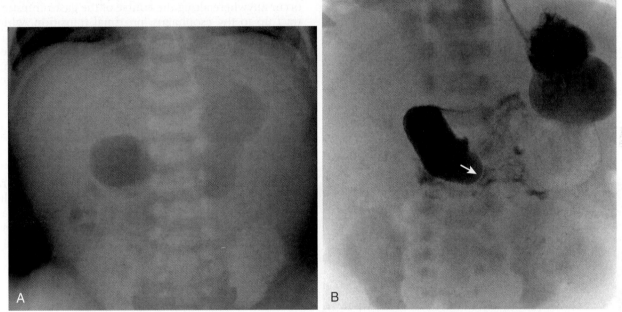

Fig. 4.7 Duodenal web. (A) Radiograph of the abdomen showing "double-bubble"-like dilation of proximal duodenum with gas in distal bowel loops. (B) UGI showing a duodenal web (*arrow*) outlined by contrast in the distended proximal duodenum and adjacent nondistended duodenum.

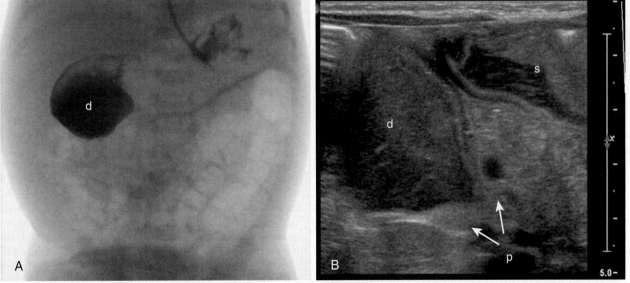

Fig. 4.8 Annular pancreas. (A) Dilated proximal duodenum in a patient with annular pancreas. (B) Ultrasound of the abdomen in the same patient shows distention of the proximal duodenum, surrounded by pancreatic tissue. *d*, duodenum; *p*, pancreas; *s*, stomach.

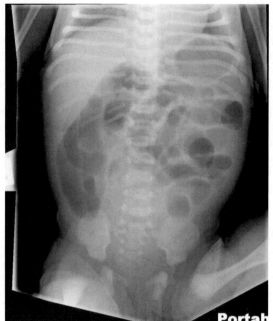

Fig. 4.9 Distal obstruction. Radiograph of the abdomen in a neonate with bilious emesis shows multiple, tense-appearing, dilated loops of bowel. This distal obstruction was secondary to extensive colonic aganglionosis.

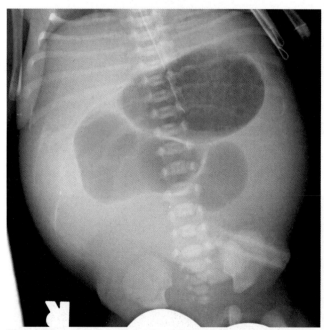

Fig. 4.10 Jejunal atresia. Dilated duodenum and proximal small bowel without distal bowel gas. Linear calcifications in the flanks are secondary to in utero perforation with meconium peritonitis.

HIRSCHSPRUNG DISEASE

Hirschsprung disease causes 15% to 20% of bowel obstructions in newborns, occurring in 1/5000 live births. It may be missed in the newborn period and present later in childhood. The myenteric plexus of the autonomic nervous system normally migrates from proximal to distal along the length of the gut; in Hirschsprung disease, migration does not progress normally all the way to the rectum. The noninnervated bowel is unable to relax and normally propagate peristaltic waves, causing a functional obstruction. This is evaluated on contrast enema by locating a transition zone between the typically normal-caliber bowel distal to the point of obstruction and the dilated bowel proximally. This transition zone usually occurs in the rectosigmoid region, causing a reversal of the normal rectosigmoid ratio. Instead of the rectum being larger than the sigmoid (Fig. 4.15), the obstructed sigmoid dilates and is larger in caliber than the rectum (Fig. 4.16). The bowel at and distal to the transition zone requires surgical excision because functional peristalsis cannot be restored to noninnervated bowel. Because the transition zone can occur anywhere along the course of the gastrointestinal tract up to the esophagus, proximal transition, which is not compatible with life, occasionally occurs. Total colonic Hirschsprung disease can be difficult to detect with contrast enema, because no caliber change may be seen. In these cases the colon may have a "question mark" configuration.

Bilious Vomiting in Older Infants and Children

Midgut malrotation can cause bilious vomiting beyond the newborn period from either Ladd bands or volvulus and should not be excluded from the differential diagnosis in older infants. The other incompletely obstructing proximal duodenal lesions may also present beyond the newborn period, as can Hirschsprung disease.

■ Nonbilious Vomiting

If the vomiting is nonbilious, the age of the patient and character of the vomiting episodes are important. The ACR Appropriateness Criteria on Vomiting in Infants divide nonbilious vomiting into two categories: infant between 2 weeks and 3 months with new-onset vomiting vs otherwise healthy infant.

Is the Vomiting Projectile and New in Onset (Suspected Pyloric Stenosis)?

The most pressing surgical cause of nonbilious vomiting in young infants aged 4 to 12 weeks is hypertrophic pyloric stenosis (HPS). Classically this presents in 6-week-old, firstborn, male children with projectile vomiting. Some may have failure to thrive, dehydration, and metabolic disturbances from frequent vomiting of acidic gastric contents. Not all patients, however, present with these suggestive criteria. In this setting the study of choice is abdominal US to rule out HPS (see ACR Appropriateness Criteria). If the initial study is inconclusive, a repeat examination may be warranted after several days to a week if symptoms persist, because

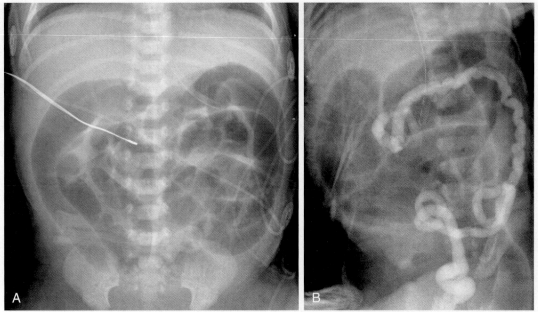

Fig. 4.11 Ileal atresia. (A) Distal obstruction: radiograph of the abdomen showing multiple dilated loops of bowel. (B) Microcolon on contrast enema.

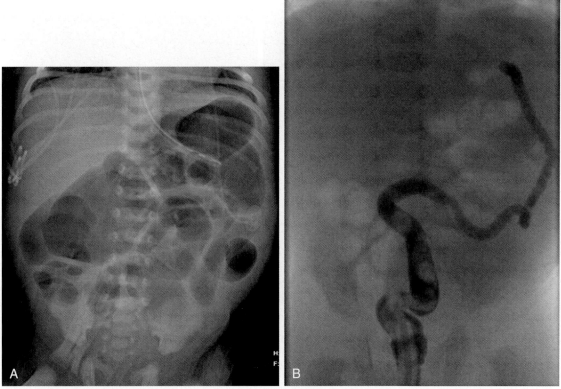

Fig. 4.12 Colonic atresia. (A) Radiograph of the abdomen showing multiple dilated loops of bowel. (B) Contrast enema showing distal microcolon on enema; contrast could not be refluxed proximal to the splenic flexure.

pyloric stenosis progresses with time. A UGI series may also be performed but is less desirable because of the radiation.

HPS is seen in 2 to 5/1000 live births in Caucasians of Northern European descent. It is decreased in Caucasians of Indian descent and further decreased in Black and Asian populations. Incidence is increased in first-degree relatives of patients with HPS. Although its etiology remains unclear, failure of pyloric muscle relaxation and increased production of growth factors leading to muscle hypertrophy have been postulated as causative factors (Fig. 4.17).

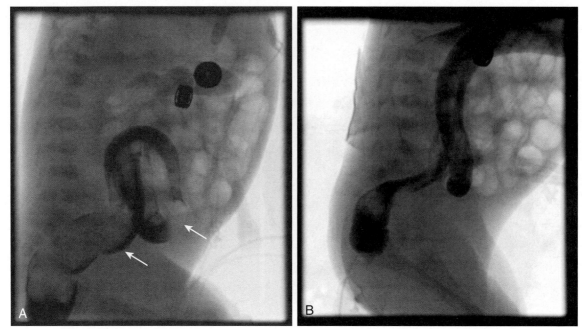

Fig. 4.13 Functional immaturity of the colon. (A) Contrast enema showing filling defects (*arrows*) in the distal colon. Rectosigmoid ratio is normal. (B) These meconium "plugs" were evacuated during the contrast enema.

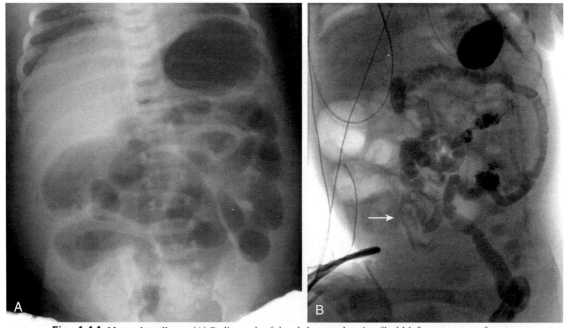

Fig. 4.14 Meconium ileus. (A) Radiograph of the abdomen showing "bubbly" appearance of meconium in the right flank. (B) Contrast enema showing proximal dilated loops of bowel, multiple filling defects from meconium in ileum (*arrow*), and a microcolon. Contrast in stomach and small bowel from UGI series requested by surgery.

Otherwise Healthy Infant (Suspected Uncomplicated Esophogreal Reflux)

Intermittent nonbilious vomiting is usually due to gastroesophageal reflux (GER), but may also be caused by HPS, pylorospasm, milk allergy, or gastroenteritis. GER may be further characterized as normal, minimal amounts seen in all individuals; functional, usually occurring after feeds and common in otherwise normal infants; and pathological, when associated with failure to thrive, dyspnea, coughing, choking, or other symptoms (Fig. 4.18). Pathological GER is more frequently associated with an anatomic abnormality, such as hiatal hernia or cause of proximal obstruction, and this setting is most frequently encountered in patients younger than 1 year. The gold standard for the diagnosis of GER remains evaluation with pH/impedance probes, which

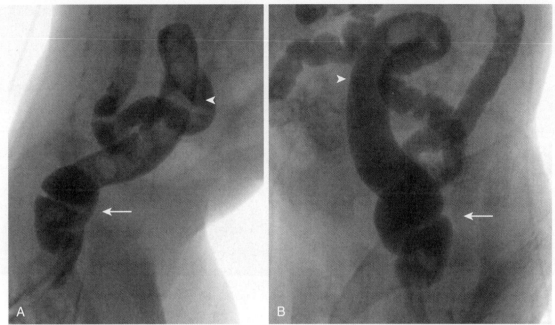

Fig. 4.15 Normal rectosigmoid ratio on enema. (A) Lateral view. (B) Anteroposterior view. *Arrows* denote rectum; *arrowheads* denote sigmoid.

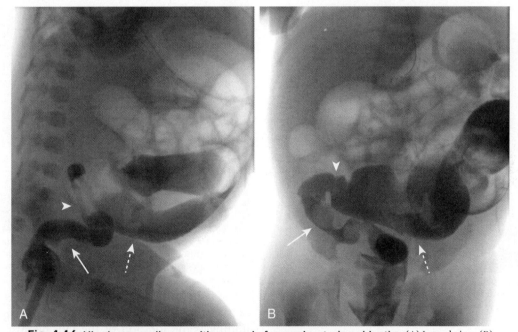

Fig. 4.16 Hirschsprung disease with reversal of normal rectosigmoid ratio. (A) Lateral view. (B) Anteroposterior view. *Arrows* denote narrow-caliber rectum; *hashed arrows* denote larger-caliber sigmoid; *arrowheads* denote radiographic transition zone.

are more sensitive than imaging assessment. Although UGI may demonstrate GER, it is less sensitive and specific than evaluation with pH/impedance probes. US can also demonstrate GER but is also less sensitive and specific. Reflux scintigraphy with Tc-99m-labeled sulfur colloid is at least as sensitive and is more specific than barium studies. However, because reflux is commonly seen in asymptomatic infants, the role of imaging in managing this scenario is less straightforward. Many clinicians request imaging simply to exclude an anatomic cause of the vomiting.

■ Imaging Techniques

Abdominal Radiograph

The supine radiograph of the abdomen should extend from the domes of the diaphragm through the pelvis. A normal bowel gas pattern in an infant consists of multiple, overlapping, air-filled loops of bowel throughout the abdomen and pelvis (Fig. 4.19). After the first 24 hours of life, air should extend through the bowel to the rectum.

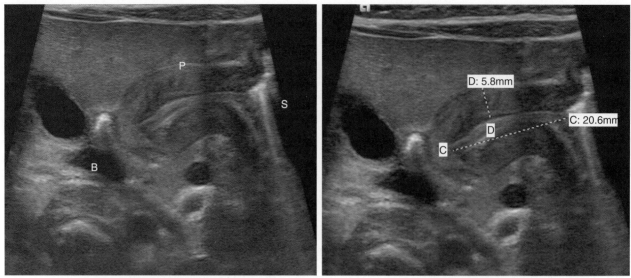

Fig. 4.17 Hypertrophic pyloric stenosis. Hypoechoic pyloric muscle is elongated and thickened. Hypertrophied echogenic mucosal folds fill the pyloric channel. *B,* Duodenal bulb; *P,* pyloric channel; *S,* stomach.

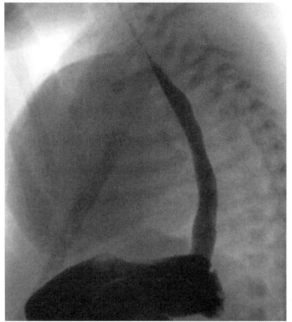

Fig. 4.18 Gastroesophageal reflux: upper gastrointestinal series showing gastroesophageal reflux to the thoracic inlet in a child with feeding intolerance after cardiac surgery.

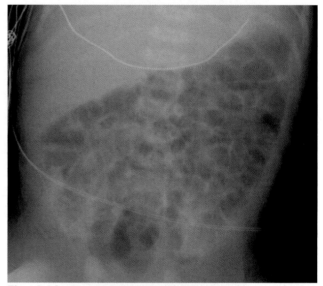

Fig. 4.19 Normal bowel gas pattern. Multiple, overlapping loops of nondistended bowel throughout the abdomen to the rectum. Appearance has been likened to chicken wire or "happy polygons."

A "double bubble" with no distal gas is seen in duodenal atresia, and generally no further imaging is required (see Fig. 4.6). Multiple dilated loops of bowel are seen in distal obstruction (see Fig. 4.9). When the radiograph has any other appearance, including both a normal or "nonspecific" bowel gas pattern that does not fit described patterns, midgut malrotation cannot be excluded, and further imaging evaluation is required in the setting of bilious vomiting.

Upper Gastrointestinal Series

In the Setting of Bilious Vomiting

A complete UGI consists of evaluation of the esophagus, stomach, and duodenum to the DJJ at the ligament of Treitz. In the setting of bilious vomiting the crucial finding is the location of the DJJ, because the goal is to exclude malrotation. Technique should therefore be optimized to maximize the likelihood of a diagnostic examination.

The steps to perform a UGI through an enteric tube for bilious vomiting are as follows:
- With enteric tube in the distal stomach, place infant in right lateral decubitus (RLD) position.
- Initially instill 5 mL contrast (typically 50% dilute, single-contrast barium sulfate oral suspension such as E-Z-Paque, Bracco; if water-soluble contrast is used, consider isosmolar agents such as iohexol [Omnipaque 180, GE Healthcare] to avoid complications if aspirated) into antrum.
- Document duodenal C loop in lateral position (bulb, down D2, then up to D4).

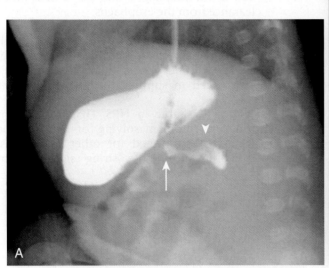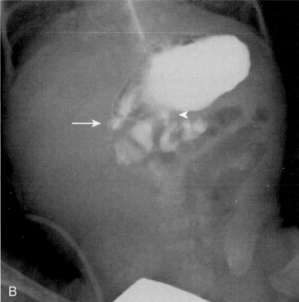

Fig. 4.20 Bedside upper gastrointestinal series. (A) Lateral view. (B) Anteroposterior view. *Arrows* denote bulb; *arrowheads* denote DJJ.

- Stomach may empty slowly; be patient and use intermittent pulsed fluoroscopy.
- Placing infant slightly prone may facilitate emptying. An additional 5 cc contrast may be instilled as needed.
- Turn infant supine (no obliquity) to document that D4 is lateral to spinous pedicles at level of the bulb (see Fig. 4.1).
  - Capturing images during the first pass of contrast is ideal.
- Esophagus and stomach can then be further evaluated as desired (see later).

In unstable neonatal intensive care unit infants, a "bedside UGI" can be performed. This consists of a scout radiograph to confirm appropriate enteric tube positioning in the distal stomach followed by a series of supine anteroposterior radiographs. In the technique described by Nayak etal. (2014), radiographs are obtained immediately after the instillation of 5 mL nonionic, isosmolar, water-soluble contrast and again at 30 seconds and 1, 3, and 5 minutes. Between radiographs the infant should be placed into RLD position if possible to promote gastric emptying. Although this is a hit or miss attempt, images may be diagnostic shiftenter(-Fig. 4.20).

Problems and Pitfalls

An overdistended stomach or adjacent small bowel loops may displace the DJJ inferiorly, leading to a false-positive diagnosis of malrotation. Similarly, an enteric tube may displace the stomach, and an enlarged kidney or spleen may also distort normal anatomy. If the stomach is not emptying, instilling an additional 5 cc contrast may be helpful, although there is some risk that overdistention of the stomach with contrast will obscure the bulb when patient is placed supine.

Rapid gastric emptying with filling of multiple small bowel loops may obscure the DJJ. When this happens, after waiting for small bowel contrast to progress further distally, additional contrast boluses can be followed through the duodenal loop. Full-strength contrast can also be used to better track a later bolus over a background of loops with contrast.

Redundant duodenal loops with a meandering course may suggest malrotation if the contrast is not followed out far enough, but the DJJ should ultimately be identified in the appropriate location (Fig. 4.21).

If the location of the DJJ is still uncertain, delayed images may document a right lower quadrant location of the cecum. Keep in mind that 20% of patients with malrotation may have a normally located cecum, and many infants normally have a high riding cecum, so normal cecal location is not diagnostic of normal proximal shiftenterrotation, and abnormal cecal location is not diagnostic of malrotation.

US may be helpful as a problem-solving technique if fluoroscopic UGI is nondiagnostic. US has recently been suggested as a primary imaging tool for malrotation, not just a problem-solving technique, and is discussed further below. This may vary by comfort level of sonographers, radiologists, and surgeons.

If all else fails, the examination may be repeated after the contrast has cleared.

In the Setting of Nonbilious Vomiting

To perform an UGI series feeding the infant by bottle:
- Puncture nipple to allow easier extraction of contrast.
- Place infant in left lateral decubitus (LLD/LPO) position and feed for several sucks (may be done in RPO position, but this is less controlled and risks the possibility of missing images of the DJJ if there is rapid gastric emptying).
  - Document lateral esophagus views.
- When contrast reaches fundus, hold feed and turn infant to RLD position to opacify duodenum.
- Proceed as described earlier to document DJJ.
- Feed in supine position for additional view of esophagus.

To assess for reflux (many feel this is not necessary, as nonvisualization of reflux during the exam does not rule out reflux):

- Instill contrast through tube or feed to distend stomach.
- Withdraw tube above gastroesophageal junction; if feeding infant, allow all contrast to enter stomach.
- Rotate infant between LLD, supine, and RLD positions to elicit reflux. The infant may also be fed water while imaging, which can elicit reflux by siphon effect.
  - Image intermittently over several minutes.
  - In our experience reflux is most frequently elicited in the RLD position.

- Describe qualitatively the following:
  - Frequency of episodes, height of barium column in the esophagus, and speed of contrast clearance from the esophagus.

To evaluate the esophagus with enteric tube:

- Pull enteric tube to the mid-esophagus and instill contrast with patient in supine and lateral or posterior oblique (swimmer's) positions.
  - Can also feed in supine and lateral positions (Fig. 4.22).

Although less desirable in HPS, UGI is occasionally performed for problem solving, or HPS may be diagnosed in UGI performed for other indications. Diagnostic findings include the "string" sign of a thin

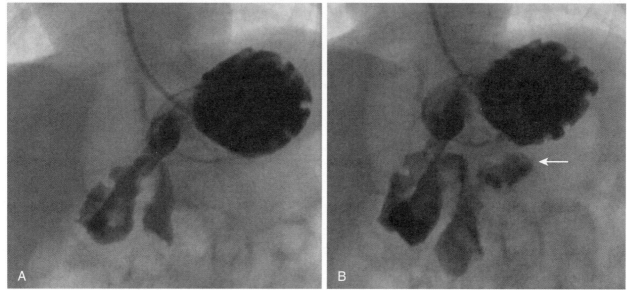

Fig. 4.21 Redundant duodenum. (A) During initial part of examination the duodenal–jejunal junction (DJJ) may not appear appropriately located. (B) Continued filling demonstrates the DJJ is located normally (*arrow*).

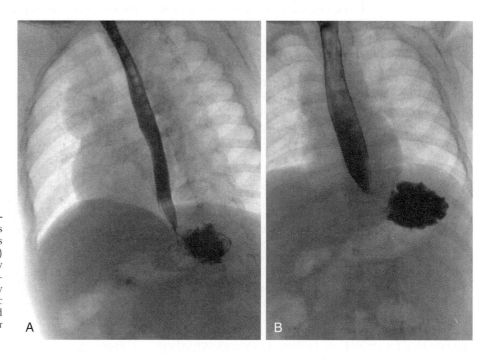

Fig. 4.22 Normal upper gastrointestinal series. The esophagus was well distended during initial swallows on this baby fed barium orally. (A) Right posterior oblique (RPO) view shows lateral view of esophagus. Contours should be smooth, with only subtle indentations from the aortic arch and heart. (B) Contours should also be smooth on the anteroposterior view.

band of contrast within the elongated pyloric channel and the "shoulder" sign of the hypertrophied pyloric channel protruding into the gastric antrum and duodenal bulb (Fig. 4.23).

Contrast Enema

When distal obstruction is present on initial radiographs and air-filled loops of bowel below the pelvis suggesting incarcerated hernia are not seen, a contrast enema is performed (Fig. 4.24). No bowel preparation is performed, because rectal stimulation may interfere with a diagnostic examination in the setting of Hirschsprung disease. A Foley catheter typically from 10 to 20 Fr is placed into the rectum. It may be taped in place, although many practitioners prefer to hold it in place manually. Choice of contrast depends on the clinical scenario. Diatrizoate meglumine and diatrizoate sodium (Gastrografin)

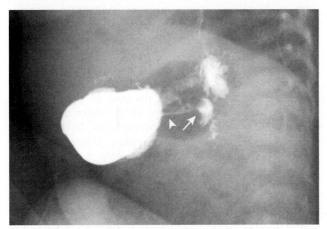

Fig. 4.23 Pyloric stenosis. Arrow denotes shoulder sign, arrowhead denotes string sign.

may be selected if meconium ileus is suspected, because the detergent nature of the agent may be therapeutic, assisting evacuation of inspissated meconium in the ileum. Alternatively, other shiftenterwater-soluble contrast agents such as used for voiding cystourethrogram (e.g., iothalamate meglumine [Cysto-Conray, Guerbet]) may be used. Barium is less commonly used and is usually reserved for patients older than 1 year. The baby is placed in the LLD position, and contrast is introduced into the rectum during fluoroscopic observation. Positioning is crucial to detect a normal rectosigmoid ratio on the lateral view, where the caliber of the rectum should be larger than that of the sigmoid. This normal ratio is lost in the setting of Hirschsprung disease (see Figs. 4.15 and 4.16). Contrast is followed proximally to the cecum if possible, the goal being to introduce contrast into the dilated loops of bowel seen on the radiograph, crossing the point of obstruction. The course, caliber, and filling of the colon are assessed to exclude functional immaturity with small left colon or meconium plug (see Fig. 4.13). Ideally contrast will reflux through the ileocecal valve in meconium ileus, demonstrating the multiple filling defects of meconium pellets (see Fig. 4.14). A postevacuation image may be obtained. If the colon is normal in appearance, an image delayed up to 24 hours may demonstrate retained contrast in the setting of Hirschsprung disease; although this may be more likely to be seen if barium was used, it is still often seen with water soluble contrast in infants.

Abdominal Ultrasound

US techniques to assess the stomach and duodenum by US have been described since the 1970s, and there has recently been renewed interest in using this modality. Sonography for proximal bowel pathology is

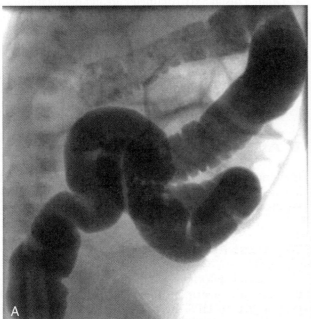
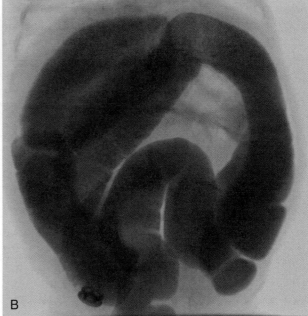

Fig. 4.24 Normal contrast enema. (A) Lateral view demonstrates normal rectosigmoid ratio. (B) Contrast can be followed proximally to the cecum.

technically challenging and operator dependent, but it can be learned with time and practice.

To Assess Midgut Malrotation and Volvulus

Documenting the presence of the third portion of the duodenum within the retroperitoneum confirms normal midgut location and fixation, precluding malrotation. Ideally infants will not be fed for 1 to 2 hours before the study, but in an urgent situation no study delay is required. A high-frequency linear or curved transducer or both is used to image the epigastric region in transverse planes with craniocaudal angulation, as well as longitudinal planes, using graded compression to displace intervening bowel gas. Initially, a midline cine clip should be obtained in the transverse plane from the level of the origins of the SMA and SMV to the bladder, if possible. If visualization at midline is limited by bowel gas despite pressure, a right-sided approach can be attempted. This clip is then repeated with color Doppler. A third clip is performed to follow the duodenum from the pylorus to as far distally as possible; as in UGI, the DJJ should be to the left of the vertebral body at the same transverse level as the duodenal bulb. Administration of 30 mL of 5% glucose by mouth or 30 mL of sterile water through an enteric tube can aid visualization of the entire course of the duodenum. A fourth clip to identify a right lower quadrant cecum and its relation to the umbilicus and iliac vessels is also useful. D3 may be collapsed or may contain fluid or gas, and should be located between the aorta and the SMA/SMV. The uncinate process of the pancreas is adjacent to D3 on the right but should not cross the midline. Jejunal veins may be seen anterior to D3 draining into the SMV. The technique initially described by Yousefzadeh et al. (2010) documents four views in the axial plane from superior to inferior: (1) the confluence of splenic vein/SMV at the level of the pancreas; (2) left renal vein crossing the aorta to join the IVC behind D3; (3) first left jejunal vein; and (4) D3

passing anterior and inferior to the left renal vein and posterior to the jejunal veins, crossing the midline adjacent to the uncinate process. In the longitudinal plane D3 is demonstrated between the SMA/SMV anteriorly and the aorta and renal vein posteriorly. Gentle pressure on the right hemiabdomen may help push jejunal loops to the left and bring the SMA anterior to the aorta in the longitudinal plane. If the examination is not diagnostic, most practitioners proceed to fluoroscopic UGI.

An adjunctive finding is the *relative positions of the SMA and SMV*. This relationship is best imaged in the midline. The SMV is normally located to the right of the SMA. If imaging from the right, the SMV should be to the right of a line drawn between the SMA and the aorta. Location of the SMV to the left of the SMA is suggestive of malrotation, although this is occasionally seen with normal rotation. Finding the SMV located ventrally to the SMA is indeterminate; although the patient may have malrotation, in most cases there is normal rotation. In addition, one-third of infants with malrotation have a normal SMA/SMV relationship. Assessment of the SMA/SMV relationship may be thus be most helpful in the setting of equivocal UGI findings.

The "clockwise whirlpool" sign in malrotation with midgut volvulus can be detected when the SMV and mesentery wrapping around the axis of the SMA create a "whirlpool" appearance that rotates in a *clockwise* direction with caudal movement of the transducer while scanning in the transverse plane (Fig . 4.25). This can be accentuated with color Doppler. A counterclockwise whirlpool is due to normal SMV branches swirling around the SMA, but this is not compatible with midgut volvulus.

Other findings suggestive of volvulus include:

- Dilatation of the proximal duodenum (distended with administered fluids) with tapering of more distal duodenum, analogous to "beaking" on UGI.
- Dilated distal SMV (diameter greater below the umbilicus than above); this is a specific finding, but is not sensitive.
- Fixed, clustered loops of midline bowel (abnormal jejunal loops).
- Thickened duodenal wall, measured after distention, and ascites are often seen in volvulus, but these findings are not statistically significant.

To Assess Gastroesophageal Reflux

Imaging in an oblique sagittal plane using the liver as a window may demonstrate GER through the lower esophageal sphincter.

To Assess Pyloric Stenosis

The normal pyloric channel is a short segment seen between the gastric antrum and the duodenal bulb (Fig. 4.26). In HPS the pyloric channel is elongated and the muscle thickness is increased; the pyloric channel mucosa is hypertrophied, giving rise to echogenic layers filling the channel, causing a channel di-

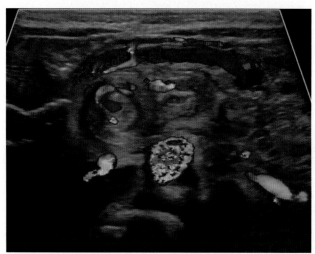

Fig. 4.25 Midgut volvulus on ultrasound. Tranverse color Doppler image through the abdomen showing clockwise rotation of the mesentery and superior mesenteric vein around the superior mesenteric artery, consistent with midgut volvulus.

ameter nearly as thick as the muscle (Fig. 4.27). The heaped-up borders of the pyloric channel are often seen protruding both into the gastric antrum and the duodenal bulb, correlating to the "shoulder" and "mushroom" signs (respectively) on UGI. Muscle thickness is best measured in the midline of the channel, because measuring too far off the midline may overestimate muscle thickness. This is avoided when the prominent central mucosa is seen in the imaging plane. Pyloric muscle thickness below 1.5 mm is normal, between 2 and 3 mm may be abnormal but is not diagnostic of pyloric stenosis, above 3 mm is suggestive of HPS, and above 4 mm is considered by most investigators to be diagnostic of HPS. Pyloric channel length of up to 14 mm may be seen without HPS, above 15 mm is suggestive of HPS, and above 18 mm is considered by most investigators to be diagnostic of HPS. That being said, measurements near 3 mm in thickness and ~15 mm in length may be caused by

pylorospasm. Objective criteria vary; accepting lower muscle thickness for HPS will increase sensitivity and decrease specificity, and vice versa. Curving of the hypertrophied pyloric muscle may limit longitudinal measurements; contiguous sections can be measured and summed to assess length more accurately. Keep in mind that the channel may curve out of the plane of view and be undermeasured.

The patient ideally should not be fed in the hour or two before the examination because a distended stomach increases the difficulty of the examination. To start, the patient is placed on their back and rolled slightly toward the right; a folded towel under the left flank can assist with positioning. This helps distribute the gastric fluid contents into the antrum. The right upper quadrant is insonated with a high-frequency, linear transducer held at an oblique angle midway between longitudinal and transverse planes. Sweeping the transducer through an angle from the right lower quadrant to the left upper quadrant optimizes visualization of the pyloric channel, which is located medial and superior to the upper pole of the right kidney and medial and inferior to the gallbladder, which serve as useful landmarks to the appropriate scan site. Varying the obliquity of the transducer may be necessary to visualize the pyloric channel. In some infants the pylorus may be more posteriorly located, especially if the stomach is distended with air or shadowing gastric contents, and supine positioning or rolling the patient toward the left may help. Insonation using the liver as a window may also allow visualization of the pylorus in challenging situations. Once the pylorus is found, the hypoechoic muscle thickness and channel length are measured. Muscle thickness should also be measured in the transverse plane, or "donut" view of the pyloric channel if possible, obtained by rotating the transducer to view the pylorus in cross section (Fig. 4.28). Observation for passage of gastric contents through

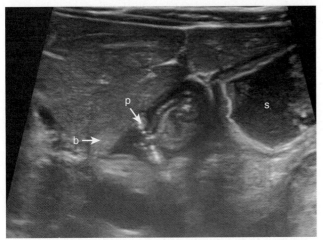

Fig. 4.26 Normal pylorus on ultrasound. *b,* bulb; *p,* pylorus; *s,* stomach.

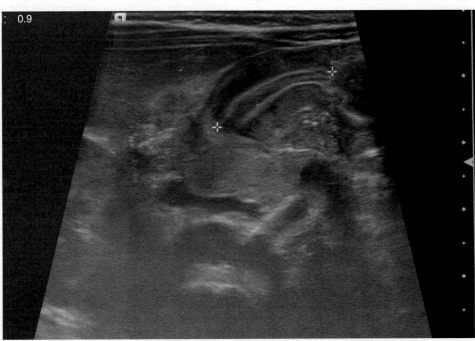

Fig. 4.27 Hypertrophic pyloric stenosis on ultrasound.

the pyloric channel is also useful, as seeing this can help distinguish between HPS and pylorospasm in the case of overlap in muscle thickness and length between these two entities. The patient can be fed glucose water to facilitate this. Pyloric stenosis is not a complete obstruction, however, so some gastric contents may pass. Extended observation also allows identification of change in the appearance of the pyloric channel; variable channel length during a single examination is more suggestive of pylorospasm (Fig. 4.29). Feeding a small volume of glucose water may also help calm an agitated infant in whom the examination is not otherwise possible.

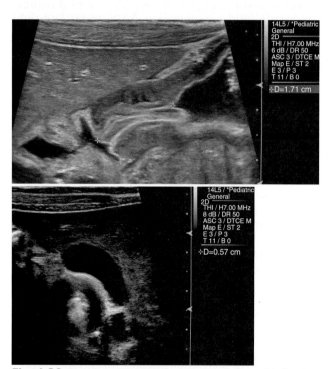

Fig. 4.28 Hypertrophic pyloric stenosis. Ultrasound in longitudinal (top) and transverse (bottom) planes.

Pitfalls When Assessing the Pylorus With US:

- The hypertrophied pyloric channel in HPS is often curved, and length can be underestimated.
- Pyloric muscle sonolucency artifact at 12 and 6 o'clock can be problematic on longitudinal imaging, leading to false undermeasurement of muscle thickness. Measuring slightly off channel midline may help minimize this. Be sure to still see the thickened mucosa in the channel.
- Off-channel imaging may cause false-positive muscle thickness measurement in the longitudinal plane; be sure to visualize thickened pyloric mucosa within the channel to avoid this.
- An overdistended stomach may prevent visualization of the pyloric channel; try rotating the patient or scanning through the liver, although it may be necessary to wait until this clears and then repeat the examination.
- A crying infant makes the examination extremely difficult, and swallowed gas may further limit visualization.
- Pylorospasm may mimic HPS. Several minutes of observation should confirm constant channel length; visualization of passage of gastric contents through the pyloric channel is more suggestive of pylorospasm, although small amounts can pass with pyloric stenosis.

■ Summary

Vomiting in infants has multiple causes. Although it may be part of the expected trials of early parenthood, careful assessment of the clinical picture and a systematic approach to imaging is crucial to detect treatable causes of vomiting in a timely manner and avoid potentially catastrophic consequences. We have discussed our approach to the questions to be asked and the imaging techniques to be used in evaluating vomiting in infants. Knowledge of the age of the infant and the character (bilious or nonbilious, projectile) and timing of onset

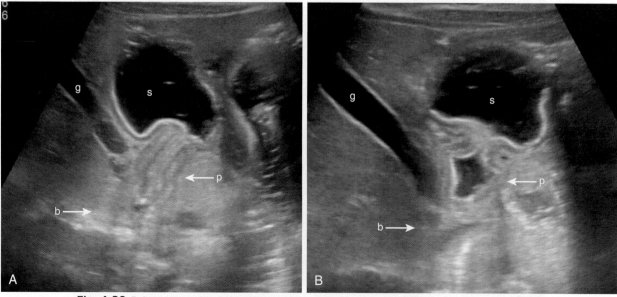

Fig. 4.29 Pylorospasm-simulating hypertrophic pyloric stenosis. Pyloric channel looks elongated (A) but clearly opens up a few minutes later (B). *b,* bulb; *g,* gallbladder; *p,* pylorus; *s,* stomach.

of symptoms is essential for selection and performance of the appropriate study. Causes of vomiting in infancy and age of presentation for different etiologies are summarized in Tables 4.1 and 4.2.

TABLE 4.1   Causes of Vomiting in Infancy

Proximal obstruction	Midgut malrotation +/− volvulus
	Duodenal atresia/web
	Annular pancreas
	Preduodenal portal vein
	Pyloric stenosis
	Pylorospasm
Distal obstruction	Hirschsprung disease
	Ileal/colonic atresia/stenosis
	Jejunal atresia/stenosis
	Meconium ileus
	Functional immaturity (meconium plug/small left colon)
	Incarcerated hernia
	Intussusception
Nonobstructing causes	Nonpathological "spitting up"
	Gastroesophageal reflux
	Formula intolerance
	Gastroenteritis
Nongastrointestinal causes	Increased intracranial pressure from tumor or trauma
	Infection
	Metabolic disorders

TABLE 4.2   Causes of Vomiting by Age

< 2 days	Midgut malrotation +/− volvulus
	Nonpathological "spitting up"
	Duodenal atresia/web
	Annular pancreas
	Preduodenal portal vein
	Hirschsprung disease
	Ileal/colonic atresia/stenosis
	Jejunal atresia/stenosis
	Meconium ileus
	Meconium plug/small left colon
	Incarcerated inguinal hernia
>2 days	Midgut malrotation +/− volvulus
	Nonpathological "spitting up"
	Pyloric stenosis
	Pylorospasm
	Gastroesophageal reflux
	Hirschsprung disease
	Duodenal stenosis/web
	Annular pancreas
	Preduodenal portal vein
	Incarcerated inguinal hernia

Bibliography

Alazraki, A. L., Rigsby, C. K., Iyer, R. S., Bardo, D. M. E., Brown, B. P., Chan, S. S., … Karmazyn, B. (1995, updated 2020). *ACR Appropriateness Criteria Vomiting in Infants*. American College of Radiology ACR Appropriateness Criteria. Available at https://acsearch.acr.org/docs/69445/Narrative/ American College of Radiology. Accessed 5/11/2021.

Applegate, K. E. (2009). Evidence-based diagnosis of malrotation and volvulus. *Pediatric Radiology, 39*(Suppl. 2), S161–S163.

Applegate, K. E., Anderson, J. M., & Klatte, E. C. (2006). Intestinal malrotation in children: A problem-solving approach to the upper gastrointestinal series. *RadioGraphics, 26,* 1485–1500.

Buonomo, C. (1997). Neonatal gastrointestinal emergencies. Imaging of the acute pediatric abdomen. *Radiologic Clinics of North America, 35*(4), 845–864.

Chao, H. C., Kong, M. S., Chen, J. Y., Lin, S. J., & Lin, J. N. (2000). Sonographic features related to volvulus in neonatal intestinal malrotation. *Journal of Ultrasound in Medicine, 19,* 371–376.

Herliczek, T. W., Raghavan, D., McCarten, K., & Wallach, M. (2011). Sonographic upper gastrointestinal series in the vomiting infant: How we do it. *Journal of Clinical Imaging Science, 1,* 19.

Hernanz-Schulman, M. (2009). Pyloric stenosis: Role of imaging. *Pediatric Radiology, 39*(Suppl. 2), S134–S139.

Maxfield, C. M., Bartz, B. H., & Shaffer, J. L. (2013). A pattern-based approach to bowel obstruction in the newborn. *Pediatric Radiology, 43,* 318–329.

Nayak, G. K., Levin, T. L., Kurian, J., Kohli, A., Borenstein, S. H., & Goldman, H. S. (2014). Bedside upper gastrointestinal series in critically ill low birth weight infants. *Pediatric Radiology, 44,* 1252–1257.

Nguyen, H. T. N., Sammer, M. B. K., Ditzler, M. G., Carlson, L. S., Somcio, R. J., Orth, R. C., … Seghers, V. J. (2021). Transition to ultrasound as the first-line imaging modality for midgut volvulus: keys to a successful roll-out. *Pediatric Radiology, 51,* 506–515. https://doi.org/10.1007/s00247-020-04913-9

Ryan, S., & Donoghue, V. (2010). Gastrointestinal pathology in neonates: New imaging strategies. *Pediatric Radiology, 40,* 927–931.

Yousefzadeh, D. K., Kang, L., & Tessicini, L. (2010). Assessment of retromesenteric position of the third portion of the duodenum: An US feasibility study in 33 newborns. *Pediatric Radiology, 40,* 1476–1484.

CHAPTER 5
Pediatric Abdominal Pain

Adina L. Alazraki and Edward J. Richer

CHAPTER OUTLINE

What Is the Role of Imaging in Abdominal Pain?, 98
How to Approach the Abdominal Radiograph in Pediatrics, 99
How to Describe the Overall Gas Pattern, 100
    Normal Gas Pattern, 100
    Ileus, 100
    Obstruction, 100
Age-Based Differential Considerations, 100
    Infants Beyond the Neonatal Period, 101
    Toddlers and School-Age Children, 101
    Older Children and Teenagers, 103
Common Diagnostic Etiologies for Abdominal Pain Across Age Groups, 103
    Malrotation With Midgut Volvulus, 103

Colonic Volvulus, 104
Intussusception, 104
Appendicitis, 106
Gastroenteritis, 108
Meckel Diverticulum, 109
Mesenteric Adenitis, 110
Urinary Tract Infection, 110
Pneumonia, 112
Pancreatitis, 113
Henoch-Schönlein Purpura, 116
Hemolytic Uremic Syndrome, 118
Inflammatory Bowel Disease, 118
Trauma, 121
Constipation, 124
Summary, 125

In pediatrics, one of the most common presenting symptoms to the pediatrician or emergency department is abdominal pain. It is a source of much consternation for parents and is often an extrapolated symptom by the parent based on how the child is behaving. Nearly one-fourth of patients younger than 15 years will have seen a physician for this problem. Abdominal pain may be defined as any discomfort that may be acute or chronic, constant or intermittent, or sudden or insidious. These variables, along with the patient's age and accompanying symptoms or signs, play a role in the subsequent work-up of the problem and help determine the path that is most appropriate for diagnosis and treatment. The differential diagnosis is broad (Table 5.1); therefore any signs, symptoms, or laboratory data that may narrow the differential are helpful. The history is crucial to arrive at a tailored diagnosis.

Scientifically, abdominal pain results from stimulation of nociceptive receptors and afferent sympathetic stretch receptors. Visceral pain is triggered by nociceptors of a hollow viscera as experienced in intestinal obstruction, appendiceal inflammation, and renal or biliary stones. Visceral pain is often referred and therefore not well localized. Parietal pain is associated with direct noxious stimuli to the parietal peritoneum, as demonstrated by tenderness at McBurney point or pain from irritation of the diaphragm. Alternatively, abdominal pain can be induced or psychosomatic in etiology, presenting as a manifestation of a psychosocial problem that may be rooted in the home or at school. These cases are the most difficult to sort out, and radiology is rarely helpful other than to exclude other demonstrable causes.

■ What Is the Role of Imaging in Abdominal Pain?

Imaging of the abdomen can help guide the clinician toward a surgical or nonsurgical approach and expedite the appropriate care of the child. The etiology for pain can be benign or gravely serious requiring immediate attention, which is part of the challenge to approaching these patients for the clinician. Unfortunately for the clinician, the spectrum of symptoms produced by these conditions can often be vague and nonspecific, and for this reason imaging plays a prominent role in the evaluation of these patients. A complete history and physical examination are necessary to direct the imaging workup. Often a screening radiograph of the abdomen is most useful to assess the need for further imaging or to determine the need for immediate surgical intervention (Table 5.2). The decision to image or not often depends on the acuity of the presenting symptom;

TABLE 5.1   Limited Age-Based Table of Common Etiologies for Abdominal Pain in Children With Secondary Associated Symptom Differential Diagnosis

2 MONTHS TO 2 YEARS	2–5 YEARS	>5 YEARS
With Fever:	**With Fever:**	**With Fever:**
Hepatitis	Appendicitis	Appendicitis
Gastroenteritis	Gastroenteritis	Gastroenteritis
Viral illness	Viral illness	Viral illness
Urinary tract infection	Pharyngitis	Pneumonia
Toxin	Hepatitis	Pancreatitis
With Vomiting:	Urinary tract infection	Pharyngitis (strep)
Adhesions	Pneumonia	Mesenteric adenitis
Incarcerated hernia	**With Vomiting:**	Cholecystitis
Intussusception	Adhesions	Hepatitis
Dietary protein allergy	Ovarian torsion	Urinary tract infection
Bloody Stool:	Toxin	**With Vomiting:**
Hemolytic uremic syndrome	**Bloody Stool:**	Diabetic ketoacidosis
Hirschsprung disease	Hemolytic uremic syndrome	Ovarian torsion
Meckel diverticulum	Intussusception	Adhesions
Other:	Henoch-Schönlein purpura	Testicular torsion
Sickle cell crisis	Meckel diverticulum	**Bloody Stool:**
Tumor	**Other:**	Hemolytic uremic syndrome
Foreign body ingestion	Constipation	Inflammatory bowel disease
Trauma (including NAT)	Sickle cell crisis	Meckel diverticulum
	Tumor	Henoch-Schönlein purpura
	Foreign body ingestion	**Other:**
	Trauma (including NAT)	Sickle cell crisis
		Constipation
		Trauma

NAT, Nonaccidental trauma.

TABLE 5.2   Primary Indications for Abdominal Radiography

1. Evaluation for and follow-up of abdominal distention, bowel obstruction, or nonobstructive ileus
2. Constipation
3. Evaluation for necrotizing enterocolitis, particularly in the premature newborn
4. Evaluation of congenital abnormalities
5. Follow-up of the postoperative patient, including detection of inadvertent retained surgical foreign bodies
6. Evaluation for and follow-up of urinary tract calculi, including assessment of lithotripsy patients
7. Search for foreign bodies
8. A preliminary radiograph before a planned imaging examination, such as fluoroscopy
9. Evaluation of the position of medical devices
10. Evaluation for pneumoperitoneum
11. Evaluation of possible toxic megacolon
12. Evaluation for bowel perforation and fractures in unstable patients after blunt trauma
13. Evaluation of a palpable mass in a child

Adapted from the ACR-SPR Practice Parameter for the Performance of Abdominal Radiography.

therefore to direct the imaging most logically, an algorithm may help direct the workup where the initial distinction is acute versus chronic. After this, the age of the patient, along with the presence or absence of fever, might mark the next branch point in the decision tree. Associated symptoms and signs will lead down directed pathways to finally arrive at a concise differential diagnosis. When the starting symptom is as broad as abdominal pain, even a directed algorithm will still result in a differential diagnosis rather than a single final answer.

■ How to Approach the Abdominal Radiograph in Pediatrics

There are many approaches to interpreting abdominal plain film, some of which are guided by catchy mnemonics. All of these have in common the goal of being systematic so as not to neglect any one aspect of the film. This can happen when there is a positive finding, the so-called satisfaction of search. Although ordering a plain radiograph is frequently a knee-jerk reflex for the clinician, it is important to understand the limitations of the examination. Not surprisingly, the plain abdominal radiograph is often as nonspecific as the presenting complaint. There is broad variability in the interpretation and agreement among radiologists. Thus the final interpretation of a "nonspecific bowel gas pattern" is often considered a nondiagnostic examination (see Box 5.1).

BOX 5.1   Mnemonics
Inside-out, outside-in
Gas, mass, bones, stones
CBA (chest, bones, abdomen)
A-A-I-I-M-M:
■ Adhesions
■ Appendicitis
■ Intussusception
■ Inguinal hernia
■ Malrotation
■ Miscellaneous (Meckel, tumor, duplication, etc.)

■ How to Describe the Overall Gas Pattern

Many terms are used in the radiology lexicon to describe both specific and nonspecific gas patterns. Radiologists should be familiar with the various descriptions, their implied meanings, and the interpreted meaning by the referring doctor.

Normal Gas Pattern

When evaluating the bowel by radiograph, we are looking at the gas pattern, because the air interface with the adjacent tissue is really what is being imaged. Normal position of the bowel is the first assessment. The stomach typically contains air and is located in the left upper quadrant. The small bowel is often central and should be relatively uniform where it is air filled (Fig. 5.1). One should be careful in using adult criteria for bowel obstruction, such as dilation of bowel loops longer than 3 cm, because this may lead to underdiagnosis in children. Average bowel diameter in infants is approximately 1.2 cm at 6 months of age, increasing to 2.1 cm by 8 years of age, and reaching average adult diameter by 15 years. One should be able to see the valvulae conniventes traversing the small bowel loop in older patients, but in the young toddler and infant, these may not yet be visible. Large bowel is typically located on the periphery, and the haustral markings can be seen more widely spaced apart and partially indenting the gas-filled looped on either side (Fig. 5.2). In younger children, haustra may not be present. Depending on the timing of imaging, a variable amount

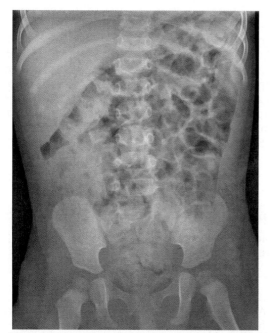

Fig. 5.1 Happy polygons. Normal bowel gas pattern on this supine radiograph showing varied polygonal shape to gas-filled nondilated bowel loops throughout the abdomen.

of formed stool may be seen in the colon. The delayed development of haustral markings and visibility of small bowel plicae can make bowel evaluation and localization of the problem in the youngest patients more difficult.

Ileus

Ileus is typically adynamic. Adynamic ileus refers to a functional or nonanatomic etiology for the obstruction of gas in the small bowel, or a functional paralysis of the bowel. Because there is no anatomic obstruction, there is no disproportionate dilation of upstream bowel. Therefore the bowel loops are either uniformly dilated or uniformly without any gas (Fig. 5.3). These patients may present asymptomatically or with signs and symptoms of an anatomic obstruction. Typical clinical settings include sepsis, trauma, and metabolic disturbances (see Box 5.2).

Obstruction

A mechanical blockage, either intrinsic or extrinsic, to the passage of air or fecal content in the bowel results in obstruction. The radiographic appearance is specific with dilated bowel loops proximal to the point of obstruction and decompressed bowel distal to that point. Conversely, in later obstruction the bowel may be fluid filled and dilation difficult to assess, thus the importance of an orthogonal view. There are often cases where variation in timing of the obstruction leads to anomalies in the gas pattern. Some experts describe the appearance of obstructed bowel loops as "sad sausages" (Fig. 5.4) in reference to their smooth, featureless appearance, in contrast with "happy polygons" (see Fig. 5.1), which describes the normal wall variability seen in nonobstructed bowel. The "string of pearls" or "string of beads" sign refers to the appearance of trapped air between the valvulae conniventes in a predominantly fluid-filled small bowel loop. These gas bubbles may appear stacked or side by side in a string. Alternatively, there may be a "stepladder" configuration of small air–fluid levels in the obstructed small bowel (Fig. 5.5; see also Box 5.3).

■ Age-Based Differential Considerations

The broad range of etiologies that may cause acute-onset abdominal pain in children overlaps across age groups, although some may be more typical than others in each age group. We will discuss each of these entities in detail, but keep in mind, many of these diagnoses may be seen in all age groups. In most cases, when a child presents with acute abdominal pain, the most pressing question is whether the child needs an operation, or can surgery be prevented in the near future by intervening/acting on an important finding.

Infants Beyond the Neonatal Period

The etiology of abdominal pain in infants between 2 months and 2 years of age may be difficult to diagnose because symptoms are largely interpreted based on physical signs. Mechanical causes for pain are the most important to exclude, most commonly, intussusception and volvulus. Less common causes of acute abdominal pain in this age group include appendicitis, sepsis, and obstruction as a result of adhesions. Although the most common causes for abdominal pain may be non-life-threatening, such as colic or enteritis, the clinician needs to maintain a high level of suspicion for less common but possibly life-threatening causes for pain in this age group, such as nonaccidental trauma.

Toddlers and School-Age Children

Abdominal pain in toddlers and young school-age children is a common problem. According to Centers for Disease Control and Prevention statistics, the incidence of children aged 0 to 4 years presenting to either the outpatient setting or the emergency department with abdominal pain was approximately 268 per 10,000 as of 2010. The causes of abdominal pain in this age group can range from the annoying but relatively benign (constipation, gastroenteritis) to life-threatening (appendicitis, intussusception). Unfortunately for the clinician, the spectrum of symptoms produced by these conditions can often be vague and nonspecific, and for this reason imaging plays an important role in the evaluation of these patients.

Right lower quadrant pain in toddlers and young children is a frequent presenting complaint, the etiologies of

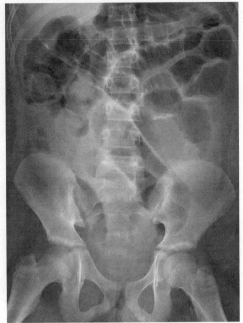

Fig. 5.3 Ileus pattern in an 11-year-old. Supine radiograph with dilated small bowel loops. Air is also present in colonic loops and in the rectum, without a transition to suggest high-grade obstruction.

BOX 5.2   When to Suspect Ileus

Clinical findings: Abdominal distention with or without obstructive symptoms (i.e., vomiting)
Imaging findings:
- Uniform air-filled distention of nondilated bowel
- Localized: sentinel dilated loop
- Presence of distal colonic gas

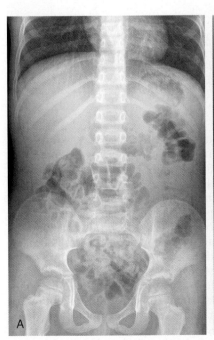
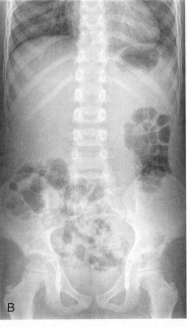

Fig. 5.2 Normal bowel gas pattern in an 11-year-old. Supine (A) and upright (B) radiographs show normal small and large bowel loops. Haustra are well developed and easy to distinguish. Small bowel loops are polygonal and varied.

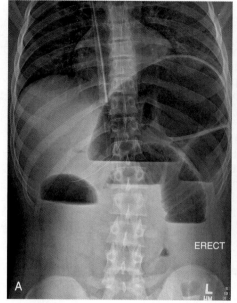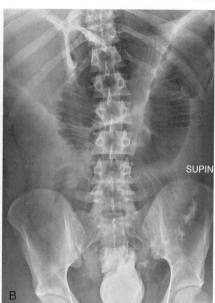

Fig. 5.4 *Sad sausages.* Upright (A) and supine (B) radiographs in a patient with small bowel obstruction. Markedly dilated bowel loops with "sad sausage" configuration. Note the prominence of the valvulae conniventes indicating small bowel.

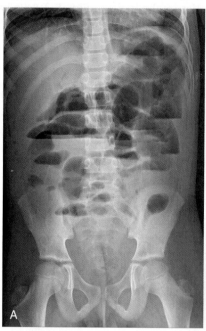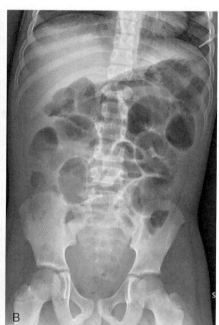

Fig. 5.5 Stepladder configuration. Upright (A) and supine (B) radiographs show dilated bowel loops with air–fluid levels and different heights, the stepladder pattern, which is highly suspicious for obstruction.

BOX 5.3   When to Suspect Obstruction

Clinical findings: Abdominal distention, pain, and vomiting
Imaging findings:
- Dilated bowel loops upstream of the transition
- Decompressed distal loops
- Air–fluid levels
- "String of pearls" sign in late obstruction
- "Sad sausages"

which range from the emergent, such as appendicitis and intussusception, to the self-limited, such as mesenteric adenitis. Evaluation often begins with radiographs, due to widespread availability, rapidity of the exam, and lack of need for patient prep or sedation. Findings on radio-

graphs are frequently nonspecific, however, which may prompt a need for more advanced imaging, such as ultrasound, computed tomography (CT), or magnetic resonance imaging (MRI). The availability of these more advanced imaging modalities varies with the facility to which the patient presents, and transfer to higher-level facilities may be needed to accomplish this imaging.

Bowel obstruction on plain radiographs can be one of the quickest methods to distinguish serious from benign conditions. Causes of bowel obstruction in young children are generally going to be those potentially requiring surgical intervention, such as appendicitis, intussusception, or Meckel diverticulum. The AAIIMM mnemonic (appendicitis, adhesions, intussusception, inguinal hernia, Meckel, malrotation) can be a helpful reminder of some of the conditions producing bowel obstructions in children.

Patient age and clinical symptoms are important to narrow the differential diagnosis when a bowel obstruction is recognized. Intussusception typically occurs in patients 3 months to 3 years of age and is typically accompanied by crampy abdominal pain, fussiness, lethargy, and, possibly, bloody stools ("currant jelly stool"). Appendicitis is seen more frequently in older pediatric patients (10–19 years old) and is associated with fever, leukocytosis, nausea/vomiting, and anorexia. In toddlers and younger children who may not be able to verbalize their symptoms, the diagnosis of appendicitis is more likely to be delayed and present with appendiceal perforation. In these patients, symptoms may include vague abdominal pain and distention, fussiness, or lethargy, in addition to fever and vomiting.

Older Children and Teenagers

The range of pathology that may present with abdominal pain in the older child age group is broad, but often can be limited by the history that is more easily obtained in these patients. Although many of the diagnoses that are imaged require cross-sectional imaging to diagnose, the abdominal plain film is again frequently a good starting point.

Important factors to consider from the history are the duration of pain, the acuity of onset of pain (versus an insidious onset), the quality of the pain, and associated symptoms, such as vomiting, diarrhea, or fever. Finally, exposures are an important piece of information that may provide an etiology for a suspected infectious cause.

Acute abdominal pain may be emergent or life-threatening, but in the majority of patients, this is not the case. The clinician is tasked with determining the urgency of pain, and the radiologist is often consulted.

We will discuss the more common causes of abdominal pain in children later in this chapter, focusing on those etiologies where radiology may play an important or diagnostic role in the workup.

■ Common Diagnostic Etiologies for Abdominal Pain Across Age Groups

Malrotation With Midgut Volvulus

Malrotation/midgut volvulus is a true life-threatening surgical emergency and should be suspected in any infant with acute-onset bilious vomiting. Although it is usually diagnosed in the neonatal period, a delayed presentation of malrotation with midgut volvulus must still be at the top of the differential diagnosis for bilious emesis in any age group. Because of its short mesentery, malrotated bowel is at risk for volvulus with secondary bowel ischemia, which can result in complete loss of the midgut and even death.

Plain radiographs are often normal, because volvulus presents early after the twisting of the bowel and there is little time for dilation of the upstream bowel. The diagnostic imaging study of choice is the upper gastrointestinal (GI) series. In a normal study the position of the duodenojejunal junction has a rigid fixed location to the left of midline, just left of the left pedicle at the same level as the duodenal bulb. This marks the fixation by the ligament of Treitz, which traverses the mesentery diagonally, also fixing the cecum in the right lower quadrant. In a well-performed upper GI series, almost any deviation from the normal examination is highly suspicious for malrotation (Fig. 5.6).

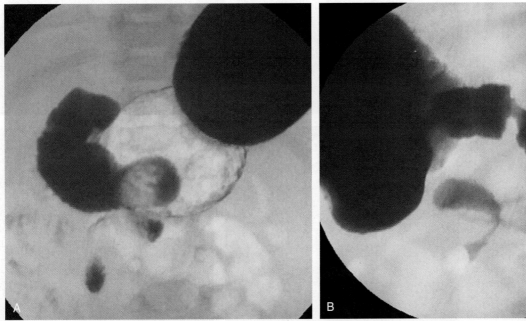

Fig. 5.6 Malrotation with midgut volvulus. Anteroposterior image (A) from an upper gastrointestinal series in a patient with bilious vomiting showing the third portion of the duodenum inferiorly displaced and a spiraling appearance of the subsequent bowel loops. Lateral image (B) redemonstrates the twisting of the bowel loops inferiorly and only mild dilation of the proximal duodenum.

When patients with malrotation/midgut volvulus present with vomiting that is not recognized as bilious, the diagnosis of pyloric stenosis may be suspected, resulting in an ultrasound of the abdomen. Sonographic findings that suggest malrotation include reversal of the position of the superior mesenteric artery and vein positions (Fig. 5.7; see Box 5.4; also refer to Chapter 4, Vomiting Infant).

Colonic Volvulus

Children with colonic volvulus typically present with continuous, severe abdominal pain and colonic dilatation. The pain in the colonic volvulus may be described as colicky, mimicking episodes of peristalsis. Vomiting may occur several days after the onset of pain. Children who have a history of colonic dysmotility or chronic constipation may as a result have a redundant sigmoid colon that can increase the possibility of volvulus (Fig. 5.8). Similarly, patients with a narrow mesenteric attachment, either congenitally or secondary to prior bowel surgery, may also be at risk for development of colonic volvulus. Cecal volvulus is uncommon in children and may be seen in patients with intestinal malrotation or abnormal fixation with adhesive bands (see Box 5.5).

Intussusception

Intussusception is a telescoping of a proximal segment of bowel (the intussusceptum) into a more distal segment (the intussuscipiens). Intussusception may involve the small intestine only (enteroenteric), small intestine and colon (ileocolic), or colon only (colocolonic). The variety that is of particular concern for the radiologist is the ileocolic intussusception because this can be

---

BOX 5.4   When to Suspect Malrotation With Midgut Volvulus

Clinical findings: Acute-onset bilious vomiting in an infant, crampy abdominal pain
Imaging findings:
- Radiograph: Typically normal bowel gas pattern; Can be dilated in late diagnosis
- UGI: malposition of the duodenojejunal junction
  Downward spiral of the duodenum/jejunum
  Abrupt cessation of contrast passage in the third portion of the duodenum
- US: reversal of the SMA/SMV, whirlpool sign

SMA, superior mesenteric artery; *SMV,* superior mesenteric vein; *UGI,* upper gastrointestinal; *US,* ultrasound.

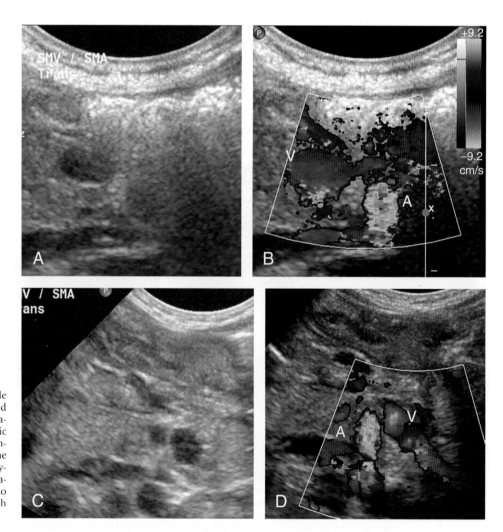

Fig. 5.7 Malrotation. Grayscale (A) and color Doppler ultrasound (B) images showing normal relationship of the superior mesenteric artery (SMA) and superior mesenteric vein (SMV). The SMV is to the right and anterior to the SMA. Grayscale (C) and color Doppler ultrasound (D) images in a patient who was vomiting showing reversal with the SMV to the left of the SMA.

reduced by a therapeutic enema performed under fluoroscopic guidance.

Ileocolic intussusception is a commonly suspected diagnosis in the infant and toddler age group. Nearly 60% of children with ileocolic intussusception are younger than 1 year, and 80% to 90% are younger than 2 years. In children 6 months to 3 years of age, ileocolic intussusception is the most common cause of intestinal obstruction. Prevalence varies by locale, and an overall prevalence is not established; however, the estimated incidence in the United States is approximately 1 in 2000 live births. There is a seasonal variation, with peaks coinciding with peaks in viral gastroenteritis in some geographic regions. This correlates with the hypothesized etiology for idiopathic ileocolic intussusception in that a preceding viral infection causes lymphoid hyperplasia or enlargement of Peyer patches (submucosal aggregated lymphoid tissue in the ileum) that serves as a lead point. In patients outside the typical age range (younger than 3 months, older than 6 years), a pathological lead point is more likely, such as a Meckel diverticulum, duplication cyst, polyp, or lymphoma.

Patients with intussusception may have a variety of symptoms, including colicky abdominal pain alternating with periods of quiescence, lethargy, bloody or "currant jelly" stools, and vomiting that may be bilious. Symptoms may be vague and insidious initially, mimicking more benign processes, such as gastroenteritis, and leading to delay in presentation.

As in many cases of abdominal pain in children, the initial evaluation of potential ileocolic intussusception is often with abdominal radiographs. Possible abnormalities detected on radiographs include a right lower quadrant soft tissue mass with or without meniscus sign, bowel obstruction, or paucity of gas within the right lower quadrant (Fig. 5.9). Radiographs have been shown to be unreliable for diagnosis of ileocolic intussusception in numerous studies, with a sensitivity of 60% and specificity of 26% for a supine abdominal radiograph, and

---

BOX 5.5   *When to Suspect Colonic Volvulus*

Clinical findings: Insidious-onset pain and distention, vomiting, constipation
Imaging findings:
- Colonic dilation
- Cecal "bascule"
- Bird beak in ascending colon
Imaging in sigmoid volvulus:
- Colonic dilation
- "Coffee bean" sign
- Absent rectal gas
- Beaking distally on contrast enema

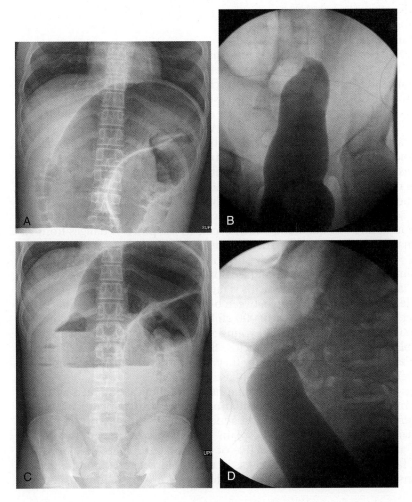

Fig. 5.8 *Sigmoid volvulus.* Supine (A) and upright (B) radiographs show a large dilated bowel loop pointing to the left shoulder and demonstrating the "coffee bean" sign. Anteroposterior (C) and lateral (D) views from contrast enema demonstrate the "bird beak" at the top of the twist.

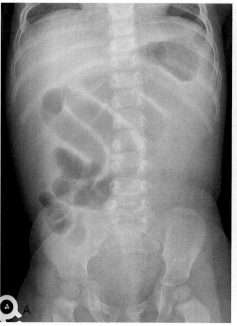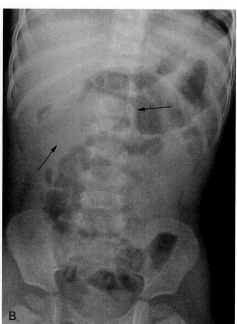

Fig. 5.9 Intussusception. Abdominal radiograph (A) demonstrates small bowel obstruction, with multiple dilated, stacked small bowel loops and absence of colorectal gas. (B) Abdominal radiograph in a different patient shows a soft tissue mass in the right upper quadrant with a "meniscus sign," in which the leading edge of the intussusception is outlined by gas in the more distal colon (*arrows*).

only 74% and 58%, respectively, for a two-view x-ray series. In fact, in up to 25% of cases, the abdominal radiographs may be completely normal. Conversely, the negative predictive value of the three-view abdominal radiograph was shown to be quite high. That is, when the presence of an air-filled cecum and an otherwise normal bowel gas pattern can be definitively seen, this may be sufficient to exclude the presence of intussusception. Radiographs are also helpful in excluding bowel perforation, a contraindication to therapeutic enema for intussusception reduction. Although radiographs are frequently obtained, the definitive presence of intussusception is rarely indisputable, and a follow-up confirmatory test is usually required.

The imaging modality of choice for diagnosis of intussusception is abdominal ultrasound. Ultrasound is readily available in most institutions, is portable, requires no patient prep or sedation, and uses no ionizing radiation. When an ileocolic intussusception is present, there is usually no diagnostic dilemma, because a large soft tissue mass is immediately evident. The classic ultrasound findings are of the "target" or "bull's-eye" sign when the intussusception is imaged in the short axis and the "pseudokidney" sign when imaged longitudinally (Fig. 5.10A–C). The alternating layers seen in the target sign represent the outer intussuscipiens, a middle layer of mesenteric fat and lymph nodes, and the inner intussusceptum. Ancillary findings that may be helpful to note include the presence of free fluid, decreased blood flow within the involved bowel segments on Doppler interrogation, and "trapped" fluid between the layers of the intussusception (see Fig. 5.10D). These findings can indicate that therapeutic enema may be difficult or unsuccessful, but they do not contraindicate the procedure.

Treatment of ileocolic intussusception is with therapeutic enema or surgery. Enema is generally attempted first because of its less invasive nature, with failures of reduction proceeding surgery. Contraindications to thera-

peutic enema include presence of bowel perforation/free air, peritonitis, or a patient in shock. Details of the performance of therapeutic enema are beyond the scope of this text (see Box 5.6).

Appendicitis

Appendicitis remains the most common cause of acute abdominal pain presenting to the emergency department among adults and children. In the United States, about 70,000 pediatric cases per year are diagnosed, with the majority of affected children in the second decade of life (10–19 years old). Appendicitis is considered a surgical emergency and can be life-threatening. If undiagnosed, it can progress to rupture and peritonitis with development of intraabdominal abscesses. Therefore early diagnosis is key to preventing morbidity from this disease. Clinically the most predictive indicator in an older child is pain that localizes from the periumbilical region to the right lower quadrant, which occurs as the process changes from visceral to parietal stimulus of pain receptors. Subsequently, patients may show abdominal wall rigidity on physical examination (see Box 5.7).

Appendicitis is rare in the infant and young child. The incidence between birth and 4 years of age is only 1 to 2 cases per 10,000 children per year. It is not uncommon for the child younger than 2 years to present with perforated appendicitis. Because of the later presentation in this age group, they are more likely to have abnormally elevated acute-phase reactants.

Plain radiographs are frequently obtained as an initial step in evaluating patients with appendicitis but are typically nondiagnostic. In a child with perforated appendicitis, plain radiographs may demonstrate an early obstructive or ileus pattern. There may be a paucity of bowel gas in the right lower quadrant because of an abscess or phlegmon. A small amount of free

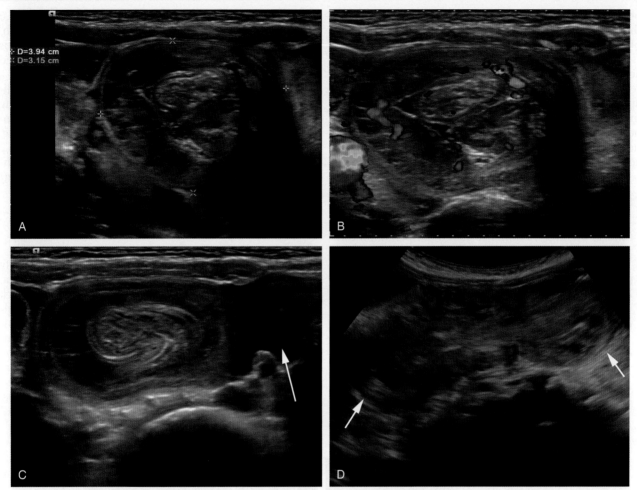

Fig. 5.10 Intussusception. Transverse grayscale ultrasound image (A) reveals a target-like lesion consistent with ileocolic intussusception. Note the relatively larger size than enteroenteric intussusceptions, as well as the presence of a layer of trapped mesenteric fat. Color Doppler ultrasound image (B) shows preserved blood flow to the intussusception. Diminished blood flow can indicate ischemia and a potentially difficult therapeutic enema. Transverse grayscale ultrasound image (C) shows free fluid is seen adjacent to the intussusception (*arrow*). Large or complex ascites may also indicate a difficult enema reduction. "Trapped" fluid within the layers of the intussusception is occasionally seen, with the same implication. Longitudinal grayscale ultrasound image (D) shows the "pseudokidney" sign (*arrows*) of an ileocolic intussusception when imaged in the longitudinal plane.

BOX 5.6   When to Suspect Intussusception

Clinical findings: Colicky abdominal pain alternating with periods of quiescence, lethargy, bloody stools, +/- bilious vomiting

Imaging findings:
- Paucity of gas in the RLQ
- Meniscus sign on the left lateral decubitus view
- Mass visualized with meniscus sign
- Bowel obstruction in an otherwise healthy 6-month-old to 3-year-old child
- "Target" or "pseudokidney" sign on ultrasound

RLQ, right lower quadrant.

---

intraabdominal air may also be seen with perforated appendicitis. The presence of a right lower quadrant calcified fecalith can be a helpful finding. Occasionally radiographs suggest an alternative diagnosis, such as basilar pneumonia with referred right lower quadrant

pain. When there is a strong clinical suspicion for appendicitis, radiographs may be supplanted in favor of other imaging modalities discussed later.

In pediatric patients in whom appendicitis is strongly suspected, abdominal ultrasound using graded compression is the modality of choice. In experienced hands, ultrasound is nearly as accurate as CT in diagnosing appendicitis, with a sensitivity and specificity of approximately 90%, with the benefit of no ionizing radiation. Ultrasound findings include a noncompressible tubular structure in the right lower quadrant, with wall thickness more than 2 mm and an overall diameter over 6 mm. Additional findings include hyperemia of the appendiceal wall, increased echogenicity of the mesenteric fat representing inflammation, presence of a shadowing appendicolith, and free fluid (Fig. 5.11A–C). In the setting of perforated appendicitis, a right lower quadrant abscess may be present, with nonvisualization of the appendix itself (see Fig. 5.11D). Ancillary findings in perforated appendicitis may include dilated, fluid bowel loops representing obstruction or ileus, reactive thickening of adjacent small or large intestine, and complex fluid.

Notably, unless a normal appendix is visualized, acute appendicitis is not specifically excluded. In this setting, depending on clinical symptoms, it may be appropriate to progress to more advanced imaging, including CT and MRI. CT is most commonly used because of its widespread availability, speed of examination, and lack of need for sedation. The CT findings of acute appendicitis are well known in both adults and children, including an enlarged appendix more than 6 mm, periappendiceal inflammatory changes, fecalith, and right lower quadrant abscess. MRI for appendicitis is available in some institutions but has not yet achieved the widespread availability or cost factor to become a first-line imaging study. MRI findings of acute appendicitis also include a dilated appendix with surrounding fluid or edema, shown as periappendiceal hyperintensity on T2-weighted fat-suppressed sequences (Fig. 5.12). Appendicoliths may be visible as foci of low T2 signal within the appendiceal lumen. Perforated appendicitis can be suggested if an organized fluid collection/abscess is present (see Box 5.8).

Gastroenteritis

Acute gastroenteritis is a clinical diagnosis generally made by the clinical symptoms of vomiting, diarrhea, and abdominal pain. Usually there is a history of a sick contact or recent exposure. The etiology is almost always viral and tends to cluster during community outbreaks. Less commonly, bacterial causes may be encountered, most commonly *Escherichia coli*, *Salmonella*, *Shigella*, and *Campylobacter*. These infections are more commonly associated with hematochezia. In the setting of recent antibiotic therapy for other infections, *Clostridioides difficile* may also be considered. Stool

---

BOX 5.7   When to Suspect Appendicitis in the Older Child

Clinical findings: Abdominal pain often periumbilical and becoming localized to the RLQ, low-grade or no fever, early-on anorexia

Imaging findings:
- Radiographs: Normal or vague ileus, +/– Paucity of gas in the RLQ, +/– Appendicolith
- US: enlarged appendix >6 mm, hyperemia, echogenic periappendiceal fat, fluid collection
- CT/MRI: enlarged, enhancing appendix >6 mm, fat stranding, fluid collection, +/– appendicolith

CT, Computed tomography; *MRI*, magnetic resonance imaging; *RLQ*, right lower quadrant; *US*, ultrasound.

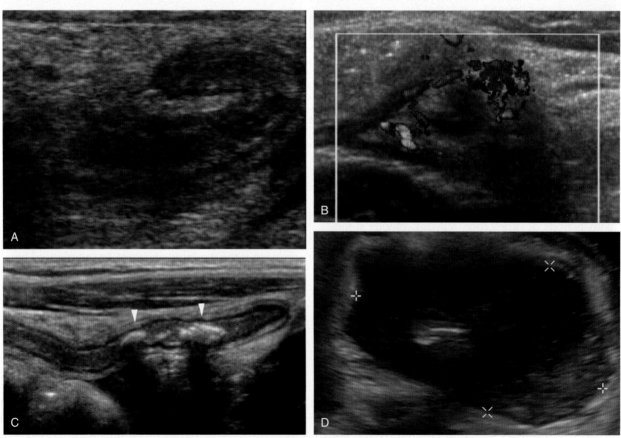

Fig. 5.11 *Appendicitis ultrasound.* (A) Abnormally dilated appendix. (B) Appendiceal wall hyperemia on color Doppler image. (C) Intraluminal appendicoliths with posterior acoustic shadowing (*arrowheads*). (D) Perforated appendicitis with abscess formation. (Courtesy Ramon Sanchez, MD)

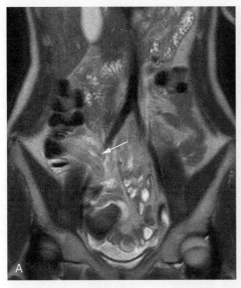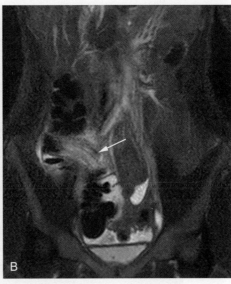

Fig. 5.12 Appendicitis magnetic resonance imaging. Coronal T2-weighted steady state free precession (SSFP) (A) and coronal short tau inversion recovery (STIR) (B) images demonstrate acute appendicitis with a dilated, T2 hyperintense appendix arising from the cecal base (*arrows*). Adjacent edema is best demonstrated on the STIR image.

BOX 5.8   When to Suspect Appendicitis

Clinical findings: Anorexia, low-grade fever, and abdominal pain
   Normal or mildly elevated white blood cell count
   Normal or mildly elevated C-reactive protein
Imaging findings:
- Radiograph findings:
  - Fecalith in RLQ
  - Paucity of gas in the RLQ
  - Ileus pattern
- Sonographic findings:
  - Noncompressible blind ending appendix >6 mm
  - Echogenic periappendiceal fat
  - Increased vascularity to the appendix
  - Abscess/phlegmon
- CT findings:
  - Appendix >6 mm
  - Fecalith
  - Periappendiceal inflammatory changes
  - Abscess
- MRI findings:
  - T2 hyperintensity within the thickened appendix/periappendiceal
  - T2 hypointense fecalith
  - Abscess/phlegmon

CT, Computed tomography; *MRI,* magnetic resonance imaging; *RLQ,* right lower quadrant.

---

cultures and fecal analysis play an important role in the workup of gastroenteritis. Imaging may not play a pivotal role in the diagnosis and is not routinely indicated, but is frequently obtained when emesis becomes profound and there is a concern for other etiology of the presenting symptoms. Emesis may be described as greenish by the parents, usually representing undigested gastric juices/acid rather than true bilious vomiting. Plain radiographs will often show air–fluid levels, usually within the colon, indicative of liquid feces (Fig. 5.13; see Box 5.9).

Meckel Diverticulum

Meckel diverticulum is the most common congenital anomaly of the GI tract, occurring in approximately 2% of the population, and is due to failure of regression of the omphalomesenteric duct, which connects the midgut to the yolk sac in utero. The diverticulum is located along the antimesenteric border of the bowel and is typically located within 100 cm of the ileocecal valve. There is no sex predilection, although complications are reported more commonly in males. Up to 60% of diverticula are lined by heterotopic mucosa, most commonly gastric (62%), followed by pancreatic (6%), or both (5%), which can contribute to some of their associated symptoms. Up to 50% of symptomatic Meckel diverticula cases present before the age of 10 years. Common presentations include painless lower GI bleeding as a result of peptic ulceration caused by the presence of heterotopic gastric mucosa, intussusception with the diverticulum serving as a lead point, and Meckel diverticulitis.

Plain abdominal radiographs in a symptomatic Meckel diverticulum may demonstrate bowel obstruction or an air–fluid level within the diverticulum. Ultrasound is commonly used in the setting of Meckel diverticulitis or inverted Meckel diverticulum with intussusception as a result of overlap with the clinical picture of acute appendicitis. Sonography of the right lower quadrant in a patient with Meckel diverticulitis may show a fluid-filled, blind-ending cystic structure connecting with bowel, showing typical ultrasound gut signature (Fig. 5.14A–C). Enteroliths may be seen within the lumen, and there may be adjacent echogenic fat or free fluid

^{99m}Tc-pertechnetate scintigraphy is the study of choice in cases of lower GI bleeding in young patients in whom the diagnosis of Meckel diverticulum is suspected. ^{99m}Tc-pertechnetate is taken up by gastric mucosa. The diagnosis can be confirmed by demonstrating a focus of uptake in the right lower quadrant corresponding to the site of a Meckel diverticulum. Following the intravenous (IV) injection of the radiotracer, real-time dynamic

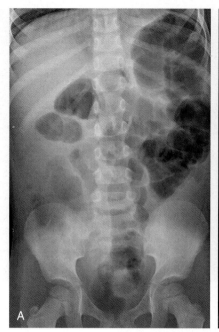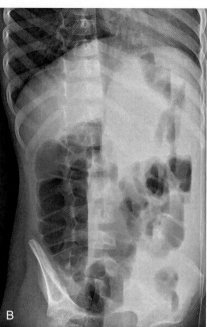

Fig. 5.13 Acute gastroenteritis in a 3-year-old. Supine (A) and left lateral decubitus (B) radiographs demonstrate scattered colonic air–fluid levels without obstruction or small bowel dilation.

BOX 5.9   When to Suspect Gastroenteritis

Clinical findings: Abdominal pain with vomiting and/or diarrhea, +/− fever or sick exposure
Imaging findings:
- Scattered colonic air–fluid levels
- No upstream dilation of small bowel

---

imaging under a gamma camera is performed for 20 minutes. Subsequently, static delayed images are obtained in frontal and lateral projections for localization at 25 to 30 minutes. It is worth remembering, however, that only 60% of Meckel will contain gastric mucosa, yielding a fairly large number of false-negative examinations (Fig. 5.15).

On CT and MRI, it may be difficult to identify the noninflamed Meckel diverticulum. A blind-ending, fluid-filled structure along the antimesenteric border of the distal small bowel may be visualized (see Fig. 5.14D). A Meckel diverticulum complicated by diverticulitis is more easily identified, with inflammatory fat stranding and free fluid surrounding the structure. Careful evaluation to exclude appendicitis would be prudent in this setting (see Box 5.10).

Mesenteric Adenitis

Mesenteric adenitis is a benign, self-limited inflammatory process of the mesenteric lymph nodes that can present with acute or chronic abdominal pain, often localizing to the right lower quadrant. Etiologies include preceding viral or bacterial GI infection (most common bacterial pathogen being *Yersinia enterocolitica*), as well as more remote infections, including group A streptococcal pharyngitis. Due to pain localizing to the right lower quadrant, imaging is often obtained to exclude acute appendicitis.

The classic appearance of mesenteric adenitis is a cluster of at least three enlarged mesenteric lymph nodes, defined as measuring at least 5 mm in short axis most commonly in the right lower quadrant, although enlarged mesenteric nodes elsewhere may also suggest the diagnosis (Fig. 5.16). It is important to note, however, that mesenteric adenitis is a diagnosis of exclusion, and careful evaluation for other sources of reactive adenopathy, such as appendicitis and inflammatory bowel disease (IBD), must be undertaken. Additional imaging findings of mesenteric adenitis include mild thickening of the terminal ileum or colon in a minority of cases and absence of abscess or phlegmon (see Box 5.11).

Urinary Tract Infection

Urinary tract infections (UTIs) are common in children and often present with abdominal pain as a major complaint, prompting imaging evaluation. UTIs may involve the lower urinary tract (cystitis) or the upper tract (pyelonephritis). In younger children and infants, the symptoms of upper and lower tract infections may be difficult to distinguish and may include fever, suprapubic tenderness, fussiness, or poor feeding. In older patients who are able to verbalize their symptoms, suggestive complaints include fever, abdominal or flank pain, and urinary symptoms, including dysuria, frequency, or incontinence. Urinalysis may show bacteriuria, pyuria, and positive leukocyte esterase and nitrites. When UTI is suspected clinically, initial imaging is typically obtained with a renal and bladder ultrasound, although it should be noted that in a large percentage of cases, no abnormalities are detected by ultrasound.

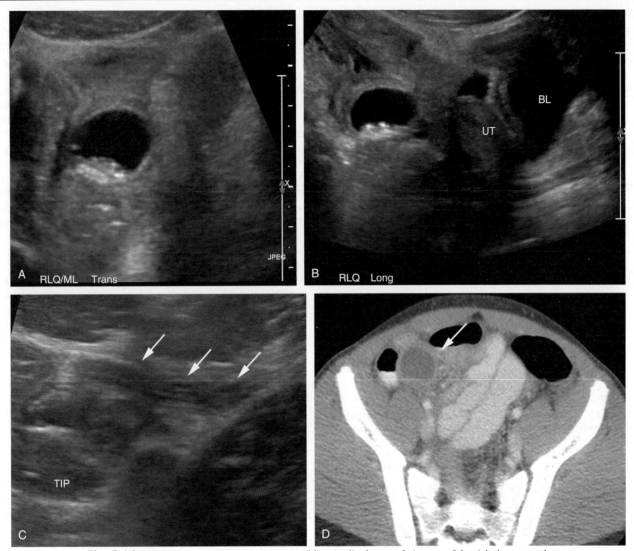

Fig. 5.14 Meckel diverticulitis. Transverse and longitudinal grayscale images of the right lower quadrant (A–C) reveal a round, cystic structure with gut signature and internal dependently layering debris that is separate from the urinary bladder, uterus, and normal appendix (*arrows*). Contrast-enhanced computed tomography (D) shows a similar cystic structure with surrounding fat stranding, consistent with Meckel diverticulitis. *BL*, bladder; *RLQ*, Right lower quadrant; *RLQ/ML*, right lower quadrant/midline; *TIP*, tip of appendix; *UT*, uterus.

In cases of uncomplicated cystitis, ultrasound may show debris within the urinary bladder, with or without bladder wall thickening. Bladder wall thickening may be focal or circumferential. A wall thickness of more than 3 mm in a well-distended bladder or more than 5 mm in a decompressed bladder is considered abnormal.

Sonographic findings in pyelonephritis are variable. The kidneys can appear normal or can be enlarged with increased echogenicity, loss of corticomedullary differentiation, and variable dilation of the collecting system. Focal pyelonephritis involving a segment of a kidney may also occur, appearing as a round or wedge-shaped, echogenic, masslike area with decreased perfusion on color or power Doppler imaging (Fig. 5.17). Mobile debris may be seen within the renal collecting system or proximal ureter. Associated thickening of the uroepithelium in the central renal pelvis may be seen. Perinephric free fluid is often visualized. In advanced cases, pyelone-

phritis may progress to frank renal abscess, with a well-defined, hypoechoic, avascular intrarenal fluid collection.

Important ultrasound findings for the radiologist to note include hydronephrosis, potentially indicating an obstructed, infected system; presence of abscess; and presence of cortical scars, which suggests prior episodes of pyelonephritis. Dilation of the distal ureter at the level of the bladder may suggest distal obstruction or vesicoureteral reflux.

CT or MRI findings of pyelonephritis can be variable. Imaging is best achieved with contrast-enhanced examinations, although if there is a contraindication to contrast, such as allergy or renal impairment, or if other pathology such as renal stones is suspected, a noncontrast study may be obtained. CT is more widely used for evaluation of pyelonephritis, but similar findings would be seen on MRI.

Noncontrast CT or MRI may show renal enlargement caused by edema, and there may be perinephric free fluid or fat stranding. T2-weighted fat-suppressed MRI sequences may demonstrate the perinephric edema and

fluid better than CT because of the superior contrast resolution of MRI and may also show wedge-shaped foci of decreased signal intensity in the renal parenchyma, as well as a decrease in renal corticomedullary differentiation that may not be perceptible on CT (Fig. 5.18). A focal lesion that is hypodense on CT or hyperintense on T2-weighted MRI sequences may reflect a developing intrarenal abscess.

Contrast-enhanced CT or MRI may show the classic striated nephrogram appearance of the renal parenchyma, with linear or wedgelike areas of hypoenhancement extending to the renal capsule. An intrarenal abscess has similar features to abscesses elsewhere, including a well-defined, near-fluid signal lesion with a peripheral rim of enhancement. Occasionally the abscess can breach the surface of the kidney and extend into the subcapsular or perirenal spaces (Fig. 5.19).

Scintigraphy plays an important role in the follow-up of UTI to evaluate for scar and assess renal function in the affected kidney. Cortical agents such as ^{99m}Tc-DMSA (dimercapto succinic acid) are still used to evaluate for scar, while ^{99m}Tc-MAG 3 (mercaptuacetyltriglycine) is the preferred agent to assess renal function and the relative contribution of each kidney to the overall function. The use of ^{99m}Tc-DMSA to evaluate for acute pyelonephritis is less common in the advent of superior ultrasound imaging and MRI with MR urography (see Box 5.12).

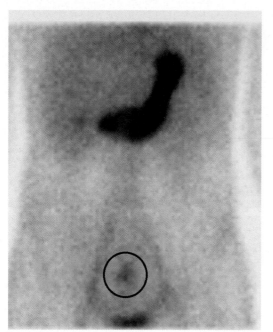

Fig. 5.15 Meckel diverticulum in an 18-month-old with history of bloody stool. Planar image from ^{99m}Tc pertechnetate scintigraphy. Faint but focal uptake appearing at the same time as uptake in the stomach confirms Meckel diverticulum in the midline.

BOX 5.10 When to Suspect Meckel Diverticulum

Clinical findings: Painless lower GI bleeding
Imaging findings:
- Blind ending tubular structure in the RLQ with a normal appendix visualized
- Antimesenteric border of distal ileum, 100 cm from ileocecal valve
- Positive Tc-pertechnetate scintigraphy

GI, gastrointestinal; *RLQ*, right lower quadrant.

Pneumonia

Referred pain from pneumonia is a well-known cause of abdominal pain in children. In a series of nearly 1200 children with acute abdominal pain, Ravichandran and Burge (1996) found pneumonia to be the diagnosis in approximately 1.5% of patients. The exact mechanism of referred pain is unclear but is presumably due to overlap of several anatomic dermatomes between the chest and abdomen. Pneumonia does not necessarily need to be in the lower lobes to induce abdominal pain, because there are cases of referred pain from middle or upper lobe pneumonias, and the site of pain may be opposite the site of pneumonia (Fig. 5.20) (see Box 5.13).

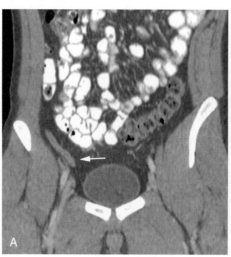
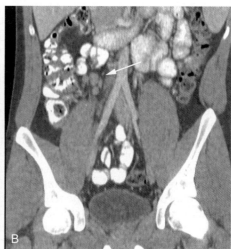

Fig. 5.16 Mesenteric adenitis. Coronal contrast-enhanced computed tomographic image (A) shows a normal appendix (*arrow*) with no adjacent inflammation. A second coronal image (B) in the same patient shows a cluster of mildly prominent right lower quadrant lymph nodes (*arrow*). The diagnosis of mesenteric adenitis was offered because no other cause for the patient's abdominal pain was evident.

Pancreatitis

Pancreatitis in children is caused by a diverse range of etiologies, in contrast with pancreatitis in adults, which is most frequently caused by cholelithiasis and alcohol use. In children, common causes of pancreatitis include

---

BOX 5.11 When to Suspect Mesenteric Adenitis

Clinical findings: Vague abdominal pain
+/– RLQ
+/– Strep positive
+/– Fever
Mesenteric adenitis is sometimes offered as a summary when prominent mesenteric and right lower quadrant lymph nodes are seen in the absence of other pathology

RLQ, right lower quadrant.

---

abdominal trauma (either accidental or nonaccidental), pancreaticobiliary system anomalies, systemic infection, and medications, although in up to 25% of cases the cause is unknown. Presenting clinical symptoms are also more variable in children than in adults, with most patients reporting abdominal pain, tenderness, and vomiting. Less commonly, patients may present with fever, hypotension, or jaundice. Laboratory values are frequently abnormal, with elevation of amylase and lipase levels.

Imaging of pancreatitis can be accomplished with ultrasound, CT, or MRI. Abdominal radiographs may be obtained initially to look for a source of abdominal pain, but they rarely demonstrate a finding specific for pancreatitis. A potential radiographic finding of acute pancreatitis is the "colon cutoff sign," which is distention of the ascending and transfer colon with abrupt narrowing at the splenic flexure. This finding is caused by pancreatic inflammation extending into the

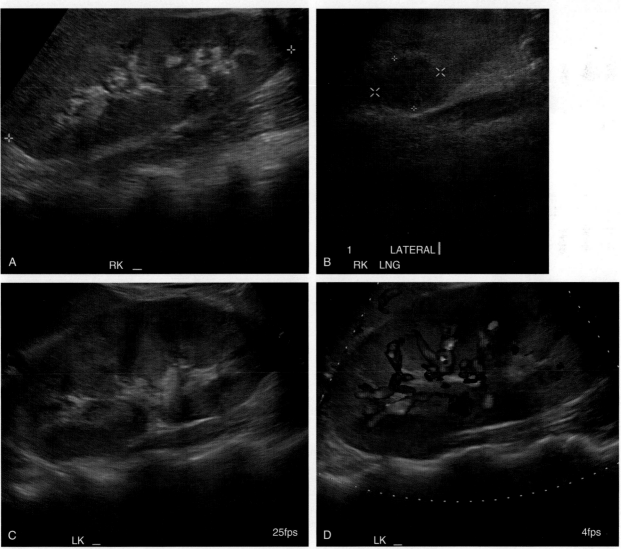

Fig. 5.17 Pyelonephritis. Longitudinal grayscale ultrasound images of the right kidney (A, B) shows mildly increased renal echotexture, being isoechoic to liver, with a focal hypoechoic lesion in the mid to lower pole. Clinically the patient had symptoms of infection, raising concern for intrarenal abscess over neoplasm or other possibilities. Grayscale and color sonography of the left kidney (C, D) reveals heterogeneous renal parenchyma with hypoechoic bands extending through the renal cortex and decreased blood flow within the lower pole.

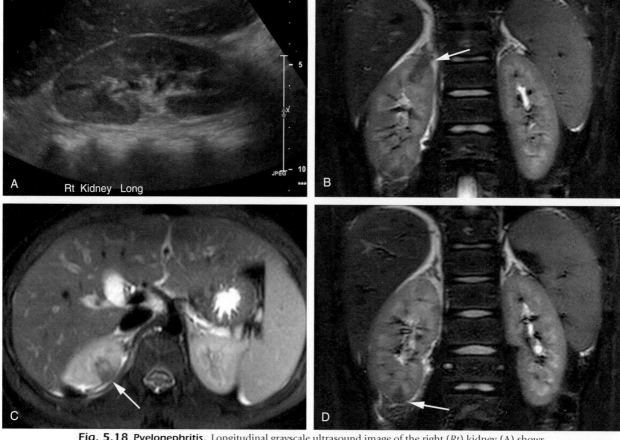

Fig. 5.18 Pyelonephritis. Longitudinal grayscale ultrasound image of the right (*Rt*) kidney (A) shows mildly increased renal echotexture, being hyperechoic to liver, without other abnormality. Coronal and axial fluid-sensitive, fat-suppressed magnetic resonance imaging (MRI) (B–D) reveal multiple wedgelike areas of decreased signal within the right renal cortex, consistent with pyelonephritis. MRI was obtained to rule out appendicitis; pyelonephritis was an unexpected finding.

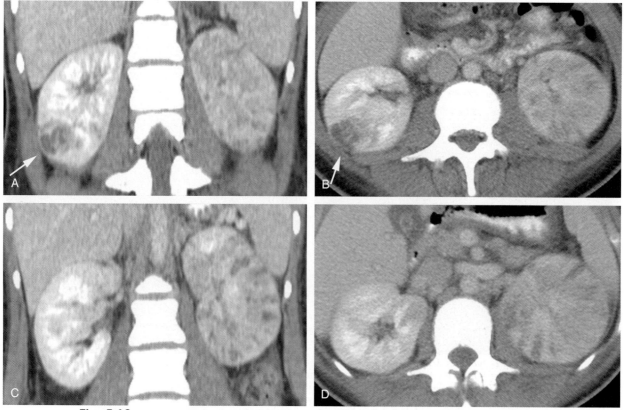

Fig. 5.19 Pyelonephritis. Coronal and axial contrast-enhanced computed tomography images (A, B) from the same patient demonstrate the heterogeneous, hypodense lesion in the mid to lower right kidney consistent with renal abscess (*arrows*). The left kidney (C, D) is diffusely enlarged and hypoenhancing relative to the right kidney secondary to edema and shows the classic striated nephrogram appearance of pyelonephritis.

phrenicocolic ligament with resultant colonic narrowing (Fig. 5.21A).

In the acute setting, ultrasound may show either focal or diffuse enlargement of the pancreas with decrease in echogenicity of the pancreatic parenchyma. Anechoic peripancreatic fluid collections may be seen, and the peripancreatic fat may be echogenic, reflecting edema. In chronic pancreatitis the gland becomes atrophic and may become echogenic and may have associated focal or diffuse calcification. The pancreatic duct also commonly enlarges. If present, fluid collections become more organized with well-defined walls compatible with pseudocysts. Sonographic evaluation can be limited by intervening bowel gas, most often within the stomach, which may obscure the pancreatic distal body and tail.

CT, despite the disadvantage of radiation exposure, is the most commonly used imaging modality in suspected pancreatitis because it gives a more comprehensive evaluation of the pancreas and any complications. Unless there is a contraindication, IV contrast material should be administered. In acute pancreatitis the gland may again appear either focally or diffusely enlarged, and there is often peripancreatic free fluid and inflammatory fat stranding (see Fig. 5.21B–D). Nonenhancing portions of the gland represent necrosis. Either free fluid

or more organized fluid collections may be present. Vascular complications sometimes occur, including pseudoaneurysm of the splenic artery or thrombosis of the splenic vein.

In chronic pancreatitis the gland becomes atrophic and may contain focal or diffuse calcifications. The pancreatic duct is often dilated. Peripancreatic fluid collections become better organized into frank pseudocysts.

MRI also can be used to evaluate pancreatitis, with the main advantage over CT being avoidance of ionizing radiation. Potential disadvantages of MRI, however, include need for sedation in younger patients and less availability than CT.

MRI findings in acute pancreatitis include focal or diffuse gland enlargement, with associated increased T2 signal intensity of the pancreatic parenchyma and surrounding fluid (Fig. 5.22). The normal pancreas normally has intrinsically bright T1 signal intensity because of a high concentration of proteinaceous enzymatic material; in acute pancreatitis, there is loss of the normal intrinsic T1 hyperintensity. Similar to CT, heterogeneous or poor pancreatic enhancement represents areas of necrosis, and vascular complications can be assessed on postcontrast sequences. MRI has the distinct advantage of allowing multiphase postcontrast assessment.

In chronic pancreatitis the gland appears atrophic and also shows decreased T1 signal reflecting diminished ability to synthesize enzymes. The pancreatic duct may be ectatic, and irregularity of the main duct and side branch ductal dilation may be seen on T2-weighted sequences because of the improved contrast

---

BOX 5.12   When to Suspect Urinary Tract Infection

Clinical findings: Fever, dysuria, urinary frequency/urgency

Imaging findings:
- Debris in the bladder
- Debris in the proximal collecting system, thickening of uroepithelium
- Hypoechoic foci in the kidney
- Enlarged kidneys
- Striated nephrogram on CT/MR
- Abscess

CT, Computed tomography.

BOX 5.13   When to Suspect Pneumonia

Clinical findings: Vague abdominal pain

Imaging findings:
- Normal bowel gas pattern
- Attention to the lung bases on KUB: look for retrocardiac or posterior costophrenic angle consolidation
- Consider chest x-ray

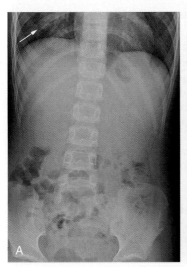
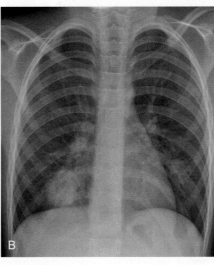

Fig. 5.20 Pneumonia. Abdominal radiograph (A) demonstrates an essentially normal examination, with no finding to explain the patient's pain. A partially imaged opacity was noted in the right lower lobe, however (*arrow*). Chest radiograph (B) reveals a rounded right lower lobe opacity consistent with round pneumonia. No other cause for the patient's abdominal pain was identified.

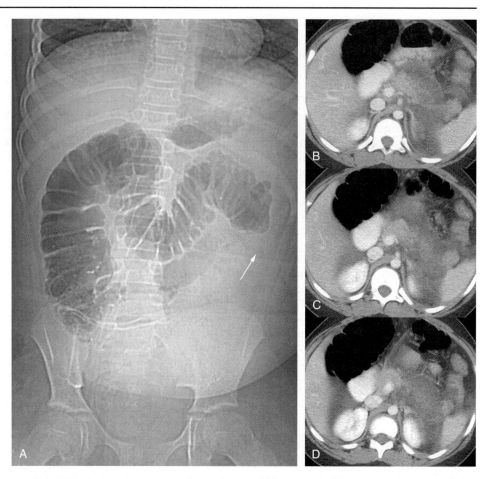

Fig. 5.21 Acute pancreatitis. Abdominal radiograph (A) shows the classic "colon cutoff sign" (*arrow*) associated with pancreatitis, caused by reactive narrowing of the descending colon secondary to retroperitoneal peripancreatic inflammation. Axial contrast-enhanced computed tomography images (B–D) reveal hypoenhancement of the distal body and tail of the pancreas with marked adjacent fat stranding and nonorganized fluid.

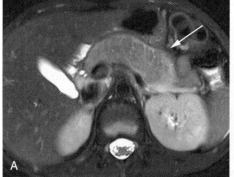 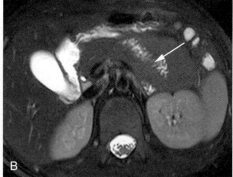

Fig. 5.22 Acute pancreatitis. Axial fluid-sensitive, fat-suppressed magnetic resonance imaging (MRI) (A) demonstrates diffuse enlargement and increased T2 signal of the pancreas (*arrow*) with mild peripancreatic edema, consistent with acute pancreatitis. Pancreatitis in this patient was medication induced. Axial STIR MRI (B) of the same patient 3 months prior demonstrates normal pancreatic size and signal intensity (*arrow*).

resolution of MRI over CT (Fig. 5.23). Pseudocysts may be present with a well-defined enhancing rim and internal fluid signal.

Magnetic resonance cholangiopancreatography (MRCP) can be a useful adjunct to standard abdominal MRI in evaluation of pancreatitis. MRCP uses heavily T2-weighted, thin-section sequences of the pancreaticobiliary system that can show potential causes of pancreatitis, including choledocholithiasis and anomalies of the biliary tree, such as choledochal cysts, long common channels, or pancreas divisum. Gallstones or calculi in the biliary tree appear as well-defined, T2 hypointense filling defects. The appearance of choledochal cysts depends on involvement of the intrahepatic versus extrahepatic bili-

ary tree and can be categorized according to the Todani classification system. Pancreas divisum is a congenital anomaly in which the dorsal pancreatic duct does not communicate with the common bile duct and does not drain into the major papilla, but rather drains separately via the minor papilla. Although controversial, some authors consider pancreas divisum to be a cause of pancreatitis (Fig. 5.24; see Box 5.14).

Henoch-Schönlein Purpura

Henoch-Schönlein purpura (HSP) is a self-limited, immunoglobulin A–mediated small vessel vasculitis.

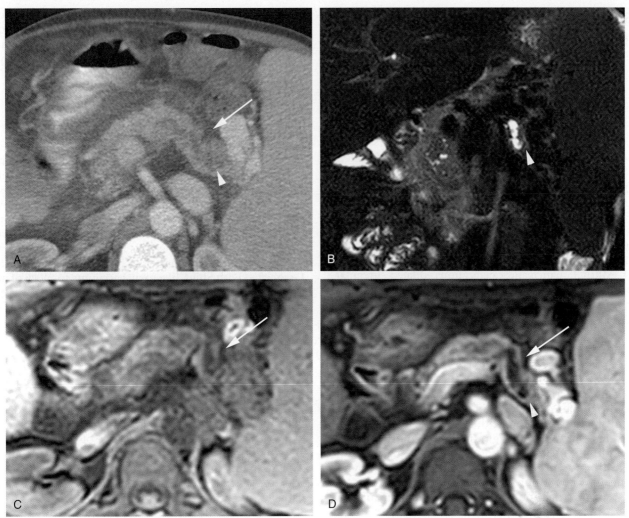

Fig. 5.23 Acute-on-chronic pancreatitis. Contrast-enhanced computed tomography image (A) shows relative atrophy of the distal body and tail of the pancreas (*arrow*) with associated pancreatic duct dilation (*arrowhead*), consistent with chronic pancreatitis. Superimposed peripancreatic fat stranding compatible with acute pancreatitis. Heavily T2-weighted MRCP image (B) in the same patient reveals the ductal dilation to better advantage (*arrowhead*), as well as the hazy pancreatic high T2 signal edema. Precontrast and postcontrast fat-suppressed T1-weighted (C, D) images show distal pancreatic atrophy, as well as decrease in the normal intrinsic high T1 signal intensity and decreased enhancement of the involved segment (*arrows*). These are additional findings of chronic pancreatitis.

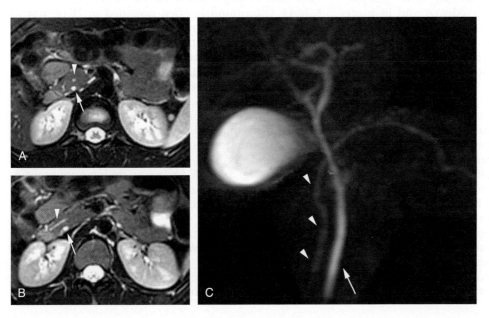

Fig. 5.24 Pancreas divisum. Axial STIR magnetic resonance images (A, B) show pancreas divisum with the common bile duct (*arrows*) draining via the major papilla and the main pancreatic duct (*arrowheads*) draining via the minor papilla. Three-dimensional reformatted image from an MRCP (C) in the same patient reveals the completely separate common bile duct (*arrow*) and main pancreatic duct (*arrowheads*).

Clinical findings:
   Abdominal pain, tenderness, vomiting
   +/− Jaundice
   Fever, elevated acute-phase reactants
   Elevated amylase/lipase
   Imaging findings:
- Normal bowel gas pattern or sentinel loop sign; colon "cutoff" sign
- US: focal or diffuse hypoechogenicity, fluid collections, ductal dilation
- CT: hypodense, hypoenhancing gland, pseudocysts
- MR: T2 hyperintense or T1 hypointense gland, edema, pseudocysts, ductal dilation or anomaly, choledocholithiasis

Chronic pancreatitis:
Imaging findings:
- MRI/CT: pancreatic calcifications, dilated, irregular pancreatic duct, atrophy of the pancreas, mature pseudocyst

CT, Computed tomography; *MRI*, magnetic resonance imaging; *US*, ultrasound.

It is characterized by triad of palpable purpura, abdominal pain, and arthritis. The disease predominantly affects children, with a peak age between 4 and 6 years, and has a slight male predominance. GI symptoms, including abdominal pain, nausea, and vomiting, occur in up to 50% of patients. GI symptoms typically follow development of the characteristic purpuric rash but may precede the rash in up to 30% of cases. GI symptoms are secondary to immunoglobulin A deposition into the intestinal small vessels, which can result in mural hemorrhage, with secondary intussusception and GI bleeding. Management of HSP is with supportive care, and the vast majority of cases resolve spontaneously.

Abdominal radiographs in HSP may show a spectrum of findings, including a normal bowel gas pattern, bowel wall thickening, or edema, and in more severe cases, with mural hematomas or intussusceptions, bowel obstruction, soft tissue masses, or even pneumoperitoneum may be seen. The radiographic findings taken in isolation, however, are not specific for the diagnosis of HSP.

Abdominal ultrasound is frequently obtained in cases of HSP because of suspicion for other entities, typically appendicitis or idiopathic intussusception. Ultrasound findings in HSP can be suggestive, but not diagnostic, of the disease. There may be segmental or diffuse thickening of small bowel loops, representing mural edema or hemorrhage; the colon is uncommonly involved (Fig. 5.25). The affected bowel is typically hypoperistaltic. Eccentric wall thickening protruding into the lumen of the bowel may represent a focal mural hematoma, with or without obstruction. Free abdominal fluid is present in 50% of cases. Intussusception may be seen in approximately 3% of patients and is most commonly ileoileal (60%) (see Fig. 5.25C). Small bowel intussusceptions can be distin-

guished by their smaller size (generally in the range of 1–2 cm in diameter) and shorter length. Fifty percent of patients will have associated renal disease, which can sonographically manifest as echogenic enlarged kidneys (see Box 5.15).

Hemolytic Uremic Syndrome

Hemolytic uremic syndrome (HUS) is characterized by the triad of renal failure, hemolytic anemia, and thrombocytopenia. The disease most frequently occurs in children younger than 5 years old, but older children, adolescents, and adults may also be affected. HUS is the most common cause of acute renal failure in infants and young children. HUS is divided into two categories, typical or atypical, based on whether it is associated with a Shiga-like toxin producing bacterial infection. Typical HUS (associated with Shiga-like toxin) accounts for 90% of all cases and is most commonly due to ingestion of *E. coli* serotype O157:H7. Atypical HUS can be sporadic or familial. The pathophysiology of HUS is development of endothelial damage and microvascular thrombi, as well as red blood cell fragmentation.

The clinical presentation of the typical form of HUS is that of a prodrome of abdominal pain, fever, gastroenteritis, or diarrhea that begins 2 to 12 days after the exposure. Diarrhea frequently becomes bloody after a few days. Subsequently, 70% of patients will experience renal failure, which is reversible in up to 80% of patients. In the atypical form of HUS, patient outcomes are worse, with a 25% mortality rate in the acute phase and 50% of survivors progressing to end-stage renal disease or brain damage.

The imaging findings of HUS are not specific for the disease; however, the astute radiologist may be the first to suggest the entity if the findings are correlated with the patient's symptoms or the presence of renal failure. Abdominal radiographs may show bowel wall thickening, especially of the colon, where the "thumbprint" sign may be present. Wall thickening can also be associated with bowel luminal narrowing or dilation (Fig. 5.26A). Ultrasound is often obtained in HUS, not to evaluate for the disease specifically, but because the symptoms may overlap with more common causes of abdominal pain in this age range, such as intussusception or appendicitis. Ultrasound will also show abnormal bowel wall thickening with hyperemia on color Doppler images (see Fig. 5.26B–C). Ascites may be present. CT and MRI are not generally obtained in the setting of HUS, but again may be performed if there is clinical concern for another disease process. Bowel wall thickening will likely be evident, particularly of the colon (see Fig. 5.26D). Again, the findings are nonspecific but, taken together with the clinical symptoms, may suggest the correct diagnosis (see Box 5.16).

Inflammatory Bowel Disease

IBD is one of the most common GI tract disorders in older children in the developed world. Crohn disease is more

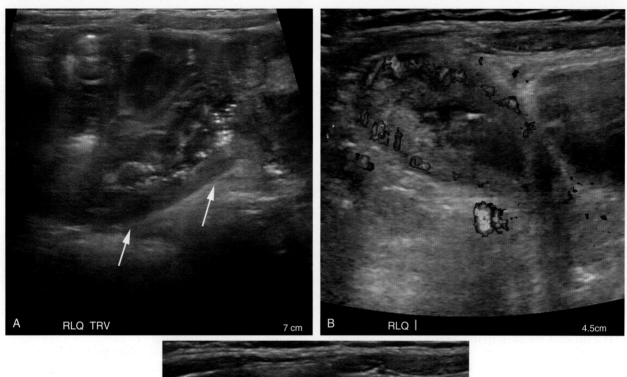

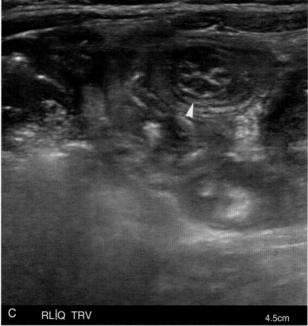

Fig. 5.25 Henoch-Schönlein purpura. (A) Transverse grayscale ultrasound image through the abdomen shows thick-walled small bowel in lower abdomen (*arrows*). Corresponding color ultrasound image (B) demonstrates intestinal wall hyperemia. Transverse grayscale ultrasound image through the right lower quadrant (C) shows an ileoileal intussusception (*arrowhead*). Note the relatively small size and absence of middle fat/lymph node layer compared with ileocolic intussusceptions in Fig. 5.10.

common than ulcerative colitis in adolescents. Adults and children may have similar clinical presentations, including abdominal pain, diarrhea, and weight loss, but there are unique secondary presenting complications in children that need attention, such as delayed puberty or growth failure. Imaging, along with endoscopy and biopsy, aids in the diagnosis.

Upper GI/small bowel follow-through for assessment of IBD was formerly the mainstay of imaging for IBD. Although images are excellent at revealing strictures and fistulas, it gives no information about addi-

tional extramural complications, such as abscess, perianal disease, or fistulae at risk (Fig. 5.27). CT with oral and IV contrast provides good visualization of the bowel lumen and wall, and it is able to provide valuable information regarding the presence or absence of abscess or bowel tethering suggestive of fistula. Recently, however, MR enterography (MRE) has become the primary imaging modality in the work-up of patients with IBD because of its lack of ionization radiation and its ability to depict both intramural and extramural complications of IBD. MRE has the ability to assess the bowel wall and lumen, to give information regarding presence of penetrating disease and/or abscess, and allows excellent visualization of the perineum to assess for perianal fistula involvement. Oral contrast and IV contrast are generally administered, but even without the oral contrast, there is still adequate visualization of the bowel to assess disease. MRE is often limited by motion, especially in the younger patient, and some institutions use glucagon to slow bowel motility during contrast-enhanced imaging. Sedation may be required, and in these patients, oral contrast may be withheld to avoid risk for aspiration.

Imaging findings of Crohn disease across modalities may range from subtle loss of mucosal features to bowel wall thickening and enhancement to frank perforation with abscess (Figs. 5.28–5.30). Other findings may include proliferation of periserosal fat with separation of bowel loops or tethering of several adjacent bowel loops with or without a fistula (the "star" sign). Patients with high-grade strictures may present with abdominal pain and obstruction on plain radiograph. Ultrasound may be the initial screen when these patients present with symptoms mimicking appendicitis, and the distinction between distal ileum and appendix may be difficult and requires an experienced sonographer (see Box 5.17).

BOX 5.15   When to Suspect Henoch-Schönlein Purpura

Clinical findings: Abdominal pain, nausea, vomiting, +/– GI bleeding, purpuric rash, hematuria, +/– elevated platelets, intussusceptive/obstructive symptoms
Imaging findings:
- Plain film: any of the following: obstruction, mass, pneumoperitoneum
- US: ileoileal intussusception, bowel wall thickening, sometimes asymmetrical
- CT/MRI: small bowel wall thickening, mural hematoma, free fluid, obstruction

CT, Computed tomography; *GI*, gastrointestinal; *MRI*, magnetic resonance imaging; *US*, ultrasound.

BOX 5.16   When to Suspect Hemolytic Uremic Syndrome

Clinical findings: Abdominal pain, fever, diarrhea, progression to renal failure, +/– elevated platelets
Imaging findings are nonspecific:
- Plain film: bowel wall thickening with "thumbprinting"; luminal narrowing
- US: bowel wall thickening, hyperemia, ascites
- CT/MRI: bowel wall thickening, free fluid, +/– obstruction

CT, Computed tomography; *MRI*, magnetic resonance imaging; *US*, ultrasound.

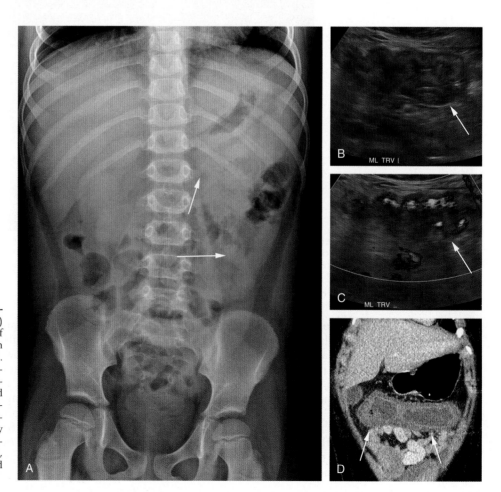

Fig. 5.26 Hemolytic uremic syndrome. Abdominal radiograph (A) shows marked wall thickening of the transverse and descending colon with luminal narrowing (arrows). Transverse grayscale and color Doppler ultrasound images of the transverse colon (B, C) reveal thickened and hyperemic colonic wall (*arrows*). Coronal reformatted contrast-enhanced computed tomography (D) scan shows similar wall thickening of the transverse colon (*arrows*), mucosal hyperenhancement, and pericolonic fat stranding.

Trauma

Trauma in the older child is usually not a mystery. These children/adolescents can usually give an historical account of an accident or other injury that may have led to the development of abdominal pain, be it minor or major. Careful evaluation for peritoneal signs on examination is important to the imaging approach. The mechanism of injury is also important to correlate the findings to the history in cases where maltreatment may be suspected. Because the pediatric abdomen has a smaller an-

teroposterior dimension and generally less intraabdominal fat, the area in which the force of an injury dissipates is smaller, making the possibility of a solid organ injury more likely. According to the Pediatric Emergency Care Applied Research Network (PECARN) in 2013, approximately 5% to 10% of children who suffered blunt trauma sustained intraabdominal injuries (Holmes etal., 2013). Further, Cooper etal. (1994), reported that mortality is directly related to the number of structures injured. Therefore imaging diagnosis is central to the predictive mortality in these patients and plays an important role in triaging the trauma patient who may present in what appears to be stable condition.

The bedside FAST (focused assessment with sonography in trauma) in the emergency department has become the sixth vital sign in these cases. It is used in the emergency department as an adjunct to the ATLS (advanced trauma life support) primary survey, and its use should not interfere with the ongoing assessment and management in the trauma bay. The procedure is traditionally performed in the supine position, and the protocol consists of four acoustic windows: pericardiac, perihepatic, perisplenic, and pelvic. Expanded FAST, or eFAST, has been developed to include limited evaluation of the lungs for pneumothorax. Additional views and recommendations to improve fluid visualization with positioning are also published. However, because there are many limitations to the study, this should not be considered a diagnostic examination. CT with IV contrast is indicated in the assessment of abdominal trauma if the patient does not require emergent operative intervention and is stable. This will allow grading of solid organ injury, which may further drive management of a stable patient (Tables 5.3 and 5.4) (Kozar, Crandall, & Shanmuganathan, 2018).

In the younger child who presents with vague symptoms of pain, vomiting, and pallor, and the history is lacking, one must always keep a heightened suspicion for nonaccidental trauma. Nonaccidental trauma is a

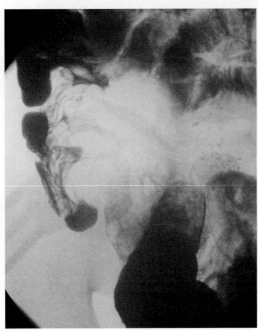

Fig. 5.27 Crohn disease. Single spot image from a small bowel follow-through series showing irregular, narrowed appearance of the terminal ileum and a somewhat narrowed appearance of the cecum.

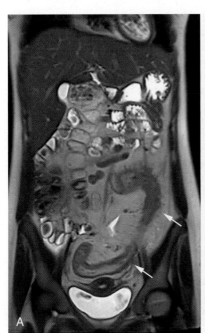
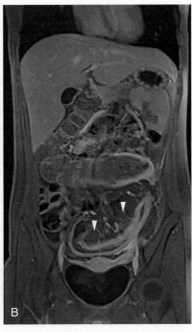

Fig. 5.28 Crohn disease on magnetic resonance imaging enterography. Coronal T2-weighted (A) and coronal T1-weighted fat-saturated postcontrast (B) images demonstrating an inflamed loop of sigmoid colon (*arrows*), emphasizing the thickened wall, creeping fat with separation of the bowel loop, prominent vasa recta (*arrowheads*), and luminal narrowing, all features of active Crohn disease.

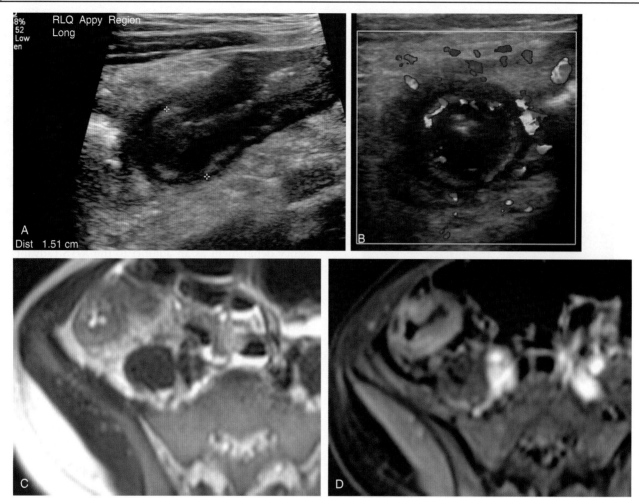

Fig. 5.29 Crohn disease mimicking appendicitis. Teenage female patient presented to the emergency department with abdominal pain and suspicion for appendicitis. Longitudinal and transverse ultrasound images (A, B) show a markedly thickened, hyperemic terminal ileum with echogenic fat surrounding the loop. Follow-up magnetic resonance imaging in the same patient shows axial T2-weighted (C) and corresponding axial T1 gradient-echo postcontrast (D) images that highlight the thickened, hyperenhancing terminal ileum and cecum.

condition that the pediatrician and pediatric radiologist always keeps in the back of their minds when the injury does not fit with the clinical history. In these patients the history is often either intentionally misleading or withheld to protect the perpetrator, or it is simply not known by the caretaker who brought the child for medical attention. The typical pattern of nonaccidental trauma in the abdomen is one of a direct blow or blunt trauma to the belly. Because the anteroposterior diameter of the pediatric abdomen is small and there is little intraabdominal fat to act as a cushion, the organs injured are most commonly the anterior liver, duodenum, and pancreas (Fig. 5.31). These organs are directly in front of the spine, which allows them to be impacted by the direct blow against a hard surface. Other abdominal organs that may be injured by direct inflicted abdominal trauma include the adrenal gland, kidney, and spleen. Liver injuries make up nearly two-thirds of solid organ injuries in nonaccidental trauma, pancreatic injury is seen in up to 17%, renal injury in 25%, and splenic injury occurs less frequently, in 9% to 26% of patients. Even though the kidneys and spleen are somewhat protected by the rib cage, adrenal injury is not infrequently a result of shear injury, and hematoma may be seen in the absence of other solid organ trauma. Hypoperfusion complex secondary to blood loss and shock may be seen and is an important predictor of poorer outcomes (Fig. 5.32). Characteristic imaging findings include flattened inferior vena cava, small-caliber aorta, and hyperenhancing dilated fluid-filled bowel loops.

Patients may present with pancreatitis, vomiting secondary to obstruction from a duodenal hematoma, shock, or vague abdominal pain. There may be some delay in presentation from the initial event, and thus laboratory findings are often the guiding impetus to image. Plain film findings may be nonspecific or show a localized ileus or obstruction. Rarely, free air may be seen from hollow viscous injury. Ultrasound can be used as a screening tool, but CT is generally indicated to assess the extent of trauma and organs involved. The role of the radiologist is to recognize a pattern of unsuspected trauma as abuse

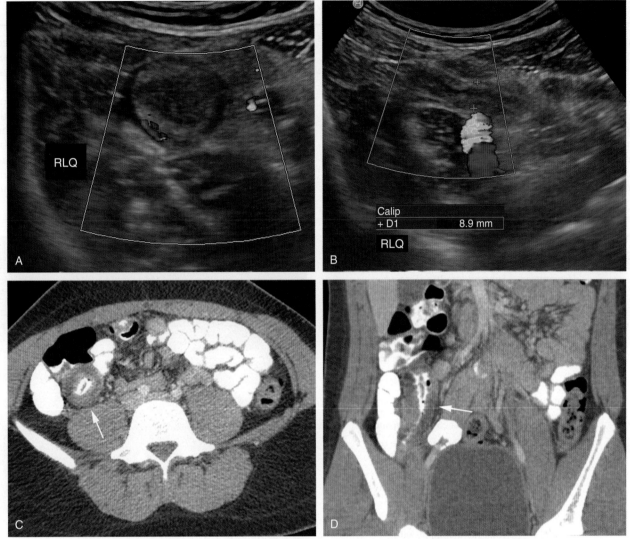

Fig. 5.30 Crohn disease mimicking appendicitis. (A, B) Transverse color Doppler ultrasound images of the right lower quadrant (RLQ) show a dilated tubular structure with mild adjacent inflammation, measuring 9 mm in diameter. This was interpreted as an inflamed appendix, although neither a blind tip nor cecal origin was demonstrated. Axial and coronal contrast-enhanced computed tomography (C, D) images reveal a thickened terminal ileum (*arrows*) consistent with Crohn disease. The appendix was normal (not shown).

BOX 5.17 When to Suspect Inflammatory Bowel Disease

Clinical findings: Abdominal pain, diarrhea (symptoms may mimic appendicitis acutely), family history of IBD, elevated acute-phase reactants

Imaging findings:

- Plain film: nonspecific, +/− obstruction or ileus
- US: thickened terminal ileum in the RLQ may mimic appendicitis
- Small bowel follow through (SBFT): thickened irregular terminal ileum, separation of bowel loops
- CT/MRI:
  - Bowel wall thickening (may be segmental or pancolonic)
  - Striated bowel wall enhancement
  - Creeping fat
  - Strictures with or without upstream dilated bowel
  - "Star sign" on MRI indicating fistula
  - Perianal fistula

CT, Computed tomography; *IBD*, inflammatory bowel disease; *MRI*, magnetic resonance imaging; *RLQ*, right lower quadrant; *US*, ultrasound.

TABLE 5.3 Liver Injury Scale

GRADE[a]	INJURY	DESCRIPTION OF INJURY
I	Hematoma	Subcapsular <10% surface area
	Laceration	Capsular tear <1 cm parenchymal depth
II	Hematoma	Subcapsular 10%–50% surface area or intraparenchymal <10 cm in diameter
	Laceration	Capsular tear 1–3 cm parenchymal depth, <10 cm in length
III	Hematoma	Subcapsular >50% surface area or expanding; intraparenchymal hematoma ≥10 cm or expanding≥
	Laceration	>3 cm parenchymal depth
IV	Laceration	Parenchymal disruption involving 25%–75% hepatic lobe or 1–3 Couinaud segments
V	Laceration	Parenchymal disruption involving >75% hepatic lobe or >3 Couinaud segments in a single lobe
	Vascular	Juxtahepatic venous injury
VI	Vascular	Hepatic avulsion

[a]Advance one grade for multiple injuries up to grade III.
From Moore, E. E., Cogbill, T. H., Jurkovich, G. J., Shackford, S. R., Malangoni, M. A., Champion, H. R. (1995). *Journal of Trauma*, 38(3):323–324.

and to be accurate and thorough in identifying and grading the injuries (see Box 5.18).

Constipation

Probably one of the most common and non-life-threatening causes for abdominal pain in children is constipation. This entity is a cause of described and perceived pain across all age groups in the pediatric population, but other more pressing causes should be exclud-

ed before the pain is attributed solely to an increased fecal burden. Typically, constipated patients present with a history of decreased stool output, and children can have severe lower abdominal pain. There may be a history of soiling and fecal incontinence in the setting of impaction or even retentive posturing and pain with stooling. On physical examination, large stool may be palpable in the rectum, and there may be a palpable abdominal mass. Plain film findings are variable, and the volume of stool within the colon at any one point in time may be misleading. However, fecal impaction and

TABLE 5.4   Splenic Injury Scale

GRADE[a]	INJURY	DESCRIPTION OF INJURY
I	Hematoma	Subcapsular <10% surface area
	Laceration	Capsular tear <1 cm parenchymal depth
II	Hematoma	Subcapsular 10%–50% surface area or intraparenchymal <5 cm diameter
	Laceration	Capsular tear 1–3 cm parenchymal depth, <5 cm in length with no involved trabecular vessel
III	Hematoma	Subcapsular >50% surface area or expanding; intraparenchymal hematoma ≥5 cm or expanding≥
	Laceration	>3 cm parenchymal depth or involving trabecular vessel
IV	Laceration	Involving segmental or hilar vessels producing major devascularization (>25% spleen)
V	Laceration	Complete shattered spleen
	Vascular	Hilar vascular injury with devascularized spleen

[a]Advance one grade for multiple injuries up to grade III.
From Moore, E. E., Cogbill, T. H., Jurkovich, G. J., Shackford, S. R., Malangoni, M. A., Champion, H. R. (1995). *Journal of Trauma*, 38(3):323–324.

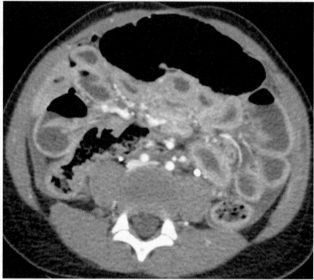

Fig. 5.32 Hypoperfusion complex. Axial contrast-enhanced computed tomography in a toddler who suffered from blunt injury found to be nonaccidental trauma showing hyperenhancing, dilated, fluid-filled bowel loops and small-caliber vessels. Also note free fluid.

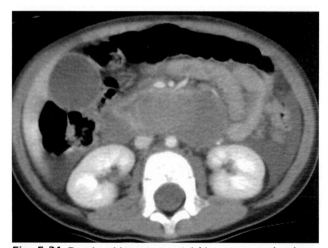

Fig. 5.31 Duodenal hematoma. Axial intravenous and oral contrast computed tomography. Increased attenuation at the midline within a dilated duodenum seen in a duodenal hematoma with associated free intraabdominal fluid in nonaccidental trauma.

BOX 5.18   When to Suspect Life-Threatening Abdominal Trauma

Clinical findings: Reported blunt injury with pain out of proportion, rigid abdomen on examination/peritoneal signs, GI bleeding, hypovolemia
Imaging findings:
- Plain film: ileus pattern, pelvic fractures
- CT: solid organ injury (important to give accurate description and grading)
  - Free air
  - Free fluid, especially complicated fluid (blood, feces)
  - Vascular injury/extravasation
Nonaccidental trauma:
  History often misleading or does not fit the injuries
Imaging findings at CT:
- Solid organ injury: liver laceration, pancreatic injury, adrenal hematoma, splenic laceration
- Duodenal hematoma or perforation

CT, Computed tomography; *GI,* gastrointestinal.

findings of bowel distention are a telling sign that there may be a more significant problem (Fig. 5.33).

Underlying causes of constipation may be explored on a nonemergent basis. In the majority of cases, constipation is either functional or behavioral, with no underlying pathology. A careful history eliciting the onset of constipation can be helpful in distinguishing behavioral from organic causative factors.

When a pathological cause of constipation is suspected, Hirschsprung disease is the most common entity. Contrast enema, typically performed with water-soluble contrast, is the test of choice. The diagnostic finding at enema is a reversed rectosigmoid index where the rectal caliber is smaller than the

upstream sigmoid colon (Fig. 5.34). The transition zone may be more proximal or distal, but can usually be ascertained. Exceptions are extreme cases, such as total colonic or ultrashort-segment Hirschsprung disease, which may be difficult to diagnose at enema and may require biopsy to make the diagnosis. Short-segment and ultrashort-segment Hirschsprung disease may be missed early on, and older children may present with a history of chronic constipation. The radiograph may show a distended sigmoid colon or redundancy of the colon. The absence of intramural ganglion cells is the gold standard to diagnose this disease, which ultimately results in abnormal lack of relaxation of the anal sphincter and failure of peristalsis. Other causes of constipation may be neurological, cerebral palsy, spinal cord disorders (including tumors that impinge on the cord), or metabolic/endocrinological (see Box 5.19).

■ Summary

Abdominal pain is a common symptom in children and imaging can be a helpful adjunct to physical and laboratory exams to evaluate for causes of abdominal pain. Imaging workups often begin with radiographs and/or ultrasound in children to reduce radiation exposure.

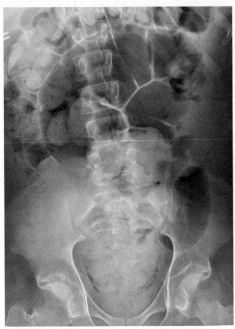

Fig. 5.33 Fecal impaction. Supine radiograph showing a large fecal bolus in the rectum with dilated redundant upstream sigmoid colon. Note formed stool throughout the remainder of the colon.

BOX 5.19   When to Suspect Constipation

Clinical findings: Abdominal pain, +/– palpable mass, firm large stool on rectal exam
Imaging findings (not specific):
• Fecal impaction
• Distended, redundant sigmoid/colon
• Obstruction, rare
• Can be seen in setting of Hirschsprung: contrast enema with inverse rectosigmoid ratio, transition zone

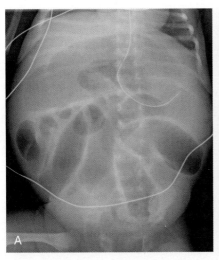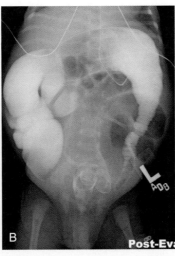

Fig. 5.34 Hirschsprung disease. Supine radiograph (A) showing dilated bowel loops with little or no rectal gas concerning for obstruction. Postevacuation supine radiograph after a barium enema (B) showing decreased caliber of the rectum and sigmoid with a transition zone in the middescending colon. Note tertiary contractions in the aganglionic segment.

Reference

Kozar, R. A., Crandall, M., Shanmuganathan, K., etal. (2018). Organ injury scaling 2018 update: Spleen, liver, and kidney. *The Journal of Trauma and Acute Care Surgery, 85*(6), 1119–1122. https://doi.org/10.1097/TA.0000000000002058. 30462622.

Bibliography

ACR–SPR Practice parameter for the performance of abdominal radiography amended 2014 (resolution 39)∗ collaborative committee members represent their societies in the initial and final revision of this practice parameter: Matthew S. Pollack, MD, FACR, Co-Chair, Barry D. Daly, MD, MB, BCh, Co-Chair, Lynn A. Fordham, MD, Leann E. Linam, MD, Daniel J. Podberesky, MD, Alexander J. Towbin, MD. https://www.acr.org/-/media/ACR/Files/Practice-Parameters/radabd.pdf. Accessed December 1, 2016.

Berger, M. Y., Tabbers, M. M., Kurver, M. J., Boluyt, N., & Benninga, M. A. (2012). Value of abdominal radiography, colonic transit time, and rectal ultrasound scanning in the diagnosis of idiopathic constipation in children: A systematic review. *The Journal of Pediatrics, 161*(1), 44–50 e1–e2.

Braithwaite, K., & Alazraki, A. (2014). Use of the star sign to diagnose internal fistulas in pediatric patients with penetrating Crohn disease by MR enterography. *Pediatric Radiology, 44*(8), 926–931.

Cooper, A., Barlow, B., DiScala, C., & String, D. (1994). Mortality and truncal injury: The pediatric perspective. *Journal of Pediatric Surgery, 29*(1), 33–38.

Daneman, A., & Robben, S. G. (2010). An approach to imaging the acute abdomen in the pediatric population. In J. Hodler, G. K. Von Schulthess, & C. L. Zollikofer (Eds.), *Diseases of the abdomen and pelvis* (pp. 167–173). Springer.

Daneman, A., & Willi, U. (2006). An approach to imaging the acute abdomen in pediatrics. In J. Hodler, G. K. Von Schulthess, & C. L. Zollikofer (Eds.), *Diseases of the abdomen and pelvis* (pp. 33–39). Springer.

Edwards, D. K. (1980). Size of gas-filled bowel loops in infants. *American Journal of Roentgenology, 135*, 331–334.

Elsayes, K. M., Menias, C. O., Harvin, H. J., & Francis, I. R. (2007). Imaging manifestations of Meckel's diverticulum. *American Journal of Roentgenology, 189*, 81–88.

Garfunkel, L. (2002). *Abdominal pain, pediatric clinical advisor (pp. 4–7).* Mosby, Inc.

Hampson, F. A., & Shaw, A. S. (2010). Assessment of the acute abdomen: Role of the plain abdominal radiograph. *Reports in Medical Imaging, 3*, 93–105.

Haworth, E. M., Hodson, C. J., Joyce, C. R. B., Pringle, E. M., Solimano, G., & Young, W. F. (1967). Radiological measurement of small bowel calibre in normal subjects according to age. *Clinical Radiology, 18*, 417–421.

Hernandez, J. A., Swischuk, L. E., & Angel, C. A. (2004). Validity of plain films in intussusception. *Emergency Radiology, 10*, 323–326.

Holmes, J. F., Lillis, K., Monroe, D., etal. (2013). Identifying children at very low risk of clinically important blunt abdominal injuries. Pediatric Emergency Care Applied Research Network (PECARN). *Annals of Emergency Medicine, 62*(2), 107–116.

Hooker, R. L., Hernanz-Schulman, M., Yu, C., & Kan, J. H. (2008). Radiographic evaluation of intussusception: Utility of left-side-down decubitus view. *Radiology, 248*(3), 987–994.

Hrabovsky, E. (1996). Acute and chronic abdominal pain. In R. Kliegman (Ed.), *Practical strategies in pediatric diagnosis and therapy* (pp. 258–279). W.B. Saunders Co.

Hryhorczuk, A. L., Mannix, R. C., & Taylor, G. A. (2012). Pediatric abdominal pain: Use of imaging in the emergency department in the United States from 1999 to 2007. *Radiology, 263*(3), 778–785.

Lane, W. G., Dubowitz, H., Langenberg, P., & Dischinger, P. (2012). Epidemiology of abusive abdominal trauma hospitalizations in United States children. *Child Abuse & Neglect, 36*(2), 142–148.

Macari, M., Hines, J., Balthazar, E., & Megibow, A. (2002). Mesenteric adenitis: CT diagnosis of primary versus secondary causes, incidence, and clinical significance in pediatric and adult patients. *American Journal of Roentgenology, 178*, 853–858.

Mandeville, K., Chien, M., Willyerd, F. A., Mandell, G., Hostetler, M. A., & Bulloch, B. (2012). Intussusception: Clinical presentations and imaging characteristics. *Pediatric Emergency Care, 28*(9), 842–844.

Manson, D. (2004). Contemporary imaging of the child with abdominal pain or distress. *Paediatrics and Child Health, 9*(2), 93–97.

Moore, E. E., Shackford, S. R., Pachter, H. L., McAninch, J. W., Browner, B. D., Champion, H. R., etal. (1989). Organ injury scaling: Spleen, liver, and kidney. *The Journal of Trauma, 29*(12), 1664–1666.

Perret, R. S., & Kunberger, L. E. (1998). Case 4: Cecal volvulus. *American Journal of Roentgenology, 171*(3), 855 859, 860.

Putnam, L. R., John, S. D., Greenfield, S. A., Kellagher, C. M., Austin, M. T., Lally, K. P., etal. (2015). The utility of the contrast enema in neonates with suspected Hirschsprung disease. *Journal of Pediatric Surgery, 50*(6), 963–966.

Ravichandran, D., & Burge, D. M. (1996). Pneumonia presenting with acute abdominal pain in children. *British Journal of Surgery, 83*, 1707–1708.

Rothrock, S. G., & Pagane, J. (2000). Acute appendicitis in children: Emergency department diagnosis and management. *Annals of Emergency Medicine, 36*(1), 39–51.

Samuel, M., Boddy, S. A., Nicholls, E., & Capps, S. (2000). Large bowel volvulus in childhood. *Australian and New Zealand Journal of Surgery, 70*, 258.

Salati, U., Mcneill, G., & Torreggiani, W. C. (2011). The coffee bean sign in sigmoid volvulus. *Radiology, 258*(2), 651–652.

Sheybani, E. F., Gonzalaz-Araiza, G., Kousari, Y. M., Hulett, R. L., & Menias, C. O. (2014). Pediatric nonaccidental abdominal trauma: What the radiologist should know. *RadioGraphics, 34*(1), 139–153.

Shuman, W. P., Ralls, P. W., Balfe, D. M., Bree, R. L., DiSantis, D. J., Glick, S. N., etal. (2000). Imaging evaluation of patients with acute abdominal pain and fever. *American College of Radiology. ACR Appropriateness Criteria. Radiology, 215*(Suppl. l), 209–212.

Stranzinger, E., DiPietro, M. A., Teitelbaum, D. H., & Strouse, P. J. (2008). Imaging of total colonic Hirschsprung disease. *Pediatric Radiology, 38*, 1162–1170.

van den Berg, M. M., Benninga, M. A., & Di Lorenzo, C. (2006). Epidemiology of childhood constipation: A systematic review. *American Journal of Gastroenterology, 101*(10), 2401.

CHAPTER 6
Abdominal Masses in Children

Benjamin Taragin, Sonali Lala, and Jenna Le

CHAPTER OUTLINE

How Should Abdominal Masses in the Pediatric
   Population Be Imaged?, 127
How Should a Differential Diagnosis Be
   Approached?, 128
Abdominal Masses in Neonates/Infants, 128
   Renal Masses: Hydronephrosis, Cystic Renal
      Diseases, and Renal Neoplasms, 128
   Hydronephrosis, 128
   Cystic Renal Diseases, 128
   Renal Neoplasms, 129
   Adrenal Masses, 130
   Ovarian and Uterine Masses, 130
Gastrointestinal Tract Masses, 131
   Hepatobiliary Masses: Infantile Hepatic
      Hemangiomas, Hepatoblastomas, Mesenchymal
      Hamartomas, and Choledochal Cysts, 131
   Infantile Hepatic Hemangioma, 131
   Hepatoblastoma, 132

Mesenchymal Hamartoma of the Liver, 132
   Choledochal Cyst, 133
   Bowel-Related Masses: Enteric Duplication Cysts and
      Meconium Pseudocysts, 133
   Enteric Duplication Cyst, 133
   Meconium Pseudocyst, 135
Miscellaneous Abdominal Masses, 135
   Lymphatic Malformations, 135
   Infradiaphragmatic Pulmonary Sequestration, 135
   Sacrococcygeal Teratoma, 135
Abdominal Masses in Children Older Than 1 Year, 136
   Renal Masses, 136
   Neuroblastoma, 140
Hepatic Masses: Hepatoblastoma, Hepatocellular
   Carcinoma, Undifferentiated Embryonal Sarcoma,
   and Angiosarcoma, 140
Germ Cell Tumors, 142
   Rhabdomyosarcoma and Other Sarcomas, 144
Lymphoma, 144

Abdominal masses in children present with variable symptoms, including abdominal pain, abdominal distention, and palpable mass on physical examination. Palpable abdominal masses are a common presenting problem on pediatric outpatient services. Although many pediatric patients ultimately have benign causes for their palpable abdominal masses, such as constipation (in fact, up to 3% of all pediatric outpatient visits are thought to be secondary to constipation), there is a subset of patients who have more significant underlying disease. In addition, malignant masses may present with constitutional symptoms or symptoms related to metastatic disease.

After reasonable measures have been undertaken to exclude benign causes, including collecting a detailed clinical history and performing a physical examination, appropriate imaging should be directed by the physical examination findings, relevant history, and laboratory test abnormalities. Ultrasound (US), with its lack of ionizing radiation, ease of acquisition, and user-friendly environment, is the first-line modality for imaging of most abdominal masses. If the US demonstrates an abdominal mass, additional cross-sectional imaging should be performed. Magnetic resonance imaging

(MRI) is often preferred over computed tomography (CT) because it does not subject the patient to radiation. Notably, patients may require sedation for MRI, and if this is not feasible, CT is an alternative modality.

■ How Should Abdominal Masses in the Pediatric Population Be Imaged?

Properly supervised US should be able to demonstrate greater than 90% of intraabdominal masses of the solid organs. Technically limiting factors, such as bowel gas, constipation, and patient agitation, can limit the utility of US. In those cases, rescanning after addressing the underlying limitation may be helpful.

In addition, US can help the radiologist plan proper additional imaging based on the appearance of the abnormality, its vascularity, and its relationship to other structures. In patients with negative US who are still highly likely to have underlying pathology, as well as patients with positive US who need further diagnostic imaging, imaging with CT with contrast or MRI without and with intravenous contrast can be the appropriate follow-up examination. Abdominal CT is fast and extensively available but has ionizing radiation, whereas MRI has improved soft tissue resolution but is often less available and may necessitate sedation because of the longer examination time. Other examinations may subsequently be needed for staging and evaluation for potential metastatic disease (such as chest CT or F-18 FluoroDeoxyGlucose Positron Emission Tomography-CT (F-18 FDG PET-CT)).

■ How Should a Differential Diagnosis Be Approached?

The combination of patient age, location of mass, and imaging appearance will narrow down the differential diagnosis significantly. Pathologies are often different in neonates/infants compared with older children, and although there may be mild overlap in age of presentation, individualized differential diagnoses for those age groups may be helpful.

■ Abdominal Masses in Neonates/ Infants

In children younger than 1 year, the vast majority of abdominal masses are benign; in fact, approximately 80% are not even neoplastic but instead are developmental or inflammatory in etiology. When focusing on neonates (i.e., children <1 month old), roughly 75% of palpable abdominal masses arise from the genitourinary tract, including kidneys, adrenal glands, bladder, and reproductive system.

Renal Masses: Hydronephrosis, Cystic Renal Diseases, and Renal Neoplasms

Hydronephrosis
Hydronephrosis, the most common etiology of an abdominal mass in a neonate, often presents as a palpable flank mass. Major causes include uretero-pelvic junction (UPJ) obstruction, posterior urethral valves, UVJ obstruction, vesicoureteral reflux, neurogenic bladder, and prune belly. Because hydronephrosis is such a common entity, it is discussed in detail in a dedicated chapter in this book (see Chapter 8, Imaging Approach to Urinary Tract Dilation).

Cystic Renal Diseases
Cystic renal diseases in the neonate include, but are not limited to, multicystic dysplastic kidney (MCDK) and autosomal dominant and autosomal recessive polycystic kidney disease. Whereas inherited cystic disease affects both kidneys, MCDK is a nonhereditary condition that is thought to develop secondary to a congenital complete obstruction at the ureteropelvic junction. Although MCDK is usually unilateral, patients with MCDK have a 20% to 50% chance of having other concurrent contralateral renal anomalies, for example, a UPJ obstruction or vesicoureteral reflux.

When cystic renal disease is suspected, US is the first-line imaging study. The typical sonographic appearance of a MCDK is a kidney replaced by multiple noncommunicating cysts and dysplastic-appearing intervening thin parenchyma (Fig. 6.1); compensatory hypertrophy of the contralateral kidney will generally be seen, particularly as the infant grows. In some cases, it can be challenging to differentiate MCDK from unilateral hydronephrosis. In these cases, functional imaging with Tc-99m-MAG3 scintigraphy can be considered as a follow-up study to US. On scintigraphy, an MCDK will show no renal function, whereas a hydronephrotic kidney will usually show at least a small amount of renal function.

Autosomal dominant polycystic kidney disease will often not present until the child is older; however, macrocysts in a neonate should prompt a discussion of this entity with the referring clinician to evaluate family members because greater than 90% of these cases are inherited.

Autosomal recessive polycystic kidney disease will appear as markedly enlarged and diffusely echogenic kidneys as a result of tubular ectasia (Fig. 6.2). Small renal cysts or areas of severe tubular ectasia may be seen; other times, only diffusely increased echogenicity is seen because the cystic spaces may be too small to resolve via US and instead will appear echogenic because of increased surface interfaces.

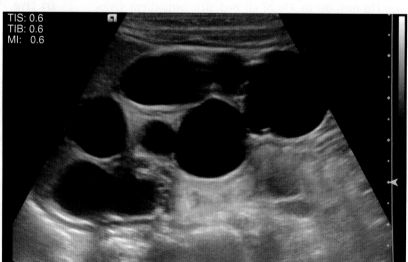

Fig. 6.1 Multicystic dysplastic kidney in a neonate with a history of a cystic right kidney on prenatal imaging. Longitudinal grayscale image of the right renal fossa showing a conglomerate of cysts with no normal intervening.

Renal Neoplasms

The most common renal neoplasm in children younger than 1 year is mesoblastic nephroma. Other renal neoplasms, such as Wilms tumor, are relatively rare in neonates and occur more frequently between the ages of 1 and 11 years. Wilms tumor will be discussed in greater depth later in this chapter.

Mesoblastic nephroma affects boys more often than girls. The mean age at diagnosis is 3 months. Ninety-five percent of cases are benign. Ten percent of patients will have a prenatal history of polyhydramnios. Patients typically come to medical attention when they are found to have a palpable abdominal mass; other clinical findings, such as hypertension and hypercalcemia, are rare. On US (either prenatal or postnatal) a mesoblastic nephroma will appear as a large, predominantly solid renal mass measuring from 5 to 30 cm in length. The mass is typically fairly homogeneous in echotexture. Generally speaking, hemorrhage and necrosis are absent except in the rare malignant form.

Once US has demonstrated a solid renal mass, further workup with contrast-enhanced MRI or CT is indicated (Fig. 6.3). On cross-sectional imaging, mesoblastic nephroma is often noted splaying the renal calyces. On MRI, it is T1 hypointense and T2 hyperintense to adjacent renal parenchyma, a nonspecific appearance shared by many renal masses. It is crucial to evaluate for renal vein involvement. The radiologist should also look carefully for metastases to lymph nodes and/or lung (the latter is better demonstrated on CT), because these can be seen in the rare malignant form. Mesoblastic nephroma cannot be definitively differentiated from Wilms tumor on imaging, and nephrectomy is the standard of care. After nephrectomy, either US or MRI can be performed at intervals for postsurgical surveillance as clinically indicated.

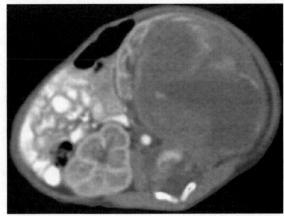

Fig. 6.3 Mesoblastic nephroma in 6-month-old infant with a palpable abdominal mass and hypercalcemia on laboratory testing. Contrast-enhanced computed tomography scan of the abdomen shows a large heterogeneous hypoattenuating mass arising from the left kidney.

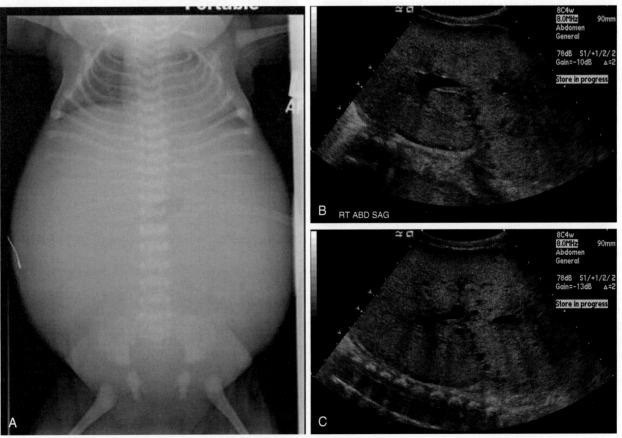

Fig. 6.2 Autosomal recessive polycystic kidney disease in 7-day-old neonate with decreased urine output and palpable abdominal masses. Single anteroposterior view of the chest and abdomen (A) shows centralized location of the stomach, absence of bowel gas, and bulging of the flanks. Longitudinal grayscale images of the right (B) and left (C) show markedly enlarged and echogenic kidneys containing innumerable small subcentimeter cysts.

Adrenal Masses

The most common solid malignant neoplasm in neonates/infants is neuroblastoma, a "small round blue cell tumor" arising from premature neuroectodermal cells and affecting 1 in 10,000 individuals. Although neuroblastoma can arise from sympathetic nervous stem cells anywhere in the body, most neuroblastomas in infants arise in the abdomen, usually from the adrenal medulla. The median age at presentation is 1 year 10 months, although some cases can be congenital. Symptoms can include diaphoresis, flushing, and diarrhea. Laboratory findings include high urine levels of catecholamine metabolites, such as homovanillic acid and vanillylmandelic acid. Pathologically, *N-Myc* gene amplification within tumor cells is associated with worse prognosis.

Imaging is crucial for accurate diagnosis and staging of neuroblastoma. Imaging evaluation typically begins with US, where neuroblastoma appears as a heterogeneous, predominantly solid mass often located superior to and separate from the kidney (Fig. 6.4A). Calcifications, cystic components, hemorrhage, and/or necrosis may be present. Neuroblastoma can be quite large at the time of diagnosis, often traversing the midline, surrounding vascular structures, and displacing the bowel. When the neuroblastoma is small, an important mimic is adrenal hemorrhage, which will not have internal vascularity on color Doppler and will decrease in size on follow-up ultrasounds, whereas neuroblastoma will have internal Doppler flow and typically stay the same size or enlarge on short-term follow-up. Another important mimic is infradiaphragmatic pulmonary sequestration (IPS), especially when the lesion is located in the left suprarenal fossa. Infradiaphragmatic sequestration is discussed in detail later in the Miscellaneous Abdominal Masses section.

Further cross-sectional imaging with MRI or CT is performed at the time of diagnosis for detection of imaging-defined risk factors (IDRFs). MRI is a sensitive modality for assessing the presence of local invasion, especially paraspinal/spinal involvement, and metastases (Fig 6.4B). Lymph node, osseous, and liver metastases are more common sites of involvement, whereas lung and brain metastases are generally seen only in advanced disease. MRI also demonstrates the relationship between the tumor and adjacent blood vessels, which may be in contact with, flattened by, or encased by tumor. On MRI, neuroblastoma will appear as a T1-hypointense, slightly T2-hyperintense mass with heterogeneous enhancement that encases, rather than displaces, adjacent structures. If MRI is not clinically feasible, CT can be performed as an alternative.

Necessary additional imaging at the time of diagnosis includes I-123 *meta*-iodobenzylguanidine (MIBG) scan, which can be used to identify primary uptake, as well as cortical bone, bone marrow, and soft tissue metastases. Important auxiliary imaging modalities for staging neuroblastoma include Technetium

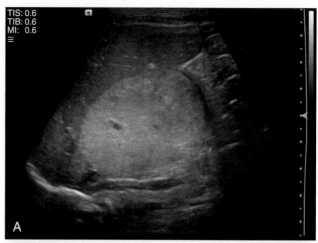

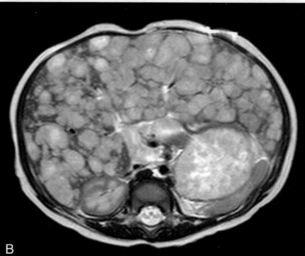

Fig. 6.4 Metastatic neuroblastoma in a 3-month-old infant presenting with a firm and distended abdomen. Longitudinal (A) grayscale image of the left upper quadrant shows an echogenic suprarenal mass. Axial T2-weighted image (B) through the abdomen shows the known left suprarenal mass, as well as innumerable hepatic masses, confirmed to be metastatic neuroblastoma by liver biopsy.

(99mTc) medronic acid (Tc-99m-MDP) bone scan, which can be used to evaluate for cortical bone metastases.

Ovarian and Uterine Masses

Ovarian masses in neonates are usually benign; most, in fact, are cysts. The first-line imaging modality for the evaluation of neonatal ovarian masses is US. Not only can US characterize an ovarian mass as either a simple cyst, complex cyst, or a solid mass, but it can also help determine whether there is associated ovarian torsion. Small simple cysts are safe to follow with US, whereas large simple cysts should be referred to a surgeon for possible excision because of the risk for torsion. Complex cysts can be treated with aspiration or excision. Excision is recommended for all solid masses.

The most common uterine abnormality that causes a palpable abdominal mass is hydrometrocolpos, which occurs when maternal hormones stimulate endometrial secretions that cannot be excreted because of the presence of an imperforate hymen, vaginal atresia, or persistent urogenital sinus. Hydrometrocolpos is generally easy to identify on US, with fluid distention of the vagina causing an ovoid hypoechoic structure, often with posteriorly layering proteinaceous debris (Fig. 6.5).

■ Gastrointestinal Tract Masses

Hepatobiliary Masses: Infantile Hepatic Hemangiomas, Hepatoblastomas, Mesenchymal Hamartomas, and Choledochal Cysts

Infantile Hepatic Hemangioma
Infantile hepatic hemangiomas (IHHs) are the most frequently occurring benign liver mass in the neonatal

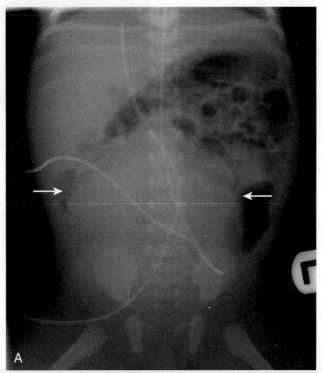

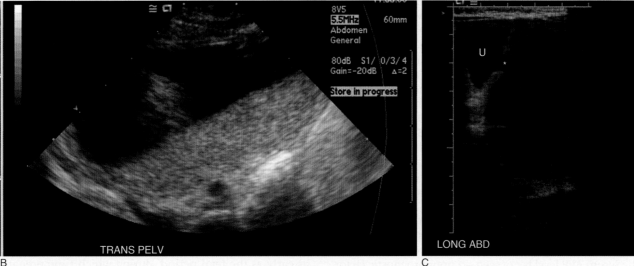

Fig. 6.5 Hydrometrocolpos in a 0-day-old neonate with ambiguous genitalia and abdominal distention. Single anteroposterior view of the abdomen (A) shows a central abdominal-pelvic soft tissue mass (*arrow*). Transverse grayscale ultrasound image (B) shows that the mass corresponds to a vagina distended with fluid and debris. Longitudinal grayscale ultrasound image (C) through the mid-abdomen shows fluid distending the cervix (*asterisk*) and extending into the uterus. The patient had a subsequent genitogram confirming the presence of a persistent urogenital sinus, explaining the cause for hydrometrocolpos.

age group. In the literature an important distinction has been made between congenital hemangiomas and infantile hemangiomas (IHs). IHs appear shortly after birth, stain positive for Glucose transporter 1 (GLUT-1), and rapidly proliferate before undergoing a slow spontaneous involution within the first decade of life.

Patients may present with a palpable right upper abdominal mass. Alternatively, they may present with symptoms of congestive heart failure (if the IHH causes significant arteriovenous shunting) or thrombocytopenia (if the IHH causes platelet sequestration). Because there is an association between IHH and cutaneous IH, patients with more than five cutaneous IHs will undergo an abdominal US to assess for the presence of IHH and other visceral hemangiomas. Unlike patients with hepatoblastomas, patients with IHH have serum alpha-fetoprotein (AFP) levels that, when age-adjusted using a pediatric nomogram, are normal.

The sonographic appearance of IHHs is often a hypoechoic mass, but IHHs may also be hyperechoic, or of mixed echogenicity. On grayscale images, large vessels may be seen coursing through the vessels, and with color Doppler, IHHs will demonstrate avid vascularity. They can be solitary or multifocal. If there is significant arteriovenous shunting secondary to an IHH, the celiac artery may be enlarged, with tapering of the abdominal aorta inferior to the celiac axis.

Contrast-enhanced MRI can be obtained for further workup if the diagnosis is still unclear. IHHs will be T1-hypointense and markedly T2-hyperintense. Large flow voids can be seen coursing through the lesion. While in their proliferative phase, IHHs demonstrate rapid and intense arterial phase enhancement (Fig. 6.6). If imaged during involution, arterial enhancement may be variable and less robust.

Because the majority of IHHs involute spontaneously without the need for medical treatment (propranolol, steroids, interferon, or vincristine), embolization, or surgery, it is reasonable to follow them with serial USs.

Hepatoblastoma

Hepatoblastoma is the most common primary liver malignancy in children. Although the peak age of diagnosis is 1.5 to 2 years, this tumor is sometimes diagnosed in infants. Hepatoblastoma is relatively rare: whereas, say, neuroblastoma affects approximately 100 in 1 million individuals, hepatoblastoma affects only 13 in 1 million individuals. Risk factors include familial adenomatous polyposis, Beckwith-Wiedemann syndrome, and premature birth. Most of the time hepatoblastoma can be palpated on physical examination. Important laboratory findings include a serum AFP level that, when age-adjusted using a pediatric nomogram, is elevated; this can be used to help distinguish a hepatoblastoma from an IHH. In 10% of patients with hepatoblastoma, the expected increase in the serum AFP level is not seen—a poor prognostic factor.

As with the other neonatal/infant liver tumors, imaging workup begins with US, which will often show heterogeneous, mixed echogenicity mass or masses with a mean primary size of 10 cm. A heterogeneous appearance is due to variable internal hemorrhage, necrosis, and/or coarse calcification (Fig. 6.7A).

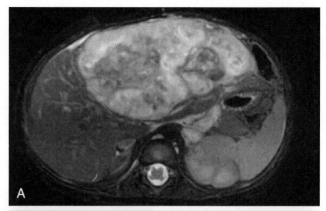

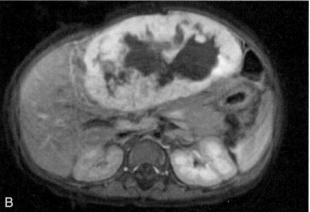

Fig. 6.6 Infantile hepatic hemangioma in a 6-month-old with hepatomegaly. Axial T2-weighted image (A) shows a large T2 hyperintense mass in the left lobe of the liver. Postcontrast T1-weighted fat-suppressed imaging (B) shows nodular peripheral avid enhancement, typical of large infantile hepatic hemangiomas.

MRI or CT of the abdomen is performed for staging, using the PRETEXT (Pre-Treatment EXTent of tumor) system, describing extent of tumor in the liver, degree of vascular involvement, and extrahepatic and metastatic disease A CT scan of the chest is needed to evaluate for lung metastases, the most common site of metastatic involvement.

MRI of hepatoblastoma will demonstrate a heterogeneous T1-hypointense and T2-hyperintense hypoenhancing mass (see Fig. 6.7B–D). Foci of T1 hyperintensity and T2 hypointensity may be present and compatible with hemorrhage and/or calcification.

Mesenchymal Hamartoma of the Liver

Mesenchymal hamartoma is the second most often encountered benign liver mass in the neonatal population. Mesenchymal hamartoma is a nonneoplastic mass consisting of disordered hepatic tissue, including hepatocytes, epithelium-lined bile ducts, connective stroma, and venous channels. They are almost never seen in patients older than 2 years and are sometimes diagnosed as early as the fetal period, during which time prenatal US may reveal a cystic-and-solid liver lesion that may cause mass effect on the lungs and adjacent blood vessels occasionally resulting in hydrops.

In the postnatal period, imaging workup also begins with US, on which mesenchymal hamartoma cystic-and-solid liver mass with a prominent cystic component

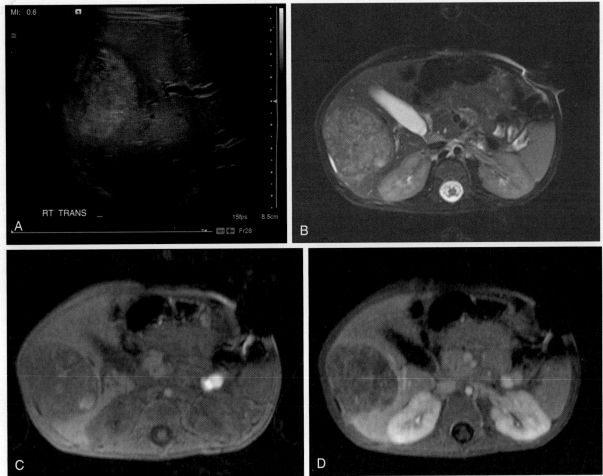

Fig. 6.7 Hepatoblastoma in an 11-month-old with a history of Beckwith-Wiedemann syndrome and increasing alpha-fetoprotein. Transverse grayscale ultrasound image (A) of the liver shows a heterogeneous but echogenic mass in the right lobe. Axial T2-weighted image (B) shows the mass to be heterogeneously hyperintense to hepatic parenchyma; axial three-dimensional T1-weighted gradient recalled echo image (C) shows a hypointense mass with small hyperintense foci consistent with hemorrhage; postcontrast axial three-dimensional T1-weighted gradient recalled echo image (D) demonstrates hypoenhancement of the mass relative to hepatic parenchyma.

is frequently divided into numerous locules by thin septations. Cysts may be macrocystic or microcystic. Microcystic lesions can mimic solid masses.

MRI can be useful in assisting with surgical planning. On MRI, mesenchymal hamartoma will appear as a well-demarcated liver mass whose solid component is T2 hypointense, while its cystic component(s) is strongly T2 hyperintense. The solid component shows variable enhancement on postcontrast images (Fig. 6.8).

Choledochal Cyst
A choledochal cyst is defined as a congenital cystic dilatation of the extrahepatic and/or intrahepatic biliary tree. It is often an incidental imaging finding and can be seen during prenatal imaging but may present with symptoms such as a palpable abdominal mass, abdominal pain, or jaundice.

Sonography shows a cystic mass in the porta hepatis communicating with the biliary tree. Other cystic lesions that may be encountered in the region of the porta hepatis include enteric duplication cysts and lymphatic malformations (LMs). If US is equivocal, MRCP can be performed because it can clearly demonstrate continuity between the cyst and the biliary tree. An abrupt caliber change will be seen between the cyst and the normal bile ducts that connect to it. If there is persistent uncertainty about whether the lesion represents a choledochal cyst (communicates with the biliary tree) or an enteric duplication cyst (does not communicate with the biliary tree), MRI with a hepatobiliary contrast agent may be performed to answer this question (Fig. 6.9).

Choledochal cysts are treated with surgical resection and hepaticojejunostomy for symptom relief, as well as for the heightened risk for infection, stones, and (in the long term) malignancy if left untreated.

Bowel-Related Masses: Enteric Duplication Cysts and Meconium Pseudocysts

Enteric Duplication Cyst
Enteric duplication cysts are benign cystic structures that are most commonly found at the mesenteric border of the jejunum or ileum, although they theoretically can

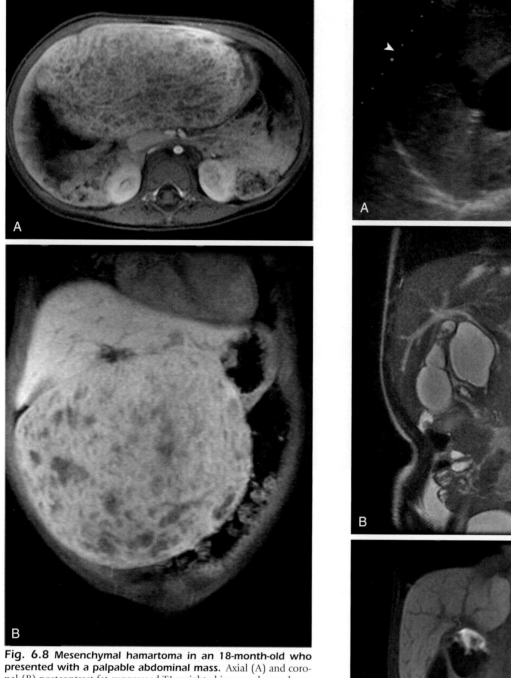

Fig. 6.8 Mesenchymal hamartoma in an 18-month-old who presented with a palpable abdominal mass. Axial (A) and coronal (B) postcontrast fat-suppressed T1-weighted images show a large, heterogeneously enhancing exophytic mass with small avascular cystic spaces.

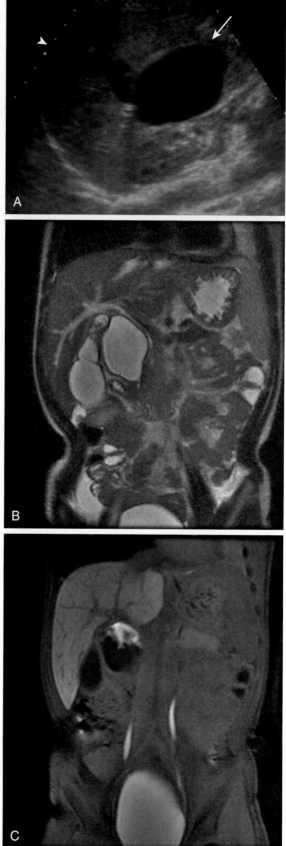

Fig. 6.9 Choledochal cyst in a 1-year-old. Oblique grayscale ultrasound image (A) depicts an ovoid anechoic mass in the porta hepatis. Coronal T2-weighted image (B) shows a T2-hyperintense mass in the porta hepatis. After gadoxetate disodium administration, a delayed coronal T1-weighted image (C) demonstrates filling of the T2-hyperintense mass in the porta hepatis, confirming the diagnosis of a type I choledochal cyst.

form at any location along the gastrointestinal tract from the esophagus to the anus. They may or may not communicate with the bowel segment with which they share a wall. Duplication cysts are often discovered incidentally, but may occasionally cause complications such as bowel obstruction, volvulus, or intussusception. In a minority of cases, they contain gastric mucosa, which can lead to hemorrhage or perforation.

On US, they appear as round, oval, or tubular cystic structures whose defining feature is the sonographic gut signature: a five-layered lining consisting of alternating hyperechoic and hypoechoic lines representing mucosa

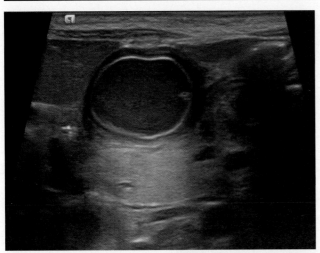

Fig. 6.10 Gastric duplication cyst in 1-day-old neonate with prenatal history of intraabdominal cystic mass. Transverse grayscale ultrasound image shows a cystic mass in the right upper quadrant. The wall of the mass has "gut signature."

(the echogenic innermost layer), muscularis mucosa, submucosa, muscularis propria, and serosa (the echogenic outermost layer) (Fig. 6.10).

Meconium Pseudocyst
Meconium pseudocysts are due to intrauterine/perinatal bowel perforation with resultant leakage of meconium into the peritoneum, with subsequent walling off of the meconium and fluid. Patients at increased risk for development of meconium pseudocysts include infants with cystic fibrosis and Hirschsprung disease and infants of diabetic mothers. In these patients, meconium is more likely to become inspissated in the bowel, leading to bowel perforation and spillage of meconium into the peritoneal cavity. Meconium pseudocysts typically contain fluid with proteinaceous debris, with associated calcifications from inflammatory reaction to meconium.

On plain radiographs a meconium pseudocyst will appear as a soft tissue density with rim calcification (Fig. 6.11A). US may be helpful for delineating the relationship of the pseudocyst to adjacent structures, as well as confirming calcifications and defining cystic nature (see Fig. 6.11B–C).

■ Miscellaneous Abdominal Masses

Lymphatic Malformations

LMs are benign masses of lymphatic tissue that are separate from the central lymphatic system. LMs develop during fetal life and may be evident on prenatal imaging. The majority (95%) will become clinically evident by 2 years of life. They can be located anywhere in the body. In the abdomen, they may be related to the omentum ("omental cysts"), the mesentery ("mesenteric cysts"), or the retroperitoneum. When in the abdomen, patients can present with abdominal pain, abdominal distention, and/or bowel obstruction.

On US, LMs will appear as cystic septated mass of variable size. They can be macrocystic, with cystic spaces measuring more than 2 cm; microcystic, with cystic spaces measuring less than 2 cm; or mixed. Internal debris and fluid-fluid levels may be seen if there is superimposed infection or hemorrhage. Although US is an excellent imaging modality for assessment of LMs, its depth of penetration and field of view can be a limitation when evaluating an LM, because these lesions can be large and are often insinuating lesions that do not respect anatomic boundaries.

MRI can demonstrate the true extent of an LM and may be obtained before treatment. On MRI, LMs will appear as T2-hyperintense, T1-hyperintense lesions with enhancing septations. Fluid–fluid levels with associated T1 hyperintensity may be seen in the setting of infection or hemorrhage.

Infradiaphragmatic Pulmonary Sequestration

IPSs make up 2% to 15% of all extralobar pulmonary sequestrations. Like other pulmonary sequestrations, IPSs consist of nonfunctioning lung parenchyma that does not communicate with the tracheobronchial tree and is supplied by systemic (rather than pulmonary) arteries. Because they are extralobar, they are invested in their own pleura. Some are associated with other congenital anomalies, such as a diaphragmatic hernia or bronchogenic cyst.

IPSs are frequently detected on routine prenatal US. Virtually all IPSs are located on the left. Because IPSs are most often suprarenal in location, the most important differential consideration is neuroblastoma. On US, an IPS may appear as a homogeneously echogenic mass superior to the left kidney and separate from both the kidney and the adrenal gland. This is in contradistinction to neuroblastomas, which are often inseparable/arise from the adrenal gland. The homogeneously echogenic appearance of IPSs can also be used to distinguish them from neuroblastomas, because neuroblastomas usually contain cysts, areas of hemorrhage, or calcification that give them a heterogeneous appearance. In addition, IPS appears during the secondary trimester, whereas neuroblastoma appears during the third trimester. On Doppler evaluation of an IPS, an abnormal feeding artery can sometimes be seen arising from the aorta. CT angiography depicts systemic arterial supply to best advantage (Fig. 6.12).

Sacrococcygeal Teratoma

In neonates the most common location of a teratoma is the sacrococcygeal region. Three-quarters of sacrococcygeal teratomas (SCTs) are found in neonates. The incidence is higher in girls. Approximately one-quarter of SCTs are malignant, with the likelihood of malignancy increasing with increasing age. In addition, SCTs that are diagnosed in fetuses tend to have a poorer prognosis

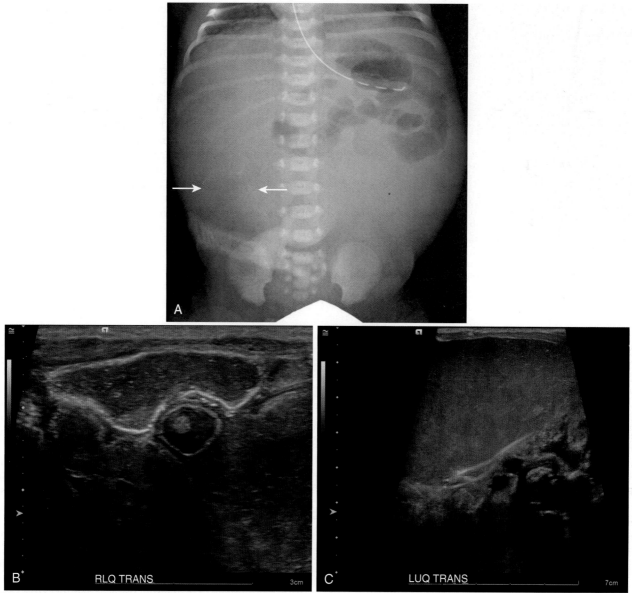

Fig. 6.11 Meconium pseudocyst in a 0-day-old neonate. Anteroposterior view of the abdomen (A) shows paucity of bowel gas in the lower abdomen with mass with rim calcification in the right lower quadrant (*arrows*) consistent with a meconium pseudocyst. A transverse grayscale ultrasound image (B) of the right lower quadrant shows a complex fluid collection in the right lower quadrant with peripheral calcification confirming the presence of a meconium pseudocyst. Additional transverse grayscale ultrasound image (C) of the left lower quadrant shows another large complex fluid collection. Intraoperative findings included a mid-small bowel perforation, meconium, and abundant inflammatory adhesions.

than those diagnosed in neonates. SCTs may be associated with sacral and anorectal malformations (Currarino's triad).

When detected on prenatal imaging, SCT appears as a large heterogeneous mass, frequently with calcifications. Polyhydramnios and hydrops may also be seen. The presence of predominantly cystic components generally heralds a better outcome.

After the child is born, MRI should be performed to delineate the tumor's location and extent (Fig. 6.13). SCTs can be grouped into four types based on their location and extent, with type IV (the completely intrapelvic type) having the worst prognosis, thought to be due to later detection. MRI is also useful for preoperative evaluation of the tumor's relationship to adjacent vasculature,

as well as for assessment of liver and lymph node metastases. CT is more sensitive than MRI for lung metastases.

■ Abdominal Masses in Children Older Than 1 Year

Renal Masses

The majority of pediatric renal masses in children older than 1 year are Wilms tumors, which make up more than 80% of pediatric renal masses. Wilms tumors have an incidence peaking at 3 to 4 years of age and usually present before 5 years of age. It most commonly

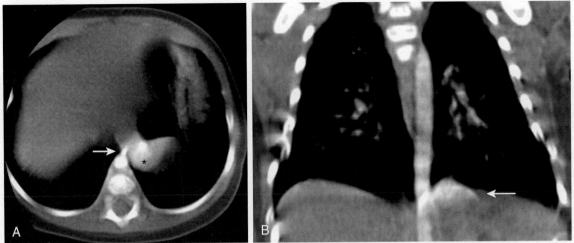

Fig. 6.12 Infradiaphragmatic extralobar pulmonary sequestration in a 6-month-old with prenatal history of left suprarenal mass. Axial contrast-enhanced computed tomography angiography (CTA) image (A) through the chest and upper abdomen shows an avidly enhancing mass (*asterisk*) with arterial supply arising from the proximal abdominal aorta (*arrow*). On the coronal contrast-enhanced CTA image (B) of the chest the mass appears to be located inferior to the left medial hemidiaphragm. Intraoperative findings revealed that the extralobar sequestration was within the diaphragm.

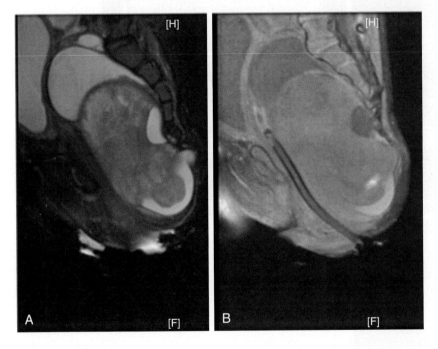

Fig. 6.13 Sacrococcygeal teratoma in a 4-year-old girl. Sagittal T2-weighted fat-suppressed image (A) shows a presacral predominantly mixed solid and cystic mass. Sagittal postcontrast T1-weighted image (B) demonstrates enhancement of the solid components.

presents as a palpable abdominal mass and rarely presents with flank pain or hematuria. The presence of a palpable mass should prompt sonographic evaluation of the kidneys. It is important to note that definitive differentiation of Wilms tumor from other renal masses requires histological analysis.

On sonography, Wilms tumor appears as a solid, intrarenal, heterogeneous mass with associated hemorrhage and necrosis, deforming the normal renal architecture. Careful color and spectral Doppler waveform analysis can demonstrate tumor thrombus in the renal vein and inferior vena cava. Typical CT appearance of Wilms tumor is large heterogeneous mass with areas of necrosis. On MRI the tumor demonstrates low signal intensity on T1-weighted images and high signal inten-

sity on T2-weighted images. MRI is especially useful for detection of tumor thrombus (Fig. 6.14). In addition to detecting tumor thrombus, the primary goals of cross-sectional imaging also include detection of nodal and hepatic metastases and detection of synchronous tumor in the contralateral kidney, because 6% of Wilms tumor cases are bilateral at the time of diagnosis due to the presence of nephrogenic rests or primitive renal blastema.

Nephroblastomatosis refers to the presence of multiple nephrogenic rests, which may undergo malignant transformation into Wilms tumor. Diffuse nephroblastomatosis will manifest sonographically with bilateral nephromegaly and multiple renal masses of mixed echogenicity (Fig. 6.15A–B). On MRI, nephrogenic rests

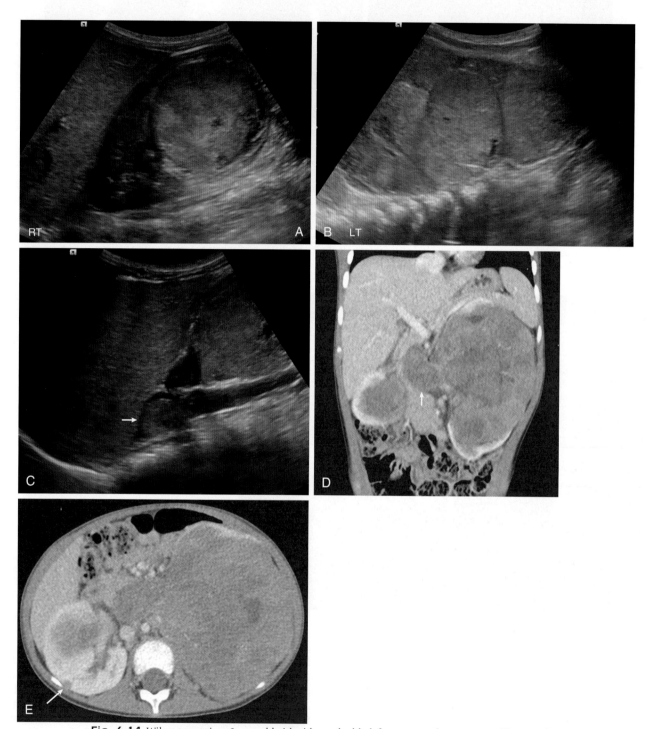

Fig. 6.14 Wilms tumor in a 3-year-old girl with a palpable left upper quadrant mass and hematuria. Longitudinal grayscale ultrasound image of the right (A) and left (B) kidneys demonstrates bilateral solid renal masses. Longitudinal grayscale ultrasound image (C) through the inferior cava shows tumor thrombus (*arrow*). Coronal contrast-enhanced computed tomography (CT) image (D) through the abdomen shows bilateral renal masses and tumor thrombus extending from the left renal vein to the inferior vena cava (*arrow*). Axial contrast-enhanced CT image (E) through the abdomen shows a subcentimeter hypoattenuating lesion in the posterior cortex of the right kidney, likely a nephrogenic rest.

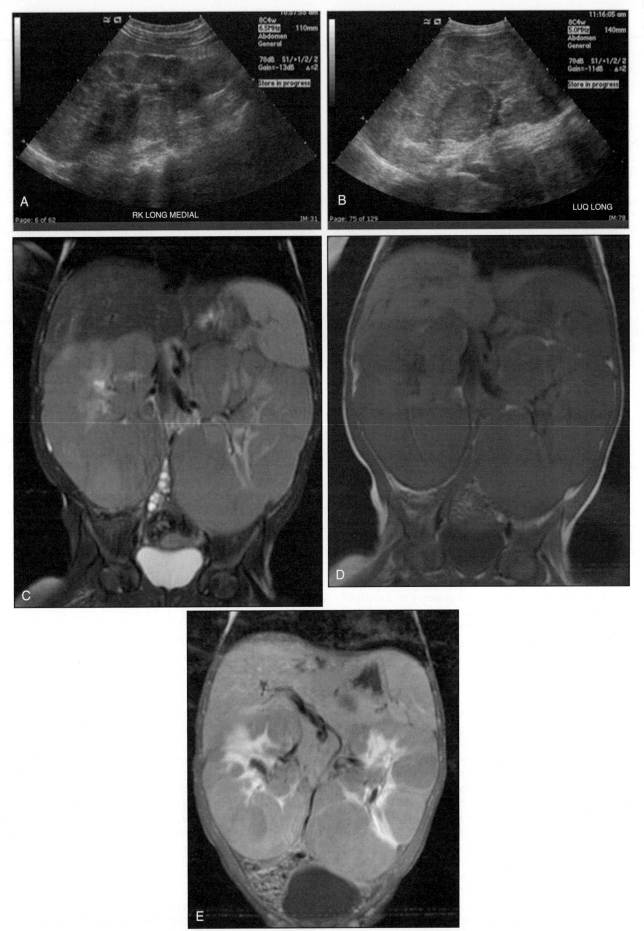

Fig. 6.15 Nephroblastomatosis in an 11-month-old with constipation. Longitudinal grayscale ultrasound images of the right (A) and left (B) kidneys show multiple renal masses of mixed echogenicity. Coronal T2-weighted fat-suppressed image (C) demonstrates multiple T2 hypointense masses that are also hypointense on coronal T1-weighted imaging (D) and hypoenhancing relative to renal parenchyma on postcontrast coronal T1-weighted fat-suppressed image (E).

appear as T1- and T2-hypointense masses that enhance to a lesser degree than normal renal parenchyma (see Fig. 6.15C–E).

The use of chest CT in evaluation of pulmonary metastases and staging of Wilms tumor is controversial. Although CT has been shown to be more sensitive in the detection of pulmonary nodules compared with chest radiography, it remains uncertain whether detection of these nodules improves outcomes.

Although many pediatric renal tumors appear similar to Wilms tumor, close attention to the sonographic appearance and the clinical history can point the radiologist in the right direction. For example, a subcapsular fluid collection associated with the solid renal mass is more indicative of a rhabdoid tumor. Renal cell carcinomas may present in the pediatric population; however, these are often small and not always sonographically apparent. In a patient with a history of either sickle cell trait or sickle cell (SC) disease, renal medullary carcinoma should be considered. Certain features seen on contrast-enhanced imaging may help differentiate Wilms tumor from other renal masses. Renal cell carcinoma is best seen on CT and MRI, which demonstrate a heterogeneous intra-renal mass (heterogeneous because of hemorrhage and necrosis) with a small amount of enhancement (Fig. 6.16). A subcapsular fluid collection and tumor lobules with intervening necrosis or hemorrhage and surrounding calcification are suggestive of a rhabdoid tumor (Fig. 6.17). Notably, concurrent brain metastases or primary brain tumors are associated with rhabdoid tumor, and brain MRI should be performed in patients with suspected or confirmed rhabdoid tumor. Clear cell sarcoma is virtually indistinguishable from Wilms tumor on cross-sectional imaging but is rarely associated with vascular invasion and often has osseous metastases. Renal medullary carcinoma occurs in patients with sickle cell trait and appears as a centrally located, heterogeneous mass with areas of hemorrhage and necrosis often invading the renal sinus causing caliectasis.

Neuroblastoma

Neuroblastomas may arise anywhere along the sympathetic nerve chain or in the adrenal medulla, with approximately two-thirds of lesions arising in the abdomen and two-thirds of those lesions arising from the adrenal medulla. Abdominal neuroblastomas otherwise commonly occur in the paravertebral sympathetic chain or presacral area. Ninety percent of neuroblastoma cases occur in patients between 1 and 5 years of age. Neuroblastoma can present with abdominal pain and distention and with nonspecific constitutional symptoms, but also with paraneoplastic syndromes. It can be occasionally noted incidentally on US or radiographs. The approach to, and imaging appearance of, neuroblastoma has been discussed in detail in the Abdominal Masses in Neonates/Infants section.

■ Hepatic Masses: Hepatoblastoma, Hepatocellular Carcinoma, Undifferentiated Embryonal Sarcoma, and Angiosarcoma

The most common hepatic tumor in children is hepatoblastoma, with the majority of cases presenting before 2 years and 90% of cases presenting before age 5 years. Patients may present with nonspecific symptoms and an enlarging abdomen. In 10% to 20% of cases, pulmonary metastases are present at the time of diagnosis. Hepatoblastoma also metastasizes to bone, brain, lymph nodes, eyes, and the ovaries. The imaging approach to hepatoblastoma has been discussed previously in the Abdominal Masses in Neonates/Infants section and is not significantly changed for older children.

Hepatocellular carcinoma (HCC) occurs in older children (age 10–14 years), and nearly 50% of them have predisposing conditions, including hepatitis B, glycogen storage disease, and tyrosinemia. Patients may present with weight loss, abdominal pain and distention, fever, and loss of appetite. AFP levels are elevated (except in cases of fibrolamellar HCC). In the setting of a hepatic mass and hepatomegaly, two less common tumors, undifferentiated embryonal sarcoma (UES) and angiosarcoma (AS), should also be considered as possible diagnoses. Patients with UES are usually younger (age 6–10 years) and have a normal AFP. Patients with AS often present with coagulopathy and abnormal blood cell counts accompanied by hepatomegaly.

Sonography is the first-line imaging modality in the setting of hepatomegaly to establish the presence or absence of a hepatic lesion. The sonographic appearance of HCC is variable: it may appear either hypoechoic, isoechoic, or hyperechoic; smaller lesions are usually hypoechoic. A hypoechoic halo may be seen if a tumor capsule is present, whereas an infiltrative tumor will distort the normal hepatic architecture. Larger lesions may appear heterogeneous because of areas of hemorrhage or necrosis. Doppler interrogation is useful for demonstrating arterial flow to the lesion and for evaluation of possible tumor thrombus. UES is seen as a large solid mass, isoechoic to hypoechoic relative to liver, with anechoic spaces within (secondary to necrosis or hemorrhage). Sometimes the lesion may be predominantly anechoic. An HCC that has undergone cystic degeneration may also have this appearance. AS can have a variable imaging appearance: on US it may appear as multiple nodules, a large mass, or as a diffusely heterogenous liver. Contrast-enhanced, multiphase MRI or CT is optimal for further characterization of liver lesions.

On both CT and MR, HCC will demonstrate early arterial enhancement with progressive equilibration on the portal venous phase. If a tumor capsule is present, it will demonstrate delayed enhancement. On MR the lesion is often heterogeneous due to the presence of fat, necrosis, hemorrhage, and calcification. The presence of a nonenhancing, T2-hypointense central scar is consistent with typical imaging appearance of fibrolamellar HCC.

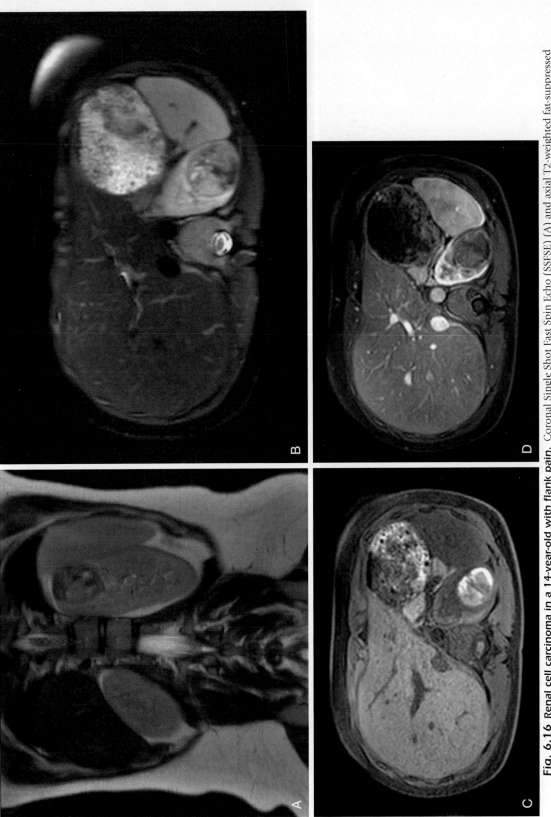

Fig. 6.16 Renal cell carcinoma in a 14-year-old with flank pain. Coronal Single Shot Fast Spin Echo (SSFSE) (A) and axial T2-weighted fat-suppressed (B) images show a heterogeneously hypointense mass at the upper pole of the left kidney. Axial precontrast three-dimensional (3D) T1-weighted gradient recalled echo image (C) shows intrinsic T1 shortening consistent with hemorrhage. Axial postcontrast 3D T1-weighted gradient recalled echo image (D) shows mild predominantly peripheral enhancement with a central region of hypoenhancement.

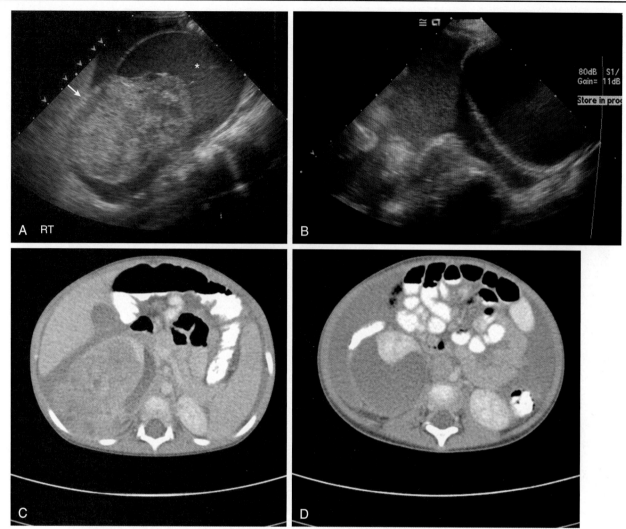

Fig. 6.17 **Rhabdoid tumor in a 22-month-old with abdominal distention, anemia, and thrombocytopenia.** Longitudinal grayscale ultrasound image (A) of the right renal fossa shows a solid mass arising from the right kidney (*arrow*) and subcapsular fluid collection (*asterisk*). Longitudinal grayscale ultrasound image (B) through the pelvis shows debris fluid in the pelvis concerning for hemoperitoneum. Two axial contrast-enhanced computed tomography images (C, D) through the abdomen show a heterogeneous but hypoattenuating mass arising from the midposterior pole of the right kidney, a large subcapsular fluid collection compressing the renal parenchyma, and large-volume ascites.

Contrast-enhanced imaging of an UES will demonstrate a lesion predominantly filled with fluid with areas of soft tissue peripherally or forming septa. There may be an enhancing peripheral rim corresponding to a pseudocapsule. On MR the pseudocapsule will appear hypointense on T1- and T2-weighted images. Focal areas of T1 hyperintensity and T2 hypointensity may be seen, corresponding to regions of hemorrhage. The peripheral and solid portions of the mass will enhance after administration of gadolinium.

CT of an AS will demonstrate hypoattenuating nodules with foci of hyperattenuation and areas of early and heterogeneous enhancement, which can sometimes be centrally located and persist on delayed imaging. On MR the lesion will be low in signal intensity relative to liver on T1-weighted images and heterogeneously hyperintense on T2-weighted images. Fluid levels or dark septa may be seen because of hemorrhage. On postcontrast imaging the lesion will demonstrate progressive heterogeneous enhancement, without central filling (Fig. 6.18).

■ Germ Cell Tumors

Germ cell tumors occur most frequently within the gonads but may also present in the pineal region, neurohypophysis, mediastinum, pelvis, and retroperitoneum. Germ cell tumors are classified as either seminomatous or nonseminomatous (mixed germ cell tumor, choriocarcinoma, yolk sac tumor, and teratoma). For the purposes of this chapter, we will focus our discussion on retroperitoneal germ cell tumors, which may be either a primary lesion or a secondary, metastatic lesion. Clinically, patients may present with a variety of symptoms: abdominal pain, back pain, gastrointestinal or genitourinary symptoms, or leg swelling secondary to lymphatic obstruction. Elevated AFP (particularly in the case of a malignant teratoma) and beta-Human chorionic gonadotropin (HCG) levels may be present.

Retroperitoneal extragonadal germ cell tumors are typically seen in the midline, between T6 and S2. A more midline location is suggestive of a primary rather

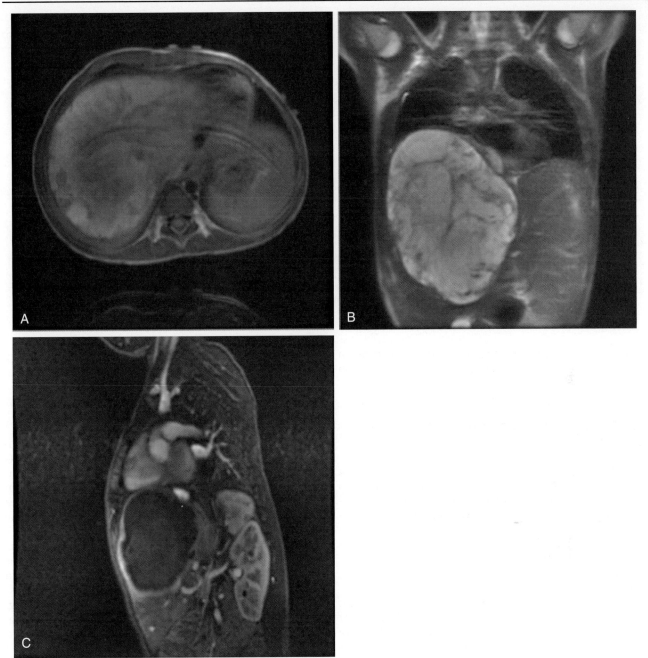

Fig. 6.18 Hepatic angiosarcoma in a 5-year-old. Axial precontrast T1-weighted fat-suppressed image shows (A) a large heterogeneous mass replacing the liver parenchyma. Coronal T2-weighted image (B) shows the mass to be T2 hyperintense. Sagittal postcontrast T1-weighted image (C) demonstrates peripheral enhancement.

than a metastatic lesion. Seminomas will appear as homogeneous solid-appearing masses that are often large and lobulated and have enhancing fibrous septations. There may be ringlike calcifications within the mass. Conversely, nonseminomatous germ cell tumors will have a heterogeneous appearance with areas of hemorrhage or necrosis and enhancement (Fig. 6.19). Flow-related signal voids may be present in areas of vascularity. The presence of a retroperitoneal germ cell tumor should prompt investigation for a possible remote primary site. Notably, sometimes a primary tumor may not be seen because of primary tumor regression.

Teratomas are the third most common retroperitoneal tumor in children (after neuroblastoma and Wilms tumor). There is a bimodal distribution to presentation. They may be classified as either mature or immature (in immature teratomas, greater than 10% of the tissue is undifferentiated). Imaging of mature teratomas demonstrates a largely cystic lesion with fat and calcification. Villiform solid portions, known as Rokitansky protuberances, are frequently seen. Thickening of the wall or the presence of a cauliflower-like projection is suggestive of malignant transformation.

Imaging of immature teratomas demonstrates a largely solid mass with areas of fat and calcification.

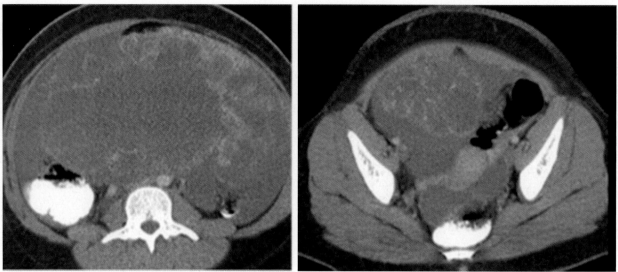

Fig. 6.19 Malignant germ cell tumor in a 15-year-old who presented with a 2.5-month history of abdominal pain and distention and an elevated serum alpha-fetoprotein level. Contrast-enhanced computed tomography shows a large, complex solid-and-cystic mass occupying the lower abdomen and pelvis, with surrounding ascites.

Cystic areas may also be present, and distinguishing an immature from a mature teratoma is often difficult on imaging.

Rhabdomyosarcoma and Other Sarcomas

The most common soft tissue sarcoma among children is rhabdomyosarcoma, which can be differentiated into two types, embryonal and alveolar. Rhabdomyosarcomas are associated with various clinical syndromes, including neurofibromatosis type 1, Beckwith-Wiedemann syndrome, and Li-Fraumeni syndrome. Rhabdomyosarcoma most commonly occurs in the head and neck region, followed by the genitourinary tract, extremities, and other sites, including the retroperitoneum, gastrointestinal tract, biliary tree, pancreas, or omentum. Clinical presentation can vary based on the location of the tumor; however, the rapid growth of sarcomas may result in neurovascular compromise. If metastatic disease is present, patients may present with generalized symptoms, such as fatigue, weight loss, and abnormal cell counts.

MR is the mainstay of imaging in abdominal/pelvic rhabdomyosarcoma. However, if sonography of rhabdomyosarcoma is performed, it will demonstrate a heterogeneous, well-defined, somewhat hypoechoic mass with internal vascularity. On contrast-enhanced MR, rhabdomyosarcoma appears as a predominantly T1- and T2-hypointense mass with heterogeneous enhancement (Fig. 6.20). Occasionally the tumor may be predominantly cystic. Hemorrhagic foci and regions of necrosis may be present. Once a histological diagnosis has been confirmed, further evaluation with chest CT, imaging of local lymph nodes, and bone scan are performed to assess for metastatic disease.

Other soft tissue sarcomas that may occur in the abdomen, although uncommon, include liposarcoma, fibrosarcoma, and leiomyosarcoma and have imaging features related to their histopathological elements.

■ Lymphoma

Lymphoma makes up 10% to 15% of all childhood cancers. Although Hodgkin disease (HD) typically presents with nodal or splenic involvement, non-Hodgkin lymphoma (NHL) typically presents extranodally. Children with intraabdominal involvement may present with a variety of symptoms secondary to mass effect from the tumor, including inferior vena cava obstruction, intestinal obstruction, intussusception, and ureteral obstruction. Histological evaluation is required for diagnosis of lymphoma; however, imaging plays a major role in evaluating the location and extent of disease.

US plays a large role in the initial evaluation and diagnosis of a child with symptoms secondary to lymphoma. US provides an evaluation of the abdominal viscera and lymph nodes. Although it is limited by bowel and bone interference, US may be particularly advantageous in evaluating retroperitoneal structures because of the lack of retroperitoneal fat in children. US is also superior to CT in evaluation of the female pelvis. In both HD and NHL, lymphomatous involvement of retroperitoneal lymph nodes may be present. Sonography may demonstrate a mass along the aorta and inferior vena cava or bilateral masses in the prevertebral region. Progressive disease may demonstrate encasement of the aorta and inferior vena cava, or encasement of the mesenteric vessels and root of the mesentery.

Splenic involvement in both HD and NHL may present as splenomegaly, or as single or multiple hypoechoic nodules. The liver may be involved (more commonly in NHL than in HD), in which case sonography would demonstrate hepatomegaly with multiple anechoic or hypoechoic nodules. It is worth noting, however, that both splenomegaly and hepatomegaly are nonspecific

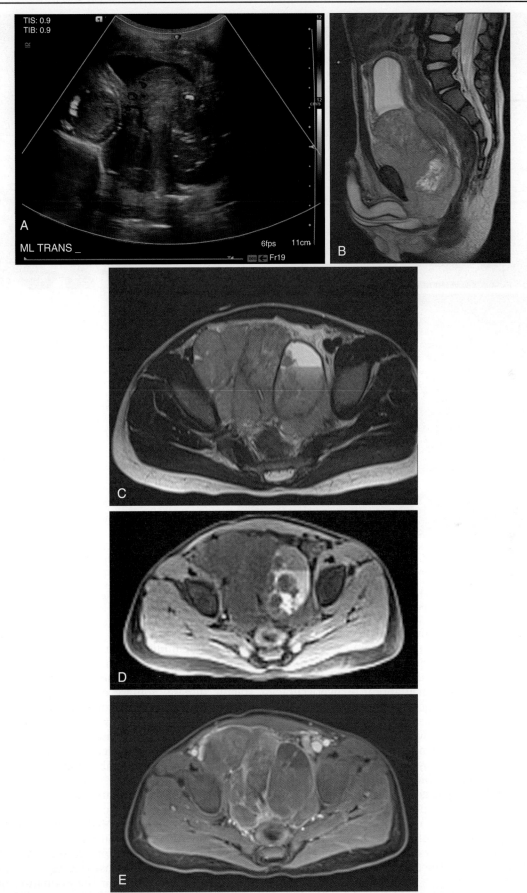

Fig. 6.20 Rhabdomyosarcoma in a 3-year-old boy with urinary retention. Transverse ultrasound image (A) through the pelvis demonstrates a mass with calcification indenting on or within the urinary bladder. Sagittal (B) and axial (C) T2-weighted images show a predominantly T2-hypointense mass centered in the prostate and urinary bladder base, extending into the urinary bladder. A fluid–fluid level is seen, secondary to hemorrhage. Axial precontrast three-dimensional (3D) T1-weighted gradient recalled echo image (D) shows hyperintense foci with a fluid–fluid level confirming the presence of hemorrhage. Postcontrast 3D T1-weighted gradient recalled echo image (E) demonstrates mild and heterogeneous enhancement.

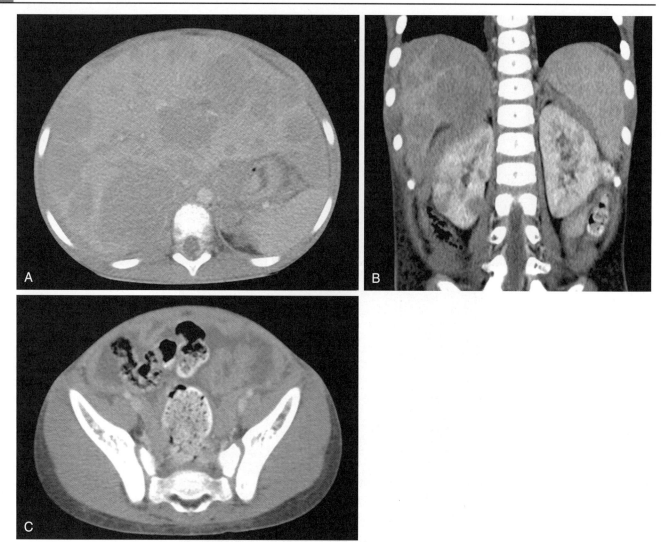

Fig. 6.21 Burkitt lymphoma in a 5-year-old with hepatomegaly. Axial contrast-enhanced computed tomography (CT) image (A) through the abdomen shows hepatomegaly with multiple hypoattenuating solid lesions throughout the hepatic parenchyma. Coronal contrast-enhanced CT image (B) through the abdomen demonstrates hepatic lesions but also several hypoattenuating solid lesions in both kidneys. Axial contrast-enhanced CT image (C) through the pelvis shows nodular peritoneal thickening and ascites consistent with peritoneal involvement.

findings: patients may have organ enlargement without lymphomatous infiltration, and vice versa.

Children with abdominal NHL commonly present with gastrointestinal involvement. Lymphomatous involvement of the bowel may appear as hypoechoic bowel wall thickening with loss of stratification on US. Alternatively, it may appear as a complex or hypoechoic mass associated with the bowel, with areas of necrosis, which appear anechoic. Primary renal lymphomas are rare; however, the kidneys may be a secondary site of disease, in which case hypoechoic or anechoic renal masses may be present on US. The gonads may be involved in disseminated disease. The presence of a hypoechoic ovarian mass or a confluent mass occupying the pelvis should suggest ovarian involvement. Hyperemia, discrete hypoechoic nodules, or diffuse replacement of the testicle by a hypoechoic structure may be seen in testicular lymphoma.

CT is particularly useful in the delineation of intraabdominal lymph nodes and any involvement of abdominal viscera. CT findings mirror the aforementioned sonographic findings. As on US, confluent retroperitoneal masses may be seen, sometimes encasing major vessels. CT is likely superior to US in the evaluation of splenic disease. Solitary or multiple low-attenuation, nonenhancing splenic lesions may be seen. Similar findings may be seen in the liver. Omental caking and ascites may be seen in the case of peritoneal involvement (Fig. 6.21). Infiltrated bowel will demonstrate soft tissue attenuation with minimal enhancement and marked bowel wall thickening.

F-18 FDG PET is currently used in children with HD to determine disease stage and to plan radiation therapy. Because childhood NHL demonstrates high cure rates with use of chemotherapy alone, the detection of small-bulk disease is not necessary, and PET should not be performed for disease staging in this population. However, PET is useful for the evaluation of response to therapy. It is important to note that FDG avidity may result from nonmalignant and malignant processes.

Bibliography

Balassy, C., Navarro, O. M., & Daneman, A. (2011). Adrenal masses in children. *Radiologic Clinics of North America, 49*(4), 711–727.

Brisse, H. J., McCarville, M. B., Granata, C., Krug, K. B., Wootton-Gorges, S. L., Kanegawa, K., F0BC International Neuroblastoma Risk Group Project, et al. (2011). Guidelines for imaging and staging of neuroblastic tumors: Consensus report from the International Neuroblastoma Risk Group Project. *Radiology, 261*(1), 243–257.

Chandler, J. C., & Gauderer, M. W. (2004). The neonate with an abdominal mass. *Pediatric Clinics of North America, 51*(4), 979–997.

Choyke, P. L., Hayes, W. S., & Sesterhenn, I. A. (1993). Primary extragonadal germ cell tumors of the retroperitoneum: Differentiation of primary and secondary tumors. *RadioGraphics, 10*(6), 1365–1375.

Chung, E. M., Lattin, Jr, G. E., Cube, R., Lewis, R. B., Marichal-Hernández, C., Shawhan, R., et al. (2011). From the archives of the AFIP: Pediatric liver masses: Radiologic-pathologic correlation. Part 2. Malignant tumors. *RadioGraphics, 31*(2), 483–507.

Faingold, R., Albuquerque, P. A., & Carpineta, L. (2011). Hepatobiliary tumors. *Radiologic Clinics of North America, 49*(4), 679–687.

Gatcombe, H. G., Assikis, V., Kooby, D., & Johnstone, P. A. S. (2004). Primary retroperitoneal teratomas: A review of the literature. *Journal of Surgical Oncology, 86*(2), 107–113.

Geller, E., & Kochan, P. S. (2011). Renal neoplasms of childhood. *Radiologic Clinics of North America, 49*(4), 689–709.

George, A., Mani, V., & Noufal, A. (2014). Update on the classification of hemangioma. *Journal of Oral and Maxillofacial Pathology, 18*, S117–S120.

Golden, C. B., & Feusner, J. H. (2002). Malignant abdominal masses in children: Quick guide to evaluation and diagnosis. *Pediatric Clinics of North America, 49*(6), 1369–1392.

Kalenahalli, K. V., Garg, N., Goolahally, L. N., Reddy, S. P., & Iyengar, J. (2013). Infradiaphragmatic extralobar pulmonary sequestration: Masquerading as suprarenal mass. *Journal of Clinical Neonatology, 2*(3), 146–148.

Kissane, J. M., & Dehner, L. P. (1992). Renal tumors and tumor-like lesions in pediatric patients. *Pediatric Nephrology, 6*(4), 365–382.

Marwede, D., Tillig, E. R., & Hirsch, W. (2008). Imaging findings and differential diagnosis of infradiaphragmatic pulmonary sequestration. *Pediatrics International, 50*(6), 821–823.

McCarville, M. B. (2001). Rhabdomyosarcoma in pediatric patients: The good, the bad, and the unusual. *American Journal of Roentgenology, 176*(6), 1563–1569.

Navarro, O. (2011). Soft tissue masses in children. *Radiologic Clinics of North America, 49*(6), 1235–1259.

Peterson, C. M., Buckley, C., Holley, S., & Menias, C. O. (2012). Teratomas: A multimodality review. *Current Problems in Diagnostic Radiology, 41*(6), 210–219.

Rajiah, P., Sinha, R., Cuevas, C., Dubinsky, T. J., Bush, W. H., Jr., & Kolokythas, O. (2011). Imaging of uncommon retroperitoneal masses. *RadioGraphics, 31*(4), 949–976.

Ranganath, S. H., Lee, E. Y., & Eisenberg, R. L. (2012). Focal cystic abdominal masses in pediatric patients. *American Journal of Roentgenology, 199*(1) W1–W16.

Rha, S., Byun, J., Jung, S., Chun, H. J., Lee, H. G., & Lee, J. M. (2003). Neurogenic tumors in the abdomen: Tumor types and imaging characteristics. *RadioGraphics, 23*(1), 29–43.

Shah, R. U., Lawrence, C., Fickenscher, K. A., Shao, L., & Lowe, L. H. (2011). Imaging of pediatric pelvic neoplasms. *Radiologic Clinics of North America, 49*(4), 729–748.

Towbin, A. J., Meyers, R. L., Woodley, H., Miyazaki, O., Weldon, C. B., Morland, B., et al. (2018). 2017 PRETEXT: Radiologic staging system for primary hepatic malignancies of childhood revised for the Paediatric Hepatic International Tumour Trial (PHITT). *Pediatric Radiology, 48*(4), 536–554.

Van Rijn, R. R., Wilde, J. C., Bras, J., Oldenburger, F., McHugh, K. M. C., & Merks, J. H. M. (2008). Imaging findings in noncraniofacial childhood rhabdomyosarcoma. *Pediatric Radiology, 38*(6), 617–634.

Wells, R. G., & Sty, J. R. (1990). Imaging of sacrococcygeal germ cell tumors. *RadioGraphics, 10*(4), 701–713.

SECTION 3

Genitourinary

CHAPTER 7
Scrotal Pain and Swelling

Amy W. Lai

CHAPTER OUTLINE

Imaging Techniques, 151
Ultrasound Examination Protocol, 151
   What Should I Do If I Cannot Document Flow in
     the Testicles of a Small Child?, 152
   Anatomy and Normal Ultrasound Appearance, 152
Diagnostic Workup, 152
Image Interpretation, 154
   Does the Patient Have Pain?, 154
   Twisted Spermatic Cord, 154
   Nontwisted Spermatic Cord With Normal Testicular
     Vascularity, 155

Nontwisted Spermatic Cord and Increased
   Vascularity, 161
Nontwisted Spermatic Cord and Decreased
   Vascularity, 162
Painless Scrotal Swelling, 163
   Extratesticular Cystic Lesions, 163
   Extratesticular Solid Lesions, 165
   Intratesticular Cystic Lesions, 166
   Intratesticular Solid Lesions, 166
Summary, 170

When a child presents with scrotal pain and swelling, the most important determination is between surgical and nonsurgical causes of the symptoms. This often cannot be differentiated with certainty from the physical examination and clinical history. Imaging can, therefore, be crucial to management.

The term *acute scrotum* refers to sudden-onset scrotal pain, erythema, and/or swelling. The most common causes of acute scrotum are torsion of the spermatic cord, torsion of testicular/epididymal appendages, and epididymitis/epididymo-orchitis. These entities are treated in different ways: surgery for spermatic cord torsion, conservative management for testicular/epididymal appendiceal torsion, and potentially antibiotics for epididymitis. Common causes for the nonacute scrotum include painless scrotal swelling or mass. For nonacute scrotal presentations, imaging can determine the compartment and likely cause of the abnormality, guiding management.

■ Imaging Techniques

Scrotal ultrasound with Doppler is the first-line imaging technique for evaluating the child with scrotal pain and swelling. It is widely available and inexpensive, offers high sensitivity and specificity, requires no radiation, and is a relatively quick examination, avoiding the need for anesthesia.

In the past, technetium-99m scrotal scintigraphy was used to distinguish ischemia from infection. It was well established and predictable, especially in adults. In practice, it is now rarely used because of longer examination times, decreased availability, radiation exposure, and diminished diagnostic capability in young children, who have small genitalia that are difficult to image.

Advanced imaging with magnetic resonance imaging has limited application, especially acutely, given long examination time and limited availability. It does offer lack of ionizing radiation and occasionally can be helpful as an ancillary study in equivocal cases.

■ Ultrasound Examination Protocol

The patient should be supine, with a towel between the thighs lifting and supporting the scrotum. A large amount of warm gel is used to minimize pressure on the skin. High-frequency linear-array transducers are recommended (15-8 MHz for neonates; 8-5 MHz in older boys). The asymptomatic side is evaluated first to optimize ultrasound settings and to allow accurate assessment of the symptomatic side. It is also paramount to obtain a midline grayscale and color Doppler image including both testicles, allowing for a side-by-side comparison of the right and left testicular parenchyma, paratesticular tissues, and vascularity, which should be symmetric. In addition, real-time evaluation of the spermatic cord should be performed along its length in the transverse and longitudinal planes.

The testes should be evaluated in at least two planes, with central, medial, and lateral longitudinal images, as well as superior, mid, and inferior transverse images. Each testicle should be measured in three planes, and a volume should also be calculated. Color Doppler images, including spectral Doppler waveforms, allow evaluation of perfusion. Power Doppler can be used

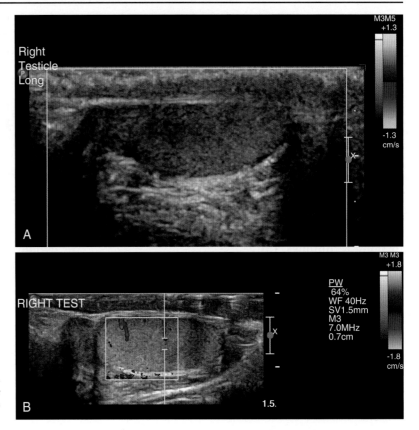

Fig. 7.1 Optimizing Doppler. Initial color Doppler image (A) of the testicle shows limited vascularity of the testicle. Color Doppler was optimized by decreasing the size of the color interrogation box (B).

to increase sensitivity to blood flow. The epididymides should be evaluated, with the head, body, and tail imaged if possible. Scrotal skin thickness and any palpable abnormality should be directly imaged. Additional maneuvers (Valsalva or upright positioning) can be considered.

What Should I Do If I Cannot Document Flow in the Testicles of a Small Child?

It is often challenging to get flow within the testicles of infants and small children. Often the children are not resting still or comfortably, which causes Doppler artifact. Occasionally the emergency department physicians may need to give medication to make a child more comfortable for the examination to be performed. If initial attempts at documenting vascularity to the testicles are not successful, color Doppler and spectral Doppler waveform analysis can be optimized by using a higher-frequency probe or decreasing color box interrogation dimensions (Fig. 7.1).

Anatomy and Normal Ultrasound Appearance

The scrotum is divided into two halves, each containing a testis, epididymis, and spermatic cord. The testis is surrounded by the tunica albuginea, a strong, fibrous connective tissue layer. A fold of this tunica forms the mediastinum of the testis. The tunica vaginalis covers the tunica albuginea and is composed of an outer parietal and inner visceral layer. A small amount of fluid is normally present within the layers. The epididymis is composed of a head, body, and tail, and it is located at the posterolateral aspect of the testis.

Both testes should have a similar volume and shape on grayscale imaging, with smooth echotexture and medium echogenicity. Blood flow on color Doppler should be symmetric. The testicular mediastinum is seen as hyperechoic linear band along the long axis of the testis (Fig. 7.2). The epididymides should have the same or slightly increased echogenicity as the testes, with a triangular or pyramidal head. The spermatic cords are visualized as slightly hypoechoic tubular structures that course through the inguinal canal (Fig. 7.3).

The ultrasound appearance of the scrotum differs in young children compared with adults. The testicles are slightly more hypoechoic in children, with slight increase in echogenicity as the child approaches puberty. The mediastinum may be less visible. The epididymal body and tail can be difficult to see in young children, with only the epididymal head visible along the upper pole of the testis. Finally, the intratesticular vessels can be difficult to visualize with the use of color Doppler in young children.

■ Diagnostic Workup

During the imaging workup of scrotal pain and/or swelling, abnormalities can be divided into intratesticular, extratesticular, and nonscrotal (Table 7.1).

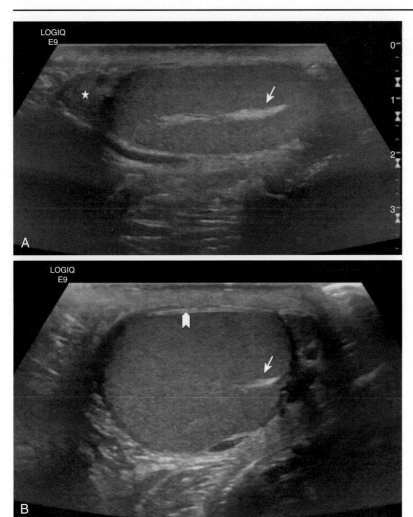

Fig. 7.2 Normal testicular anatomy. Longitudinal (A) and transverse (B) images of a normal left testis demonstrate smooth medium echogenicity. The epididymal head (*star*) has a triangular configuration at the superior pole of the testicle. The echogenic line in the middle of the testis is the mediastinum (*arrow*), a reflection of the tunica albuginea, which manifests as two parallel echogenic lines (*arrowhead*).

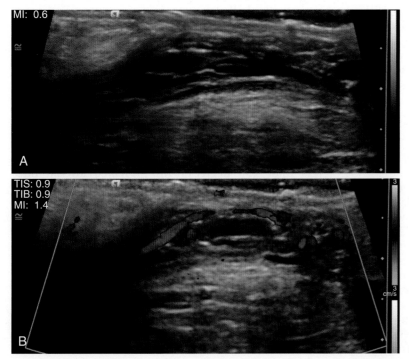

Fig. 7.3 Normal spermatic cord. Grayscale (A) and color Doppler (B) longitudinal images of the spermatic cord. The normal spermatic cord courses straight through the inguinal canal.

TABLE 7.1   Differential Diagnosis of Scrotal Pain and Swelling

INTRATESTICULAR	EXTRATESTICULAR, INTRASCROTAL	NONSCROTAL
Testicular torsion	Torsion of testicular appendages	Renal stone
Trauma	Abnormality of the processus	Appendicitis
• Hematocele	• Vaginalis	Abdominal/pelvic mass
• Fracture	• Hernia	
• Rupture	• Hydrocele	
Epididymitis	Epididymal cyst/spermatocele	
Epididymo-orchitis	Paratesticular mass: rhabdomyosarcoma	
Testicular mass		
Congenital abnormality	Inflammation	
• Asymmetry	• Cellulitis	
• Polyorchidism	• Idiopathic scrotal edema	
• Testicular ectopia	• Vasculitis/Henoch-Schönlein purpura	
	• Idiopathic scrotal fat necrosis	

Intratesticular abnormalities include testicular torsion, trauma, inflammation, masses, and congenital variants. Extratesticular abnormalities include torsion of testicular appendages, epididymitis, epididymal cysts or spermatoceles, hernias, hydroceles, varicoceles, paratesticular masses, and superficial skin lesions. Nonscrotal causative factors for pain include referred pain from renal stones, appendicitis, abdominal or pelvic masses, or neurological issues. These can be considered if the scrotal ultrasound is normal.

■ Image Interpretation

When interpreting a scrotal ultrasound, a few critical questions should be posed to guide us to the correct the diagnosis.

Does the Patient Have Pain?

If the answer is yes, then the differential diagnosis for acute scrotum should be considered (Box 7.1).

Although the acute scrotum can be assessed based on scrotal compartment, an alternative diagnostic pathway focuses first on the appearance of the spermatic cord, followed by an assessment of testicular vascularity (Table 7.2). This is to emphasize the importance of spermatic cord assessment in the setting of acute scrotum.

Twisted Spermatic Cord

The sole diagnosis in the setting of a twisted spermatic cord is *testicular torsion.*

Twisting of the spermatic cord first causes venous and then arterial obstruction. The degree of testicular ischemia is determined by the duration of torsion, as well as the degree of twist, which can range from 180 to 720 degrees.

In the pediatric population, testicular torsion most often occurs in adolescents. Typical presentation in children includes acute-onset scrotal pain, with inguinal and scrotal swelling. One-third of patients will present with nausea and vomiting.

Most cases of testicular torsion arise in patients with an anatomic abnormality known as the "bell-clapper" deformity. Normally, the tunica vaginalis surrounds the

BOX 7.1   Acute Scrotum

Extratesticular
Torsion of the appendix testis
Epididymitis
Hernia
Inflammation
Cellulitis
Idiopathic scrotal edema
Vasculitis/Henoch-Schönlein purpura
Idiopathic scrotal fat necrosis

Intratesticular
Testicular torsion
Trauma
Orchitis and Epididymo-orchitis
Vasculitis

anterior and inferior aspect of the testicle. The epididymis and spermatic cord insertion are not covered by the tunica vaginalis, serving as a point of mesenteric fixation. In the bell-clapper deformity, the tunica extends superior to the spermatic cord, enveloping the epididymis and spermatic cord, allowing increased mobility and twisting of the testis within the tunica. Many of these patients with bell-clapper deformities experience recurrent bouts of acute-onset unilateral pain with spontaneous resolution secondary to incomplete or spontaneously resolving torsion (Box 7.2).

Definitive sonographic evidence of torsion is complete loss of blood flow to the affected testis (Fig. 7.4A). However, with partial testicular torsion the cord twists less than 450 degrees with preserved arterial flow, which may be diminished or even normal relative to the contralateral normal side (Figs. 7.5A and 7.6A), making this a challenging diagnosis. This underscores the value of real-time spermatic cord assessment. In the setting of complete or partial testicular torsion the spermatic cord can have a target, doughnut, or whirlpool appearance depending on the angle of the transducer relative to the point of the torsion (Figs. 7.5B–C and 7.6B). This so-called whirlpool sign is the most sensitive and specific sign for complete and partial testicular torsion. The spermatic cord can also be enlarged and edematous.

TABLE 7.2 Differential diagnosis of acute scrotum based on the appearance of the spermatic cord and testicular vascularity

BOX 7.2 Torsion-Detorsion Sequence or Intermittent Testicular Torsion: What to Look For

Clinical history: recurrent bouts of acute-onset scrotal pain with spontaneous resolution
Spermatic cord abnormality
- Edematous spermatic cord
- +/– Whirlpool appearance

Testicular vascularity
- Normal
- Increased
- Decreased

Scrotal pseudomass located superior to the testicle
Epididymal enlargement and hyperemia

*Important: Patients with torsion-detorsion sequence can present with imaging findings similar to epididymo-orchitis because of reactive hyperemia. Findings that can distinguish torsion-detorsion from epididymo-orchitis include:
1. Twisted spermatic cord (if present)
2. Pseudomass
3. Resolution of symptoms after detorsion

Additional imaging features include normal and symmetric volumes and echogenicity in the first 1 to 3 hours of onset of symptoms. Subsequently the testis becomes edematous and hypoechoic, with development of peritesticular hyperemia and edema. There may be an associated hydrocele and scrotal thickening. The affected testis may have an unusual lie, in which the testicle has a transverse configuration in the longitudinal plane (Fig. 7.4B) (Box 7.3).

In torsion-detorsion sequence or intermittent testicular torsion, testicular blood flow may be decreased, normal, or increased (post-ischemic hyperemia) (Fig. 7.7A–B). Additional findings that support the diagnosis of torsion-detorsion include a boggy, edematous spermatic cord and a pseudomass located superior to the testicle (Fig. 7.7C). A whirlpool sign or twist of the cord may be present if complete detorsion has not occurred. The epididymis may also be enlarged and hyperemic (Fig. 7.7C).

If the spermatic cord is not twisted, an assessment of the testicular vascularity can assist in the differential diagnosis.

Testicular torsion is a surgical emergency. Time is of the essence, with testicular salvage more likely in patients who are detorsed within 4 to 6 hours, and testicular viability dramatically worsened with surgery performed beyond 12 to 24 hours.

Nontwisted Spermatic Cord With Normal Testicular Vascularity

When the spermatic cord is not twisted and the vascularity of the testicle on the side of the patient's pain is normal, primary diagnostic considerations include torsion of a testicular appendage and epididymitis. Other entities to consider include torsion-detorsion sequence and extratesticular causes of pain related to the scrotal

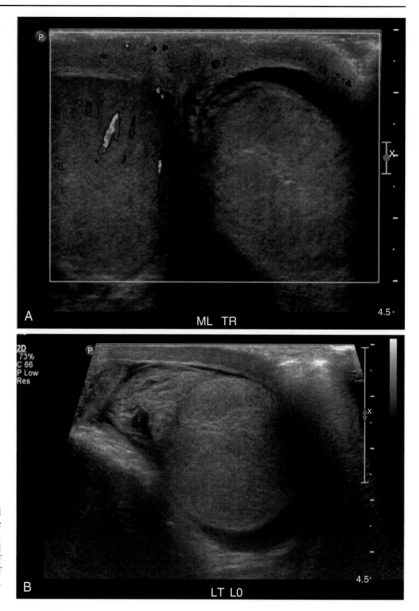

Fig. 7.4 Acute testicular torsion. Eleven-year-old boy with 1 hour of left groin pain. Midline transverse color Doppler image (A) demonstrates an enlarged, heterogeneous left testis with absent vascularity and small left hydrocele. Longitudinal grayscale image of the left testicle (B) shows an abnormal orientation of the testicle, where on this longitudinal image the testicle has a transverse configuration.

skin, such as scrotal cellulitis, idiopathic scrotal edema, and scrotal edema secondary to Henoch-Schönlein purpura (HSP) and Kawasaki disease. Idiopathic scrotal fat necrosis is an uncommon extratesticular cause of pain.

Torsion of the testicular appendages occurs in prepubertal boys. It is the most common cause of acute scrotum in boys 7 to 14 years old. Differentiation of appendiceal torsion from testicular torsion is important because management consists of bed rest and nonsteroidal anti-inflammatory agents rather than surgical exploration.

Testicular appendages are best seen when outlined by scrotal fluid (Fig. 7.8). These pedunculated vascularized tissues are remnants of the embryonic mesonephric and paramesonephric ducts. The appendix testis, also known as the hydatid of Morgagni, is a structure isoechoic to the testis, present in the groove between the epididymis and testis. The appendix epididymis is found at the head of the epididymis. The appendix of the epididymal tail is less commonly identified.

Any of these appendages may twist on their pedicle, leading to ischemia of the appendage. Patients may present with gradual or sudden intense pain, localized at the upper pole of the testis. Clinically, a highly specific physical finding called the "blue dot" sign may be seen, consisting of a firm nodule superior to the testis with bluish discoloration of the overlying skin.

Ultrasound imaging reveals a round, avascular, often reticulated extratesticular mass, usually at the upper pole of the testis, with variable echogenicity depending on the duration of symptoms (Fig. 7.9). The adjacent epididymis is enlarged hyperemic. There may also be edema and hyperemia of the testicle with ongoing duration of symptoms (Fig. 7.10). There may also be a reactive hydrocele and scrotal skin thickening. Importantly, the spermatic cord is not twisted.

Epididymitis has two peaks of prevalence: younger than 2 years and older than 6 years of age. Noninfectious etiologies of epididymitis include trauma, reflux of sterile urine, ectopic insertion of a ureter into a seminal ves-

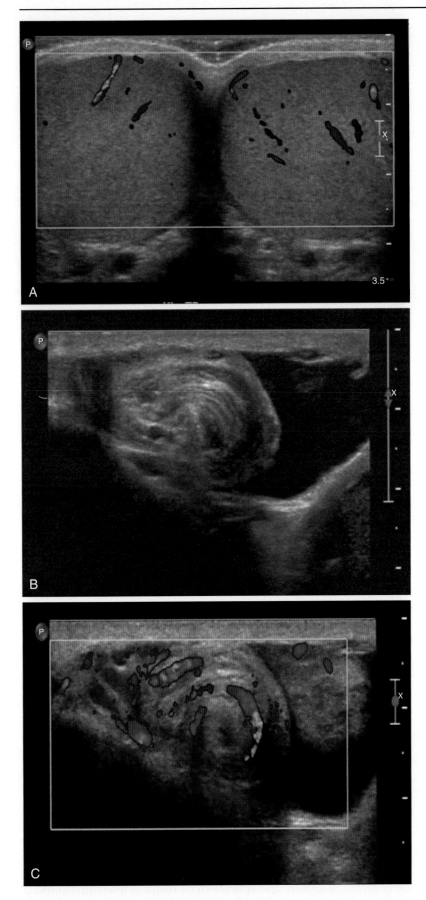

Fig. 7.5 Partial testicular torsion. A 16-year-old boy presented to the emergency department with acute-onset left testicular pain for 90 minutes. Midline transverse color Doppler image (A) shows slightly decreased vascularity of the right testicle relative to the left. Grayscale (B) and color Doppler (C) images through the right spermatic cord show twisting or a "whirlpool" appearance of the spermatic cord, consistent with partial testicular torsion. The patient was found to have a partial torsion and a bell-clapper deformity intraoperatively.

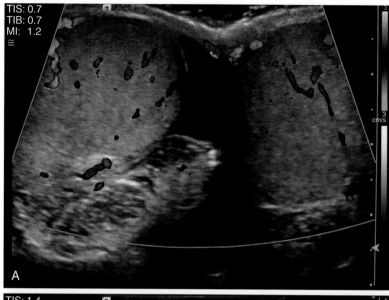

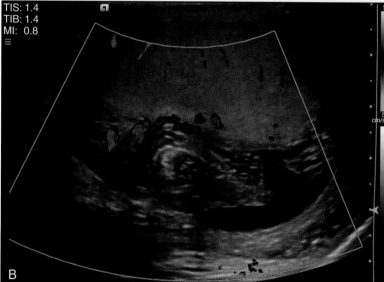

Fig. 7.6 Partial testicular torsion. A 13-year-old boy presented to clinic with 2 hours of acute right testicular pain. Midline transverse color Doppler image demonstrates symmetric vascularity of the right and left testicles (A). Longitudinal color Doppler image of the right testicle (B) shows a "whirlpool" configuration of the right spermatic cord, consistent with partial testicular torsion.

BOX 7.3   Testicular Torsion: What to Look For

Spermatic cord abnormality
- Enlargement and edema
- Target, doughnut, or whirlpool appearance
- Hypoechoic, hyperechoic, or heterogeneous

Asymmetric testicular vascularity
- Complete loss of blood flow to the affected side
- Diminished vascularity

Testicular size and echogenicity
- Enlargement
- Decreased echogenicity

Abnormal testicular orientation
Peritesticular hyperemia and edema
Hydrocele
Scrotal skin thickening

icle or epididymis, reactive changes to adjacent torsion of the testis or of the testicular appendages, and vasculitides, including HSP and Kawasaki disease. Infectious causative agents, such as urinary tract infections, are more common in older patients. The infection usually originates in the bladder or prostate gland and spreads to the epididymis, finally reaching the testis. Epididymitis may also be secondary to viral infection and postviral inflammation. In adolescents, sexually transmitted diseases must also be considered.

Children younger than 2 years with epididymitis should be evaluated for genitourinary anomalies. Known associations include imperforate anus, posterior urethral valves, ectopic ureter, ectopic vas deferens, Müllerian duct cyst, neurogenic bladder, bladder exstrophy, voiding dysfunction, and vesicoureteral reflux. A renal ultrasound is

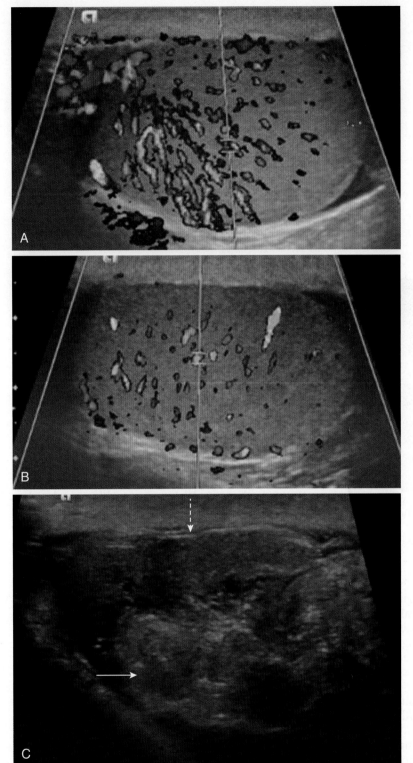

Fig. 7.7 Torsion-detorsion sequence. An 18-year-old boy presented to the emergency department with 2 hours of acute right testicular pain. At the time of imaging, however, he reported resolution of symptoms. Longitudinal color Doppler images of the right (A) and left (B) testicles show asymmetric increased vascularity of the right testicle, the side of his pain. Grayscale image through the right epididymis (C) shows enlargement of the epididymis (*dashed arrow*) and an echogenic pseudomass adjacent to the head of the epididymis (*arrow*). The findings of increased vascularity of the affected testicle, edematous epididymis, and pseudomass, with clinical history, support the diagnosis of torsion-detorsion sequence, or intermittent testicular torsion.

a good first-line study, with a voiding cystourethrogram to follow as clinically indicated.

Imaging features of epididymitis include an enlarged, hypervascular epididymis and a normal spermatic cord (Fig. 7.10B–C). Rarely blood flow to the testis may be decreased when edema from epididymitis compromises testicular blood flow. A reactive hydrocele and scrotal skin thickening are associated findings.

Imaging features of epididymitis may not point to the underlying etiology. In these cases, clinical history and features can be helpful. Acute infectious epididymitis may present with fever, dysuria, and laboratory evidence of leukocytosis or urinary tract infection. Epididymitis secondary to HSP may present with concurrent lower-extremity purpuric rash or arthritis. Epididymitis as a complication of Kawasaki disease should present with

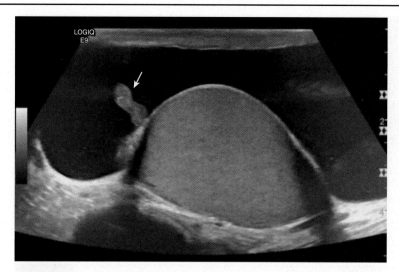

Fig. 7.8 Hydrocele and appendix testis. Ultrasound of a newborn with scrotal swelling shows a right hydrocele surrounding the testicle. The appendix testis is seen arising from the superior pole of the testicle (*arrow*). Note the posterior attachment of the testicle to the tunica vaginalis.

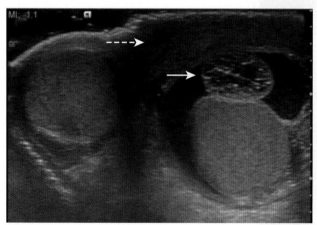

Fig. 7.9 Torsion of the appendix testis. A 5-year-old presented to the emergency department with left scrotal pain. Midline transverse image shows a reticulated structure (*arrow*) adjacent to the superior pole of the left testicle, consistent with torsion of the appendix testis. There is also scrotal skin thickening (*dashed arrow*) and a small hydrocele (arrowhead).

history of high-grade fever and may present with concurrent conjunctival injection and oropharyngeal changes.

As stated earlier, *torsion-detorsion sequence,* or intermittent testicular torsion, may present sonographically with a nontwisted spermatic cord, if complete detorsion has occurred. Blood flow to the affected side can be normal after detorsion.

The cause of acute scrotum may be limited to the scrotal skin. Etiologies include acute idiopathic scrotal edema, HSP, and cellulitis.

Acute idiopathic scrotal edema is less frequent than epididymitis, testicular torsion, or appendiceal torsion, but it is an important consideration in acute scrotum. The cause is not completely known but is hypothesized to be secondary to a hypersensitivity reaction. Clinically, patients present with scrotal pain and discomfort. Pain can be severe. On physical examination there is unilateral or bilateral scrotal erythema and swelling that can extend to the perineum and the inguinal regions. This benign, self-limited condition is managed with nonsteroidal anti-inflammatory drugs and antibiotics and tends to resolve in 3 to 5 days.

On ultrasound, there is thickening of the scrotal skin, which may be homogeneous or striated in appearance. The "fountain sign" describes the pronounced vascularity seen on transverse color Doppler images (Fig. 7.11). Importantly, the testes and paratesticular tissues are normal in volume, grayscale appearance, and vascularity. The spermatic cords are normal. Small hydroceles may be present.

Henoch-Schonlein purpura (HSP) is a systemic small-vessel immunoglobulin A–mediated vasculitis usually affecting patients younger than 20 years. Thirty percent of patients with HSP will present with scrotal symptoms of pain and swelling. In addition to epididymitis and epididymo-orchitis, other scrotal manifestations of HSP include isolated scrotal edema and, rarely, spermatic cord edema and hematoma. Although the classic presentation is that of a lower-extremity rash with abdominal pain and arthritis, we should keep in mind that scrotal symptoms can occur simultaneous with or precede other clinical findings.

Kawasaki disease is a small- to medium-vessel vasculitis that clinically presents with conjunctival inflammation, lymphadenitis, high fever not responsive to antibiotics, oral inflammation (strawberry tongue), and palmar erythema and desquamation. Scrotal involvement can occur, which can include epididymitis, epididymo-orchitis, orchitis, and isolated scrotal edema.

Idiopathic scrotal fat necrosis is a benign entity seen only in children. There is no intrascrotal fat in a normal adult man. Prepubescent boys have fatty tissue in the scrotum. The fat normally regresses during puberty, and the blood supply becomes tenuous during this process. Superimposed cold-related vasoconstriction may be enough to cause the fat to become ischemic. The typical patient is an overweight prepubescent boy with recent exposure to cold, usually through swimming. Patients report mild to moderate pain (never severe), with a usual duration of 2 to 3 days before seeking treatment. There are typically no urinary symptoms, systemic symptoms, or history of trauma.

Ultrasound imaging reveals bilateral echogenic scrotal masses separate and inferior to the testes, with posterior acoustic shadowing. On occasion, involvement may be unilateral. The testes and epididymides are

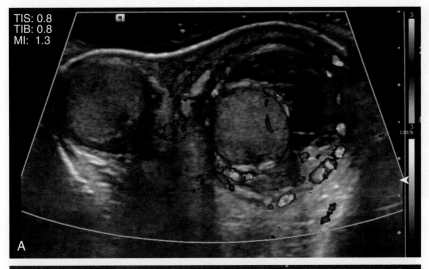

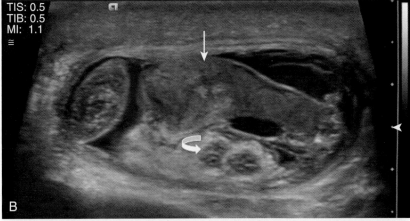

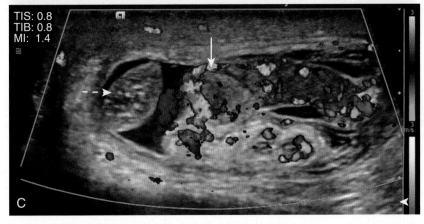

Fig. 7.10 Torsion of the appendix testis with reactive epididymitis and orchitis. A 7-year-old boy presented with left scrotal pain and swelling. A midline transverse color Doppler image (A) shows a small complex left hydrocele, with increased vascularity of the left paratesticular tissues and left tunica albuginea. Longitudinal grayscale (B) and color Doppler (C) images though the epididymis show epididymal enlargement and hyperemia (*arrow*). An avascular reticulated structure is seen adjacent to the epididymal head consistent with torsion of the appendix testis (*dashed arrow*). Note the edema of the spermatic cord (*curved arrow*).

normal in grayscale and Doppler appearance. The scrotal wall is usually normal but may be erythematous or edematous.

Nontwisted Spermatic Cord and Increased Vascularity

When the spermatic cord is not twisted, and there is increased vascularity of the testicle on the side of the patient's pain, primary diagnostic considerations include epididymo-orchitis, orchitis, torsion-detorsion sequence, and torsion of a testicular appendage.

When considering the differential diagnosis for *epididymo-orchitis*, one can refer to the differential diagnosis for epididymitis. Epididymal inflammation and infection can result in subsequent testicular inflammation and infection. Sonographic features of epididymo-orchitis are similar to those of epididymitis, with the exception that the affected testicle will be hyperemic. With ongoing inflammation, the testicle may become heterogeneous. Rarely, intratesticular abscess may develop. In addition, severe epididymo-orchitis can result in testicular infarction secondary to compromise of blood flow as a result of increased testicular pressure (Box 7.4).

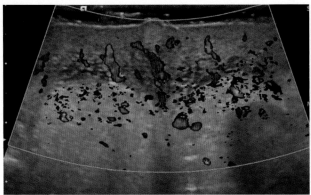

Fig. 7.11 Idiopathic scrotal edema. A 6-year-old with exquisite bilateral scrotal pain and swelling. Midline transverse color Doppler image of the testicle shows marked scrotal skin swelling with increased vascularity.

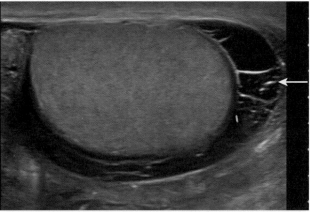

Fig. 7.12 Hematocele. The patient fell off a ladder 4 days ago. Longitudinal grayscale images of the left hemiscrotum. A complex fluid collection with septations is present within the scrotal sac, consistent with a subacute hematocele.

BOX 7.4	Epididymitis and Epididymo-orchitis: What to Look For

Epididymis
- Enlarged
- Hyperemic
- Hypoechoic, hyperechoic, or heterogeneous

Testicular vascularity
- Normal
- Increased if orchitis

Reactive hydrocele

Scrotal skin thickening

Etiology:
1. Systemic symptoms: infectious causes, vasculitis
2. Trauma: traumatic epididymitis
3. Reactive: torsion of testicular appendage
4. Presentation <2 years of age: ectopic insertion of ureter

Isolated *orchitis* in the pediatric population is less common than epididymitis and epididymo-orchitis. It is usually secondary to viral infection (Epstein-Barr virus, adenovirus, coxsackie virus, and mumps). Isolated orchitis may also be secondary to Kawasaki disease.

Torsion-detorsion sequence, or intermittent testicular torsion, may present sonographically with a nontwisted spermatic cord and testicular and epididymal hyperemia. The presence of both epididymal and testicular hyperemia may lead to the diagnosis of epididymo-orchitis; however, the presence of a boggy and edematous cord, as well as the clinical absence of pain at the time of imaging, should point to the correct diagnosis of torsion-detorsion.

Nontwisted Spermatic Cord and Decreased Vascularity

When the spermatic cord is not twisted and there is decreased vascularity of the testicle on the side of the patient's pain, diagnostic considerations include scrotal trauma, for which the correct history should be elicited, and testicular infarction, which can be secondary to epididymitis, epididymo-orchitis, orchitis, and trauma.

Scrotal trauma can be blunt or penetrating, and can result in hematocele, hematoma, testicular fracture, testicular rupture, epididymitis, and posttraumatic torsion and hernias. Although diagnosis is simplified in the setting of a clear clinical history, children, especially younger children, may be unable to provide a reliable history. Minor trauma is common in children.

A *hematocele* is a posttraumatic, avascular scrotal fluid collection between the visceral and parietal tunica vaginalis. In the acute setting, it is hyperechoic due to blood products. Over time the blood products evolve, and the fluid becomes hypoechoic, sometimes with low-level echoes or fluid–fluid levels. Chronic hematoceles may demonstrate septations (Fig. 7.12).

Testicular hematomas are avascular focal collections. They may be single or multiple and variable in size and echogenicity (Fig. 7.13). In the acute setting, they may be isoechoic to testicular parenchyma, and therefore suspected hematomas should be reassessed 12 to 24 hours after initial evaluation. If superinfected, they may develop a hyperemic rim. Testicular hematomas should be followed to resolution because of the risk of infection and necrosis. Large intratesticular hematomas are explored and drained to prevent pressure necrosis and atrophy. In addition, focal testicular lesions should be followed until resolution to exclude tumor.

Testicular fracture sonographically appears as a linear hypoechoic band extends across the parenchyma. The overall testicular contour remains smooth, and the normal ovoid shape of the testicle is maintained. Assessment of vascularity is important. Testicular fracture is treated conservatively when vascularity is normal. Decreased or absent flow is a sign of ischemia and an indication for surgery.

Testicular rupture is the most severe manifestation of testicular trauma and can lead to ischemic necrosis, abscess formation, and posttraumatic autoimmune infertility. Emergent surgery is indicated, which allows for testicular salvage and prevention of complications in most cases. The tunica albuginea, which is normally seen as two parallel hyperechoic lines surrounding the testis, is disrupted, and testicular contour becomes irregular and bulges into the scrotal sac. Testicular echotexture becomes heterogeneous and may contain focal hypoechoic or

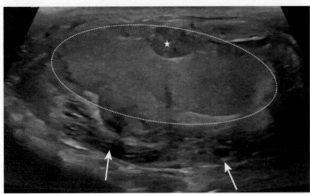

Fig. 7.13 Testicular hematoma. Eighteen-year-old with testicular trauma. Longitudinal images of the right testicle. Dotted line outlines the testis. There is subcapsular hematoma (*star*) and paratesticular hematoma (*arrows*). (Image courtesy Summer Kaplan, MD, Children's Hospital of Philadelphia)

hyperechoic collections representing infarct and hematoma. The testis may demonstrate increased, decreased, or complete lack of blood flow. In practice, a large hematocele may obscure visualization of the tunica albuginea, and therefore surgical exploration is indicated in cases of strong clinical suspicion of testicular rupture.

Notably, testicular trauma can result in epididymitis and testicular torsion because of forceful cremasteric contraction in patients with a bell-clapper deformity.

Painless Scrotal Swelling

If the patient does not have pain, then the differential diagnosis for painless scrotal swelling should be considered (Box 7.5). The differential diagnosis can be further narrowed based on scrotal compartment (extratesticular or intratesticular) and by sonographic appearance ("cystic" versus solid).

Extratesticular Cystic Lesions
By far, the most common cause of painless scrotal swelling is *hydrocele*. It is an abnormal collection (>1–2 mL) of fluid between the visceral and parietal layers of the tunica vaginalis. Hydroceles in neonates are usually congenital and related to a patent processus vaginalis.

Sonographically a hydrocele appears as anechoic fluid collection surrounding the anterolateral testis (Fig. 7.8). On occasion, low-level swirling echoes may be seen, related to protein aggregation or cholesterol crystals. It should not have a mass effect on the testis.

A spectrum of congenital hydroceles may be seen, depending on the closure of the processus vaginalis. The communicating hydrocele involves a completely open processus vaginalis, with fluid freely extending between the abdominal and scrotal cavities. In the funicular hydrocele, the portion of the processus closest to the testis closes, but communication with the abdominal cavity persists. In the encysted hydrocele (also known as the spermatic cord cyst), the processus vaginalis closes above the testis but below the internal inguinal ring, trapping fluid at the spermatic cord, with no communication between the abdominal and scrotal cavities (Fig. 7.14). A rare entity is the abdominoscrotal hydrocele, in which a large scrotal hydrocele extends through the inguinal canal

---

BOX 7.5   Painless Scrotal Swelling

Extratesticular
Cystic
Hydrocele
Hernia[a]
Epididymal cyst
Spermatocele
Varicocele

Solid
Paratesticular mass
Meconium periorchitis
Polyorchidism
Testicular ectopia

Intratesticular
Cystic
Epidermoid cyst (note: can appear solid)
Cystic dysplasia of the rete testis

Solid
Testicular tumor
Testicular size asymmetry

[a]May present with pain.

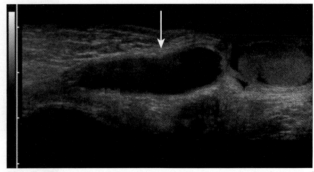

Fig. 7.14 Encysted hydrocele of the cord. Longitudinal image of the left inguinal region in an 8-week-old with a palpable left groin lesion shows a fluid collection (*arrow*) located above the testicle and contained within the inguinal canal, consistent with a hydrocele of the cord.

into the abdomen, creating an hourglass or dumbbell appearance.

Most congenital hydroceles resolve without treatment by 2 years of age. However, spermatic cord and abdominoscrotal hydroceles are usually managed surgically.

Hydroceles in older children and adolescents are usually secondary to inflammation, torsion, trauma, or tumor. A new hydrocele in an older child that is not associated with obvious trauma or inflammation can be a sign of paratesticular rhabdomyosarcoma, and careful evaluation for soft-tissue nodularity should be performed.

Indirect inguinal hernias, with herniation of bowel, omentum, and/or mesentery through a patent processus vaginalis may present with painless swelling. Inguinal hernias are more common in premature infants, because the processus vaginalis has not yet fused. Right-sided hernias are more common, because the right processus vaginalis closes later than the left. The physical examination is often sufficient to diagnose the hernia. Ultrasound is used in cases of inconclusive physical examination, acute scrotum, and to evaluate for contralateral hernia.

Ultrasound images reveal a tubular fluid- or air-filled structure with peristalsis, sometimes with surrounding fluid. If abdominal fat is involved, the mass may appear complex and echogenic.

Patients may present with pain in the setting of the strangulation. An akinetic dilated loop of bowel is a spe-cific sign of strangulation and is an indication for urgent surgery. Pain may also ensue if there is significant mass effect on the testicle, with alteration of blood flow to the testicle (Fig. 7.15).

Epididymal cysts and *spermatoceles* may come to medi-cal attention as palpable lesions. They have an identical

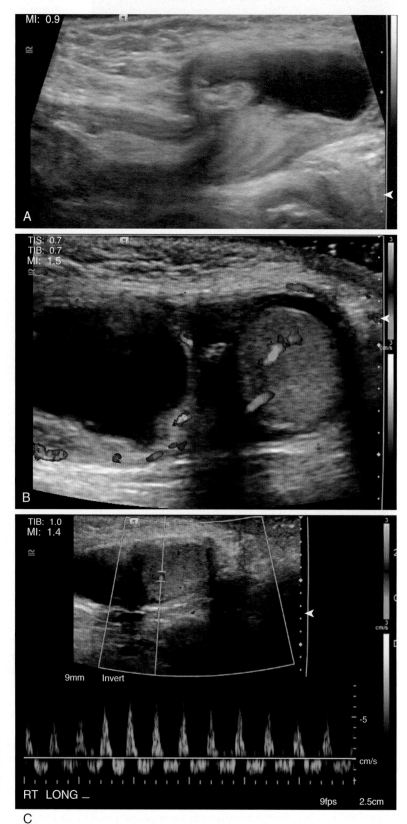

Fig. 7.15 Inguinal hernia. A 3-year-old presented to the emergency department with acute-onset right scrotal pain and swelling. Longitudinal images of the right groin (A) and right hemiscrotum (B) show a loop of bowel extending into the right inguinal canal and right hemiscrotum with mass effect on the right testi-cle with resultant vascular compromise, as shown by reversal of diastolic flow (C).

sonographic appearance, consisting of a simple or septated thin-walled, anechoic or hypoechoic lesion with no internal vascularity and increased through transmission. Epididymal cysts can be seen anywhere along the epididymis. Spermatoceles occur after puberty and are present only at the epididymal head.

Varicoceles are seen in adolescents and young adults. They consist of abnormal dilation of the spermatic cord pampiniform plexus veins. Patients may present with scrotal swelling and sometimes a sensation of pain or heaviness, worse when upright or straining. Grayscale imaging demonstrates multiple tortuous, tubular, anechoic structures along the spermatic cord, measuring greater than 3 mm. These dilated veins demonstrate blood flow with color Doppler imaging that augments with Valsalva maneuver (Fig. 7.16).

Assessment of testicular volumes is important, because the size of the testicle ipsilateral to the varicocele can have a decreased volume. Treatment is controversial and usually reserved for cases that are symptomatic, bilateral, or involve testicular growth arrest or abnormal semen analysis. Care should be taken in patients with right-sided, sudden-onset, or nonreducible varicoceles. These may be caused by a retroperitoneal neoplasm obstructing the testicular vein drainage into the renal vein on the left or inferior vena cava on the right. In this setting, renal sonography would be recommended for further assessment.

Extratesticular Solid Lesions

As in adults, most paratesticular masses are benign. *Paratesticular rhabdomyosarcoma*, however, is an import-

ant exception and is the most common extratesticular tumor in children. Paratesticular rhabdomyosarcomas originate from mesenchymal tissues of the spermatic cord, epididymis, testis, and testicular tunics. Most present in the first two decades of life, with peak incidence in the 1- to 5-year age range.

The clinical presentation is usually short in duration, with a few weeks of unilateral, painless scrotal swelling without fever. Metastases at presentation are fairly common, with lymph node metastases seen in a third of cases, and hematogenous metastases to the lungs, liver, and bone marrow seen in 20% of cases.

Ultrasound imaging demonstrates a hypervascular, hypoechoic, or hyperechoic solid mass that surrounds or invades the epididymis and testis (Fig. 7.17). There may be an associated hydrocele.

Other rare paratesticular tumors include lymphoma and neuroblastoma (Fig. 7.18).

Meconium periorchitis can present as soft hydrocele in a neonate but also as a hard palpable painless mass in neonates and young children as old as 5 years. It is the result of in utero bowel perforation with passage of meconium through a patent processus vaginalis. Meconium incites an inflammatory process with subsequent peritesticular calcification. Characteristic sonographic findings of meconium periorchitis include one or more calcified intrascrotal extratesticular masses (Fig. 7.19A). Calcifications can also be seen along the course of the spermatic cord. Sonographic findings can raise suspicion for other paratesticular aggressive lesions, such

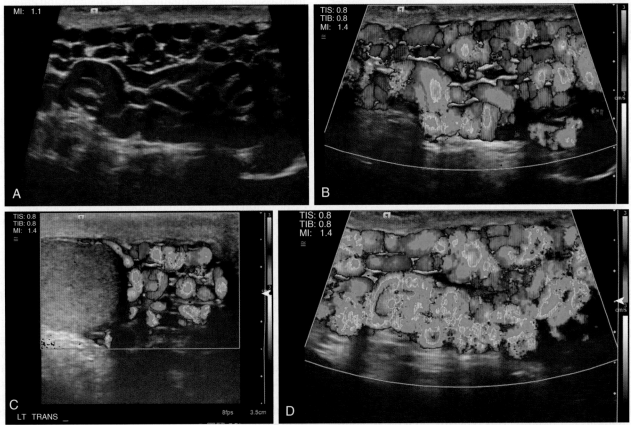

Fig. 7.16 Varicocele. A 17-year-old boy presented for imaging after his pediatrician felt a palpable lesion along the lateral aspect of the left hemiscrotum on physical examination. Longitudinal grayscale image (A) demonstrates several dilated tubular structures along the lateral aspect of the left hemiscrotum, which fill in with color Doppler imaging (B, C). With Valsalva maneuver, there is augmentation of flow (D).

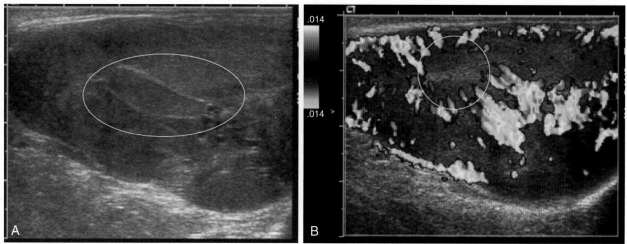

Fig. 7.17 Paratesticular rhabdomyosarcoma. A 3-year-old boy with scrotal swelling. Longitudinal grayscale (A) and color Doppler images (B) reveal a large vascular mass surrounding the testicle. The testicle can be identified by the echogenic line representing the tunica albuginea (*oval*) in (A) and the mediastinum testes (*circle*) in (B).

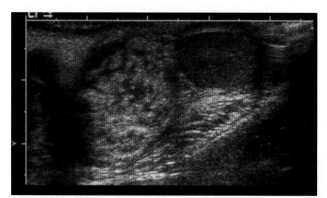

Fig. 7.18 Neuroblastoma. A 2-year-old boy presented to the emergency department with painless left scrotal swelling. An echogenic mass is seen superior to the left testicle (*arrow*). A biopsy revealed neuroblastoma.

as rhabdomyosarcoma and neuroblastoma; however, imaging of the upper abdomen may demonstrate meconium peritonitis with punctate peritoneal calcifications supporting the diagnosis of meconium periorchitis (Fig. 7.19B). Patients with meconium periorchitis should be evaluated for cystic fibrosis because of the association between in utero bowel perforation and cystic fibrosis.

Developmental variants can also present as painless scrotal enlargement and unilateral scrotal mass. Polyorchidism, secondary to abnormal division of the genital ridge resulting in multiple testes on one side of the scrotum, more commonly left sided, can also present as a unilateral mass. The supernumerary testis is usually smaller than the normal testes, but typically has a similar grayscale appearance. Testicular ectopia, secondary to abnormal descent of a testicle, results in two testicles in the same hemiscrotum or ipsilateral inguinal canal.

Intratesticular Cystic Lesions

The most common benign testicular neoplasm is the epidermoid cyst, a lesion composed of keratinized squamous epithelium. This typically presents in young adults. This entity is called a cyst but has a variable appearance and may appear solid. The most characteristic appearance is of a well-defined, avascular mass with an "onion skin" appearance of alternating hypoechoic and hyperechoic rings (Fig. 7.20).

Cystic dysplasia of the rete testis has an appearance similar to tubular ectasia of the rete testis seen in adults, but it arises from a developmental failure of fusion between the efferent ducts and the rete testis rather than obstruction. Ipsilateral renal anomalies, such as renal agenesis, multicystic dysplastic kidney, and renal dysplasia, are common associated abnormalities. The rete testis and efferent ducts dilate with subsequent parenchymal atrophy. On imaging, multiple small cysts are located at the mediastinum (Fig. 7.21). The appearance can mimic testicular microlithiasis or a cystic neoplasm, such as a teratoma. Mucoid-filled cysts can mimic a solid mass. The presence of an associated renal anomaly is helpful in differentiating cystic dysplasia of the testes from a solid mass.

Other cystic testicular lesions, including intratesticular simple cysts, tubular ectasia of the rete testis, tunica albuginea cyst, intratesticular varicocele, and intratesticular spermatocele, are seen more often in adults than in children. Intratesticular cysts are problematic because they can be difficult to differentiate from cystic neoplasms. If a cystic lesion has any solid components and does not have classic imaging features of an epidermoid cyst, it must be considered malignant until proven otherwise.

Intratesticular Solid Lesions

The typical presentation of a *testicular tumor* is as a hard, painless scrotal mass. On occasion the presenting symptom can be a sensation of fullness or heaviness in the lower abdomen and scrotum. Pain is a less common presenting symptom, seen in only 10%, and typically seen in association with hemorrhage or infarction. Testicular tumors are much less common in children than in adults. The incidence in children has been reported at 0.5 to 2 per 100,000 children, accounting for about 1% of all pediatric solid tumors. There are two peaks of prevalence: before 3 years of age and after puberty.

Testicular tumors include germ cell and nongerm cell tumors. Germ cell tumors include seminoma, embryonal

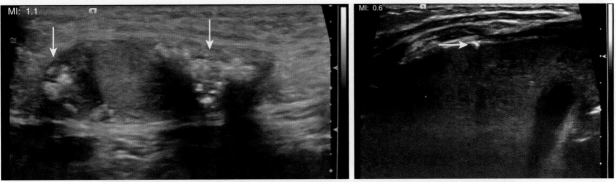

Fig. 7.19 Meconium periorchitis. A 3-month-old boy presented with a hard palpable right scrotal mass. After evaluation at an outside institution, the mother was told that her son would need an orchiectomy for this mass. Longitudinal grayscale image (A) shows several echogenic foci (*arrows*), some associated with posterior acoustic shadowing, along the superior and inferior aspect of the testicle. Abdominal ultrasound (B) shows a calcification along the liver (*arrow*). Sonographic findings are consistent with meconium periorchitis.

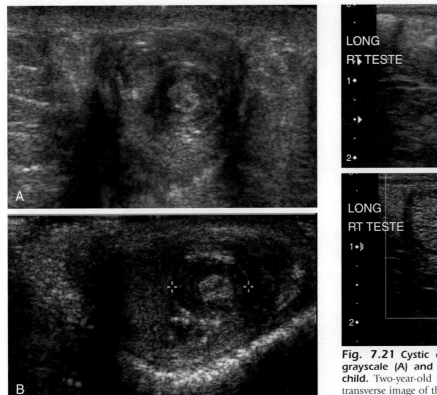

Fig. 7.20 Epidermoid cyst. Transverse (A) and longitudinal (B) images of the left testicle show an intratesticular ovoid lesion consisting of alternating hyperechoic and hypoechoic rings. Image features are typical of an epidermoid cyst.

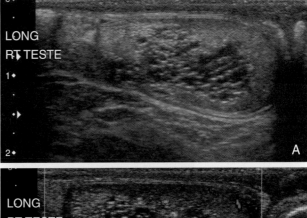

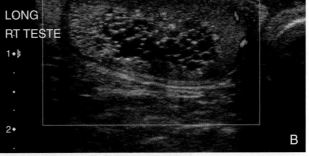

Fig. 7.21 Cystic dysplasia of the rete testis. Longitudinal grayscale (A) and color doppler (B) images in a 7-year-old child. Two-year-old with painless right scrotal swelling. Midline transverse image of the scrotum (A) shows marked asymmetrical enlargement of a heterogeneous right testicle. Longitudinal grayscale (B) and color Doppler (C) images of the right testicle show a slightly hyperechoic intratesticular mass (*arrows*) that is hypervascular. Pathology revealed a yolk sac tumor.

carcinoma, yolk sac tumor, choriocarcinoma, teratoma, and mixed germ cell tumor. Nongerm cell tumors include sex cord and stromal tumors, lymphoma/leukemia, and metastases from neuroblastoma, Wilms tumors, and retinoblastoma. In children, the most common testicular neoplasm by far is the yolk sac tumor, representing 80% of all pediatric testicular neoplasms, followed by teratomas and stromal tumors. Teratomas are benign in prepubertal boys. Seminomas are not seen in prepubertal boys.

Sonographic features of yolk sac tumor are typically a large homogenous mass, replacing much of the testicular parenchyma. Color Doppler imaging demonstrates marked hyperemia (Fig. 7.22). Teratomas appear as mixed solid and cystic lesions, with occasional calcifications (Fig. 7.23).

When bilateral intratesticular solid masses are present, lymphoma and leukemia are the primary diagnostic considerations. Although lymphoma represents only 5% of testicular tumors, it is the most common cause of bilateral testicular masses. Leukemia can affect the testes as a site of recurrence, because the testes can serve as a sanctuary from chemotherapy, as a result of the blood–testis barrier. Sonographic findings include focal or diffuse hypoechoic or hyperechoic masses, which can be unilateral or bilateral, often with testicular enlargement. Blood flow is increased at site of leukemic infiltration (Fig. 7.24).

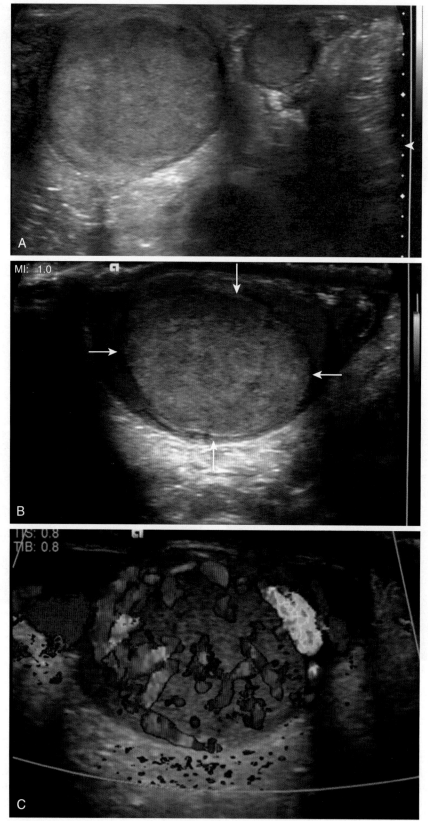

Fig. 7.22 Yolk sac tumor. A 2-year-old with painless right scrotal swelling. Midline transverse image of the scrotum (A) shows marked asymmetric enlargement of a heterogeneous right testicle. Longitudinal grayscale (B) and color Doppler (C) images of the right testicle show a slightly hyperechoic intratesticular mass (*arrows*) that is hypervascular. Pathology revealed a yolk sac tumor.

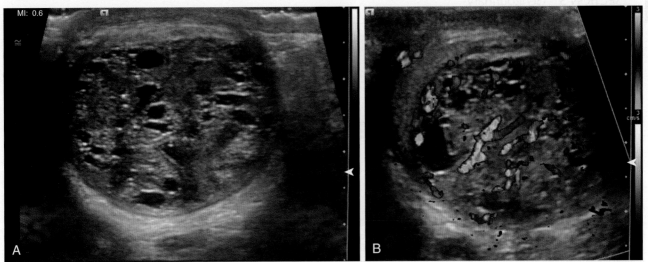

Fig. 7.23 Teratoma. A 2-year-old boy presented to the emergency department with painless scrotal swelling. Longitudinal (A) and transverse color Doppler (B) images show a mixed solid and cystic vascular intratesticular mass. An orchiectomy was performed; pathology revealed a teratoma.

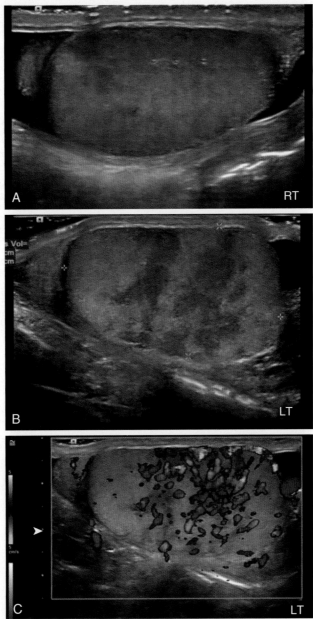

Fig. 7.24 Leukemia. A 14-year-old boy presenting to the emergency department for scrotal fullness and heaviness. Longitudinal grayscale images of the right and left testicles (A, B) show heterogeneity of both testicles. More well-defined hypoechoic bands are seen in the left testicle, with increased vascularity on color Doppler imaging (C).

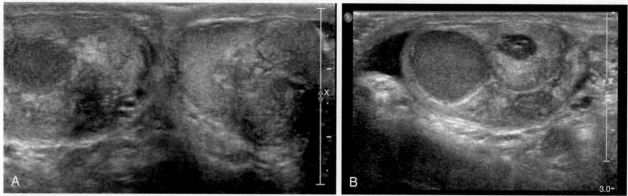

Fig. 7.25 **Testicular adrenal rests.** A 15-year-old boy with hypertension, short stature, and history of precocious puberty. On physical examination the endocrinologist noted enlarged testicles bilaterally, leading to a scrotal ultrasound. Midline transverse grayscale image (A) and longitudinal grayscale image of the right testicle (B) demonstrate multiple hypoechoic, isoechoic, and hyperechoic intratesticular masses. A differential diagnosis of lymphoma, leukemia, and tuberculosis was provided. Endocrine workup revealed 11β-hydroxylase deficiency. Testicular lesions were attributed to testicular adrenal rests in the setting of long-standing untreated congenital adrenal hyperplasia.

A rare but known cause of bilateral testicular masses are testicular adrenal rest tumors seen in patients with congenital adrenal hyperplasia and occasionally Cushing syndrome. Adrenal rests are trapped in the gonads during development and enlarge in response to elevated adrenocorticotropic hormone, creating testicular adrenal rest tumors. The lesions are typically multiple, bilateral, and can be hyperechoic, isoechoic, or hypoechoic with associated hyperemia (Fig. 7.25). Lesions are typically centered around the mediastinum. The clinical history is important in suggesting this diagnosis.

■ Summary

In conclusion, scrotal pain and swelling are a common complaint with many possible causes, some of which require surgical management. Ultrasound imaging in combination with clinical history can be a powerful guide to the most appropriate treatment for the child. In the setting of acute scrotum, real-time assessment of the spermatic cord is necessary to make the correct diagnosis, particularly in cases of partial and intermittent testicular torsion.

Bibliography

Applegate, K. E. (2009). Evidence-based diagnosis of malrotation and volvulus. *Pediatric Radiology, 39*(Suppl. 2), S161–S163.

Applegate, K. E., Anderson, J. M., & Klatte, E. C. (2006). Intestinal malrotation in children: A problem-solving approach to the upper gastrointestinal series. *RadioGraphics, 26*, 1485–1500.

Buonomo, C. (1997). Neonatal gastrointestinal emergencies. *Radiol Clin North Am, 35*(4), 845–864.

Chao, H. -C., Kong, M. -S., Chen, J. -Y., Lin, S. J., & Lin, J. N. (2000). Sonographic features related to volvulus in neonatal intestinal malrotation. *J Ultrasound Med, 19*, 371–376.

Herliczek, T. W., Raghavan, D., McCarten, K., & Wallach, M. (2011). Sonographic upper gastrointestinal series in the vomiting infant: How we do it. *J Clin Imaging Sci, 1*, 19.

Hernanz-Schulman, M. (2009). Pyloric stenosis: Role of imaging. *Pediatric Radiology, 39*(Suppl. 2), S134–S139.

Maxfield, C. M., Bartz, B. H., & Shaffer, J. L. (2013). A pattern-based approach to bowel obstruction in the newborn. *Pediatric Radiology, 43*, 318–329.

Nayak, G. K., Levin, T. L., Kurian, J., Kohli, A., Borenstein, S. H., & Goldman, H. S. (2014). Bedside upper gastrointestinal series in critically ill low birth weight infants. *Pediatric Radiology, 44*, 1252–1257.

Raske etal. (August 2015). ACR appropriateness criteria vomiting in infants up to 3 months of age. https://www.jacr.org/article/S1546-1440(15)00443-3/fulltext

Ryan, S., & Donoghue, V. (2010). Gastrointestinal pathology in neonates: New imaging strategies. *Pediatric Radiology, 40*, 927–931.

Yousefzadeh, D. K., Kang, L., & Tessicini, L. (2010). Assessment of retromesenteric position of the third portion of the duodenum: An US feasibility study in 33 newborns. *Pediatric Radiology, 40*, 1476–1484.

CHAPTER 8

Imaging Approach to Urinary Tract Dilation

Jeanne S. Chow

CHAPTER OUTLINE

How Do We Evaluate Urinary Tract Dilation?, 171
  Ultrasound, 171
  Dynamic Renal Scintigraphy, 175
  Magnetic Resonance Urography, 177
  Tests for Vesicoureteral Reflux: Voiding
    Cystourethrogram, Radionuclide Cystogram, and
    Contrast-Enhanced Voiding Urosonography, 178
  Computed Tomography, 179

Differential Diagnosis and Treatment, 179
  Hydronephrosis: Ureteropelvic Junction Obstruction
    (UPJO), 180
  Hydroureteronephrosis: Obstruction, Reflux, or
    Both, 180
  Duplex Kidneys, Ectopic Ureters, and Ureteroceles, 182
  Bladder Outlet Obstructions: Neurogenic Bladder,
    Posterior Urethral Valves, a Posterior Urethral
    Valve Mimic, and Prune Belly Syndrome, 186

Key point: Distinguishing normal from pathological causes of urinary tract dilation (UTD) is one of the most important topics in pediatric uroradiology. Most etiologies of UTD in children are congenital.

Understanding UTD is one of the primary indications for radiological evaluation of the urinary tract in fetuses and children. Most causes of UTD in children are congenital and are first detected in utero. Routine antenatal ultrasound (US) has led to the detection of UTD of 1% to 2% of fetuses. Many of these children are followed after birth. However, 70% to 80% of fetal UTD resolves and requires no further imaging. Thus distinguishing the normal appearance, the abnormal appearance, and the causes of abnormal UTD is an important subject in pediatric uroradiology.

This chapter outlines the normal appearance of the urinary tract, the congenital causes of abnormal UTD, and the tests used in distinguishing the causes and severity of disease. The common treatments, medical and surgical, will also be described so that the radiologist can be familiar with the outcomes of their diagnoses.

Many descriptive terms have been used to describe UTD, including hydronephrosis, hydroureter, hydroureteronephrosis, pyelectasis, pelviectasis, and caliectasis. Grading systems are also used in children that have been popularized by the Society of Fetal Urology, European Society of Pediatric Radiologist, and the Onen system. However, not all of these descriptive systems are applied to fetuses.

In 2014, practitioners in all fields caring for fetuses and infants with UTD formed a new UTD system to try to standardize descriptions in fetuses and infants (Fig. 8.1). This system uses the following criteria to describe and grade the appearance of the urinary tract: anterior-posterior renal pelvic diameter, pelvic dilation, calyceal dilation (with a distinction between central and peripheral calyces), ureteral dilation, bladder appearance, and renal parenchymal appearance. In utero, the amniotic fluid quantity is also an important factor (Nguyen et al., 2014; Chow et al., 2017; Nguyen, Phelps, Coley, Rhee, & Chow).

■ How Do We Evaluate Urinary Tract Dilation?

Key point: US is the screening test of choice of the child's urinary tract. Additional tests provide functional information.

Ultrasound

US is the screening test of choice of the urinary tract because it is readily available, inexpensive, and emits no ionizing radiation, a particular concern in children. Most postnatal USs to follow up prenatal hydronephrosis are performed in the first month of life, at least 48 hours after birth. Normal newborn oliguria in the first few days of life can cause underdistention of the urinary tract, and the appearance of the urinary tract at that time may falsely underestimate the degree of dilation. If the suspected prenatal abnormality is severe enough to be treated shortly after birth, such as posterior urethral valves (PUVs) in boys, then earlier imaging may be warranted.

UTD Classification System

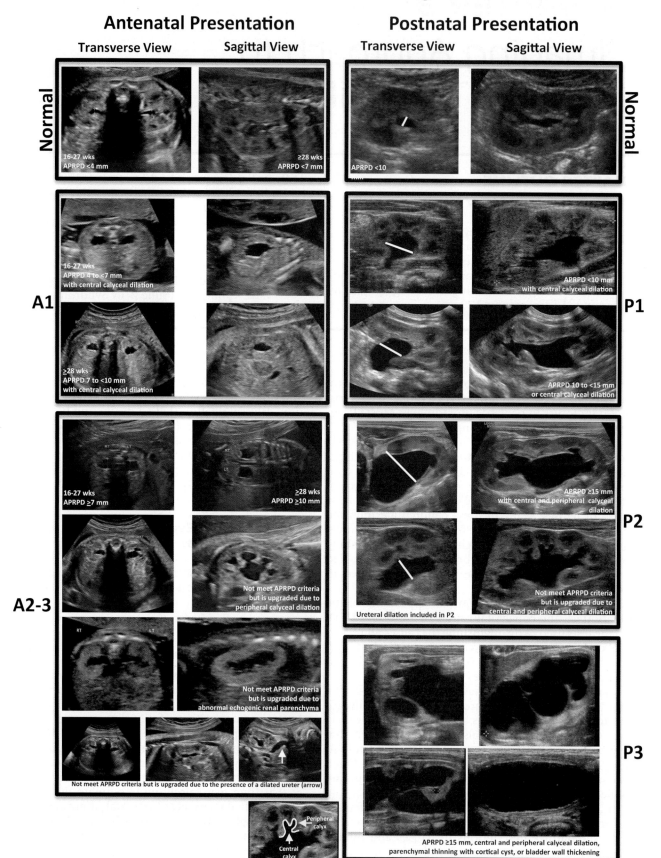

Antenatal Presentation

Transverse View   Sagittal View

Postnatal Presentation

Transverse View   Sagittal View

Normal

16-27 wks
APRPD <4 mm

≥28 wks
APRPD <7 mm

APRPD <10 mm

Normal

A1

16-27 wks
APRPD 4 to <7 mm
with central calyceal dilation

≥28 wks
APRPD 7 to <10 mm
with central calyceal dilation

APRPD <10 mm
with central calyceal dilation

APRPD 10 to <15 mm
or central calyceal dilation

P1

A2-3

16-27 wks
APRPD ≥7 mm

≥28 wks
APRPD ≥10 mm

Not meet APRPD criteria
but is upgraded due to
peripheral calyceal dilation

Not meet APRPD criteria
but is upgraded due to
abnormal echogenic renal parenchyma

Not meet APRPD criteria but is upgraded due to the presence of a dilated ureter (arrow)

APRPD ≥15 mm
with central and peripheral calyceal
dilation

Ureteral dilation included in P2

Not meet APRPD criteria
but is upgraded due to
central and peripheral calyceal dilation

P2

Peripheral
calyx

Central
calyx

APRPD ≥15 mm, central and peripheral calyceal dilation,
parenchymal thinning with cortical cyst, or bladder wall thickening

P3

Fig. 8.1 Urinary tract dilation (UTD) wall chart. The UTD-P classification system is based on six postnatal (P) ultrasound (US) findings: (1) anteroposterior renal pelvic diameter (APRPD), (2) calyceal dilation with distinction between central and peripheral calyceal dilation postnatally, (3) renal parenchymal thickness, (4) renal parenchymal appearance, (5) bladder abnormalities, and (6) ureteral abnormalities. Normal values are also defined. The UTD classification system distinguishes whether findings are antenatal (A) or postnatal (P). The higher the number, the more severe are the findings. Thus UTD A1 represents mild antenatal urinary tract dilation, and UTD P3 represents severe urinary tract dilation and/or other abnormalities, such as renal hyperechogenicity or a thick bladder wall after birth. Grading is based on the most severe finding. Because abnormalities of the urinary tract are more subtle and difficult to visualize in a fetus than in a child, there are only three antenatal categories (normal, UTD A1, UTD A2–3) and four postnatal categories (normal, UTD P1, UTD P2, and UTD P3). (Reprinted with permission from Journal of Pediatric Urology.)

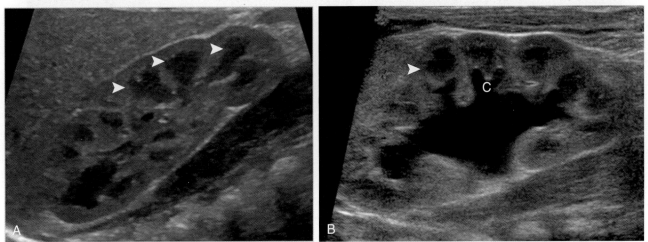

Fig. 8.2 (A, B) Hypoechoic pyramid versus dilated calyx: normal medullary pyramids in the newborn period appear hypoechoic and should not be confused for the dilated calyces of urinary tract dilation. Residual hypoechogenicity may persist through childhood. (A) The normal appearance of the hypoechoic pyramids (*arrowheads*) in a 2-week-old referred for prenatal hydronephrosis. (B) A patient with dilation of the peripheral calyces (C) adjacent to the normal hypoechoic pyramids (*arrowhead*).

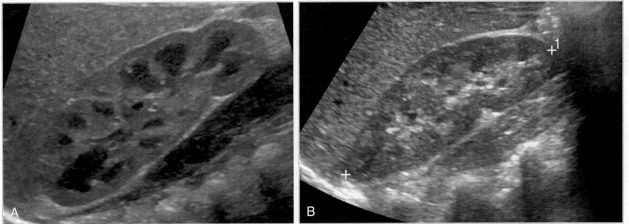

Fig. 8.3 Normal ultrasound (US) of the kidneys at different ages. Sagittal US images of the kidney in two different patients shows the progression of appearance of the kidney from infancy to later in childhood. (A) In neonates the kidneys are lobulated in contour because of normal fetal lobation, with hypoechoic renal pyramids. (B) Later in childhood, the contour of the kidney becomes smooth. The renal pyramids are not as hypoechoic, and the echogenicity of the renal parenchyma is more homogeneous.

The normal kidneys in the newborn period have a characteristic appearance that is different from the adult kidney. The medullary pyramids are hypoechoic, and this should not be confused for dilation of the renal calyces (Fig. 8.2). Later, the hypoechoic pyramids become more homogeneous with the surrounding renal parenchyma, and the kidneys assume a more "adult appearance" (Fig. 8.3). The normal renal parenchyma in a newborn has a variety of appearances. Unlike adults where the echogenicity of the kidney is normally less than that of the

liver or spleen, the normal newborn renal parenchyma can be hypoechoic, isoechoic, or hyperechoic relative to the liver or spleen (Fig. 8.4). Normal hyperechoic parenchyma is especially common in newborns and premature infants.

It is important to distinguish a normal amount of fluid within the urinary tract from abnormal quantities of fluid. Because the function of the urinary tract is to drain the urine, fluid is normally present. The normal measurements of the renal pelvis measured in the

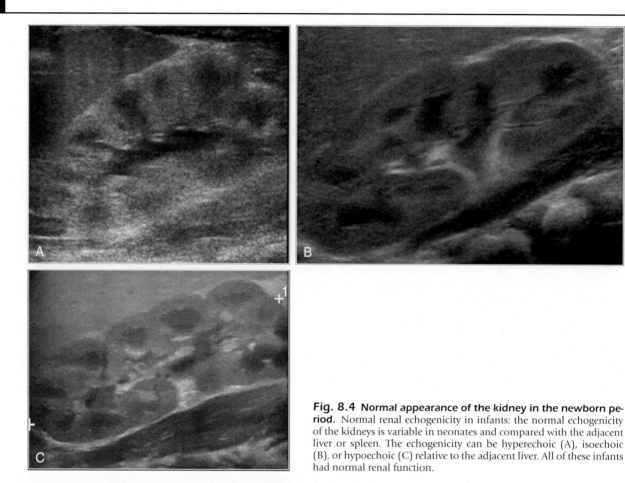

Fig. 8.4 Normal appearance of the kidney in the newborn period. Normal renal echogenicity in infants: the normal echogenicity of the kidneys is variable in neonates and compared with the adjacent liver or spleen. The echogenicity can be hyperechoic (A), isoechoic (B), or hypoechoic (C) relative to the adjacent liver. All of these infants had normal renal function.

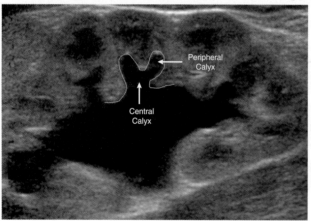

Fig. 8.5 This image demonstrates the difference between location of the central and peripheral calyces, an important distinction when using the urinary tract dilation (UTD) grading system in infants. The central calyx is located closer to the pelvis. The terms *central* and *peripheral calyces*, rather than *major* and *minor calyces*, are used to describe the urinary tract because the term *major calyceal dilation* could be have two meanings: one that the major calyx is dilated, or the second that there is severe calyceal dilation. The terms *central* and *peripheral* also clearly describe the location.

transverse plane or anteroposterior renal pelvis diameter (APRPD) is normally less than 10 mm. The average measurement increases slightly with age and with a full urinary bladder. When the calyces become dilated, especially peripheral calyces, the dilation becomes more abnormal (Fig. 8.5). The greater the degree of UTD, the

more potentially abnormal is the urinary tract. However, a normal urinary tract on US does not exclude pathology, particularly vesicoureteral reflux (VUR; Fig. 8.6) (Kenney, Negas, & Miller, 2002).

Unless careful attention is paid to the ureters, these structures are frequently not seen by US. Occasionally the normal ureter is seen to be slightly distended by urine because of a normal peristaltic wave. Normal ureteral jets of urine are seen intermittently through the ureteral orifices and into the bladder. A normal ureter measures 4 mm or less in diameter. The more dilated the ureter, the more likely it is that there is an abnormality causing the dilation (Vivier, Augdal, & Avni, 2018; Zelenko, Coll, Rosenfield, & Smith, 2004; Kljucvesek, Battleino, Tomazic, & Kersnik Levart, 2012) (Fig. 8.7).

Lower urinary tract abnormalities can lead to hydroureteronephrosis. For example, boys with urethral obstruction caused by PUVs may have UTD from either reflux or ureterovesical junction obstruction in the presence of an incompetent ureteral orifice. Reflux is caused by increased intravesical pressure. The same pressure over time also causes bladder wall hypertrophy, which can result in ureterovesical junction obstruction. Occasionally the ureter may both reflux and be obstructed. Often the effect of bladder outlet obstruction is different in one ureter than the other. Thus carefully examining the bladder or urethra is crucial to understanding the cause of UTD. A normal bladder

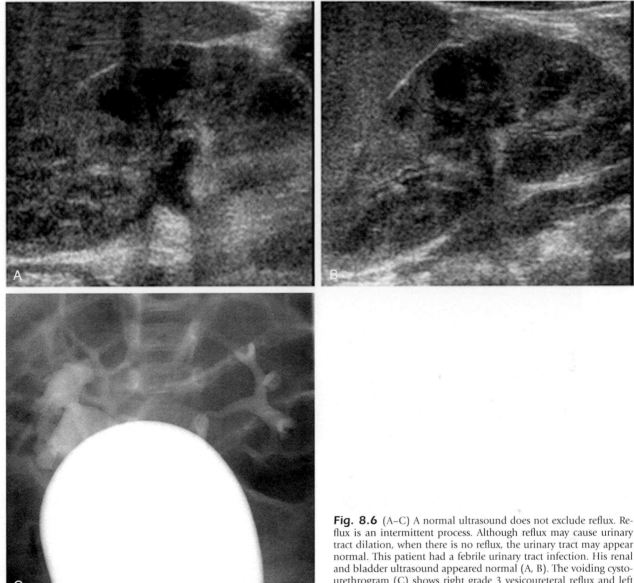

Fig. 8.6 (A–C) A normal ultrasound does not exclude reflux. Reflux is an intermittent process. Although reflux may cause urinary tract dilation, when there is no reflux, the urinary tract may appear normal. This patient had a febrile urinary tract infection. His renal and bladder ultrasound appeared normal (A, B). The voiding cystourethrogram (C) shows right grade 3 vesicoureteral reflux and left grade 2 vesicoureteral reflux.

wall is smooth (Fig. 8.8). When hypertrophy occurs, the bladder wall becomes trabeculated (Fig. 8.9).

The goals of imaging are not only to visualize the urinary tract but also to help determine which conditions are pathological and may result in deterioration of renal function. The greater the degree of UTD, the more likely it is that there is an abnormality that is causing it, typically obstruction.

After an US determines that the urinary tract is abnormally dilated, additional tests (dynamic renal scintigraphy, cortical scintigraphy, magnetic resonance urography [MRU], fluoroscopic voiding cystourethrography, and radionuclide cystography) distinguish obstructed urinary tracts from those with reflux and measure the degree of renal functional impairment. When ultrasound contrast agents are injected intravenously (IV) or infused intravesically, US can serve as a functional study as well.

Dynamic Renal Scintigraphy

Dynamic renal scintigraphy and diuresis renography are commonly used tests to assess UTD to help assess UTD by assessing the degree of obstruction. Dynamic renal scintigraphy is performed with the radiopharmaceutical ^{99m}Tc-mercaptoacetyltriglycine (^{99m}Tc-MAG3), which is excreted by active renal tubular transport. ^{99m}Tc-diethylene-triamine-pentacetic acid is a less commonly used alternative to ^{99m}Tc-MAG3.

Dynamic renal scintigraphy depends on the rapid excretion of radiopharmaceuticals through the kidney. This requires three steps: (1) renal perfusion and cortical uptake of ^{99m}Tc-MAG3, (2) cortical transit of ^{99m}Tc-MAG3 into the renal collecting system, and (3) excretion of ^{99m}Tc-MAG3 through the urinary collecting system. Imaging and quantitative measurement of each of these

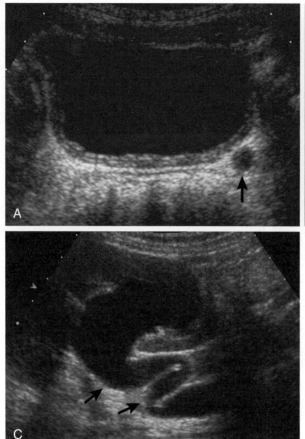

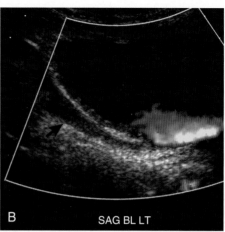

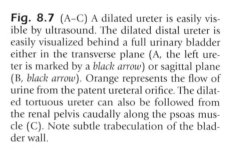

Fig. 8.7 (A–C) A dilated ureter is easily visible by ultrasound. The dilated distal ureter is easily visualized behind a full urinary bladder either in the transverse plane (A, the left ureter is marked by a *black arrow*) or sagittal plane (B, *black arrow*). Orange represents the flow of urine from the patent ureteral orifice. The dilated tortuous ureter can also be followed from the renal pelvis caudally along the psoas muscle (C). Note subtle trabeculation of the bladder wall.

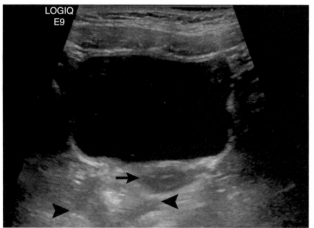

Fig. 8.8 This baby girl has a normal-appearing bladder. The wall is smooth and thin. The bladder is a good acoustic window for structures posterior to the bladder, including the ureter. The ureters are not visualized and thus thought to be normal. The normal uterus (*arrow*) and rectum (*arrowheads*) are also well visualized because of the bladder serving as an acoustic window.

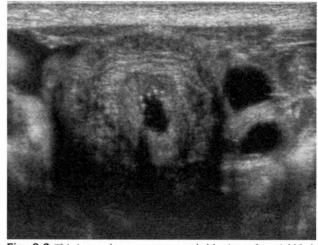

Fig. 8.9 This image demonstrates remarkable circumferential bladder wall thickening in a patient with posterior urethral valves. The distal left ureter is dilated and lateral to the bladder.

steps provides information about renal function. The pattern of cortical uptake, which is measured during the first 2 minutes of the study, can identify regions of cortical hypoperfusion or scar, as well as provide a measure of differential (left versus right) renal function. Although this provides approximate differential function, a renal cortical scan (typically dimercaptosuccinic acid (DMSA)) provides more accurate indication of differential renal function. The rate of cortical transit, normally 3 to 6 minutes, is an indicator of renal function. The rate and pattern of ^{99m}Tc-MAG3 excretion is used to assess collecting system drainage. Delayed drainage may indicate collecting system obstruction, but also may occur with low urine flow or in a markedly dilated collecting system. With diuresis renography, urine flow is increased, typically with IV saline infusion and IV administration of furosemide, to help distinguish collecting system obstruction from other causes of delayed collecting system drainage (Fig. 8.10).

Several patient factors can confound interpretation of the studies. Infants, especially those younger than 1 month, have functionally immature kidneys, which may delay cortical uptake and excretion of radiopharmaceuticals. In older children, impaired renal function can slow urinary excretion of radiopharmaceutical and limit evaluation of the urinary collecting system.

Recent administration of radiographic contrast may transiently diminish radiopharmaceutical excretion.

Cortical scintigraphy does not evaluate UTD directly, but it does measure functioning renal tissue. The amount of functional renal tissue is an important parameter in helping to determine the management of the child.

Magnetic Resonance Urography

MRU has the combined benefit of clearly depicting anatomic structures, showing the uptake and excretion of

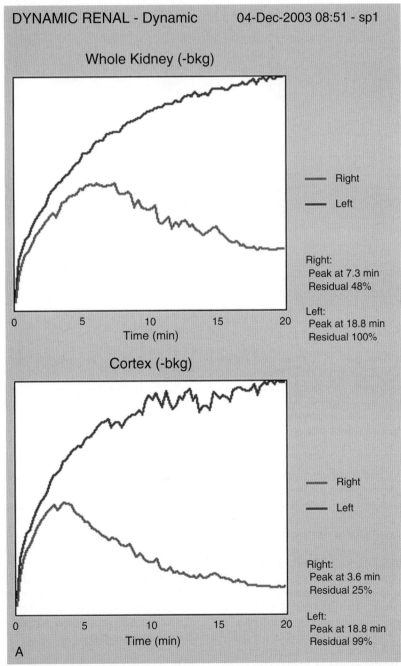

Fig. 8.10 (A, B) Mercaptoacetyltriglycine (MAG3) study shows obstruction as evidenced by delayed excretion of contrast and abnormal emptying of the urinary tract after diuresis in the left kidney compared to the normal right kidney.

Continued

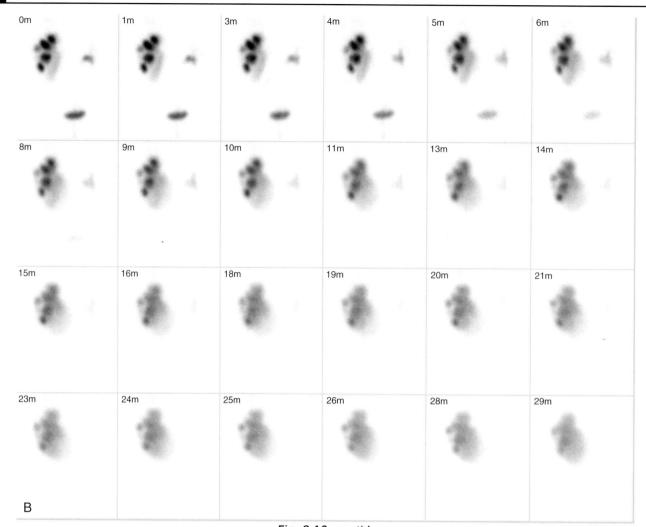

B

Fig. 8.10, cont'd

contrast through the urinary tract over time, and calculating parameters to show differential renal function. To assess function, like the diuretic renography, the patient needs an IV line for hydration, contrast administration, and a diuretic challenge. The main limitation of this technique is the need to keep the patient still for the relatively lengthy examination (45 minutes). This may necessitate sedation.

Static noncontrast T1 and fluid-sensitive sequences depict the anatomic appearance of the urinary tract beautifully in three dimensions. The fluid-sensitive sequences show dilation of the urinary tract and clearly show the sites and causes of obstruction (Fig. 8.11A).

During dynamic imaging with contrast enhancement, the perfusion, concentration, and excretion by the kidney can be seen and measured through changes in signal intensity over time. The differential renal function between the kidneys is measured by the degree of contrast enhancement. The Patlak number, an indirect measure of glomerular filtration rate, is a surrogate for renal function and can be measured by MRU. This study also has the advantage of showing the anatomy of the renal vessels, including crossing vessels, which may lead

to ureteropelvic junction obstruction (UPJO; see Fig. 8.11B).

MRU is helpful in predicting which patients may regain renal function after surgery. If a dilated urinary tract shows normal drainage after hydration and administration of a diuretic, the system is considered compensated. In kidneys with compensated hydronephrosis, surgery does little to improve the function of the kidney. However, if high flow rates result in inadequate drainage of the urinary tract during MRU, the system is considered decompensated. In these patients, successful surgery will improve the function of the kidney.

Tests for Vesicoureteral Reflux: Voiding Cystourethrogram, Radionuclide Cystogram, and Contrast-Enhanced Voiding Urosonography

VUR occurs when there is abnormal retrograde flow of urine from the bladder up into the ureter, renal pelvis, or calyces. Reflux, especially high-grade reflux, can cause

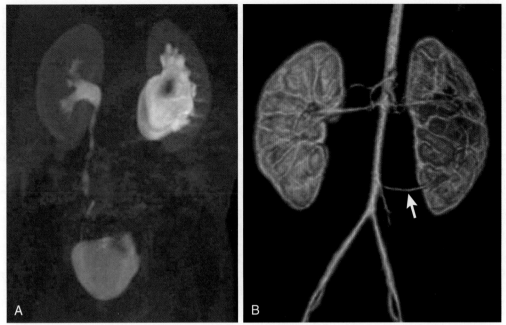

Fig. 8.11 (A, B) This 10-year-old boy had intermittent abdominal pain and was found to have hydronephrosis on ultrasound. (A) Late contrast-enhanced images demonstrate a dilated left renal pelvis and calyces with swirling of the contrast within the pelvis. The right urinary tract appears normal. (B) Magnetic resonance angiography shows the anomalous renal artery (*arrow*), which is causing the ureteropelvic junction obstruction. (Images courtesy Dr. Damien Grattan Smith)

UTD. Three tests are available to evaluate for reflux: the fluoroscopic voiding cystourethrogram (VCUG), the radionuclide cystogram (RNC), and the contrast-enhanced voiding urosonography (ceVUS) (Fig. 8.12). Each of these tests is performed similarly but use different contrast agents.

For each test, contrast is instilled into the bladder, typically through a urethral catheter, until the patient voids. This process is visualized under fluoroscopy (VCUG), a gamma camera in nuclear medicine (RNC), or by US (ceVUS). If contrast refluxes into the ureter, renal pelvis, or calyces, there is VUR. The contrast used in VCUG contains iodine; in RNC the radiopharmaceutical is ^{99m}Tc-pertechnetate; and for ceVUS, it is a microbubble contrast agent. The greater the reflux, the higher is the grade. Reflux is graded in a 1 to 5 scale by VCUG and a 1 to 3 scale by RNC (Fig. 8.13).

Reflux is an intermittent phenomenon. Most patients with reflux, especially low-grade reflux, do not have hydronephrosis and may have a normal renal US. US is a poor screening test for reflux. Thus the only reliable methods of showing reflux are one of the three methods described earlier. Reflux can cause dilation of the urinary tract, especially when it is severe (see Fig. 8.12A). Findings are classically intermittent, with UTD occurring only during the reflux.

The VCUG and ceVUS have the advantage of showing greater anatomic detail of the kidney, bladder, and urethra than the RNC. The main disadvantage of the RNC and the VCUG is the radiation dose. When done with proper technique and low-dose pulse fluoroscopy, VCUG doses are low and equivalent to a few days of background radiation. Doses of RNC studies are even lower. Given the lack of ionizing radiation which allows for continuous imaging through multiple cycles of filling and voiding, and the exquisite sensitivity to detect

a small amount of refluxing ultrasound contrast agent, ceVUS is more sensitive for the detection of reflux compared to VCUG and now the current recommended study (Ntoulia, Aguirre Pascual, & Back).

Computed Tomography

Unlike for adults, where computed tomography (CT), often in multiphase studies, is the screening study of the urinary tract, concerns of radiation make US the primary screening study of choice for children. However, if the CT is performed using the latest dose-reduction protocols and tailored to the size of the patient, very low doses can be achieved.

CT is rarely used to evaluate children with congenital UTD. The main use of CT in children is to evaluate for nephroureterolithiasis after a screening US to further evaluate stone disease. A CT angiogram may be helpful in assessing whether a crossing vessel is the cause of a UPJO.

■ Differential Diagnosis and Treatment

The following section describes the common and uncommon causes of UTD. The most common cause of congenital pathological UTD is obstruction at either the ureteropelvic junction or ureterovesical junction. As is true for all congenital anomalies, the severity of obstruction ranges from mild to severe. The purpose of imaging studies is not only to show the abnormality but also to try to predict which anomalies require further treatment. Typically, treatment is warranted if the problem results in renal dysfunction. Many causes of UTD require no treatment, only observation.

VUR can cause UTD independently or can occur concomitantly with obstruction. Thus patients with dilated urinary tracts are frequently worked up for reflux. In these patients with dilated urinary tracts the absence of reflux implies that the dilation is due to obstruction. Occasionally both reflux and obstruction coexist.

The following is a description of entities that cause UTD, from most to least common.

Key points: The most common "pathological" cause of hydronephrosis is UPJO. Hydroureteronephrosis can be caused by obstruction (mainly primary megaureter), VUR, or both.

Hydronephrosis: Ureteropelvic Junction Obstruction (UPJO)

The most common pathological cause of prenatal and postnatal UTD is a UPJO. A UPJO is typically caused by a congenital narrowing of the renal pelvis at the junction of the proximal ureter. Depending on the degree of obstruction, this leads to dilation of the renal pelvis and calyces. Rarely, UPJO is caused by a renal crossing vessel, typically an artery going to the lower pole of the kidney that kinks the ureteropelvic junction (see Fig. 8.11).

Typically, after US raises suspicion for UPJO and the reflux study is normal, diuretic renography or MRU is used to show the degree of obstruction to help determine whether surgery is needed. Surgical intervention occurs if there are obstructive parameters measured by renography, decompensated hydronephrosis by MRU, or decline in renal function over time (Fig. 8.14). If the obstructed kidney has little parenchyma, a DMSA scan is used to quantify the function, to see if the amount of function is worth preserving.

If the UPJO is causing functional impairment of the kidney, a Hynes-Anderson pyeloplasty (Fig. 8.15) is performed to relieve the obstruction. If the UPJO does not appear to be causing obstruction by diuretic renography, has parameters of compensated hydronephrosis by MRU, or does not appear to cause functional impairment, the kidney may be watched by imaging for change. In fact, much congenital UTD is watched, rather than operated on.

Hydroureteronephrosis: Obstruction, Reflux, or Both

The most common causes of dilation of the renal pelvis, calyces, and ureter (or hydroureteronephrosis) is either primary megaureter, reflux or both.

Primary megaureter is the most common cause of congenital ureterovesical junction obstruction. The orthotopic distal ureter is functionally obstructed and causes dilation of the ureter above it and, to a lesser degree, the renal pelvis and calyces (Fig. 8.16). Because 70% to 80% of cases improve with time and cause no functional impairment of the kidney, primary megaureter is typically followed by imaging, mainly US, and rarely requires surgery. It is important to know that the natural history of primary megaureter is spontaneous improvement so that unnecessary operations are prevented. Less commonly, UVJO can be associated with ectopic ureteral insertions, either from ureters arising from the upper pole of a duplex kidney or a single system ectopic ureter (see later).

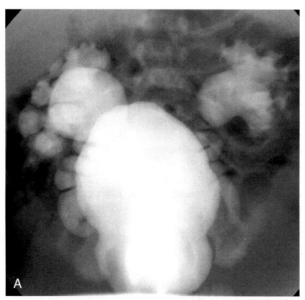

Fig. 8.12 (A–C) These three images depict the appearance of different studies that diagnose vesicoureteral reflux (VUR). Reflux can cause dilation of the urinary tract. (A) Voiding cystourethrogram (VCUG) demonstrates bilateral high-grade VUR and a dilated urinary bladder. When there is cycling of urine in the bladder because of high-grade reflux, the ureters and bladder dilate, called the megacystis-megaureter association.

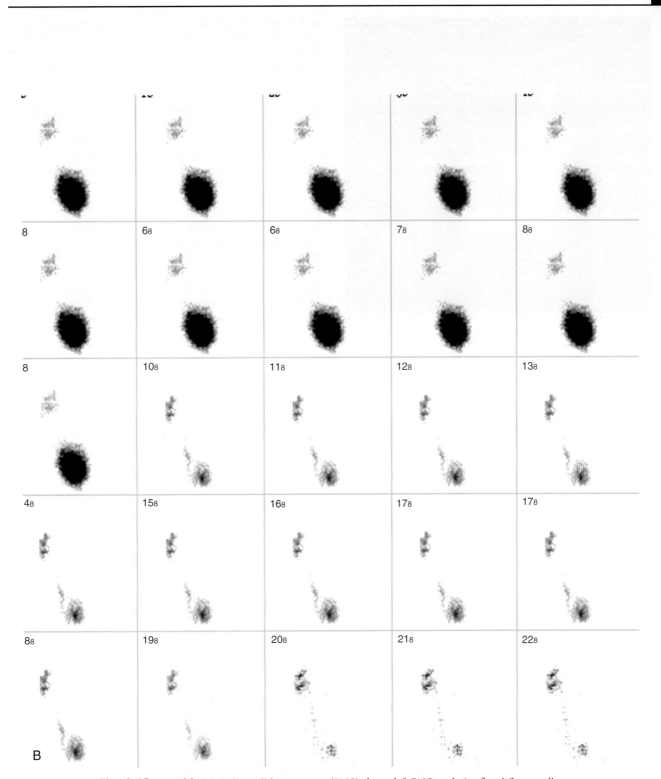

Fig. 8.12, cont'd (B) Radionuclide cystogram (RNC) shows left RNC grade 3 reflux. When grading reflux, a 1 to 3 system is used in nuclear medicine, where a 1 to 5 system is used with fluoroscopic VCUGs, with lower numbers representing lower grades of reflux.

Continued

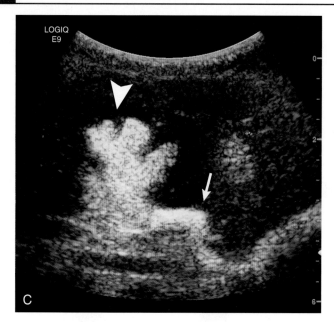

Fig. 8.12, cont'd (C) Contrast-enhanced voiding urosonography (ceVUS; left with *arrow*): sagittal image of the left kidney during a ceVUS in a newborn with prenatal hydronephrosis demonstrates high-grade reflux into the left kidney. The echogenic contrast fills the dilated pelvis, calyces (*arrowhead*), and ureter (*arrow*).

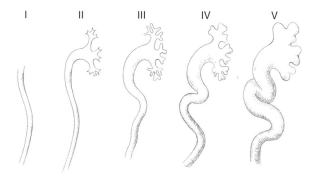

GRADES OF REFLUX

Fig. 8.13 The International Reflux Study grading system of vesico-ureteral reflux for voiding cystourethrograms shows the appearances of the five grades, from mild (grade 1) to severe (grade 5). (Image courtesy Dr. Robert Lebowitz, MD)

In the rare circumstance in which surgery is required, the dilated ureter is tapered and reimplanted into the bladder, a combined surgery called *megaureter tapering and ureteral reimplantation* (Fig. 8.17). Usually surgery is unnecessary unless the degree of dilation increases or renal function declines. If the urinary tract appears decompensated by MRU, then surgery may also be considered.

VUR can also cause hydroureteronephrosis. VUR occurs when there is retrograde flow of urine from the bladder, up the ureter, and into the renal pelvis and calyces. Reflux may be primary, and caused by an abnormality at the ureterovesical junction, or secondary, as a result of other causes. Reflux is diagnosed by RNC, VCUG, or ceVUS (described earlier). When reflux

is bilateral or severe on one side, the refluxed urine cycles from the bladder to the ureters repeatedly such that the ureters dilate and the bladder enlarges. This phenomenon is called the *megacystis megaureter association* (see Fig. 8.12A). Because reflux is intermittent, hydroureteronephrosis associated with reflux is intermittent or changing. When a patient with reflux is not refluxing, the urinary tract often appears normal. Many patients with reflux have a normal renal US.

It is important to distinguish reflux from reflux coexisting with obstruction because the treatment is different. Reflux may be associated with UPJ or UVJ obstruction. The hallmarks of reflux and obstruction on VCUG are hesitation, dilution, and retention of contrast. The refluxed contrast will hesitate before passing the obstruction, will appear diluted beyond the obstruction because the contrast is mixing with trapped urine, and will be retained proximal to the obstruction after the rest of the urinary tract has drained (Fig. 8.18).

The most common causes of secondary reflux are bladder diverticula and bladder outlet obstruction. Periureteral (also known as Hutch) diverticula may enlarge near the ureterovesical junction, incorporating the adjacent ureter, and lead to reflux (Fig. 8.19). This phenomenon is intermittent. If a patient has increased intravesical pressure because of bladder outlet obstruction, either congenital, neurogenic, or acquired, the increased intraluminal pressure may lead to VUR.

The natural history of primary reflux is that most low-grade reflux resolves with time, especially when initially diagnosed at a young age. The higher the grade of reflux, the less likely the reflux will resolve spontaneously. The most common treatments offered to patients with primary reflux are antibiotics, endoscopic submucosal injection of Deflux (hyaluronic acid/dextranomer; Salix Pharmaceuticals, Bridgewater, New Jersey), and ureteral reimplantation. Prophylactic antibiotics are prescribed to prevent urinary tract infections while the reflux resolves. Deflux is the most common substance which is injected submucosally below the ureteral orifice to narrow the distal ureterovesical junction to prevent reflux. Deflux mounds appear as masses on US and occasionally calcify, mimicking malignancies (Fig. 8.20) or distal ureteral calculi (Fig. 8.21) to those unfamiliar with this method of treating reflux.

The definitive surgical correction of VUR is ureteral reimplantation. There are many different methods to perform this procedure. The basic principle is that the submucosal ureteral tunnel is lengthened to prevent reflux. The ureters may be reimplanted on the same side as the original ureteral orifice or on the opposite side, as in the Cohen cross-trigonal ureteral reimplantation technique (Fig. 8.22). If the ureter is dilated, it may be tapered before reimplantation, like the surgery to fix primary megaureter.

Duplex Kidneys, Ectopic Ureters, and Ureteroceles

Less common causes of UTD are related to duplex kidneys, ectopic ureters, and ureteroceles.

Urine typically drains from a kidney into a single ureter. Less commonly the kidney may have two separate ureters: one draining the upper pole and the other draining the lower pole. In patients with complete ureteral duplication the upper pole ureter is ectopic. The Weigert-Meyer rule describes that the upper pole ureteral orifice of a duplex kidney is ectopic. This upper pole ureter may be obstructed at the ureterovesical junction leading to hydroureteronephrosis (Fig. 8.23). The upper pole ureter inserts medial and inferior to the ureteral orifice in the bladder in boys and girls (Fig. 8.24). In girls the ectopic pathway is such that the ureter may insert into the urethra, vagina, and perineum. In boys the ectopic ureter may insert into

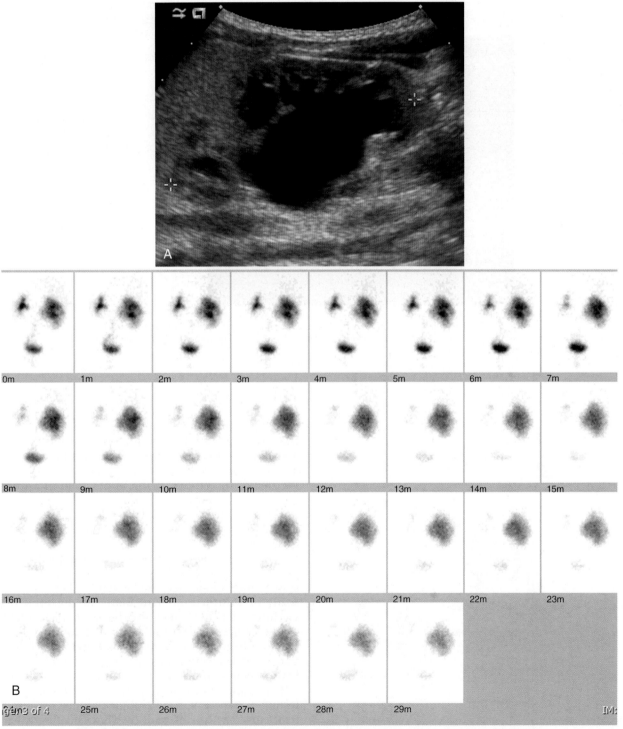

Fig. 8.14 (A–D) This newborn had prenatal hydronephrosis. (A) Sagittal ultrasound image of the right kidney demonstrates a dilated renal pelvis, central calyces, and peripheral calyces and renal parenchymal thinning (urinary tract dilation [UTD] P3). There was no dilation of the ureter. The left kidney appeared normal (not shown).

Continued

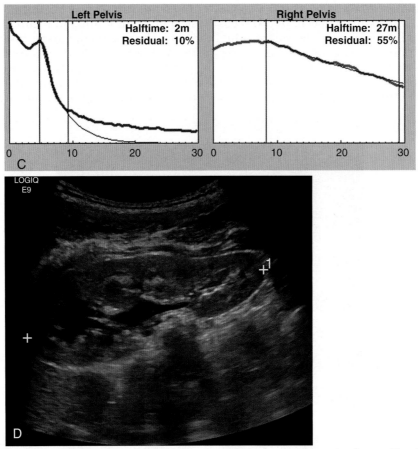

Fig. 8.14, cont'd (B, C) Diuresis renography shows delayed contrast excretion from a dilated right renal pelvis. The half-time is 27 minutes, which is delayed and consistent with obstruction. This patient underwent pyeloplasty. (D) The postoperative ultrasound shows marked improvement in the degree of urinary tract dilation.

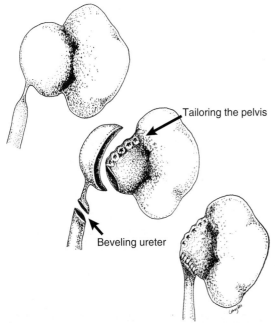

Fig. 8.15 This image shows the method of performing the Hynes-Anderson pyeloplasty used to repair a ureteropelvic junction obstruction. The stenotic segment, and often a portion of the renal pelvis, are removed, and the beveled ureter is reanastomosed to the renal pelvis. (Image courtesy Dr. Robert Lebowitz, MD)

the urethra above the urinary sphincter and even into the ejaculatory ducts and branching structures. These same sites of ectopic ureteral insertion also occur in the rarer single system ectopic ureter. The renal tissue associated with the ectopic ureter may be dysplastic, and the degree of dysplasia is directly correlated with the degree of ectopia. If the upper pole of a duplex kidney is extremely dysplastic and diminutive, the lower pole may be confused for a single system kidney. Rarely, upper pole ureters may also dilate because of reflux.

The lower pole ureter is the analog to the ureter of a single system kidney. The lower pole collecting system may dilate because of reflux (Figs. 8.25 and 8.26) or obstruction, particularly at the ureteropelvic junction. There may also be incomplete ureteral duplication such that the upper and lower pole ureters join to form a common distal ureter. A UVJO, in that situation, would cause both upper and lower pole hydroureteronephrosis.

It is important to distinguish UTD of a single collecting system or part of a duplex kidney because the treatment may be different. By US, evaluating whether the dilation occurs centrally within the kidney typically implies that there is a single collecting system. If the dilation is eccentric, then it may be associated with

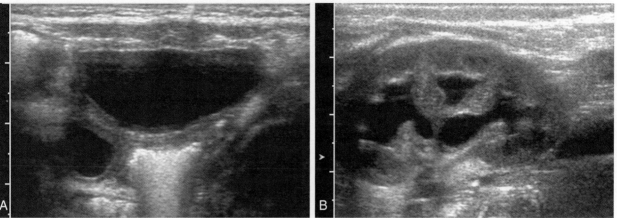

Fig. 8.16 (A, B) This infant with prenatal hydronephrosis was found to have a dilated right ureter (A) and dilated renal pelvis and calyces (B) or urinary tract dilation [UTD] P2. The voiding cystourethrogram (VCUG) was normal. Because the site of ureteral insertion appeared to be normal, this patient presumably had primary megaureter. The dilation resolved with time, and this patient needed no surgery.

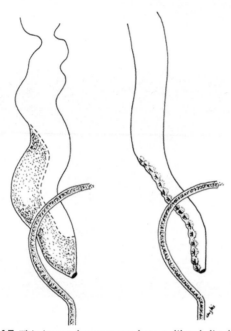

Fig. 8.17 This image demonstrates how a dilated distal ureter is tapered before reimplantation. The shaded portion of the ureter (left image) is removed to taper the distal ureter. This tapered ureter is then reimplanted into the bladder (right image). (Image courtesy Dr. Robert Lebowitz, MD)

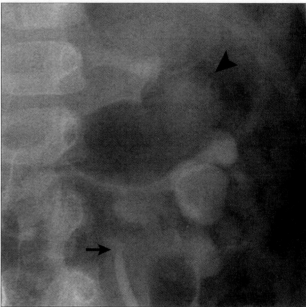

Fig. 8.18 This 10-year-old had intermittent flank pain and a urinary tract infection. Voiding cystourethrogram (VCUG) demonstrates reflux into the left ureter with hesitation at the ureteropelvic junction (UPJ) (*arrow*). Contrast is dilute within the dilated collecting system and was retained there on delayed images (*arrowhead*). This patient has reflux and concomitant UPJ obstruction. Reflux cannot be graded using the 1 through 5 scale because the dilation of the calyces reflects the obstruction, not just the reflux.

either the upper or lower pole of the kidney. It is always important to consider that a kidney may not have a single collecting system.

If a patient has complete ureteral duplication and one of the ureters needs to be reimplanted because of either reflux or ureterovesical junction obstruction, the adjacent ureter shares blood supply and is typically reimplanted as well. This is referred to as a common sheath ureteral reimplantation. If the moiety associated with the dilated ureter is so poorly functioning that it is deemed not worthy of preserving, a partial nephrectomy may also be performed. Although DMSA is more accurate than MAG-3 for determining differential renal function, it is of limited availability. MRU is an alternative to providing accurate functional information.

A ureterocele is a focal dilation of the intravesical portion of the distal ureter. This focal dilation can be associated with obstruction at the ureteral orifice and thus hydroureteronephrosis. In girls, ureteroceles are typically associated with the ectopic upper pole of a duplex kidney (Fig. 8.27). In boys, ureteroceles are typically associated with single system kidneys, called *simple ureteroceles*.

The distal orifice is incised and enlarged to relieve the obstruction caused by the ureterocele. This often relieves

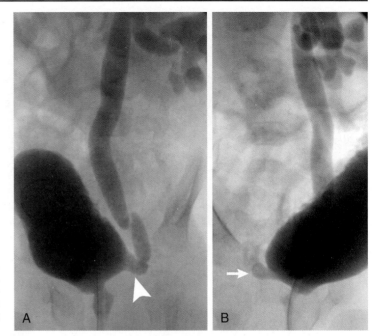

Fig. 8.19 (A, B) This newborn had prenatal hydronephrosis. (A) The postnatal ultrasound shows left grade 3 vesicoureteral reflux. The left ureter inserts into a diverticulum (*arrowhead*). (B) Near the right ureterovesical junction, there is a periureteral or Hutch diverticulum (*arrow*). There is no right reflux.

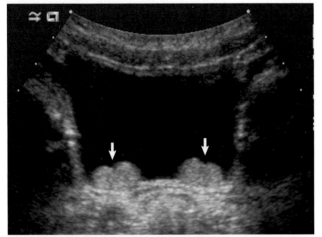

Fig. 8.20 This 11-year-old girl had bilateral grade 2 reflux and underwent bilateral Deflux injections. A transverse view of the bladder demonstrates bilateral bilobed echogenic mounds at the ureterovesical junctions (*arrows*), the site of the submucosal injections.

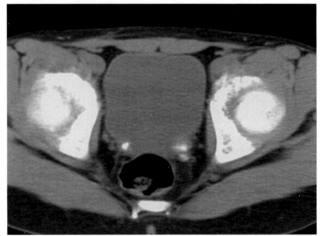

Fig. 8.21 This 10-year-old presented with abdominal pain and hematuria. An axial image from a noncontrast computed tomography scan demonstrates bilateral hyperdensities at the ureterovesical junctions that were thought to represent bilateral ureterolithiasis at the ureterovesical junctions. However, this patient was treated with Deflux, and these represent calcified Deflux mounds.

obstruction but also results in VUR. The ureterocele may also be excised, and then the ureter is reimplanted. Like other duplex kidneys with a poorly functioning moiety (typically the upper pole), a partial nephrectomy rather than a ureteral reimplantation may be the surgery of choice.

Bladder Outlet Obstructions: Neurogenic Bladder, Posterior Urethral Valves, a Posterior Urethral Valve Mimic, and Prune Belly Syndrome

Increased intravesical pressure caused by bladder outlet obstructions may also cause hydroureteronephrosis ei-

ther as result of reflux or ureterovesical obstruction, or, rarely, both. The increased intravesical pressure caused by the obstruction results in reflux if the ureteral orifice is also abnormal. Chronic obstruction leads to hypertrophy and trabeculation of the bladder wall. This thickened bladder wall may lead to ureterovesical junction obstruction. Rarely, both reflux and obstruction occur in the same ureter. The effect of bladder outlet obstruction can be asymmetrical, and reflux may be present in one ureter and obstruction in the other. Chronic reflux or obstruction can lead to scarring and renal damage.

Even normal pressure from a full bladder can lead to dilation of the urinary tract (Fig. 8.28). Thus if UTD is associated with a full bladder, the bladder should be emptied and the urinary tract re-evaluated.

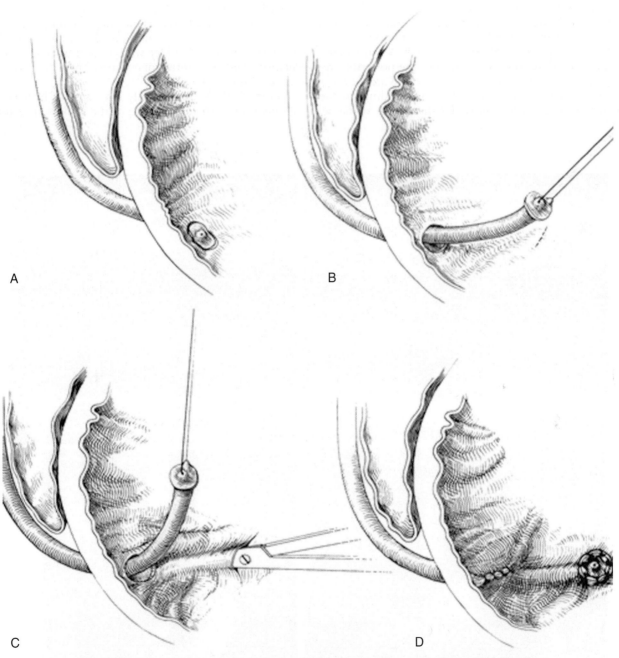

A

B

C

D

Fig. 8.22 During a Cohen cross-trigonal ureteral reimplantation, the ureter is dissected free from the bladder wall (A). A horizontal submucosal tunnel is created, and the distal ureter is pulled through this tunnel so that the orifice is now on the contralateral side (B, C). The ureter is secured into place (D). (Image courtesy Dr. Robert Lebowitz, MD)

The most common congenital anomaly that causes increased bladder outlet resistance is due to bladder sphincter dyssynergia in patients with spinal cord abnormalities, the most common of which is spina bifida. Clean intermittent catheterization allows for these children to empty their bladder on a regular basis and decreases hydroureteronephrosis and subsequent damage to the kidneys.

Congenital narrowing of the urethra is far more common in boys than in girls. The most common cause in boys is posterior urethral valves (PUV). PUVs are located at the base of the verumontanum in the posterior urethra. A voiding cystourethrogram or ceVUS are the diagnostic studies of choice for PUVs. Depending on the degree of obstruction caused by these slips of tissue,

there is resultant bladder outlet obstruction, bladder wall thickening and trabeculation, and hydroureteronephrosis, similar to those with neurogenic bladder. The combination of a thick-walled bladder and hydroureteronephrosis in a boy should prompt the consideration of PUVs. The dilated posterior urethra and bladder form a "keyhole" appearance. This diagnosis can also be suggested in utero (Fig. 8.29).

The treatment of PUVs is transurethral incision. After successful transurethral incision, the dilation of the posterior urethra, bladder wall thickening and trabeculation, and hydroureteronephrosis begin to decrease almost immediately.

Prune belly is an extremely rare cause of hydroureteronephrosis. The appearance of the urinary tract may

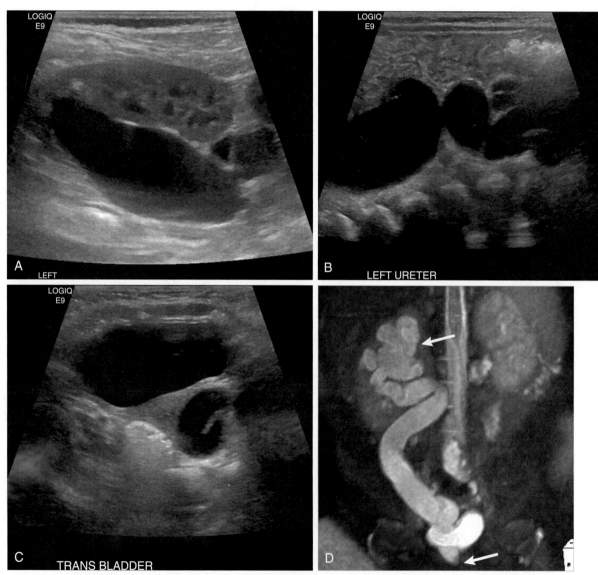

Fig. 8.23 (A–E) Ultrasound images of duplex kidneys by US (A–C) and MRU (D) and DMSA (E) demonstrating the Weigert Meyer Rule. Sagittal US image of the left kidney demonstrates the left upper pole pelvis is eccentrically positioned in the kidney and very dilated (A). The ureter is seen to be dilated in the sagittal plane (B) and transverse plane (C) to the level of the bladder. Magnetic resonance urography (D) shows a duplex right kidney with the ureter inserting ectopically below the base of the bladder. When there is complete ureteral duplication, the upper pole ureter is ectopic and may be obstructed, as in these examples.

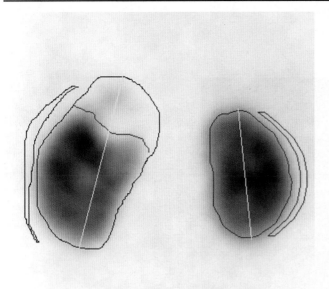

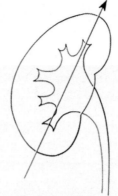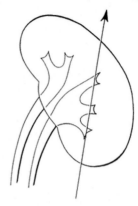

Fig. 8.25 The lower pole of a duplex kidney may reflux, leading to hydroureteronephrosis. By voiding cystourethrogram (VCUG), reflux into the lower pole ureter is distinguished from reflux into a single system ureter by the axis of the calyces. Note that the normal axis of the calyces is toward the contralateral shoulder. The axis of the calyces in lower pole relux is to the ipsilateral shoulder. (Images are courtesy of Robert Lebowitz, MD.)

Posterior View			
	Left Kidney	**Upper**	**Lower**
Ratios(%)	54.7	2.3	52.4
Length (cm)	6.5		
E			

Fig. 8.23, cont'd (E) DMSA shows the poor renal function (2%) of the upper pole of a left duplex kidney. This is the same patient as the ultrasound example. The more ectopic the ureter, typically the more dysplastic and poorly functioning is the associated moiety.

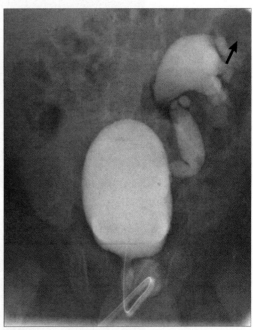

Fig. 8.26 The lower pole of a duplex kidney may reflux, leading to hydroureteronephrosis. By voiding cystourethrogram (VCUG), reflux into the lower pole ureter is distinguished from reflux into a single system ureter by the axis of the calyces. In lower pole reflux the axis of the calyces is toward the ipsilateral shoulder, as shown by the *arrow*.

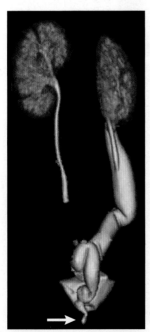

Fig. 8.24 This oblique view from the posterior projection demonstrates that the dilated upper pole ureter ends ectopically below the bladder base. The power of MRU is the clear anatomical delineation of the genitourinary system, in addition to providing functional information. (Images courtesy Dr. Damien Grattan Smith.)

mimic that of severe PUVs. However, the physical examination is different. These patients have marked deficiency of the abdominal musculature manifested in a wrinkly, prunelike appearance of the anterior abdominal wall. This abdominal muscle deficiency, coupled with marked dilatation of the ureters and cryptorchidism, is the hallmarks of prune belly syndrome. The etiology of this condition is unknown but is thought to be due to abnormalities of the mesenchyme early in gestation.

Additional genitourinary anomalies include urachal diverticula and patency and dilation of the urethra or

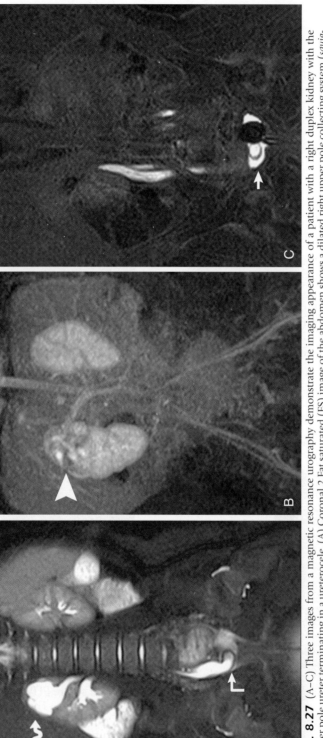

Fig. 8.27 (A–C) Three images from a magnetic resonance urography demonstrate the imaging appearance of a patient with a right duplex kidney with the upper pole ureter terminating in a ureterocele. (A) Coronal 2 Fat saturated (FS) image of the abdomen shows a dilated right upper pole collecting system (*squiggly arrows*) that ends in a ureterocele (*curved arrow*). (B) Early postcontrast dynamic images show delayed excretion of contrast in the upper pole (*arrowhead*), because of the obstruction caused by the ureterocele. (C) The delayed postcontrast-enhanced image shows contrast within the ureterocele and bladder (*arrow*). (Images courtesy Dr. Damien Grattan Smith.)

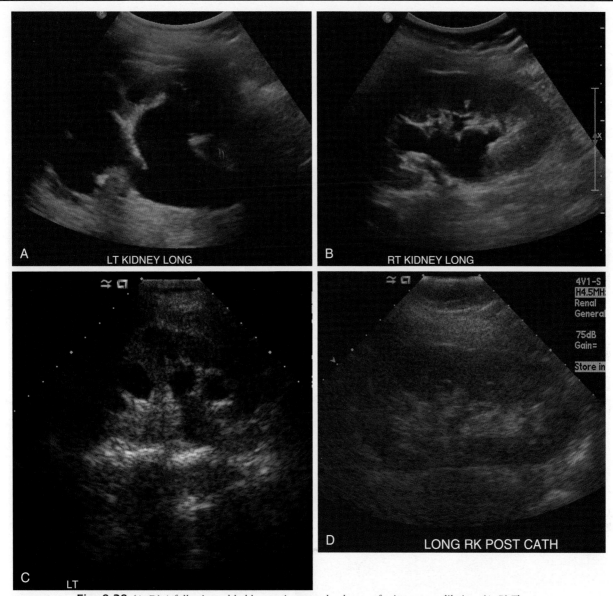

Fig. 8.28 (A–D) A full urinary bladder can increase the degree of urinary tract dilation. (A, B) The severely dilated left and mildly dilated right renal pelvis and calyces when the bladder is full. The degree of dilation decreased to mild on the left (C) and becomes normal on the right (D) after voiding.

megalourethra. An absence of prostatic tissue makes the posterior urethra appear dilated, and thus the appearance of a dilated posterior urethra can be confused with patients who have posterior urethra valves, with the important distinction of having no valves in patients with prune belly (Fig. 8.30).

In this chapter, the common and uncommon causes of congenital UTD are described. Although obstruction and VUR are the most common causes of dilation, radiologists should also be aware of the less common causes, including ectopic ureters or bladder outlet obstruction in boys.

■ **Acknowledgments**

I am grateful to Robert Lebowitz, Rhonda Johnson, and Jane Choura for their invaluable help in preparing this chapter and, always, for their friendship.

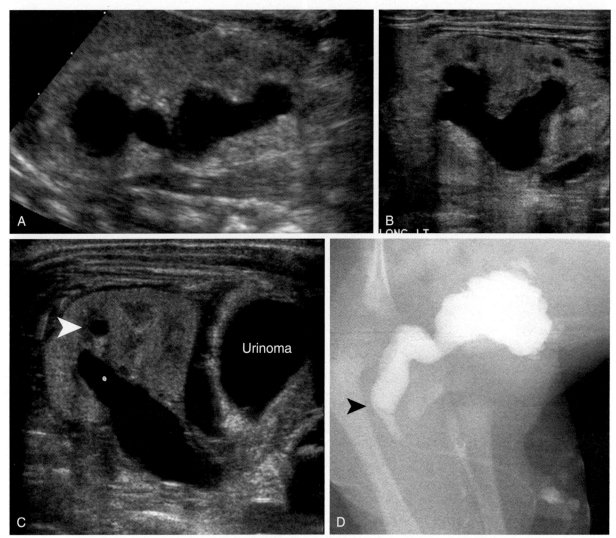

Fig. 8.29 (A–D) Posterior urethral valves can cause hydroureteronephrosis in boys. This baby boy with severe posterior urethral valves has bilateral dilation of the renal pelvis and calyces (A, right; B, C, left). Both kidneys are echogenic with small cortical cysts representative of dysplasia (arrowhead). Near the left kidney there is free fluid and a urinoma, secondary to forniceal rupture. The voiding cystourethrogram (VCUG) (D) demonstrates the posterior urethral valves (*black arrowhead*), a dilated posterior urethra, and a severely thickened bladder with trabeculations.

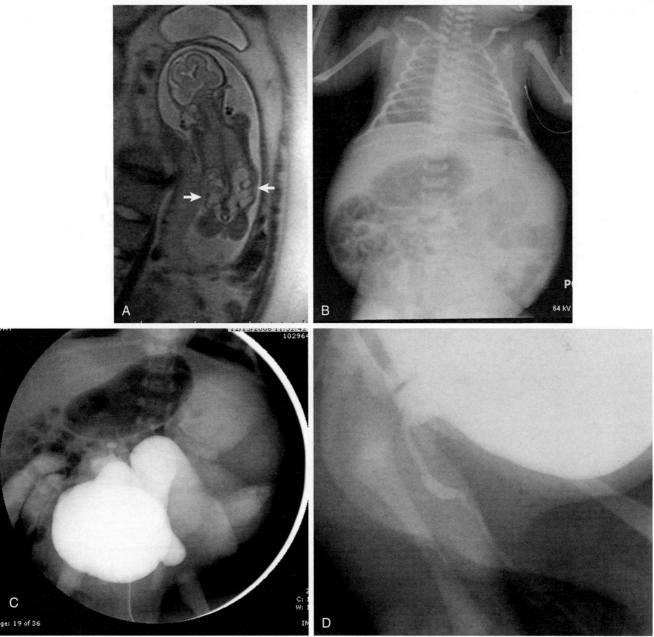

Fig. 8.30 (A–D) Patients with prune belly syndrome have severe hydroureteronephrosis; some imaging findings are similar to that of patients with posterior urethral valves. On prenatal magnetic resonance imaging the ureter, renal pelvis, and calyces are severely dilated (A, *arrows*). After the child is born, there is a wrinkly appearance of the anterior abdominal wall. The kidneys, ureter, and bladder (KUB) (B) show the flaccid abdomen as a result of the lack of normal abdominal wall musculature. This patient has bilateral severe reflux into tortuous ureters (C). When the patient voids, the posterior urethra is dilated, but there are no posterior urethral valves (D).

References

Chow, J. S., Koning, J. L., Back, S. J., Nguyen, H. T., Phelps, A., & Darge, K. (2017). Classification of pediatric urinary tract dilation: The new language. *Pediatric Radiology, 47*(9), 1109–1115.

Kenney, I. J., Negas, A. S., & Miller, F. N. (2002). Is sonographically demonstrated mild distal ureteric dilatation predictive of vesicoureteric reflux as seen on micturating cystourethrography? *Pediatric Radiology, 32*(2), 175–178. https://doi.org/10.1007/s00247-001-0615-1

Kljucvesek, D., Battleino, N., Tomazic, M., & Kersnik Levart, T. (2012). A comparison of echo-enhanced voiding urosonography with X-ray voiding cystourethrography in the first year of life. *Acta Paediatrica, 101*(5), 235–239. https://doi.org/10.1111/j.1651-2227.2011.02588.x

Nguyen, H. T., Phelps, A., Coley, B., Rhee, A., & Chow, J. (2021). Update on the urinary tract dilation (UTD) classification system: clarifications, review of the literature, and practical suggestions. *Pediatric Radiology.* In Press.

Nguyen, H., Benson, C., Bromley, B., Campbell, J., Chow, J., Coleman, B., & Stein, D. (2014). Multidisciplinary concensus on the classificatin of prenatal and postnatal urinary tract dilation (UTD classification system). *Journal of Pediatric Urology, 10*(6), 982–989. https://doi.org/10.1016/j.jurol.2014.10.002

Ntoulia A., Aguirre Pascual E., Back S.J., Contrast-enhanced voiding urosonography: Vesicoureteral reflux evaluation. *Pediatric Radiology.* In Press.

Vivier, P. H., Augdal, T. A., & Avni, F. E. (2018). Standardization of pediatric uroradiological terms: a multidisciplinary European glossary. *Pediatric Radiology, 48*(2), 291–303. https://doi.org/10.1007/s00247-017-4006-7

Zelenko, N., Coll, D., Rosenfield, A. T., & Smith, R. C. (2004). Normal ureter size on unenhanced helical CT American. *Journal of Radiology, 182*(4), 1039–1041. https://doi.org/10.2214/ajr.182.4.1821039

Bibliography

Barbosa, J. A., Chow, J. S., Benson, C. B., Yorioka, M. A., Bull, A. S., Retik, A. B., et al. (2012). Postnatal longitudinal evaluation of children diagnosed with prenatal hydronephrosis: Insights in natural history and referral pattern. *Prenatal Diagnosis, 32,* 1242–1249.

Corteville, J. E., Gray, D. L., & Crane, J. P. (1991). Congenital hydronephrosis: Correlation of fetal ultrasonographic findings with infant outcome. *American Journal of Obstetrics and Gynecology, 165,* 384–388.

Fernbach, S. K., Maizels, M., & Conway, J. J. (1993). Ultrasound grading of hydronephrosis: Introduction to the system used by the Society for Fetal Urology. *Pediatric Radiology, 23,* 478–480.

Jones, R. A., Grattan-Smith, J. D., & Little, S. (2011). Pediatric magnetic resonance urography. *Journal of Magnetic Resonance Imaging, 33,* 510–526.

Lebowitz, R. L., & Blickman, J. G. (1983). The coexistence of ureteropelvic junction obstruction and reflux. *American Journal of Roentgenology, 140,* 231–238.

Meyer, J. S., & Lebowitz, R. L. (1992). Primary megaureter in infants and children: A review. *Urologic Radiology, 14,* 296–305.

Nelson, C. P., Johnson, E. K., Logvinenko, T., & Chow, J. S. (2014). Ultrasound as a screening test for genitourinary anomalies in children with UTI. *Pediatrics, 133,* e394–e403.

Nguyen, H. T., Benson, C. B., Bromley, B., Campbell, J. B., Chow, J., Coleman, B., et al. (2014). Multidisciplinary consensus on the classification of prenatal and postnatal urinary tract dilation (UTD classification system). *Journal of Pediatric Urology, 10*(6), 982–998.

Onen, A. (2007). An alternative grading system to refine the criteria for severity of hydronephrosis and optimal treatment guidelines in neonates with primary UPJ-type hydronephrosis. *Journal of Pediatric Urology, 3,* 200–205.

Papadopoulou, F., Ntoulia, A., Siomou, E., & Darge, K. (2014). Contrast-enhanced voiding urosonography with intravesical administration of a second-generation ultrasound contrast agent for diagnosis of vesicoureteral reflux: Prospective evaluation of contrast safety in 1,010 children. *Pediatric Radiology, 44,* 719–728.

Riccabona, M., Avni, F. E., Blickman, J. G., Dacher, J.-N., Darge, K., Lobo, M. L., et al (2009). Imaging recommendations in paediatric uroradiology. Minutes of the ESPR uroradiology task force session on childhood obstructive uropathy, high-grade fetal hydronephrosis, childhood haematuria, and urolithiasis in childhood. ESPR Annual Congress, Edinburgh, UK, June 2008. *Pediatric Radiology, 39,* 891–898.

Schaeffer, A. J., Kurtz, M. P., Logvinenko, T., McCartin, M. T., Prabhu, S. P., Nelson, C. P., et al. (2016). MRI-based reference range for the renal pelvic anterior-posterior diameter in children ages 0-19 years. *British Journal of Radiology, 89*(1067), 20160211.

Swenson, D. W., Darge, K., Ziniel, S. I., & Chow, J. S. (2014). Characterizing upper urinary tract dilation on ultrasound: A survey of North American pediatric radiologists' practices. *Pediatric Radiology, 45*(5), 686–694.

Zerin, J. M., Ritchey, M. L., & Chang, A. C. (1993). Incidental vesicoureteral reflux in neonates with antenatally detected hydronephrosis and other renal abnormalities. *Radiology, 187,* 157–160.

CHAPTER 9
Pelvic Pain

Paula Dickson

CHAPTER OUTLINE

What Imaging Modality Is Best to Assess Pelvic Pain?, 195

What to Do With an Ovarian Cyst?, 195

When to Suspect Ovarian Torsion, 196

What to Do With a Paraadnexal Cyst, 199

Imperforate Hymen and Müllerian Duct Anomalies, 200

Pelvic Inflammatory Disease, 203

Ectopic Pregnancy, 204

What to Do With Chronic Pelvic Pain, 205

Endometriosis, 205

Pelvic Congestion, 208

Summary, 208

Pelvic pain in a preadolescent or adolescent girl can be a diagnostic challenge. Ovarian causes, including torsion of the ovary, ovarian cysts, and paraovarian cysts, must be distinguished from nonovarian diagnoses, such as appendicitis, renal calculi, urinary tract infection, and even intussusception in younger children. Because ovarian or fallopian tube torsion are emergent situations, rapid diagnosis is key.

■ What Imaging Modality Is Best to Assess Pelvic Pain?

Ultrasound is the most useful imaging modality for evaluating the ovaries. A transabdominal approach is typically performed in adolescence. A full bladder is necessary for optimized transabdominal pelvic ultrasound. In the optimized setting the ovaries are well visualized, and the study is quick. If the patient is unable to drink, bolus intravenous fluids can be given, or if emergent diagnosis is necessary, a Foley catheter can be placed. Transabdominal ultrasound is also the modality of choice for evaluating the appendix, so in a female patient with right lower quadrant/pelvic pain, concomitant focused abdominal and pelvic ultrasounds can be performed. Computed tomography (CT) or magnetic resonance imaging (MRI) may be used if more information is needed after ultrasound.

■ What to Do With an Ovarian Cyst?

Pelvic pain can be caused by an enlarging ovarian cyst, hemorrhage into a cyst, rupture of a cyst, or ovarian torsion caused by a cyst (Box 9.1). In postpubertal fe-

males, follicle-stimulating hormone causes one or more Graafian follicles to emerge with a diameter of 1.0 to 2.5 cm in preparation for ovulation. Once an oocyte is released, the Graafian follicle is transformed into a corpus luteum cyst, which remains for 14 days unless the egg is fertilized. If ovulation does not occur and the Graafian follicle continues to enlarge, or if a corpus luteum cyst fails to involute, then a functional/pathological cyst will result. A functional cyst is distinguished from a follicle by size, with follicles measuring less than 3 cm and functional cysts measuring greater than 3 cm. The literature does not indicate a size at which ovarian cysts become symptomatic. There is also controversy regarding the size of an ovarian cyst, and its risk for causing torsion. Some articles cite 5 cm cysts as more likely to be associated with torsion, and some believe that the risk for torsion increases if the cyst is greater than 8 to 9 cm.

Functional cysts can be simple or hemorrhagic. A simple cyst is unilocular with anechoic fluid. A hemorrhagic cyst occurs as a result of bleeding into a follicular cyst or more often into a corpus luteum cyst. The corpus luteum is lined with thin-walled vessels that can rupture. Most hemorrhagic cysts that are imaged are complex in appearance with a septated fishnet pattern caused by fibrin strands (Figs. 9.1–9.3), fluid–debris levels, or a retracting internal clot (Figs. 9.4 and 9.5). This appearance is thought to represent a subacute cyst, with an acutely hemorrhagic cyst potentially seen as an isoechoic cyst or a cyst with an internal fluid–fluid level. A hemorrhagic cyst can rupture with significant intraperitoneal hemorrhage causing pain with a decline in hematocrit. Blood is then demonstrated within the pelvis as complex free fluid. Hemorrhagic cysts can have a more homogenous appearance, mimicking a solid mass, but with increased through transmission (Fig. 9.6) and

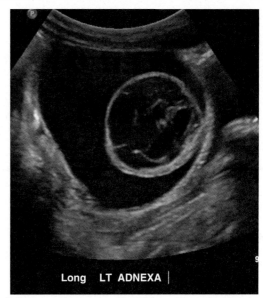

Fig. 9.3 Hemorrhagic cyst with a fishnet pattern inside a large cyst with no visible ovarian parenchyma.

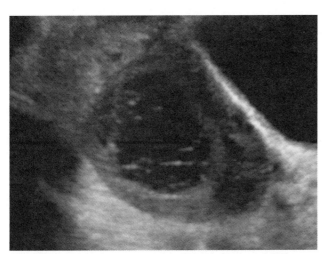

Fig. 9.1 Hemorrhagic cyst with a fishnet pattern within a normal ovary.

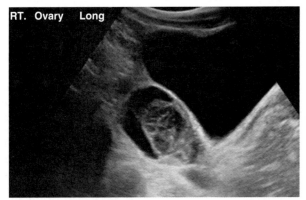

Fig. 9.2 Hemorrhagic cyst with fibrin stranding in a fishnet pattern on longitudinal sonographic image in a 14-year-old girl with pelvic pain.

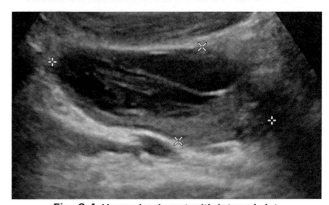

Fig. 9.4 Hemorrhagic cyst with internal clot.

acoustic enhancement. A hemorrhagic cyst can be confused with a teratoma or cystic neoplasm, tuboovarian abscess, ectopic pregnancy, or appendiceal abscess. MRI has been suggested to further evaluate the ovarian parenchyma and to distinguish between these etiologies when necessary (Box 9.2).

Simple and hemorrhagic cysts between 3 and 5 cm should resolve within one to two menstrual cycles and should be followed with ultrasound on days 5 to 10 (follicular phase) of the subsequent menstrual cycle to ensure resolution. Hemorrhagic cysts will become

anechoic over time. Ninety percent of cysts spontaneously resolve.

Ovarian cysts larger than 5 cm are less likely to regress, although the majority do regress in 2 to 3 months or two to three menstrual cycles. There are no definite pediatric guidelines for the length of follow-up, although some advocate for allowing 8-12 weeks for resolution. Oral contraceptives for the treatment of functional cysts are not considered to be beneficial. If the decision is made to operate because of size, symptoms, or persistence of the cyst, laparoscopy with excision of the cyst and sparing of the remainder of the ovary is usually recommended. Fenestration of the cyst has a recurrence rate of 5% to 8%. Aspiration is not recommended with a recurrence rate of 33% to 84%.

■ When to Suspect Ovarian Torsion

Ovarian torsion occurs primarily in adolescents and young women. The classic presentation is severe lower abdominal, pelvic, or groin pain with nausea and vomiting. The pain can be intermittent and recurrent because

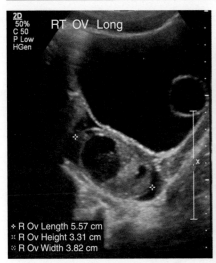

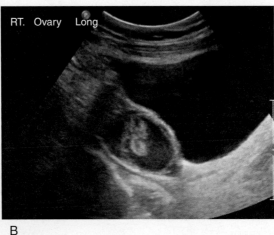

Fig. 9.5 Hemorrhagic cysts with internal clot in two different patients (A and B). The cysts obscure normal ovarian architecture.

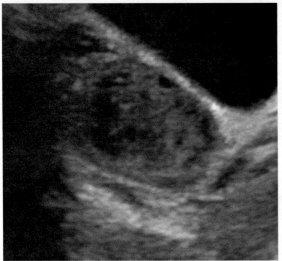

Fig. 9.6 Hemorrhagic cyst that is solid in appearance with through transmission.

| BOX 9.2 | When to Suspect Pelvic Pain as a Result of an Ovarian Cyst |

When ultrasound imaging detects:
Simple ovarian cyst (defined as >3 cm)
Hemorrhagic cyst
Large amount of free fluid within the pelvis suggesting rupture of a simple cyst
Hemorrhagic cyst with echogenic free fluid and decreased hematocrit

of torsion and detorsion. Studies have found that fever and white count are less elevated, and pain is more localized with ovarian torsion than with appendicitis. Torsion results when the ovary partially or completely rotates around its vascular pedicle, which first compromises lymphatic and venous flow. The ovary then becomes congested with eventual arterial obstruction and subsequent infarction and necrosis. Adnexal torsion is usually unilateral with 60% of torsions involving the

right ovary hypothesized to be caused by the protective nature of the sigmoid colon filling the left pelvis.

Torsion can involve a normal ovary or an ovary associated with a cyst or mass. Torsion of a normal ovary is more likely to occur in the pediatric population than the adult population because of the laxity and elongation of the supporting ligaments in the younger population, which allows increased mobility of the ovary. The uteroovarian ligament, which attaches the ovary to the uterus, shortens with age. A cyst or mass within an ovary can act as a fulcrum causing the ovary to twist upon itself or to swing around its pedicle. The suspensory ligament or infundibulopelvic ligament attaches the ovary to the pelvic sidewall and contains the ovarian vessels. The mesovarium is spread between the ovary and the fallopian tube so that when the ovary twists, the tube may also be involved in the torsion (Diagram 9.1).

It can be difficult to determine whether an ovarian cyst is causing pain primarily or if secondary torsion has occurred, causing the pain (Fig. 9.7). One of the more challenging diagnostic dilemmas occurs when a hemorrhagic cyst or mass occupies the ovary and obscures the normal parenchyma, causing the ovary to appear complex. The differential includes ovarian torsion or a nontorsed ovary containing a hemorrhagic cyst or mass (Figs. 9.8 and 9.9). A complex ovary can also be caused by a tubo-ovarian abscess or rarely an ectopic pregnancy. Often torsion cannot be excluded when a complex ovary is imaged. Clinical presentation may be helpful in determining whether surgery is warranted.

A benign teratoma is the most common ovarian mass associated with torsion (Box 9.3). The presence of a teratoma may cause symptoms without torsion (Fig. 9.10). When a radiograph is obtained for abdominal pain, assessment of the pelvis should include a search for calcifications that may indicate the presence of a teratoma (Fig. 9.11). If pelvic calcifications are present, an ultrasound is performed to confirm a mass and to evaluate the ovary for signs of torsion (Fig. 9.12). By ultrasound, echogenic foci representing calcifications, hair, and fat can be seen within the teratoma. The echogenic foci may appear as a mural nodule or dermoid plug, or as

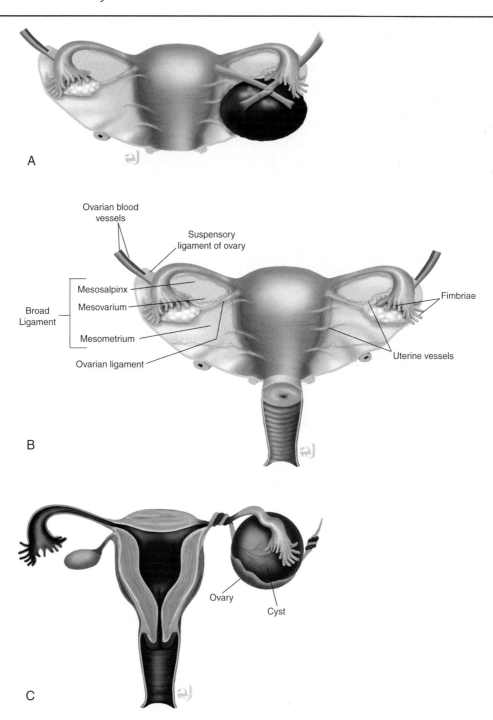

A

Ovarian blood
vessels

Suspensory
ligament of ovary

Mesosalpinx

Mesovarium

Broad
Ligament

Mesometrium

Ovarian ligament

Fimbriae

Uterine vessels

B

Ovary

Cyst

C

DIAGRAM 9.1

central masses (Fig. 9.13). Shadowing can occur because of matted sebum and hair or calcifications, and it can obscure a portion of the mass. A teratoma can appear anechoic if mostly composed of sebum or serous fluid, or can appear solid if mostly composed of teeth, cartilage, hair, and fat. The teratoma can be large, filling the abdomen with nonvisualization of the normal ovary or ovaries (Fig. 9.14). If ascites is present, an immature, malignant teratoma should be suspected (Fig. 9.15).

The most reliable sign of torsion is enlargement of the ovary (Boxes 9.4 and 9.5). The torsed ovary may be 5 to 6 times the size of the normal ovary (Fig. 9.16). In a study by Linam et al. (2007), an adnexal volume of <20 ml is one of the few findings that excluded adnexal torsion in menarchal females. Small uniform follicles aligned around the periphery of an enlarged ovary are another sign of torsion seen in up to 75% of cases. The peripheral location of follicles is theorized to be due to vascular congestion with central parenchymal/stromal edema (Fig. 9.17). Peripheral follicles are not specific for torsion and can be seen with polycystic ovary disease (Fig. 9.18). A torsed ovary may also move to

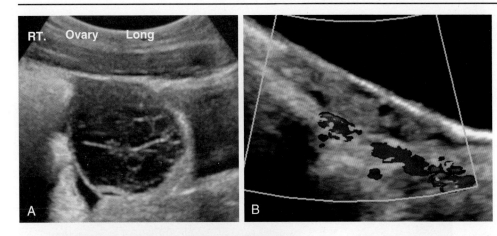

Fig. 9.7 Hemorrhagic cyst (A) that resolved 3 months later (B) in a 14-year-old with pelvic pain.

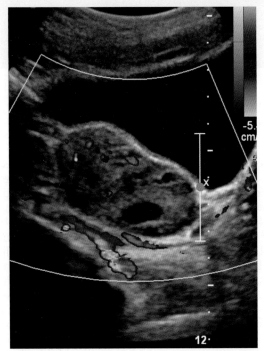

Fig. 9.8 Enlarged complex ovary with color flow in a 12-year-old with intense pelvic pain. Surgery revealed torsed ovary containing hemorrhagic cyst.

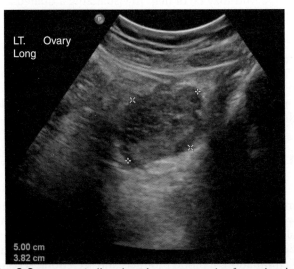

Fig. 9.9 Asymmetrically enlarged ovary concerning for torsion, but surgery revealed hemorrhagic cyst occupying the ovary without torsion.

> **BOX 9.3   Pelvic or Abdominal Pain With Pelvic Calcification**
>
> Think teratoma with possible ovarian torsion.

an extraadnexal position in the cul-de-sac, in the midline or superior to the uterus (Fig. 9.19). Some radiologists advocate sweeping through the adnexa with color Doppler looking for a twisted vascular pedicle, a positive whirlpool sign. Although this is a specific sign of torsion, it is difficult to detect. Blood flow to the ovary is not reliable. Arterial flow can be demonstrated even when the ovary is torsed because venous flow is occluded before arterial flow and because of the dual arterial blood supply to the ovaries from the uterine and ovarian arteries. Color Doppler flow has been reported in about 65% of torsed ovaries in children and does not entirely exclude torsion (Fig. 9.20). Increased compensatory flow can be seen if the ovary has torsed and detorsed. The absence of flow is suggestive of torsion but can also be caused by technical factors. Use of high-frequency probes and small Doppler sampling box may be helpful to optimize color Doppler flow.

MRI may be helpful if further characterization is needed. Fast spin-echo T2-weighted images are best for demonstrating peripherally displaced follicles in an enlarged ovary (Fig. 9.21). Nonenhancement of the ovary is helpful in diagnosing torsion, although as with ultrasound, enhancement can occur with torsion. The whirlpool sign with a twisted vascular pedicle is specific but not often seen. The uterus may deviate toward the side of the torsion. A mass within the ovary may be better defined with MRI than with ultrasound. Findings with CT are similar, although a nonenhancing ovary is easier to distinguish from a nonenhancing cyst on MRI.

■ What to Do With a Paraadnexal Cyst

A fimbrial cyst or hydatid cyst of Morgagni is a rare cause of pelvic pain but should be considered when an adnexal or midline cyst is observed separate from the ovary. The cyst is attached to the fimbriated end of the fallopian tube by a pedicle and can cause torsion of the tube. Torsion of the fallopian tube without an abnormality

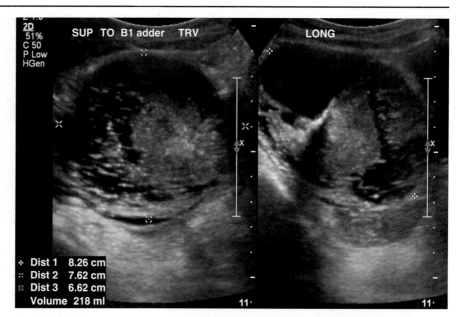

Fig. 9.10 Benign teratoma with shadowing calcification on longitudinal image discovered in a 12-year-old premenarchal patient with pelvic pain. No torsion was found during surgery.

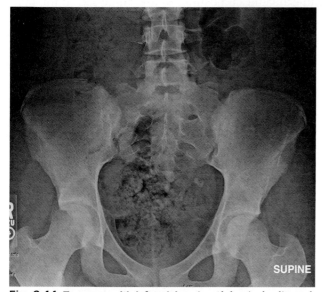

Fig. 9.11 Teenager with left pelvic pain. Abdominal radiograph demonstrates calcification in left pelvis. Benign teratoma with torsion was found at surgery.

of the ovary is referred to as isolated fallopian tube torsion (IFTT) (Box 9.6). The fimbrial cysts are remnants of the müllerian (paramesonephric) and wolffian (mesonephric) ducts. Paraovarian cysts are another type of paraadnexal cyst that originate from the parovarium of the broad ligament. The torsed cyst is often superior to the uterus or in the cul-de-sac. A change in position of the cyst within the pelvis on sequential ultrasounds increases the consideration that the cyst has caused the fallopian tube to twist. A CT may be helpful to better visualize the location of the cyst and to confirm that the cyst is separate from the ovaries (Figs. 9.22 and 9.23). By CT the uterus may be deviated toward the side of the torsion. An adjacent dilated, fluid-filled tube, if present, helps confirm the diagnosis but is rarely demonstrated. MRI may be helpful in visualizing the dilated fallopian tube. Paraadnexal cysts can also twist on themselves at

the neck of the cyst or may rupture, causing pain (Fig. 9.24). A paraadnexal cyst is not affected by the hormonal cycle and will not vary in size with the menstrual cycle. These cysts are rarely neoplastic.

Isolated tubal torsion also occurs without an associated fimbrial cyst. Hydrosalpinx is one etiology and is due to obstruction of the fimbrial end of the tube possibly secondary to a congenital malformation of the tube or adjacent pelvic infections causing obstruction. It has been suggested that as menses approaches, ovarian and tubal function are activated, resulting in hydrosalpinx, which can then twist. An elongated mesosalpinx, adhesions, adnexal venous congestion, and pelvic inflammatory disease are other causes. Ultrasound may reveal a fluid-filled tubular structure that may be folded on itself and appear C- or S-shaped. The sonographic appearance of the dilated fallopian tube often has internal pseudoseptations from the longitudinal folds along the fallopian tube (Fig. 9.25). Color Doppler is not useful because of the dual blood supply to the tube. As noted earlier, MRI may be of help in visualizing a dilated tube that may be positioned in the midline.

Isolated tubal torsion occurs most often in young adolescent girls between 12 and 15 years old. Symptoms are pelvic pain with nausea and vomiting (Box 9.7). IFTT is rare and difficult to diagnose but must be kept in mind so that surgery is timely. Laparoscopy is performed with excision of the cyst and salvage of the fallopian tube, if possible.

■ Imperforate Hymen and Müllerian Duct Anomalies

Imperforate hymen may present with pelvic pain and/or abdominopelvic distension and presents in neonatal life or in peripubertal age. The complete hymen is the most common cause of vaginal obstruction, causing accumulation of blood products and secretions, secondary distension of the vagina, and often mild distention

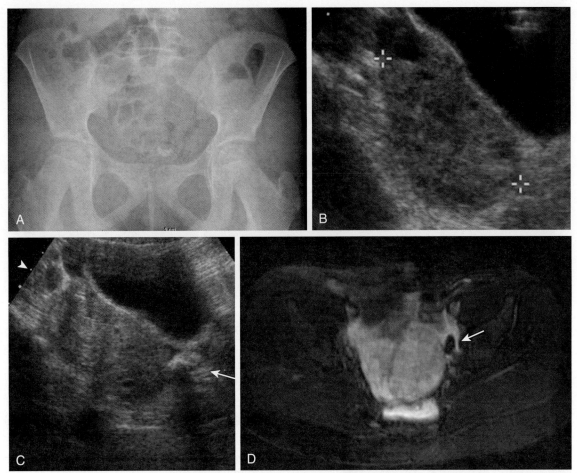

Fig. 9.12 Calcification in the left pelvis of an 11-year-old with pelvic pain (A). Ultrasound (B and C) and magnetic resonance imaging (D) reveal an enlarged right ovary with separate calcification (*arrow*). At surgery, the right ovary was acutely torsed with an atrophic and calcified left ovary, presumably as a result of prior torsion.

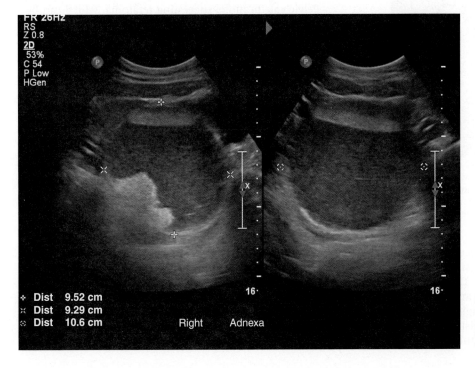

Fig. 9.13 Patient with 2 weeks of pain. Ultrasound demonstrates right adnexal mass with layering echogenicities and mural nodule. A benign dermoid causing a 720-degree twist was found with a purple ischemic ovary and tube.

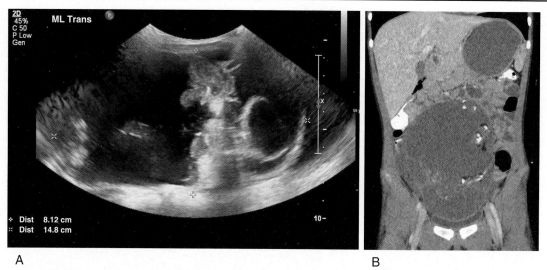

A   B

Fig. 9.14 Large teratoma, the majority of which is anechoic with echogenic central masses by ultrasound (A), and a dermoid plug by computed tomography (B). The ovaries could not be distinguished from the mass but were the assumed origin.

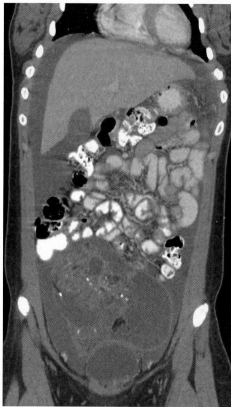

Fig. 9.15 Large septated cystic teratoma with calcifications and a large amount of ascites in a patient with lower abdominal and pelvic pain. Pathology was benign mature teratoma, but the mass recurred with the diagnosis of primitive neuroectodermal tumor. An immature teratoma should be suspected if ascites is present.

BOX 9.4   Pelvic Pain With Imaging of Enlarged Ovary Compared With Contralateral Side

Think ovarian torsion.

BOX 9.5   When to Suspect Pelvic Pain as a Result of Ovarian Torsion

Enlarged ovary is the most reliable sign—compare with contralateral side
Enlarged ovary with small, uniform peripheral follicles
Complex adnexal mass with nonvisualization of normal tissue
Positioning of the ovary in the midline, superior to the uterus or in the cul-de-sac
Twisted vascular pedicle—whirlpool sign
Pelvic calcifications suggesting teratoma, which can be a cause of torsion
Additional findings by MRI/CT
    Deviation of the uterus toward the side of torsion
    Nonenhancement of affected ovary on postcontrast MRI or CT
Doppler flow is unreliable and should not sway your decision based on other findings
CT, Computed tomography; *MRI,* magnetic resonance imaging.

---

of the uterus called *hydrometrocolpos* or *hematometrocolpos.* The vagina may become surprisingly large and often demonstrates a fluid–debris level. The distended vagina will be seen between the bladder and rectum; however, if large enough, the distended vagina may displace/efface them. The uterus does not distend as much as the vagina because of myometrial stiffness.

Although many female patients with müllerian duct anomalies (MDAs) will be asymptomatic, there are categories of MDA that can present with pelvic pain as a result of vaginal or hemivaginal obstruction, cervical obstruction, or a rudimentary uterine horn with functioning endometrium. A full discussion of MDAs is out of the scope of this chapter; however, an included diagram depicting the categories of MDA and their multiple variants may help elucidate their characteristics (Fig. 9.26). The reader may reference review articles that outline the many variations of MDA (e.g., Patton et al., 2004; Troiano & McCarthy, 2004).

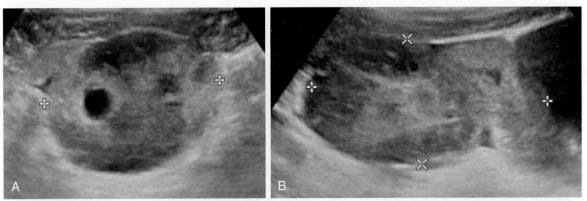

Fig. 9.16 Enlarged right ovary (A, B) with a volume of 127 cc compared with the contralateral ovary with a volume of 7 cc (not shown). Surgery demonstrated an enlarged blackened ovary torsed 720 degrees.

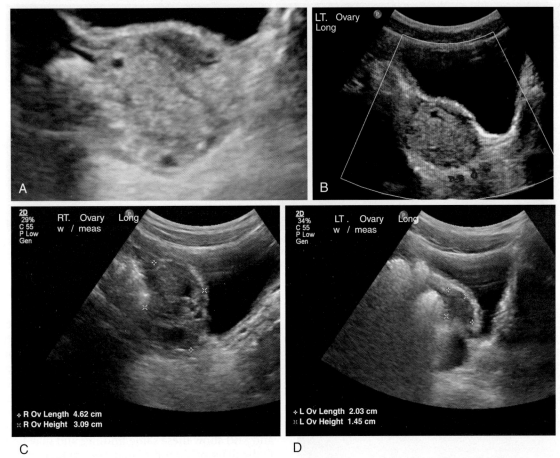

Fig. 9.17 Enlarged left ovary with peripheral follicles found to be torsed in an 11-year-old with left pelvic pain (A). The ovary was detorsed and left in place. The ovary torsed again 2 months later and was again detorsed (B). Four months later the patient experienced right pelvic pain. The right ovary had torsed (C), and the left ovary had atrophied (D).

If the patient has already started menstruation but also appears to have an obstruction of the vagina and uterus on ultrasound, the diagnosis may be an MDA known as obstructed hemivagina with ipsilateral renal agenesis in a patient with two separate vaginal and uterine cavities (such as uterus didelphys, bicornuate uterus with longitudinal vaginal septum, or complete septate uterus with vaginal septum) with one obstructed and one patent outflow tract (Fig. 9.27). Many patients with MDA have renal anomalies, the most common of which is renal agenesis ipsilateral to the vaginal/uterine anomaly. Work-up of MDA should include an assessment of the entire genitourinary system, beginning with ultrasound followed by MRI.

■ Pelvic Inflammatory Disease

Pelvic inflammatory disease with pyosalpinx and tuboovarian abscess can overlap with the appearance of

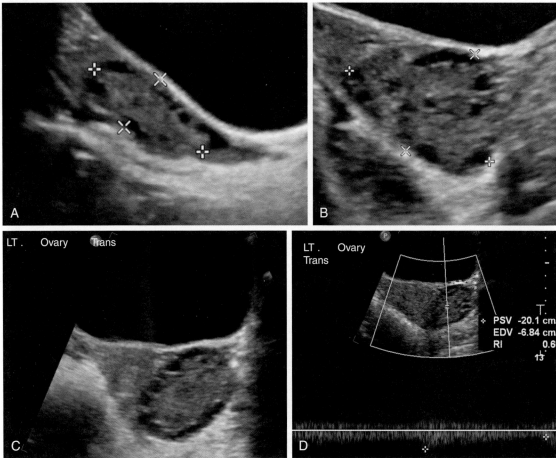

Fig. 9.18 A 15-year-old with recurrent left abdominal and pelvic pain. Peripheral follicles noted in both the right ovary (A) and the left ovary with enlargement of the left ovary (B, C). Polycystic ovary syndrome (PCOS) with left ovarian torsion was suspected, although flow was present in the left ovary (D). Torsion and PCOS were confirmed.

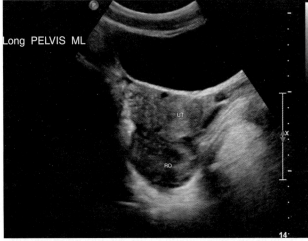

Fig. 9.19 Torsed ovary that has flipped into the cul-de-sac.

ovarian torsion, IFTT, and complicated ovarian cysts (Box 9.8). Fever and an elevated white blood cell count help guide the diagnosis, but imaging can be helpful in diagnosis and management. Ultrasound demonstrates uterine and ovarian enlargement, indistinctness of the uterus, endometrial fluid and complex free fluid in the pelvis. With pyosalpinx, the fallopian tubes are dilated with thick walls and filled with debris. Thickened endosalpingeal folds within the tube give a "cogwheel" appearance. If the infection progresses to a tuboovarian abscess, a complex cystic adnexal mass is present with no distinguishable ovarian tissue. Hyperemia of the thickened tube and tuboovarian abscess is demonstrable with color Doppler. The disease is often bilateral. CT and MRI show these same findings and may help solidify the diagnosis. Multiplanar T2-weighted images delineate dilated fluid-filled fallopian tubes. Increased signal on T2-weighted images, diffusion-weighted images, and contrast-enhanced T1-weighted images may help distinguish tuboovarian abscesses from other ovarian causes of pelvic pain.

■ Ectopic Pregnancy

An ectopic pregnancy should be considered and searched for in postmenarchal females with pelvic pain, particularly if associated with vaginal bleeding. A complex mass between the ovary and the uterus is the most common finding. An ectopic can also appear as a tubal ring without central features, a tubal ring with a yolk

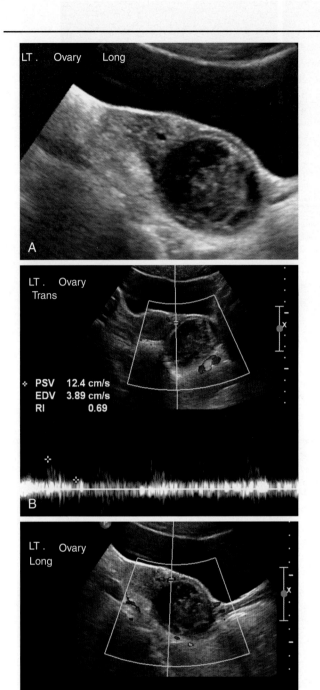

Fig. 9.20 Large hemorrhagic ovarian cyst (A) with arterial (B) and venous flow (C) present within the small amount of visualized surrounding ovary, but torsion was found at surgery.

sac, or a tubal ring containing a yolk sac and embryo. Only 1% of ectopic pregnancies are within the ovary, so a complex ovarian mass is unlikely to represent an ectopic pregnancy. A thick-walled corpus luteum cyst can mimic an ectopic pregnancy. If scanning with an endovaginal probe, pressure may be applied to the ovary to determine whether the mass moves with the ovary or separate from the ovary. An associated pseudosac is occasionally visible by ultrasound located centrally in the uterine endometrium. A pseudosac is an intrauterine fluid collection that is a hormonal response to an ectopic pregnancy. This is opposed to an intrauterine gestational sac that is eccentrically located in the endometrium. Ectopic pregnancies can also be implanted in the interstitial or intramyometrial portion of the fallopian tube or in the cervix.

■ What to Do With Chronic Pelvic Pain

Chronic pelvic pain is defined as nonmenstrual pain that continues for at least 6 months. The differential for chronic pelvic pain in adolescent girls includes endometriosis and pelvic congestion syndrome. Endometriosis occurs in approximately 10% of postmenarchal females and in 60% to 70% of adolescents with chronic pelvic pain not controlled with medical management. Surgery is often necessary for diagnosis. Pelvic congestion syndrome is characterized by dilated pelvic and ovarian veins seen on imaging studies without another cause for the pain. This syndrome is usually seen in the adult population but has been reported in the pediatric literature.

■ Endometriosis

Endometriosis is not commonly an imaging diagnosis in the pediatric age, although occasionally small implants can be found on endoscopy for extreme pelvic pain. The majority of ectopic endometrial tissue occurs in the ovaries, but implants are also found in the uterosacral ligaments, peritoneum, surface of the uterus, fallopian tubes, rectosigmoid colon, and bladder. Although small implants and deep pelvic endometriiosis are best identified by MRI ultrasound is the modality of choice to distinguish an ovarian endometrioma from a complex ovarian cyst. On ultrasound, low-level internal echoes within an ovarian cyst represent cyclic bleeding giving a homogeneous, ground-glass appearance, hence the name "chocolate cyst" given to these entities. An echogenic bright focus in the wall can be seen and is specific for an endometrioma (Box 9.9). Endometriomas may have an irregular border, and they demonstrate no vascular flow. Endometriomas may appear more complex with septations or fluid–fluid levels and resemble a hemorrhagic cyst or neoplasm. They are often multiple and bilateral and are stable in appearance, whereas hemorrhagic cysts evolve.

MRI is helpful in distinguishing an endometrioma from other ovarian masses because of the signal characteristics of the blood products. An endometrioma will be hyperintense on T1-weighted images and hypointense on T2-weighted images, distinguishing it from cysts, abscesses, or neoplasms. The hypointensity and loss of signal on T2-weighted images is due to concentrated blood products and is termed *T2 shading*. The loss of signal may be complete, heterogeneous, or a fluid–fluid level with hypointense and hyperintense T2 signal.

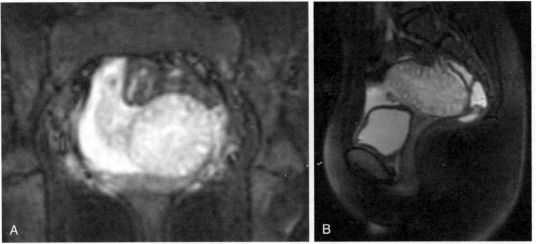

Fig. 9.21 Coronal (A) and sagittal (B) magnetic resonance imaging T2-weighted images demonstrate an enlarged ovary with peripheral follicles.

BOX 9.6   When to Suspect Pelvic Pain as a Result of a Paraadnexal Cyst or Isolated Fallopian Tube Torsion

Midline cyst superior to bladder or in cul-de-sac
Cyst adjacent to but separate from ovary
Adnexal cyst changing in position between examinations
Dilated tubular structure in adnexa or midline
Pelvic pain, which may be localized, associated with nausea and vomiting

---

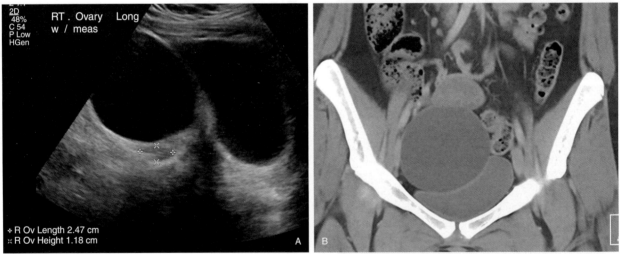

Fig. 9.22 A 10 cm paraadnexal cyst imaged with ultrasound adjacent to a normal right ovary in a 14-year-old girl with right lower quadrant pain (A). The pain increased, and a subsequent computed tomography scan shows the cyst to be repositioned in the midline inferior to an enlarged right ovary containing peripheral cysts (B). Surgery revealed a torsed right ovary and cyst.

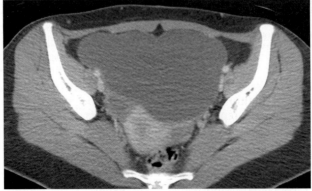

Fig. 9.23 Midline cyst separate from the ovaries in a teenager with pelvic pain. Surgery revealed a torsed paraadnexal cyst. Recognizing that a midline cyst in a female can be a torsed para-adnexal cyst is important to provide the possibility of detorsion with salvage of the tube and ovary.

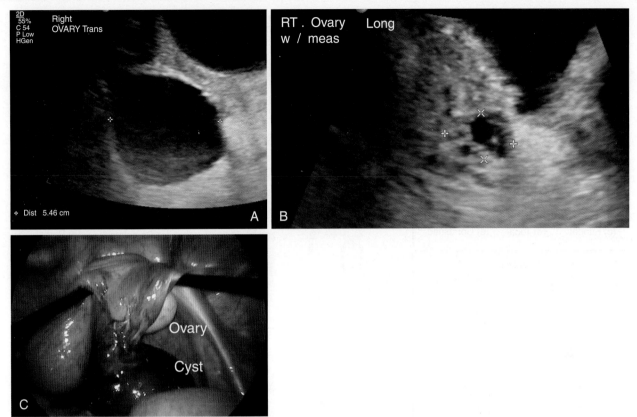

Fig. 9.24 A 13-year-old premenarchal patient with a 3-month history of unexplained intermittent vomiting. Abdominal pain finally accompanied the vomiting and was thought to be viral, until the pain localized to the right groin. Ultrasound reveals a 5.5-cm cyst with debris (A) adjacent to a normal right ovary (B). Surgery found a purple hemorrhagic fimbrial cyst torsed on itself at its neck (C). The fimbriae were edematous with a normal tube and ovary. The cyst was drained and removed in pieces laparoscopically.

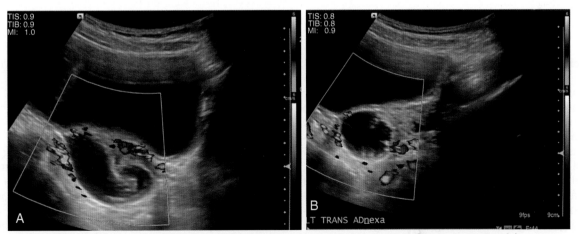

Fig. 9.25 A 10-year-old girl presented to the emergency department with acute-onset pelvic pain. Ultrasound reveals a fluid-filled C-shaped structure (A) containing small pseudoseptations (B). Laparoscopy revealed an isolated tubal torsion.

BOX 9.7   Pelvic pain with cyst adjacent to ovary or in midline

Think paraadnexal cyst causing torsion of the fallopian tube.

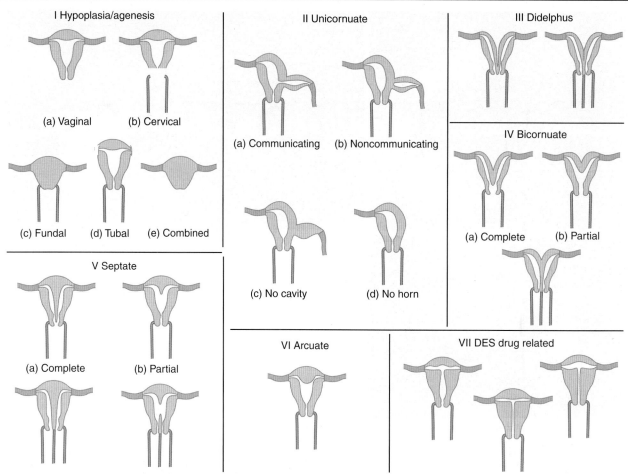

Fig. 9.26 Classification of müllerian duct anomalies. *DES*, diethylstilbestrol.

■ Pelvic Congestion

In pelvic congestion syndrome, dilated tortuous pelvic veins are present adjacent to the ovaries and uterus with a diameter greater than 6 mm. Reversed flow or slow flow may be demonstrated, as well as dilated myometrial veins communicating with bilateral pelvic varices. CT and MRI are helpful to further visualize pelvic varices, as well as to visualize dilated ovarian veins. Reversal of flow in the ovarian veins is also demonstrated by cross-sectional imaging. Before treatment, ovarian vein venography is performed with findings including ovarian vein diameter >10 mm, varices adjacent to the uterus and ovaries, and filling of the pelvic veins across the midline. Transcatheter embolotherapy is the usual treatment, with 65% to 85% of women having some improvement in pelvic pain (Box 9.10).

■ Summary

The exact cause of pelvic pain can be challenging in females. Transabdominal sonography is the primary imaging modality for pelvic pain in the pediatric population. Optimized technique, knowledge of normal uterus and ovarian appearance, reference to normal ovarian sizes and attention to ovarian symmetry are important. Although it may be difficult to be definitive in the setting of pelvic pain with an ovarian mass or cyst, the possibility of torsion must be considered and communicated.

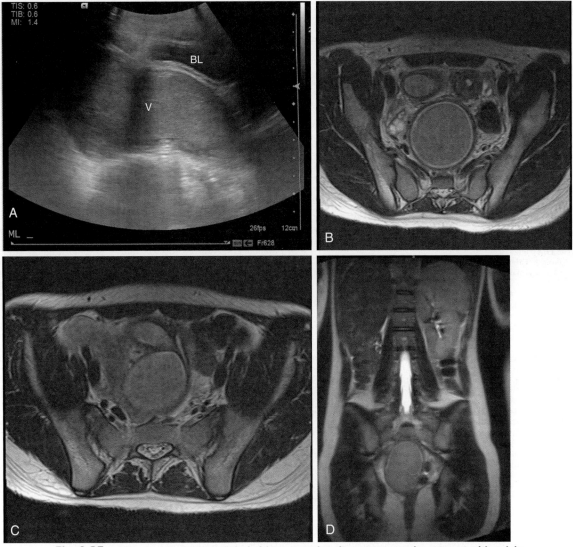

Fig. 9.27 A 12-year-old postmenarchal girl presented to the emergency department with pelvic pain. Longitudinal grayscale image through the pelvis (A) demonstrates a dilated vagina (V) containing hypoechoic blood products posterior to the bladder (BL). Axial oblique T2-weighted images through the pelvis (B, C) reveal two widely splayed uterine horns and an obstructed right hemivagina and right uterine horn consistent with a uterine didelphys with an obstructing vaginal septum. Image through the kidney (D) shows right renal agenesis, ipsilateral to the side of uterine didelphys and vaginal obstruction.

BOX 9.8 When to Suspect Pelvic Pain as a Result of Pelvic Inflammatory Disease

Enlargement and indistinctness of the uterus
Enlargement of the ovaries
Dilated, hyperemic, thickened, debris-filled tubular structures
Cogwheel appearance of dilated tubes
Complex adnexal masses with increased Doppler flow and increased signal on T2-weighted and enhanced T1-weighted images
Bilateral findings
Fever and leukocytosis

BOX 9.9 When to Suspect Pelvic Pain as a Result of an Endometrioma

Nonvascular cyst with low-level echoes and a ground-glass appearance
Punctate echogenic focus in the wall of the cyst
Multiple and bilateral cysts
Hyperintense on T1-weighted images and hypointense or loss of signal on T2-weighted images

BOX 9.10 When to Suspect Pelvic Pain as a Result of Pelvic Congestion

Pelvic varices near the ovaries and uterus
Dilated ovarian veins
Reversal of flow in ovarian veins
Reversal of flow or slow flow in pelvic varices
Filling of pelvic veins across the midline

Bibliography

Antony, J. (2011). *Hemorrhagic ovarian cyst: A sonographic perspective.* ObGyn. net https://www.contemporaryobgyn.net/view/hemorrhagic-ovarian-cyst-sonographic-perspective.

Benjaminov, O., & Atri, M. (2004). Sonography of the abnormal fallopian tube. *American Journal of Roentgenology, 183*(3), 737–742.

Boukaidi, S. A., Delotte, J., Steyaert, H., et al. (2011). Thirteen cases of isolated tubal torsions associated with hydrosalpinx in children and adolescents, proposal for conservative management: Retrospective review and literature survey. *Journal of Pediatric Surgery, 46*(7), 1425–1431.

Brandt, M. L., & Helmrath, M. A. (2005). Ovarian cysts in infants and children. *Seminars in Pediatric Surgery, 14*(2), 78–85.

Chang, H. C., Bhatt, S., & Dogra, V. S. (2008). Pearls and pitfalls in diagnosis of ovarian torsion. *RadioGraphics, 28*(5), 1355–1368.

Chiou, S.-Y., Lev-Toaff, A. S., Masuda, E., Feld, R. I., & Bergin, D. (2007). Adnexal torsion. *J Ultrasound Med., 26*, 1289–1301.

Duigenan, S., Oliva, E., & Lee, S. I. (2012). Ovarian torsion: Diagnostic features on CT and MRI with pathologic correlation. *American Journal of Roentgenology, 198*(2), W122–W131.

Frates, M. C., Doubilet, P. M., Peters, H. E., & Benson, C. B. (2014). Adnexal sonographic findings in ectopic pregnancy and their correlation with tubal rupture and human chorionic gonadotropin levels. *Journal of Ultrasound in Medicine, 33*(4), 697–703.

Garel, L., Dubois, J., Grignon, A., Filiatrault, D., & Van Vliet, G. (2001). US of the pediatric female pelvis: A clinical perspective. *RadioGraphics, 21*(6), 1393–1407.

Ghonge, N. P., Lall, C., Aggarwal, B., & Bhargava, P. (2015). The MRI whirlpool sign in the diagnosis of ovarian torsion. *Radiology Case Reports, 7*(3), 731.

Harmon, J. C., Binkovitz, L. A., & Binkovitz, L. E. (2008). Isolated fallopian tube torsion: Sonographic and CT features. *Pediatric Radiology, 38*(2), 175–179.

Jain, K. A. (2002). Sonographic spectrum of hemorrhagic ovarian cysts. *Journal of Ultrasound in Medicine, 21*(8), 879–886.

Kao, L. Y., Scheinfeld, M. H., Chernyak, V., Rozenblit, A. M., Oh, S., & Dym, R. J. (2014). Beyond ultrasound: CT and MRI of ectopic pregnancy. *American Journal of Roentgenology, 202*(4), 904–911.

Kuhn, J.P., Slovis, T.L., Haller, J.O., & Caffey, J. (2004). Caffey's pediatric diagnostic imaging. Mosby.

Linam, L., Darolia, R., Naffaa, L. N., Breech, L. L., O'Hara, S. M., Hillard, P. J., & Huppert, J. S. (2007). US findings of adnexal torsion in children and adolescents: size really does matter. *Pediatric Radiology, 37*, 1013–1019. https://doi.org/10.1007/s00247-007-0599-6. In this issue.

Lourenco, A. P., Swenson, D., Tubbs, R. J., & Lazarus, E. (2013). Ovarian and tubal torsion: Imaging findings on US, CT, and MRI. *Emergency Radiology, 21*(2), 179–187.

Mandade, K., Yadav, V., Singh, S., Dp, B., & Deshpande, S. (2014). Bilateral parovarian cyst complicated with torsion in 12yrs girl: Case report. *JDMS, 13*(1), 89–91.

Merlini, L., Anooshiravani, M., Vunda, A., et al. (2008). Noninflammatory fallopian tube pathology in children. *Pediatric Radiology, 38*(12), 1330–1337.

Özcan, C., Çelik, A., Özok, G., Erdener, A., & Balık, E. (2002). Adnexal torsion in children may have a catastrophic sequel: Asynchronous bilateral torsion. *Journal of Pediatric Surgery, 37*(11), 1617–1620.

Patton, P. E., Novy, M. J., Lee, D. M., & Hickok, L. R. (2004). The diagnosis and reproductive outcome after surgical treatment of the complete septate uterus, duplicated cervix and vaginal septum. *American Journal of Obstetrics and Gynecology, 190*(6), 1669–1675.

Pomeranz, A. J., & Sabnis, S. (2004). Misdiagnoses of ovarian masses in children and adolescents. *Pediatric Emergency Care, 20*(3), 172–174.

Poonai, N., Poonai, C., Lim, R., & Lynch, T. (2013). Pediatric ovarian torsion: Case series and review of the literature. *Canadian Journal of Surgery, 56*(2), 103–108.

Potter, A. W., & Chandrasekhar, C. A. (2008). US and CT evaluation of acute pelvic pain of gynecologic origin in nonpregnant premenopausal patients. *RadioGraphics, 28*(6), 1645–1659.

Schmitt, E. R., Ngai, S. S., Gausche-Hill, M., & Renslo, R. (2013). Twist and shout! Pediatric ovarian torsion clinical update and case discussion. *Pediatric Emergency Care, 29*(4), 518–523.

Siegel, M.J. (2011). Pediatric sonography. Lippincott Williams & Wilkins.

Smith, C. J., Bey, T., Emil, S., Wichelhaus, C., & Lotfipour, S. (2008). Ovarian teratoma with torsion masquerading as intussusception in 4-year-old child. *Western Journal of Emergency Medicine, 9*(4), 228–231.

Tessiatore, P., Guanà, R., Mussa, A., et al. (2012). When to operate on ovarian cysts in children? *Journal of Pediatric Endocrinology & Metabolism, 25*(5–6), 427–433.

Troiano, R. N., & McCarthy, S. M. (2004). Müllerian duct anomalies: Imaging and clinical issues. *Radiology, 233*(1), 19–34.

Wassong, C., Shah, B., Kanayama, M., Bjarnason, H., & Milla, S. S. (2011). Radiologic findings of pelvic venous congestion in an adolescent girl with angiographic confirmation and interventional treatment. *Pediatric Radiology, 42*(5), 636–640.

Yilmaz, E., Usal, C., Kovanlikaya, A., & Karabay, N. (2001). Sonographic and MRI findings in prepubertal adnexal hemorrhagic cyst with torsion. *Journal of Clinical Ultrasound, 29*(3), 200–202.

Zolton, J. R., & Maseelall, P. B. (2013). Evaluation of ovarian cysts in adolescents. *Open Journal of Obstetrics and Gynecology, 3*(7), 12–16.

MSK

CHAPTER 10
Imaging the Limping Child

Shreya Mozer and Sarah Dantzler Bixby

CHAPTER OUTLINE

What Imaging Modalities Are Useful for Working Up a Limp in a Pediatric Patient?, 213
What Is the Utility of Radiographs?, 214
What Is the Utility of Sonography?, 215
Is There a Role for Bone Scans?, 218
Is There a Role for Computed Tomography?, 218
When to Consider Magnetic Resonance Imaging?, 219
How Does the Patient's Age Affect Imaging Workup?, 221
How to Image a Child With Suspected Trauma, 221
    Radiographs in the Setting of Trauma, 221
    Suspected Trauma in Newly Ambulating Child: The Toddler Fracture, 222

What to Do in Young Children With Suspected Trauma but Unreliable Histories?, 224
How to Image a Child With Suspected Infection, 224
How to Approach a Child With No History of Trauma and No Signs of Infection, 229
How to Approach a Child With Subacute or Chronic Limp, 231
Does the Presence of Pain Help?, 231
What Conditions Present With Pathological Fractures?, 232
Summary, 233

The observation that a child has a limp is not a diagnosis, but rather a manifestation of an underlying problem. A limping child has altered gait, which may or may not also be antalgic. This is a commonly encountered phenomenon in pediatric medicine, and ~4% of all pediatric patient visits are related to acute onset of limp or refusal to ambulate. The causes of limp in childhood are many and span a broad range of etiologies including, but not limited to, congenital abnormalities, infection, trauma-related injury, neoplastic conditions, neuromuscular disease, and vascular insult. A proper clinical history and physical examination are crucial for narrowing down an otherwise extensive differential. Certain physical examination findings or maneuvers may assist in tailoring an appropriate differential diagnosis. For instance, observation of circumduction during gait suggests an ankle or foot problem. Similarly, absence of or decreased ability to internally rotate the hip raises concern for Legg-Calvé-Perthes (LCP) or slipped capital femoral epiphysis (SCFE). A Trendelenburg gait in which the pelvis tilts downward and away from the affected hip as a result of weakening of the contralateral gluteus medius muscle is associated with unilateral developmental hip dysplasia, SCFE, and LCP.

Despite having adequate clinical history and the aid of physical examination maneuvers, often a single cause cannot be isolated. The clinical history is not always easily elucidated from young children, and there may be overlapping or confounding clinical features. In many of these instances, imaging plays a crucial role in narrowing the differential diagnoses from a broad list of various entities to a more focused concern. This is important not only for arriving at the correct diagnosis but also for recognizing potential life- or limb-threatening entities that require immediate intervention.

■ What Imaging Modalities Are Useful for Working Up a Limp in a Pediatric Patient?

A variety of diagnostic imaging modalities may be useful for the assessment of the various causes of limp in a child. Imaging may be targeted to the lower extremities, pelvis, or spine depending on what is felt to be most contributing to the altered gait. Plain radiographs are generally the most frequent, initially used imaging modality. Plain radiographs are widely available, straightforward to perform, relatively low cost, and well suited to demonstrate many osseous abnormalities that cause a limp without need for further imaging. Sonography is another vital imaging tool in children, particularly when assessing for joint effusions. Magnetic resonance imaging (MRI), computed tomography (CT), and bone scintigraphy are imaging modalities that may be useful depending on the specific clinical features and differential diagnoses under consideration. The role of imaging should be to aid in diagnosis in the context of relevant

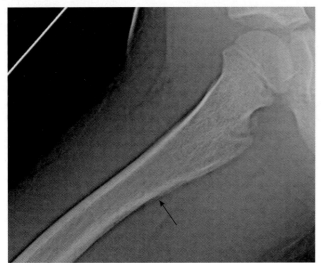

Fig. 10.1 Lateral radiograph of the right femur in a 4-year-old girl with fever and limp demonstrates subtle periosteal reaction and cortical irregularity along the posterior proximal femoral diaphysis (*arrow*). Magnetic resonance imaging later confirmed the diagnosis of osteomyelitis.

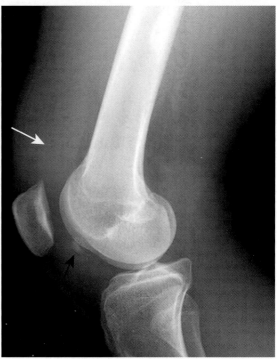

Fig. 10.2 Lateral radiograph of the right knee in a 16-year-old boy with knee swelling and limp demonstrates large joint effusion (*white arrow*). There is also a loose bony fragment in the joint space (*black arrow*) related to a displaced osteochondral fracture.

history and physical examination findings, as well as to separate benign from more aggressive entities that require urgent attention. In addition, the radiologist should help guide appropriate imaging depending on the available clinical information with the primary goal of promoting patient safety by expediting a correct diagnosis while minimizing radiation exposure.

■ What Is the Utility of Radiographs?

In most situations the initial imaging approach to the limping child will be to obtain plain radiographs of the area in question. Radiographs are most useful in screening for traumatic causative factors, such as fractures, to assess the overall anatomy, positioning and morphology of the bones, and to ensure normal growth and development. Focal bone lesions, periosteal new bone formation indicative of underlying fracture or lesion, areas of bone infection or neoplasm (Fig. 10.1), and avascular necrosis are conditions that may be identified based on radiographic features alone. Radiographs may also detect large joint effusions, although they should not be relied on for screening (Fig. 10.2). Occasionally soft tissue masses with or without calcification may be detected on radiographs because of obliteration of normal soft tissue planes (Fig. 10.3).

When the limping child is able to identify a focal area of concern, at least two orthogonal views of the anatomic area should be obtained. These often include anteroposterior (AP) and lateral radiographs of the area of concern. Additional views may be necessary depending on the anatomic area or the initial findings. Mortise views in the setting of ankle pain or oblique views of the tibia in suspected toddlers' fracture may increase diagnostic yield. In younger children (generally younger than 4 years) or in patients unable to localize the area of concern, initial radiographs can be focused on the tibia/fibula, because a toddler fracture is the most commonly seen abnormality (see American College of Radiology appropriateness criteria in Milla et al. [2012]). Comparative radiographs of the contralateral limb will increase radiation exposure and are usually not necessary in routine imaging. If radiographs are considered indeterminate or subtle findings are detected with unclear significance, imaging of the contralateral side may be helpful in select cases to rule out normal developmental variations (Fig. 10.4).

Hips are the exception to the routine practice of unilateral imaging of the affected side. When hip pathologies are under consideration, AP and frog-leg lateral views are obtained of both hips together. The normal side may serve as a normal control with regard to the developmental ossification pattern of the acetabulum and proximal femur, and also to evaluate for other pelvic processes such as avulsion injuries (Fig. 10.5) and sacroiliac joint disease that are made more conspicuous by the asymmetry with the unaffected side. Frog-leg lateral views are obtained with the limb flexed both at the knee and the hip approximately 30 to 40 degrees and with the hip externally rotated 45 degrees. The frog-leg views are more sensitive than AP views for detection of entities such as SCFE (Fig. 10.6) and LCP (Fig. 10.7). The initial AP film should include the entire pelvis without gonadal shielding to assess other pelvic anatomy, including the sacrum and sacroiliac joints. The frog-leg view should use gonadal shielding to minimize exposure to radiosensitive organs.

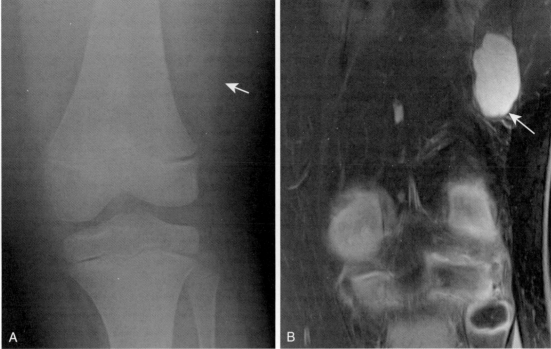

Fig. 10.3 (A) Anteroposterior radiograph of the left knee on a 9-year-old boy with "funny walking" demonstrates a subtle soft tissue mass in the lateral aspect of the distal thigh (*arrow*). (B) Coronal Proton Density-weighted sequence with fat suppression of the left knee in a 9-year-old boy demonstrates a lobular mass with increased signal (*arrow*) that represents a synovial sarcoma.

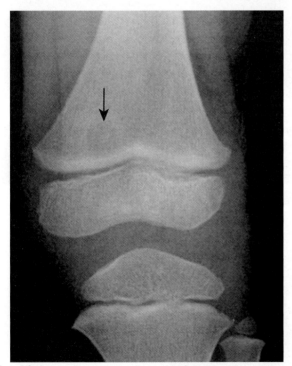

Fig. 10.4 Anteroposterior radiograph of the knee in a 3-year-old boy with limp demonstrates a rounded lucency in the medial femoral condyle (*arrow*) consistent with a "cortical desmoid," a normal variant.

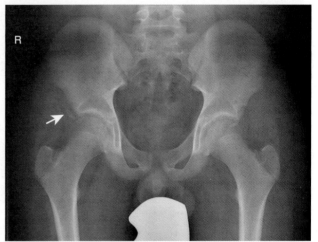

Fig. 10.5 Anteroposterior view of the pelvis in a 13-year-old boy with altered gait and right hip pain demonstrates an avulsion fracture of the right anterior inferior iliac spine (*arrow*).

■ What Is the Utility of Sonography?

Sonography is a widely implemented imaging modality in pediatric imaging because of lack of ionizing radia-

tion and capability for dynamic real-time imaging. Pediatric patients are particularly well suited to ultrasound because of their relatively small body habitus, which allows for improved image resolution. Images can also be acquired without the use of sedation by relying on methods of patient distraction to encourage cooperation during the examination. Although osseous structures with dense cortical bone are suboptimally assessed with ultrasound, the surrounding soft tissues are often depicted beautifully. In the neonatal period when the cartilaginous femoral head has not yet ossified, ultrasound is the imaging modality of choice for early diagnosis of developmental hip dysplasia (Box 10.1; Fig.

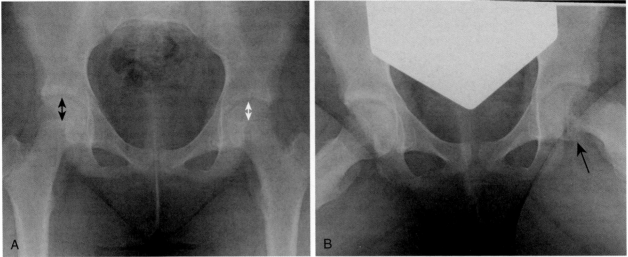

Fig. 10.6 (A) Anteroposterior radiograph of the pelvis in an 11-year-old with left hip pain and limp demonstrates decreased height of the left femoral head (*white arrow*) compared with the right (*black arrow*). (B) Frog-leg lateral radiograph of the hips in an 11-year-old with left hip pain demonstrates mild posteromedial displacement of the femoral head with respect to the neck (*black arrow*) in keeping with mild slipped capital femoral epiphysis.

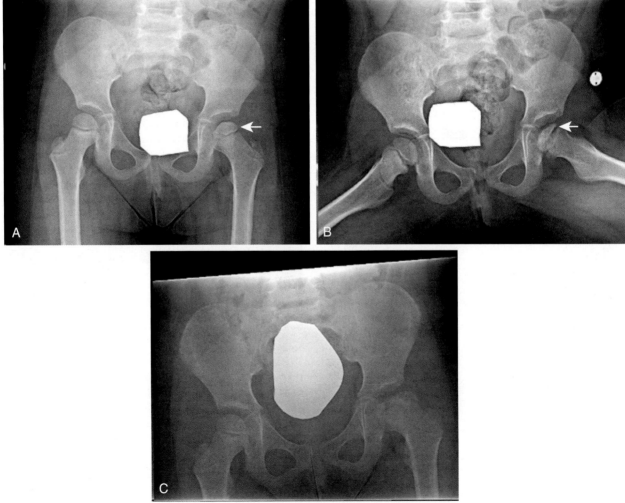

Fig. 10.7 (A) Anteroposterior (AP) radiograph of the pelvis in a 4-year-old girl with limp and pain demonstrates a relatively small left femoral head (*arrow*). (B) Frog-leg view of the pelvis shows subtle subchondral lucency anterolaterally (*arrow*). (C) AP view of the pelvis in the same patient 2 years later showing flattening and fragmentation of the left capital femoral epiphysis and broadening of the left proximal femoral metaphysis.

10.8A–B). After the age of 6 months, imaging diagnosis is typically made by radiography (see Fig. 10.8C). Radiographs will show increased acetabular angle (typically greater than 30 degrees) and subluxed or dislocated hip. The proximal femoral epiphysis of the affected hip is typically smaller than the contralateral normal hip.

BOX 10.1   Developmental Dysplasia of the Hip

May develop before or after birth

Femoral head may migrate out of joint secondary to joint laxity or acetabular underdevelopment

Screening ultrasound in the United States indicated in setting of abnormal newborn physical examination or risk factor (family history, torticollis, breech delivery, clubfoot, twin)

Left hip more commonly affected

Sonographic evaluation consists of both static and dynamic maneuvers through a lateral imaging approach with coronal and transverse planes

Ultrasound has much greater sensitivity compared with radiographs for detecting small fluid collections in the joints and soft tissues. Ultrasound is the study of choice for evaluation of joint effusions, particularly hip effusions, either in the setting of aseptic (transient synovitis) or septic arthritis (Fig. 10.9). Synovial thickening and hyperemia can also be readily identified on ultrasound in the setting of synovitis. Ideally, assessment for a hip effusion should be performed with a high-frequency linear array transducer, oriented in a sagittal plane along the axis of the femoral neck anteriorly. Imaging of the contralateral hip is imperative to assess for bilateral involvement and for accentuation of unilateral effusion. Bilateral effusions may suggest systemic arthritic disease over septic arthritis. The adjacent soft tissue structures may also be interrogated with ultrasound to evaluate for myositis or soft tissue fluid collections such as abscess.

Some authors propose the use of ultrasound to follow disease in patients with known juvenile idiopathic arthritis (JIA). This will be discussed in further detail toward the end of the chapter.

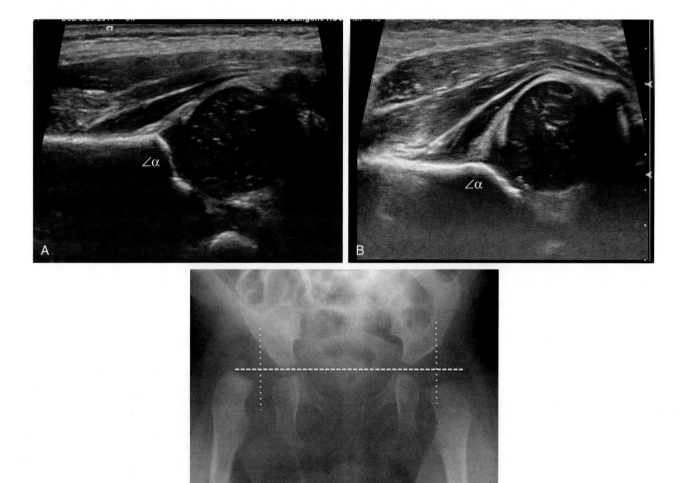

Fig. 10.8 (A) Coronal image of the left hip in an infant shows normal left coverage with an alpha angle of greater than 60 degrees. (B) Coronal imaging of the right hip in an infant with hip dysplasia shows lateral subluxation of the hip with an alpha angle of less than 60 degrees. (C) Radiograph of the pelvis demonstrates increased right acetabular angle and a small right capital femoral epiphysis. The right capital femoral epiphysis is positioned in the superolateral quadrant created by the intersecting Hilgenreiner line (*dashed line*) and Perkin line (*dotted line*). The normal left capital femoral epiphysis is positioned in inferomedial quadrant.

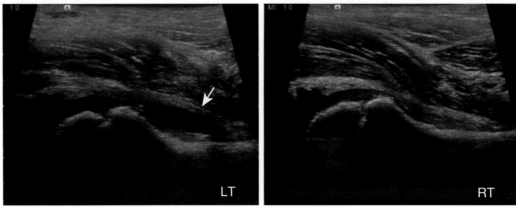

Fig. 10.9 Longitudinal ultrasound image through the right and left hips hip in a 7-year-old boy with limp demonstrates moderate left joint effusion (*arrow*).

■ Is There a Role for Bone Scans?

Bone scans may be used to isolate causes of limp in young children (younger than 5 years) especially in the setting of nonlocalizing symptoms on physical examinations. Perhaps one of the best implementations of bone scans in pediatric patients is in the evaluation of suspected stress fractures, especially involving the tarsal bones. Other fractures, such as the classic toddler fracture of the tibia, can also be seen with slightly increased sensitivity on bone scan compared with plain radiographs (Fig. 10.10), although radiographs remain the initial first-line approach because of their lower cost and decreased radiation dose. In addition to their potential utility in the evaluation of stress fractures, bone scans have other applications, including identifying primary bone tumors and metastatic disease, separating cellulitis from osteomyelitis and prosthetic loosening in patients with orthopedic hardware, assessing for osteoid osteoma, and assessing bone viability (infarction versus avascular necrosis), to name a few.

Bone scans are considered second-line imaging studies in the setting of trauma when radiographs fail to demonstrate suspected fractures. Radiographically occult fractures are often visible on bone scintigraphy. Similarly, bone scans are more sensitive than radiographs for detecting osteomyelitis, diskitis, avascular necrosis, bone infarcts, and bone neoplasms.

Traditional bone scanning agents are technetium-labeled diphosphonates, namely ^{99m}Tc-methylene diphosphonate (MDP). Diphosphonates are useful agents because these have rapid renal excretion and high target-to-nontarget ratios. Imaging may consist of only a single delayed skeletal phase or three-phase imaging, depending on the indication and concern. The three phases are generally performed in the setting of infection/inflammation and demonstrate an initial angiographic (blood flow) phase, blood pool (soft tissue) phase, and delayed (skeletal) phase with chemisorption of the agent on the bone. These various phases not only demonstrate bony abnormalities but can also detect pathology in the soft tissues, such as cellulitis.

A newer agent, ^{18}F sodium fluoride (^{18}F-NaF) is an analogue for hydroxyl ion in the bone matrix and is another useful bone-imaging agent due to its high initial extraction efficiency. An ^{18}F-NaF bone scan detects areas of altered osteogenic bone activity. With both rapid bone uptake and clearance, there is a high bone-to-background ratio much like traditional ^{99m}Tc-MDP. However, this is coupled with higher imaging resolution of positron emission tomography (PET) scanners, which are used to detect ^{99m}Tc tracer accumulation. As a compounded result, PET/CT ^{18}F-NaF bone scans have better anatomic and spatial resolution than the traditional MDP bone scans and are acquired over much shorter durations after tracer injections. These newer bone scans have not replaced traditional ^{99m}Tc-MDP imaging, however, because of higher costs and increased radiation doses. In indications where higher-resolution imaging is beneficial, for example, evaluating adolescent back pain or in nonaccidental trauma with equivocal radiographs, ^{18}F-NaF is preferred over ^{99m}Tc-MDP bone scans (Fig. 10.11).

■ Is There a Role for Computed Tomography?

In general, CT scanning is performed uncommonly and judiciously in the limping child because of the potentially harmful effects of ionizing radiation. In the particular scenario of initial presentation of a child with a limp, CT has a limited role. If a complex fracture is present, CT may be beneficial in preoperative planning, especially if there are concerns for intraarticular extension of fracture lines or concerns for loose bodies within the joint. CT may also be beneficial in instances where osteoid osteoma is on the differential to assess for lucent nidus with central calcification (Fig. 10.12; Box 10.2). CT scans may also show osteopenia early in the course of tibial stress fractures. In cases where limping is due to referred pain because of spinal or paraspinal processes, CT of the lumbosacral spine or pelvis may be beneficial to assess for psoas abscess or bony destruction in vertebral body osteomyelitis, or assess for raging appendicitis, which may lead secondarily to muscle spasms and contractures. Lastly, CT scans of the ankles are routinely performed in cases of altered gait and pes planus deformity to assess for underlying tarsal coalition as a mechanical cause.

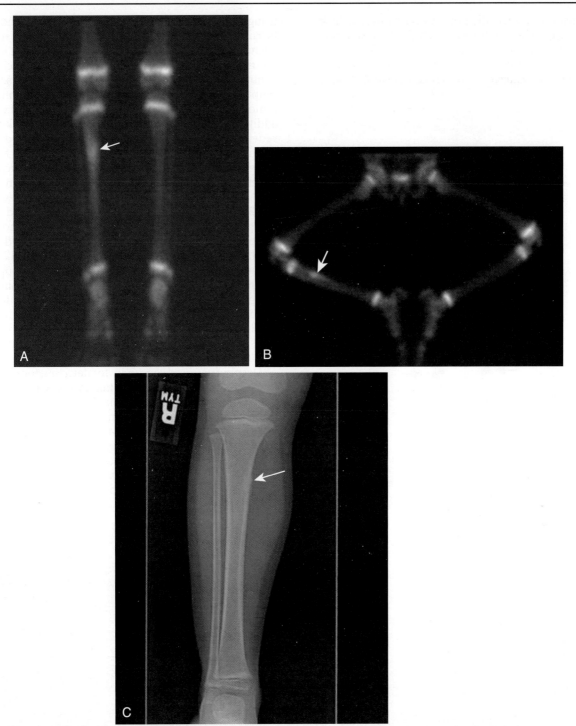

Fig. 10.10 (A) Planar anteroposterior (AP) view of the lower legs from a ^{99m}Tc-methylene diphosphonate (MDP) bone scan in a 3-year-old girl with limp after falling off the monkey bars demonstrates abnormal increased uptake in proximal right tibia (*arrow*). (B) Planar lateral views of the lower legs from a ^{99m}Tc-MDP bone scan in a 3-year-old girl with limp after falling off the monkey bars demonstrates abnormal increased uptake in proximal right tibia (*arrow*). (C) AP radiograph in a 3-year-old girl with limp after falling off the monkey bars confirms proximal tibial fracture (*arrow*).

■ When to Consider Magnetic Resonance Imaging?

Like ultrasound, MRI does not require the use of ionizing radiation. MRI is superior to ultrasound at imaging osseous structures and also provides a more global evaluation of the area of concern. The variety of different imaging sequences in MRI allows for tailored protocols that address specific clinical questions and increase diagnostic certainty, making MRI an exceptional tool in evaluation of many pediatric conditions that cause a limp. The drawbacks of MRI are that it is expensive, relatively time consuming, and often difficult to perform in younger patients without the use of anesthesia. Contrast administration is usually not necessary but may be beneficial in certain conditions, such as the evaluation of infection, tumor, or synovitis.

When osteomyelitis is high on the differential and precise anatomic localization is not possible, whole-body MRI

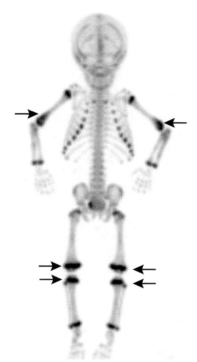

Fig. 10.11 Planar image of the whole body from a ¹⁸F sodium fluoride positron emission tomography scan in a 9-month-old girl with concern for child abuse demonstrates multiple areas of increased tracer uptake corresponding to multiple fractures.

using coronal fluid-sensitive fat-suppressed sequences may be considered to identify areas of abnormal bone marrow edema or soft tissue abnormalities. MRI can detect intraosseous, subperiosteal, or soft tissue abscesses, especially on contrast-enhanced sequences. Even with the presence of limp or localizable involvement, multifocal osteomyelitis is more likely to be detected by large initial field of view. In addition, less common causes of limp, such as diskitis and vertebral body osteomyelitis, may not be detected unless the field of view is expanded. A screening, wide-field-of-view MRI of the lower extremities may be beneficial in a variety of different clinical scenarios, particularly in a child who is cooperative and does not require anesthesia (Fig. 10.13). For instance, a patient diagnosed with and undergoing treatment for septic arthritis of the hip who is not responding to antibiotics may have an associated osteomyelitis or soft tissue abscess. MRI may facilitate diagnosis in these patients and direct them toward more appropriate treatment. In addition, in patients with puzzling clinical presentations where fractures have been excluded on radiographs and infection is not considered likely based on clinical factors, other soft tissue injuries such as tendinosis or tendon tear, ligament injury, muscular strains, or articular cartilage damage are best assessed by MRI.

Despite increased sensitivity for detecting focal marrow lesions or areas of marrow edema, whole marrow infiltrative or replacement processes may be difficult to appreciate if the abnormality is diffuse and uniform in appearance. For this reason, it is important to take note of the marrow signal characteristics on individual imaging sequences to ensure that marrow signal is following the expected pattern. In most ambulatory or school-age patients undergoing MRI imaging, it would be reasonable to expect the

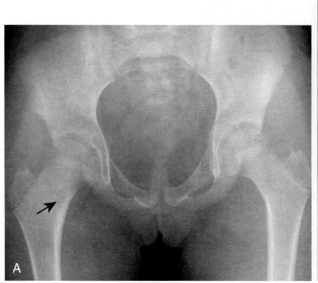

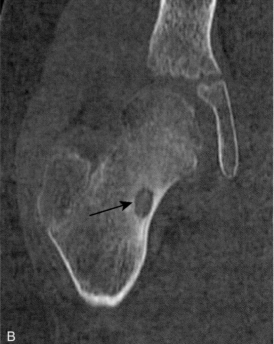

Fig. 10.12 (A) Anteroposterior radiograph of the pelvis in an 8-year-old girl with right hip pain and limp for 1 year demonstrates a focal lucent lesion at the inferior aspect of the right femoral neck (*arrow*). (B) Coronal reformatted image of a computed tomography scan of the pelvis in an 8-year-old girl with right hip pain and limp for 1 year demonstrates the osteoid osteoma at the inferior aspect of the right femoral neck (*arrow*).

BOX 10.2   Osteoid Osteoma

Benign bone tumor less than 1.5 cm
  Most common between age 4 and 25 years, and three times more common in males
  Femur and tibia are the most common locations
  Lesions do not grow, but incite large amount of surrounding reactive bone
  Patients present with dull, aching pain unrelated to activity that can become severe at night

BOX 10.3   Leukemia

Usually affects children between 2 and 10 years of age
  Most common malignancy in children between 1 and 4 years of age
  ~40% of children with acute lymphoblastic leukemia present with bone pain confined to a single limb
  May have nearly normal hematological values if bone pain is presenting symptom
  Radiographic signs may include clear metaphyseal bands, lytic or sclerotic bone lesions, or periosteal elevation (although radiographs are often normal)

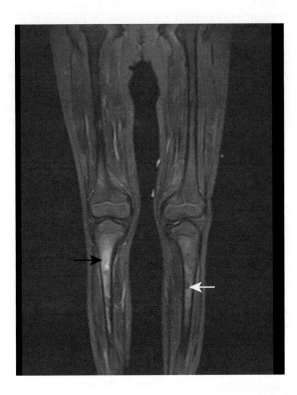

Fig. 10.13 Coronal STIR large field of view sequence through the lower extremities in a 7-year-old boy with sepsis, fevers, and lower-extremity pain demonstrates an area of osteomyelitis in the right tibia (*black arrow*) and signal abnormality in left tibia (*white arrow*) related to prior intraosseous catheter.

diaphysis of the long bones to demonstrate fatty marrow signal, which is bright on T1-weighted sequences and dark when fat suppression techniques are applied. If the marrow appears dark on T1-weighted images or bright on fluid-sensitive sequences with fat suppression, a diffuse marrow process, such as a lymphoproliferative disorder, must be considered, for example, leukemia or lymphoma (Box 10.3). Also, MRI lacks the fine spatial resolution of CT and may obscure tiny abnormalities, such as the nidus in an osteoid osteoma. Secondary signs of disease may be helpful in these patients, such as geographic marrow edema, cortical thickening, or synovitis (when the lesion is intraarticular).

■ How Does the Patient's Age Affect Imaging Workup?

Much like other pediatric disorders, patient age affects the diagnostic approach to the child with a limp. It may

be helpful to categorize patients into one of three categories when determining which imaging studies will be most helpful in the workup of the limping child: young children (younger than 4 years), older children (older than 4 years but younger than 10 years), and adolescents (older than 10 years). A subcategory of young children includes infants, those younger than 1 year and not yet ambulating but who may present with altered morphology, decreased tone, or delayed developmental milestones that suggest and precede later onset of gait abnormalities. In neonates and infants, congenital, metabolic, and/or endocrine derangements may present in this manner, although infection, trauma (including nonaccidental injury; Box 10.4), and tumor also remain on the differential.

In younger children the broad differential diagnosis for a limp includes trauma, toxic synovitis, osteomyelitis, septic arthritis, developmental hip dysplasia (DDH), leg-length discrepancy, and inflammatory arthritis (JIA) (Box 10.5). In older children, trauma, toxic synovitis, osteomyelitis, and septic arthritis remain high on the differential, and LCP disease also becomes a serious consideration. In adolescents, trauma, sports-related injuries (stress fractures), osteomyelitis, septic arthritis, SCFE, chondromalacia, and neoplasm are higher on the differential. Infection and trauma are common processes that affect all patient populations regardless of age.

■ How to Image a Child With Suspected Trauma

Radiographs in the Setting of Trauma

Far and away the most common cause of acute limp in children is trauma. Up to 20% of children younger than 5 years who present with an acute limp will have a fracture(s). Younger children are more likely to present with fractures involving the physes. Unlike adult bones, pediatric bones behave differently because of the presence of the physis (growth plate), a cartilaginous structure that serves as the site for longitudinal bone growth (Box 10.6). The physis is a relatively weak region of the musculoskeletal system that is prone to injury. In comparison, the ligamentous and capsular structures of children are generally stronger than the physes and less prone to injury. In adolescents with fused physes, ligaments and

BOX 10.4   Child Abuse

Radiographic skeletal survey for diagnosis of child abuse includes the following separate radiographs:
- AP and lateral all appendicular bones
- AP and lateral skull
- Lateral thoracic and lumbar spine
- Lateral cervical spine (separate)
- AP chest (+/– oblique ribs)
- AP abdomen
- AP pelvis

Coned-down views may be added at discretion of radiologist.

High-specificity injuries include:
- CMLs
- Multiple and posterior rib fracture
- Scapular fractures
- Sternal fractures

In select instances, whole-body ^{18}F-NaF PET bone scans may supplement (but never replace) initial skeletal survey. ^{18}F-NaF PET bone scans may be more sensitive for rib fractures but have lower sensitivity for CMLs.

Mimics of abuse include normal developmental variants, rickets, Menkes disease, and osteogenesis imperfecta.

AP, Anteroposterior; *CML,* classic metaphyseal lesion; *^{18}F-NaF PET,* ^{18}F-sodium fluoride positron emission tomography.

BOX 10.5   Leg-Length Discrepancy

Caused by previous injury, prior infection, arthritis, hemihypertrophy, neurological conditions, or bone dysplasia.

Conditions that can cause limb shortening or hypertrophy include neurofibromatosis type 1, multiple hereditary osteochondromatoses, and Ollier disease.

Mild discrepancies may be physiological and do not require treatment.

Larger discrepancies may be treated surgically with epiphysiodesis of the longer limb or lengthening osteotomy of the shorter leg.

BOX 10.6   Physeal Fractures

Physis is involved in 15%–30% of long-bone fractures in children.

Physeal cartilage is weaker than surrounding bones and ligaments.

Salter-Harris classification system is the most widely used, based on the extent of involvement of the physis, metaphysis, and epiphysis.

Salter-Harris type II fracture is the most common physeal fracture, consisting of fracture through both physis and metaphysis.

tendons hence become the weaker structures of the musculoskeletal system. Adolescent children are more likely to sprain ligaments or dislocate joints, while younger children are more likely to fracture through the bony physis. The types of fracture seen in children are also more variable than those encountered in adult bone as pliable bones demonstrate more bending-, bowing-, or buckling-type fracture deformities (Fig. 10.14).

Radiographs are usually all the imaging that is required for diagnosis of fracture, especially when unified with certain clinical findings, such as point tenderness or gross morphological deformity. In such instances, radiographs detect approximately 97% of the lower-extremity fractures in children aged 1 to 15 years. When these associated clinical features are absent or not elicited, radiographs are less likely to yield a diagnosis of fracture.

If plain radiographs are normal in the initial evaluation of limp in the setting of trauma and no alarming clinical features are present (fever, elevated white blood cell [WBC] count, erythrocyte sedimentation rate [ESR], C-reactive protein [CRP]), conservative management is often recommended. If suspicion for fracture is high despite initially normal radiographs, appropriate immobilization followed by repeat radiographs in 10 to 14 days will show a healing response at the sites of previously occult fractures, thereby increasing the fracture conspicuity. Treating the patient for a presumed fracture and repeat radiographs may be especially beneficial if the patient has persistent pain and limp in addition to a history of trauma.

As mentioned earlier, older children (typically >10 years of age) and adolescents are more likely to present with sprains and/or ligamentous injuries. Among these, ankle sprains are the most common cause of limp. Other traumatic-type injuries can result in microtrauma or overuse syndromes, such as stress fractures (Fig. 10.15), shin splints, Osgood-Schlatter, Sever disease (Fig. 10.16), and chondromalacia patellae.

Suspected Trauma in Newly Ambulating Child: The Toddler Fracture

The classic toddler fracture, considered a type I toddler fracture, is a nondisplaced spiral fracture of midshaft of the tibia (Fig. 10.17A). The fracture line is often occult and is best seen on oblique views (Box 10.7).

A type II toddler fracture results from knee hyperextension, a mechanism that differs from the classic type I injury. The type II lesion is also usually more conspicuous than type I and occurs in the upper tibia (see Fig. 10.14) or, less frequently, distal femur. Radiographically, there are three components to the fracture that consist of a buckle fracture deformity of the anterior upper tibial cortex, which can also be accompanied by increased concavity of the tibial tubercle notch (best seen on lateral view), anterior tilting of the epiphyseal plate, and a radiographically hairline fracture of upper tibia that may be accompanied by a buckle fracture along the medial or lateral tibial cortex.

Clinical history, laboratory results, and physical examination findings aid in diagnosis of toddler fractures. In cases where physical examination findings, history, and plain films are equivocal, a bone scan may offer more definitive diagnosis with sensitivity approaching near 100%. Similarly, MRI has sensitivity near 100%,

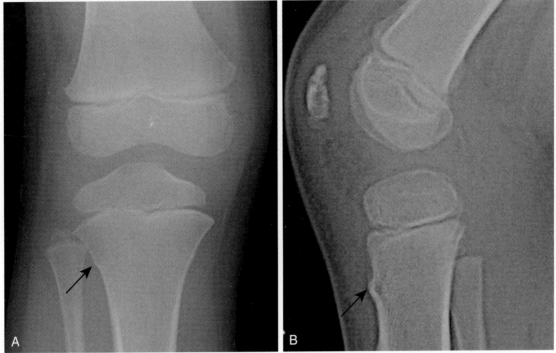

Fig. 10.14 (A) Anteroposterior and (B) lateral radiographs of the knee in a 6-year-old girl with pain after fall demonstrates buckling of the lateral and anterior cortex of the tibia (*arrows*). This fracture pattern is often seen in trampoline injuries.

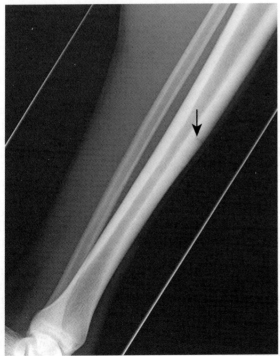

Fig. 10.15 Lateral radiograph of the left tibia in a 17-year-old boy with pain and limp demonstrates a stress fracture within the anterior tibial cortex (*arrow*).

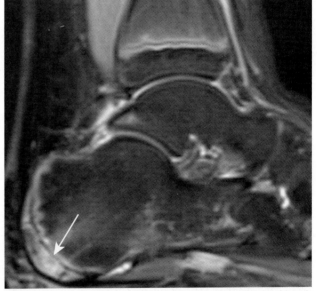

Fig. 10.16 Sagittal STIR image of the ankle in a 12-year-old with heel pain and limp demonstrates abnormal marrow signal within the calcaneal apophysis (*arrow*) consistent with Severs apophysitis.

although relatively lengthy acquisition times and potential need for sedation may make the study prohibitive. Alternatively, radiographically occult toddler's fractures may be followed with short-interval repeat radiographs that will demonstrate signs of healing in up to 85% of the cases (see Fig. 10.17B). Radiographic features of a healing toddler fracture include cortical thickening or irregularity, periosteal reaction, and/or sclerotic bands. There are other stress fractures associated with the initiation of walking, such as fractures of the cuboid and calcaneus, all of which are also toddler-type fractures and should be considered in any newly ambulating young child (Fig. 10.18). For this reason, radiographs of the tibia should be extended to include the ankle and midfoot when toddler fractures are high on the differential.

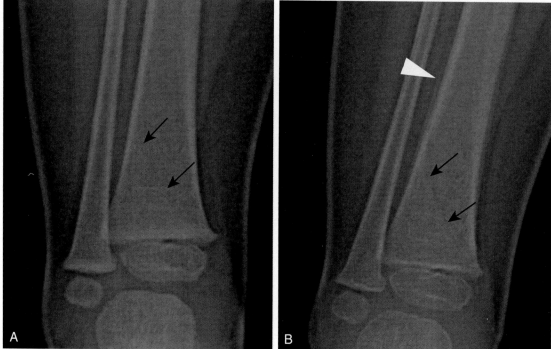

Fig. 10.17 (A) Anteroposterior (AP) radiograph of the tibia coned to the ankle in an 18-month-old girl with limp demonstrates a faint, oblique lucency in the distal tibial diametaphysis (*black arrows*). (B) AP radiograph of the tibia coned to the ankle in an 18-month-old girl 2 weeks after injury demonstrates a faint, oblique lucency in the distal tibial diametaphysis (*black arrows*) and new periosteal bone formation (*white arrowhead*) indicative of healing fracture.

BOX 10.7   Toddler Fracture

Occurs in young ambulatory children (9 months to 3 years)
  Spiral or oblique fracture of the distal shaft of the tibia
  Fracture occurs as a result of a twisting injury
  May be occult on initial radiographs; oblique views may be helpful, as well as follow-up radiographs in 10–14 days to detect signs of healing
  Nondisplaced cuboid fracture is another form of toddler fracture; may appear occult initially on radiographs with subtle focal sclerosis 1–2 weeks after injury

---

What to Do in Young Children With Suspected Trauma but Unreliable Histories?

Generally, children younger than 4 years are often unable to provide reliable clinical histories. In these younger children, diagnostic imaging is crucial to patient management because ascertaining an accurate history is challenging and often unrealistic. Physical examination findings may also be challenging if the trauma is occult and if the child is crying inconsolably and apprehensive of the examining physician. Laboratory information should still be obtained in these patients in conjunction to imaging.

Excluding the congenital issues contributing to a limp (which often present in infants younger than 1 year), the most common causes in this age group include trauma, infection, and tumor, in order of decreasing frequency. In addition to the classic toddler fractures, other traumatic-type fractures encountered in younger children include distal tibial torus fractures, "bunk-bed" fractures (Fig. 10.19), and plastic-bending fractures of the fibula. The torus or buckle fracture of distal tibia involves the cortex and is often accompanied by an angulated component. The angulation results from additional mechanisms superimposed on the axial loading forces, such as either hyperextension, hyperflexion, or varus or valgus forces.

Bunk-bed fractures are the result of landing on a hyperflexed forefoot with the dissipation of the landing energy through the base of the first metatarsal or cuboid bones. When the cuboid bone is involved, there are no visible fracture lines in younger children, but instead a subtle region of increased density may be seen on radiographs (see Figs. 10.18 and 10.19). In older children a fracture line may be present.

Lastly, plastic bending fractures of fibula are additional causes for limps in the younger child. After the forearm structures (radius and ulna) and clavicle, fibula is the next most commonly encountered bone to demonstrate plastic bending-type injuries. This manifests as increased inward bending of the fibula. Normally, both fibulae demonstrate some mild degree of inward bowing, so care must be taken not to confuse this with normal variation. Comparative views are often necessary for this diagnosis.

■ How to Image a Child With Suspected Infection

In the setting of fever (≥38.5°C or 101°F), elevated WBC count (>12,000 WBCs/µL), elevated CRP (>2.00 mg/dL),

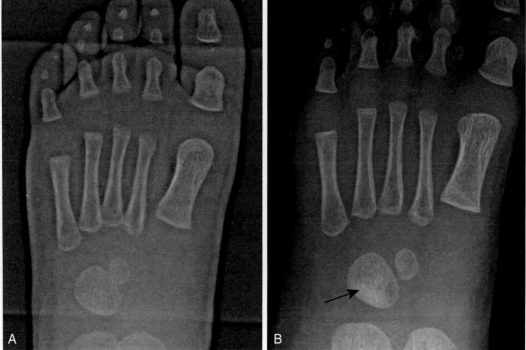

Fig. 10.18 (A) Anteroposterior (AP) radiograph of the foot in an 18-month-old girl with acute-onset limp reveals a normal appearance of the cuboid. (B) AP radiograph of the foot in an 18-month-old girl 2 weeks later reveals a band of sclerosis within the proximal cuboid consistent with a healing fracture (*arrow*).

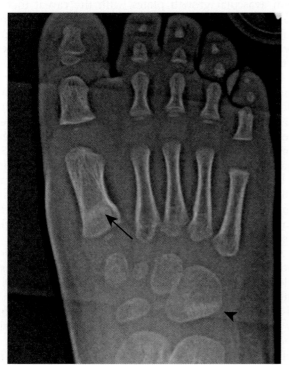

Fig. 10.19 Anteroposterior radiograph of the right foot in a 22-month-old boy with limp demonstrates band of sclerosis (*arrow*) in the base of the first metatarsal with mild angulation of the lateral cortex in keeping with a healing buckle fracture, commonly termed "bunk-bed" fracture in this location. Band of sclerosis in the proximal cuboid (*arrowhead*), consistent with a healing cuboid fracture.

and/or elevated ESR (>40 mm/h), infection should be high on the differential diagnosis, especially when four or more of these features are present. The most common causes for infectious limp in a child include septic arthritis, osteomyelitis, discitis, myositis, and paraspinal infections, such as psoas abscess. Other entities that may have some overlapping features but are not infectious include transient synovitis, Langerhans cell histiocytosis, leukemia, osteosarcoma, and osseous metastases.≥µ

When clinical and laboratory evidence favor infection as the leading cause of limp, septic arthritis of the hip should be high on the differential. Septic arthritis is an orthopedic emergency and is the most common cause of severe, monoarticular pain in a child. Delay in diagnosis may lead to irrevocable damage, including avascular necrosis and arthrosis. A targeted ultrasound can be performed quickly and efficiently to assess for the presence of a hip effusion, as well as for effusions in other joints that may be of concern, including the knee or ankle. Sonographic findings in septic arthritis are nonspecific and include the presence of joint fluid, which may appear anechoic or contain echogenic debris. Color Doppler evaluation may reveal nonspecific hyperemia of the surrounding synovium. There may also be associated soft tissue swelling. A needle aspiration is often directly performed after sonography if clinical suspicion is high, to prevent delay in diagnosis (Box 10.8).

If an MRI is performed, T2-weighted fluid-sensitive sequences demonstrate a hyperintense joint effusion and often additional hyperintense signal in the adja-

---

BOX 10.8   Septic Arthritis

Bacterial infection of the joint, most common causative agent is S. aureus

Most commonly monoarticular, with knee, hip, and ankle most frequently encountered joints

Distention of joint may result in ischemia or infarction of epiphysis

Proteolytic enzymes in infected joint fluid destroy cartilage

Joint aspiration necessary to determine whether fluid is infected

Prompt surgical intervention necessary to avoid joint damage

BOX 10.9   Osteomyelitis

Most commonly bacterial, with S. aureus being the most common organism

Hematogenous spread most common route of infection in children

Usually affects vascularized metaphyses of long bones

Fastest growing bones most commonly affected: distal femur, proximal tibia, proximal humerus, and distal radius

Sonographic findings of subperiosteal abscess and magnetic resonance imaging findings of marrow alterations precede radiographic changes

Complications include fracture, premature physeal closure and growth disturbance, joint destruction, and venous thrombosis

---

BOX 10.10   Magnetic Resonance Imaging Approach to Suspected Lower-Extremity Infection in Young Children

Initial large field of view coronal STIR or T2-weighted sequence with fat suppression from pelvis to ankles (may require several coils and composition of images)

Focused examination over area of abnormality identified on initial sequence

- Coronal T1
- Axial T2-weighted image with fat suppression
- Sagittal Inversion Recovery

Postcontrast imaging if necessary (particularly for soft tissue abscess)

---

cent subchondral bone. Postcontrast sequences demonstrate enhancement of the synovium, which is often also thickened, and enhancement of the subchondral bone (in the region of bone marrow edema). There may be associated soft tissue enhancement or a soft tissue abscess. In rare cases where a foot joint is involved, an appreciable joint effusion may not be seen either with sonography or via MRI.

Osteomyelitis may accompany septic arthritis, especially in children younger than 2 years, because the metaphyses in certain locations, namely, proximal femur and distal tibia, extend into the joint (Box 10.9). When septic arthritis of the hip or ankle is encountered in an infant, MRI should be strongly considered to assess for concurrent osteomyelitis (Box 10.10).

If the initial ultrasound is negative for an effusion and infection remains high on the differential, osteomyelitis without associated septic arthritis should be considered. In such instances, further imaging evaluation should be performed with either MRI or scintigraphic bone scan. MRI is preferred unless the risk for sedation for the MRI scan is high. When clinical suspicion and imaging features suggest osteomyelitis, *Staphylococcus aureus* is the most common causative agent. In children the most common route of infection is hematogenous spread, although direct inoculation and local extension from contiguous infection (e.g., cellulitis) also may result in osteomyelitis (Fig. 10.20).

In children between the ages of 2 and 16 years, osteomyelitis most often occurs in the metaphyses of the long bones or metaphyseal equivalents near the apophyses of the ilium and greater trochanter, or adjacent to growth centers, such as the ischiopubic synchondrosis and triradiate cartilage of the hip. These regions are more prone to infection because of the relatively rich vascular supply, and the capillaries present in these areas lack phagocytic cell lining. Bacteria have easier access into marrow, especially in the setting of concurrent septic arthritis. In contrast with the metaphyses, epiphyses are relatively resistant to hematogenous spread due to protection from avascular growth plates, with the caveat that in children younger than 18 months, persistent transphyseal vessels make this population susceptible to epiphyseal osteomyelitis even when no infection is present within the metaphysis.

Plain radiographs are often normal in the setting of osteomyelitis, especially early in the course of infection because radiographic findings typically lag behind clinical features of infection by at least 7 to 10 days. Nuclear medicine bone scans are much more sensitive for detecting infection. Bone scans are able to detect as little as 5% change in bone turnover (typically, radiographs require at least 30% loss of mineralization before changes are visible). Bone scans become sensitive within 24 hours of symptom onset and are potentially even more effective than MRI given that a larger region can be imaged with ease when symptoms are poorly localized.

A scintigraphic bone scan in the setting of infection should be performed with imaging in three phases (blood flow, blood pool, and delayed phase). A positive study should demonstrate increased tracer activity in all three phases. Although there may be some variability in the findings on all three phases, increased activity in delayed or skeletal phase must always be present to make the diagnosis of osteomyelitis. In some circumstances, three-phase imaging may not be feasible. In these instances, only delayed imaging is necessary. It is important to note that regardless of whether symptom onset is early or late, initial radiographs of the extremity must be available for correlation with bone scan findings. In patients with limp, it is not unusual to see diffusely increased radionuclide uptake in the normal, contralateral limb compared with the symptomatic

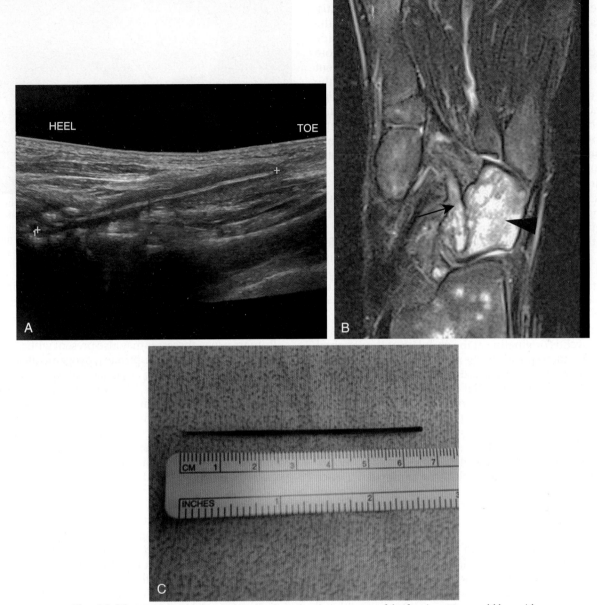

Fig. 10.20 (A) Sagittal ultrasound image along the plantar aspect of the foot in a 12-year-old boy with pain and limp demonstrates a linear foreign body in the soft tissues of the foot denoted by the calipers. (B) Coronal footprint fluid-sensitive fat-suppressed image from magnetic resonance imaging of the foot on the same patient demonstrates the linear foreign body (*arrow*) adjacent to the cuboid bone (*arrowhead*), which is diffusely abnormal in signal secondary to osteomyelitis. (C) Photograph of the splinter removed from the patient's foot.

limb. Correlation with history of trauma, presence of erythema, and ESR and CRP values is also beneficial. In rare instances a bone scan may demonstrate "cold" osteomyelitis. This relative photopenia is thought to be due to decreased blood flow resulting from elevated bone pressures, or perhaps due to vascular thrombosis or bone infarcts. Initially "cold" photopenic osteomy-elitis can become "hot" on later scans because dynamic changes in bone lead to intense tracer accumulation.

The role of other nuclear medicine tests for infection, such as WBC scintigraphy, is generally limited in the set-ting of osteomyelitis. WBC scans are more laborious and require blood withdrawal before the start of study. These scans can be considered in more complex situations, such as those in patients who have surgical hardware.

Osteomyelitis in neonates behaves somewhat differ-ently than in older children. Neonatal osteomyelitis is often hard to detect given that there are often no com-pelling signs of infection, such as fever or leukocytosis. Decreased motion in a limb or swelling may be the only signs of underlying osteomyelitis. Neonatal osteomyeli-tis is seen more commonly in low-birth-weight infants, premature infants, or infants with other antecedent illnesses, umbilical artery catheter placement, or other invasive procedures. Given the presence of persistent transphyseal vessels that penetrate the growth plate, metaphyseal osteomyelitis can infect the epiphyses and also extend into joint spaces, leading to septic arthritis. In addition, the periosteum is loosely adherent to the bone in infants, allowing the infection to spread outside of the bone and into the surrounding soft tissues more easily than in older children. When neonates present with a soft tissue abscess intimately associated to the adjacent bone, this finding should be considered a sign of underlying osteomyelitis. For this reason, ultrasound may be helpful in this population of patients to evaluate for joint effusions and soft tissue abscesses that may be present in the setting of osteomyelitis. Neonates also are more prone to multifocal osteomyelitis than older children.

As a general rule, there is little to no role for CT in the setting of osteomyelitis given that CT does not allow for imaging of the bone marrow.

Although rarer than other causes of childhood infection, discitis is an important diagnosis to consider in a child with a limp, especially in the setting of buttock or lateral thigh pain. Approximately 75% of the cases of discitis in children affect the lumbar or lumbosacral spine and occur predominantly from hematogenous spread. In adults, spinal infection typically manifests as osteomyelitis originating at the endplate of the vertebral body and then spreads to the disc. In children, however, discitis precedes vertebral body osteomyelitis. These tendencies are related to normal developmental changes in the vascular anatomy. In neonates, arterioles are present in the cartilage canals of the developing vertebral endplate. These form rich anastomoses with the arteries within the intervertebral disc. Over time, these connections begin to involute. By adolescence and adulthood, only end arteries persist within the endplates. Hence rich blood supply in the neonatal and infancy period predisposes to discitis. This same blood supply is also efficacious, as with proper treatment, patients generally have good outcomes.

The presenting features of discitis are often nonspecific, usually with more insidious onset of back pain that may radiate into the scrotum or perineum. The patient may refuse to bear weight or ambulate. There may be loss of lower back flexion and the normal lumbar lordosis as a result of contractures and spasms of the psoas and other paravertebral muscles. The hip is often irritated if held in extension. Blood work is often negative, delaying diagnosis. Initial radiographs are often negative or demonstrate subtle abnormalities. Usually the earliest radiographic sign is seen with concomitant infection of the vertebral endplate within 2 to 8 weeks of symptom onset. There is loss of endplate definition with irregularity and sometimes erosive changes. Additional narrowing and erosive changes within the disc space may also be present. Healing is characterized by sclerosis along the affected margins.

Early detection is best achieved via MRI, although bone scintigraphy is also more sensitive than plain radiography and can demonstrate changes within 1 to 2 days of infection onset. MRI is not only sensitive but also specific in the setting of spinal infection. Typical findings include T2-weighted hyperintense signal within the intervertebral disc and in the adjacent ver-

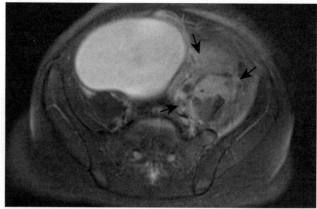

Fig. 10.21 Axial T2-weighted image with fat suppression through the lower abdomen of a 25-month-old girl with limp and pain and with normal radiographs of the entire lower extremity and normal hip ultrasound demonstrates an abscess within the left psoas muscle (*arrows*).

tebral body. There are often abundant changes in the adjacent paravertebral tissues, including paravertebral psoas abscesses. Additional spread into the spinal canal can present with epidural disease.

Primary psoas abscesses may also present with referred hip pain. In patients with primary pyogenic abscess of the psoas sheath, the hips are usually flexed as a result of psoas muscular spasm. This may be from primary pyomyositis originating within the muscle or secondary spread of infected fluid into the muscle from adjacent suppurative external iliac lymphadenitis or infection of the adjacent gastrointestinal (e.g., appendicitis) or genitourinary tracts. Diagnosis is based on clinical suspicion and imaging. In suitable patients, sonography is an effective tool to assess for asymmetrical thickening of the psoas muscle with or without liquefaction. Although radiographs may demonstrate obliteration of the normal psoas shadow, findings are generally less specific. In patients with suboptimal acoustic windows, a dedicated CT or MRI scan through the desired area can be performed to assess for inflammatory changes and fluid collections (Fig. 10.21). Alternatively, CT abdomen/pelvic imaging may be essential in cases where secondary psoas infection is suspected from primary abdominal or pelvic pathology, such as enteritis. Needle aspiration may guide antibiotic therapy, although the most commonly isolated organism is *S. aureus*.

It is important to note that primary psoas pyogenic abscesses are a separate entity from the cold abscesses of tuberculous spondylitis, which manifest secondary to primary spinal involvement.

Lyme disease, a spirochete infection transmitted by a tick acting as the vector, may also present with arthritis and limp. Although there are both early and late stages of the infection, the majority of patients lack the classic erythema migrans rash (annular "bulls-eye" rash) and constitutional symptoms, leading to a delay in diagnosis. Although Lyme disease is an endemic condition in the northeast and mid-Atlantic regions of the United States, the entity has both increased in frequency and become more widespread throughout the country. Children younger than 10 years are particularly vulnerable to infection, and fewer than 20% will present with erythema migrans. Unlike the later stages of adult infections that commonly present with neurological symptoms, children in subacute to later phases commonly present with oligoarticular arthritis, particularly of the knee. Other frequently encountered joints include the hip, ankle, elbow, and wrist.

Laboratory values and aspiration of joint fluid may fail to separate Lyme arthritis from septic arthritis, because serum ESR and CRP and joint fluid WBC values may overlap values encountered with septic arthritis. Radiographs are nonspecific and may demonstrate signs of a joint effusion. Although plain radiographic features and clinical presentation may overlap with septic and other arthritides, certain MRI findings favor Lyme arthritis, and imaging may serve as the first clue toward Lyme as the etiology of limping and joint pain. MRI features favoring Lyme include the presence of myositis, lymphadenopathy (particularly in cases involving the knee with enlarged popliteal nodes), and absence of subcutaneous edema. In contrast, septic arthritis is less likely to present with myositis and lymphadenopathy, but it is much more likely to show subcutaneous edema. This subcutaneous edema is postulated to result from concurrent cellulitis in bacterial infections. Both Lyme and septic arthritis demonstrate synovial inflammation and hyperemia, and both may additionally demonstrate hemarthrosis. Thus Lyme should especially be on the differential in a child who has visited or lived in endemic regions of the United States and presents with features of both synovitis and myositis, especially in the setting of constitutional symptoms or more insidious onset.

■ How to Approach a Child With No History of Trauma and No Signs of Infection

When traumatic and infectious causes of limp have been excluded on the basis of history and physical examination, there are several common pediatric diagnoses that must be considered. The imaging work-up will largely depend on whether the pain/limp can be localized to a particular area, which would allow a more focused and directed imaging approach. When a child presents with a limp with clinical signs and symptoms referable to the hip, there are specific pediatric conditions that must be considered, many which can be evaluated quite easily with radiographs and/or ultrasound.

One of the most common and benign entities that should be considered in this category is toxic or aseptic synovitis. Generally, toxic synovitis affects children between the ages of 3 and 10 years who generally are not acutely febrile or infectious appearing during the time of presentation (Box 10.11). There is usually a preceding history of respiratory illness 2 weeks before the onset of limp, and the symptomology may reflect an immune-mediated response or viral synovitis. Although radiographs may demonstrate widening of the medial joint space of the affected hip, effacement of the surrounding soft tissue borders, or sometimes even slight demineralization of the affected proximal femoral metaphysis,

---

BOX 10.11 Toxic Synovitis

Most commonly seen in children <8 years old
  Presenting symptoms include limp, thigh/groin pain, and limited range of motion
  Believed to be viral in etiology
  Hip ultrasound demonstrates joint effusion without capsular thickening
  Resolves spontaneously in ~1 week without treatment

---

ultrasound is the imaging method of choice. Ultrasound is highly sensitive to detect the presence of a joint effusion with extremely low false-negative results. Bone scans have little role in the diagnosis because of their low specificity. If performed, however, bone scintigraphy generally demonstrates early findings of decreased tracer uptake. In later stages because of hyperemic response, there may be increased tracer accumulation.

Septic arthritis is the major differential diagnosis to exclude. This may be on the basis of clinical history, examination findings, and laboratory values. In general, patients with transient synovitis are afebrile, nontoxic, and have less pain and restricted range of motion compared with septic arthritis. More stringent criteria for separating the two entities include the widely used Kocher criteria. This four-point scoring tool is based on the following entities, with one point awarded for each of the criterion: non–weight bearing on the affected side, ESR higher than 40 mm/h, fever above 38.5°C, and WBC count greater than 12,000 cells/mm³. When all four findings are present, the likelihood of septic arthritis is 99.6%; when three of the four findings are present, the likelihood is 93.1%. When only one finding is present, the likelihood precipitously declines to 3.0%. When two of the findings are present, the likelihood is 40.0%. In these more intermediary instances, needle aspiration of joint fluid may distinguish transient synovitis from septic arthritis.

Although joint aspiration remains the gold standard in distinguishing between transient synovitis and septic arthritis, MRI may be considered in a suitable patient, that is, a patient who is able to tolerate the examination without additional risk for sedation or prolonged wait time. Transient synovitis is isolated to the joint space. If MRI indicates any evidence of abnormal marrow signal, for instance, hyperintense signal on fat-suppressed T2-weighted images in the adjacent bone marrow, septic arthritis or osteomyelitis should be considered. In addition, if corresponding decreased perfusion is seen in the subjacent epiphysis (generally, proximal femoral epiphysis in scenarios involving the hip joint) on contrast-enhanced fat-suppressed T1-weighted sequences, these findings strongly support septic arthritis over transient synovitis.

Another common, atraumatic, noninfectious cause of limp is Legg-Calvé-Perthes (LCP) disease (Box 10.12). LCP is an idiopathic osteonecrosis that results in a growth disturbance of the capital femoral epiphysis. Children with LCP typically present with antalgic gait or hip pain that may be referred to the knee. LCP typically presents with limited hip movement, especially during internal rotation and abduction. Although the age of presentation may range from 2 to 14 years, it classically peaks around 5

BOX 10.12   Legg-Calvé-Perthes Disease

Most common in children between 4 and 10 years of age
  Affects boys five times more often than girls
  Caused by temporary loss of vascularity to the femoral head
  Early radiographic changes include anterolateral subchondral fissure/fracture and femoral head sclerosis
  Treatment consists of both conservative and surgical measures

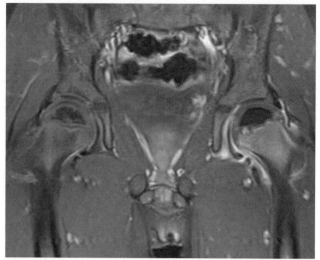

Fig. 10.22 Coronal T1-weighted image with fat suppression after gadolinium administration demonstrates lack of enhancement of the flattened femoral head on the left, with metaphyseal cystic change and synovial enhancement consistent with Perthes disease.

to 6 years of age and is five times more common in boys. Up to 15% of the cases are bilateral, although both femoral heads are rarely affected at the same time.

Radiographs are the first-line imaging modality for detection of LCP. On radiographs, findings include loss of the normal spherical femoral head with flattening, fragmentation, and sclerosis (see Fig. 10.7). The affected joint space may appear widened. In subacute and chronic phases the width of the femoral neck may increase and the femoral head may become demineralized. Ensuing coxa plana and coxa magna deformities may be seen (see Fig. 10.7C).

MRI may be valuable in early detection of disease before manifestations are apparent on radiographs. MRI is most sensitive when it is performed with contrast to assess for hypoperfusion of the affected side (Fig. 10.22). In the very early stages, unenhanced MRI studies may often appear normal. MRI is preferred over bone scan for this indication given the lack of radiation and more precise delineation of the extent of femoral head involvement. MRI also helps separate LCP from other (rarer) epiphyseal lesions, such as multiple epiphyseal dysplasia, spondyloepiphyseal dysplasia, and Meyer dysplasia. MRI also plays a role in prognosticating outcome and assessing for complications. Although approximately 60% to 70% of hips will spontaneously heal without any significant long-term consequences, most common long-term sequelae, including secondary femoroacetabular impingement and osteoarthritis and its early changes, are well depicted by MRI.

Slipped capital femoral epiphysis (SCFE) is the most common hip abnormality in adolescents (Box 10.13). The cause is a nontraumatic shearing fracture through the proximal femoral physis that leads to posterior and medial slippage of the femoral epiphysis relative to the femoral neck. The diagnosis of SCFE requires urgent reduction and pinning, and if undiagnosed, SCFE may lead to early osteoarthritis.

Most commonly SCFE presents with hip pain, although referred knee pain is another common feature. The pain is rather insidious. SCFE is more common in males, African Americans, and obese children. Patients with endocrine problems, such as hypothyroidism, panhypopituitarism, or hypogonadism, are also at an increased risk and often present at an earlier age.

SCFE is primarily diagnosed via radiographs. Bilateral imaging is critical so that the hip in question can be compared with the unaffected side. Up to one-third of the cases are bilateral, which may be synchronous or asynchronous. Classic radiograph findings include

BOX 10.13   Slipped Capital Femoral Epiphysis

Most common adolescent hip disorder
  Age range 8–15 years
  Shearing injury along proximal femoral physis with posterior displacement of femoral head
  Patients present with groin, thigh, or knee pain and limited internal rotation and flexion
  Risk factors include obesity, growth spurt, hypothyroidism, growth hormone supplementation

widening of the physis, demineralization and decreased height of the proximal femoral epiphysis, and increased radiodensity of the affected proximal metaphysis (Fig. 10.6). On the AP view a line drawn along the lateral margin of the femoral neck ("Klein line") may fail to intersect the femoral head on the affected side or may intersect the femoral head to a lesser degree (by ≥2 mm) than on the unaffected side.

SCFE may present at different stages because of its insidious onset. In the earliest "preslip phase," patients present with less than 2 to 3 weeks of pain. Radiographs generally demonstrate physeal widening and osteopenia. There is no actual displacement of the femoral head. MRI studies performed during this time period demonstrate loss of the normal high signal intensity in the proximal metaphysis on T1-weighted sequences and marrow edema surrounding the proximal femoral physis. In the "acute-on-chronic phase," the most common stage of presentation, patients present with hip pain after relative minor trauma. There is often a history of several weeks of antecedent hip pain. "Chronic phase" SCFE presents with more than 3 weeks of hip/knee pain. Radiographs demonstrate physeal widening, as well as sclerosis and irregularity surrounding the physis. There may be additional remodeling of the femoral neck.

Juvenile idiopathic arthritis (JIA) is a noninfective autoimmune process that results in synovial inflammation

BOX 10.14 Juvenile Idiopathic Arthritis

Most common rheumatological pathology in children and adolescents, by definition those <16 years of age

Autoimmune, noninfective inflammation of joints characterized by synovial inflammation

Classification depends on number of joints involved, other symptoms, family history, and serology

Symptoms are nonspecific: lethargy, decreased activity, and often limp, especially in younger children

Common areas of involvement include knee, ankle, wrist, and small hand/foot joints, also spine, sacroiliac joints, shoulders, hip, and jaw

X-rays generally show chronic findings

US and MRI can guide therapy because of ability to detect acute inflammation

- Contrast-enhanced MRI is most sensitive for detecting synovitis
- US is much more sensitive than x-rays for joint effusions and synovial thickening and is particularly helpful to image small joints of hands and feet

MRI, Magnetic resonance imaging; *US*, ultrasound.

(Box 10.14). It is rarely diagnosed in the acute stage, in part because the definition requires symptoms persisting for longer than 6 weeks. JIA is also a diagnosis of exclusion. By definition, JIA occurs in children younger than 16 years. It is the most common rheumatological disorder in children and is often bilateral, although not always symmetrical. JIA initially presents with large effusions and inflammatory changes of the synovium, including hypertrophy and hyperemia. Later findings include bony erosions and cartilage destruction. End-stage untreated JIA may result in bony ankylosis. Like SCFE and other causes of limp with a more insidious onset, the pain is usually less severe and debilitating than seen with acute fractures. There are additional clues that point to a rheumatological etiology, including the presence of morning stiffness and improvement of pain and limited mobility with activity. JIA is an important diagnosis to consider in patients with recurrent episodes of altered gait, particularly when signs and symptoms are centered around large joints.

Imaging serves as an important tool not only in the initial diagnosis but also in monitoring for additional sites of involvement, assessing for active inflammation, and monitoring response to therapy. Clinical history and physical examination may be deficient in fully delineating the areas of involvement, because inflammation may be subclinical until there are more serious and sometimes irreversible changes, such as bony erosions.

Radiography alone is suboptimal for early detection of disease because bone findings occur late in the disease process. Although periosteal reaction may occasionally be seen early in the course of disease on radiographs, findings are nonspecific. Much of the radiographic findings are seen only with long-standing involvement and include joint space narrowing and subluxations, erosions, growth disturbances, osteopenia, and signs of soft tissue swelling. Both ultrasonography and MRI are helpful for assessing for active inflammation and detecting erosive/destructive osseous changes. When joint effusions are present, a contrast-enhanced MRI separates the thickened, proliferative synovial tissue seen in JIA from an associated joint effusion. Both fluid and synovium appear bright on fluid-sensitive sequences, but the inflamed synovium will enhance avidly after contrast administration, whereas the fluid will not. MRI is also the only imaging modality that will detect bone marrow edema.

Ultrasound is also effective at detecting thickened synovium in a cooperative child, and it requires no sedation. Common sonographic findings in JIA include the presence of a joint effusion, thickened and hyperemic synovium, and/or the presence of fluid surrounding the tendon sheaths indicative of tenosynovitis or enthesitis. Both color and power Doppler evaluation are important components of sonographic evaluation, because the presence of increased vascularity helps assess for active inflammation. Ultrasound can also detect bursal inflammation and synovial cysts and is especially useful in imaging small peripheral joints. Within 1 week of effective steroidal or other systemic therapy, sonography can demonstrate treatment response, such as reduction in size of joint effusions, synovial thickness, and synovial hyperemia.

■ How to Approach a Child With Subacute or Chronic Limp

As noted earlier, JIA should be considered on the differential for a child with intermittent, recurrent, or long-standing symptoms. This diagnosis should be high on the differential for any child with a limp that persists for greater than 3 weeks, who does not appear toxic or with infectious-type findings to suggest septic arthritis or osteomyelitis. Other chronic etiologies of limp include mechanical disturbances, such as leg-length discrepancy, overuse syndromes, apophysitis, and other systemic illnesses, whether rheumatological or neoplastic. A detailed discussion of all such entities is beyond the scope of this chapter. However, a few other key systemic considerations that may present with limp while involving various other parts of the body include chronic noninfectious osteomyelitis (Box 10.15) and Langerhans cell histiocytosis.

Although most chronic entities are generally more benign in presentation, certain red flags should raise suspicion and demand more immediate attention (Box 10.16). This includes the presence of nighttime pain and symptoms that awaken the child from sleep. Although benign neoplastic conditions, such as osteoid osteomas, could have this presentation, primary malignant bone tumors, including osteosarcoma, Ewing sarcoma, leukemia, lymphoma, and osseous metastases, may also have similar features. In such instances the presence of chronicity or long-standing systems should not falsely lend itself toward benign diagnoses or differentials.

■ Does the Presence of Pain Help?

The presence of pain is a helpful clinical marker in the limping child, because the pain helps direct attention toward the affected area and hastens accurate diagnosis. The nature and character of the pain may also help

BOX 10.15   Chronic Noninfectious Osteomyelitis

Rare autoinflammatory disorder in children, girls affected more often than boys

Patients present with bone pain with fever and multiple bone lesions

Common locations include metaphyses of long bones, clavicle, and shoulder

Associated dermatological manifestations: psoriasis, acne, pustules on the palms of hands and feet

Bone lesions lytic in the early phase and sclerotic in the late phase

Treatment includes medical management (nonsteroidal anti-inflammatory drugs, bisphosphonates, steroids)

BOX 10.16   Red Flags

Very young (<2 years old) with septic arthritis: consider concurrent osteomyelitis

Ill, febrile, and non–weight bearing with restricted hip movements because of pain

Nighttime symptoms that awaken child from sleep, loss of appetite or weight loss: consider neoplastic processes

Multifocal joint involvement: not always rheumatological or infectious, consider malignancy

Diffuse bone marrow abnormality may be missed without appropriate T1-weighted imaging: consider lymphoproliferative etiologies

Negative imaging of supposed region of pain may be a result of referred pain: search elsewhere when suspicion is high

Radiographic findings and physical examination findings out of proportion for given history: raise concern for nonaccidental trauma

BOX 10.17   Chronic Regional Pain Syndrome

Characterized by prolonged pain that may be constant and/or severe

Rare in children younger than 10 years

Chronic pain involving a single limb usually after trauma or injury to that limb

May be associated with skin changes, abnormal sweating, and nail and hair changes

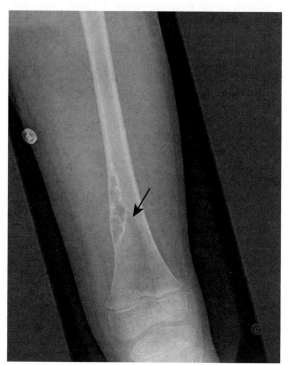

Fig. 10.23 Anteroposterior radiograph of the distal femur in an 8-year-old boy with pain and limp demonstrates a nondisplaced fracture (*arrow*) through a benign lesion (nonossifying fibroma) in the distal femoral metaphysis.

narrow the differential diagnosis. Localized, severe pain immediately after a traumatic event points to fracture or soft tissue injury as the cause of the limp. If there is no history of trauma but the pain is severe and reproducible, it suggests a possible infectious cause, such as osteomyelitis or septic arthritis. Pain that is more chronic and worse with activity suggests stress-related conditions, such as stress fractures or overuse syndromes (shin splints, tendinosis/tendinopathy, and hypermobility syndromes). Pain that improves with activities and is worse in the morning suggests rheumatological conditions. Intermittent or transient pain can be seen in the setting of JIA, LCP, SCFE, Osgood-Schlatter disease, and transient synovitis. Pain that is out of proportion to history can be seen as reflex sympathetic dystrophy, also known as complex regional pain syndrome (Box 10.17). Bilateral thigh or leg pain may be related to myositis. Strange or migratory pain patterns may be seen in patients with metabolic or hematological conditions, such as sickle cell disease or leukemia. Lastly, one must be wary of referred pain that may be misleading. For example, children with SCFE, LCP, and osteoid osteoma or other hip conditions may experience referred pain to the knee. It is important to keep in mind that hip conditions may manifest in children as referred knee pain.

■ What Conditions Present With Pathological Fractures?

Both benign and malignant osseous lesions can lead to pathological fractures. This includes benign pathologies, such as unicameral bone cysts, nonossifying fibromas (Fig. 10.23), and fibrous dysplasia, as well as aggressive lesions, such as osteosarcoma and Ewing sarcoma (Fig. 10.24). In addition, any process that leads to localized or diffuse bony demineralization may lead to a pathological fracture, including disuse osteopenia, vitamin deficiency, or osteogenesis imperfecta as examples.

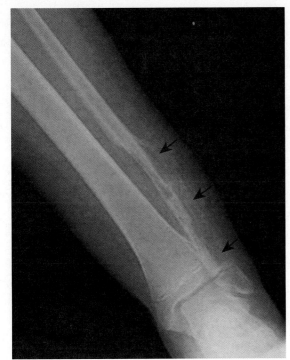

Fig. 10.24 Anteroposterior radiograph of the left ankle/lower leg in an 11-year-old girl with leg pain and limp demonstrates permeative bone destruction in the distal fibula (*black arrows*) corresponding to the site of Ewing sarcoma.

■ Summary

There are a variety of conditions that may present as a limp in a child. Elucidating the cause of the limp is a challenging task for the clinicians caring for the patient, particularly in the very young child who is not capable of verbalizing symptoms. Helpful clues may be elicited by means of a thorough clinical history, including the events immediately leading up to presentation, as well as physical examination findings and pertinent laboratory markers. A history of trauma is helpful in narrowing the differential diagnosis, particularly when the limp is accompanied by pain focused in a particular area. Symptoms and signs of infection prompt a more aggressive search for evidence of osteomyelitis or septic arthritis, conditions that demand immediate or urgent treatment/intervention. In the absence of trauma or infectious symptoms, the age of the patient can help narrow the differential diagnosis given that the various pediatric conditions that may cause limp do not affect all ages of children with equal frequency (Table 10.1). Particular attention to the nature of the pain, when pain is present, may also help narrow the differential diagnosis. Although there is no one specific algorithm that defines the approach to every child, the principles proposed in this chapter should help guide the imaging work-up of the limping child toward a definitive diagnosis.

TABLE 10.1 Common Differential Diagnoses for Limp Based on Various Factors, Including Chronicity, Clinical Signs and Symptoms, and Patient Age (Not Comprehensive)

CHRONICITY	CLINICAL SIGNS/SYMPTOMS	DIFFERENTIAL DIAGNOSIS
Acute	Trauma/injury	Young child <4 years: toddler fracture tibia, cuboid, metatarsal
		Child 4–12 years: physeal fractures, overuse syndromes
		Adolescent: 12+ years
		Ligamentous injury, overuse syndromes, apophysitis, chondromalacia
	Infection/inflammation	Toxic synovitis, septic hip, osteomyelitis, pyomyositis, discitis, psoas abscess
	Nontraumatic/noninfectious	SCFE, LCP, leukemia
Chronic	Localizing signs/symptoms	Neoplasm (benign or malignant), CNO, JIA, myositis
	Nonlocalized	DDH, leg-length discrepancy, leukemia/lymphoma, JIA

CNO, Chronic noninfectious osteomyelitis; *JIA,* juvenile idiopathic arthritis; *LCP,* Legg-Calvé-Perthes; *SCFE,* slipped capital femoral epiphysis.

Bibliography

Aronson, J., Garvin, K., Seibert, J., Glasier, C., & Tursky, E. A. (1992). Efficiency of the bone scan for occult limping toddlers. *Journal of Pediatric Orthopaedics, 12,* 38–44.
Barkin, R. M., Barkin, S. Z., & Barkin, A. Z. (2000). The limping child. *Journal of Emergency Medicine, 18*(3), 331–339.
Baskett, A., Hosking, J., & Aickin, R. (2009). Hip radiography for the investigation of nontraumatic, short duration hip pain presenting to a children's emergency department. *Pediatric Emergency Care, 25,* 78–82.
Boles, C. A., & El-Khoury, G. Y. (1997). Slipped capital femoral epiphysis. *RadioGraphics, 17,* 809–823.
Bomer, J., Klerx-Melis, F., & Holscher, H. C. (2014). Painful paediatric hip: Frog-leg lateral view only!. *European Radiology, 24,* 703–708.
Brown, R., Hussain, M., McHugh, K., Novelli, V., & Jones, D. (2001). Discitis in young children. *The Journal of Bone & Joint Surgery, 83,* 106–111.
de Moraes Barros Fues, P. M., Meves, R., & Yamada, H. H. (2012). Spinal infections in children: A review. *International Orthopaedics, 36,* 387–395.

Dillman, J. R., & Hernandez, R. J. (2009). MRI of Legg-Calve-Perthes disease. *American Journal of Roentgenology, 193,* 1394–1407.
DiPoce, J., Jbara, M. E., & Brenner, A. I. (2012). Pediatric osteomyelitis: A scintigraphic case-based review. *RadioGraphics, 32,* 865–878.
Dwek, J. R. (2011). The radiographic approach to child abuse. *Clinical Orthopaedics and Related Research, 469*(4), 776–789.
Ecklund, K., Vargas, S., Zurakowski, D., & Sundel, R. P. (2005). MRI features of Lyme arthritis in children. *American Journal of Roentgenology, 184,* 1904–1909.
Flynn, J. M., & Widmann, R. F. (2001). The limping child: Evaluation and diagnosis. *Journal of the Americal Academy of Orthopaedic Surgeons, 9*(2), 89–98.
Green, D. W., Mogekwu, N., Scher, D. M., Handler, S., Chalmers, P., & Widmann, R. F. (2009). A modificiation of Klein's line to improve sensitivity of the anterior-posterior radiograph in slipped capital femoral epiphysis. *Journal of Pediatric Orthopedics, 29,* 449–453.
Jain, N., Sah, M., Chakraverty, J., Evans, A., & Kamath, S. (2013). Radiological approach to a child with hip pain. *Clinical Radiology, 68,* 1167–1178.

Kadambari, D., & Jagdish, S. (2000). Primary pyogenic psoas abscess in children. *Pediatric Surgery International, 16*, 408–410.

Karmazyn, B., Kleinman, M. B., Buckwalter, K., Loder, R. T., Siddiqui, A., & Applegate, K. E. (2006). Acute pyomyositis of the pelvis: The spectrum of clinical presentations and MR findings. *Pediatric Radiology, 36*, 338–343.

Kemp, A. M., Butler, A., & Morris, S. (2006). Which radiological investigations should be performed to identify fractures in suspected child abuse? *Clinical Radiology, 61*(9), 723–736.

Kleinman, P. (1998). *Diagnostic imaging of child abuse.* St. Louis, MO: Mosby Inc.

Kwack, K. -S., Cho, J. H., Lee, J. H., Cho, J. H., Oh, K. K., & Kim, S. Y. (2007). Septic arthritis versus transient synovitis of the hip: Gadolinium-enhanced MRI finding of decreased perfusion at the femoral epiphysis. *American Journal of Roentgenology, 189*(2), 437–445.

Leung, A. K., & Lemay, J. F. (2004). The limping child. *Journal of Pediatric Health Care, 18*(5), 219–223.

Leventhal, J. M., Thomas, S. A., Rosenfield, N. S., & Markowitz, R. I. (1993). Fractures in young children. Distinguishing child abuse from unintentional injuries. *American Journal of Diseases of Children, 147*(1), 87–92.

Merten, D. F., & Carpenter, B. L. (1990). Radiologic imaging of inflicted injury in the child abuse syndrome. *Pediatric Clinics of North America, 37*(4), 815–837.

Mettler, F. A., & Guiberteau, M. J. (2012). Skeletal system. In F. A. Mettler, & M. J. Guiberteau (Eds.), *Essentials of nuclear medicine imaging* (6th ed.) (pp. 271–314). Philadelphia, PA: Elsevier Saunders.

Milla, S. S., Coley, B. D., Karmazyn, B., Dempsey-Robertson, M. E., Dillman, J. R., Dory, C. E., et al. (2012). ACR appropriateness criteria limping child: Ages 0-5 years. *Journal of the American College of Radiology, 9*(8), 545–553.

Ramos, P. C., Ceccarelli, F., & Jousse-Joulin, S. (2012). Role of ultrasound in the assessment of juvenile idiopathic arthritis. *Rheumatology, 51*, vii10–vii12.

Rivara, F. P., Parish, R. A., & Mueller, B. A. (1986). Extremity injuries in children: Predictive value of clinical findings. *Pediatrics, 78*, 803–807.

Sawyer, J. R., & Kapoor, M. (2009). The limping child: A systemic approach to diagnosis. *American Family Physician, 79*(3), 215–224.

Singer, J. I. (1985). The cause of gait disturbance in 425 pediatric patients. *Pediatric Emergency Care, 1*, 7–10.

Smith, E., Anderson, M., & Foster, H. (2012). The child with a limp: A symptom and not a diagnosis. *Archives of Disease in Childhood - Education and Practice, 97*, 185–193.

Stauss, J., Hahn, K., Mann, M., & Palma, D. (2010). Guidelines for paediatric bone scanning with 99mTc-labelled radiopharmaceuticals and 18F-fluoride. *European Journal of Nuclear Medicine and Molecular Imaging, 37*(8), 1492–1493.

Swischuk, L. E. (2007). The limping infant: Imaging and clinical evaluation of trauma. *Emergency Radiology, 14*, 219–226.

Umans, H., Liebling, M. S., Moy, L., Haramati, N., Macy, N. J., & Pritzker, H. A. (1998). Slipped capital femoral epiphysis: A physeal lesion diagnosed by MRI, with radiographic and CT correlation. *Skeletal Radiology, 27*(4), 139–144.

CHAPTER 11
Skeletal Dysplasias

Neena A. Davisson, Adina L. Alazraki, Shailee Lala, and Sarah Sarvis Milla

CHAPTER OUTLINE

Skeletal Dysplasias With Predominant Skull
 Involvement, 236
Extremities: Dysplasias With Prominent Diaphyseal
 Involvement, 239
Extremities: Dysplasias With Prominent Metaphyseal
 Involvement, 240
Extremities: Dysplasias With Prominent Epiphyseal
 Involvement, 240
Skeletal Dysplasias With Thoracic Involvement, 241
Skeletal Dysplasias With Pelvic Involvement, 242

Skeletal Dysplasias With Major Involvement of the
 Spine, 242
Skeletal Dysplasias With Extraosseous Organ
 Involvement, 242
Skeletal Dysplasias With Decreased Bone Mineral
 Density, 244
Skeletal Dysplasias With Increased Bone Mineral
 Density, 246
Mimickers of Skeletal Dysplasias, 246
Summary, 253

Skeletal dysplasias are bone and cartilage disorders that result in abnormal skeletal development and often, short stature. Skeletal dysplasias and syndromes with bony involvement are not uncommonly seen in pediatric populations. The differential diagnosis of dysplasias includes more than 450 heritable disorders. Early and accurate diagnosis of skeletal dysplasia/syndrome is essential to determining prognosis, receiving appropriate treatment and management of associated complications, and obtaining referral to genetic counseling for future family planning. This chapter will describe a radiological approach to diagnosing skeletal dysplasia using a working algorithm, while illustrating the classic features of many common and visually classifiable skeletal syndromes and dysplasias. Several rare but well-described "Aunt Minnie" diagnoses will be reviewed as well.

When there is a clinical suspicion for a diffuse skeletal syndrome or dysplasia, most evaluations begin with a skeletal survey for osseous abnormalities and a genetics consultation. Dedicated neuroimaging may occur if clinical suspicion for craniosynostosis (computed tomography) or neurological disorder, such as developmental delay or seizures (magnetic resonance imaging). Skeletal surveys performed for evaluation of dysplasias are similar to those for abuse, except the oblique rib radiographs are not performed, and the long bones may be imaged together (femur with tibia/fibula, humerus with radius/ulna, or entire limbs if child is small). Dedicated skull, chest, pelvis, and spine radiographs are also obtained.

Multiple classification systems have been used to characterize skeletal dysplasias; in this chapter, the mnemonic "HELPS ME" will be used to highlight all of the features to evaluate or comment about in the work-up of a skeletal dysplasia, including bones most commonly involved: head (skull), extremities, length, pelvis, spine, mineralization, and extra clinical information. The systematic approach and what to look for follows.

The *head* should be evaluated on anteroposterior and lateral views of the skull. Analysis should include evaluation of the sutures, including width, evidence of premature fusion or craniosynostosis, and/or presence of a large fontanelle. Specific evaluation for the presence of frontal bossing, Wormian bones (intrasutural bones), midface hypoplasia, and teeth abnormalities should be made. The contour of the skull should be evaluated for lytic lesions, "Lückenschädel" appearance (thinning of the skull), or "copper beaten skull" deformities (gyral impressions seen throughout the skull vault). The sella shape and presence of external auditory canals also should be carefully examined and may be better evaluated on computed tomography.

When evaluating the *extremities*, the part of the individual long bone that is abnormal should be included in the analysis: the epiphysis, metaphysis, or diaphysis. Look for stippling, delayed ossification, epiphyseal flattening, metaphyseal widening/cupping, bowed diaphyses, and fractures, old and new (Fig. 11.1). Keep in mind that fractures of different ages can be indicative of non-accidental trauma; however, multiple age-indeterminate fractures are also hallmark features of osteogenesis imperfecta, which is a diagnosis of exclusion.

Simultaneously, the *length* of the dominant extremity part involved should be evaluated. Portions of the limbs involved can be classified as acromelic (involving the hands or feet), mesomelic (involving the forearm, tibia/fibula), or rhizomelic (involving the humerus or femur). Additional evaluation for extra digits or fusions, radioulnar synostosis, and/or absent bones should be noted. Special attention should also be made for hypoplastic or absent clavicles/scapulae, shortened ribs, and narrow thorax.

The *pelvis* is also frequently affected by skeletal dysplasias, making observation of the iliac, ischium, pubis, and acetabulum pertinent to the work-up of these syndromes. Certain skeletal dysplasias are associated with pathognomonic "tombstone" iliac bones. The presence of lacy crests or "Mickey Mouse" iliac bones also help narrow the differential diagnosis. Defective development or complete absence of the pubic bones is also characteristic of certain skeletal dysplasias. Trident or horizontal acetabula can offer clues to certain skeletal dysplasias or syndromes as well.

The *spine* should be carefully evaluated because vertebral anomalies are commonly seen in skeletal dysplasias. The shape of the vertebral bodies (e.g., platyspondyly, bullet-shaped, beaked), presence of fusion or segmentation (i.e., butterfly segmentation) anomalies, as well as agenesis or dysgenesis of the vertebral bodies should be evaluated. Curvatures of the spine should be included in this analysis.

Mineralization or density of the bones should be considered in the work-up of skeletal dysplasias and syndromes. Undermineralization, undertubulation (expanded metaphyses, Erlenmeyer flask deformities), and bone age can give insight into categorization of dysplasias/syndromes as well.

Extra clinical information, such as clinically noted facial dysmorphias, ophthalmological involvement, hearing loss, genetic testing, presence of extraskeletal organ involvement (e.g., cardiac, renal, hepatosplenomegaly, brain malformation), growth/developmental delay, and metabolic/laboratory aberrations, are pertinent for accurate diagnosis and treatment of skeletal dysplasias/syndromes. Consideration of "mimickers" of skeletal dysplasias may fall within the diagnostic differentials as well, including, but not limited to, rickets, scurvy, Blount disease, and physiological bowing.

The following sections will review the most common diagnoses and the rare but classic radiographic appearance of skeletal dysplasias.

■ Skeletal Dysplasias With Predominant Skull Involvement

Craniosynostosis is a condition in which the fibrous sutures in the skull prematurely fuse, affecting the growth pattern of the skull. Craniosynostosis is usually isolated to one suture and idiopathic; however, the presence of multiple suture involvement, particularly bilateral coronal craniosynostosis, may suggest syndromic association. The most common syndromes associated with craniosynostosis include Apert, Crouzon, Pfeiffer, Muenke, Saethre-Chotzen, and Antley-Bixler. Most of these conditions are due to mutations on fibroblast growth factor

receptor (FGFR) genes, most commonly *FGFR2*, with additional genetic mutations in *FGFR1* gene in Pfeiffer, *FGFR3* in Crouzon and Muenke, and *TWIST1* gene in Saethre-Chotzen. Individuals affected by these syndromic disorders typically have exophthalmos and midface hypoplasia. Associated issues include sleep apnea, airway compromise, and hydrocephalus. Several of these are also termed acrocephalosyndactylies because of additional hand/foot malformations. Apert syndrome is also known as type I acrocephalosyndactyly and has an incidence of 1 in 65,000 to 80,000 pregnancies. Patients with Apert syndrome have characteristic soft tissue and osseous syndactyly ("hoof" hand/foot) (Fig. 11.2).

Crouzon syndrome is also characterized by premature craniosynostoses. It has a similar incidence at approximately 1 in 62,500 pregnancies and is associated with a bifid uvula in addition to exophthalmos and midface hypoplasia. It is associated with Chiari type I malformations and cervical spine fusion. It is not frequently associated with limb abnormalities.

Saethre-Chotzen, or type III acrocephalosyndactyly, is the most common craniosynostosis syndrome and affects 1 in 25,000 to 50,000 individuals without predilection for male or female sex. The craniosynostosis typically occurs in the coronal plane, and syndactyly of two or three digits of the hand is typical. There is a characteristic appearance of the ears with a small pinna and prominent superior and/or inferior crus. Individuals with this syndrome also characteristically have ptosis. Cardiac anomalies are associated with Saethre-Chotzen syndrome. Mutations in the *TWIST1* gene located on chromosome 7p21 are inherited in an autosomal dominant pattern and lead to this characteristic syndrome.

Pfeiffer syndrome, or type V acrocephalosyndactyly, is characterized by proptosis, brachydactyly (particularly broad thumbs/great toes), and maxillary hypoplasia in addition to craniosynostosis and syndactyly. It arises from mutations in the *FGFR1* gene on chromosome 8 or the *FGFR2* gene on chromosome 10. There are three types of Pfeiffer syndrome, with type 1 being the classic syndromal appearance, with individuals having normal intelligence; types 2 and 3 have poorer prognosis with severe neurological compromise and proptosis, respectively.

Severe multisutural fusions can cause a "cloverleaf" skull deformity, which has been associated with many syndromes, including Crouzon, Pfeiffer, and Carpenter, as well as type II thanatophoric dysplasia.

Cleidocranial dysostosis is a skeletal dysplasia with distinct skull involvement and is characterized by incomplete intramembranous ossification of certain skeletal structures. Cranial manifestations include multiple Wormian bones, frontal bossing, brachycephaly, high arched palate, and supernumerary teeth (Fig. 11.3). The clavicles and pubic bones are often shortened or absent. The vertebral column (mild and long bones) may also be affected. The thorax is often affected with a narrowed, bell-shaped appearance, which can lead to respiratory distress in severe cases. There is abnormal development of the ear structures, which can cause hearing loss in some cases. A majority of patients with cleidocranial

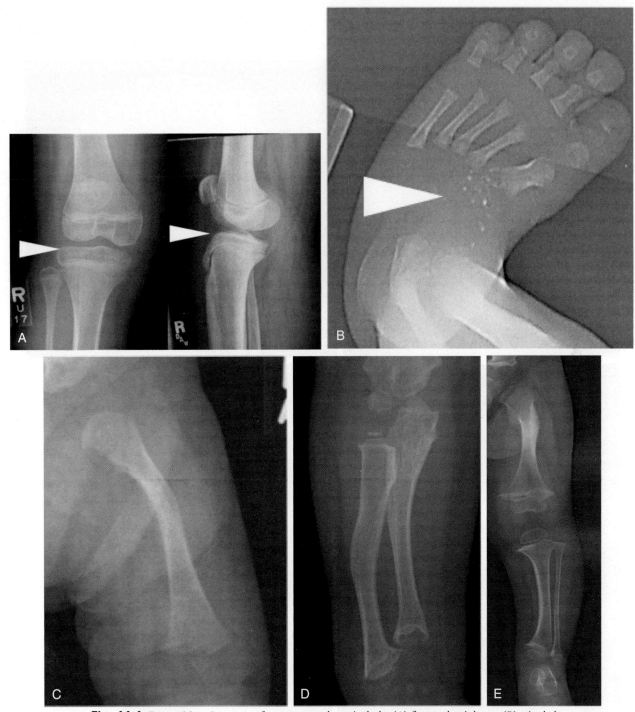

Fig. 11.1 Extremities. Important features to evaluate include: (A) flattened epiphyses, (B) stippled epiphyses, (C) diaphyseal bowing, (D) metaphyseal cupping, and (E) metaphyseal widening.

dysostosis have a mutation in the *RUNX2* gene on chromosome 6, with an autosomal dominant inheritance pattern. Approximately 30% of patients do not have an identified causal mutation.

Pyknodysostosis, or Toulouse-Lautrec syndrome, is characterized by osteosclerosis and short stature. Patients present with delayed closing of cranial sutures and frontal/occipital bossing, short broad hands, and multiple long bone fractures after minimal trauma. It is

a lysosomal disorder due to a deficiency of cathepsin K, which is necessary for normal osteoclast function. Radiographically, there is evidence of delayed bone age, aplasia of the terminal phalanges, Wormian bones, proptosis, prognathism, vertebral segmentation anomalies (primarily upper cervical and lower lumbar), and hypoplastic clavicles. The abnormality is on the *CTSK* gene on chromosome 1 and is inherited in an autosomal recessive pattern.

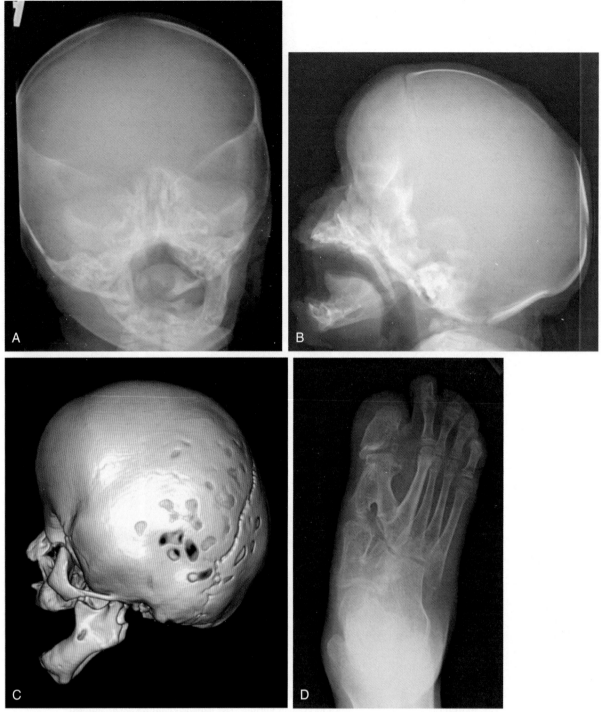

Fig. 11.2 Acrocephalosyndactyly. Frontal (A) and lateral (B) views of the skull in a patient with Apert syndrome showing bicoronal craniosynostosis with upward distortion of the lateral orbits "harlequin eyes." (C) Three-dimensional computed tomography skull reformatting in a patient with Apert syndrome and bicoronal synostosis. (D) Osseous and soft tissue fusion of digits in the foot of another patient with Apert syndrome.

Multiple syndromes involve facial development, such as Goldenhar syndrome; although sometimes referred to as hemifacial microsomia, it may manifest as a bilateral condition and is a severe manifestation along the oculo-auriculo-vertebral spectrum characterized by abnormalities of the eyes, ears, and vertebrae. Patients manifest with underdevelopment of the affected facial bones with otic hypoplasia, preauricular appendages,

and ipsilateral microphthalmia. It occurs sporadically with a slight male predominance and an incidence of 1 in 3000 to 5000 births.

Facial underdevelopment is Pierre Robin sequence, which is characterized by mandibular micrognathia, glossoptosis (retraction of the tongue), and a high or U-shaped palate. Severe micrognathia may lead to airway obstruction and hypoxia. Robin sequence occurs in 1 in

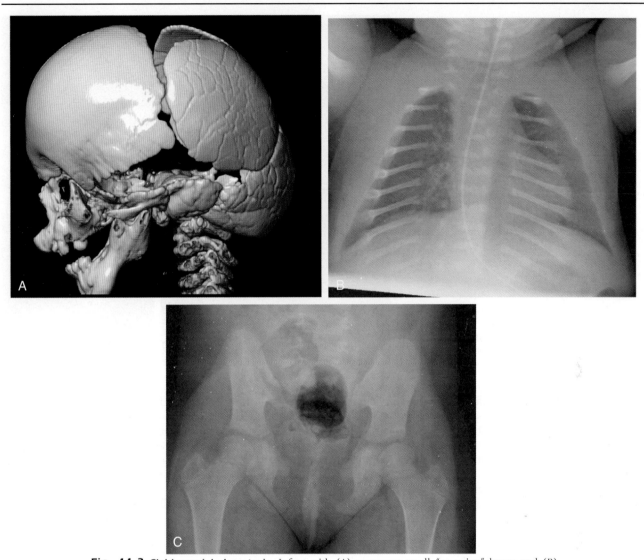

Fig. 11.3 *Cleidocranial dysostosis.* Infant with (A) numerous small "wormian" bones and (B) absence of the clavicles with shortened appearance of the ribs. (C) Pelvic radiograph from a different, older patient demonstrates absent ossification of the pubic bones.

8500 births. DNA mutations near the *SOX9* gene are thought to be the inciting genetic cause of the disorder. Nongenetic causes, such as oligohydramnios and in utero restriction, are speculated to result in isolated Pierre Robin sequence because of jaw growth restriction.

■ Extremities: Dysplasias With Prominent Diaphyseal Involvement

Thanatophoric dysplasia is the most common lethal skeletal dysplasia with an incidence of 1 in 25,000 to 50,000 births. It results from a mutation in the *FGFR3* gene on chromosome 4p16 and occurs sporadically. There are two subtypes: type I is associated with "telephone receiver"–shaped femurs (Fig. 11.4), while type II is characterized by a "cloverleaf skull" and milder limb shortening. The proximal long bones are typically shortened, giving a rhizomelic appearance, with bowing and metaphyseal flar-

ing. The iliac bones are hypoplastic, and there may be "trident acetabula," as well as platyspondyly. The thorax may be narrowed with shortened ribs and small scapulae. The condition is lethal within a few hours of birth secondary to respiratory failure or brainstem compression from a narrowed foramen magnum.

Bent bone dysplasias predominantly affect the diaphyses. They are syndromes characterized by lower extremity bowing, hypoplastic scapulae, dysplastic acetabula and iliac bones, and dislocated hip and knee joints. Campomelic dysplasia, meaning "bent limb" in Greek, is a bent bone dysplasia characterized by a hypoplastic mandible, cephalad angulation of the clavicles, hypoplastic scapulae, and rib anomalies (i.e., 13 pairs) (Fig. 11.5). It is attributed to a mutation in the *FGFR2* gene and has an incidence of 1 in 200,000 births with an autosomal recessive inheritance. It is a relatively lethal disorder, causing death in up to 97% of patients within the first year of life caused by respiratory failure.

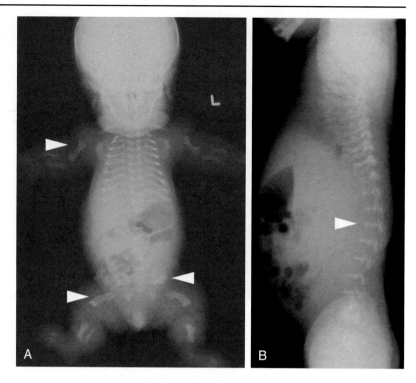

Fig. 11.4 Thanatophoric dysplasia. (A) Telephone-receiver long bones, rhizomelia, trident acetabula and, narrow thorax and (B) platyspondyly.

Isolated bent bone dysplasias also can be seen in neurofibromatosis type 1 (NF1), also known as von Recklinghausen disease, which primarily involves bowing of the tibia and fibula (Fig. 11.6). This may progress to resorption of bone at the maximal site of bowing usually between the mid and distal thirds of the diaphysis and, subsequently, characteristic pseudarthrosis most commonly seen in the tibia and fibula. *NF1* gene on chromosome 17 encodes a tumor suppressor in the Ras/Mitogen-Activated Protein Kinase pathway. Fifty percent of cases are inherited in an autosomal dominant pattern, with the remaining half occurring sporadically. Diagnosis of NF1 must have two of the following: greater than six café au lait spots, at least two neurofibromas or one plexiform or optic nerve glioma, distinctive osseous lesions, at least two iris hamartomas, axillary or inguinal freckling, and a primary relative with NF1. There is an association with learning disabilities (45%), numerous types of neoplasm, rib notching, and limb hemihypertrophy.

■ Extremities: Dysplasias With Prominent Metaphyseal Involvement

Achondroplasia is the most common type of short-limbed dwarfism (1 in 20,000), caused by a mutation in the *FGFR3* gene. Eighty percent of cases occur sporadically, while the remaining 20% of cases have an autosomal dominant inheritance pattern. Characteristic features included rhizomelic shortening and metaphyseal widening, vertebral column anomalies (e.g., exaggerated lumbar lordosis, posterior vertebral body scalloping,

narrowing interpedicular distance), flattened acetabula and rounded iliac bones ("tombstone" appearance), and oval, lucent femurs ("ice-cream scoop" appearance) (Fig. 11.7). Affected individuals have normal intelligence. Hypochondroplasia is a similar entity that presents later in life with milder clinical/radiographic findings.

Metaphyseal chondrodysplasia, Schmid type is a mild skeletal dysplasia due to a mutation in type X collagen (*COL10A1* gene), which causes cupping of the metaphyses, similar to that seen in rickets.

■ Extremities: Dysplasias With Prominent Epiphyseal Involvement

Multiple epiphyseal dysplasia is a skeletal dysplasia with predominant epiphyseal involvement. It is characterized by delayed and irregular ossification centers, flattened epiphyses, thin lateral tibial epiphyses, double-layered patella, hypoplastic tibial and femoral condyles with shallow intercondylar notches. It is inherited in an autosomal dominant pattern (Fig. 11.8).

The chondrodysplasia punctata group is a heterogeneous group of skeletal dysplasias characterized by epiphyseal calcific deposits and calcific stippling of cartilage and periarticular soft tissues (Fig. 11.9). There are both rhizomelic and nonrhizomelic forms, which can be inherited in a variety of ways, including X-linked dominant or recessive and autosomal dominant or recessive. The rhizomelic form may be lethal. Mimickers of skeletal dysplasias with stippled epiphyses also can be seen in children of mothers who were taking warfarin and consuming alcohol during pregnancy.

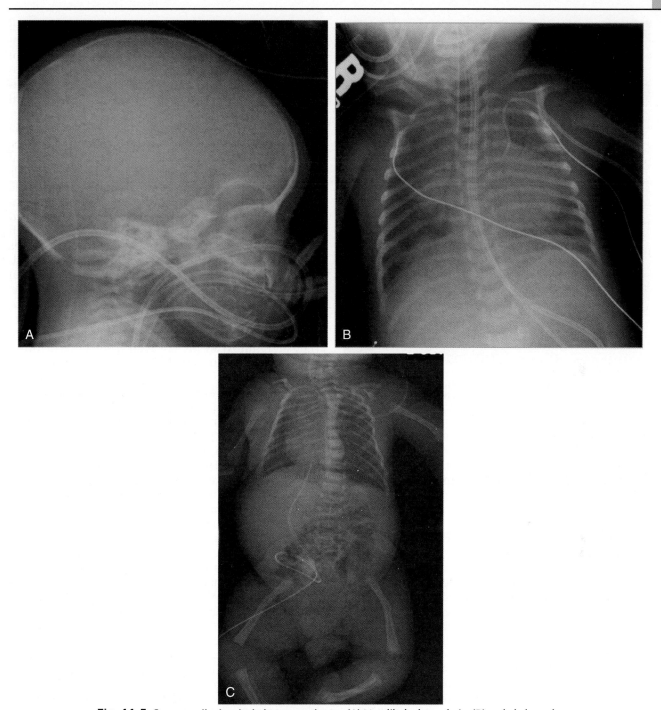

Fig. 11.5 Campomelic dysplasia in two patients. (A) Mandibular hypoplasia, (B) cephalad angulation of the clavicles and hypoplastic scapulae, and 13 paired ribs and (C) angulated femurs.

■ Skeletal Dysplasias With Thoracic Involvement

When thinking about skeletal dysplasias, one must not forget to evaluate the thorax for shortened ribs. For example, asphyxiating thoracic dysplasia, or "Jeune syndrome," is a short-limb skeletal dysplasia associated with a "bell-shaped" chest secondary to pulmonary hypoplasia and "handlebar" clavicles (Fig. 11.10). There are characteristic shortened distal limbs, flared iliac bones, and trident acetabula, and there is a strong association with cystic renal disease. Jeune syndrome is seen in 1 out of 70,000 births and is inherited in an autosomal recessive pattern.

Another short rib polydactyly syndrome is Ellis von Creveld syndrome, which is associated with a narrow thorax/short ribs, mesomelic limb shortening, and postaxial polydactyly (Fig. 11.11). The forearms and lower legs are predominantly affected in this shortened limb syndrome. There may also be bowing

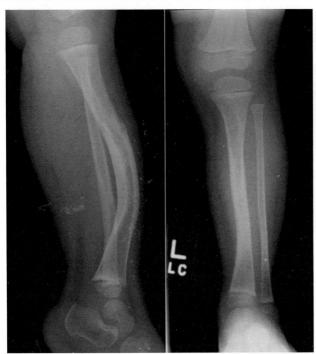

Fig. 11.6 Neurofibromatosis. Distinctive "anterolateral" tibial bowing that may progress to or present as pseudoarthrosis, typically within the first year of life, as a result of mesodermal dysplasia.

of the femora and humerii and shortening of the fibulae. More than 50% of patients will have a cardiac anomaly, most often an atrial septal defect. More than half of affected individuals have a mutation in *EVC* or *EVC2* genes.

■ Skeletal Dysplasias With Pelvic Involvement

Several skeletal dysplasias have pelvic involvement. Tombstone iliac bones, characterized by flattened acetabula and rounded iliac bones, were previously mentioned as a characteristic of achondroplasia. A Mickey Mouse pelvis, or outward flaring of the iliac wings, can be seen in Down syndrome, or trisomy 21. Small iliac wings with broad, lacy crests (Fig. 11.12) are seen in Dyggve-Melchior-Clausen syndrome, which is also associated with short-trunked dwarfism, mental retardation, platyspondyly with notched end plates, lateral displacement of capital femoral epiphyses, and accessory ossification centers in the first metacarpals and proximal and middle phalanges. Smith-McCort syndrome is similar to Dyggve-Melchior-Clausen syndrome, but patients have normal neurological function.

■ Skeletal Dysplasias With Major Involvement of the Spine

Close evaluation of vertebral body shape should be made in the work-up of skeletal dysplasias. To begin, spondylometaphyseal dysplasia is characterized by shortening of the spine and lower limbs. The vertebral bodies are typically flattened in appearance (platyspondyly) (Fig. 11.13). Per the name, there is irregularity of the metaphyses (i.e., "cupping and fraying"), predominantly involving the lower extremities, as well as shortened femoral necks. It is inherited as an autosomal dominant syndrome.

Spondyloepiphyseal dysplasia is a skeletal dysplasia that involves the spine and proximal epiphyseal centers. Similar to spondylometaphyseal dysplasia, the vertebral bodies are flattened in appearance. These individuals have a short neck with predominant involvement of the cervical and lumbar spine, including atlantoaxial instability, craniovertebral junction stenosis, and exaggerated lumbar lordosis. The proximal limbs are short with underdeveloped proximal epiphyses. These patients have a short trunk with protruding abdomen and waddling gate. There is association with myopia, retinal hemorrhage, hearing loss, and nephrotic syndrome. Spondyloepiphyseal dysplasia is due to abnormal synthesis of type II collagen. There are two types: congenita and tarda. Congenita occurs when the abnormalities (i.e., short limbs) are present at birth and tarda deformities (i.e., short trunk) become more apparent in adolescence.

Kniest dysplasia is a rare type II collagenopathy caused by a mutation in the *COL2A1* gene. It is characterized by dumbbell-shaped femurs, nonossified flattened epiphyses, platyspondyly, metaphyseal flaring, absent ossification of the public bones, kyphoscoliosis, and micromelia (Fig. 11.14). There is a strong association with hearing and vision loss. Kniest dysplasia has an incidence of 1 in 1 million people and is inherited in an autosomal dominant fashion. There is no predilection for male or female sex.

Metatropic dysplasia is characterized by rhizomelic shortening of the extremities, tibial bowing, severe platyspondyly, narrow chest, kyphoscoliosis, hypoplastic ilia with narrow sacrosciatic notches, and trident acetabula/horizontal acetabular roof. Patients are typically born with a narrow chest and short extremities with a coccygeal tail in some cases. Joint contractures and kyphoscoliosis can manifest within the first year of life. The kyphoscoliosis typically worsens over time, with the torso appearing comparably shorter compared with the limbs. These phenotypic changes over time are how this syndrome got its fitting name *metatropos*, meaning "changing patterns" in Greek.

■ Skeletal Dysplasias With Extraosseous Organ Involvement

The mucopolysaccharidoses are the classic lysosomal disorder with deposition of glycosaminoglycans (GAG) proteins causing skeletal abnormalities, hepatosplenomegaly, and often with neurological findings. Other disorders with skeletal and organ involvement include gangliosidosis and sialidosis/galactosialidosis.

There are multiple types of mucopolysaccharidoses with eight variants often reviewed: type I with mild vari-

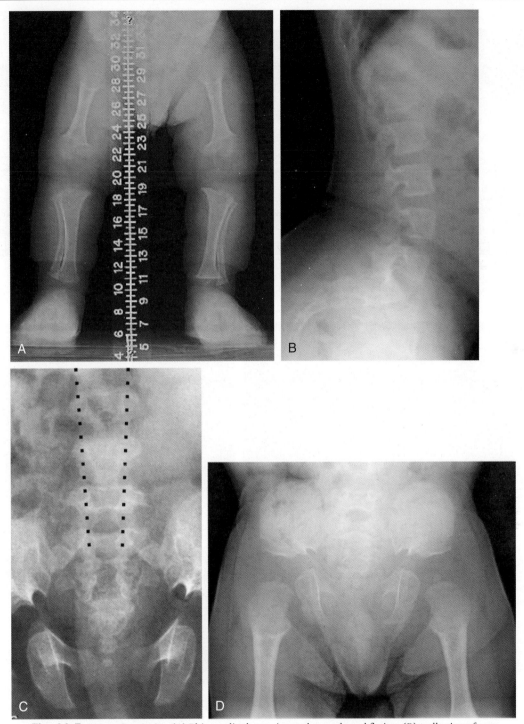

Fig. 11.7 Achondroplasia. (A) Rhizomelic shortening and metaphyseal flaring, (B) scalloping of posterior vertebral bodies with prominent lumbosacral kyphosis, (C) progressive narrowing of the interpediculate distances, and (D) "ice-cream scooper" proximal femoral metaphyses, and "tombstone" iliac wings.

ant Scheie syndrome (I-S) and more severe Hurler (I-H) syndrome, Hunter (II), San Filippo (III) and Morquio (IV), Maroteaux-Lamy (VI), Sly (VII), and Natowicz (IX) syndromes. Of these syndromes, all are autosomal recessive, except for type II Hunter, which is X linked. Due to the deposition of the GAG proteins in bones and organs, the mucopolysaccharidosis are classically characterized by broad ("oar-shaped") ribs, short clavicles, pointed proximal metacarpals (trident hands), vertebral body beaking, and mixed osteopenia and sclerosis (Fig. 11.15). Skull findings include J-shaped (enlarged) sella turcica and a narrow foramen magnum. The spectrum of neuroimaging findings also includes prominent perivascular spaces (Fig. 11.16), white matter signal abnormalities (particularly Hunter/Hurler), and various degrees and patterns of craniocervical junction narrow-

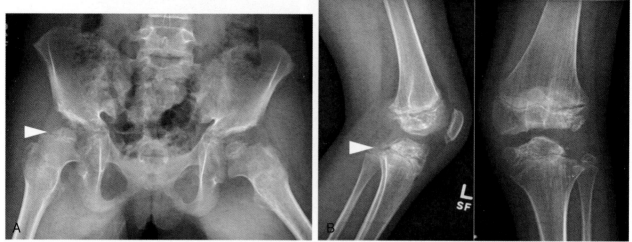

Fig. 11.8 Multiple epiphyseal dysplasia, or Fairbank disease. (A) Delayed and irregular ossification of the capital femoral epiphyses, and (B) bilateral flattened, dysplastic distal femoral, and proximal tibial epiphyses with shallow intercondylar notch.

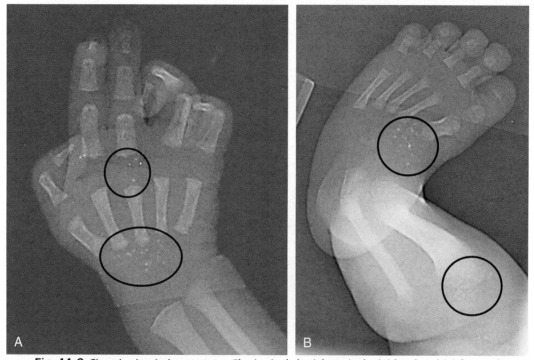

Fig. 11.9 Chondrodysplasia punctata. Classic stippled epiphyses in the (A) hand, and (B) foot, and tibia with periarticular soft tissue calcifications as well.

ing and vertebral body abnormalities. Spinal abnormalities often include vertebral body beaking (anteroinferior beaking with Hunter/Hurler), and bullet-shaped vertebral bodies are often seen in Morquio syndrome. Flat and broad cervical vertebra with cervical canal stenosis is often seen in Morquio syndrome.

Morquio syndrome (type IV mucopolysaccharidosis) is associated with atlantoaxial subluxation, goblet-shaped flared iliac wings, and metaphyseal flaring of the long bones. These abnormalities are a result of excess keratan sulfate that accumulates in various tissues, including cartilage, the nucleus pulposus of intervertebral disks, and corneas. Patients have normal intelli-

gence. Estimated incidence is 1 in 40,000, and expected life expectancy is 30 to 40 years, with cervical myelopathy as the common cause of death.

■ Skeletal Dysplasias With Decreased Bone Mineral Density

In the assessment of skeletal dysplasias the bone mineral density must be taken into account. The most common skeletal dysplasia with decreased bone mineral density is osteogenesis imperfecta, which occurs in 1 of 12,000 to 15,000 births. It is caused by defects in

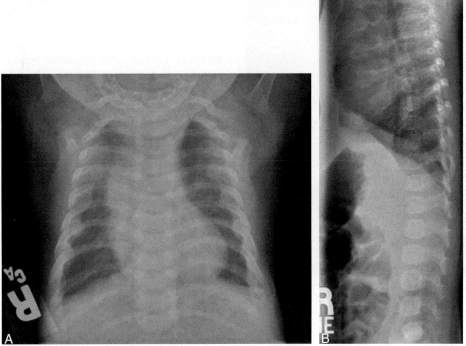

Fig. 11.10 Jeune syndrome, or asphyxiating thoracic dysplasia. (A) Narrow transverse diamteter of the chest with pulmonary hypoplasia, and (B) small anteroposterior diameter of the chest as a result of short ribs with widening of ribs anteriorly and prominent costochondral junctions.

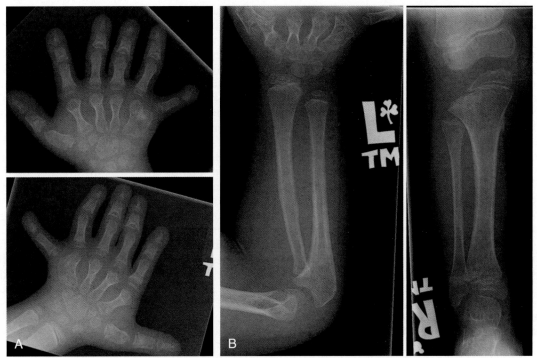

Fig. 11.11 Ellis von Creveld, or chondroectodermal dysplasia. One of the short ribs polydactyly syndromes with (A) bilateral postaxial polydactyly in the hands and (B) characteristic mesomelic limb shortening typically involving forearms and lower legs. Note fibular shortening and dysplastic epiphyses secondary to cartilage dysplasia.

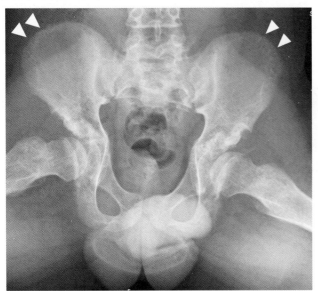

Fig. 11.12 Patient with Dyggve-Melchior-Clausen (DMC) syndrome, a rare spondylo-epi-metaphyseal dysplasia, with unique "lacy" iliac crests, as well as acetabular abnormalities. Similar radiographic features are seen in the associated allelic variant Smith McCort syndrome (SMC); however, SMC does not have the microcephaly and intellectual disability seen in DMC.

the *COL1A1* and *COL1A2* genes and is a disorder of type I collagen production. Classic clinical features include blue sclera, osteoporosis with abnormal bone fragility, multiple fractures, dentinogenesis imperfecta, hearing impairment, ligamentous laxity and hypermobile joints, easy bruising, and short stature. There is characteristic cortical thinning of bones and callous formation involving age-indeterminate fractures (Fig. 11.17). Given a history of multiple healed/healing fractures and deformed bones, be sure to rule out nonaccidental trauma as the etiology of multiple fractures of different ages. There are multiple types of osteogenesis imperfecta, ranging from mild (type I) to severe (type III) and lethal (type II).

Hypophosphatasia is another skeletal condition characterized by decreased bone mineral density. It is caused by deficient serum alkaline phosphatase activity due to a mutated *ALPL* gene. It ranges in severity, some of which can be lethal in the perinatal (100% of cases) and infantile (up to 50% of cases) subtypes. Radiographically, hypophosphatasia is characterized by bowing of long bones, osteoporosis, irregular metaphyses, craniosynostosis, and looser zones ("Milkman lines," "pseudofractures," "cortical infractions") (Fig. 11.18).

■ Skeletal Dysplasias With Increased Bone Mineral Density

Osteopetrosis is a skeletal dysplasia characterized by sclerotic bone formation secondary to defective osteo-clast function. There are two main types: infantile type, which is the most severe, resulting in death in up to 70% of patients by age 6 years; and adult type, which is benign. The infantile type is inherited in an autosomal recessive pattern, and the adult type is inherited in an autosomal dominant fashion. Radiographically, bones have a "hair-on-end" appearance and appear dense/sclerotic (Fig. 11.19). There is oftentimes a "bone-in-bone" appearance, and metaphyseal bands may be present. The vertebrae take on a "sandwich-like" appearance with central lucency and surrounding sclerosis, and long bones may resemble an "Erlenmeyer flask."

■ Mimickers of Skeletal Dysplasias

In the evaluation of skeletal dysplasias, physicians must also consider alternative diagnoses, including, but not limited to, vitamin deficiencies, nonaccidental trauma, and normal developmental changes. For purposes of this chapter, we will consider the differential diagnoses for leg bowing (Fig. 11.20). For example, rickets, a condition caused by vitamin D deficiency, can cause leg bowing secondary to weakened bone, and results in abnormal configuration of the metaphyses characterized by fraying (indistinct margins), splaying (widening of the metaphyseal ends), and/or cupping (concavity of the metaphysis). Radiologists may be able to identify Harris growth arrest lines parallel to the metaphysis, which would signify prior rickets. Classically, there is a "rachitic rosary" appearance of the anterior ribs caused by expansion and nodularity at the costochondral joints.

Pathological bowing is also seen in scurvy, a condition caused by vitamin C deficiency. Patients are at risk of increased bleeding tendency, impaired wound healing, and osteoporosis (poor collagen synthesis). Radiographically, lucent metaphyseal bands are present ("Trümmerfeld zone"), and there may be cupping of the metaphysis caused by metaphyseal spurs. Unlike rickets, the costochondral junction is angular with a sharper step-off.

Painless leg bowing is also seen in Blount disease, which results as a growth disturbance of the medial proximal tibial metaphysis. There are infantile, juvenile, and adolescent forms, with the infantile form being the most common. The adolescent form is strongly associated with obesity and is typically unilateral and post-traumatic. Blount disease is thought to result from early compressive forces on the proximal tibial physis leading to a relative lack of growth along the medial tibial growth plate, giving the metaphysis a beaklike appearance. The adjacent epiphysis is oftentimes wedge-shaped, fragmented, or absent.

Lastly, physiological bowing is a common developmental condition that causes normal age-related exaggerated angulation at the knee joint. The metaphyses are otherwise normal.

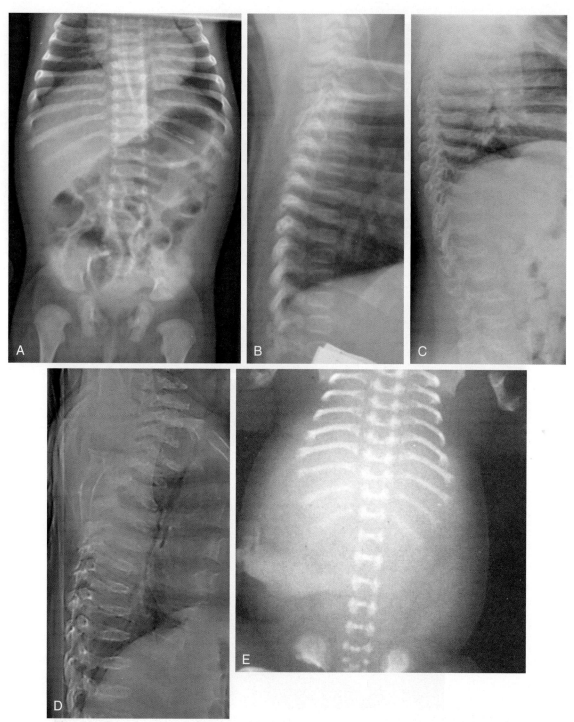

Fig. 11.13 Varying degrees of platyspondyly: (A) Kniest dysplasia, (B) spondyloepiphyseal dysplasia, (C) spondylometaphyseal dysplasia, (D) metatropic dysplasia, and (E) thanatophoric dysplasia.

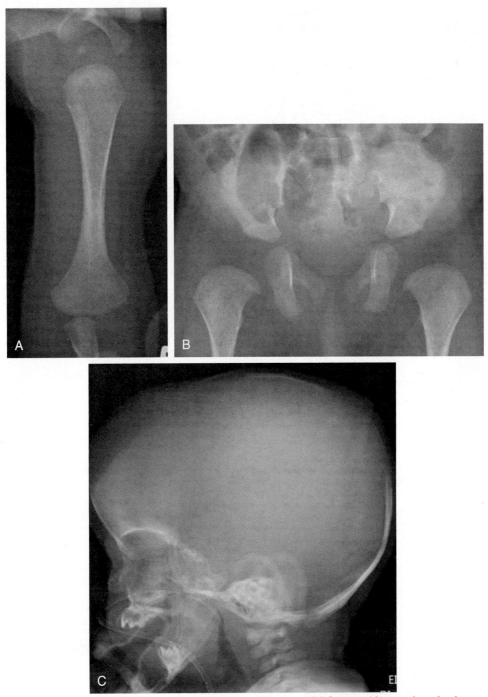

Fig. 11.14 Kniest dysplasia. (A) Dumbbell-shaped humerus, (B) femurs with metaphyseal enlargement and (C) frontal bossing.

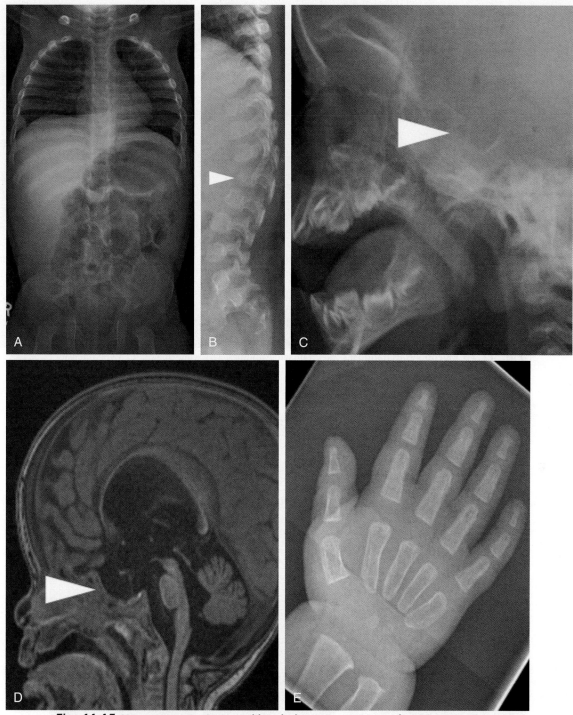

Fig. 11.15 Mucopolysaccharidoses. Although there are variations to features seen in the various mucopolysaccharidoses, shared radiographic features include: (A) "paddle/oar-shaped" ribs, (B) vertebral body abnormalities (Hurler syndrome shown, with different vertebral manifestations in variants), (C) radiographic and (D) magnetic resonance imaging demonstration of broad and deep J-shaped sella, and (E) hand radiograph with "pointed" proximal metacarpals.

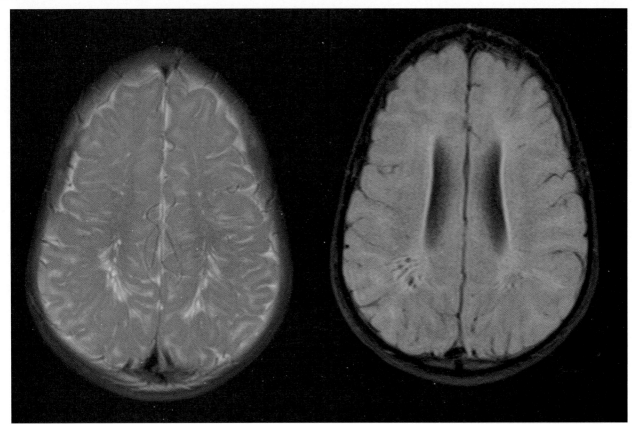

Fig. 11.16 Mucopolysaccharidoses. Neuroimaging findings: (A) white matter T2 hyperintensity with prominent perivascular spaces can be seen in Hurler (I-H), (B) spinal findings consistent with Hurler, and (C, D) Morquio (IV) syndrome.

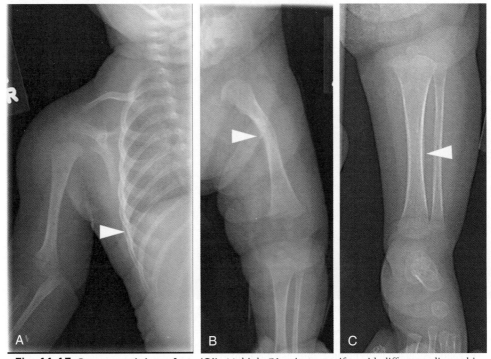

Fig. 11.17 Osteogenesis imperfecta (OI). Multiple OI variants manifest with different radiographic severity. Mild forms may present with a solitary fracture or subtle fractures in varying states of healing. An example of fractures in an infant: (A) healing rib fracture, (B) femoral periosteal reaction, (C) tibial stress, and (D) distal radius buckle fracture. Severe forms are detected in utero or at birth with (E) obvious fractures and deformities.

Continued

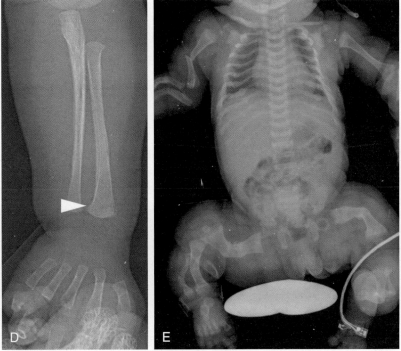

Fig. 11.17, cont'd

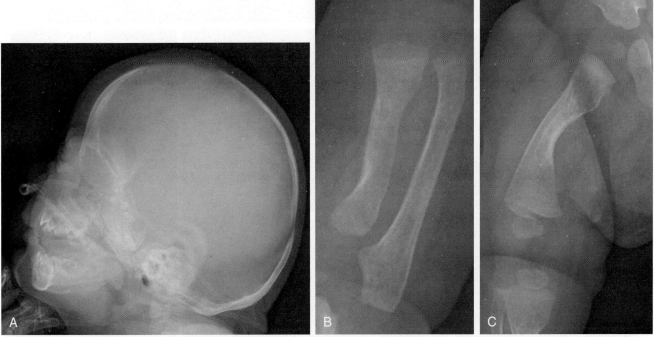

Fig. 11.18 Hypophosphatasia. (A) Lateral skull radiograph showing mild osteopenia, large fontanelle, and widened sutures, (B) irregular, metaphyseal cupping and (C) bowed diaphyses in the long bones.

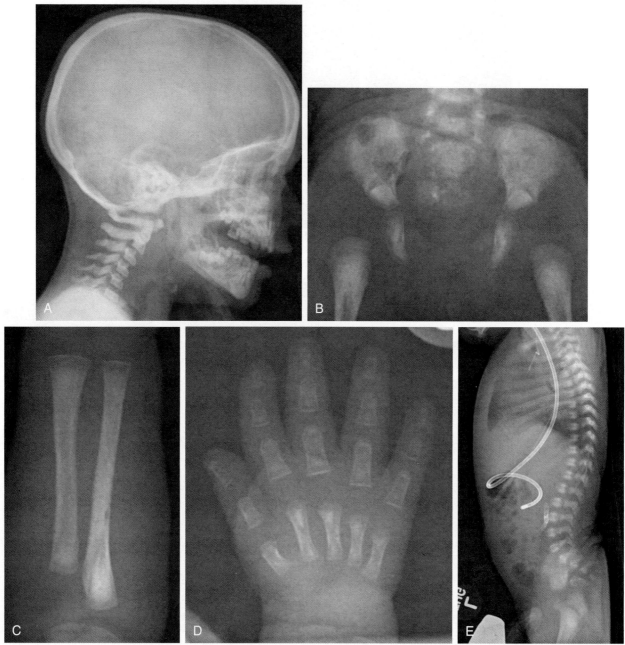

Fig. 11.19 Osteopetrosis. Defective osteoclast function results in sclerotic bone formation. (A) Lateral skull radiograph showing a sclerotic calvarium, (B–D) "bone-in-bone," appearance with metaphyseal lucent bands in the pelvis, forearm and hand, and (E) "sandwich-like" vertebra.

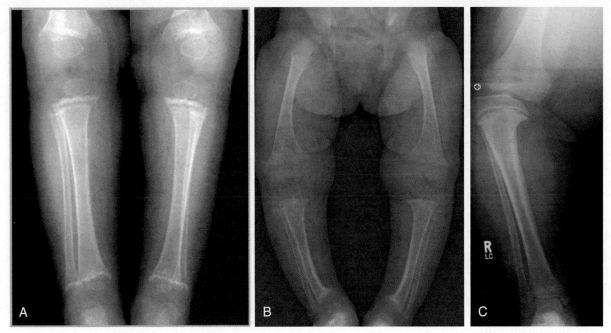

Fig. 11.20 *Mimickers.* (A) Lucent metaphyseal bands in scurvy, (B) metaphyseal widening and fraying in rickets and (C) proximal medial metaphyseal beaking in Blount disease.

■ Summary

In summary, the radiographic appearance of bony abnormalities in the setting of skeletal dysplasia is very broad, and there are many overlapping features. In the work-up of skeletal dysplasias/syndromes, alternative diagnoses must be considered and a thorough genetic evaluation pursued. The mnemonic HELPS ME can be used to systematically approach the radiographic evaluation of skeletal dysplasias to narrow the differential and more promptly make an accurate diagnosis, which is essential for proper treatment and management of complications.

Bibliography

Cormier-Daire, V. (2008). Spondylo-epi-metaphyseal dysplasia. *Best Practice & Research Clinical Rheumatology, 22*(1), 33–44.

Governale, L. S. (2015). Craniosynostosis. *Pediatric Neurology, 53*(5), 394–401.

Krakow, D. (2015). Skeletal dysplasias. *Clinics in Perinatology, 42*(2), 301–319.

Nicolas-Jilwan, M., & AlSayed, M. (2018). Mucopolysaccharidoses: Overview of neuroimaging manifestations. *Pediatric Radiology, 48*(10), 1503–1520.

Panda, A., Gamanagatti, S., Jana, M., & Gupta, A. K. (2014). Skeletal dysplasias: A radiographic approach and review of common non-lethal skeletal dysplasias. *World Journal of Radiology, 6*(10), 808–825.

Sawh-Martinez, R., & Steinbacher, D. M. (2019). Syndromic craniosynostosis. *Clinics in Plastic Surgery, 46*(2), 141–155.

Spranger, J. W., Brill, P. W., & Poznanski, A. K. (2002). *Bone dysplasias: An atlas of genetic disorders of skeletal development* (2nd ed.). München: Urban & Fischer Verlag.

Taybi, H., & Lachman, R. (2007). *Radiology of syndromes, metabolic disorders, and skeletal dysplasias*. Philadelphia: Mosby Elsevier.

CHAPTER 12
Approach to Pediatric Foot

Sarah J. Menashe and Mahesh Thapa

CHAPTER OUTLINE

Laying the Groundwork, 254
  Technique, 254
  Basic Anatomy, 254
The Normal Foot: Lines and Positions to Know, 254
Terminology, 256
  Heel Terminology, 256
    Equinus Position, 256
    Calcaneus Position, 256
  Hindfoot Terminology, 256
    Valgus, 256
    Varus, 256

Plantar Arch Terminology, 256
Forefoot Terminology, 256
  Adduction (Varus) and Abduction (Valgus), 256
  Inversion (Forefoot Varus and Supination) and
    Eversion (Forefoot Valgus and Pronation), 257
Important Pathologies and Radiographic Findings, 258
  Congenital Talipes Equinovarus (Clubfoot), 258
  Metatarsus Adductus, 258
  Skewfoot, 259
  Flatfoot (Planovalgus), 261
  Congenital Vertical Talus, 262
  Tarsal Coalition, 262
Summary, 262

The pediatric foot can be complex, from both clinical and imaging perspectives. Acquired and congenital diseases can affect the foot, especially during early childhood development. Because radiographs are often first line in imaging, having an appreciation for the normal appearance of the developing foot and, similarly, what can go wrong, is paramount.

■ Laying the Groundwork

Technique

When imaging the foot, weight-bearing views (or simulated weight-bearing views in infants or nonambulatory patients) help evaluate the foot in its functional state. Both dorsoplantar (anteroposterior projection [AP]) and lateral views should be obtained, each with the tibia as perpendicular to the plain of the film as possible. Other views for more specific abnormalities may be required (e.g., the Harris view in suspected talocalcaneal coalition). However, initial imaging with these orthogonal views will help direct you toward more specialized views, as needed (Thapa, Pruthi, & Chew, 2010).

Basic Anatomy

The foot is divided into three sections: the hindfoot, the midfoot, and the forefoot. The hindfoot is composed of the talus and calcaneus. The midfoot is composed of the cuboid, navicular, and cuneiforms. The forefoot includes the metatarsals and phalanges.

At birth, the talus, calcaneus, cuboid, metatarsals, and phalanges are partially ossified. The navicular is the last bone to ossify (range, 9 months to 5.5 years).

A key point to keep in mind is that all of the bones of the foot have muscular attachments, *except* the talus. Because many foot deformities are related to underlying neurological or neuromuscular diseases, many of the bones of the foot are subject to changes in the setting of muscle or tendinous tension, and as a result can be anomalously positioned. The talus, however, is not so affected. As such, when analyzing foot abnormalities, one can typically assume that the talus is correctly positioned and can therefore evaluate the remaining bones of the foot with respect to their relationship with the talus (Ozonoff, 1992).

■ The Normal Foot: Lines and Positions to Know

Heel alignment is best evaluated on the weight-bearing lateral view of the foot by assessing the tibiocalcaneal angle. The tibiocalcaneal angle is the angle between a vertical line through the axis of tibia and a line paralleling the axis of the calcaneus. The normal tibiocalcaneal angle measures between 55 and 90 degrees (Fig. 12.1). In addition, a tangential line along the inferior surface or through the middle of the calcaneus will highlight a normal slight anterior dorsiflexion of 20 to 30 degrees.

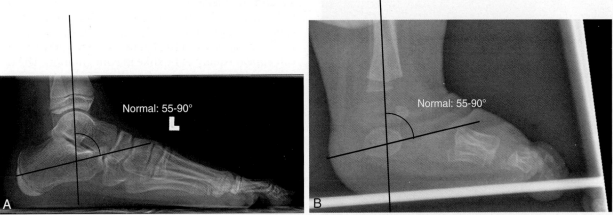

Fig. 12.1 Normal heel alignment. Lateral weight-bearing view of the foot in an adolescent (A) and lateral simulated weight-bearing view of the foot in a neonate (B) showing normal heel alignment. The tibiocalcaneal angle is assessed by drawing a vertical line through the axis of the tibia and a line parallel to the plantar aspect of the calcaneus. With normal heel alignment, the normal tibiocalcaneal angle measures between 55 and 90 degrees.

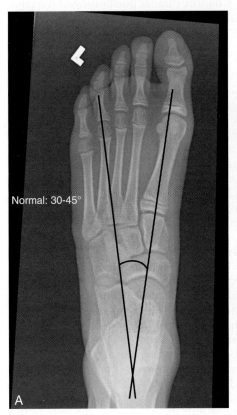
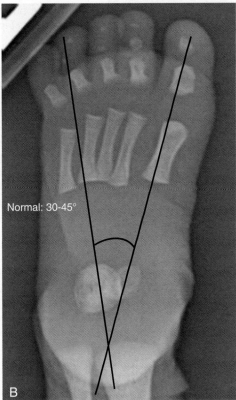

Fig. 12.2 Normal hindfoot alignment. Anteroposterior projection (AP) weight-bearing radiograph of the foot in an adolescent (A) and AP-simulated weight-bearing radiograph of the foot in a neonate (B) showing normal hindfoot alignment. On an AP view the midtalar line, drawn parallel to the medial surface of the talus, extends through the medial base of the first metatarsal. The midcalcaneal line, drawn parallel to the lateral surface of the calcaneus, extends through the base of the fourth metatarsal. With normal hindfoot alignment the talocalcaneal angle measures between 30 and 45 degrees.

When evaluating hindfoot alignment on the AP projection, the midcalcaneal line is drawn parallel to the lateral cortical surface of the calcaneus and normally intersects the base of the fourth metatarsal. The midtalar line is drawn parallel to the medial cortical surface of the talus and normally passes through or just medial to the base of the first metatarsal. A normal hindfoot will have a talocalcaneal angle of 30 to 45 degrees (Fig. 12.2).

On the lateral view, hindfoot alignment is evaluated by drawing a tangential line along the inferior surface or through the middle of the calcaneus, and the midtalar line through the mid talus, which normally courses though or parallel to the shaft of the first metatarsal. A normal hindfoot will have a lateral talocalcaneal angle of 35 to 50 degrees (Fig. 12.3). The normal navicular will be positioned directly opposite the talus. Talonavicular subluxation can often indicate hindfoot malalignment.

The plantar arch is assessed on the lateral weight-bearing film. In a normal weight-bearing foot the midline axis of the talus runs through the midline axis of the first metatarsal (Fig. 12.4).

Finally, one should also keep in mind that on an AP view of the foot, the metatarsal bases should overlap just slightly. As described later, the amount of overlap can change with forefoot alignment abnormalities.

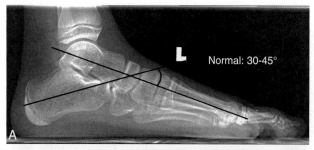

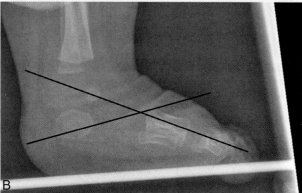

Fig. 12.3 Normal hindfoot alignment. Lateral weight-bearing radiograph of the foot in an adolescent (A) and lateral simulated weight-bearing radiograph of the foot in a neonate (B) showing normal hindfoot alignment. On the lateral projection the midtalar line, drawn through the axis of the talus, is parallel to the shafts of the metatarsals. At the intersection of the midtalar line and the midcalcaneal line is the lateral talocalcaneal angle, which measures between 35 and 50 degrees with normal hindfoot alignment.

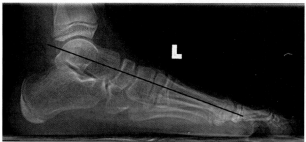

Fig. 12.4 Normal plantar arch. Lateral weight-bearing radiograph of the foot showing a normal plantar arch. In a normal plantar arch a line drawn through the midtalus with course through the midaxis of the first metatarsal.

■ Terminology

Specific terms are used to describe foot abnormalities, and as such, becoming familiar with them is necessary for accurate characterization of any abnormalities (Tables 12.1 and 12.2).

Heel Terminology

Equinus Position
Equinus positioning describes plantar flexion of the calcaneus such that its anterior aspect is depressed. With equinus positioning of the calcaneus, the tibiocalcaneal angle measures greater than 90 degrees (Fig. 12.5). Note that equinus position can also refer to fixed plantar flexion of the entire foot.

Calcaneus Position
Calcaneus positioning describes dorsiflexion of the calcaneus such that there is elevation of the anterior aspect of the calcaneus. On the lateral projection the calcaneus can appear square or boxlike in configuration. The tibiocalcaneal angle measures less than 55 degrees.

Hindfoot Terminology

Valgus
Hindfoot valgus deformity describes lateral deviation of the axis of the calcaneus and the midcalcaneal line; the axis of the talus and the midtalar line appears medially deviated relative to the first metatarsal on the AP view and the navicular, if ossified, is displaced laterally relative to the talus (Fig. 12.6B). On the AP projection the talocalcaneal angle will measure greater than 45 degrees.

On the lateral view the talus will appear more vertical than normal - with more plantar positioning of the talus - and the talocalcaneal angle will measure greater than 50 degrees (Fig. 12.7B).

Varus
Hindfoot varus deformity describes medial displacement of the axis of the calcaneus and the midcalcaneal line; the axis of the talus and the midtalar line will be laterally deviated relative to the first metatarsals, and the navicular will be displaced medially relative to the talus (see Fig. 12.6C). On the AP projection, there will be superimposition or near-parallel orientation of the calcaneus and talus, and the talocalcaneal angle will measure less than 30 degrees. On the lateral projection the calcaneus and talus will have a near-parallel configuration (see Fig. 12.7C).

Plantar Arch Terminology

Pes planus deformity describes flattening of the plantar arch, the apex of which is formed by the junction of the metatarsals and calcaneus. The calcaneus will be more horizontal than usual. On a lateral view a line drawn through the midtalus will course inferior relative to the midline axis of the first metatarsal (Fig. 12.8). This finding will be exaggerated in *rocker-bottom deformity*. In rocker-bottom deformity the plantar arch is convex at its apex, or inverted (Fig. 12.9).

In *pes cavus* deformity, there is increased height of the plantar arch, with dorsiflexion of the anterior end of the calcaneus and plantar flexion of the metatarsal heads. A line drawn through the midtalus on the lateral view will course superior relative to the midline axis of the first metatarsal (Fig. 12.10).

Forefoot Terminology

Adduction (Varus) and Abduction (Valgus)
Adduction and abduction are best evaluated on the AP projection and describe the anomalous positioning of the metatarsals with respect to the midline of the body. Although the metatarsal shafts are flexible

TABLE 12.1   Heel, Hindfoot, and Arch Alignment Abnormalities

TERMINOLOGY	DEFINITION	PROJECTION ON WHICH BEST EVALUATED	ASSOCIATIONS
Equinus	Plantar flexion of the calcaneus (anterior end depressed)	Lateral	Clubfoot Congenital vertical talus
Calcaneus	Dorsiflexion of the calcaneus (anterior end elevated)	Lateral	Pes cavus
Valgus	Lateral deviation of the calcaneus/midcalcaneal line	Anteroposterior	Flatfoot Skewfoot Congenital vertical talus
Varus	Medial deviation of the calcaneus/midcalcaneal line	Anteroposterior	Clubfoot
Pes cavus	Increased concavity/height of the plantar arch	Lateral	Primary condition Clubfoot correction, neuromuscular disease Local trauma
Pes planus	Flattening of plantar arch	Lateral	Flexible planovalgus Cerebral palsy Tarsal coalition
Rocker-bottom deformity	Convexity of plantar arch	Lateral	Congenital vertical talus Oblique talus Severe cerebral palsy with hindfoot valgus Partially or incorrectly treated clubfoot

TABLE 12.2   Forefoot Alignment Abnormalities

TERMINOLOGY	DEFINITION	PROJECTION ON WHICH BEST EVALUATED	ASSOCIATIONS
Adduction/Varus	Angulation of the metatarsal heads, as a unit toward midline	AP	Congenital clubfoot Skewfoot Metatarsus adductus
Abduction/Valgus	Angulation of the metatarsal heads, as a unit away from the midline	AP	
Inversion (varus and supination)	Medial rotation of the metatarsals (sole of the foot faces medial)	AP and lateral	Congenital clubfoot Metatarsus adductus
Eversion (valgus and pronation)	Lateral rotation of the metatarsals (sole of the foot faces lateral)	AP and lateral	Cerebral palsy Congenital vertical talus

AP, Anteroposterior.

and can have variable appearances and subject to patient cooperation, the positioning the metatarsal bases should remain in constant alignment to the distal tarsal row.

Malalignment will therefore affect the metatarsals as a unit: in forefoot adduction or varus the metatarsals pivot at the tarsal-metatarsal joints in the plane of the foot toward the midline (Fig. 12.11). In forefoot abduction or valgus the metatarsal pivot at the tarsal-metatarsal joints away from the midline (Fig. 12.12). There is no inversion or eversion by definition.

Inversion (Forefoot Varus and Supination) and Eversion (Forefoot Valgus and Pronation)

Forefoot inversion describes metatarsal rotation such that the plantar aspect of the foot is turned medially. On lateral radiographs the metatarsals lose their normal overlapping configuration and instead appear like rungs on a ladder (also known as stair-step configuration),

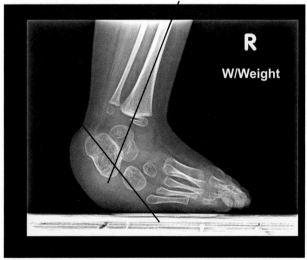

Fig. 12.5 Equinus. Lateral weight-bearing radiograph of the foot. There is plantar flexion of the calcaneus and a tibiocalcaneal angle measuring greater than 90 degrees, consistent with equinus.

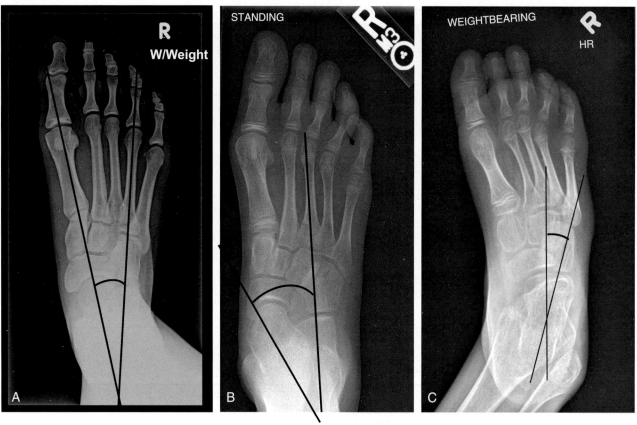

Fig. 12.6 *Hindfoot alignment, anteroposterior projection (AP).* AP weight-bearing radiographs of normal (A), valgus (B), and varus (C) hindfoot alignment. With normal hindfoot alignment the midtalar line courses through the first metatarsal, and the midcalcaneal line courses through the fourth metatarsal. With valgus alignment of the hindfoot (B) the midtalar line extends medial to the first metatarsal, with a resultant increased talocalcaneal angle, measuring greater than 45 degrees. With varus alignment of the hindfoot (C), there is overlap of the talus and calcaneus. The midtalar line extends far lateral to the base of the first metatarsal, and the midcalcaneal line extends lateral to the base of the fourth metatarsal. There is a decreased talocalcaneal angle, measuring less than 30 degrees.

with the first metatarsal highest and the fifth metatarsal lowest. On the AP projection, there is increased overlap of the metatarsal bases.

Forefoot eversion describes metatarsal rotation such that the plantar aspect of the foot is turned laterally. The associated radiographic manifestations include ladder-like appearance again seen on the lateral view (although the reverse of inversion, where the fifth metatarsal is now the highest) and increased separation of the metatarsal bases on the AP projection.

■ Important Pathologies and Radiographic Findings

Congenital Talipes Equinovarus (Clubfoot)

Clubfoot is one of the most common disorders of foot alignment with an incidence of 1 in 1000 live births. Fifty percent of cases are bilateral. The condition has many associations and possible causes, including underlying central nervous system abnormal-

ities, ligamentous laxity, and abnormal intrauterine positioning.

Radiographic findings include:
1. equinus of the hindfoot, with an increased tibiocalcaneal angle (lateral view)
2. hindfoot varus with a near-parallel orientation of the talus and the calcaneus (lateral view) and a decreased talocalcaneal angle (AP view)
3. forefoot varus and inversion with medial displacement of the metatarsals at the tarsal-metatarsal joints (AP view) (Fig. 12.13)

Metatarsus Adductus

Metatarsus adductus is the most common congenital foot abnormality with an incidence of 1 to 3 per 1000 live births. It is thought to be secondary to intrauterine packing and compression. Notably, up to 10% of patients with metatarsus adductus will have concurrent hip dysplasia.

Radiographic findings include:
1. normal heel alignment
2. normal hindfoot alignment

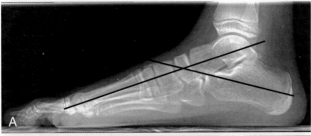

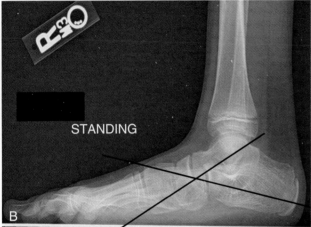

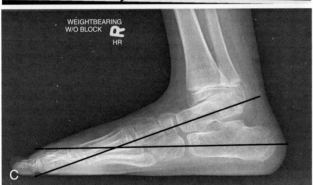

Fig. 12.7 Hindfoot alignment, lateral projection. Lateral weight-bearing radiographs of normal (A), valgus (B), and varus (C) hindfoot alignment. With normal hindfoot alignment (A), the midtalar line parallels the axis of the metatarsals, and the talocalcaneal angle measures between 35 and 50 degrees. With hindfoot valgus (B), there is slight plantar positioning of the talus and an increased talocalcaneal angle, measuring greater than 50 degrees. With varus alignment of the hindfoot (C), there is a near-parallel orientation of the talus and the calcaneus.

3. forefoot varus and inversion with medial displacement of the metatarsals at the tarsal-metatarsal joints (Fig. 12.14)

Skewfoot

Skewfoot is also called the Z-shaped or S-shaped foot. It is a rare disorder of foot alignment. It can be considered to be a severe form of metatarsus adductus or a type of pes planus deformity characterized by both rigid forefoot varus and hindfoot valgus.

Radiographic findings include:
1. normal heel alignment
2. hindfoot valgus, with the axis of the talus directed medially, increased talocalcaneal angle, and lateral

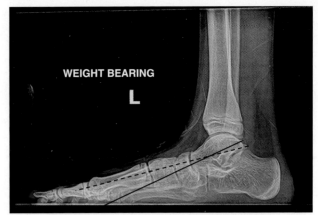

Fig. 12.8 Pes planus. Lateral weight-bearing view of the foot. The plantar arch is flattened, and there is slight plantar flexion of the anterior aspect of the calcaneus. A line drawn through the midaxis of the talus (*solid line*) courses inferior relative to a line drawn through the midline axis of the first metatarsal (*dashed line*).

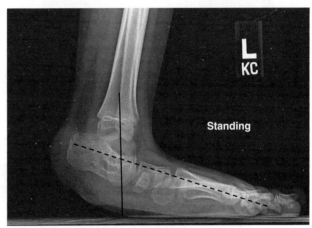

Fig. 12.9 Rocker-bottom deformity. Lateral weight-bearing view of the foot. The plantar arch is inverted. A line drawn through the midaxis of the talus (*solid line*) has a near-vertical course and is significantly inferior to a line drawn though the midline axis of the first metatarsal (*dashed line*).

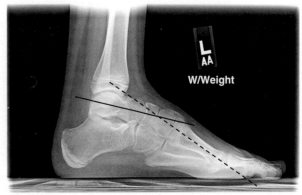

Fig. 12.10 Pes cavus. Lateral weight-bearing view of the foot. There is a high plantar arch, with dorsal positioning of the anterior aspect of the calcaneus. A line drawn through the midaxis of the talus (*solid line*) courses superior relative to a line drawn through the midline axis of the first metatarsal (*dashed line*).

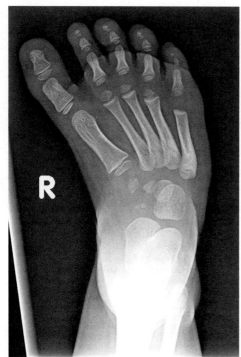

Fig. 12.11 Forefoot varus. Anteroposterior projection (AP) weight-bearing view of the foot. There is medial deviation of the metatarsals at the level of the tarsometatarsal joints toward the midline of the body.

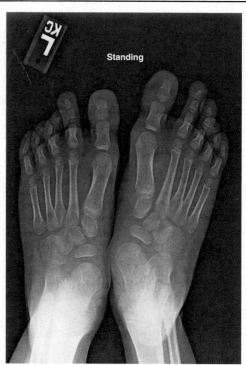

Fig. 12.12 Forefoot valgus. Anteroposterior projection (AP) weight-bearing views of the both feet. There is lateral deviation of the right metatarsals at the level of the tarsometatarsal joints.

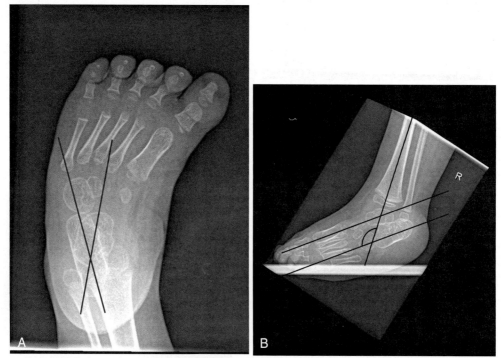

Fig. 12.13 Congenital talipes equinovarus (congenital clubfoot). Anteroposterior projection (AP) (A) and lateral (B) weight-bearing views of the foot. On the AP view, there is adduction (forefoot varus) and inversion of the forefoot with medial displacement of the metatarsals at the tarsometatarsal joints and increased overlap at the metatarsal bases. There is also hindfoot varus. The lateral view shows an equinus deformity of the heel with a tibiocalcaneal angle greater than 90 degrees and near-parallel orientation of the talus and the calcaneus (abnormal talocalcaneal angle). The "stair-step" configuration of metatarsals is due to forefoot inversion.

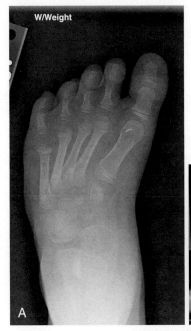

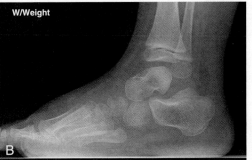

Fig. 12.14 Metatarsus adductus. Anteroposterior projection (AP) (A) and lateral (B) weight-bearing views of the foot. On the AP view, there is medial displacement of the metatarsals at the tarsometatarsal joints. On the lateral view, there is a stair-step configuration of the metatarsals. There is normal hindfoot alignment.

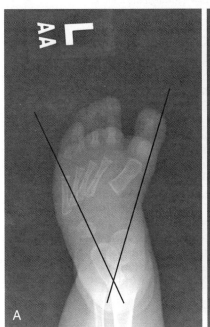

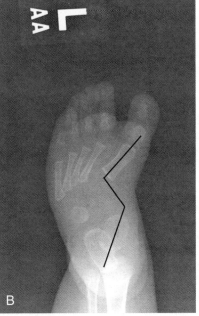

Fig. 12.15 Skewfoot. Anteroposterior projection (AP) weight-bearing radiographs of the foot. There is hindfoot valgus with medial displacement of the midtalar line. (A) There is also forefoot varus, with medial deviation of the metatarsals at the tarsometatarsal joints. When a line is drawn connecting the midtalar line and a line through the first axis of the first metatarsal, the characteristic "backward Z" is formed (B).

subluxation of the navicular relative to the talus on the AP view
3. forefoot varus with medial displacement of the metatarsals at the tarsal-metatarsal joints (Fig. 12.15)

Flatfoot (Planovalgus)

Planovalgus deformity describes a pronated flatfoot, an abnormality that can be an isolated finding or one associated with specific clinical entities. Until midchildhood, flattening of the arch, or flexible flatfoot, is considered normal as the arch develops. Although its asymptomatic

persistence into later years may represent normal variation as well, it is more commonly seen in overweight individuals. In contradistinction, rigid flatfoot is often the result of underlying pathology related to tarsal coalition, neurological diseases, or tight heel cord.

Radiographic findings of planovalgus include:
1. normal heel alignment
2. hindfoot valgus with increased talocalcaneal angle on the AP and lateral views
3. normal talonavicular alignment on the lateral view
4. normal forefoot alignment
5. flattened plantar arch (Fig. 12.16)

In cases of flexible pes planovalgus the plantar arch reconstitutes with non–weight bearing.

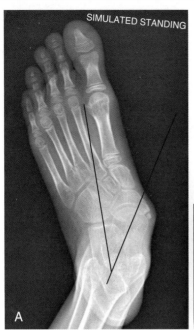
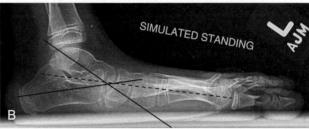

Fig. 12.16 Pes planovalgus. Anteroposterior projection (AP) (A) and lateral (B) weight-bearing radiograph of the foot. There is hindfoot valgus. On the lateral projection a line drawn through the midaxis of the talus (*solid line*) courses inferior relative to a line drawn through the midline axis of the first metatarsal (*dashed line*).

Congenital Vertical Talus

Congenital vertical talus is the most severe type of rigid flatfoot. It is characterized by fixed dorsal dislocation of the talonavicular joint with rigid heel equinus. Clinically, congenital vertical talus will result in a rocker-bottom deformity with a convex plantar arch. Possible causes include intrinsic abnormalities of skeletal muscle, muscle imbalance, and intrauterine compression. Sixty percent of patients with congenital vertical talus have associated conditions, including myelomeningocele, arthrogryposis, and aneuploidy.

Radiographic findings include:

1. heel equinus, with an increased tibiocalcaneal angle
2. hindfoot valgus with medial deviation of the axis of the talus and an increased talocalcaneal angle on the AP view
3. near-vertical orientation of the talus on the lateral view with dorsal dislocation of the navicular
4. forefoot valgus relative with lateral deviation of the metatarsals at the tarsometatarsal joints (Fig. 12.17)

In patients younger than 3 years, the navicular is unossified. The position of the navicular can be inferred by the location of the cuneiforms and the metatarsal bases. In addition, the cuboid can serve as a substitute for the unossified navicular, because the cuboid may be positioned anterior to the dorsal aspect of the talus in congenital vertical talus (Figs. 12.17A and 12.18B).

When maximal plantar flexion lateral radiographs are obtained, talonavicular dissociation persists in the setting of congenital vertical talus (see Fig. 12.18). If the navicular dislocation is reducible with maximal plantar flexion, the diagnosis is oblique talus.

Tarsal Coalition

Pain or decreased motion may be the initial presentation for abnormal bony or fibrous attachments between the tarsal bones, most commonly, the calcaneus, talus, and navicular. Due to the different stresses and altered mechanics, there are imaging features on radiographs that can suggest the diagnosis of tarsal coalition. On the lateral radiograph, elongation of the anterior calcaneal process, or the "anteater sign," suggests calcaneonavicular coalition (Fig. 12.19A). The curvilinear continuity formed by posterior curve of the talar dome and the posterior inferior aspect of the sustentaculum tali, or continuous C sign, suggests talocalcaneal coalition (Fig. 12.19B). Upward extension of the anterior superior talus, or a talar beak, can suggest calcaneonavicular or talocalcaneal coalition (Fig. 12.19C). Oblique radiographs of the foot may show an osseous calcaneonavicular coalition or irregularity and sclerosis at the calcaneonavicular joint, as can be seen in fibrous or cartilaginous coalition (Fig. 12.19D).

■ Summary

Foot alignment and malformations may initially appear complex; however, it becomes manageable when broken down into basic evaluations: heel alignment, hindfoot alignment, and forefoot alignment. Additional evaluation of the talar configuration and arch will complete the evaluation.

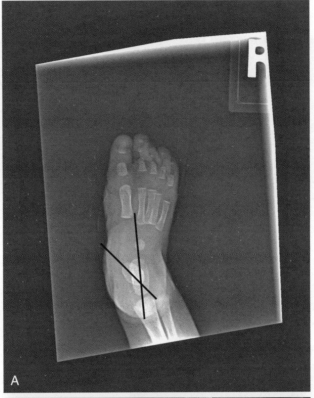

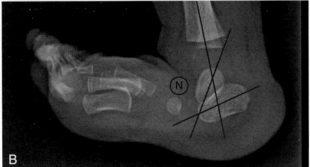

Fig. 12.17 Congenital vertical talus: anteroposterior projection (AP) (A) and lateral (B) weight-bearing radiographs of the foot. AP radiograph shows forefoot eversion, with decreased overlap of the metatarsal bases, and hindfoot valgus. On the lateral view, there is equinus, with plantar flexion of the calcaneus, and increased tibiocalcaneal angle. There is hindfoot valgus, with an increased talocalcaneal angle. There is dissociation of the talus from the cartilaginous navicular (*N*). The cuboid is located anterior to the dorsal aspect of the talus.

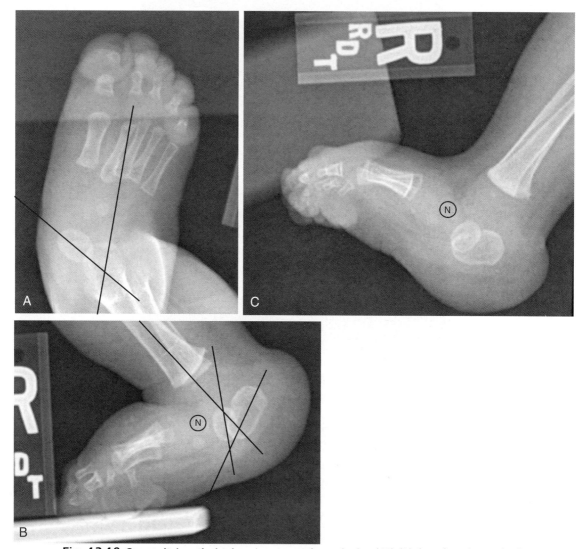

Fig. 12.18 Congenital vertical talus. Anteroposterior projection (AP) (A), lateral maximum dorsi-flexion (B), and plantarflexion (C) views of the foot. On the AP view, there is marked hindfoot valgus. On the lateral view, with dorsiflexion and plantarflexion, there is fixed talonavicular dissociation, consistent with congenital vertical talus. *N* denotes the approximate location of the cartilaginous navicular. The cuboid is located anterior to the dorsal aspect of the talus.

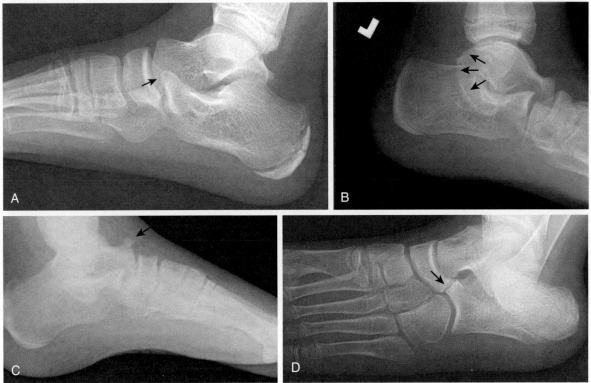

Fig. 12.19 Coalition. (A) Elongation of the anterior calcaneal process on the lateral view, often referred to as the "anteater sign" suggesting calcaneonavicular coalition. (B) Curvilinear continuity formed by the posterior curve of the talar dome and the posterior inferior aspect of the sustentaculum tali, also known as "continuous C sign" in this patient with talocalcaneal coalition. (C) Upward extension of the anterior superior talus, or "talar beak." (D) Oblique radiograph of the foot showing sclerosis and irregularity of the anterior process of the calcaneus and the lateral navicular with decreased joint space in this patient with fibrous calcaneonavicular coalition.

Bibliography

Crim, J. R., & Kjeldsberg, K. M. (2004). Radiographic diagnosis of tarsal coalition. *American Journal of Roentgenology, 182*, 323–328.

Jeans, K. A., Erdman, A. L., Jo, C. H., & Karol, L. A. (2016). A longitudinal review of gait following treatment for idiopathic clubfoot: Gait analysis at 2 and 5 years of age. *Journal of Pediatric Orthopedics, 36*, 565–571.

Maldjian, C., Hofkin, S., Bonakdarpour, A., Roach, N., & McCarthy, J. J. (1999). Abnormalities of the pediatric foot. *Academic Radiology, 6*, 191–199.

Ozonoff, M. B. (1992). *Pediatric orthopedic radiology* (2nd ed.). Philadelphia: W.B. Saunders.

Sadeghi-Demneh, E., et al. (2015). Flatfoot in school-age children: Prevalence and associated factors. *Foot & Ankle Specialist, 8*, 186–193.

Stolzman, S., Irby, M. B., Callahan, A. B., & Skelton, J. A. (2015). Pes planus and paediatric obesity: A systematic review of the literature. *Clinical Obesity, 5*, 52–59.

Thapa, M. M., Pruthi, S., & Chew, F. S. (2010). Radiographic assessment of pediatric foot alignment: Review. *American Journal of Roentgenology, 194*, S51–S58.

CHAPTER 13
Approach to Pediatric Elbow

Kiery Braithwaite

CHAPTER OUTLINE

Part 1: Imaging Basics, 267
What Are the Standard Radiographic Views of the Pediatric Elbow?, 267
When Are Additional Views Helpful?, 267
When Are Other Imaging Modalities Useful?, 267
Part 2: Approach to the Pediatric Elbow Radiograph: FOOL Checklist, 267
F: Fat Pads: Joint Effusion = Fracture (Most Likely), 267
What Is the Significance of the Posterior Fat Pad Sign?, 267
What Is the Significance of the Anterior Fat Pad?, 268
What If Positive Fat Pad and No Fracture Line Is Identified?, 268
O: Overt Findings and Outlines, 268
O: Ossification Centers, 268
What Is the Significance of CRITOE?, 268
When Is CRITOE Most Useful?, 268
Are There Any Variants of CRITOE?, 268
L: Lines, 269
What Is the Anterior Humeral Line?, 269
What Is the Radiocapitellar Line?, 270
Are There Any Exceptions to the Anterior Humeral Line?, 270
Are There Any Exceptions to the Radiocapitellar Line?, 270
Part 3: Acute Pediatric Elbow Injuries, 270
Radial Head Subluxation (Nursemaid's Elbow), 270
What Is the Role of Imaging in Radial Head Subluxation? What If the Clinician Suspects Radial Head Subluxation But the Radiographs Are Normal?
Can Radial Head Subluxation Occur in Infants 6 Months and Younger?, 271
Common Pediatric Elbow Fractures, 271

Supracondylar Fracture Overview, 272
Lateral Condyle Fracture Overview, 272
Medial Epicondyle Fracture Overview, 274
Radial Neck Fracture Overview, 275
Less Common Pediatric Elbow Fractures, 275
Transphyseal Distal Humerus Fracture Overview, 275
Radial Head Fracture Overview, 276
Olecranon Fracture Overview, 276
Pediatric Elbow Dislocation, 276
Posterior Dislocation Overview, 277
Radial Head Dislocation Overview, 277
Which Fractures Should Raise Suspicion of an Associated Dislocation?, 277
Part 4: Congenital and Posttraumatic Deformities Worth Mentioning, 278
What Is Congenital Proximal Radioulnar Synostosis?, 278
What Is the Supracondylar Process?, 279
What Is the Fishtail Deformity?, 280
Part 5: Chronic Elbow Injuries in the Athletic Child, 280
What Is Little League Elbow?, 280
Little League Elbow, Medial Compartment: Medial Epicondylitis/Apophysitis, 281
Is "Little League Elbow" Seen in Other Sports?, 283
Lateral Compartment: Juvenile Osteochondritis Dissecans, 283
What Is Juvenile Osteochondritis Dissecans?, 283
What Other Sports Predispose Adolescent Athletes to Osteochondritis Dissecans of the Elbow?, 283
Posterior Compartment: Persistence of the Olecranon Physis, 283
What Is Panner Disease?, 283
Summary, 284

The elbow is complex in its multiple articulations, which allow for flexion and extension, as well as supination and pronation. Imaging of the pediatric elbow is deceptively simple: two conventional radiographic orthogonal views are all that is required to diagnose most pediatric elbow fractures. The challenge lays in the radiographic interpretation of a joint with evolving os-sification whose appearance changes significantly as the child's skeleton matures.

Elbow injuries are quite common in childhood; pediatric elbow fractures account for approximately 15% of all childhood fractures. The child's upper extremity is central to their development, permitting babies to feed themselves and explore their environment. As a toddler

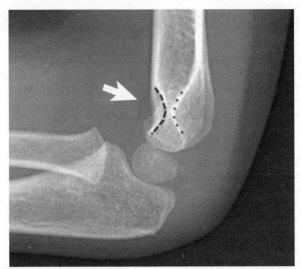

Fig. 13.1 Normal fat pads on lateral elbow radiograph. Normal anterior fat pad (*arrow*) hugs the anterior cortex of the distal humerus with normal lack of visualization of the posterior fat pad in this 4-year-old boy. The coronoid fossa (*dashed line*) and olecranon fossa (*dotted line*) form an hourglass configuration on an appropriately positioned lateral radiograph.

and young child, the upper extremity plays an essential role in the child's ability to play and climb, simultaneously protecting them during falls. In adolescence the elbow has vital functions in many popular sports. Patterns of injury change as the child evolves from a curious toddler discovering their world to the monkey bar champion of the elementary-school playground, from first gymnastics classes and little league games to playing on competitive traveling teams.

■ Part 1: Imaging Basics

What Are the Standard Radiographic Views of the Pediatric Elbow?

Anteroposterior (AP) and lateral projections are the standard radiographic views obtained in the evaluation of the pediatric elbow. The AP view is performed in full extension, with the forearm supinated. The lateral view is acquired with the elbow flexed at 90 degrees, the forearm in neutral position, with the wrist in a true lateral position, thumb up. Obtaining a *true* lateral is essential for accurate interpretation. Recognizing the hourglass or figure-of-eight morphology of the distal humerus is a quick technique for confirming adequate positioning of the lateral radiograph (Fig. 13.1).

When Are Additional Views Helpful?

Oblique views can occasionally be helpful for specific injuries, including lateral condyle and medial epicondyle fractures. Comparison views of the contralateral elbow are occasionally helpful, particularly in the case

BOX 13.1   FOOL Checklist

- F = fat pads
- O = overt findings and outlines
- O = ossification centers
- L = lines

of distinguishing a fracture from an ossification variant. In the majority of cases, however, additional views are not necessary.

When Are Other Imaging Modalities Useful?

When additional imaging evaluation is required, ultrasound and/or magnetic resonance imaging (MRI) is often the next imaging modality. Ultrasound is user/technologist and site dependent. The use of ultrasound, however, should always be considered, particularly in younger children who may require sedation for MRI. MRI is most commonly used in athletes with chronic repetitive injuries, although radiographs should always be acquired first. For traumatic injuries, acute or chronic, MRI is typically performed either without contrast or after arthrography. Indications for MRI with intravenous contrast include evaluation for infection, inflammatory arthritis, and/or masses. Computed tomography (CT) is rarely indicated.

■ Part 2: Approach to the Pediatric Elbow Radiograph: FOOL Checklist

Conventional radiography is the primary imaging tool used for the accurate diagnosis and management of children with elbow injuries. The unique and evolving radiographic appearance of the pediatric elbow can be challenging. Outlined here is an approach that aims to improve diagnostic accuracy and prevent one from looking like a "FOOL" (Box 13.1).

F: Fat Pads: Joint Effusion = Fracture (Most Likely)

Displacement of the fat pads indicates the presence of a joint effusion. A positive fat pad sign indicates high likelihood for fracture.

What Is the Significance of the Posterior Fat Pad Sign?

Presence of a posterior fat pad sign is always abnormal. The posterior fat pad is anatomically positioned within the intercondylar depression (olecranon fossa) of the distal humerus, and in the normal elbow it is obscured by overlying bone on the lateral radiograph (see Fig. 13.1). In the presence of a joint effusion the posterior fat pad is displaced posteriorly, allowing for its visualization (Fig. 13.2). The presence of a posterior fat pad raises significant suspicion for a fracture.

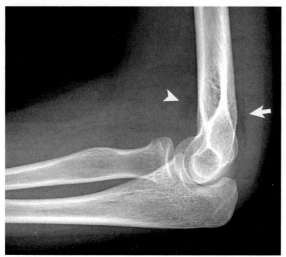

Fig. 13.2 Joint effusion with abnormal fat pads on lateral radiograph. Displaced anterior fat pad ("sail sign") (*arrowhead*) with abnormal visualization of posterior fat pad (*arrow*).

What Is the Significance of the Anterior Fat Pad?

Presence of the anterior fat pad can be normal or abnormal. The anterior fat pad is normally visualized in all patients. Ordinarily it hugs the anterior cortex of the distal humerus (see Fig. 13.1). It too can be displaced by a joint effusion, and in this setting is often more prominent or elevated ("sail sign") away from the anterior cortex of the distal humerus (see Fig. 13.2). Determining whether an anterior fat pad sign is present is a less reliable and more subjective tool than the posterior fat pad sign.

What If Positive Fat Pad and No Fracture Line Is Identified?

In the setting of trauma, the presence of a joint effusion as evidenced by displacement of the fat pads, is highly suspicious for fracture. In a retrospective study, joint effusions were identified in 91 percent of pediatric patients with elbow fractures. The presence of a displaced posterior fat pad should therefore prompt a rigorous, magnified search for any subtle fracture. Even if no fracture is identified on initial radiographs, most patients with isolated post traumatic joint effusions are treated as probable occult fractures with posterior elbow splinting and follow-up.

O: Overt Findings and Outlines

First the forest, then the trees: Always evaluate for obvious soft tissue injuries and obvious fractures and/or dislocations. This is akin to the physical examination and sets pretest probability of an abnormality. For example, patients with medial epicondyle avulsion fractures typically present with marked medial soft tissue swelling. Even if a fracture is not initially detected, the abnormal soft tissue swelling prompts a closer inspection. Occasionally, honing in on a small osseous finding may distract from the bigger picture. Soft tissue swelling and inflammatory stranding are important to note, particularly because radiologists often do not examine

---

the child and may have a limited history. Use soft tissue clues to get a general gestalt of whether the study is normal or abnormal.

After general characterization of the forest, scrutinize individual trees. Trace outlines of each bone, particularly the distal humerus and proximal radius, for any subtle contour deformities and/or buckle fractures. Examples of subtle abnormalities seen in common fractures include subtle cortical disruptions in supracondylar and lateral condyle fractures and mild cortical buckling of the proximal radius in radial neck fractures.

O: Ossification Centers

Radiographic evaluation of the pediatric elbow is unique due to the variable appearance of the ossification centers about the elbow, which undergo transformation from cartilaginous at birth, progressively ossifying, and subsequently fusing during childhood and adolescence.

What Is the Significance of CRITOE?

There are six centers of secondary ossification in children. At birth, these centers are all cartilaginous, and therefore not visible by plain radiography until they begin to ossify. The age at which ossification and fusion occur varies, but fortunately the sequence of ossification is predictable: Capitellum, Radial head, Internal (medial) epicondyle, Trochlea, Olecranon, External (lateral) epicondyle (CRITOE). Familiarity with this pattern is critical to the interpretation of pediatric elbow radiographs (Boxes 13.2 and 13.3) (Fig. 13.3).

Knowing the exact age at which ossification occurs is less important than sequence, with both ethnic and sex variability. A general rule of thumb used by some is 1-3-5-7-9-11 years. Girls ossify and fuse earlier than boys by an average of 2 years.

When Is CRITOE Most Useful?

If the sequence of CRITOE is abnormal, this raises suspicion for a traumatic avulsion fracture with displacement. This is most commonly seen with medial epicondyle avulsion fractures that may displace into the medial joint space, mimicking a trochlear ossification center. Thus, if a "trochlear" ossification center is identified without a medial epicondyle, the "trochlea" is most likely an avulsed medial epicondyle fragment.

Are There Any Variants of CRITOE?

Variants of CRITOE are rare but have been reported. One of the more common ossification sequence variants includes the appearance of the medial epicondyle before the radial head, more commonly in girls (CIRTOE) (Fig. 13.4). Case reports also include the olecranon before the trochlea (CRIOTE). In these rare cases, comparison with the contralateral elbow may be useful when the clinical history and imaging findings are not congruent. However, normal development can also be asymmetrical.

L: Lines

The anterior humeral line (AHL) and the radiocapitellar line (RCL) confirm normal alignment of the elbow. Disruption of either line is suspicious for fracture and/or dislocation. Remember that proper positioning of the elbow is paramount to avoiding pitfalls, particularly the lateral view; otherwise, the use of these lines can be misleading. In addition, both the AHL and RCL are less reliable in infants and toddlers, related to small and possibly eccentric ossification centers seen during early stages of physiologic ossification.

What Is the Anterior Humeral Line?
The AHL is a vertical line drawn parallel to the anterior cortex of the distal humerus on the lateral radiograph. This line normally bisects the middle third of the capitellum (Fig. 13.5A). Disruption of this line is suggestive, but not pathognomonic, for a supracondylar fracture (see Fig. 13.5B).

BOX 13.3 CRITOE Pearls

1. Ossification centers appear and fuse earlier in girls than boys.
2. Capitellum ossifies first, often by 6 months of age, and is typically well formed by 1 year of age in both girls and boys.
3. Lateral epicondyle ossifies last, typically by 10–12 years of age.
4. Medial epicondyle is the last ossification center to fuse to the distal humerus, typically during mid to late teenage years.
5. Trochlea, lateral epicondyle, and olecranon have multiple ossification centers and can normally appear fragmented or irregular.
6. Variants include CIRTOE and CRIOTE.

CRITOE, Capitellum, Radial head, Internal (medial) epicondyle, Trochlea, Olecranon, External (lateral) epicondyle.

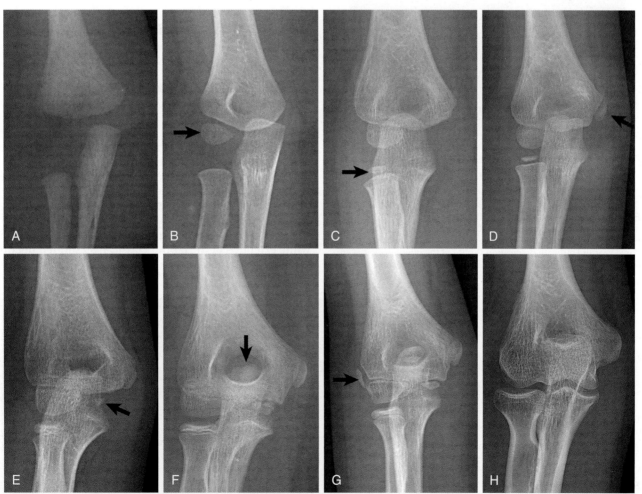

Fig. 13.3 CRITOE (Capitellum, Radial head, Internal [medial] epicondyle, Trochlea, Olecranon, External [lateral] epicondyle): normal sequence of ossification on sequential anteroposterior elbow radiographs. (A) Infant with no epiphyseal or apophyseal ossification. (B) Capitellum (*arrow*). (C) Radial head (*arrow*). (D) Internal (medial) epicondyle (*arrow*). (E) Trochlea (*arrow*). (F) Olecranon (*arrow*). (G) External (lateral) epicondyle (*arrow*). (H) Skeletal maturity with fusion of ossification centers.

What Is the Radiocapitellar Line?

The RCL is a vertical line drawn parallel through the central shaft of the proximal radius toward the elbow on both the AP and lateral views (Fig. 13.6). The RCL should intersect the capitellum on both radiographic views, but it has been shown to be more reliable on the lateral view. Studies have demonstrated that the RCL is most accurate when drawn along the central shaft of the radial neck, rather than the proximal radial diaphysis, because of the mild normal angulation at the proxi-mal radial metaphyseal–diaphyseal junction. The radial neck landmark should be used for both lateral and AP views. An abnormal RCL is characteristic of a radial head dislocation, as can be seen in the Monteggia fracture/ dislocation. It is also abnormal in displaced lateral condyle fractures. Both of these fractures are described and illustrated in more detail later.

Are There Any Exceptions to the Anterior Humeral Line?

Proper positioning is paramount. A true lateral view is particularly necessary for the diagnostic accuracy of AHL. In younger children (<2.5 years old) the AHL may not be as reliable, frequently crossing the anterior third of the capitellum.

Are There Any Exceptions to the Radiocapitellar Line?

Studies validating the RCL have shown it to be reliable in 84% to 95% of children. It is most accurate on lateral radiographs and in older children (>5 years old). This may be explained by the fact that the ossification pattern of the capitellum in growing children begins in an eccentric location. As described earlier, reliability is most consistent when drawn parallel to the radial neck.

■ Part 3: Acute Pediatric Elbow Injuries

Radial Head Subluxation (Nursemaid's Elbow)

Radial head subluxation is one of most common acute pediatric orthopedic injuries. The injury is unique to children, with most occurring in toddlers (peak inci-dence 2–3 years old). The injury has several colorful nicknames, including nursemaid's elbow, pulled elbow, supermarket elbow, and temper tantrum elbow. The typical mechanism of injury occurs when a caretaker ("nursemaid") pulls a young child's pronated forearm while extended at the elbow, classically a sudden tug on the child's arm, perhaps to prevent a fall. The left arm is

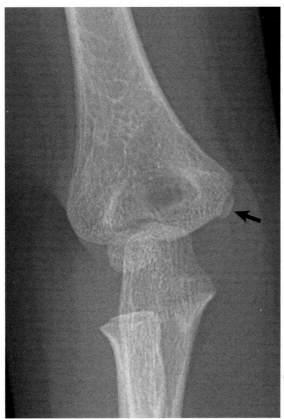

Fig. 13.4 Ossification variant CIRTOE instead of CRITOE: Capitel-lum, Internal [medial] epicondyle, Radial head, Trochlea, Olecranon, External [lateral] epicondyle] on anteroposterior elbow radiograph. Three-year-old girl with ossification variant of the internal/medial epi-condyle (*arrow*) appearing/ossifying before the radial head.

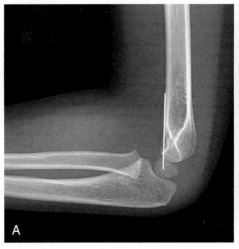
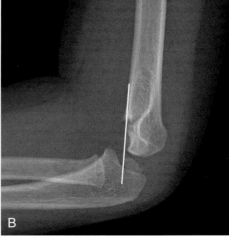

Fig. 13.5 Anterior humer-al line (AHL) on lateral radio-graphs (lines). (A) Normal AHL. (B) Disrupted AHL in a 3-year-old boy with a supracondylar fracture.

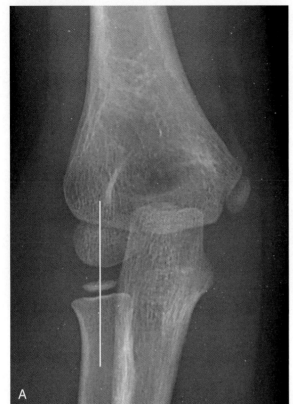

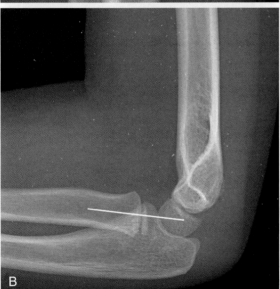

Fig. 13.6 Normal radiocapitellar line (*lines*) on both anteroposterior (A) and lateral (B) radiographs. A line drawn along the midshaft of the radial neck should intersect the capitellum on both views.

affected more frequently, attributed to right hand dominance of caretakers. The sudden traction on the arm results in disruption of the annular ligament from its periosteal attachment to the radial head; the detached annular ligament then interposes between the radial head and capitellum. The annular ligament attachment is weak in young children, becoming stronger in later childhood, thus explaining the preponderance of this injury in toddlers. The second most common mechanism of injury is a fall.

BOX 13.4   Radial Head Subluxation

- Most common pediatric elbow injury, often not requiring imaging
- Toddlers: most commonly 1–4 years old
- Classic mechanism (50%): sudden longitudinal pull on child's arm by parent/caretaker
- Most common presentation: refuses to use arm, usually in an otherwise happy child, no or minimal focal tenderness or swelling
- Radiographs: typically normal; sometimes disruption of the radiocapitellar line

The chief complaint in children presenting to the emergency department in a retrospective review by Schunk (1990) was "not using the arm," with the majority of children described as in a good mood (81% of cases). In most cases, reduction maneuvers by an experienced clinician either with supination/flexion or hyperpronation techniques can be performed in an office setting or in the emergency department without sedation. With successful reduction the child's symptoms usually immediately resolve. Recurrent subluxations can occur (Box 13.4).

What Is the Role of Imaging in Radial Head Subluxation? What If the Clinician Suspects Radial Head Subluxation But the Radiographs Are Normal?

In the majority of cases, radial head subluxation is diagnosed clinically. Radiographs are typically not necessary if the history and physical examination are consistent with the diagnosis. Indications for imaging include atypical presentation, focal pain and/or tenderness, swelling, and/or inability to reduce. In these cases, imaging is useful to exclude other causes of elbow pain, such as fracture.

Radiographs are normal in most cases with a history of nursemaid's elbow/radial head subluxation, because the injury is often reduced before imaging. However, occasionally RCL displacement is identified with lateral subluxation of the radial head on the AP view and/or posterior subluxation on the lateral view. Joint effusions can be seen. Imaging does not change treatment, management, or outcome of radial head subluxation.

Can Radial Head Subluxation Occur in Infants 6 Months and Younger?

Yes, although this is rare. Typical history in this younger age group includes pain after either a pull/lift during play or while rolling over. The latter mechanism is thought to be secondary to the forearm getting trapped under the baby's body, simulating a tug.

Common Pediatric Elbow Fractures

Pediatric elbow fractures are common, accounting for approximately 15% of all childhood fractures (Boxes 13.5 and 13.6).

BOX 13.5   Most Common Pediatric Elbow Fractures

1. Supracondylar
2. Lateral condyle
3. Medial epicondyle avulsion
4. Radial neck

BOX 13.6   Less Common Pediatric Elbow Fractures

- Medial condyle
- Lateral epicondyle
- Radial head
- Olecranon apophyseal avulsion fractures (50% occur in osteogenesis imperfecta)

Supracondylar Fracture Overview

The supracondylar fracture accounts for 50% to 70% of all pediatric elbow fractures. The majority occur from a fall on an extended arm, commonly occurring in active toddlers and elementary-school children.

Typically, supracondylar fractures are most apparent on the lateral radiograph, although often identified on the AP view as well. With hyperextension, the distal humerus fractures across an area of relative weakness, demarcated by the "hourglass configuration" of the distal humerus seen on lateral radiographs, formed by the coronoid and olecranon fossa. When the child falls with arm extended, force on the distal humerus hinges against the olecranon, frequently resulting in posterior angulation/displacement of the distal fracture fragment. The degree of posterior displacement governs classification and treatment. Nondisplaced fractures can be subtle; always checking the AHL, particularly in the presence of a joint effusion, often aids in the detection of a subtle fracture. Gartland type 1 fractures are nondisplaced and are treated conservatively with casting (Fig. 13.7). Gartland type 2 fractures are displaced with intact posterior cortex (Fig. 13.8A). Gartland type 3 fractures are displaced with disruption of the posterior cortex (see Fig. 13.8B). Gartland type 2 and 3 fractures often require operative reduction and percutaneous pinning.

Rarely, supracondylar fractures occur from a flexion-type mechanism, typically from a direct blow to a flexed elbow. In these cases the distal fracture fragment may be anteriorly displaced.

Complications of supracondylar fracture include neurovascular compromise, residual deformity, and rarely, compartment syndrome. About 10% to 15% of patients present with neuropraxia, most commonly involving the anterior interosseus and median nerves. Fortunately, the majority of nerve injuries are stretch injuries, often transient, and rarely require treatment. Compartment syndrome is a rare but serious complication that mandates emergent surgery. Studies have shown that children with brisk capillary refill and warm pink hands even in the setting of diminished radial pulses are unlikely to have a true compartment syndrome (Box 13.7).

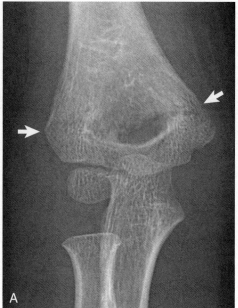

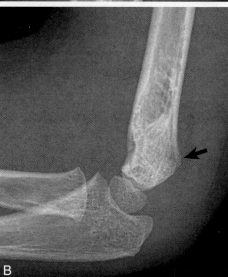

Fig. 13.7 Supracondylar fracture, Gartland type 1: 6-year-old girl with elbow pain and swelling after fall. (A) Anteroposterior radiograph with lucent fracture line (*arrows*) traversing the distal humerus. (B) Lateral radiograph demonstrates joint effusion with displacement of anterior and posterior fat pads with subtle fracture line disrupting the posterior cortex (*arrow*).

Lateral Condyle Fracture Overview

Another common pediatric elbow fracture is the lateral condyle fracture, accounting for approximately 20% of elbow fractures. The mechanism of injury is typically a fall on an outstretched hand (FOOSH). Patients often present with more superficial lateral bruising and swelling than those with supracondylar fractures.

Nondisplaced lateral condyle fractures are notoriously subtle and can be easily missed or misclassified (Fig. 13.9). Fundamental to this fracture is its lateral metaphyseal involvement (Salter-Harris type II) and possible intraarticular extension (Salter-Harris type IV) (Fig. 13.10). The distal extension of fracture is typically not radiographically visible, as it involves the still-cartilaginous portion of the distal humerus before it ossifies. Often it is the

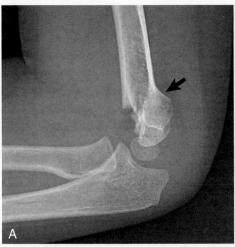
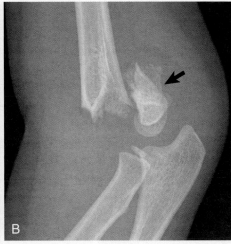

Fig. 13.8 Supracondylar fractures. Gartland type 2 (A) and Gartland type 3 (B) supracondylar fractures (*arrows*) on lateral views of the elbow.

BOX 13.7   Supracondylar Fracture

- Typical age 3–10 years
- Most common mechanism: hyperextension injury, fall on an outstretched hand
- Radiographs: joint effusion, disruption of anterior humeral line, subtle cortical disruption distal humerus on anteroposterior and/or lateral images, and/or posterior buckling/angulation/displacement of distal fragment
- Gartland classification: determines management
  1. Type 1: no displacement
  2. Type 2: distal fragment is angulated/displaced posteriorly, but the posterior humeral cortex is maintained, functioning as a hinge
  3. Type 3: complete displacement

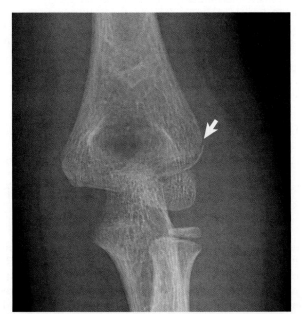

Fig. 13.9 Nondisplaced lateral condyle fracture on anteroposterior view of elbow. Six-year-old girl with subtle cortical disruption of the lateral cortex (*arrow*) after a fall consistent with a lateral condyle fracture.

distance between the humerus and the fracture fragment that suggests Salter-Harris type II or IV classification. The true extent is better characterized by MRI, although MRI is rarely indicated, as it does not typically alter management determined from radiographs.

On AP radiographs an oblique or horizontal fracture line traverses the distal lateral metaphysis or physis and then extends vertically toward the distal articular surface. Evaluating for subtle cortical lucency and/or cortical disruption of the lateral condyle on AP views aids in detecting nondisplaced or minimally displaced fractures. The fracture can often be better delineated by an internal oblique radiograph. When a lateral condyle fracture is suspected, some authors recommend obtaining four views of the elbow, adding internal and external oblique views to the standard AP and lateral images.

Reporting displacement is important because it governs treatment. Displaced (≥2 mm) fractures typically require reduction and surgical fixation. The less common, nondisplaced fractures are treated with immobilization and splinting. However, close interval radiographic follow-up is recommended, because late displacement has been reported which may necessitate surgical reduction and fixation.

The Jakob classification of lateral condyle fractures characterizes the distance/displacement and rotation of the fracture. A Jakob type 1 fracture has less than 2-mm displacement of the fracture fragment and no definite extension to articular surface. A Jakob type 2 fracture has 2- to 4-mm displacement, with fracture extension to the articular surface. A Jakob type 3 fracture has greater than 4 mm of displacement with rotation of the distal fracture fragment.

The Milch classification characterizes lateral condyle fractures with respect to the position of the distal fracture line in the coronal plane. The classification system affects prognosis, but not treatment. Classification by conventional radiographs is often not possible because the distal fracture line is often not evident due to nonossified cartilage. In the coronal plane a Milch type 1 fracture extends through the capitellar ossification center. However, if it crosses medially into the trochlear groove, it is a Milch type 2 fracture.

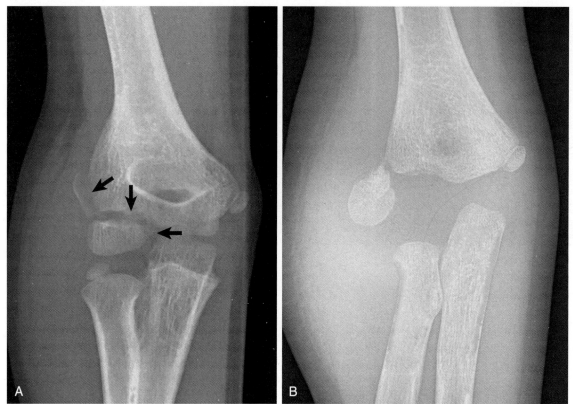

Fig. 13.10 *Displaced lateral condyle fractures on anteroposterior elbow radiographs.* (A) Seven-year-old boy with displaced lateral condyle fracture; displacement allows for improved visualization of this Salter-Harris type IV fracture as evidenced by lateral cortical disruption, physeal widening, and extension through the medial border of the capitellar epiphysis (*arrows*). (B) Four-year-old girl with a significantly displaced lateral condyle fracture. Note lateral soft tissue swelling in both cases.

Complications of lateral condyle fractures include nonunion, cubitus varus/valgus, and fishtail deformity. Nonunion, although generally rare in all pediatric elbow fractures, is most common when there is injury to the lateral condyle. Nonunion typically presents with cubitus valgus, which can be complicated by ulnar nerve palsy, as a result of stretching of the nerve (Box 13.8).

Medial Epicondyle Fracture Overview

The most common apophyseal elbow injury in children is the medial epicondyle fracture (Fig. 13.11). Other less common apophyseal injuries include the olecranon and lateral epicondyle fractures. An important unifying pearl to remember for pediatric apophyseal elbow fractures is the association with *MORE* fractures, coined by Little (2014) (Box 13.9).

Medial epicondyle fractures typically occur in an older age group (7–15 years age) than classic supracondylar and lateral condyle fractures. Fifty percent of fractures are associated with pediatric elbow dislocations, which may spontaneously reduce before imaging. Whenever elbow dislocation is encountered, one should remember to always comment specifically on the position of the medial epicondyle.

Medial epicondyle avulsion fractures occur from a valgus stress causing traction on the flexor-pronator muscle group, which inserts onto the medial epicondyle.

BOX 13.8   Lateral Condyle Fracture

- Typical age 5–10 years; however, can be seen outside this age range
- Classic mechanism: fall on an outstretch hand
- Radiographs: joint effusion, cortical lucency/disruption lateral condyle on anteroposterior, disruption of anterior humeral line, and/or radiocapitellar line if displaced
- Pearls
  - Fractures can often be subtle.
  - Prominent lateral bruising can be clue.
  - Internal oblique radiograph may be helpful.
  - Intraarticular fracture, typically Salter-Harris type IV, can lead to growth deformity.
  - Fracture displacement >2 mm typically requires reduction and fixation.
  - Nondisplaced fractures require close follow-up because late displacement may occur.

Frequently occurring in adolescent athletes, patients often report feeling a sudden pop followed by pain. The normal medial epicondyle apophysis is located posterior to the distal humerus on the lateral view. Avulsed fragments are often displaced anteriorly and inferiorly and may also be entrapped into the ulnar humeral joint space (Fig. 13.12). The CRITOE mnemonic aids in dis-

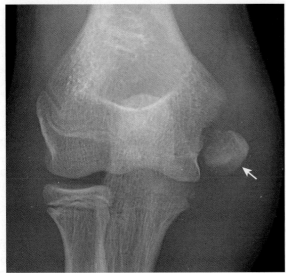

Fig. 13.11 *Medial epicondyle avulsion fracture on anteroposterior elbow radiograph.* Thirteen-year-old boy who hyperextended his elbow during wrestling. Medial and inferior displacment of the avulsed medial epicondyle (*arrow*) from the parent bone with associated marked overlying soft tissue swelling.

BOX 13.9   MORE: Apophyseal Elbow Fractures Associated With Other Fractures

- M = medial epicondyle
- O = olecranon
- R = radial head/neck
- E = external (lateral) epicondyle

---

tinguishing an avulsed medial epicondyle fracture fragment from the normal trochlea. Significant medial soft tissue swelling is often a clue. Because the medial epicondyle is extraarticular, a joint effusion is not always present.

Fractures displaced more than 5 mm require operative reduction and internal fixation. Displacement, however, is often underestimated on conventional frontal and lateral radiographs. An internal oblique view can be useful for more accurately determining the amount of displacement (Box 13.10).

Radial Neck Fracture Overview

Radial neck fractures account for approximately 5% to 10% of elbow fractures in children and occur at a wide variety of ages (Fig. 13.13). The radial neck is equivalent to the proximal radial metaphysis. Pediatric radial neck fractures are typically sustained from fall onto an outstretched hand. Displaced radial neck fractures are associated with a second fracture in up to 50% of patients, and thus a judicious search for additional fractures is recommended. Commonly associated fractures include olecranon, proximal ulna, and supracondylar fractures. Treatment is dictated by the degree of displacement and angulation, using the Judet classification. Fractures with greater than 30 degrees of angulation (Judet types III and IV) require reduction (Box 13.11).

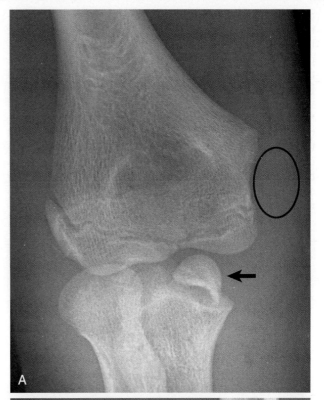
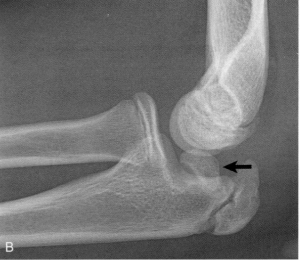

Fig. 13.12 *Displaced medial epicondyle avulsion fracture.* Thirteen-year-old boy who fell on outstretched hand while playing football. Apparent lack of an internal/medial epicondyle (*circle*) on anteroposterior (AP) (A) radiograph with presence of ossified trochlear, olecranon, and lateral epicondyle ossification center violates CRITOE checklist. Medial epicondyle is displaced into the medial joint space on both AP (A) and lateral (B) radiographs (*arrows*).

Less Common Pediatric Elbow Fractures

Transphyseal Distal Humerus Fracture Overview

Transphyseal distal humeral fractures are uncommon and radiographically challenging,. Transphyseal fractures can be associated with traumatic birth injuries, trauma, as well as child abuse. These fractures occur in newborns, infants, and young children (<2–3 years of age), at a time when the distal humeral epiphysis is often mostly or completely cartilaginous. Thus the fracture line may not be apparent on radiographs. Further, displaced transphyseal fractures mimic elbow dislocation, the latter of which is exceedingly rare in young children (Fig. 13.14). If capitellar ossification has begun, then vigilant attention to the RCL aids in the diagnosis of transphyseal fracture by confirming maintained radiocapitellar alignment (Fig. 13.15). A second clue is that these fractures are often displaced posteriorly and medially, rather than the classic posterolateral elbow dislocation. This will radiographically manifest as posterior and medial displacement of the radius and ulna with respect to the distal humerus.

MRI or ultrasound may be necessary to confirm a transphyseal fracture, particularly in infants. More than 50% of transphyseal fractures are secondary to child abuse, and thus warrant further investigation. Other mechanisms include FOOSH and birth-related trauma.

Radial Head Fracture Overview
Radial head fractures are rarely identified in children, but when present are usually seen in older children/adolescents involved in higher-energy activities, such as skateboarding. Adolescent athletes (baseball, gymnastics) are susceptible to stress injuries to the radial head, including osteochondritis dissecans (OCD).

Olecranon Fracture Overview
Olecranon fractures are uncommon fractures in children, almost always accompanying other injuries, most commonly radial neck fractures and dislocations. Isolated olecranon fractures are rare. Olecranon apophyseal fractures, although rare, are associated with osteogenesis imperfecta approximately 50% of the time.

Most olecranon fractures are subtle, nondisplaced, or minimally displaced. Be wary of the normal olecranon ossification center, which can normally be bipartite, eccentric, or diffusely sclerotic. As children mature, the orientation of the olecranon physis can vary from transverse to oblique.

Pediatric Elbow Dislocation

Although the most common joint to dislocate in childhood, elbow dislocations account for only 3% to 5%

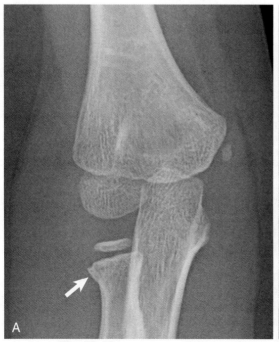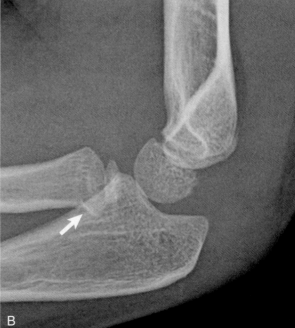

Fig. 13.13 Radial neck fracture. Five-year-old boy who fell off playground slide. Subtle buckling of the proximal radial metaphysis (*arrows*) on anteroposterior (A) and lateral (B) radiographs. Abnormal displacement of fat pads noted on lateral view consistent with traumatic joint effusion.

BOX 13.11   Radial Neck Fracture

- Wide variety of ages
- Most common mechanism: fall on an outstretch hand
- Radiographs: can be subtle, radial neck buckling, contour deformity
- Imaging pearl: look for second fracture (up to 50%)
- Judet classification of radial neck fractures (based on anteroposterior radiograph):
  - I: nondisplaced or horizontal shift of epiphysis
  - II: <30 degrees angulation
  - III: 30–60 degrees angulation
  - IVa: 60–80 degrees angulation
  - IVb: >80 degrees angulation or complete dislocation of epiphysis

of all pediatric elbow injuries. Posterior and radial head dislocations occur most frequently in children. An associated fracture is the rule and should prompt one to always search for additional fractures. Missing subtle dislocations can be avoided by always checking the RCL.

Posterior Dislocation Overview
Posterior dislocation of the radius and ulna is the most common pediatric elbow dislocation, typically postero-laterally (Fig. 13.16). Rare in children younger than 10 years, the majority of posterior elbow dislocations occur in adolescence, with a peak incidence at 12 to 13 years of age. Malalignment in posterior elbow dislocation is easily recognizable, whereas accompanying associated fractures can be more elusive. A careful search for a con-comitant avulsion of the medial epicondyle should be undertaken, as this may require surgical management. Coronoid process and radial neck fractures are also common fractures associated with posterior elbow dis-location (Box 13.12).

Radial Head Dislocation Overview
Radial head dislocations occur both in younger children and adolescence, with a mean age of 7 to 8 years. Again, associated fractures are the rule. Radial head disloca-tion with fracture of the proximal third of the ulna, also known as the Monteggia fracture-dislocation, occurs both in children and in adults (Fig. 13.17). The Bado classification system is based on the direction of radial head dislocation, most commonly anterior, but can also be lateral and, rarely, posterior. Slight variants to the tra-ditional Monteggia have been described in children, in-cluding the Hume variant, which comprises anterior ra-dial head dislocation with an olecranon fracture. Other pediatric variants of Monteggia include ulnar greenstick and bowing/plastic deformities (Fig. 13.18), as well as proximal radius fractures (rather than dislocation) and isolated radial neck fractures with radiocapitellar dislo-cation (Box 13.13).

Missing subtle dislocations can be avoided by always checking the RCL in both the AP and lateral projections, especially in the setting of proximal ulna and olecranon fractures.

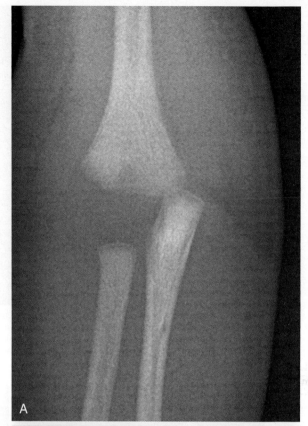
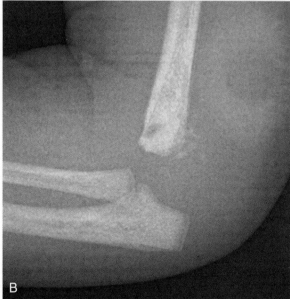

Fig. 13.14 Transphyseal fracture on anteroposterior (A) and lateral (B) elbow radiographs. Eight-day-old infant will not move left arm since birth; there is a history of difficult delivery. Displaced transphy-seal fracture mimics medial (A) and posterior (B) dislocation, but age of patient and medial rather than lateral displacement are clues to the diagnosis of transphyseal fracture.

Which Fractures Should Raise Suspicion of an Associated Dislocation?
Fractures associated with elbow dislocation include frac-tures of the proximal third ulnar diaphysis, olecranon, coronoid (anterior aspect proximal ulna) and avulsion of medial epicondyle.

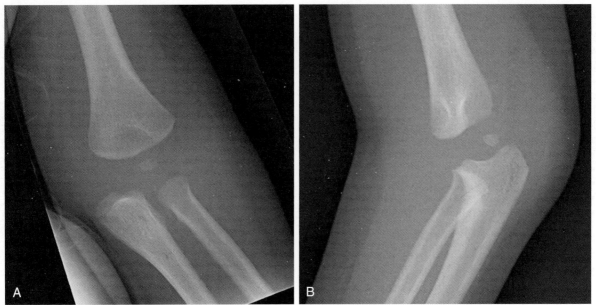

Fig. 13.15 Transphyseal fracture. Seventeen-month-old boy who fell off chair landing directly on elbow. Radiocapitellar alignment is maintained on both anteroposterior (A) and lateral (B) views, distinguishing this displaced transphyseal fracture from dislocation. Injury was witnessed by multiple adults; child advocacy consulted but felt no additional work-up was necessary.

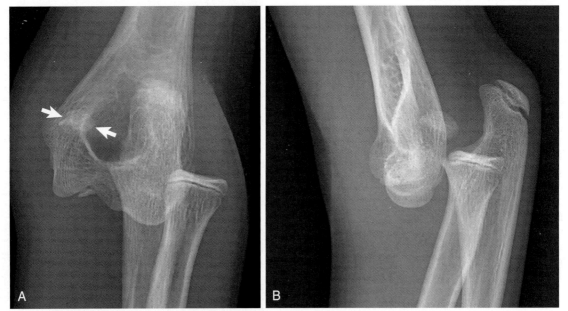

Fig. 13.16 Posterior elbow dislocation, with medial epicondyle avulsion fracture. Eleven-year-old girl who fell on outstretched hand at cheer practice. Anteroposterior (A) and lateral (B) radiographs demonstrate typical lateral (A) and posterior (B) elbow dislocation with avulsed medial epicondyle fracture (*arrows*).

BOX 13.12   Posterior Elbow Dislocation

- Most common in adolescents
- Typically posterolateral
- Pearl: find additional fractures, most frequently associated with medial epicondyle avulsion fractures
- Pitfall: transphyseal fractures in infants and young children may mimic posterior dislocation (child abuse association)

■ **Part 4: Congenital and Posttraumatic Deformities Worth Mentioning**

What Is Congenital Proximal Radioulnar Synostosis?

Congenital proximal radioulnar synostosis is a rare upper limb malformation that typically involves chronic

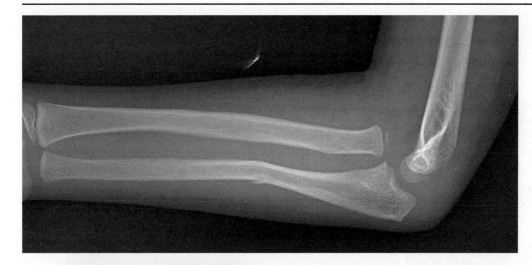

Fig. 13.17 Monteggia fracture dislocation. Lateral forearm radiograph in 4-year-old girl demonstrates typical Monteggia injury pattern with proximal ulna fracture and associated radial head dislocation, as evidenced by disruption of radiocapitellar line.

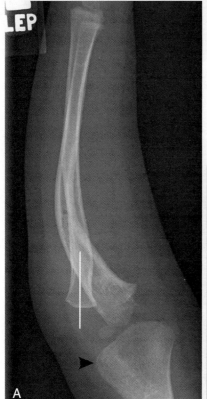

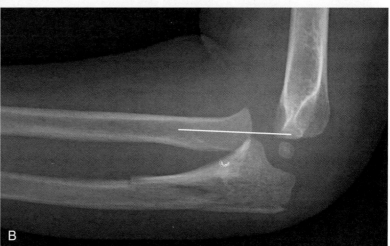

Fig. 13.18 Pediatric variant Monteggia fracture dislocation. Anteroposterior (A) and lateral (B) radiographs in a 2-year-old boy with pediatric variant Monteggia injury pattern with greenstick/bowing fracture of proximal ulna and associated radial head dislocation, as evidenced by disruption of radiocapitellar line on both views (*lines*). A subtle lateral condyle fracture (*arrowhead*) is also identified on the AP view (A).

BOX 13.13   Pediatric Variants of Monteggia Fracture/Dislocation

- Radial head dislocation with proximal ulnar bowing deformity/fracture
- Radial neck fracture with greenstick fracture proximal ulnar metaphysis
- Hume fracture: radial head dislocation with olecranon fracture

---

posterior dislocation of the radial head with fusion of the proximal radius and ulna (Fig. 13.19). Symptoms vary from mild to severe, often with limited ability to supinate. It can be seen in syndromes and skeletal dyspla-sias, but is more frequently a sporadic, isolated anomaly. The anomaly is often bilateral.

What Is the Supracondylar Process?

The supracondylar process is an anatomic variant osseous excrescence from the distal humerus with a typical radiographic appearance (Fig. 13.20). It has also been called an "avian spur" and is the osseous origin of the "ligament of Struthers" connecting the supracondylar process to the medial epicondyle, described by John Struthers, a contemporary of Charles Darwin. It is typically asymptomatic and of no clinical significance in

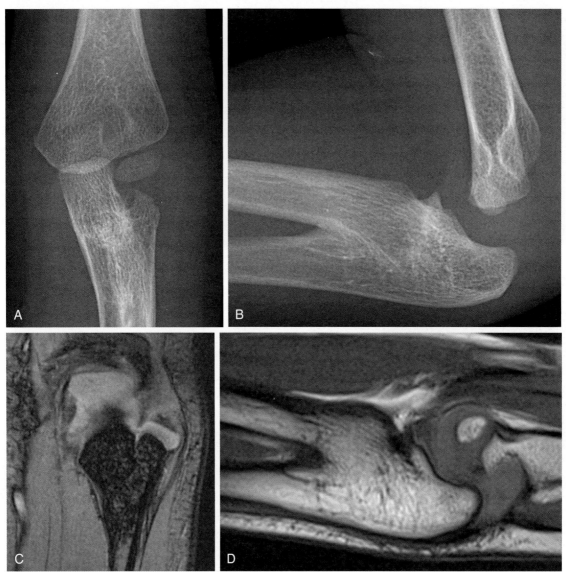

Fig. 13.19 Congenital radioulnar synostosis. Three-year-old boy with inability to pronate the forearm. Conventional anteroposterior and lateral radiographs (A, B) and subsequent coronal T2 gradient-echo (C) and sagittal T1 (D) magnetic resonance images both demonstrating complete osseous fusion of the proximal radius and ulna resulting in posterior positioning of the radial head.

the pediatric population. A small triangular, bony protuberance projects from the anteromedial distal humeral shaft, usually incidentally noted on the lateral film. It can mimic an osteochondroma but classically points toward the joint space, rather than away. Rarely it may fracture or be associated with median nerve neuralgia.

What Is the Fishtail Deformity?

Fishtail deformity is a rare, delayed complication of a variety of pediatric elbow fractures, often presenting with pain years after initial injury (Fig. 13.21). Characterized by a concave central deformity of the distal humerus on AP radiographs, it is the result of incomplete ossification and/or bony resorption of the lateral trochlea from a vascular injury. It is most commonly seen after supracondylar fractures because of the high incidence of this fracture type; however, it occurs in a higher percentage of patients with lateral condyle fractures.

■ Part 5: Chronic Elbow Injuries in the Athletic Child

In the United States the majority of sports-related elbow injuries in children are related to the popular sports of baseball and gymnastics. Overuse injuries in these sports are common and can manifest with acute and/or chronic symptoms.

What Is Little League Elbow?

The term "Little League elbow" refers to a characteristic spectrum of injuries that occur in skeletally immature, overhead-throwing athletes, most typically baseball pitchers. Although the term "Little League elbow" is classically associated with medial epicondylitis, the spectrum of injuries can include lateral OCD and less commonly posterior compartment abutment/impingement injuries, such as olecranon apophysitis. The mech-

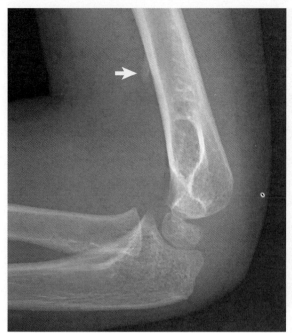

Fig. 13.20 Supracondylar process. Five-year-old with midulnar fracture (not shown). Lateral elbow radiograph with incidental small triangular protuberance (*arrow*), the supracondylar process, typically of no clinical significance. Supracondylar process typically points toward the joint space, which distinguishes it from an osteochondroma.

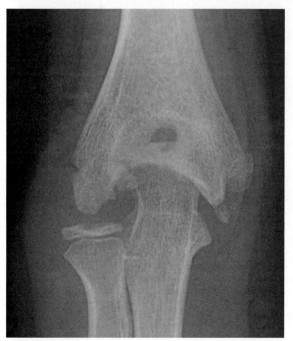

Fig. 13.21 Fishtail deformity. Six-year-old girl with fishtail deformity of the distal humerus on anteroposterior elbow radiograph. Patient had history of type 3 supracondylar fracture of elbow at age 5 years (not shown), previously treated with open reduction and internal fixation.

anism of chronic repetitive trauma in these patients is coined *valgus extension overload* and may result in injuries to the medial, lateral, and/or posterior compartments of the elbow. The mechanics of throwing a baseball during pitching results in medial distraction and simultaneous lateral compression forces to the flexed elbow.

BOX 13.14   Little League Elbow

1. Age: classically 10–14 years old
2. Typically dominant arm of baseball players, typically pitchers
3. Classic mechanism: chronic repetitive stress with repetitive valgus extension in throwing athlete
4. Signs and symptoms
   a. Medial and/or lateral pain; less commonly posterior pain
   b. Medial instability
   c. Medial epicondyle swelling, tenderness to palpation
5. Radiographs: can be normal or abnormal
   a. Medial = medial epicondylitis (irregular ossification, sclerosis, and apophyseal widening), fragmentation medial epicondyle inferiorly, overgrowth of the medial epicondyle and medial crest of proximal ulna
   b. Lateral = capitellar OCD (typically older children)
   c. Less commonly trochlear and olecranon OCD, olecranon apophysitis, olecranon stress fractures

Maximum valgus stress occurs during the cocking and accelerating phase of the throwing motion. Although the mechanism of pitching stays relatively constant over time, patterns of injury change over time as the areas of relative weakness in the growing skeleton evolve as the patient progresses from preadolescence through puberty, eventually reaching skeletal maturity. Patterns of injury can be divided classically into medial and lateral compartments, as follows (Box 13.14).

Little League Elbow, Medial Compartment: Medial Epicondylitis/Apophysitis

Medial compartment injuries in Little League elbow most commonly include stress-related changes to the medial humeral epicondyle and injuries to the anterior band of the medial ulnar collateral ligament (UCL) either at its proximal or distal attachment.

The classic medial epicondylitis, also coined *traction apophysitis*, associated with Little League elbow, is due to chronic tensile stress to the medial epicondyle, which is cartilaginous at birth but during childhood progressively ossifies and eventually fuses to the parent bones. The medial epicondyle begins to ossify on average around 5 to 7 years of age and fuses around 14 to 17 years of age. As the secondary physis of the medial epicondyle apophysis undergoes progressive endochondral ossification, the newly mineralized bone is more susceptible to trauma. Medial epicondylitis/apophysitis is thought to result from chronic repetitive stress to the newly mineralized subchondral bone at the bone–cartilage interface. The pathophysiology and radiographic changes are similar to other chronic injures to the primary physis of the proximal humerus in Little League shoulder or the distal radius in gymnast's wrist, except that it is occurring along the secondary circular physis of the medial epicondyle.

Although radiographs can often be normal, abnormalities identified by plain film in medial epicondylitis

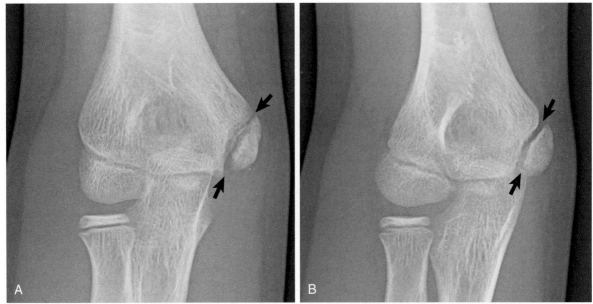

Fig. 13.22 Little League elbow, medial epicondylitis on anteroposterior (A) and oblique (B) elbow radiographs. Eleven-year-old male right-handed baseball pitcher with persistent medial right elbow pain. Both views both demonstrate abnormal widening between the medial epicondyle and parent bone (*arrows*) consistent with medial epicondylitis.

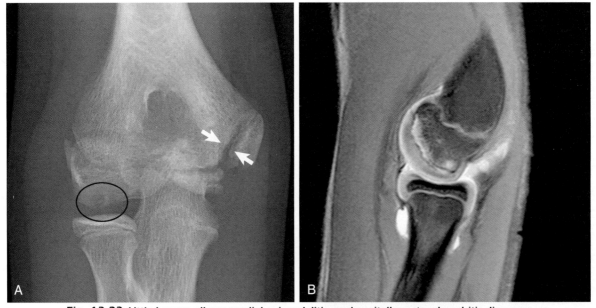

Fig. 13.23 Little League elbow, medial epicondylitis, and capitellar osteochondritis dissecans (OCD). Thirteen-year-old male baseball player with chronic elbow pain plays a variety of positions. (A) Anteroposterior radiographs demonstrate changes of medial epicondylitis (*arrows*), as well as abnormal lucency and irregularity of the capitellum consistent with changes of juvenile OCD (*circle*). (B) Sagittal T2 fat suppressed magnetic resonance image after arthrogram shows typical changes of capitellar OCD.

include widening of the medial epicondyle apophysis, irregular ossification, and/or fragmentation of the medial epicondyle, as well as abnormal sclerosis (Figs. 13.22 and 13.23A). Comparison with the contralateral elbow may be helpful.

As the patient approaches skeletal maturity, and the medial epicondyle begins to fuse to the parent bone, this portion of the bone becomes stronger and less susceptible to microtrauma as ossification has now matured. Continued medially tensile forces with pitching may now manifest as injuries to the medial UCL, with tears either of the ligament itself or at its proximal and distal bony attachments. Small avulsion fractures may occur along the inferior medial epicondyle or distally at its insertion into the ulna at the sublime tubercle. Mechanism and chronic injury pattern mirrors that seen in the adolescent knee, with chronic stress along the proximal and distal attachment sites of the patellar tendon, known respectively as Sinding-Larsen-Johannson and Osgood-Schlatter diseases.

Chronic stress may also manifest as bony overgrowth of the medial epicondyle and/or medial ulnar crest because of chronic hyperemia. Although osseous changes can be seen by plain radiography, they may be subtle and may not demonstrate the full extent of injury. MRI with arthrography can often more completely evaluate the extent of cartilage, osseous, and soft tissue injury, as well as identify chondral or osteochondral loose bodies, particularly in a child who does not improve with conventional treatment.

Is "Little League Elbow" Seen in Other Sports?

Similar injury patterns to those seen in Little League Elbow are seen in children participating in other overhead throwing sports, including, but not limited to, football, volleyball, javelin, and water polo.

Lateral Compartment: Juvenile Osteochondritis Dissecans

In the lateral compartment, compression forces occur across the radiocapitellar joint during the late cocking and early acceleration phase of throwing. Chronic repetitive trauma to the lateral elbow of the dominant arm in adolescent baseball players (particularly pitchers) can result in osteochondritis dissecans (OCD) of the capitellum.

What Is Juvenile Osteochondritis Dissecans?

Juvenile OCD is a disease unique to the pediatric patient, occurring typically in preteen and teen years (12–17 years of age) before physeal closure. The chondro-osseous junction is uniquely vulnerable during periods of rapid growth, as seen in during puberty/adolescence. The vascular anatomy of the capitellum in particular makes it more susceptible to ischemia. The pathophysiology of juvenile OCD seen in the pediatric knee can be applied to smaller epiphyseal centers elsewhere in the pediatric skeleton, including the capitellum of the elbow. Chronic repetitive stress leads to disruption of blood supply to the structurally vulnerable, newly formed metaphyseal-equivalent bone underlying the circular/secondary physis within the epiphysis. This results in injury to the immature, recently ossified subchondral bone and articular surface. In the elbow, OCD most frequently affects the capitellum and, to a lesser extent, the trochlea, radial head, and olecranon.

OCD of the capitellum can be subtle by plain radiography, reported to be approximately 60% sensitive. When OCD is suspected, obtaining an AP image with 45 degrees of flexion along with standard AP and lateral radiographs may improve sensitivity. Plain film findings of OCD include bony rarefaction/radiolucency, articular surface flattening and/or fragmentation with demarcating sclerosis, and displaced fragments/loose bodies. The anterior aspect of the capitellum is the most common site of OCD in baseball players secondary to the mechanics of pitching, as the elbow is typically flexed at the time of maximum valgus stress. MRI is often performed in patients with OCD because the stability of these injuries often affects treatment and outcome (see Fig. 13.23).

What Other Sports Predispose Adolescent Athletes to Osteochondritis Dissecans of the Elbow?

The lateral compartment of the elbow is also susceptible to OCD in adolescent athlete gymnasts and weight lifters due to chronic compressive forces seen across the radiocapitellar compartment. In these sports, compressive forces occur from repetitive, axial loading with hyperextension, such as with tumbling in gymnastics. Both wrestlers and gymnasts are susceptible to bilateral injuries because both upper extremities undergo similar stress; however, injuries may present asynchronously.

In gymnasts the chronic compressive forces to the capitellum occurs with the elbow in extension (handstands); thus the site of chronic trauma is classically in the load-bearing central and posterior aspect of the capitellum.

Posterior Compartment: Persistence of the Olecranon Physis

Chronic stress injuries to the olecranon apophysis can result in changes similar to those described earlier in the medial epicondyle apophysis, including stress fractures, fragmentation, and overgrowth. Persistence of the olecranon physis is often misinterpreted as persistence of a "normal" apophysis by plain film, but it is rather a true stress fracture occurring in an area where the apophysis is not normally present (Fig. 13.24). Comparison views with the contralateral elbow can be useful to distinguish normal ossification variants and olecranon stress fractures. In addition, there can be change in the orientation of the olecranon apophyseal plane on the lateral radiograph, changing from normally oblique to more vertical, which would favor an evolving stress fracture.

What Is Panner Disease?

Panner disease is an osteochondrosis of the humeral capitellum. The pathophysiological changes and resulting radiographic findings seen in Panner disease are similar to those seen in the proximal femoral head with Legg-Calve-Perthes. Panner disease is theorized to be secondary to global ischemia of the developing capitellum, which has a precarious vascular supply. This is in contradistinction to the focal, microsubchondral ischemia secondary to chronic microtrauma/stress that results in juvenile OCD. The two conditions, though, are likely on the same spectrum of disease, although they differ by their age of presentation, mechanism of injury, anatomic involvement, and prognosis.

Panner disease occurs in younger patients (<10 years old) and is traditionally described in children without a history of chronic repetitive trauma. Panner disease commonly affects the dominant elbow, potentially related to a less severe form of chronic trauma than is typically seen with adolescent athletes. Another distinguishing feature is its typical involvement of the entire capitellum. The prognosis in Panner disease is excellent,

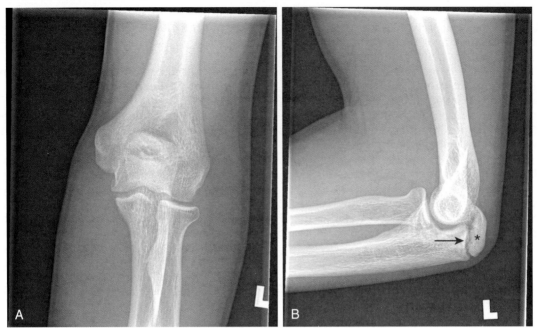

Fig. 13.24 Olecranon stress fracture. Sixteen-year-old pitcher with severe posterior elbow pain. Anteroposterior (A) and lateral (B) radiographs show fusion of the ossification centers of the capitellum, radial head, internal epicondyle, trochlea, and lateral epicondyle. Vertically oriented lucency (*arrow*) and associated osseous fragment (*asterisk*) are consistent with olecranon stress fracture rather than the normal olecranon apophysis.

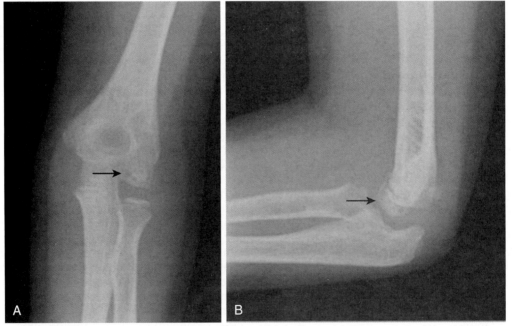

Fig. 13.25 Panner disease. Eight-year-old boy with left elbow pain. Anteroposterior (A) and lateral (B) radiographs of the left elbow show mixed sclerosis and lucency throughout the capitellum (*arrows*) consistent with Panner disease.

and the disease is usually self-limiting. Findings on conventional radiography can be subtle but include demineralization, subchondral lucency, articular flattening, fragmentation, and abnormal sclerosis of the capitellum (Fig. 13.25). Loose osteochondral bodies are rarely seen in Panner disease. MRI is useful to confirm more subtle radiographic findings

■ Summary

Understanding the normal anatomic development of the pediatric elbow, combined with the use of the FOOL mnemonic, will improve diagnostic accuracy and interpretation of elbow radiographs in children (Boxes 13.15 and 13.16).

BOX 13.15   Review of FOOL Checklist

1. F = fat pads
   a. Normal: small triangle of low density along anterior humerus
   b. Abnormal (effusion): uplifted anterior fat pad or visualized posterior fat pad
2. O = overt injuries and outlines
   a. Soft tissues (can help focus search for possible fracture)
   b. Outlines (looking for subtle cortical fractures and angulation deformities, particularly distal humerus and proximal radius)
3. O = ossification centers
   a. CRITOE (specifically looking for avulsion of medial epicondyle)
4. L = lines
   a. Anterior humeral line (abnormal in displaced supracondylar or lateral condylar fractures)
   b. Radiocapitellar line (abnormal in subluxation or dislocation of proximal radius)

CRITOE, Capitellum, Radial head, Internal (medial) epicondyle, Trochlea, Olecranon, External (lateral) epicondyle.

BOX 13.16   Final Pearls

- Supracondylar fracture: most common
- Lateral condylar fracture: can be subtle, scrutinize lateral cortical edge on anteroposterior view
- Medial epicondyle avulsion fracture: abnormal CRITOE; commonly associated with elbow dislocations
- Radial neck fracture: 50% have second fracture, commonly olecranon, proximal ulna, or supracondylar
- Transphyseal fracture: mimic of posterior dislocation in infant, consider child abuse
- Olecranon fracture: almost always associated with other fractures
- Posterior dislocation: look for medial epicondyle avulsion fracture
- Monteggia fracture/dislocation: if proximal ulna fracture, scrutinize radiocapitellar line

CRITOE, Capitellum, Radial head, Internal (medial) epicondyle, Trochlea, Olecranon, External (lateral) epicondyle.

Bibliography

Alison, M., Azoulay, R., Bogdana, T., et al. (2009). Imaging strategies in paediatric musculoskeletal trauma. *Pediatric Radiology, 39*(Suppl. 3), S414–S421.

Bancroft, L. W., Pettis, C., Wasyliw, C., et al. (2013). Osteochondral lesions of the elbow. *Seminars in Musculoskeletal Radiology, 17,* 446–454.

Davis, K. W. (2010). Imaging pediatric sports injuries: Upper extremity. *Radiologic Clinics of North America, 48*(6), 1199–1211.

Dwek, J. R., & Chung, C. B. (2013). A systematic method for evaluation of pediatric sports injuries of the elbow. *Pediatric Radiology, 43*(Suppl. 1), S120–S128.

Elliott, A. M., Kibria, L., & Reed, M. H. (2010). The developmental spectrum of proximal radioulnar synostosis. *Skeletal Radiology, 39,* 49–54.

Fader, L. M., Laor, T., Eismann, E. A., et al. (2014). MR imaging of capitellar ossification: A study in children of different ages. *Pediatric Radiology, 44,* 963–970.

Frumkin, K. (1985). Nursemaid's elbow: A radiographic demonstration. *Annals of Emergency Medicine, 14,* 690.

Grayson, D. E. (2005). The elbow: Radiographic imaging pearls and pitfalls. *Seminars in Roentgenology, 40*(3), 223–247.

Iyer, R. S., Thapa, M. M., Khanna, P. C., et al. (2012). Pediatric bone imaging: Imaging elbow trauma in children-a review of acute and chronic injuries. *American Journal of Roentgenology, 198,* 1053–1068.

Jaimes, C., Chauvin, N. A., Delgado, J., et al. (2014). MR imaging of normal epiphyseal development and common epiphyseal disorders. *RadioGraphics, 34*(2), 449–471.

Kijowski, R., & Tuite, M. J. (2010). Pediatric throwing injuries of the elbow. *Seminars in Musculoskeletal Radiology, 14*(4), 419–429.

Kunkel, S., Cornwall, R., Little, K., et al. (2011). Limitations of the radiocapitellar line for assessment of pediatric elbow radiographs. *Journal of Pediatric Orthopedics, 31,* 628–632.

Leonidou, A., Pagkalos, J., Lepetsos, P., et al. (2012). Pediatric Monteggia fracture: A single-center study of the management of 40 patients. *Journal of Pediatric Orthopedics, 32,* 352–356.

Little, K. J. (2014). Elbow fractures and dislocations. *Orthopedic Clinics of North America, 45*(3), 327–340.

Marshall, K. W. (2014). Overuse upper extremity injuries in the skeletally immature patient: Beyond little league shoulder and elbow. *Seminars in Musculoskeletal Radiology, 18*(5), 469–477.

Narayanan, S., Shailam, R., Grottkau, B. E., et al. (2015). Fishtail deformity—a delayed complication of distal humeral fractures in children. *Pediatric Radiology, 45*(6), 814–819.

Nimkin, K., Kleinman, P. K., Teeger, S., et al. (1995). Distal humerus physeal injuries in child abuse: MR imaging and ultrasonographic findings. *Pediatric Radiology, 25,* 562–565.

Ramirez, R. N., Ryan, D. D., Williams, J., et al. (2014). A line drawn along the radial shaft misses the capitellum in 16% of radiographs of normal elbows. *Journal of Pediatric Orthopedics, 34,* 763–767.

Schunk, J. E. (1990). Radial head subluxation: Epidemiology and treatment of 87 cases. *Annals of Emergency Medicine, 19,* 1019.

Shrader, M. W. (2008). Pediatric supracondylar fractures and pediatric physeal elbow fractures. *Orthopedic Clinics of North America, 39,* 163–171.

Zbojniewicz, A. M., & Laor, T. (2014). Imaging of osteochondritis dissecans. *Clinical Journal of Sport Medicine, 33,* 221–250.

CHAPTER 14
Imaging Approach to Pediatric Bone Lesions

Michael Baldwin

CHAPTER OUTLINE

Systematic Approach, 287
Patient Age, 287
    Infants and Toddlers (<5 Years of Age), 287
    Children (5–10 Years of Age), 287
    Adolescents (10–20 Years of Age), 288
Host Bone, 288
    Longitudinal Plane of the Host Bone, 288
    Axial Plane of the Host Bone, 289

Host Bone Reaction, 290
    Legion Margins/Patterns of Bone Destruction, 290
    Matrix and Mineralization, 292
    Soft Tissue Component, 292
Single or Multiple Lesions, 292
    Infants and Toddlers (<5 Years of Age), 292
    Children (5–10 Years of Age), 298
    Adolescents (10–20 Years of Age), 299
Summary, 312

"Knowledge is power...knowledge is safety...knowledge is happiness."

—*Thomas Jefferson*

Bone lesions are a frequently encountered diagnostic challenge faced by radiologists in the evaluation of pediatric and adolescent patients. Up to 42% of all bone lesions are detected in the first two decades of life, including benign and malignant neoplasms. Nine percent of bone lesions occur in the first decade of life, and approximately 33% in the second.

More than half of all childhood bone neoplasms are benign, with metastatic neuroblastoma being the most common malignant bone lesion occurring in the first two decades of life. The radiologist's primary goal when encountering a bone lesion in a radiographic examination of a pediatric or adolescent patient is to generate a succinct, logical differential diagnosis based on the imaging characteristics and available clinical information.

A critical component for the generation of an accurate differential diagnosis is distinguishing aggressive osseous lesions from benign "do not touch" lesions and tumor-like lesions, which can be reactive or developmental in etiology.

Aggressive primary bone neoplasms are rare in infants and toddlers but account for a significant proportion of childhood malignancies. The most common primary malignant bone lesions in school-aged children and adolescents are osteosarcoma and Ewing sarcoma (ES). These aggressive pediatric bone malignancies require further evaluation with cross-sectional imaging, as well as image-guided or surgical biopsy.

The most common true benign bone neoplasms in children and adolescents are osteochondroma, osteoid osteoma, osteoblastoma, enchondroma, chondromyxoid fibroma (CMF), and chondroblastoma.

The most common benign tumor-like bone lesions in childhood and adolescence are fibroxanthomas (fibrous cortical defect, nonossifying fibroma [NOF]), simple (unicameral) bone cyst (UBC), aneurysmal bone cyst (ABC), distal femoral cortical irregularity, fibrous dysplasia (FD), and Langerhans cell histiocytosis (LCH).

Radiographs remain the primary imaging modality for the initial evaluation of pediatric bone lesions. Radiographs provide several key characteristics of a lesion, including: (1) a lesion's location within the host bone; (2) lesion-host bone interface/zone of transition; (3) host bone reaction to the lesion; (4) lesion matrix production; and (5) potential cortical destruction and resulting secondary soft tissue mass.

These key radiographic imaging features, in conjunction with the patient's chronological age, remain the cornerstones in the differentiation of aggressive and nonaggressive pediatric bone lesions and tumor-like conditions, as well as the generation of an accurate and concise differential diagnosis.

The correct radiographic interpretation of pediatric bone lesions is important because classic benign, nonaggressive pediatric osseous lesions require neither additional cross-sectional imaging work-up nor subsequent biopsy.

Many aggressive and nonaggressive bone neoplasms occur in specific age groups. In addition, certain pediatric osseous lesions frequently occur in characteristic host bones of the axial and appendicular skeleton, as well as specific segments within these host bones. Therefore the patient's chronological age, host bone, and lesion location within the particular affected host bone are critical factors in the imaging evaluation of pediatric and adolescent bone lesions.

Additional clinical information can also prove invaluable in the imaging evaluation of bone lesions in young patients. The presence or absence of fever, white blood cell count, differential, and erythrocyte sedimentation rate (ESR) are also important pieces of clinical information that can assist in honing the differential diagnosis of a pediatric bone lesion. White blood cell count and ESR are often elevated in the setting of osteomyelitis but can also be elevated in acute leukemia, lymphoma, ES, and LCH.

Cross-sectional imaging with magnetic resonance imaging (MRI) and/or computed tomography (CT) can provide additional valuable imaging evaluation of a bone lesion if the diagnosis remains uncertain after the initial radiographic examination. MRI evaluation is critical for the evaluation of potential skip lesions, soft tissue extension, integrity of adjacent neuromuscular structures, initial staging, and preoperative planning for malignant osseous lesions. CT, with its high spatial resolution, can provide additional information regarding a lesion's potential internal matrix production, associated cortical erosion/disruption, or risk for potential pathological fracture.

Nuclear medicine bone scintigraphy also has a role in the evaluation of metastatic disease and/or multifocal processes, but these examinations are nonspecific. Bone scans are positive for lesions that stimulate reactive new bone formation when technetium-99m-methylene diphosphonate (MDP) is adsorbed onto newly incorporated hydroxyapatite. Lytic lesions, such as LCH, associated with bone destruction are better evaluated with radiographic skeletal surveys. Positron emission tomography (PET)-CT and MIBG (metaiodobenzylguanidine) nuclear medicine scintigraphy are additional useful modalities for the staging and posttherapy surveillance imaging of neuroblastoma.

The goal of this chapter is to put forth a systematic imaging approach for the generation of an accurate, concise differential diagnosis for pediatric and adolescent bone lesions based on the combination of characteristic imaging features of these lesions and vital corroborative clinical information.

In addition, this chapter aims to assist the radiologist in recommending the most effective imaging work-up of pediatric and adolescent bone lesions, as well as finalizing the diagnosis and defining the extent of disease.

■ Systematic Approach

The proper imaging evaluation of pediatric bone lesions requires answering the following diagnostic questions (Box 14.1).

BOX 14.1   Key Clinical Questions To Be Answered

1. What is the age of the patient?
2. What is the involved host bone?
3. What segment of the host bone is affected?
4. What is the host bone reaction to the lesion?
5. Is the lesion unifocal or part of a multifocal process?

BOX 14.2   Three Age Groups in the Imaging Evaluation of Pediatric Bone Lesions

Infants and toddlers: <5 years of age
Children: 5–10 years of age
Adolescents: 10–20 years of age

BOX 14.3   Aggressive Lesions in Infants and Toddlers

Acute leukemia
Multifocal Langerhans cell histiocytosis
Metastatic lesions secondary to neuroblastoma
Osteomyelitis

■ Patient Age

The chronological age of the affected patient is a vital piece of information in the imaging evaluation of pediatric bone lesions. Osseous lesions demonstrate a propensity for affecting certain age ranges in young patients. Establishing the age of the affected child is extremely helpful in beginning to formulate an accurate differential diagnosis.

The age ranges that have been used in the imaging evaluation of pediatric bone lesions are: *infants and toddlers* (<5 years of age), *children* (5–10 years of age), and *adolescents* (10–20 years of age). Specific bone lesions demonstrate peak occurrence rates within these age ranges. Thus the chronological age of an affected patient is critical in narrowing the differential diagnosis of an encountered bone lesion (Box 14.2).

Infants and Toddlers (<5 Years of Age)

Primary bone malignancies are extremely rare in infants and toddlers. For example, ES is rarely encountered before the age of 5 years. The differential diagnoses of aggressive bone lesions in infants and toddlers are acute leukemia, multifocal LCH, metastatic lesions secondary to neuroblastoma, and osteomyelitis (Box 14.3).

Children (5–10 Years of Age)

The differential diagnoses for aggressive bone lesions in children (5–10 years old) are ES, monostotic LCH, and osteomyelitis (Box 14.4).

BOX 14.4   Aggressive Lesions in Children

Ewing sarcoma
Monostotic Langerhans cell histiocytosis
Osteomyelitis

BOX 14.5   Aggressive Lesions in Adolescents

Osteosarcoma
Ewing sarcoma
Acute leukemia
Primary lymphoma of bone
Osteomyelitis

BOX 14.6   Nonaggressive Lesions in Adolescents

Fibroxanthoma
Osteochondroma
Simple/Unicameral bone cyst
Aneurysmal bone cyst
Chondroblastoma
Fibrous dysplasia
Osteoid osteoma/Osteoblastoma
Enchondroma
Chondromyxoid fibroma
Periosteal/Juxtacortical chondroma

BOX 14.7   Spine Lesions

Vertebral Body
    Hemangioma
    Metastasis
    Lymphoma
Posterior Vertebral Elements
    Osteoid osteoma/Osteoblastoma
    Aneurysmal bone cyst

BOX 14.8   Calcaneal Lesions

Simple/Unicameral bone cyst
Aneurysmal bone cyst
Chondroblastoma
Giant cell tumor
Pseudolesion
Intraosseous lipoma

BOX 14.9   Rib Lesions

Metastasis
Langerhans cell histiocytosis
Fibrous dysplasia
Ewing sarcoma
Lymphoma
Osteosarcoma

BOX 14.10   Lesions Within the Epiphysis

Osteomyelitis (<18 months of age)
Chondroblastoma (open physis)
Giant cell tumor (closed physis, extending from the metaphysis)
Osteoid osteoma (Trevor-Fairbank disease)

Adolescents (10–20 Years of Age)

The differential diagnoses for an aggressive osseous lesion in adolescents (10–20 years of age) are osteosarcoma, ES, leukemia, primary lymphoma of bone (PLB), and osteomyelitis (Box 14.5).

The differential diagnoses for nonaggressive osseous lesions in the adolescent age range (10–20 years of age) are extensive, including fibroxanthoma (fibrous cortical defect, NOF), osteochondroma, UBC, ABC, chondroblastoma, FD, osteoid osteoma/osteoblastoma, enchondroma, CMF, and periosteal/juxtacortical chondroma (Box 14.6).

■ Host Bone

Pediatric bone lesions demonstrate a pattern of occurrence within specific host bones. Bone neoplasms and tumor-like lesions have a propensity for development within regions of rapid bone growth and remodeling. Thus lesions tend to occur near the ends of long tubular bones in growing patients. For example, osteosarcoma commonly develops within the metaphyses of the distal femur and proximal tibia in the region of the knee. Osteosarcoma also occurs within the proximal metaphyses of the humerus, which are all regions of rapid bone growth.

Hemangiomas commonly occur in vertebral bodies and are the most common radiolucent lesion of the spine. Other osseous lesions also demonstrate a proclivity for occurring in the spine, such as osteoid osteoma, osteoblastoma, and ABC. However, these lesions occur within the posterior vertebral elements (Box 14.7).

Radiolucent lesions can occur in the calcaneus of young patients, an epiphyseal equivalent. The differential diagnosis for a radiolucent calcaneal lesion in a young patient includes a UBC, ABC, chondroblastoma, giant cell tumor (GCT), and pseudolesion (Box 14.8).

FD, LCH, ES, lymphoma, and osteosarcoma can develop in the ribs of young patients (Box 14.9). However, a healing fracture must be considered in the formulation of a differential diagnosis of any pediatric rib lesion.

Longitudinal Plane of the Host Bone

Pediatric and adolescent bone lesions also typically occur within certain regions along the longitudinal axis of the host bone (Fig. 14.1).

For example, chondroblastomas classically occur in the epiphysis and epiphyseal equivalents of long bones. Rarely, epiphyseal osteochondroma-like lesions can occur within long bones in the setting of Trevor-Fairbank disease (dysplasia epiphysealis hemimelica) (Box 14.10).

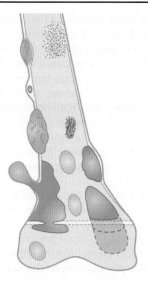

Fig. 14.1 **Field theory of bone tumor locations within the longitudinal axis of host bones.** (Modified from Koeller, K. K., Levy, A. D., Woodward, P.J., et al. [Eds.]. [2004]. *Radiologic-pathology, Vol 2: Musculoskeletal, neuroradiologic, and pediatric radiologic pathology correlations* [3rd ed.]. American Registry of Pathology, Armed Forces Institute of Pathology; and Courtesy Stephen T. Slota, PhD, University of Connecticut School of Medicine.)

Benign UBCs and ABCs, as well as osteochondroma and enchondroma, most commonly occur in the metaphases of long bones. These nonaggressive lesions can demonstrate subsequent migration away from the physes as young patients continue to grow.

GCTs, which can occur in adolescents and young adults, are classically centered in the metaphysis of long tubular bones with subsequent extension into the epiphysis after physeal closure. Osteomyelitis most commonly occurs in the metaphysis of long bones because of the presence of stagnant, slow-flowing blood within multiple looping blood vessels and sinusoids in this region.

Osteosarcoma most commonly occurs in the metaphysis of long bones as well. Therefore the differential diagnosis of an aggressive metaphyseal lesion in a long tubular bone in the second decade of life should include infection and osteosarcoma. Benign fibroxanthomas (fibrous cortical defect/NOFs), as well as CMFs, classically occur in the metaphysis and diametaphysis of long bones (Box 14.11).

FD, osteofibrous dysplasia (OFD), and enchondromas can occur in the diametaphysis of long bones. FD and OFD also can occur in the diaphysis of long bones. Small round blue cell malignancies, such as PLB, acute leukemia, and ES, also occur in the diametaphysis and diaphysis of long bones (Box 14.12).

Axial Plane of the Host Bone

Pediatric bone lesions also demonstrate patterns of occurrence with respect to the axial plane of the host bone. Lesions can be located centrally or eccentrically within the medullary cavity of the host bone. In addition, lesions also can occur within cortical or juxtacortical locations relative to the axial plane of the host bone.

BOX 14.11   Lesions Within the Metaphysis

Benign
Fibroxanthoma: Fibrous cortical defect/nonossifying fibroma
Enchondroma
Simple/Unicameral bone cyst (central)
Aneurysmal bone cyst (eccentric)
Osteochondroma
Osteomyelitis
Giant cell tumor (extending into the epiphysis if physis is closed)
Osteoid osteoma

Malignant
Metastasis
Primary lymphoma of bone
Osteosarcoma

BOX 14.12   Lesions Within the Diametaphysis and Diaphysis

Benign
Fibrous dysplasia
Osteofibrous dysplasia
Enchondroma

Malignant
Metastasis
Primary lymphoma of bone
Acute leukemia
Ewing sarcoma

BOX 14.13   Central Intramedullary Location

Enchondroma
Fibrous dysplasia
Simple/Unicameral bone cyst

BOX 14.14   Eccentric Intramedullary Location

Nonossifying fibroma
Chondromyxoid fibroma
Aneurysmal bone cyst
Giant cell tumor

Notably, periosteal lesions arise from the deep (cambium) layer of the periosteum and separate the periosteum from the subjacent cortex. Parosteal lesions arise from the outer (fibrous) layer of the periosteum and grow exophytically without elevating the subjacent periosteum from the cortex.

The differential diagnosis of an intramedullary lesion can therefore be narrowed by the identification of the epicenter of these lesions. Central intramedullary lesions of long bones include enchondroma, FD, and UBC (Box 14.13).

Eccentric intramedullary lesions include NOF, CMF, ABC, and GCT (Box 14.14).

Cortically based lesions include fibrous cortical defect and osteoid osteoma (Box 14.15). Juxtacortical lesions

Fibrous cortical defect
Osteoid osteoma

Periosteal/Juxtacortical chondroma
Osteochondroma

include osteochondroma, periosteal/juxtacortical chon-droma, as well as periosteal and parosteal osteosarcoma, which are rare in young patients (Box 14.16).

■ Host Bone Reaction

The evaluation of the type of periosteal reaction and periosteal new bone formation, or lack thereof, gener-ated by a host bone in response to the presence of a bone lesion can assist the radiologist in narrowing the differential diagnosis. Periosteal reaction is a nonspecif-ic response by the host bone to the underlying lesion. As the periosteum is irritated, and potentially raised or disrupted by a bone lesion, the host bone forms new bone in an attempt to contain the lesion.

Pediatric and adolescent bone lesions incite rela-tively early periosteal reactions because the periosteum in young patients demonstrates looser attachment to the underlying host bone in comparison with adults. Aggressive and nonaggressive osseous lesions demon-strate a high degree of overlap in the morphology of periosteal reactions they elicit. Of note, prior studies have demonstrated aggressive osseous lesions can result in benign or no periosteal reactions. Conversely, aggres-sive morphologies of periosteal reaction do not confirm the presence of an underlying aggressive malignancy.

In general the morphology of the resulting periosteal reaction and the density of the periosteal new bone for-mation, although nonspecific, are indicators of the rate of growth of the inciting osseous lesion. Slowly expand-ing, nonaggressive bone lesions typically result in a lack of periosteal reaction or dense, thick periosteal new bone formation from the host bone. Benign forms of periosteal new bone formation can demonstrate a con-tinuous single layer or solid morphologies (Fig. 14.2).

Rapidly growing, aggressive bone lesions classically result in lower-density periosteal new bone formation because the parent bone has less time to lay down new bone to contain a rapidly expanding lesion. Aggressive morphologies of periosteal reaction are spiculated in perpendicular hair-on-end and radial sunburst patterns. These forms of periosteal reaction are due to periosteal new bone formation along innumerable Sharpey fibers, which connect the periosteum to the subjacent cortex.

Lamellated or "onion skin" and disrupted periosteal new bone formation "Codman triangle" morphologies also occur in the setting of aggressive osseous lesions. Osteosarcoma and ES can result in these types of perios-teal new bone formation. Notably, nonmalignant pro-cesses such as osteomyelitis and thalassemia also can result in aggressive forms of periosteal reaction (Fig. 14.3).

Legion Margins/Patterns of Bone Destruction

The margin/zone of transition formed between an os-seous lesion and the host bone can be helpful to the radiologist in the generation of a differential diagnosis. The type of margin can indicate the lesion growth rate. The pattern of bone destruction and subsequent lesion margin can be described as geographical, moth-eaten, or permeative.

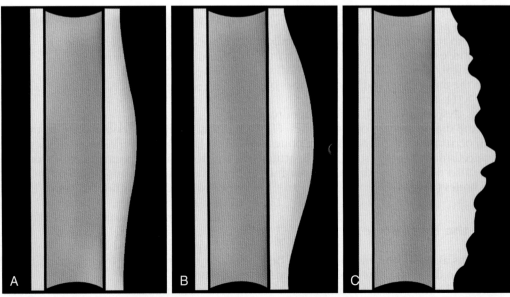

Fig. 14.2 Nonaggressive forms of periosteal reaction: (A) thin; (B) thick; and (C) thick, irregular. (Modified from Wu, J. S., & Hochman, M. G. [2012]. *Bone tumors: A practical guide to imaging.* Springer; and Courtesy Stephen T. Slota, PhD, University of Connecticut School of Medicine.)

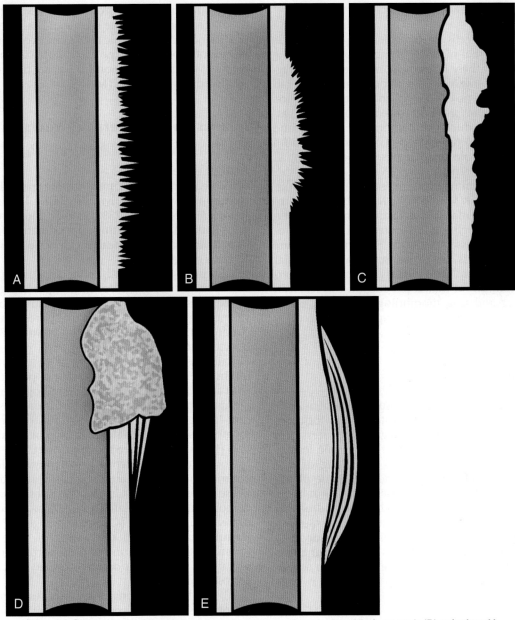

Fig. 14.3 Aggressive forms of periosteal reaction: **(A)** spiculated/hair-on-end; **(B)** spiculated/ sunburst; **(C)** disorganized; **(D)** Codman triangle; and **(E)** lamellated/onion skin. (Modified from Wu, J. S., & Hochman, M. G. [2012]. *Bone tumors: A practical guide to imaging.* Springer; and Courtesy Stephen T. Slota, PhD, University of Connecticut School of Medicine.)

Geographical bone destruction almost always results in well-defined margins and is generally present in the setting of a single discrete lytic lesion that is often well circumscribed with or without a sclerotic border. Geographical lesions tend to be nonaggressive and are almost always benign. Nonaggressive osseous lesions that result in geographical bone destruction include NOFs, bone cysts, enchondromas, FD, and chondroblastomas.

"Moth-eaten" and permeative patterns of bone destruction indicate that a bone lesion is more aggressive and often malignant. Aggressive bone destruction often results in multiple ill-defined lytic defects with poorly defined margins ("moth-eaten" appearance).

Permeative bone destruction permeates through the bone and can be difficult to visualize on radiographs; therefore MRI is extremely helpful in the imaging evaluation of a subtle permeative lytic lesion. Aggressive osseous lesions that can result in these forms of bone destruction include osteosarcoma, ES, osteomyelitis, and LCH.

The effect of an osseous lesion on the overlying cortex of the host bone also can be informative in the generation of a differential diagnosis. Cartilaginous lesions such as enchondromas are associated with endosteal scalloping. FD also can result in mild medullary expansion and endosteal scalloping. ABCs can result in prominent endosteal scalloping and cortical expansion.

Matrix and Mineralization

The mesenchymal cells of bone lesions produce the characteristic internal matrices of these neoplasms. The internal matrix of these lesions can be osseous, cartilaginous, fibrous, or myxoid. Bone neoplasms are generally named for the type of internal matrix they produce. Osseous lesions can produce a mixture of matrix patterns, such as FD, which can demonstrate osseous and cartilaginous matrix production. CMF produces both chondroid and myxoid matrix types. In contrast, not all lesions produce a matrix, such as ES and GCTs.

Osseous matrix mineralization results in a cloudlike, fluffy, or ivory density within bone lesions. Lesions producing an osseous matrix can form immature woven bone or mature lamellar bone. Osteosarcoma can produce both types of osseous matrix. FD forms immature woven bone, which is less dense than mature lamellar bone, resulting in the "ground-glass" density characteristic of FD. Chondroid matrix production can result in the classic arc and ring morphology. However, chondroid matrix also can exhibit a stippled or flocculent appearance.

Soft Tissue Component

In general the presence of a soft tissue component associated with an osseous lesion indicates underlying cortical disruption in the setting of an aggressive process. Soft tissue mass components associated with bone lesions can be evaluated for on radiographs by looking for variable densities and effacement of normal tissue planes within the soft tissues adjacent to the affected host bone. In addition, the presence of mineralization and/or matrix production within the juxtacortical soft tissues can indicate the presence of an underlying soft tissue mass component. Follow-up intravenous contrast-enhanced MRI should be performed of a bone lesion if an associated soft tissue mass is suspected.

■ Single or Multiple Lesions

Multiple osseous lesions in a young patient indicate the presence of an underlying systemic disease or syndrome predisposing to the development of bone lesions. Primary bone neoplasms tend to be monostotic. A young patient demonstrating constitutional symptoms and multiple lytic bone lesions should be considered for acute leukemia, multifocal osteomyelitis, or metastatic neuroblastoma. ES with metastases, primary bone lymphoma (PBL), or multifocal LCH should also be considered depending on the age of the patient. Notably, patients with sickle cell are at increased risk for hematogenously disseminated multifocal osteomyelitis, particularly secondary to encapsulated organisms such as *Salmonella*.

Multiple lucent "brown tumors" can also be present in the setting of underlying hyperparathyroidism. FD and LCH can demonstrate a polyostotic distribution, as described earlier. Polyostotic FD can occur in the setting of McCune-Albright syndrome (MAS). Multiple enchondromas are present in the setting of Maffucci syndrome or Ollier disease. Multiple NOFs can occur in the setting of neurofibromatosis type I and Jaffe-Campanacci syndrome. Multiple osteochondromas are present in multiple hereditary exostoses (MHE).

Infants and Toddlers (<5 Years of Age)

Acute Leukemia

Acute leukemia is the most common malignancy of childhood, with acute lymphoblastic leukemia representing approximately 75% of cases, and acute myelogenous leukemia representing approximately 15% to 20% of pediatric cases. The peak incidence is between 2 and 10 years of age.

Children present with bone or joint pain, limp, soft tissue swelling, and/or arthralgias. Fatigue secondary to anemia, fever, petechiae, bleeding, and hepatosplenomegaly also can be present at presentation. These children also can demonstrate an elevated ESR, thrombocytopenia, and neutropenia.

Radiographs are often normal or can have subtle findings (Fig. 14.4A). Forty percent of pediatric patients with acute leukemia demonstrate radiographic findings. Diffuse osteoporosis can be present or classic radiolucent "leukemic lines," which occur in the metaphysis of long bones adjacent to the zone of provisional calcification (ZPC), which often remains intact.

Poorly defined osteolytic metaphyseal lesions can occur with a "moth-eaten" or permeative appearance. These lesions can result in aggressive periosteal reactions demonstrating lamellated, spiculated, and/or interrupted morphologies (Codman triangle). Pathological fractures can occur in the setting of these aggressive lesions in the background of osteoporosis. Juxtacortical soft tissue masses can occur secondary to cortical and periosteal disruption.

T1-weighted imaging demonstrates confluent T1-hypointense regions secondary to replacement of normal marrow by leukemic infiltrates (Fig 14.4B). This T1-hypointense signal will correlate with patchy or diffuse marrow edema secondary to marrow infiltration. These hypercellular leukemic marrow infiltrates can demonstrate restricted diffusion, as well as intermediate to bright enhancement. Bone scans will demonstrate increased radiotracer uptake in foci of osseous leukemic involvement; however, bone scans may underestimate the extent of disease. PET-CT and whole-body MR can accurately assess for diffuse systemic involvement and treatment response.

Multifocal Langerhans Cell Histiocytosis

LCH is a disorder characterized by clonal proliferation of S100-positive dendritic cells. The current classification of LCH is currently based on disease extent, and may be single-system (unifocal or multifocal) and multi-system, with or without risk organ involvement (spleen, liver, or bone marrow). Ninety percent of cases of LCH present before the age of 15 years.

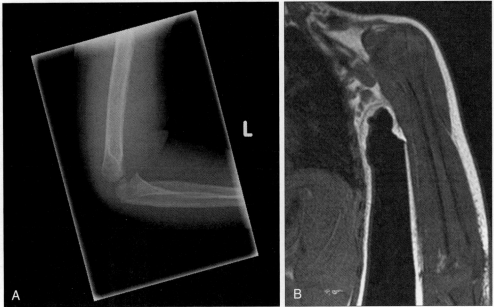

Fig. 14.4 Leukemia. (A) "Moth-eaten" appearrance of the distal humerus with associated periosteal reaction. (B) Coronal T1-weighted image though humerus showing abnormal T1 marrow signal, with complete absence of fatty marrow, consistent with marrow replacement. Note the splenomegaly and the enlarged axillary lymph nodes.

The peak incidence of multisystem disease is less than 3 years of age

The skeletal system is involved in 80% to 90% of cases, which rarely occurs in a unifocal form in infants and toddlers. Osseous lesions will most commonly involve the calvarium and classically demonstrate well-defined round or lobulated "punched-out" lesions without sclerotic rims (Fig. 14.5A). These lesions can exhibit "beveled" edges due to asymmetric involvement of the inner and outer tables of the calvarium. Flat bones are affected most commonly, with the skull, mandible, ribs, pelvis, and scapula being common sites of osseous involvement. Longs bones and vertebrae are affected less commonly by LCH, with vertebral lesions occurring most frequently in the thoracic and lumbar spine.

Vertebra plana secondary to a lytic lesion centered within a vertebral body is a classic finding in pediatric LCH spine involvement with secondary kyphosis and/or scoliosis. The adjacent disks and posterior elements are rarely involved. A diminutive soft tissue mass component relative to the degree of vertebral body destruction is characteristic of LCH spinal involvement. The differential diagnosis for a lytic spinal lesion in an infant or toddler with fever and leukocytosis should include acute leukemia, LCH, and osteomyelitis.

LCH skeletal lesions within the appendicular skeleton will demonstrate variable radiographic appearances depending on the phase of disease and subsequent treatment effects. Lesions are more commonly radiolucent than sclerotic and can exhibit geographical or permeative bone destruction with variable margins (see Fig. 14.5B–C). Aggressive and nonaggressive periosteal reactions can be present in the setting of LCH lesions. In addition, soft tissue masses can occur overlying lytic lesions, simulating an aggressive malignancy. LCH lesions most commonly occur in the metaphyses or diaphyses of long bones (see Fig. 14.5D–E).

A button sequestrum, a sclerotic focus within a lucent lesion, can occur. In addition, the floating tooth sign is a classic finding in the setting of mandibular involvement of LCH secondary to destruction of the dense lamina dura.

Radiographic skeletal surveys, F-18 fluorodeoxyglucose (^{18}F-FDG)-PET/CT, and whole-body short-tau inversion recovery (STIR) MRI can be used to evaluate for multifocal LCH and monitor treatment response. These osseous lesions demonstrate variable radiotracer uptake with common false negatives on nuclear medicine bone scans which have a lower sensitivity than radiographic skeletal surveys. Notably, these osseous lesions can demonstrate decreased radiotracer uptake with a surrounding halo of increased uptake, particularly in the calvarium.

Whole-body STIR MRI can assess for multifocal osseous and extraskeletal disease. Notably, MRI is more sensitive than radiographs or bone scan in the detection of multifocal lesions. However, STIR imaging is not effective at distinguishing acute from residual disease.

^{18}F-FDG-PET/CT is highly sensitive for active LCH lesions; however, it is less sensitive than MRI for vertebral involvement. In addition, ^{18}F-FDG/CT results in a higher radiation dose than the other imaging modalities. This radiation dose can be lowered with the use of lesion-selective CT imaging, as well as the utilization of PET/MR fusion. Thus PET/MR fusion will likely prove to be the most efficacious modality for multifocal lesion detection and treatment monitoring in the future.

Metastatic Neuroblastoma

Neuroblastoma is a malignant neoplasm of sympathetic chain primitive neural crest cells and is the most common extracranial solid malignancy in childhood

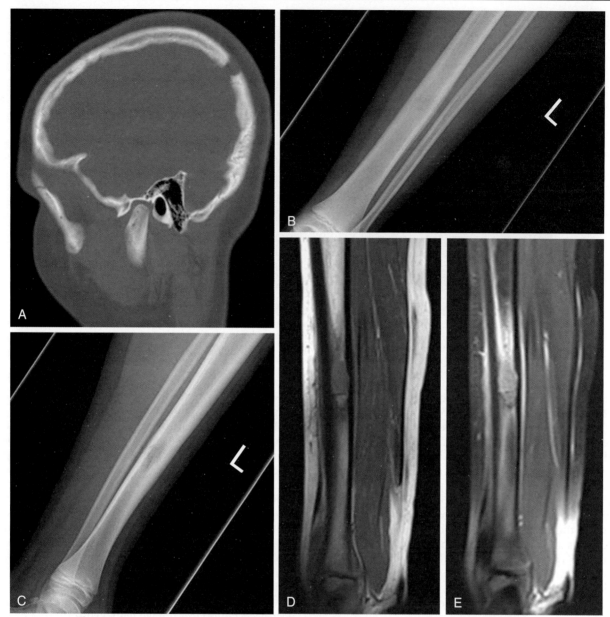

Fig. 14.5 Langerhans cell histoicystosis. (A) "Punched-out" lesion of the calvarium on a parasagital CT image of the head. (B–C) Radiolucent intramedullary diaphyseal lesions. (D) Sagittal T1-weighted-image showing an ill-defined, intramedullary, middiaphyseal lesion with pathological T1-hypointense signal. (E) Sagittal T2-weighted-image showing prominent surrounding reactive marrow edema. (Courtesy Tessa Balach, MD.)

with a median age at diagnosis of 15 to 17 months. Primary neuroblastoma can occur anywhere along the sympathetic chain from the neck to the pelvis, most commonly within the adrenal glands.

Metastases are present at diagnosis in 50% to 60% of cases of neuroblastoma. The most common sites of metastatic disease are bone, lymph nodes, liver, and soft tissues. Neuroblastoma is the most common primary malignancy resulting in metastatic bone disease in young children.

Neuroblastoma osseous metastatic lesions can manifest as focally destructive cortical lesions and/or intramedullary lesions and are the most common cause of aggressive metaphyseal lesions in young children

(Fig. 14.6A–B). Notably, extensive metastatic marrow disease can be present with little radiographic change.

Cortical lesions can present as lytic or sclerotic lesions resulting in cortical destruction and aggressive periosteal reaction. However, metastatic lesions are usually osteolytic and may result in metaphyseal radiolucent lesions resembling leukemia. Multiple lytic lesions demonstrating a permeative pattern of bone destruction may occur within the calvarium. Vertebral collapse can occur secondary to lytic vertebral metastatic lesions.

Metastatic bone lesions demonstrate uptake of I-123 MIBG with a sensitivity and specificity of approximately 90%. MIBG scintigraphy is useful for diagnosis, staging,

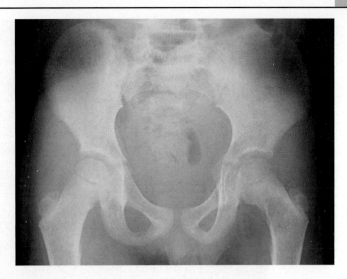

Fig. 14.6 Neuroblastoma. Lytic lesion within the inferomedial aspect of the left femoral neck. (Courtesy Tessa Balach, MD.)

and posttreatment follow-up imaging. MIBG uptake can demonstrate cortical and intramedullary osseous metastatic disease.

^{18}F-FDGPET/CT and technetium (Tc)-99m-methylene diphosphonate (MDP) bone scans are extremely useful in the evaluation of non-MIBG avid metastatic neuroblastoma. PET demonstrates a high sensitivity for soft tissue and osseous metastatic lesions, although less than MIBG. Tc-99m-MDP radiotracer also demonstrates uptake within cortical and intramedullary metastatic lesions on nuclear medicine bone scan. Notably, cortical bone lesions demonstrate increased radiotracer uptake relative to intramedullary marrow metastatic disease on nuclear medicine bone scans.

Osteomyelitis

Osteomyelitis can present as a monostotic or multifocal process with potential articular involvement and generalized sepsis. Approximately 20% of cases of multifocal osteomyelitis occur in newborns. Osteomyelitis most commonly occurs in the metaphyses of long bones as a result of slow blood flow through looping metaphyseal venules in this region (Fig. 14.7A).

The femur, tibia, and humerus represent the most common host bones. Sites of osseous infection also occur within metaphyseal equivalents, such as adjacent to synchondroses and apophyses. Osteomyelitis also can occur within the short bones of the hands and feet, pelvis, and spine.

Hematogenous bacterial seeding is the most common source of infection, with *Staphylococcus aureus* representing the causative organism in 80% to 90% of pediatric cases followed by multiple streptococcal species. Pediatric patients with osteomyelitis can present with fever, pain/irritability, and soft tissue swelling; however, patient presentation is often nonspecific. The ESR, C-reactive protein, and white blood cell count should be elevated in the setting of osteomyelitis. Notably, the femoral neck is the most common site of osteomyelitis in infants, with concomitant septic arthritis of the hip frequently occurring because of transphyseal blood flow.

Juxtacortical and/or periarticular soft tissue edema is the earliest radiographic finding. This soft tissue edema can manifest as displacement and/or effacement of adjacent fat planes, as well as reticulation of overlying subcutaneous fat. Osteolysis and periosteal reaction generally is radiographically visible within 7 to 14 days of the inciting infection. Bone destruction can demonstrate an aggressive permeative pattern with variable periosteal reaction.

Subacute, focal intraosseous infection can result in the development of a Brodie abscess. These bony lesions are radiolucent intraosseous cavities filled with purulent debris surrounded by a sclerotic rim containing vascularized granulation tissue and reactive new bone formation. This rim of vascularized granulation tissue demonstrates higher T1 signal intensity relative to the abscess cavity, which is isointense to skeletal muscle, called the *penumbra sign*. This penumbra of peripheral vascularized granulation tissue enhances with postcontrast MRI sequences, assisting the radiologist in differentiating a Brodie abscess from aggressive and benign bone lesions (Fig. 14.7B-D).

In addition, on T1-weighted imaging, osteomyelitis generally lacks a well-defined margin with the adjacent normal fatty/yellow marrow, unlike most osseous malignancies. Subperiosteal T1 bright fat globules secondary to cortical disruption and marrow fat necrosis is also indicative of osteomyelitis and not an aggressive osseous malignancy.

The presence of an adjacent joint effusion should raise the concern of associated septic arthritis, which most commonly occurs in neonates and infants. Septic arthritis will classically demonstrate a complex joint effusion, thickened hyperemic synovium, adjacent marrow edema, and juxtaarticular intramuscular and soft tissue edema.

Nuclear medicine bone scan is highly sensitive and will demonstrate increased radiotracer uptake in the angiographic, blood pool, and delayed phases. Bone scans can be used to evaluate for the presence of multiple sites of osteomyelitis. However, MRI is the most sensitive and specific modality for detection of

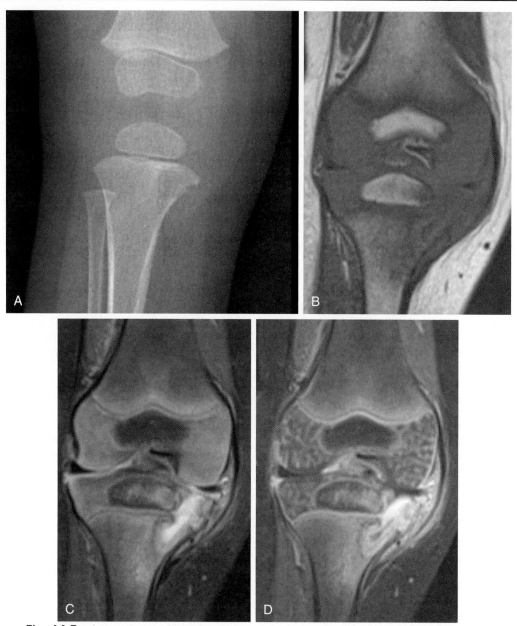

Fig. 14.7 Subacute osteomyelitis (A) Focal lucency in the proximal tibial metaphysis with adjacent cortical destruction. The patient presented with 10 days of knee swelling and pain, with low grade fevers. (B–D) Coronal T1- and T2- and post-contrast T1-weighted imaging shows a fluid filled lesion with a an enhancing T1-hyperintense rim (penumbra sign), extending into the epiphyseal cartilage, consistent with subcacute osteomyelitis with a Brodie abscess.

early osteomyelitis and the potential complications thereof.

Chronic osteomyelitis is generally sclerotic or mixed lytic and sclerotic in radiographic appearance. Chronic focal osseous infection can result in the formation of a cloaca, a radiolucent drainage tract extending from the medullary cavity through the overlying cortex. A sequestrum also can occur, which is a radiodense/sclerotic piece of necrotic intramedullary bone secondary to a lack of adequate blood supply within the region of infection.

Subperiosteal purulent debris can also elevate and strip the periosteum from the surface of the underlying cortex of the host bone. This chronically elevated

periosteum can generate a sheath of new bone, or involucrum, encasing the affected host bone. Marked cortical thickening also can occur in the setting of chronic osteomyelitis, called *Garré sclerosing osteomyelitis*.

Infantile Myofibromatosis

Infantile myofibromatosis presents in infancy, with 90% of cases diagnosed before 2 years of age. This process represents solitary (myofibroma) or multiple (myofibromatosis) which are benign fibrous neoplasms composed of clusters of spindled myofibroblastic cells that demonstrate a high rate of spontaneous regression.

Myofibromatosis can involve the bones, skin, muscle, and viscera. Most of these lesions occur within

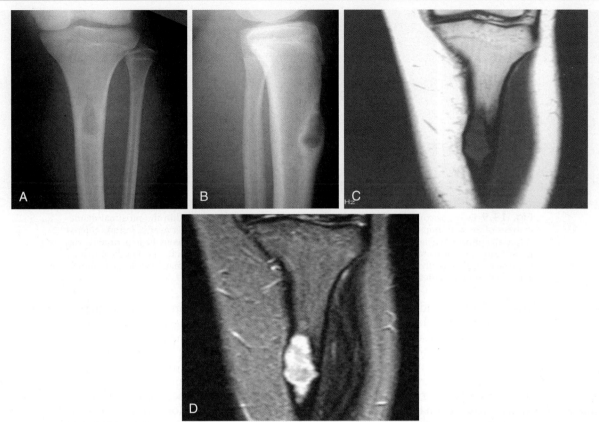

Fig. 14.8 Osteofibrous dysplasia. (A–B) Geographical, "bubbly," multilobulated lesion within the anterior cortex of proximal diaphysis of the left tibia on AP and lateral radiographs of the tibia and fibula. (C) Geographic lobulated lesion with a thin sclerotic margin is seen on T1-weighted imaging. There is no periosteal reaction. (D) No surrounding marrow edema is seen on T2-weighted imaging. (Courtesy Tessa Balach, MD.)

the skin, subcutaneous tissues, and muscles with associated osseous involvement. Affected patients can present with extensive musculoskeletal involvement, which demonstrates a high rate of spontaneous resolution over 1 to 2 years. Solid visceral involvement indicates a worse prognosis in patients with multicentric disease, with the lungs, gastrointestinal tract, heart, and liver being the most commonly affected viscera.

Myofibromas are solitary solid soft tissue masses in newborns that can present with concomitant red-purple cutaneous nodules. Myofibromatosis represents multiple, relatively symmetrical, soft tissue masses with associated well-defined, eccentric, geographical radiolucent lesions centered within the metaphyses and metadiaphyses of the appendicular skeleton with associated cortical loss and expansile remodeling. Secondaray periosteal reaction is generally absent or can occur in a benign, solid morphology.

These soft tissue masses exhibit variable sonographic characteristics and are generally well marginated; however, they can form large infiltrating nodules or plaques. Myofibromas can demonstrate heterogeneous calcification with central cystic regions with central hypovascularity and associated bizarre cortical remodeling of adjacent bones. These soft tissue masses exhibit T1-hypointense and usually T2-hyperintense signal with peripheral enhancement on MRI.

Osteofibrous Dysplasia

Osteofibrous dysplasia (OFD) is a fibroosseous lesion that primarily affects the anterior cortex of the proximal diaphysis and metadiaphysis of the tibia, but it can also involve the fibula in early childhood. Fifty percent of cases occur in the first 5 years of life with extremely rare occurrence of OFD after skeletal maturation. OFD is usually painless and can present with progressive deformity of the leg of a young child.

OFD contains variable fibroblast proliferation, osteoid, collagen fibers, and trabeculae in variable shapes and spatial orientation rimmed with osteoblasts. Notably, OFD demonstrates an absence of long bony spicules that are typical of FD. In addition, FD does not exhibit the presence of active osteoblasts.

OFD lesions are usually centered within the anterior cortex of the proximal tibia but may extend posteriorly within the medullary canal (Fig. 14.8A–B). OFD lesions are generally geographic, multilobulated masses with sclerotic margins. The majority of these lesions are lytic, with approximately 40% demonstrating a ground-glass matrix. The associated cortex is expanded and thickened with no associated periosteal reaction. Multifocal or elongated, confluent lesions can occur. OFD can result in an anterior bowing deformity and can result in pseudarthrosis formation after pathological fracture.

MRI demonstrates cortical expansion in approximately 60% of cases. Frank cortical destruction and

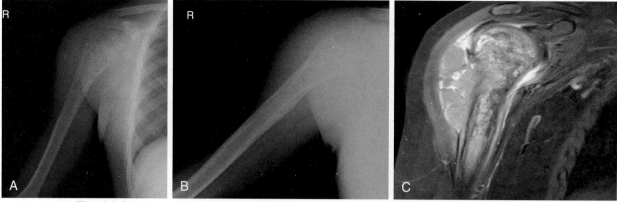

Fig. 14.9 Ewing sarcoma. (A–B) Ill-defined, permeative lesion centered within the proximal diametaphysis of the right humerus on AP and lateral radiographs. (C) Ill-defined, permeative lesion centered within the proximal metaphysis of the right humerus demonstrating heterogeneous T2-hyperintense signal and surrounding reactive marrow edema. Cortical destruction along the lateral aspect of the proximal humeral metaphysis with a prominent associated soft tissue mass component. Small reactive glenohumeral joint effusion. (Courtesy Tessa Balach, MD.)

associated soft tissue mass formation are rare. These lesions can demonstrate rare intralesion fat and cystic regions. They exhibit intense contrast enhancement with no associated soft tissue edema and/or enhancement in the absence of a pathological fracture (Fig. 14.8C–D).

OFD is on a histological spectrum with OFD-like adamantinoma and adamantinoma. OFD-like adamantinoma demonstrates identical imaging characteristics of OFD. OFD-like adamantinoma is also histologically identical to OFD, except it contains additional small nests of epithelial cells. OFD cannot be reliably differentiated with adamantinoma based solely on imaging characteristics; however, OFD usually occurs in younger patients.

In addition, cortical destruction and/or an associated soft tissue mass in an older child associated with a lesion similar in appearance to OFD should raise the concern of adamantinoma. Image-guided biopsy can determine where a lesion of concern lies on this histological spectrum as adamantinoma.

Children (5–10 Years of Age)

Ewing Sarcoma

ES is an aggressive, small, round, blue cell malignancy that can arise from bone or soft tissues. ES is the second most common primary bone malignancy in children after osteosarcoma. This malignancy is part of the ES family of tumors, which also contains primitive neuroectodermal tumor, Askin tumors, and extraosseous ES. ES occurs in Caucasians six to nine times more frequently than African Americans.

Eight-five percent of these lesions within the ES family demonstrate the t(11;22)(q24;q12) translocation. These highly cellular lesions are composed of sheets of small, round, blue cells. Affected patients can present with fever, leukocytosis, anemia, and elevated sedimentary rate, which can mimic the clinical presentation of osteomyelitis and acute leukemia. These patients can also present with local pain and swelling with a tender/palpable mass.

ES commonly presents radiographically as a large, ill-defined, highly aggressive intramedullary lesion with expansile remodeling within a long bone. ES most commonly occurs in the legs and pelvis, with 94% occurring in the diaphyses or diametaphyses of long bones. These intramedullary lesions are typically central in location within the diaphyses and more eccentric within the metadiaphyses of long bones (Fig. 14.9A–B). Rarely, these lesions can arise from peripheral periosteal or subperiosteal locations that carry a relatively favorable prognosis.

ES occurs with greater frequency within flat bones, such as the pelvis, scapula, and ribs, than other primary bone malignancies. ES also occurs within the chest wall in approximately 16% of cases, which is the most common site of extraosseous disease and results in nonspecific well-circumscribed soft tissue masses. Metastases most commonly occur within the lungs, with approximately 25% of patients demonstrating metastatic disease at the time of presentation. Local and regional lymph node involvement can also occur.

ES lesions exhibit a permeative or moth-eaten pattern of cortical bone destruction secondary to tumor infiltration through the Haversian canals. This cortical destruction results in multiple associated aggressive morphologies of periosteal reaction, including lamellated onion skin, spiculated, and sunburst patterns with reactive periosteal new bone formation laid down along Sharpey fibers superficial to the destroyed cortex.

Frank periosteal disruption can result in Codman triangle formation. Large soft tissue masses can occur secondary to ES osseous lesions (Fig. 14.9C). These soft tissue masses can be disproportionately large relative to the amount of bone destruction. Notably, ES results in no ossified tumor matrix production; therefore secondary soft tissue involvement can be radiographically occult due to the lack of soft tissue mineralization. Sclerosis can occur in approximately 25% of these aggressive osseous lesions secondary to bone necrosis.

MRI is most effective at demonstrating ES tumor margins, with T1-weighted images being the most effective in the evaluation of the extent of osseous lesions, as well as possible intraarticular involvement and skip metastatic lesions. Joint to joint imaging of the involved host bone should be performed to exclude skip lesions. ES osseous lesions will demonstrate T1-hypointense signal secondary to marrow replacement by these aggressive cellular lesions. The spatial relationship of extraosseous soft tissue involvement with respect to neurovascular structures also must be established, which is best evaluated with multiaxial precontrast and postcontrast sequences.

ES lesions demonstrate nonspecific heterogeneous T2-hyperintense signal and heterogeneous enhancement with postcontrast imaging. ES lesions can demonstrate restricted diffusion in hypercellular regions with changes in apparent diffusion coefficient (ADC) values proving helpful for the monitoring of tumor treatment response. Changes in contrast enhancement characteristics are also helpful in determining the response to chemotherapy.

CT evaluation of the chest is the most effective manner to evaluate for pulmonary metastatic disease. Tc-MDP bone scan will demonstrate intense radiotracer uptake in primary and secondary ES bone lesions. ES lesions also demonstrate ^{18}F-FDG avidity, which is also useful for the staging of disease and response to therapy.

Monostotic Langerhans Cell Histiocytosis

Approximately 66% to 75% of musculoskeletal cases of LCH are unifocal and monostotic. Approximately 70%, occur within the flat bones of the axial skeleton, including the calvarium, pelvis, and ribs. The vertebral bodies are involved in approximately 10% of cases. As mentioned earlier, lytic calvarial lesions with beveled edges, which may contain sclerotic sequestra and vertebra plana, are classic findings in LCH.

Monostotic lesions can also occur within the appendicular skeleton. The femur, tibia, and humerus represent the most common long bone hosts. These lesions most commonly occur within the diaphyses and metaphyses of long bones and rarely within the epiphyses.

These monostotic lesions can demonstrate a highly aggressive radiographic appearance. They are generally permeative, nongeographical lesions with a lack of well-defined margins. These lesions can incite aggressive periosteal reactions from the host bone with cortical breakthrough and subsequent secondary soft tissue mass formation, all findings that can be seen in the setting of aggressive osseous malignancies. Notably, monostotic LCH can demonstrate extremely rapid progression, which can help differentiate these lesions from a malignancy or osteomyelitis.

Mature monostotic LCH lesions generally demonstrate a more geographical, less aggressive appearance. Continuous, smooth periosteal reaction with endosteal scalloping secondary to mild medullary expansion and no associated soft tissue mass can be seen with more mature LCH osseous lesions.

LCH lesions demonstrate nonspecific T1-hypointense signal and heterogeneous T2-hyperintense signal with fluid-sensitive sequences. Postcontrast imaging can demonstrate heterogeneous intramedullary enhancement and heterogeneous enhancement within any

soft tissue mass associated with these bone lesions. Therefore image-guided percutaneous or surgical biopsy is required for diagnosis.

Adolescents (10–20 Years of Age)

Osteosarcoma

Osteosarcoma is the most common primary bone neoplasm in children and young adults. Seventy to eighty-five percent of these lesions represent conventional high-grade intramedullary osteosarcoma in young patients. These patients present with pain and possible palpable mass. Approximately 55% to 80% of cases occur in the region of the knee within the metaphyses of the distal femur or proximal tibia. Seventy-five percent of these metaphyseal lesions will demonstrate extension within the adjacent epiphysis. Less common sites of occurrence of osteosarcoma are the proximal humerus, flat bones of the axial skeleton, and vertebral bodies.

Rare multicentric synchronous osteosarcomas can occur in children (5–10 years of age). These multicentric lesions carry an extremely poor prognosis and represent approximately 1% of all cases of osteosarcoma. Further, the rare high-grade surface variant of osteosarcoma can occur in the adolescent age group (10–20 years of age). This peripheral variant of osteosarcoma with minimal intramedullary involvement manifests as a partially mineralized soft tissue mass with destruction of the underlying cortex. These lesions demonstrate a periosteal reaction along their margins. Notably, the telangiectatic and superficial parosteal and periosteal variants of osteosarcoma rarely occur in the pediatric and adolescent populations.

Conventional intramedullary osteosarcomas present as poorly defined intramedullary lytic and sclerotic lesions with indistinct margins and a wide zone of transition. These aggressive lesions demonstrate a mixture of bone destruction and new bone formation secondary to cloudy osteoid matrix production in 90% of cases. Osteosarcomas result in frank or permeative moth-eaten cortical destruction with secondary aggressive periosteal reaction that can demonstrate a classic sunburst morphology and/or Codman triangle (Fig. 14.10A–B).

T1-weighted imaging is the most effective MRI sequence for determining the margins of these aggressive osseous lesions (Fig. 14.10C). Joint to joint MRI of the entire host bone should be performed to exclude skip metastatic lesions. Targeted small field-of-view MRI imaging of the primary osseous lesion should also be performed to evaluate for potential involvement of the physis and the adjacent joint space and neurovascular structures. Skip lesions and transarticular lesions occur in approximately 2% to 6% of cases.

Osteosarcomas are T1-hypointense secondary to marrow replacement and heterogeneous osteoid matrix production. Heterogeneous T1-hyperintense signal can also occur secondary to intralesion hemorrhage. These lesions are hyperintense on fluid sensitive sequences (see Fig. 14.10D–E). Notably, fluid–fluid levels within the lesions should raise concern for multiloculated

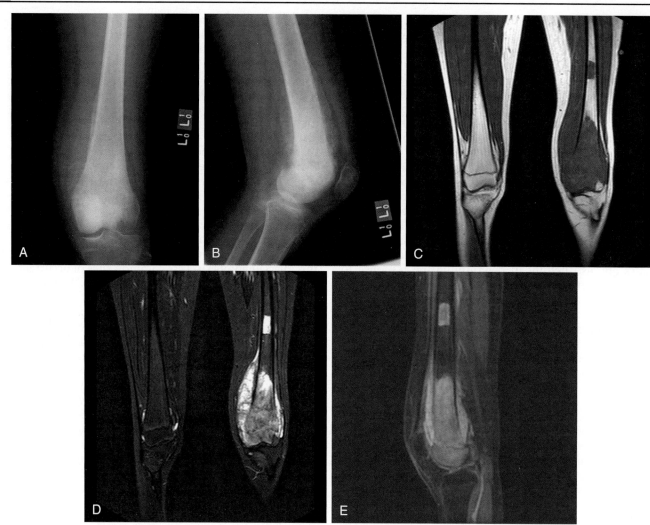

Fig. 14.10 Osteosarcoma. (A) Ill-defined, heterogeneously sclerotic, intramedullary lesion centered within the distal left femoral metaphysis on an AP radiograph of the knee. Associated periosteal reaction along the medial aspect of the distal femoral metaphysis with extraosseous osteoid matrix, indicating cortical and periosteal disruption and an associated developing soft tissue component. (B) Periosteal elevation is present along the anterior and posterior aspects of the distal femur with osteoid matrix streaming along Sharpey fibers subjacent to the elevated periosteum. (C) Coronal T1-weighted image through the distal femurs shows T1-hypointense signal and medullary expansion within the distal left femoral metaphysis. A middiaphyseal skip lesion is also present in the left femur. (D) Coronal T2-weighted fat-suppressed image shows heterogeneous T2-hyperintense signal associated with the distal left femoral intramedullary lesion. This sequence clearly demonstrates the developing extraosseous matrix production elevating the periosteum along the medial and lateral aspects of the distal left femur. The skip lesion also demonstrates T2-hyperintense signal. (E) Contrast-enhanced sagittal T1-weighted fat-supressed image shows heterogeneous intramedullary and extraosseous enhancement associated with the distal left femoral lesion. This sequence also clearly demonstrates the developing enhancing extraosseous matrix production elevating the periosteum along the anterior and posterior aspects of the distal left femoral metaphysis. The skip lesion also demonstrates enhancement. (Courtesy Tessa Balach, MD.)

intralesion hemorrhage, which can occur in the setting of the rare telangiectatic osteosarcoma variant.

Highly cellular components, regions of hemorrhage, and regions of necrosis will result in heterogeneous restricted diffusion within the lesions. ADC values with serial MRI examinations can be used to monitor lesion response to neoadjuvant chemotherapy. These lesions will also demonstrate heterogeneous enhancement with multiaxial postcontrast sequences.

Sonographic evaluation of these lesions can demonstrate echogenic osteoid matrix within juxtacortical soft tissue masses, as well as cortical destruction/disruption

and periosteal elevation. Ultrasound can also evaluate for mass effect and/or invasion of adjacent neurovascular structures, including potential intravascular extension of tumor thrombus. Diagnosis of the primary bone lesion is confirmed with image-guided percutaneous or surgical biopsy.

Tc-99m MDP bone scan demonstrates intense metabolic activity within primary and metastatic osteosarcoma lesions. [18]F FDG-PET also demonstrates intense metabolic activity within conventional osteosarcoma and metastatic lesions, which can assist in differentiating necrosis and positive neoadjuvant chemotherapy

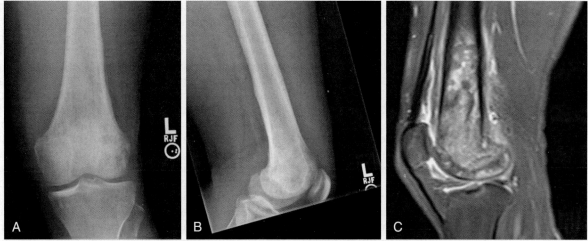

Fig. 14.11 Primary lymphoma of bone. (A–B) Heterogeneous, ill-defined, intramedullary lesion centered within the distal left femoral metaphysis. (C) Contrast-enhanced sagittal T1-weighted fat supressed image showing heterogeneous, ill-defined, intramedullary enhancement centered within the distal left femoral metaphysis with irregular cortical destruction along the posterior aspect of the distal femur. Large reactive joint effusion with associated synovial enhancement indicative of concomitant synovitis. (Courtesy Tessa Balach, MD.)

response. A chest CT is also performed at diagnosis to assess for pulmonary metastatic disease, which is present in 15% to 20% of patients at the time of presentation.

Primary Lymphoma of Bone

Primary lymhoma of the bone (PLB) can rarely occur in the adolescent population. Solitary or multifocal osseous lymphoma primarily occurs within the long bones of the lower extremities and humerus, with the proximal metadiaphysis of the femur representing the most common site of occurrence. However, these lesions can also occur within flat bones of the axial skeleton and spine in approximately 25% of cases.

These osseous lesions can present at a single skeletal site with or without regional lymph node involvement. Alternatively, polyostotic lymphoma of bone can present without visceral and/or nodal involvement. Notably, osseous metastatic disease secondary to non-Hodgkin lymphoma is much more common in young patients than PLB.

PLB lesions often demonstrate subtle radiographic findings. Osseous lymphoma lesions are typically lytic with wide zones of transition secondary to permeative bone destruction and no associated matrix production (Fig. 14.11A–B). Sclerotic reactive bone can be present, with approximately 15% of these lesions exhibiting a sclerotic intramedullary sequestrum.

These lesions can incite endosteal and cortical thickening. If cortical disruption is present, it is generally radiographically occult. Indeed, a prominent juxtacortical soft tissue mass secondary to an adjacent permeative intramedullary lytic lesion with no radiographic evidence of an associated cortical defect is indicative of primary osseous lymphoma. These lesions can result in minimal periosteal reaction, which can exhibit a lamellated morphology. In general, radiographs tend to underestimate host bone involvement secondary to primary osseous lymphoma.

CT can better demonstrate the presence of a sequestrum and/or subtle cortical disruption associated with these lesions. CT is also helpful for evaluation of the chest, abdomen, and pelvis for possible visceral involvement and lymphadenopathy. The presence of visceral involvement and remote lymphadenopathy helps to differentiate secondary lymphomatous osseous involvement from PLB.

MRI clearly defines potential extensive radiographically occult marrow involvement secondary to PLB. These intramedullary lesions are typically T1-hypointense and T2-hyperintense. Serpiginous intramedullary permeative bone destruction interposed between regions of normal intramedullary bone is characteristic of primary osseous lymphoma (Fig. 14.11C).

As described earlier, soft tissue extension is disproportionately extensive relative to the degree of subtle cortical disruption associated with PLB. Only approximately 28% of cases demonstrate frank cortical disruption with MRI. A circumferential soft tissue mass that permeates through the periosteum and cortex is a characteristic MR finding of PLB. In addition, Tc-99m MDP and gallium-67 scans can be used to evaluate for polyostotic disease.

Osteochondroma

Benign osteochondromas are thought to arise from displaced physeal cartilage of long bones; therefore these lesions are most commonly found along the surfaces of the metaphyses of long bones, adjacent to the physes. These lesions tend to migrate away from the closing physes into the metadiaphyses as the host bone grows in length.

Osteochondromas are the most common nonaggressive bone lesions in the pediatric and adolescent population. These benign lobulated sessile or pedunculated exostoses are believed to result from displaced physeal cartilage, which herniates through the periosteal bone cuff along the margins of the physis during endochondral ossification. Therefore these exostoses represent developmental lesions and are not true neoplasms.

Osteochondromas usually present in the second decade of life as a painless incidental finding along the metaphyseal surface of a long bone (Fig. 14.12A). These lesions usually cease to grow at skeletal maturation. Subsequent regression after skeletal maturation is rarely reported.

Osteochondromas that demonstrate continued increase in size and/or increasing discomfort should raise concern for malignant transformation, which is extremely rare in skeletally immature patients. Of note, these lesions can occur in 6% to 12% of patients who received radiation therapy at a young age with a mean latency of 5 to 12 years. Malignant transformation rates are not increased in radiation-induced osteochondromas.

Common sites of occurrence of osteochondromas include the proximal and distal femur, proximal tibia, and humerus, with approximately 35% of these benign lesions occurring in the region of the knee. Osteochondromas can also occur within the feet, scapula, ribs, pelvis, and, rarely, within the spine. Subungual exostoses are broad, sessile osteochondromas centered under the nailbeds of the hands and feet. These lesions most commonly occur in the great toe.

Symptomatic presentation of these lesions is usually secondary to irritation of the adjacent muscles, tendons, nerves, and/or blood vessels. Adventitial bursa formation can occur secondary to inflammation overlying the hyaline cartilage cap of these exostoses. Occasionally, pedunculated osteochondromas can fracture, resulting in acute pain. Pseudoaneurysm formation secondary to mass effect exerted on an adjacent artery is rare and most commonly occurs in the popliteal artery. Osteochondromas within the spine can rarely result in cord compression. In addition, an osteochondroma arising from a rib can potentially present with a hemothorax or pneumothorax.

Approximately 80% of osteochondromas are monostotic. However, multiple osteochondromas can occur in the setting of multiple hereditary exostosis (MHE), which usually presents before 10 years of age. MHE demonstrates autosomal dominant inheritance with incomplete penetrance, with approximately 10% of cases occurring spontaneously (Fig. 14.12B–C). Patients with MHE present with growth disturbances secondary to the formation of multiple exostoses, resulting in limb length discrepancies, pseudo-Madelung deformities, and coxa valga. Notably, patients with MHE have a 1% to 5% lifetime risk for malignant degeneration to chondrosarcoma versus approximately 1% risk for malignant degeneration secondary to solitary osteochondromas.

Dysplasia epiphysealis hemimelica (Trevor-Fairbank disease) represents epiphyseal or epiphyseal equivalent osteochondroma-like lesions. Multiple exostoses are present in multiple bones of a single extremity in this condition, usually isolated to the medial or lateral aspects of a joint(s). Trevor-Fairbank disease usually presents before 15 years of age, with approximately 75% of cases occurring in boys. The legs, most notably the foot

and ankle, are a classic site of occurrence with secondary limb deformity resulting in mechanical symptoms. The epiphyses of the involved bones will demonstrate asymmetrical prominence and surface contour irregularity secondary to evolving multiple exostosis formation.

Radiographs are usually diagnostic in the imaging evaluation of osteochondromas. These lesions demonstrate corticomedullary continuity with the underlying host bone. Osteochondromas can manifest as broad-based lobulated sessile protuberances and narrow, bulbous pedunculated exostoses with an overlying hyaline cartilage cap. Pedunculated lesions have a thin stalk of attachment to the medullary cavity and cortex of the underlying host bone. These pedunculated osteochondromas usually point away from the adjacent joint as a result of traction as the host bone continues to elongate through endochondral ossification. Chondroid mineralization may be visualized within the cartilage cap.

Sonographic evaluation of osteochondromas can confirm cortical continuity of these protuberant lesions. Ultrasound can also evaluate the overlying hyaline cartilage cap, as well as the adjacent soft tissues, to evaluate for mass effect on adjacent blood vessels and potential adventitial bursa formation. Osteochondromas can result in vascular compression, occlusion, or pseudoaneurysm formation, most commonly of the popliteal artery.

MRI of osteochondromas can definitively illustrate flowing corticomedullary continuity with the underlying host bone with T1-weighted imaging (Fig. 14.12D). The overlying hyaline cartilage cap is hyperintense on fluid-sensitive sequences. Notably, the thickness of this cartilage cap is not predictive of malignant potential in skeletally immature patients. However, increasing thickness of the articular cartilage cap in a symptomatic osteochondroma is concerning for potential evolving malignant degeneration.

Fat-suppressed T2-weighted images are helpful in the evaluation of soft tissue complications of osteochondromas, such as adjacent adventitial bursa formation. Associated nerve compression will result in heterogeneous intramuscular edema and subsequent gradual muscle atrophy adjacent to osteochondromas. The hyaline cartilage cap will demonstrate variable enhancement with postcontrast MRI (see Fig. 14.12E).

Vascular compression can result in stenosis, occlusion, or pseudoaneurysm formation. MR angiography, or CT angiography with its high spatial resolution, can be used in the evaluation of suspected vascular compromise secondary to osteochondromas.

Fibrous Dysplasia

FD is a developmental dysplasia of bone formation and does not represent a true bone neoplasm. FD occurs secondary to a defect in osteoblastic differentiation and maturation leading to expanding intramedullary osseous lesions. These lesions represent metaplasia of normal intramedullary bone to immature woven trabecula and long spicules within an avascular, low cellular fibrous stroma. Microscopically these irregular trabeculae within the fibrous stroma exhibit a "Chinese letters" or "alphabet soup" appearance. FD is more

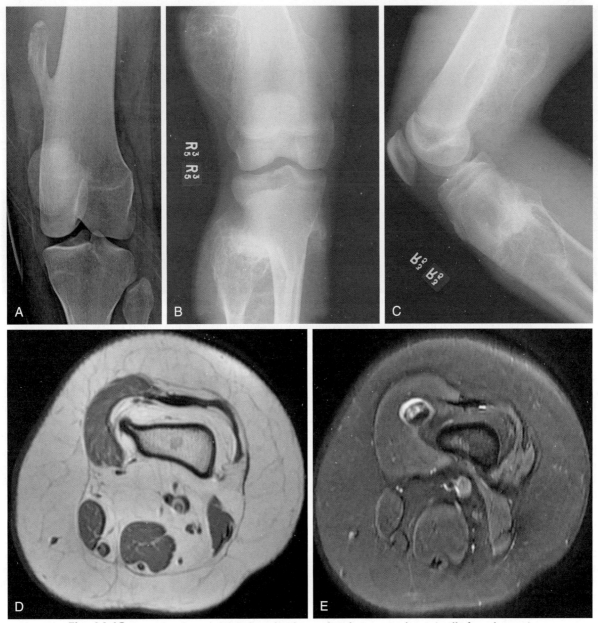

Fig. 14.12 Osteochondroma. (A) Pedunculated osteochondroma extends proximally from the proximal metadiaphysis of the distal left femur. (B–C) Multiple sessile and pedunculated exostoses throughout the region of the right knee in a patient with multiple hereditary exostoses. (D) Axial T1-weighted image demonstrates a pedunculated osteochondroma extending from the medial aspect of the distal left femur. This image demonstrates the lesion's confluence with the host bone's cortex and medullary cavity. (E) Axial T2-weighted fat supressed image shows lesion's T2-hyperintense cartilaginous cap. (Courtesy Tessa Balach, MD.)

common in girls than boys and most commonly presents in adolescents.

Seventy to eighty percent of FD cases are monostotic, and polyostotic cases tend to be unilateral in distribution, which can lead to limb-length discrepancy in approximately 70% of cases. The majority of patients with polyostotic disease are symptomatic by the age of 10 years. If FD occurs within the proximal femur, it can result in a varus bowing deformity of the femoral neck, classically described as a "shepherd's crook" appearance. FD can also result in anterior bowing of the tibia and protrusio acetabuli secondary to weakening of the

involved host bone. Pain and pathological fractures can occur secondary to these bowing deformities. Rarely, FD will undergo malignant degeneration to fibrosarcoma, chondrosarcoma, or osteosarcoma, which is more common in polyostotic and syndromic cases of FD.

McCune-Albright syndrome (MAS) is caused by a somatic mutation in the *GNAS1* gene and represents a subtype of polyostotic FD. MAS is more common in girls, representing 3% to 5% of all FD cases. MAS manifests as the classic triad of polyostotic FD, endocrine dysfunction, and cutaneous hyperpigmented "café-au-lait" skin lesions, which typically do not cross midline. These

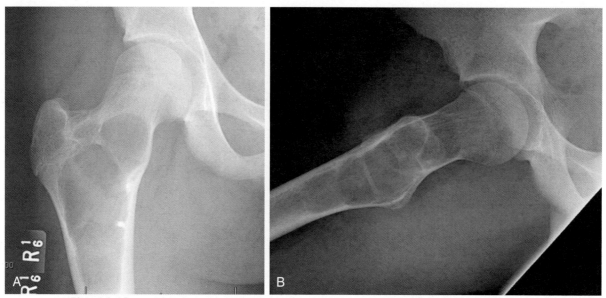

Fig. 14.13 Fibrous dysplasia. (A–B) Medullary expansion and ground-glass matrix throughout the distal right femoral neck, intertrochanteric region, and the proximal right femoral metadiaphysis. No associated pathological fracture and/or gross deformity of the proximal femur at this time. (Courtesy Tessa Balach, MD.)

café-au-lait lesions classically exhibit irregular margins with a "coast of Maine" morphology, versus the more regular "coast of California" morphology that occurs in the setting of neurofibromatosis type I. Patients with MAS can present with sexual precocity, hyperthyroidism, diabetes mellitus, hyperparathyroidism, or acromegaly. Mazabraud syndrome is extremely rare in children, characterized by polyostotic FD and multiple intramuscular myxomas.

Medullary expansion is generally most prominent secondary to FD lesions within the skull base and maxillofacial bones. Most cases of craniofacial FD are polyostotic. Bilateral FD of the mandible is inherited in an autosomal dominant pattern secondary to a defect in the c-Abl-binding protein SH3BP2, which results in a "cherubic" facial appearance. Hearing loss also can occur in craniofacial FD secondary to temporal bone involvement. Proptosis and cranial nerve impingement also can occur secondary to orbital and skull base foraminal involvement, respectively.

FD usually manifests as monostotic central geographical intramedullary lesions with variable medullary expansion within the diaphysis of long bones, most commonly the femur and tibia (Fig. 14.13A–B). These lesions often demonstrate thin, sclerotic margins and can extend within the metaphysis and occasionally to the epiphysis after physeal closure. FD also can occur within the pelvis and ribs. FD, like OFD, also can occur within the anterior cortex of the tibia.

FD radiographically presents as nonaggressive geographical intramedullary lesions. The majority of FD lesions demonstrate a mildly sclerotic "ground-glass" matrix relative to the amount of abnormal immature intramedullary woven bone within the lesion. However, lesions within the bony pelvis often demonstrate a more lytic bubbly appearance. Conversely, lesions within the base can exhibit dense sclerosis. CT evaluation, with its high spatial resolution, is usually reserved for lesions involving the skull base and maxillofacial structures for thorough evaluation of the orbits, skull base foramina, and inner ear structures.

These intramedullary lesions usually demonstrate T1-and T2-hypointense internal signal depending on the amount of underlying internal irregular woven bone. Internal regions of cystic change may be present on fluid-sensitive sequences. A T1-, T2-hypointense rind can form if cystic change is present within these lesions.

FD lesions demonstrate variable heterogeneous internal enhancement and may result in secondary ABC formation. Nuclear medicine bone scan will demonstrate variable radiotracer uptake within these lesions. Image-guided core needle biopsy is diagnostic for these lesions.

Chondroblastoma

Chondroblastomas are uncommon painful benign bone lesions composed of closely packed immature chondroblasts within a heterogeneous matrix containing scattered mature cartilage and giant cells. These painful lesions incite a marked surrounding inflammatory response resulting in marrow and soft tissue edema, as well as reactive joint effusions. Chondroblastomas can present secondary to pain, stiffness, swelling, and/or limping in the second decade of life. Most of these lesions occur within the epiphyses of long tubular bones with metaphyseal extension in approximately 50% of cases. Chondroblastomas most commonly occur within the epiphyses of the proximal tibia, proximal and distal femur, and proximal humerus. These lesions also occur in apophyses and epiphyseal equivalents, such as the patella, talus, calcaneus, tarsals, and carpals. Secondary ABC formation can occur in approximately 30% of cases.

Radiographically, chondroblastomas manifest as eccentric, geographical, lucent epiphyseal lesions within a long bone (Fig. 14.14A). Thirty to fifty percent of these

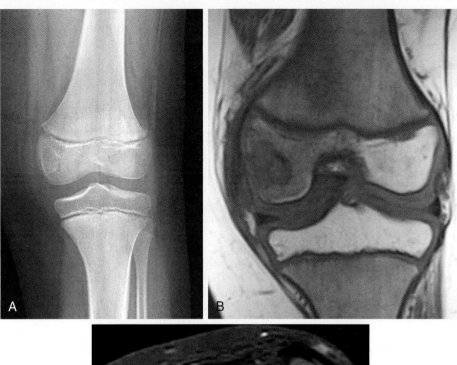

Fig. 14.14 Chondroblastoma. (A) Lucent lesion with sclerotic margins in the medial distal femoral epiphysis; (B) Coronal T1-weighted image shows a T1-hypointense lesion; (C) Axial T2-weighted fat supressed imaged shows signficant surround marrow edema and adjacent soft tissue edema.

lesions will demonstrate an internal matrix containing chondroid "rings and arcs" and exhibit thin sclerotic smooth or multilobulated borders. Medullary expansion can occur; however, the overlying cortex is usually intact. Bubbly, expansile remodeling can occur in the setting of secondary ABC formation. Solid, nonaggressive periosteal reaction can also occur along the adjacent metaphysis.

CT is generally reserved for image-guided biopsy and will demonstrate the calcified internal chondroid matrix. Chondroblastomas exhibit heterogeneous T1 internal signal with T1-hypointense signal within the peripheral rim. Heterogeneous internal T2-hyper- and -hypointense signal can be present secondary to heterogeneous calcification, hemosiderin deposition, and solid components. The thin peripheral rim will demonstrate T2-hypointense signal. Perilesional marrow, periosteal, and soft tissue edema are characteristic of these lesions (Fig. 14.4C). Chondroblastomas demonstrate heterogeneous internal enhancement, as well as enhancement of

the aforementioned perilesional marrow and soft tissue edema with postcontrast MRI.

Reactive joint effusions are present in approximately 50% of chondroblastomas. Multiple intralesion fluid–fluid levels indicate the formation of a secondary ABC, which occurs in approximately 15% to 30% of cases. Chondroblastomas rarely undergo malignant degeneration; however, benign lung metastases can occur. The differential diagnosis for a radiolucent epiphyseal lesion in a young patient is chondroblastoma, LCH, osteomyelitis, osteoblastoma, and GCT, after physeal closure.

Enchondroma

Enchondromas are benign, predominantly hypocellular, avascular chondroid neoplasms composed of foci of intramedullary hyaline cartilage thought to be secondary to focal failure of normal periphyseal endochondral bone formation. These chondroid lesions migrate within the metaphyses and diametaphyses with continued longitudinal growth of the host bone. Enchondromas

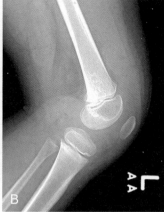
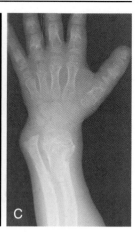

Fig. 14.15 Enchondroma. (A–B) Geographical, intramedullary, "bubbly" nonaggressive lesion within the distal left femoral metaphysis. (C) Deformation of the distal forearm and phalanges secondary to multiple expansile intramedullary enchondromas in this patient with Ollier disease. (Courtesy Tessa Balach, MD.)

become increasingly common with age, with a peak incidence within the third decade of life. These nonaggressive lesions are commonly asymptomatic and incidentally discovered; however, enchondromas can be painful, and secondary pathological fractures can occur.

These nonaggressive geographical central lesions commonly occur in the metaphyses of long bones with the proximal humerus, proximal and distal femur, and proximal tibia representing the most common sites of occurrence. However, approximately 50% of enchondromas occur within the small bones of the hands and feet. Indeed, enchondromas represent approximately 80% of primary bone tumors of the hand in pediatric patients.

Although these benign neoplasms are geographical, they rarely demonstrate a sclerotic rim radiographically. The chondroid matrix may exhibit multiple morphologies, including the classic rings and arcs appearance. However, the chondroid matrix may be extremely subtle or absent radiographically (Fig. 14.15A–B). Endosteal scalloping can occur secondary to these lesions, most notably if they are eccentrically located within the medullary cavity. Rare malignant transformation should be considered if endosteal scalloping involves greater than two-thirds of the overlying cortex and extends over two-thirds of the lesion.

Cortical disruption does not occur in the absence of a pathological fracture or rare malignant degeneration to chondrosarcoma. Periosteal reaction also will not occur in the absence of pathological fracture or malignant degeneration. Notably, malignant degeneration to chondrosarcoma is exceedingly rare in young patients with a solitary enchondroma.

Enchondromas exhibit a lytic, expansile, bubbly appearance when they occur in the small bones of the hands and feet. The chondroid matrix is most commonly subtle or absent within these peripheral lesions, which are the most common neoplasm of small tubular bones. These enchondromas may enlarge with age and exhibit increased matrix mineralization.

Ollier disease (enchondromatosis) is a nonhereditary disorder of cartilage proliferation that is more common in boys and results in enchondroma formation within multiple bones. Ollier disease most commonly affects the hands; however, any bone with a physis can

be affected (see Fig. 14.15C). These enchondromas are bilateral and asymmetrical and can result in striking hand deformities. The multiple intramedullary lucent lesions are usually expansile with thinned overlying cortex. They can also interfere with adjacent physeal function, leading to limb shortening.

Maffucci syndrome is a nonhereditary enchondromatosis associated with multiple vascular malformations within the soft tissues, which are predominantly venous in origin. Multiple calcified phleboliths will be present in these soft tissue vascular masses. The risk for malignant transformation to chondrosarcoma is significantly elevated in patients with Ollier and Maffucci syndromes; however, malignant transformation remains extremely rare in children.

Enchondromas demonstrate low-to-intermediate signal on T1-weighted imaging, heterogeneously hyperintense on T2-weighted imaging, typical of chondroid lesions, and may contain foci of normal internal fatty marrow. The internal chondroid matrix, if present, will result in heterogeneous T2-hypointense signal. These benign lesions will also demonstrate thin peripheral and septal enhancement following contrast administration. Internal solid enhancing components are indicative of malignant degeneration. Notably, enchondromas may show increased radiotracer uptake with Tc-99m-MDP bone scan, unless very small in size.

Fibroxanthomas (Fibrous Cortical Defect/ Nonossifying Fibroma)

Fibroxanthomas are the second most common bone lesion in young patients and are composed of spindle cells in a collagenous matrix often demonstrating a swirling storiform pattern with a variable number of lipid-bearing xanthomatous cells and hemosiderin pigment-laden histiocytes. Fibrous cortical defects (FCDs) and NOFs are histologically identical and considered the same lesion. In general, lesions smaller than 2 cm are called *fibrous cortical defects*, while lesions greater than 2 cm are called *NOFs*.

These masses are most commonly detected incidentally and generally considered to be developmental in etiology rather than representing true neoplasms and represent "do not touch" lesions that can be diagnosed radiographically with no additional imaging and/or

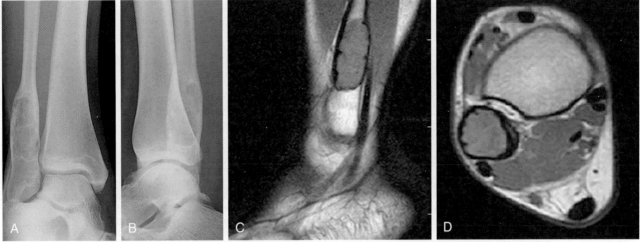

Fig. 14.16 Fibroxanthoma. (A–B) Geographical, "bubbly," nonaggressive lesion that results in medullary expansion of the distal right fibula with no associated cortical disruption or periosteal reaction. (C–D) Sagittal and axial T1-weighted images show an expansile T1-hypointense lesion with a thin surrounding rim of sclerosis and no associated cortical disruption or periosteal reaction. (Courtesy Tessa Balach, MD.)

biopsy. They are usually asymptomatic and rarely result in associated pathological fractures. However, large lesions can result in dull, vague discomfort. These lesions most commonly occur in the first two decades of life, occur in boys more than girls, and usually spontaneously involute and heal. Rarely, these lesions persist into adulthood.

Multiple NOFs can be seen in the seen in the setting of Neurofibromatosis type I. In addition, Jaffe-Campanacci syndrome is characterized by disseminated NOFs of the long bones and mandible, multiple café-au-lait spots, mental retardation, ocular malformations, hypogonadism, cryptorchidism, and cardiovascular anomalies.

FCDs and NOFs commonly occur within the cortex of the metaphyses of the distal femur and proximal tibia, as well as the distal tibia. The overlying cortex can be thinned and expanded secondary to these lesions; however, frank cortical disruption occurs only in the setting of an associated pathological fracture. These lesions can migrate within the metadiaphyses of these long bones with continued longitudinal bone growth. These lesions are cortically based except when they occur in gracile bones, such as the fibula and ulna, in which the entire width of the bone can be occupied by the lesion. FCDs and NOFs also tend to be more central in location when they are prominent in size.

FCDs and NOFs are classically geographical, lytic lesions with thin, sclerotic margins. The margins are most commonly smooth in contour and can become multilobulated as these lesions increase in size. The long axis of the lesion is typically aligned with the long axis of the host bone (Fig. 14.16A–B). They demonstrate a thicker, more sclerotic margin as they begin to heal, sclerose, and involute. Eventually, they become entirely sclerotic and may entirely remodel to normal bone.

If MRI is performed, these lesions typically demonstrate T1-hypointense signal internally. The peripheral rim of reactive sclerosis will demonstrate greater

T1-hypointensity (see Fig. 14.16C–D). These lesions exhibit heterogeneous internal T2 signal depending on the variable amounts of fibrous tissue and hemosiderin within these lesions. T2-hypointense septa can be present within these lesions with fluid-sensitive sequences. These lesions do not incite reactive marrow edema unless associated with a pathological fracture. Avid peripheral and septal enhancement may be present. No cortical disruption or associated soft tissue mass should be present secondary to FCDs and NOFs.

These masses can have minimal to mild radiotracer uptake with Tc-99m-MDP bone scans. Intense radiotracer uptake can occur in the setting of healing of these lesions. ^{18}F-FDG-avidity is variable, and be intense which can mimic malignancy.

Chondromyxoid Fibroma

CMF represents a rare benign lobulated cartilage neoplasm composed of fibrous, myxoid, and chondroid tissues. CMFs most commonly occur in the second decade of life with a male predominance. Approximately 60% of these lesions occur within the metaphyses and diaphyses of long bones, with the metaphysis of proximal tibia representing the most frequent site of occurrence. CMFs also occur within the tubular bones of the hands and feet, as well as the flat bones of the axial skeleton. The iliac wing is the most common site of CMF occurrence within the flat bones.

CMFs are eccentric, geographical, radiolucent intramedullary lesions with sclerotic margins. As described earlier, these neoplasms most commonly occur within the metaphysis of the proximal tibia and can extend to the subarticular zone of the epiphysis. The long axis of these masses is parallel with the long axis of the host bone. These lesions are multilobulated with associated medullary and cortical expansion with secondary overlying cortical thinning, which can result in a bubbly appearance. Pseudotrabeculations occur within these masses, which can appear radiographically as internal

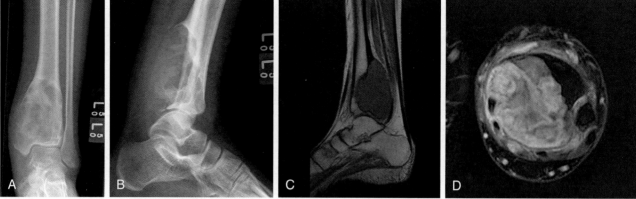

Fig. 14.17 Chondromyxoid fibroma. (A–B) Markedly expansile, "bubbly" lesion centered within the distal left tibial metaphysis with associated prominent cortical thinning and no associated aggressive periosteal reaction or evidence of a soft tissue mass component. (C) Sagittal T1-weighted image shows homogenous T1-hypointnese lesion centered within the posterior aspect of the distal left tibial metaphysis with associated prominent overlying cortical thinning and no associated aggressive periosteal reaction or evidence of a soft tissue mass component. (D) Contrast-enhanced axial T1-weighted fat-supressed image demonstrates heterogeneous internal enhancement of the lesion centered within the posterior aspect of the distal left tibial metaphysis. (Courtesy Tessa Balach, MD.)

septations (Fig. 14.17A–B). These lesions rarely result in an associated soft tissue mass component. No periosteal reaction occurs secondary to these nonaggressive benign lesions in the absence of pathological fracture.

On MRI, CMFs are generally T1-isointense with heterogeneous internal T1-hyperintense foci and a T1-hypointense sclerotic margin. These multilobulated masses can be T2-hyperintense centrally with peripheral intermediate T2-hyperintensity or diffusely and homogeneously T2-hyperintense. CMFs exhibit peripheral nodular or diffuse enhancement with hypoenhancement of the peripheral rim. Image-guided percutaneous biopsy can be performed for definitive histological diagnosis of these lesions.

Distal Femoral Avulsive Irregularity

Distal femoral avulsive irregularity can develop along the posteromedial aspect of the distal metaphysis in the region of the attachments of the medial head of the gastrocnemius and aponeurosis of the adductor magnus. This incidental finding can raise concern for an aggressive osseous lesion within the distal femur if the radiologist is not aware of this benign entity.

This focal avulsive cortical irregularity is commonly asymptomatic and incidentally discovered on lateral knee radiographs in the second decade of life. This finding is likely secondary to chronic cortical microtrauma due to repetitive traction on the posteromedial supracondylar region of the distal femur at the origin of the medial head of the gastrocnemius. This chronic avulsive microtrauma can result in focal cortical irregularity and possible interruption with adjacent cortical thickening. The deep margin of this focal cortical irregularity commonly demonstrates a concave contour with heterogeneous reactive sclerosis. In addition, solid periosteal reaction and cortical thickening can be present along the margins of this focal irregularity.

Radiographs of the contralateral knee can assist in making this diagnosis because these lesions are bilateral

in greater than 25% of cases. MRI of the distal femur can provide further imaging evaluation if necessary. A thin T1- and T2-hypointense rim is classically present along the anterior deep aspect of the focal cortical irregularity immediately deep to the origin of the medial head of the gastrocnemius. Minimal surrounding marrow edema can be present. The periosteum overlying these lesions remains intact with no associated juxtacortical soft tissue mass.

The lack of an associated soft tissue mass and aggressive periosteal reaction morphologies, as well as the location within the distal posteromedial aspect of the femur, should indicate to the radiologist the benign nature of this lesion. Focal reactive bone formation with collagenous fibrous tissue at the avulsion site can mimic an aggressive malignancy if a biopsy is performed. Therefore this self-limited finding is a "do not touch lesion."

Osteoid Osteoma/Osteoblastoma

Osteoid osteoma is a benign osteoblastic mass (nidus) of interlaced trabeculae of osteoid within a fibrovascular stroma with a prominent surrounding zone of reactive sclerosis. Osteoid osteomas are the third most common benign bone neoplasm in young patients, primarily occurring within Caucasian males. Notably, prostaglandin E_2 is markedly elevated within the nidus, which results in vasodilation and the classic insidious nocturnal pain associated with these lesions. This pain is successfully decreased with nonsteroidal antiinflammatory drugs in approximately 75% of cases. Nonsteroidal antiinflammatory drugs can also expedite lesion healing and regression over the course of years. However, image-guided therapy is definitive if the entire nidus is successfully ablated.

Osteoid osteomas most commonly present in the second decade of life. These lesions do not demonstrate malignant degeneration and have limited growth potential. They can result in angular long bone overgrowth secondary to hyperemia.

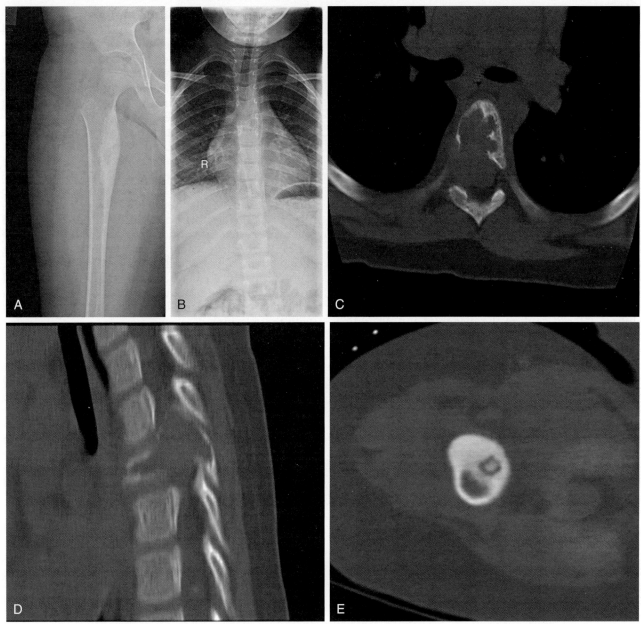

Fig. 14.18 Osteoid osteoma. (A) Focal, geographical, radiolucent lesion within the medial cortex of the proximal right femoral metaphysis with adjacent exuberant fusiform cortical thickening. (B) Radiolucent, bubbly lesion within the T6 vertebra with associated vertebral body height, most notably within the right side of the vertebra. (C–D) Low-attenuation, multilobulated lesion, with a thin, narrow zone of transition centered within the right side of the T6 vertebra on this noncontrast CT image. (E) Well-circumscribed low-attenuation cortically based lesion contains a high-attenuation nidus. This lesion is surrounded by exuberant fusiform cortical thickening on this non-contrast-enhanced axial CT image. (Courtesy Tessa Balach, MD.)

Osteoid osteomas are cortically based in 70% to 80% of cases and most commonly occur within the diaphyses and metaphyses of the long bones of the lower extremities. The femur and tibia are the most sites followed by the phalanges of the hands and feet. The single most common site of occurrence is the femoral neck (Fig. 14.18A). Less frequently, these masses occur in intramedullary and subperiosteal locations within the epiphysis or epiphyseal equivalents. Osteoid osteomas also can occur within the posterior elements of the spine.

Intraarticular lesions involving the hip can result in pain, limp, and decreased range of motion. Spine lesions can result in a painful scoliosis with the spine concavity occurring toward the side of the lesion in 50% to 60% of cases.

Osteoblastomas are nearly histologically identical to osteoid osteoma; however, these lesions are larger, with niduses greater than 1.5 cm in diameter. Osteoblastomas also occur later in life, with the majority presenting in the second and third decades. Forty percent of osteoblastomas occur in the spine and typically result in less frequent pain and reactive bone formation. These spine lesions are often expansile, typically occurring within the posterior elements, and can extend anteriorly within the vertebral body (Fig. 14.18B). They appear as a well-circumscribed, expansile mass with a narrow zone of transition and surrounding reactive sclerosis. Neurological symptoms can occur secondary to compression of the cord and/or exiting nerve roots (Fig. 14.18C–D). Another characteristic location of osteoblastomas is the neck of the talus. Secondary ABC development can occur in 10% to 15% of cases.

The nidus of osteoid osteomas can be difficult to visualize radiographically because of the small size of these lesions. If visualized, osteoid osteomas appear radiographically as a partially calcified round or ovoid radiolucent nidus with prominent surrounding cortical and intramedullary sclerosis. Intramedullary and intraarticular osteoid osteomas generate less surrounding reactive sclerosis. Periosteal reaction can occur and manifests as smooth, solid morphology that can be remote from the site of an intraarticular lesion.

Focused CT evaluation is highly effective in the evaluation of osteoid osteomas due to its high spatial resolution. CT can confirm the diagnosis and determine the anatomical location of the nidus, which facilitates follow-up image-guided or surgical treatment. The nidus appears as a round or ovoid low-attenuation focus with possible central heterogeneous calcification. Surrounding cortical thickening, as well as overlying smooth solid periosteal reaction, is well visualized with CT imaging (see Fig. 14.18E). CT is also used for image-guided radiofrequency ablation, laser photocoagulation, or cryoablation of osteoid osteomas. Surgical and image-guided treatment is effective in approximately 90% of cases.

MRI appearances are variable, due to differing degrees of mineralization within the nidus. For example, unmineralized nidus is intermediate to high in signal intense on T2-weighted imaging. Heterogeneous mineralization within the nidus results in T1- and T2-hypointense signal. Additionally, the nidus can exhibit a target appearance on T2-weighted imaging with central T2-hypointense signal secondary to mineralization surrounded by T2-hyperintense signal as a result of unmineralized fibrovascular stroma and a peripheral T2-hypointense rim secondary to surrounding reactive sclerosis. Osteoid osteomas incite prominent surrounding marrow, periosteal, and soft tissue edema. Indeed, the degree of prominent surrounding reactive marrow edema can potentially obscure a small nidus. Prominent marrow edema within the femoral neck can be indicative of an intraarticular osteoid osteoma. A reactive joint effusion and synovitis also occur with intraarticular and periarticular osteoid osteomas. With contrast admintration, the nidus enhances avidly, and a to greater degree than the surrounding marrow.

On Tc-99m-MDP bone scans, osteoid osteomas will appears as a a focus of intense radiotracer uptake within the nidus surrounded by rim of less intense radiotracer uptake, representing the "double density" sign. Single-photon emission CT increases the sensitivity for detection of subtle spinal osteoid osteomas. The sensitivity of bone scan for the detection of an osteoid osteoma is approximately 100%.

Periosteal (Juxtacortical) Chondroma

Periosteal chondromas are rare lobulated chondroid surface lesions that most commonly arise from the surfaces of the metaphyses of long bones. These benign neoplasms are histologically similar to enchondromas. Periosteal chondromas can be symptomatic with patients presenting with pain and swelling of the affected extremity in the second decade of life.

These lesions most commonly occur along the metaphyses of the proximal humerus and femur in approximately 70% of cases. These nonaggressive neoplasms also can arise from the phalanges of the hands and feet (Fig. 14.19A). Radiographically these surface lesions result in saucerization of the underlying cortex of the host bone with associated marginal sclerosis. Periosteal chondromas also classically incite dense periosteal reaction and cortical buttressing along the proximal and distal aspects of these lesions. Approximately 75% of lesions exhibit mineralized internal chondroid matrix production. Notably, an adjacent soft tissue mass can be present associated with these lesions.

These lobulated masses demonstrate nonspecific iso-intense to hypointense internal T1 signal with heterogeneous, predominantly peripheral enhancement with multiaxial precontrast and postcontrast T1-weighted sequences (see Fig. 14.19B). These neoplasms also exhibit hyperintense T2 internal signal with fluid-sensitive sequences (see Fig. 14.19C). Notably, intramedullary extension and marrow edema are present in approximately 20% of cases. Further, irregular soft tissue margins also occur in approximately 30% of cases.

Periosteal chondromas should be surgically excised because periosteal chondrosarcoma, periosteal osteosarcoma, parosteal osteosarcoma, and high-grade surface osteosarcoma can all demonstrate similar radiological appearances and sites of occurrence.

Unicameral Bone Cyst

UBCs are benign fluid-filled intramedullary cystic lesions containing serous and/or serosanguinous fluid that are not true neoplasms. They are lined by a thin membrane of loose vascular connective tissue with partial septa that may contain hemosiderin, reactive bone, osteoclast-like giant cells, and fibrous material. The term *unicameral* is a misnomer because these lesions can demonstrate internal septa, loculations, and inhomogeneous fluid contents.

These lesions most commonly present in the second decade of life and are three more times more common in boys. UBCs are usually asymptomatic unless complicated by a pathological fracture. Approximately 70% of these cysts present with pain secondary to an acute pathological fracture. Indeed, these lesions are the most common cause of pathological fractures in pediatric patients.

These cysts are classically located centrally within the metaphyses of long bones, most commonly the proximal humerus, proximal femur, and proximal tibia. UBCs also can occur within the pelvis and calcaneus in older patients. Many of these lesions resolve spontaneously as patients approach skeletal maturity.

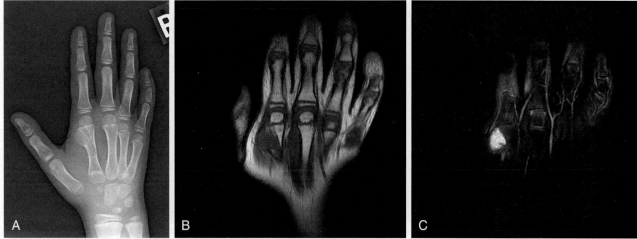

Fig. 14.19 Juxtacortical chondroma. (A) Geographical lesion demonstrates homogeneous T1-isointense signal centered along the radial cortex of the second metacarpal with no associated aggressive periosteal reaction or evidence of a soft tissue mass component on this T1 non-fat-saturated image. (C) Geographical lesion demonstrates fairly homogeneous enhancement centered along the radial cortex of the second metacarpal with no associated enhancing adjacent marrow edema or enhancing soft tissue mass component. (Courtesy Tesssa Balach, MD.)

Simple bone cysts arise centrally within the medullary cavity of the metaphyses of long bones. The long axis of these lesions is parallel with the long axis of the host bone. These geographical lesions have thin sclerotic margins and may contain pseudotrabeculations or septa. Mild circumferential medullary expansion with overlying cortical thinning is also associated with these lesions.

No cortical disruption or periosteal reaction occurs in the absence of a pathological fracture. If a fracture occurs, the resulting periosteal reaction will have benign smooth morphology. A "fallen fragment" sign may be present following pathological fracture, representing the migration of a fractured fragment of bone to a dependent position within the cyst. CT is the most effective modality for evaluating a potential pathological fracture of a UBC and secondary fallen fragment.

UBCs are non-enhancing low attenuation lesions (15 to 20 HUs). Fluid-fluid levels may be present and this, does not preclude the diagnosis of a simple bone cyst. A bubble of gas in an anti-dependent portion of the cyst can be seen in the setting of a pathological fracture, called the "rising bubble" sign.

MRI will confirm the cystic nature of these lesions, which a typically hyperintense on fluid sensitive sequences. may . Due to the presence of hemorrhage, the cyst cavity may be heterogenous and hyperintense on T1-weighted imaging. In 80% of cases, there is enhancement of the thin rim of connective tissue; a minority of UBCs enhance centrally. Septa, if present, may enhance.

Aneurysmal Bone Cyst

ABCs are benign cystic lesions composed of blood-filled cavities separated by fibrous septa. These complex cysts may arise from osseous arteriovenous malformations or venous obstruction secondary to prior trauma. ABCs most commonly occur in the first two decades of life. Seventy percent of these cysts are primary lesions, whereas secondary ABCs can arise from underlying primary osseous masses. These cysts can undergo phases of rapid growth that result in lytic bone destruction and periosteal reaction that can be concerning for an aggressive lesion. ABCs can result in pain secondary to this rapid growth and bone destruction, and pathological fractures can occur in 20% of cases.

ABCs usually arise within the metaphyses of long bones resulting in prominent medullary and cortical expansion. These lesions most commonly occur within the femur, tibia, and humerus and can migrate within the diametaphysis with continued longitudinal bone growth (Fig. 14.20A). Approximately 15% of ABCs occur within the posterior elements of the spine. These spine lesions may extend anteriorly within the vertebral body, as well as cross the intervertebral disk to involve the adjacent vertebra. Rarely, ABCs can occur within the tubular bones of the hands.

These cysts are geographical with a narrow zone of transition with intact thin sclerotic margins in approximately 60% of cases. These cysts may contain trabeculations, but internal matrix production is exceedingly rare. Periosteal reaction is variable. CT evaluation is again helpful if there is clinical concern for a pathological fracture.

ABCs exhibit multiple internal septa with MRI. Multiple fluid–fluid levels are present within ABCs secondary to different stages of internal degrading blood products, which are most prominent on multiaxial fluid-sensitive sequences (see Fig. 14.20B–C). These cysts can result in surrounding marrow and soft tissue edema. These lesions demonstrate no enhancement within the internal cystic components with post-contrast imaging; however, the fibrous septa enhance, resulting in a honeycomb appearance. Nuclear medicine bone scans will demonstrate the "donut sign" in approximately 60% of cases of ABCs, secondary to the avascular central photopenic cystic region surrounded

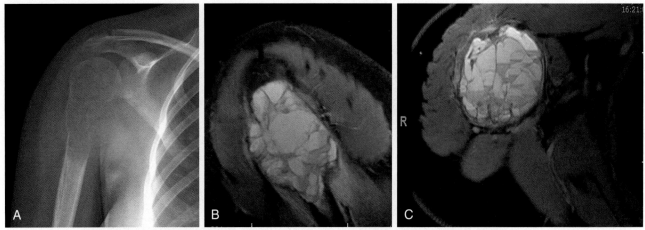

Fig. 14.20 (A) Radiolucent, "bubbly," intramedullary lesion centered within the proximal right humeral metaphysis demonstrates medullary expansion and associated overlying cortical thinning with no matrix production, aggressive periosteal reaction, or soft tissue mass component. (B) Sagittal T2 fat-saturated image demonstrates multiple fluid–fluid levels throughout an intramedullary lesion within the proximal humerus resulting in medullary expansion and associated overlying cortical thinning with no matrix production, aggressive periosteal reaction, or soft tissue mass component. (C) Axial T2 fat-saturated image demonstrates multiple fluid–fluid levels throughout an intramedullary lesion within the proximal humerus resulting in medullary expansion and associated overlying cortical thinning with no matrix production, aggressive periosteal reaction, or soft tissue mass component. (Courtesy Tessa Balach, MD.)

by increased radiotracer uptake within the peripheral marrow edema.

Notably, telangiectatic osteosarcoma can demonstrate a similar appearance as ABCs. However, telangiectatic osteosarcomas will tend to have incomplete margins with a wide zone of transition and result in focal cortical destruction with secondary soft tissue mass formation. Also, there tends to be prominent internal solid component within telangiectatic osteosarcomas.

GCTs also can demonstrate an appearance similar with ABCs. GCTs are also eccentric, metaphyseal lesions that can be as bubbly and expanded as ABCs. However, GCTs are solid neoplasms with associated internal T2-hypointense signal. Also, GCTs also tend to extend to the subchondral bone of the epiphysis after physeal closure, which is rare with ABCs. Notably, ABCs can arise secondarily from GCTs.

Secondary ABCs can arise from a GCT, osteoblastoma, chondroblastoma, and, less commonly, FD, CMF, fibroxanthoma, and solitary bone cyst.

■ Summary

A systemic approach to pediatric and adolescent bone lesions can facilitate the generation of a succinct and accurate differential diagnosis. The differential of an osseous lesion in a young patient can be significantly honed with simple consideration of the patient's age and an understanding of which bone lesions tend to occur in the different age groups and host bones of pediatric and adolescent patients.

Radiographs remain the mainstay in the imaging evaluation of bone lesions in young patients. Radiographs demonstrate many of the imaging characteristics of osseous lesions required in the formulation of an accurate differential diagnosis. However, CT and MRI, as well as nuclear medicine and ultrasound examinations, can provide additional valuable imaging information of bone lesions. Further, image-guided biopsy using ultrasound or CT can yield the final diagnosis of a bone lesion in young patients.

CHAPTER 15
Vascular Malformations

Frederic J. Bertino

CHAPTER OUTLINE

Imaging Vascular Malformations, 313
Simple Vascular Malformations, 313
Capillary Malformations, 313
Lymphatic Malformations, 314
Venous Malformations, 315

Arteriovenous Malformations, 316
Arteriovenous Fistulas, 318
Combined Vascular Malformations, 318
Anomalies of Major Named Vessels, 318
Vascular Malformations Associated With Other
    Vascular Anomalies, 318

Vascular malformations arise from disorganized angiogenesis and manifest as congenital abnormalities that may be isolated events or associated with syndromes. The International Society for the Study of Vascular Anomalies (ISSVA) recognizes vascular malformations as a separate entity from vascular tumors and classifies vascular malformations into four major groups: simple, combined, anomalies of major vessels, and those associated with other vascular anomalies. Vascular tumors, including infantile hemangioma, rapidly involuting congenital hemangioma, noninvoluting congenital hemangioma, and kaposiform hemangioendothelioma are discussed in Chapter 16.

■ Imaging Vascular Malformations

Vascular malformations may be imaged using several modalities. Ultrasound, often the first line imaging modality for a suspected vascular malformation, is helpful for the identification of superficial and deep malformations without using ionizing radiation. The added utility of color and spectral Doppler can accurately define venous and arterial anatomy, and provide nidus size and the number of feeding and draining vessels. It can also be used to assess the presence or absence of a deep venous system in affected extremities. MRI, however, is the mainstay in the imaging of most vascular malformations, owing to its superior contrast resolution and techniques providing temporal resolution. A typical protocol for imaging malformations uses conventional nonenhanced T1-weighted fast spin echo (T1W FSE), contrast-enhanced T1W FSE with fat suppression, and T2W FSE with fat suppression. Time-resolved angiographic sequences provide temporal resolution and can accurately identify abnormal arterial and venous structures and help to assess lesion enhance patterns.

Table 15.1 provides a summary of the imaging findings expected with the vascular malformations discussed in subsequent sections.

■ Simple Vascular Malformations

Simple vascular malformations are subdivided into low- and high-flow malformations. Low-flow malformations include capillary, venous, and lymphatic malformations, whereas high-flow malformations include arteriovenous malformations (AVMs) and fistulas.

■ Capillary Malformations

Capillary malformations (CM) are the most common vascular malformation and histologically present as disorganized capillary vessels embedded in the skin and subcutaneous tissues. Because of their superficial nature, CM presents as a cutaneous discoloration that is often pink-red and eponymously referred to as a port-wine stain. These lesions are frequently diagnosed on direct inspection, prompting further evaluation. CMs are infrequently imaged in isolation, with imaging often performed to identify larger vascular malformations deeper within the body. Imaging manifestations of CM may show skin or subcutaneous tissue thickening that may enhance after intravenous contrast administration. Sonographic findings of a port-wine stain are nonspecific and can demonstrate skin thickening with or without flow on color Doppler imaging.

TABLE 15.1   Summary of Imaging Findings of Vascular Malformations

| | ULTRASOUND | | MAGNETIC RESONANCE IMAGING | | |
MALFORMATION	GRAYSCALE	DOPPLER	T2W	T1W	T1W+C
Slow Flow					
Capillary	Normal Mild skin thickening	Normal-to-moderate vascular density	Mild skin thickening	Mild skin thickening	Enhancing skin lesions
Lymphatic					
Microcystic	Echogenic soft tissue thickening Ill-defined masslike tissue No large cysts	No flow within cystic spaces (if any) Possible minimal flow in tiny septa	Hyperintense due to microcystic spaces	Isointense to hypointense relative to muscle	Septal enhancement
Macrocystic	Well-defined lobulated anechoic cystic spaces +/– Fluid–fluid levels	No flow in cystic spaces +/– Flow in septa	Hyperintense fluid-filled cysts with septations Fluid–fluid levels if internal hemorrhage or infection	Isointense to hypointense relative to muscle	Septal enhancement
Venous	Compressible tubular structures +/– Fluid–fluid levels +/– Thrombi or phleboliths	Monophasic venous waveform +/– Flow depending on stagnancy of blood or thrombosed venous malformation Valsalva maneuver or compression may augment flow	Hyperintense focal or multifocal transspatial lobulated lesions Varicosities Phleboliths: low T2 Thrombi: low T2	Isointense to hyperintense relative to muscle Fat interspersed within the lesion is common No flow voids Phleboliths: low T1 Thrombi: high T1	Slow progressive enhancement on MRA No arterial component No rapid draining system
Fast Flow					
Arteriovenous	Anechoic tortuous tubular structures with central cluster (nidus)	Color signal within the anechoic spaces and nidus; mix of venous and arterial waveforms Classic high-flow, low-resistance waveform Venous waveforms may appear arterialized and show spectral broadening	Soft tissue or bone edema	Prominent flow voids with a central nidus on spin-echo sequences	Enhancement of the arterial vessels with rapid filling of draining veins on MRA Flow voids may be appreciated, as well as enhancing edematous soft tissue
Arteriovenous fistula	Vessels without central nidus	Turbulent high-flow, low-resistance waveform Yin-yang pseudoaneurysm appearance is common Arterialized draining vein is common	Soft tissue edema	Flow void without central nidus Large shunt into an arterialized large draining vein	Flow voids often seen Single feeding artery with large draining vein without central nidus on MRA

+C, with contrast; MRA, Magnetic resonance angiography; T1W, T1 weighted; T2W, T2 weighted.
Adapted from Bertino, F., Braithwaite, K. A., Hawkins, C. M., Gill, A. E., Briones, M. A., Swerdlin, R., & Milla, S. S. (2019). Congenital limb overgrowth syndromes associated with vascular anomalies. *Radiographics*, 39(2), 491–515.

■ Lymphatic Malformations

Lymphatic malformations (LM) arise from disorganized formation of endothelialized lymphatic channels that neither contribute nor connect to normal lymphatic channels. Histologically, terms such as *cystic hygroma* or *lymphangioma* are inaccurate and not favored, as the terms give a false suggestion of a vascular ("-angio-") or neoplastic ("-oma") component. LMs are subdivided into either microcystic or macrocystic groups, and some lesions may be a combination of the two entities with both microcystic and macrocystic components.

Macrocystic LMs present as fluid-filled structures greater than 1 to 2 cm and will appear hyperintense on T2-weighted imaging. Thin septations are often seen separating larger cystic spaces, and fluid–fluid levels are sometimes seen as a result of hemorrhage into a cyst (Fig. 15.1). Microcystic LMs appear to mimic "solid" masses

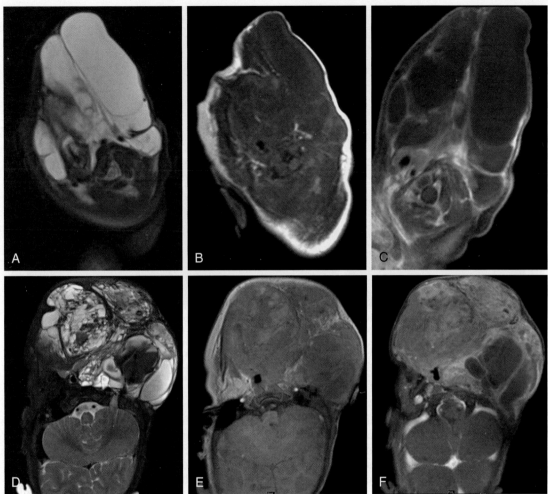

Fig. 15.1 Lymphatic malformation. Axial fat-suppressed T2-weighted (A, D), T1-weighted (B, E), and postcontrast fat-suppressed T1-weighted (C, F) images of a lymphatic malformation in a 1-day-old girl. (A–C) Images were acquired after birth and show a transspatial macrocystic lesion in the head and neck. The cystic spaces do not enhance on contrast-enhanced sequences. (D–F) Repeat examination of the same patient at 16 months of age who presented with acute enlargement of the LM. Imaging shows fluid–fluid levels in some of the cystic spaces (D), with avid contrast enhancement of thickened soft tissues/septations of the face and neck (D, E). Findings are compatible with hemorrhage into the lymphatic malformation with superinfection and cellulitis.

with lymphatic channels that are often too small to be seen. Septal enhancement on postcontrast-enhanced imaging is variable and may appear as homogeneous or slightly heterogeneous in the setting of microcystic LM. Cystic spaces should not enhance after the administration of intravenous contrast. Sonographic findings of LM correlate to the MRI findings, with large anechoic cystic spaces and septations. Microcystic lesions appear as echogenic soft tissues from the multiple reflectors of the small varying tissue interfaces between microscopic lymphatic channels and surrounding tissue (Fig. 15.2).

The most common region of the body for an LM is the head and neck, but an LM may be seen anywhere. When found in the head and neck, special considerations such as airway evaluation for patency as well as swallowing mechanics must be assessed. LMs are susceptible to superinfection and cellulitis, especially after hemorrhage into a cystic lesion. In inflammatory or hemorrhagic states, LMs increase in size and may cause airway compromise.

First line treatment of macrocystic LMs is sclerotherapy. LMs are responsive to oral sirolimus, an inhibitor of the mammalian target of rapamycin (mTOR)and are especially helpful when treating LMs and venous malformations (VMs) associated with mutations in the phosphoinositide 3-kinase/protein kinase B/mammalian target of rapamycin (*PI3K/AKT/mTOR*) pathway. Side effects of sirolimus include immunosuppression, and medical management of patients on mTOR inhibitors is best managed by hematologists with multidisciplinary care teams. Surgical excision of an LM is reserved for lesions too large to be amenable to therapy.

■ Venous Malformations

Venous malformations (VM) are low-flow malformations. These lesions may present with concomitant lymphatic channels as a combined lymphatic-venous malformation (LVM). They are dysplastic congenital anomalies

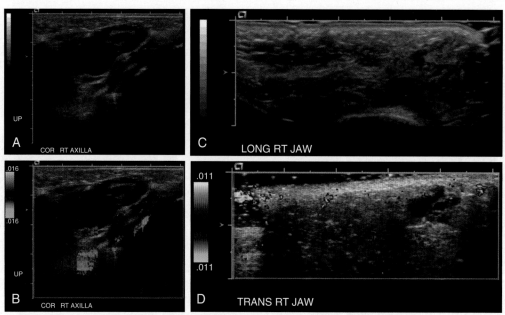

Fig. 15.2 Lymphatic malformation. Grayscale (A) and color Doppler (B) ultrasound images of a right axillary macrocystic lymphatic malformation in a 1-month-old girl showing an avascular multiseptated cystic lesion. Grayscale (C) and color Doppler (D) ultrasound images of the right jaw in a 3-year-old boy showing a microcystic lymphatic malformation. Due to innumerable small cystic interfaces with through-transmission, microcystic lymphatic malformations often appear as ill-defined echogenic masses.

that may be focal or multifocal and are sometimes trans-spatial. VMs may present as dilated venous varicosities (Fig. 15.3) or as a spongiform conglomerate of venous channels that sonographically appear as tubular-like anechoic or hypoechoic foci with either no discernable flow with color and spectral Doppler imaging, or monophasic venous flow present sometimes only after augmentation with Valsalva maneuvers, compression, or crying (Fig. 15.4). VMs are classically hyperintense on T2-weighted MRI sequences due to the slow flow within the aberrant channels; time-resolved contrast-enhanced MRA will demonstrate slow progressive filling of venous channels and delayed postcontrast imaging of a VM will characteristically demonstrate enhancement of venous channels. T1- and T2-hypointense foci within a VM represent phleboliths. Like LMs, fluid–fluid levels can be appreciated in VMs as a result of stagnant flow with hematocrit or protein layering or hemorrhage (Fig. 15.5). VMs may present radiographically with phleboliths.

VMs develop during fetal life but may or may not be clinically evident at birth. VMs grow commensurate with the patient and are also noted to grow during puberty, pregnancy, and after trauma. On physical examination, they are typically soft and compressible lesions. Patients may report pain when the lesion is in a dependent position or after thrombosis. VMs are commonly misdiagnosed as infantile hemangiomas. The natural history of a VM can be helpful to differentiate these two lesions, because an infantile hemangioma should not be present at birth. Infantile hemangiomas present shortly after birth and will undergo a phase of rapid proliferation after involution within the first decade of life. In distinction, VMs do not involute and, in fact, continue to grow, as stated previously.

Thrombophlebitis and coagulopathy are commonly associated with VMs. Clinical workup of patients with a suspected VM should include coagulation panels, including D-dimer and fibrinogen, because increases in these laboratory variables could indicate localized intravascular coagulation. Notably, acutely thrombosed VMs present as hard masses, mimicking malignancy. T1-hyperintense, T2-hypointense foci are characteristic of acute thrombi and can serve as a clue to this diagnosis.

Patients benefit from multidisciplinary care, including hematologists with anticoagulation therapies. Treatment strategies for VM favor alcohol embolization/sclerotherapy as first line and have replaced surgical excision.

■ Arteriovenous Malformations

An arteriovenous malformation (AVM) is defined as a lesion with one or more feeding arteries and draining veins around a bed of disorganized dysplastic vessels that may include smaller arteries or veins that bypass a normal capillary bed. This group of disorganized vessels is called the *nidus*. The high-flow nature of these malformations may shunt blood away from distal extremities or parts of organs and cause ischemia.

Sonographic findings show a characteristic lesion with hypoechoic channels without associated soft tissue mass. Color Doppler imaging will show hypervascularity with low-resistance arterial waveforms with spectral Doppler interrogation of arterial and venous structures (Fig. 15.6). Time-resolved contrast-enhanced MRA of high-flow malformations

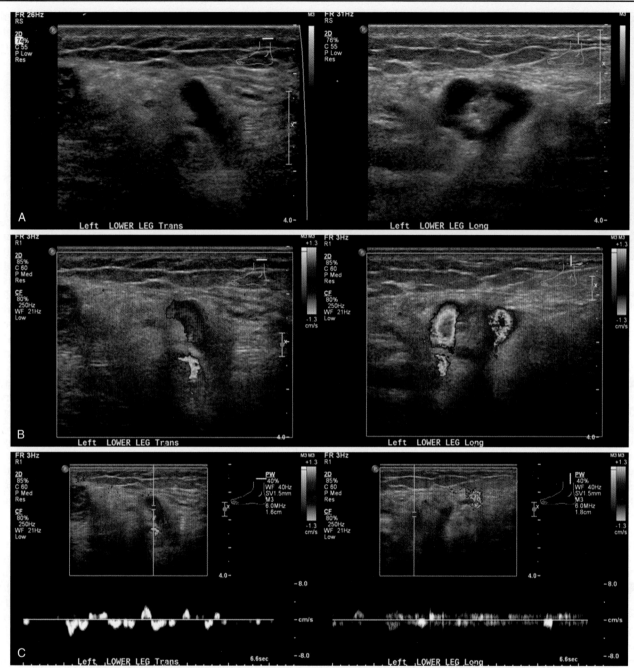

Fig. 15.3 Venous malformation. Grayscale (A), color Doppler (B), and spectral Doppler (C) images of a venous malformation in a 16-year-old boy in the left lower extremity. Imaging in similar anatomic positions on grayscale and corresponding Doppler images show anechoic tubular structures with slow flow. Venous waveforms with the ability to demonstrate respiratory variation, compressibility, and augmentation are common findings.

demonstrates arterial enhancement of vessels with prompt enhancement of venous structures to which they are connected. Flow voids on MRI are a characteristic finding of high-flow malformations (Fig. 15.7). Enhancement of the adjacent soft tissue may also be present with associated edema and fibrofatty proliferation.

Although present at birth, AVMs are not often clinically evident at that time but grow commensurate with the child and may present later in life as a pulsa-

tile painful mass with edema or ischemia of affected extremities or organs. These lesions are found in the extremities, head and neck, and pelvis. The Schobinger clinical classification scheme is used to describe the effect of an AVM on patients (Table 15.2). An additional angiographic classification system characterizes AVMs based on image fiindings (Table 15.3). Treatment options include surgical resection of an AVM; however, newer endovascular and embolic strategies allow for minimally invasive treatment.

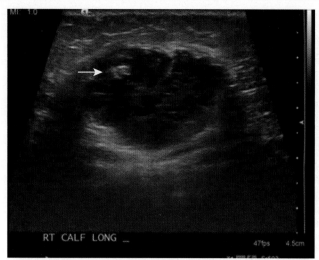

Fig. 15.4 Venous malformation. Grayscale ultrasound image of a venous malformation in a 13-month-old girl with a palpable calf mass. Spongiform venous malformations appear as a conglomerate of anechoic or hypoechoic tubular structures. Echogenic shadowing foci may be seen (*arrow*) representing phleboliths.

Arteriovenous Fistulas

Arteriovenous fistulas (AVFs) are rarely congenital and are often caused by trauma or iatrogenesis. AVFs are an abnormal direct connection of an artery to a vein without a central nidus. Examples of congenital AVFs are vein of Galen malformations and hepatic arterioportal fistulas. Similar to AVMs, AVFs will show low-resistance arterial waveforms with spectral Doppler waveform analysis (Figs. 15.8 and 15.9). Contrast-enhanced imaging demonstrates arterial and early venous enhancement.

Combined Vascular Malformations

Combined vascular malformations are defined as two or more vascular malformations found in one lesion; therefore, a multimodality approach to the diagnosis of combined vascular malformations should demonstrate these lesions as the sum of their parts. Lesions may be high or low flow, or a combination of the two. The accepted nomenclature for the description of combined vascular malformations is presented in Table 15.4 and is adapted from the ISSVA classification.

Anomalies of Major Named Vessels

Anomalies of major named vessels are also known as "channel-type" or "truncal vascular malformations" and affect lymphatics, veins, and arteries. Variations of the types of these malformations can involve abnormalities of a vessel origin, course, number, length, diameter, valves (veins), aberrant communication (AVF), and persistence of an embryonic vessel. Examples of common anomalies associated with major named vessels are shown in Fig. 15.10.

Vascular Malformations Associated With Other Vascular Anomalies

Vascular malformations associated with specific configurations of anomalies and genetic mutations may present as syndromes that follow classic phenotypes. The ISSVA classification earmarks these vascular malformation combinations separately from simple or combined malformations because many of these anomalous combinations arise specifically from somatic mutations in cellular pathways that regulate angiogenesis and soft tissue growth. For example, overgrowth syndromes associated with vascular malformations occur when somatic mutations occur in the *PI3K/AKT/mTOR* pathway. Overgrowth vascular anomaly syndromes occurring because of specific somatic mutations in *PIK3CA* result in Klippel-Trenaunay syndrome (Fig. 15.11), congenital lipomatous overgrowth, vascular anomalies epidermal nevi, spinal/scoliosis abnormalities syndrome (CLOVES) (Fig. 15.12), and megalencephaly capillary malformation syndrome. *PIK3CA* mutations may also give rise to fibroadipose vascular anomaly (FAVA), which is a painful focal soft tissue overgrowth most often occurring in the medial gastrocnemius, pathologically characterized by fatty and fibrous tissue with accompanying low-flow malformations. Neural encasement involvement in FAVA results in pain and contractures (Fig. 15.13).

Table 15.5 summarizes notable *PIK3CA*-related overgrowth syndromes (PROSs), non-PROS, and how these syndromes may be diagnosed clinically and radiologically. Patients with soft tissue overgrowth and imaging findings consistent with vascular anomalies should be recommended for genetic testing if not already performed, because the management strategies for these patients changes given the presence of somatic mutations.

PROSs and non-PROSs may increase the risk for nonvascular tumor formation, which requires appropriate clinical and imaging surveillance. Patients with phosphatase and tensin homolog (*PTEN*) mutation spectrum or *PTEN* hamartoma syndrome (PTHS) are at an increased risk for many benign and malignant tumors (colorectal cancer and polyps, thyroid cancer, uterine cancer) and should be screened per high-risk guidelines. Patients with CLOVES syndrome have been reported to have an increased risk for development of Wilms tumor, and renal ultrasound surveillance is recommended annually until the patient is at least 7 to 8 years of age. Multidisciplinary teams under the umbrella of vascular anomalies clinics are becoming more widespread, especially in pediatric health centers, and are able to provide care to patients with complex malformations and their associated comorbidities.

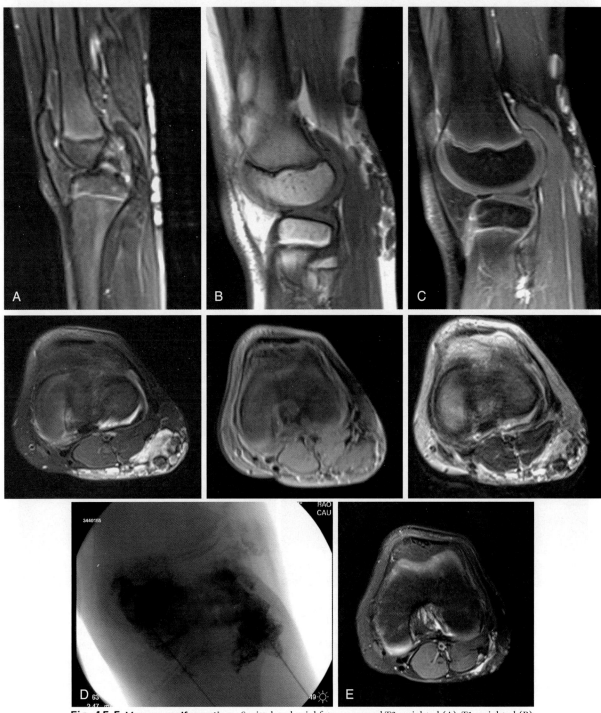

Fig. 15.5 Venous malformation. Sagittal and axial fat-suppressed T2-weighted (A), T1-weighted (B), and contrast-enhanced fat-suppressed T1-weighted (C) images of a venous malformation in a 9-year-old girl. Venous malformations are normally hyperintense on T2-weighted sequences and hyperintense to isointense to muscle on T1-weighted sequences. Slow gradual enhancement of venous malformations is typical, and fluid–fluid levels may be appreciated because of the slow-flow nature of these anomalies. Intraprocedural fluoroscopic image (D) during percutaneous sclerotherapy of the same patient with post-sclerotherapy axial T2-weighted image (E) showing reduction in size and signal of the venous malformation (compared with A).

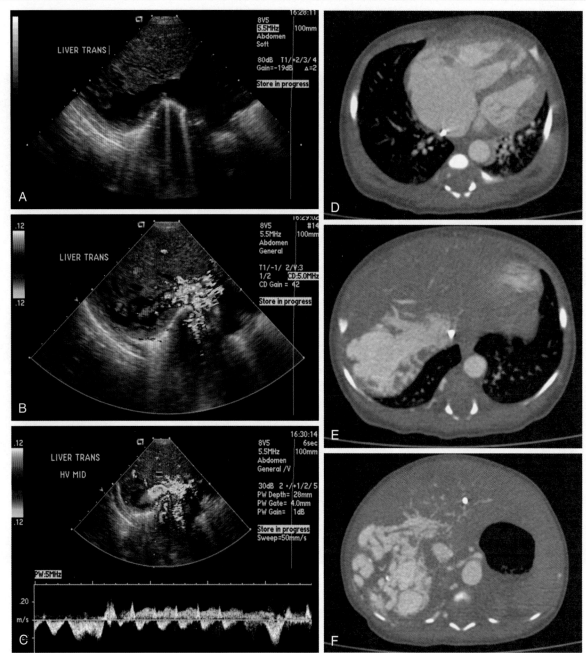

Fig. 15.6 Hepatic arteriovenous malformation. Grayscale (A) and color (B) and spectral (C) Doppler of a large hepatic arteriovenous malformation (AVM) in a 1-day-old girl. Anechoic channels (A) abruptly fill with turbulent color signal (B) with a mixed arterial and venous waveform (C) with spectral broadening suggesting turbulent, nonlaminar flow. Computed tomographic angiography of the abdomen (D–F) shows enhancing channels that drain directly into the inferior vena cava from a large hepatic venous tributary (E). Fast-flow malformations increase venous return to the heart and can result in high-output cardiac failure (D).

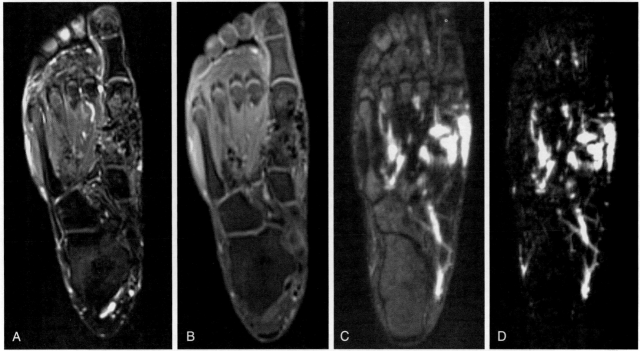

Fig. 15.7 Arteriovenous malformation. Axial fat-suppressed T2-weighted (A), axial fat-suppressed T1-weighted (B), postcontrast fat-suppressed T1-weighted (C), and subtracted time-resolved magnetic resonance angiography (D) images of the right foot in a 14-year-old girl with a large arteriovenous malformation. T1- and T2-hypointense flow voids seen on precontrast imaging around the first proximal phalanx are typical for this type of fast-flow lesion (A, B). There is marrow edema (high T2) signal within the bone. Flow voids enhance promptly after contrast administration (C, D).

TABLE 15.2   Schobinger Clinical Classification of Arteriovenous Malformations

STAGE	CLINICAL FINDINGS
Stage 1 (quiescence)	Skin warmth, discoloration
Stage 2 (expansion)	Enlargement, pulsation, bruit
Stage 3 (destruction)	Pain, ulceration, bleeding
State 4 (decompensation)	High-output cardiac failure and symptomatic hypervolemia

Adapted from Kohout, M. P., Hansen, M., Pribaz, J. J., Mulliken, J. B. (1998). Arteriovenous malformations of the head and neck: natural history and management. *Plastic and Reconstructive Surgery,* 102(3):643–654.

TABLE 15.3   Angiographic Classification of Arteriovenous Malformations

TYPE	ANATOMY
Type I	AVM ≤3 separate arteries draining to a single vein
Type II	AVM with multiple arteries draining to a single vein
Type IIIa	Multiple small AVF
Type IIIb	Multiple hypertrophied and dilated AVF in a complex network

AVF, Arteriovenous fistula; *AVM,* arteriovenous malformation. Adapted from Park, K. B., Do, Y. S., Kim, D.-I., Kim, Y. W., Shin, B. S., Park, H. S., … Lee, B.-B. (2012). Predictive factors for response of peripheral arteriovenous malformations to embolization therapy: Analysis of clinical data and imaging findings. *Journal of Vascular and Interventional Radiology,* 23(11), 1478–1486.

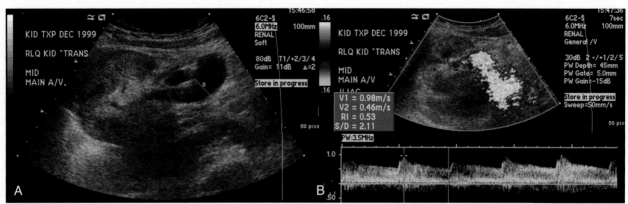

Fig. 15.8 Arteriovenous malformation. Grayscale (A) and spectral Doppler (B) ultrasound images of the right transplant kidney in the same patient in Fig. 15.7. Large anechoic tubular structure (A) likely represents an enlarged draining vein directly receiving arterial flow. Note the high-flow, low-resistance waveform with spectral broadening and color turbulence in the enlarged renal vein (B).

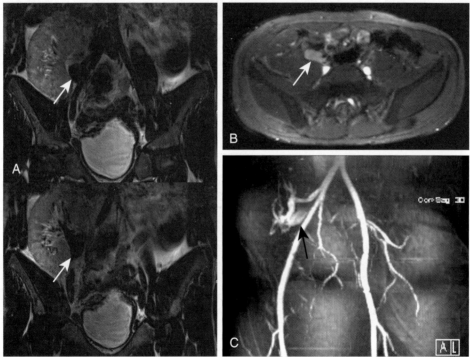

Fig. 15.9 Arteriovenous fistula. Coronal T2-weighted (A), axial fat-suppressed postcontrast T1-weighted (B), and coronal postcontrast magnetic resonance angiography maximum intensity projection (C) images of a 15-year-old boy with an iatrogenic arteriovenous fistula within a transplant renal artery and vein. Arteriovenous fistulas are often a procedural consequence and may appear as a pseudoaneurysm given the direct connection between artery and vein (*arrow*) (A). Early venous drainage (*arrow*) is appreciated on contrast-enhanced examination (B, C). There is no central nidus or tangle of vessels distinguishing this malformation from an arteriovenous malformation.

TABLE 15.4   ISSVA Nomenclature of Recognized Combined Vascular Malformations

COMPONENTS	NAME	COMBINED ABBREVIATION
CM + VM	Capillary-venous	CVM
CM + LM	Capillary-lymphatic	CLM
CM + AVM	Capillary-arteriovenous	CAVM
LM + VM	Lymphatic-venous	LVM
CM + LM + VM	Capillary-lymphatic-venous	CLVM
CM + LM + AVM	Capillary-lymphatic-arteriovenous	CLAVM
CM + VM + AVM	Capillary-venous-arteriovenous	CVAVM
CM + LM + VM + AVM	Capillary-lymphatic-venous-arteriovenous	CLVAVM

ISSVA, International Society for the Study of Vascular Anomalies.

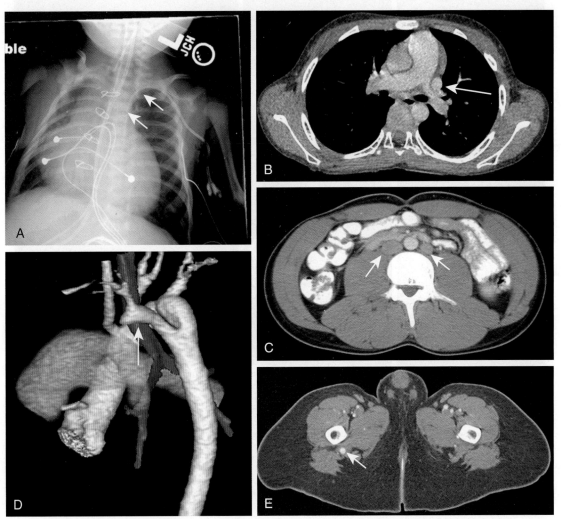

Fig. 15.10 Selected examples of vascular malformations of major named vessels in different patients. Anteroposterior radiograph of the chest (A) depicting a left superior vena cava, as indicated by the central venous catheter course (*arrows*). Axial contrast-enhanced computed tomography (CT) (B) image through the chest showing a duplicated superior vena cava (*white arrow*). Axial contrast-enhanced CT (C) image through the abdomen showing a duplicated inferior vena cava (*arrows*). Three-dimensional reconstructions from a contrast-enhanced CT angiography of chest (D) showing a right aortic arch with aberrant left subclavian vein (*arrow*) originating from a diverticulum of Kommerell. Axial contrast-enhanced CT (E) image through the pelvis showing a persistent right sciatic artery (*arrow*). This vessel may replace or provide an adjunct flow path for blood in the common iliac vessel. The external iliac artery and femoral artery may or may not be present in patients with persistent sciatic artery.

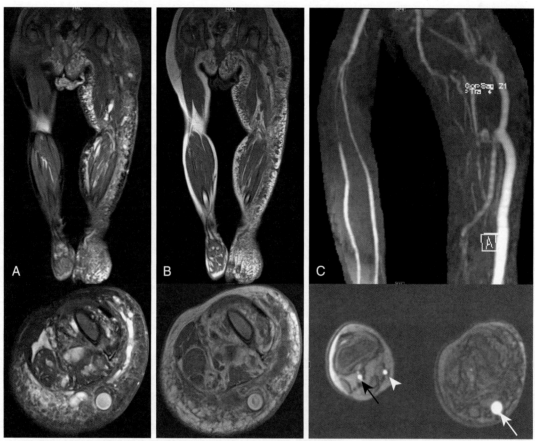

Fig. 15.11 Klippel-Trenaunay syndrome. Coronal and axial fat-suppressed T2-weighted (A), coronal and axial T1-weighted (B), and coronal and axial postcontrast magnetic resonance venography maximum intensity projections in a 5-year-old girl with Klippel-Trenaunay syndrome (KTS). Extensive venous malformations seen transspatially throughout the left lower extremity resulting in asymmetrical limb overgrowth (A, B). A large lateral embryonic vein (marginal of Servelle) is pathognomonic of KTS (C). Note the asymmetry in size of the extremities on axial images; the overgrown left limb relies solely on the lateral embryonic vein for venous drainage (C, *white arrow*) and lacks a deep venous system. The normal right lower extremity demonstrates a normal medial saphenous vein (*white arrowhead*) and popliteal vein (*black arrow*) (C).

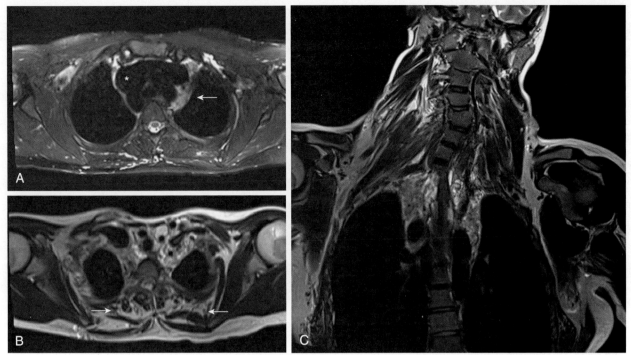

Fig. 15.12 CLOVES. Axial fat-suppressed T2-weighted (A), axial T2-weighted (B), and coronal-T2 weighted images through the chest in a 15-year-old girl with CLOVES (congenital lipomatous overgrowth, vascular malformations, epidermal nevi, scoliosis/spine anomalies) syndrome. Transspatial T2-hyperintensity in seen throughout the mediastinum (*arrow*) representing a slow-flow vascular malformation; also note the ectasia of the superior vena cava (*asterisk*) (A). There is also fatty overgrowth within the paraspinal musculature (*arrows*) (B). There is a scoliosis of the cervical spine (C) secondary to fused articular processes and facet joints from C3 to C6 (not shown).

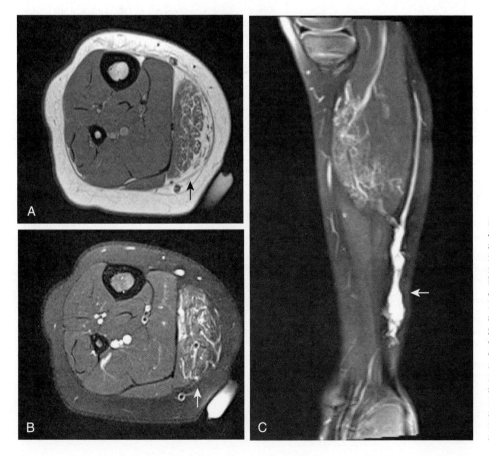

Fig. 15.13 Fibroadipose vascular anomaly. Axial T1-weighted (A), axial fat-suppressed T2-weighted, and sagittal T2-weighted images through the right lower extremity of a 6-year-old boy with new equinus contracture diagnosed with a fibroadipose vascular anomaly. T1 hyperintensity corresponding to fat is seen in the medial gastrocnemius (*arrow*) (A). Intramuscular fat is generally more conspicuous in fibroadipose vascular anomalies than in venous malformations. Mild infiltrative T2-hyperintensity is seen within the lateral gastrocnemius (*arrow*) (B). Phlebectasia is seen in the affected extremity, a common finding in patients with fibroadipose vascular anomalies (C).

TABLE 15.5 Selected Congenital Limb Overgrowth Syndromes Associated With Vascular Anomalies

SYNDROME	ISSVA CLASSIFICATION	MUTATION	KEY FEATURES
Klippel-Trenaunay syndrome (KTS)[a]	CM + VM + LM + limb overgrowth	PIK3CA	KTS triad Port-wine stain (CM) Soft tissue overgrowth Slow-flow VM or LM
CLOVES syndrome[a]	LM + VM + CM + AVM + limb overgrowth	PIK3CA	Congenital lipomatous overgrowth Slow flow Vascular malformations Epidermal nevi Scoliosis and spinal deformity Often present with slow-flow malformation Propensity for spinal AVM Increased risk for Wilms tumor
Parkes-Weber syndrome	CM + AVM + limb overgrowth	RASA1	Almost identical presentation to KTS; however, key feature is AVM development, which is not seen in KTS Patients are subject to heart failure and steal syndromes
PTEN hamartoma/Bannayan-Riley-Ruvalcaba	AVM + VM + macrocephaly + lipomatous overgrowth	*PTEN*	Hamartomatous growth and tumor syndromes Often presents with similar findings to other PROSs
Proteus syndrome	CM, VM, and/or LM + asymmetric somatic overgrowth	*AKT*	Overgrowth with gradual phenotypic change with age Cerebriform connective tissue nevus on the sole of the foot is pathognomonic

AVM, Arteriovenous malformation; *CLOVES*, congenital lipomatous overgrowth, vascular malformations, epidermal nevi, scoliosis/spine anomalies; *CM*, capillary malformation; *ISSVA*, International Society for the Study of Vascular Anomalies; *KTS*, Klippel-Trenaunay syndrome; *LM*, lymphatic malformation; *PROS*, PIK3CA-related overgrowth syndrome; *PTEN*, phosphatase and tensin homolog; *VM*, venous malformation.
Adapted from Bertino, F., & Chaudry, G. (2019). Overgrowth syndromes associated with vascular anomalies. *Seminars in Roentgenology, 54*(4), 349–358.

Bibliography

Adams, D. M., Trenor, C. C., 3rd., et al. (2016). Efficacy and safety of sirolimus in the treatment of complicated vascular anomalies. *Pediatrics, 137*(2), e20153257.

Bertino, F., Braithwaite, K. A., Hawkins, C. M., Gill, A. E., Briones, M. A., Swerdlin, R., et al. (2019). Congenital limb overgrowth syndromes associated with vascular anomalies. *RadioGraphics, 39*(2), 491–515.

Bertino, F., & Chaudry, G. (2019). Overgrowth syndromes associated with vascular anomalies. *Seminars in Roentgenology, 54*(4), 349–358.

Caux, F., Plauchu, H., Chibon, F., et al. (2007). Segmental overgrowth, lipomatosis, arteriovenous malformation and epidermal nevus (SOLAMEN) syndrome is related to mosaic PTEN nullizygosity. *European Journal of Human Genetics, 15*(7), 767–773.

Dasgupta, R., & Fishman, S. J. (2014). ISSVA classification. *Seminars in Pediatric Surgery, 23*(4), 158–161.

Fernandez-Pineda, I., Marcilla, D., Downey-Carmona, F. J., Roldan, S., Ortega-Laureano, L., & Bernabeu-Wittel, J. (2014). Lower extremity fibro-adipose vascular anomaly (FAVA): A new case of a newly delineated disorder. *Annals of Vascular Diseases, 7*(3), 316–319.

Hammill Adrienne, M., Wentzel Mary, S., Gupta, A., et al. (2011). Sirolimus for the treatment of complicated vascular anomalies in children. *Pediatric Blood and Cancer, 57*(6), 1018–1024.

Hawkins, C. M., & Chewning, R. H. (2019). Diagnosis and management of extracranial vascular malformations in children: Arteriovenous malformations, venous malformations, and lymphatic malformations. *Seminars in Roentgenology, 54*, 337–348.

Hobert, J. A., & Eng, C. (2009). *PTEN* hamartoma tumor syndrome: An overview. *Genetics in Medicine, 11*(10), 687–694.

International Society for the Study of Vascular Anomalies. Classification. Available from http://www.issva.org/classification.

Jarrett, D. Y., Ali, M., & Chaudry, G. (2013). Imaging of vascular anomalies. *Dermatologic Clinics, 31*(2), 251–266.

Jin, Y., Zou, Y., Hua, C., et al. (2017). Treatment of early-stage extracranial arteriovenous malformations with intralesional interstitial bleomycin injection: A pilot study. *Radiology, 287*(1), 194–204.

Kang, H.-C., Baek, S. T., Song, S., & Gleeson, J. G. (2015). Clinical and genetic aspects of the segmental overgrowth spectrum due to somatic mutations in PIK3CA. *The Journal of Pediatrics, 167*(5), 957–962.

Keppler-Noreuil, K. M., Rios, J. J., Parker, V. E. R., et al. (2015). *PIK3CA*-related overgrowth spectrum (PROS): Diagnostic and testing eligibility criteria, differential diagnosis, and evaluation. *American Journal of Medical Genetics. Part A, 167A*(2), 287–295.

Keppler-Noreuil, K. M., Sapp, J. C., Lindhurst, M. J., et al. (2014). Clinical delineation and natural history of the *PIK3CA*-related overgrowth spectrum. *American Journal of Medical Genetics. Part A, 164A*(7), 1713–1733.

Lackner, H., Karastaneva, A., et al. (2015). Sirolimus for the treatment of children with various complicated vascular anomalies. *European Journal of Pediatrics, 174*(12), 1579–1584.

Leslie, N. R., & Longy, M. (2016). Inherited PTEN mutations and the prediction of phenotype. *Seminars in Cell & Developmental Biology, 52*, 30–38.

Mulligan, P. R., Prajapati, H. J., Martin, L. G., & Patel, T. H. (2014). Vascular anomalies: Classification, imaging characteristics and implications for interventional radiology treatment approaches. *British Journal of Radiology, 87*(1035), 20130392.

Nosher, J. L., Murillo, P. G., et al. (2014). Vascular anomalies: A pictorial review of nomenclature, diagnosis and treatment. *World Journal of Radiology, 6*(9), 677–692.

Park, K. B., Do, Y. S., Kim, D.-I., et al. (2012). Predictive factors for response of peripheral arteriovenous malformations to embolization therapy: Analysis of clinical data and imaging findings. *Journal of Vascular and Interventional Radiology, 23*(11), 1478–1486.

Peterman, C. M., Fevurly, R. D., Alomari, A. I., et al. (2017). Sonographic screening for Wilms tumor in children with CLOVES syndrome. *Pediatr Blood Cancer, 64*(12), e26684.

Shaikh, R., Alomari, A. I., Kerr, C. L., Miller, P., & Spencer, S. A. (2016). Cryoablation in fibro-adipose vascular anomaly (FAVA): A minimally invasive treatment option. *Pediatric Radiology, 46*(8), 1179–1186.

CHAPTER 16
Approach to Pediatric Soft Tissue Masses

Craig Johnson, Michael Norred, and Christian Restrepo

CHAPTER OUTLINE

Why Imaging?, 327
Who Needs Imaging?, 327
Problem Solving: Which Modality? Which Protocol?, 327
Articular/Periarticular Mass, 328
  Is the Mass Cystic?, 328
  Does the Mass Enhance With a Gadolinium Contrast Agent?, 330
Muscle, 331

Are There Calcifications?, 331
Presentation With Torticollis?, 333
Was the Lesion Present at Birth?, 334
Is the Lesion Rapidly Growing?, 334
Nerve or Nerve Sheath, 336
Skin and Subcutaneous Fat, 338
  Is There a History of Trauma?, 338
  Does It Contain Fat?, 339
  Is It a High-Flow Vascular Lesion?, 340
  Is It a Slow-Flow Vascular Lesion?, 343
Summary, 345

■ Why Imaging?

Pediatric patients with soft tissue musculoskeletal masses encompass a wide array of pathology that ranges from benign fatty masses and self-involuting vascular tumors all the way to aggressive malignant lesions that require a multidisciplinary approach and staging before intervention is performed. Anesthesia and surgical procedures in children for histological diagnosis before imaging is performed is not without risk both in the short term from procedural complications and also potentially in the long term with the concern of long-term effect of neurological development in children secondary to certain anesthetics. Appropriate imaging not only gives the anatomic extent of the lesion and relationship to vital adjacent structures but also many times provides valuable insights into the composition and aggressiveness of the lesion, which may provide a diagnosis or greatly narrow the differential diagnosis before a procedure is decided.

■ Who Needs Imaging?

Patients who have skin manifestations of a soft tissue mass that are characteristic and diagnostic do not need further imaging unless the lesion is associated with deep invasion or ill-defined margins, such as kaposiform hemangioendothelioma (KHE), or if the lesions are felt to be metastatic from a primary source, such as a cutaneous manifestation of neuroblastoma. Typically, patients who do not have a classic history for an identifiable benign cutaneous manifestation will benefit from

imaging. In many cases, imaging will be diagnostic or at the very least will result in a differential diagnosis. In addition, imaging allows for anatomic detail regardless of which modality, which can be extremely helpful in procedural and surgical planning and also allow for a much higher degree of procedural safety.

■ Problem Solving: Which Modality? Which Protocol?

Radiographs have a limited role in soft tissue tumor evaluation in children, but in isolated circumstances can give valuable information. In addition, several advantages, such as ease of ordering and availability, the low cost, the minimal amount of ionizing radiation, and the lack of sedation need, are reasons that radiographs may be obtained in the setting of a soft tissue mass.

Ultrasound (US) is readily available and is typically the first imaging modality used to assess a soft tissue mass. US allows for a noninvasive assessment of the anatomy and for the evaluation of flow dynamics, all without exposure to ionizing radiation or the use of intravenous contrast agents. In addition, grayscale and color and spectral Doppler US may be performed as a bedside or outpatient procedure, precluding the need to transport developmentally disabled, critically ill, and unstable patients into unfamiliar beds. In addition, this method provides high spatial resolution imaging of the small vessels, calcifications, and cysts at a relatively low cost. US, however, is operator dependent and may be particularly challenging to perform and interpret in younger children. Overall, vascularity is also difficult to compare and quantify given the subjective nature and the differences in technology between different settings and machines.

Magnetic resonance imaging (MRI), with its high soft tissue contrast, is the current imaging gold standard for the evaluation of soft tissue masses in children, defining lesion diagnostic characteristics while delineating its anatomic relationships with adjacent structures. Magnetic imaging angiography (MRA) permits the noninvasive evaluation of the pediatric soft tissue masses. Some of the advantages of traditional angiography can be obtained today with MRA by using time-resolved contrast-tracking techniques. MRA still does not approach the spatial resolution and accuracy of CTA or traditional angiography, which is rarely used for diagnostic purposes today in pediatrics and is used only in conjunction with a combined planned therapeutic procedure. Because of long examination duration, MRI/MRA is often performed under sedation or general anesthesia in young children. Given recent concerns for potential neuroapoptotic effects in the brain of young patients, coaching for nonsedated examinations is encouraged. Additional limitations of MRI include its ability to detect calcifications and osseous changes that may be seen in aggressive lesions. Techniques such as diffusion-weighted imaging and dynamic contrast-enhanced imaging can be used for procedural planning on where to sample the soft tissue lesions, and in the future may be used to determine treatment response and necrosis rates. MR spectroscopy, elastography, and perfusion imaging also provide potential and promise in characterization of soft tissue masses.

Some basic technical components of the examination are relevant. Although a detailed discussion about the use of coils is out of the scope of this chapter, using the smallest possible coil for the question being asked and anatomic region being imaged is important. Likewise, each vendor and MRI machine will have different capabilities, sequence names, and software packages, so a discussion on acronyms would be of limited value. The general key is making sure the basic demographics, clinical and imaging history, reasonable differential, anatomic region for imaging, and the question to be answered are known and then to protocol the most efficient and reliable means for which to answer that question. In addition, one must remember for MR evaluation of soft tissue tumors that are visible and/or palpable that one should always consider use of a surface marker. This becomes even more important with smaller lesions, but one caveat is pressing against a compressible vascular lesion, especially venous, with the marker because this may obscure the findings. In this instance or if any question about obscuring a small superficial lesion exists, one should place a surface marker above and below the lesion.

■ Articular/Periarticular Mass

The most commonly encountered masses that involve an articular joint are cystic lesions. This includes entities such as ganglion cysts, meniscal cysts, and synovial cysts. They usually present as simple cysts. With these commonalities, they can often be difficult to distinguish from one another.

In the situation where a suspected lesion is atypical with regard to appearance (e.g., heterogeneous signal intensity on imaging), location, or that solid components are unable to be ruled out, gadolinium-based contrast material may be used. With gadolinium-based contrast a true cystic lesion will not show internal enhancement, typically only rim enhancement.

Is the Mass Cystic?

Ganglion cysts, meniscal cysts, and synovial cysts can be difficult to differentiate because of their location and similar imaging appearance on MRI. As will be a common theme, correlating clinical history with imaging is important in narrowing your differential diagnosis. On imaging, a communication with an adjacent joint or association with an effusion of the joint or tendon sheath can help determine the diagnosis. This can many times be done with a linear array transducer and close attention as to the flow direction of any internal echoes during compression, which may give the location of communication and origin.

Ganglion cysts are lesions with a dense fibrous connective tissue capsule lined with flat spindle-shaped cells. Although imaging of these lesions usually shows a simple cyst, septations may be present. Characteristics on imaging that may suggest a ganglion cyst include internal septa with peripheral fluid-filled pseudopodia that shows up as a "bunches of grapes" appearance. Typically, T1-weighted imaging of a ganglion shows intermediate to high signal intensity because of the content being either mucinous or hemorrhagic. T2-weighted sequences will show homogeneous high signal (Fig. 16.1). US will show a similar cystic appearance, and color Doppler imaging may show vascularity of the septa on low-flow settings. Although controversial, ganglion cysts are thought to arise from mucoid cystic degeneration in a collagenous structure under repetitive stress, and hence most commonly occur in the hand, wrist, and foot. The joint capsule and tendon incur the majority of the stress from repetitive activities and results in the periarticular soft tissue being prone to developing ganglia. Ganglion cysts may also occur in intraarticular, intraosseous, or periosteal locations.

Ganglion cysts are less common in children than in adults. When present, these lesions are usually asymptomatic. Management is conservative due to the tendency for ganglion cysts to spontaneously resolve, especially in the pediatric population. Repeated trauma, however, can result in progression of these masses and can lead to them becoming symptomatic or eroding adjacent bone.

Synovial cysts are commonly confused with ganglion cysts. The lesions primarily differ in that synovial cysts result from herniation of the synovial membrane through the joint capsule or fluid distention of a periarticular bursa and are thus lined by synovial cells.

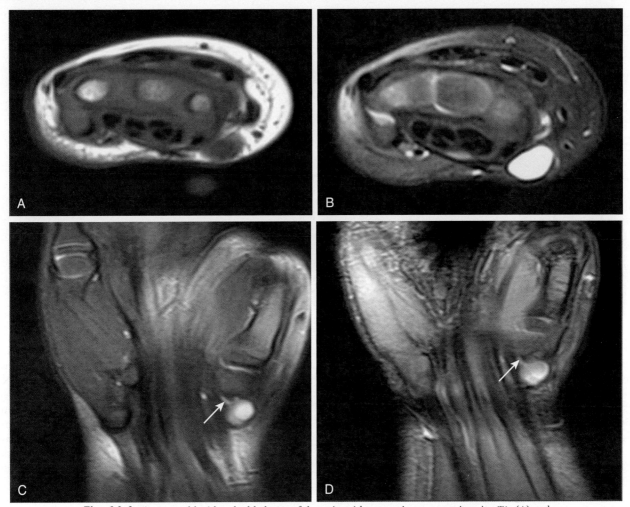

Fig. 16.1 Five-year-old with palpable lump of the wrist with magnetic resonance imaging T1- (A) and T2-weighted (B) axial images and coronal T2-weighted (C) and proton density (D) sequences showing a cystic structure adjacent to the volar midcarpal row with a thin tail (*arrow*) consistent with a ganglion cyst.

Although synovial cysts may occur in many locations, one of the most well-characterized areas is the popliteal region, where it is known as a Baker cyst. Baker cysts arise from the gastrocnemius-semimembranosus bursa and are specifically located in the medial aspect of the popliteal fossa between the medial head of the gastrocnemius muscle and the semimembranosus tendon. Complications of Baker or popliteal cysts include compression of adjacent structures, rupture, and, rarely, hemorrhage (Fig. 16.2), which have associated changes in the MR signal characteristics but classic anatomic location.

In the pediatric population, imaging of these lesions is unlikely to be associated with a joint effusion or internal derangement. Juvenile idiopathic arthritis is the primary exception to this, where popliteal cysts are shown in the majority of cases and commonly have an associated joint effusion. In children, management is normally conservative with the typical natural history being that of spontaneous involution.

Clinical history of trauma with the presentation of a mass in a joint space may suggest a meniscal cyst. These cysts occur as synovial fluid accumulates within the degenerated tissue from the injury. These cysts develop in continuity with complex meniscal tears, especially if there is horizontal cleavage. These cysts may be contained in the torn menisci as an intrameniscal cyst or may be displaced through the tear. The latter is more common and results in an expansion of the meniscocapsular margin and displacement of the capsule outward into the adjacent tissues becoming a "parameniscal cyst."

MRI shows meniscal cysts, as well as circumscribed lesions that are often described as septated fluid collections. The continuity with the horizontal cleavage or complex meniscal tear that caused their formation can often be appreciated on imaging as well. Unique features that may be seen with these lesions include low signal intensity contents on T2-weighted imaging. This finding is likely the result of water resorption by parameniscal tissue or hemorrhage. T1-weighted imaging may show these lesions as being isointense to muscle, likely because of hemorrhage or highly proteinaceous content within the cyst.

Synovial venous malformations, most frequently seen in the knee, may appear as an intraarticular cystic mass on an unenhanced MRI examination. Clues to the diagnosis include recurrent hemarthrosis and hemosiderin

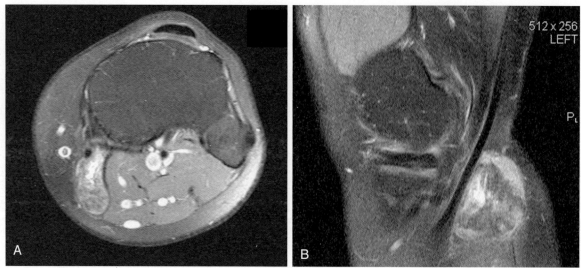

Fig. 16.2 Seventeen-year-old with painful mass of the popliteal fossa with axial (A) and sagittal (B) fat-saturated proton density sequences demonstrating heterogeneous hypointense signal between the medial gastrocnemius muscle and the semimembranosus tendon, which was found to represent a hemorrhagic popliteal (Baker) cyst.

deposition within the joint. If a synovial venous malformation is suspected, repeat contrast-enhanced MRI can be performed for diagnostic confirmation.

Does the Mass Enhance With a Gadolinium Contrast Agent?

When considering your differential for an articular mass, enhancement with gadolinium contrast can be an important differentiator from a cystic lesion. Benign tumors that may be considered include pigmented villonodular synovitis (PVNS) and giant cell tumor of the tendon sheath (GCTTS). PVNS and GCTTS are classified as benign fibrohistiocytic tumors (although there is no relationship with true histiocytes). Synovial sarcoma is an important entity to keep in mind with gadolinium-enhancing lesions due to its malignant potential.

PVNS is an idiopathic tumor of synovial origin that can occur as a diffuse or intraarticular form. This lesion can be seen in the pediatric population (usually in those older than 10 years), although it is much more prevalent in those around 20 to 50 years old. Patients have swelling and pain that develops over time; an acute presentation is rare. It most often affects the knee joint. In the knee, PVNS most commonly occurs in the Hoffa fat pad, the suprapatellar bursa, and the posteromedian synovial joint recess. Additional areas that are affected by PVNS include the ankle, hip, shoulder, and elbow. Multiple joint involvement has been reported in the pediatric population.

The difficulty in assessing some of these areas with arthroscopy (especially posteromedian synovial joint recess) highlights the importance of assessment with MRI. Findings of PVNS on MRI includes an irregularly thickened or frondlike T1- and T2-hypointense synovium (caused by hemosiderin deposition) (Fig. 16.3). The resulting low signal intensity is exaggerated by signal loss or blooming with gradient-echo or susceptibility-weighted sequences. Despite hypointensity

on T2-weighted imaging, PVNS may appear hyperintense on Short Tau Inversion Recovery (STIR) imaging. Avid enhancement after gadolinium is the norm. PVNS may be associated with joint effusions or multiseptated popliteal cyst. Bone involvement (e.g., edema, erosion) is rare in children. Although radiographs may detect any bone involvement and US may detect a large soft tissue mass and reactive effusion, the finer details, anatomy, and characterization of the articular lesions are best delineated with MRI.

Histologically, PVNS is characterized by synovial cell hyperplasia; accumulation of giant cells, macrophages, and fibroblasts; and intracellular and extracellular hemosiderin deposition. Treatment for PVNS is synovectomy. Recurrence for PVNS is estimated to be around 20% to 40%, highlighting the use of MRI in postoperative evaluation as well.

Another entity known as GCTTS is thought to be a continuation of PVNS because of their histological similarities. GCTTS has subclassifications that include a localized extraarticular, localized intraarticular (nodular synovitis), and diffuse extraarticular focus. Localized extraarticular GCTTS is the most common variant. The signal characteristics of GCTTS on MRI are similar to that of PVNS.

Synovial sarcoma, the second common pediatric soft tissue sarcoma after rhabdomyosarcoma, arises from primitive mesenchymal cells (versus synovial, despite the name). It is mostly seen in the first five decades of life. Thirty percent of cases occur in patients younger than 20 years, and it has been reported to occur in children as young as 2 years. Synovial sarcoma usually occurs in the extremities and clinically manifests as a painless, slow-growing mass that has been present for weeks to several years. Other less common clinical presentations include pain and tenderness before the mass becomes palpable, acute arthritis or bursitis, or chronic contracture.

The majority of cases of synovial sarcoma occur in a juxtaarticular location, close to the joint capsule, tendons,

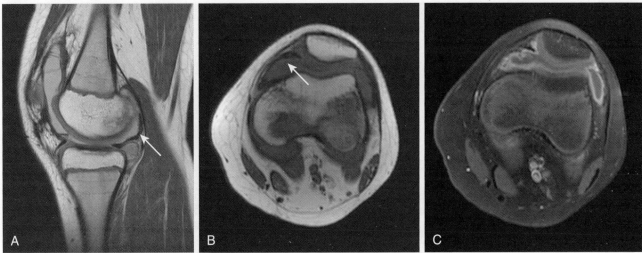

Fig. 16.3 Ten-year-old with history of knee swelling and pain with sagittal proton density sequence (A) and axial T1-weighted sequence (B) demonstrating hypointense signal of synovium and the Hoffa fat pad (*arrows*), with axial postcontrast fat-saturated image (C) demonstrating enhancing thickened synovium consistent with pigmented villonodular synovitis.

and bursa. Only a minority of cases are intraarticular. Plain films findings may include a soft tissue density and spiculated calcifications, seen in up to 30% of cases. With US, synovial sarcoma can appear as a well-defined hypoechoic vascular mass near, but not within, the joint (Fig. 16.4).

A classic MRI description of synovial sarcoma based on the most common findings is a juxtaarticular mass with a heterogeneous or triple-signal pattern (high-, intermediate-, and low-intensity areas) on T2-weighted imaging with fluid–fluid levels secondary to intralesional hemorrhage. Synovial sarcoma tends to be a well-defined mass isointense to muscle on T1-weighted images. Smaller lesions are homogenous, sometimes simulating cysts on unenhanced images. These small lesions, because of their homogenous hyperintense appearance on T2-weighted imaging and their propensity to displace, rather than infiltrate, adjacent structures, have been misdiagnosed as benign entities. Gadolinium is important in the evaluation of these masses. Unlike a cyst, these lesions will enhance.

Synovial sarcoma does often have an intimate relation to adjacent bone. About half of cases will be contiguous with bone, and about 20% will result in adjacent cortical thinning or medullary invasion, serving as a clue to the diagnosis.

■ Muscle

Despite some of the ability to make a diagnosis for most soft tissue masses, intramuscular masses lack specific diagnostic features on MRI, but clues are important for narrowing the differential diagnosis. This is especially important to keep in mind for the fibroblastic/myofibroblastic tumor group (includes nodular fasciitis, myositis ossificans [MO], fibrous hamartoma of infancy, myofibroma/myofibromatosis, fibromatosis colli, fibroma of tendon sheath, superficial fibromatosis, deep or desmoid-type fibromatosis, infantile fibrosarcoma, and

adult fibrosarcoma). Despite the limited use of MRI for diagnosis, there is still a use for defining extent of involvement. Often these entities will enhance with gadolinium contrast.

Are There Calcifications?

When calcification is present, MO is an important mass to consider. It is a localized, self-limiting, reparative lesion of muscle. Pathologically, MO has three components that include a central zone of proliferating fibroblasts, a middle zone of osteoblasts and foci of immature bone, and a peripheral layer of mature bone with trabeculae. MO is associated with a history of trauma. It can also be associated with repetitive trauma, ischemia, and inflammation. It can appear anywhere in the body, but it is usually found in the areas most associated with trauma, such as the anterior compartments of the thigh and upper extremity.

Radiographic and CT findings of MO include serpiginous calcifications 2 to 6 weeks after the traumatic event and a cleft between the calcifications and adjacent bone (Fig. 16.5).

MO follows pathological phases that change with time and correlate with imaging. The acute phase occurs during the first 2 weeks where the lesion may not be visible on T1-weighted imaging or may be poorly defined and with heterogenous signal intensity but predominantly isointense to muscle. On T2-weighted imaging, acute MO is hyperintense. Fluid–fluid levels may also be evident because of hemorrhage. There may be perilesional soft tissues edema and adjacent bone marrow edema.

The subacute phase, from 3 weeks to 6 to 8 weeks, is characterized by peripheral foci of low T1- and T2-signal intensity as a result of bone formation.

Peripheral lesion enhancement and enhancement in the edematous soft tissue may be seen during both acute and subacute phases of MO. This is important to

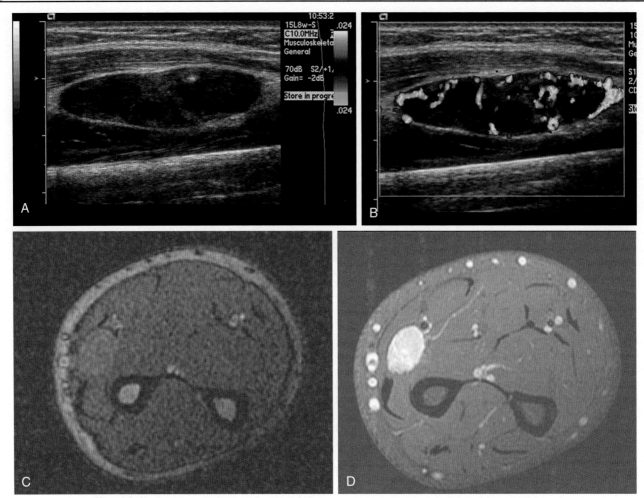

Fig. 16.4 Sixteen-year-old with growing left forearm intramuscular mass who on ultrasound has a well-circumscribed hypoechoic mass (A), which is hypervascular on color Doppler imaging (B) and axial gradient echo sequence demonstrates isointense signal to muscle (C) and postgadolinium T1-weighted fat-saturated sequence demonstrates homogeneous enhancement (D). Biopsy showed synovial sarcoma.

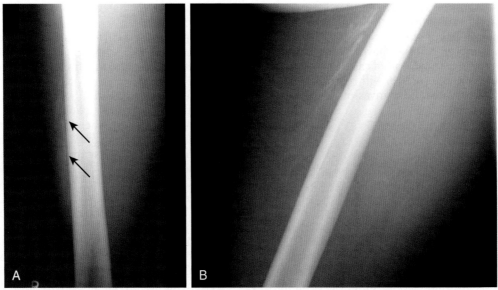

Fig. 16.5 Fifteen-year-old with football injury 1 month previously and presenting with right thigh painful mass with anteroposterior (A) and lateral (B) radiographs demonstrating serpiginous calcifications with lucent space between cortex and calcification (*arrows*) consistent with myositis ossificans.

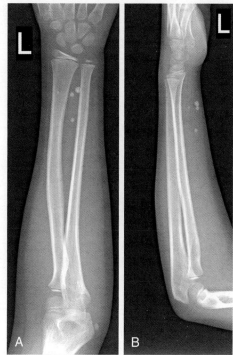

Fig. 16.6 Twelve-year-old with intermittent pain and swelling of left forearm. Anteroposterior (A) and lateral (B) radiographs of the forearm show phleboliths in the volar soft tissues consistent with a venous malformation.

consider in that these imaging findings may mimic an abscess or necrotic tumor.

Many of the aforementioned imaging findings are lost in the chronic stage. During this time (after 6–8 weeks), perilesional edema resolves and MO becomes more well defined. With progression of peripheral ossification, there is resultant more extensive low-signal intensity on all sequences. Overall, regarding MO, unenhanced CT depicts the characteristic peripheral ossification to best advantage.

Calcifications can also be seen in venous malformations in the form of phleboliths (Fig. 16.6). Venous malformations are made up of abnormal postcapillary valveless channels. There is a wide spectrum of lesions within this category, with some lesions affecting a single vessel to some affecting multiple vessels. Venous malformations are congenital but may not appear until later in childhood. Clinically, lesions are soft and compressible and have a bluish hue, but in the setting of acute thrombosis, they may be firm on physical examination, mimicking a neoplasm. When a venous malformation is suspected, the initial diagnostic modality is usually US. Venous malformations can be difficult to detect with US if a lesion is small and the child is large. In addition, it easy for a sonographer to miss a venous malformation if he or she is not careful about pressing too hard, especially with superficial lesions, which can compress the lesion, allowing it to become undetectable. Sonographic findings of a venous malformation include a compressible hypoechoic and sometimes heterogeneous lesion with no flow or monophasic low-velocity Doppler flow. Due to the absence of Doppler flow, venous malformations may be misdiagnosed as a cyst, especially when

a fluid–fluid level is seen. Fluid–fluid levels can be seen with very slow-flow venous malformations and is caused by hematocrit levels (Fig. 16.7). Valsalva maneuvers or compression of the affected body part can augment Doppler flow. Venous malformations are prone to thrombosis, and the echogenicity of thrombi depends on their chronicity. Echogenic shadowing foci representing phleboliths are again the best diagnostic clue to this diagnosis.

On MRI, venous malformations are predominantly of fluid-signal intensity on T2-weighted imaging. Low-signal foci can be observed and are related to thrombosis, septations, or phleboliths. These lesions are normally hypointense or isointense on T1-weighted imaging but may be heterogenous in cases of hemorrhage or thrombosis.

Alveolar soft part sarcoma (ASPA) is a rare slow-growing malignant tumor, usually occurring in the extremities. These masses often appear as intramuscular soft tissue masses with rich vascularity, including flow voids, and large peripheral vessels. Additional MRI characteristics of ASPA include T1 and T2 hyperintensity, avid enhancement with delayed contrast agent washout, and thick peripheral rim enhancement with central necrosis.

ASPA is usually seen in adolescents and young adults. In children, it is slightly more common in girls than in boys. On physical examination, ASPA presents as a painless mass, sometimes with pulsatility or a bruit owing to the prominent vascularity. These physical findings may lead to confusion with arteriovenous malformations (AVMs) and result in a misdiagnosis.

Metastases to the lungs, brain, and bone have been reported in up to 30% of patients at diagnosis. Treatment is surgical, with a better prognosis reported with smaller tumors, localized disease, and a younger age at diagnosis.

Presentation With Torticollis?

Twenty percent of patients with fibromatosis colli present with torticollis. Fibromatosis colli is theorized to be due to intrauterine injury to the sternocleidomastoid during the third trimester. The natural course of fibromatosis colli is benign. It is usually discovered at 2 weeks as a palpable mass, after which there is ongoing enlargement of the affected sternocleidomastoid muscle. Resolution over 4 to 8 months after conservative treatment, including physical therapy and stretching, is the norm.

US is the first-line imaging modality for suspected fibromatosis colli. US findings consist of a well-defined, unilateral fusiform enlargement of the middle or inferior third of the sternocleidomastoid muscle (Fig. 16.8). Echogenicity is variable with US, as is vascularity on color Doppler US interrogation. There is preservation of fascial planes and no surrounding inflammation or fluid collection. In cases where MRI has been used, this lesion demonstrates a fusiform enlargement and enhancement of the affected muscle without extension to adjacent tissues. Signal intensity is variable depending on the degree of fibrous and cellular tissues present.

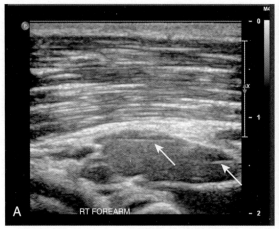
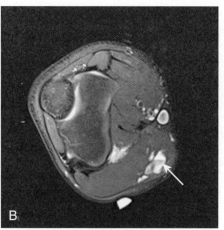

Fig. 16.7 Fourteen-year-old baseball player with right forearm mass and pain with ultrasound (A) and axial fat-saturated T2-weighted sequence (B) demonstrating intramuscular mass with slow flow indicated by fluid–fluid levels (*arrows*) and phleboliths seen on other images consistent with venous malformation.

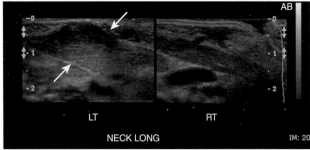

Fig. 16.8 Neonate with torticollis and comparative ultrasound showing left-sided fusiform enlargement of the sternocleidomastoid muscle (*arrows*) and smooth margins consistent with fibromatosis colli.

Was the Lesion Present at Birth?

Infantile myofibroma is the most common fibrous tumor of infancy. Most cases occur before the age of 2 years, and 60% of lesions are present at birth. These masses are characterized histologically by nodules with two distinct components: bundles of myofibroblasts and undifferentiated cells arranged around thin-walled, irregularly branching, hemangiopericytoma-like blood vessels. The arrangement suggests that there is a pathological continuum between infantile myofibroma and infantile hemangiopericytoma.

Infantile myofibroma may be solitary and multicentric. Solitary myofibromas occur almost twice as commonly in boys and occur in the head, neck, and trunk with involvement of the skin and muscle in most cases. Multicentric myofibromatosis occurs in soft tissues, bones, and viscera. Visceral involvement with myofibromatosis is associated with a poorer prognosis determined by the extent and location of the lesions, with intestinal, cardiac, and in particular lung lesions having the worst prognosis. The natural history of infantile myofibroma is spontaneous regression; however, lesions in the setting of visceral or diffuse musculoskeletal disease are the exception to this rule. Treatment for persistent masses includes excision. Multicentric lesions may be treated with chemotherapy.

Myofibromas are typically well-defined hypoechoic solid masses with US (Fig. 16.9). Central cystic necrosis with associated anechoic foci may be seen. MRI characteristics of a myofibroma include hypointense T1 signal, variable T2 signal, and peripheral enhancement. When there is osseous involvement, lytic lesions with or without sclerotic margins may be seen.

Other masses present at birth include infantile fibrosarcoma, congenital hemangiomas, and vascular malformations.

Is the Lesion Rapidly Growing?

Nodular fasciitis is a benign proliferative mesenchymal tumor that is more commonly seen in young adults but may also be seen in children. Nodular fasciitis is hypothesized to be reactive to local inflammatory processes or trauma and can occur in the upper extremities, trunk, head/neck, and lower extremities. Histologically, these masses are a manifestation of localized proliferations of plump fibroblastic/myofibroblastic cells of uncertain origin.

Patients present with a rapidly growing mass that may or may not be painful. Although the natural history of these masses is that they are fast growing, they rarely exceed 4 cm in diameter.

Imaging appearances of nodular fasciitis are variable. On US, it is generally a heterogeneous but hypoechoic mass with moderate vascularity with color Doppler imaging. Calcifications are uncommon. On MRI, nodular fasciitis is heterogeneously hyperintense on T2-weighted imaging and isointense to adjacent muscle on T1-weighted imaging. A described feature, the fascial tail sign, is a helpful clue on MRI and when seen is a linear extension of tissue from the mass along the fascia. An additional notable imaging feature is the "inverse target" appearance of nodular fasciitis, describing a peripheral rim of T2 hypointensity with central lesional

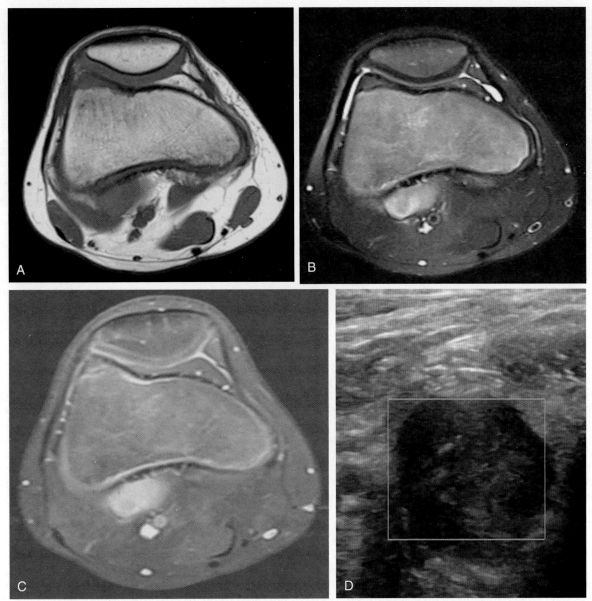

Fig. 16.9 Nine-year-old girl presents with right knee pain with T1-weighted sequence (A) demonstrating homogeneous signal isointense to muscle with heterogeneous high T2 signal on fat-saturated sequence (B) and heterogeneous enhancement on fat-saturated axial T1-weighted sequence (C). Correlating color Doppler ultrasound shows heterogeneous hypoechoic lesion with hypovascularity (D). Biopsy demonstrated myofibroma.

T2 hyperintensity. As for most intramuscular soft tissue lesions, the final diagnosis requires histology, and recurrence after local excision is rare.

Congenital infantile fibrosarcoma presents as a rapidly growing painless mass. Infantile fibrosarcoma occurs in the first 5 years of life, and one-third of cases present at birth. Most cases of infantile fibrosarcoma occur in the extremities, trunk, and head and neck region. Metastases occur in up to 10% of these cases, primarily to the lungs. Local recurrence of these masses is reported to be between 17% and 43% but has an overall better prognosis than the adult form with a greater than 80% 5-year survival rate.

Imaging is nonspecific. On MRI, infantile fibrosarcoma is a well-demarcated lesion that is isointense to muscle on T1-weighted images and heterogeneously hyperintense on T2-weighted images, with heterogeneous enhancement (Fig. 16.10).

Clinically, infantile fibrosarcoma can be confused with infantile hemangioma (IH), congenital hemangioma, or KHE because of a violaceous discoloration that is associated with phlebectatic superficial veins. Infantile fibrosarcoma may also have ulcerations that are similar to that seen in hemangioma (especially during stage of rapid proliferation), or it may be associated with DIC, which is confused for Kasabach-Merritt phenomenon seen primarily with KHE and tufted angioma. MRI may help differentiate these entities as infantile fibrosarcomas showing less homogenous contrast enhancement and absence of flow voids, characteristically seen in hemangiomas because of their avid vascularity.

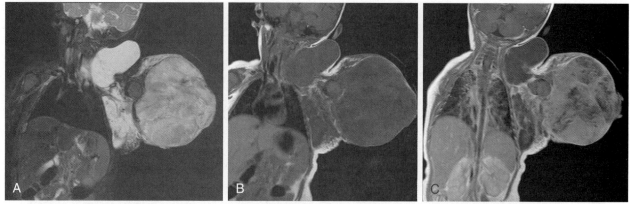

Fig. 16.10 Eight-week-old baby boy presents with rapidly increasing large left posterior back and lateral neck mass with coronal T2-weighted image (A) demonstrating mixed solid and cystic appearance, with coronal T1-weighted precontrast (B) and postcontrast (C) images demonstrating intense enhancement of the solid portions and rim enhancement of the cystic portions with biopsy demonstrating infantile fibrosarcoma.

Rhabdomyosarcoma accounts for more than 50% of soft tissue sarcomas in children. These masses are from primitive mesenchymal cells that develop into striated muscle. They can occur anywhere within the body, including areas that lack striated muscle. These most commonly occur in the head and neck and genitourinary systems, with a smaller but significant percentage occurring in the extremities. Lesions occurring in the extremities present with painless swelling and/or enlarged regional lymph nodes.

These lesions show a slight male predominance with two-thirds of children being younger than 10 years at diagnosis. These masses usually occur sporadically, although they are also found in association with Li-Fraumeni and Beckwith-Wiedemann syndromes, as well as with neurofibromatosis type I.

MRI findings for these lesions are nonspecific and can present as either well or poorly defined masses that are hypointense on T1-weighted imaging and hyperintense on T2-weighted imaging with variable enhancement patterns. There may be internal hemorrhage and/or necrosis (Fig. 16.11). Imaging of these lesions is important to establish the primary site of origin and the extent of the disease, including the detection of local lymphadenopathy because of the role these findings play in determining staging and thus treatment and prognosis.

Rhabdomyosarcomas are classified into three histological categories, including embryonal, alveolar, and pleomorphic variants. The less common alveolar subtype is seen in adolescents and young adults and more commonly found in the perineum and extremities.

■ Nerve or Nerve Sheath

Nerve sheath tumors, such as schwannomas or neurofibromas, can clinically manifest as soft tissue masses. Schwannomas are benign encapsulated nerve sheath tumors of Schwann cells. Cranial, spinal, and sympathetic nerve roots, as well as flexor surfaces of extremities (ulnar and peroneal), are most commonly affected. Histologically they appear as eccentric fusiform masses that are separate from the adjacent nerve and contain hypercellular (Antoni A) and hypocellular (Antoni B) regions. On MRI, schwannomas will appear as a fusiform T1-isointense to -hypointense and T2-hyperintense variably enhancing mass, along a peripheral nerve with a surrounding rim of fat around the tumor, known as "split-fat" sign. The fusiform appearance depicts the entering and exiting nerves and is indicative of the neurogenic origin of the tumor. On T2-weighted imaging, a "target sign" may be present (Fig. 16.12). A target sign has a hypointense to isointense center, corresponding to longitudinal bundles of residual nerve fibers or densely packed collagen fibers, and a peripheral hyperintense ring, corresponding to nonfibrillary stromal or myxoid fibers. The "fascicular sign" may also be seen on T2-weighted images, revealing multiple small ringlike structures with peripheral higher signal intensity because of the fascicular bundles. A hypointense rim marking the epineurium capsule may be evident in all MR sequences.

Neurofibroma is the most common peripheral nerve sheath tumor in children. Like schwannomas, they are a benign nerve sheath tumor made up of Schwann cells but differ in the fact that they cannot be separated from the normal nerve, requiring excision of adjacent nerves. There are three forms: localized, diffuse, and plexiform. Localized neurofibromas are well defined, encapsulated, solitary fusiform masses and are similar in imaging appearances to schwannomas. Diffuse neurofibromas are also solitary masses more common in children and are often found in the head and neck area. Plexiform neurofibromas, pathognomonic for neurofibromatosis type I, can be either superficial or deep. Their growth is characterized by the involvement of multiple fascicles of a nerve that result in a diffuse mass of thickened nerve fibers. Superficial lesions are more common and extend to the skin in a branching pattern, lacking a target sign. Deep lesions appear as multinodular masses, often referred to as a "bag of worms," and can have a target-like appearance. This target-like appearance can be mistaken for phleboliths in a venous malformation if not careful. The central and nondependent location of the foci of decreased signal intensity can be helpful to distinguish a plexiform neurofibroma from a venous malformation on unenhanced images.

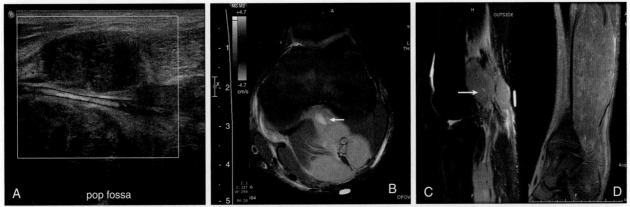

Fig. 16.11 Fifteen-year-old boy with leg mass and pain with ultrasound (A) demonstrating heterogeneous hypoechoic, hypovascular mass with axial proton density image (B) and sagittal T2 fat-saturated image (C) demonstrating hyperintense signal with focal areas of cystic/necrotic change (*arrows*) and slightly inferior sagittal postcontrast T1-weighted sequence demonstrating heterogeneous enhancement (D). Biopsy revealed alveolar rhabdomyosarcoma.

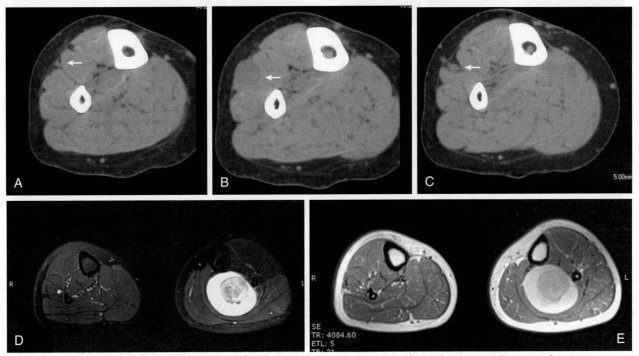

Fig. 16.12 Neurogenic tumors. Fifteen-year-old girl with right calf mass has sequential computed tomography images (A–C) demonstrating a round fusiform mass of the superficial peroneal nerve (*arrows*) with biopsy showing peripheral schwannoma and 16-year-old girl with neurofibromatosis type 1 and left leg pain with axial T1 and axial T2 fat-saturated images (D, E) consistent with a large mass of the deep peroneal nerve with a "target sign" and biopsy consistent with neurofibroma.

Malignant peripheral nerve sheath tumor (MPNST) is a high-grade sarcoma with a poor prognosis that is thought to originate from Schwann cells. Clinically, it presents in patients aged 20 to 50 years as persistent pain, neurological symptoms, and rapidly proliferating preexisting neurofibroma. It has a strong association with neurofibromatosis type I. MPNST classically affects sacrum, brachial plexus, and sciatic nerve roots. There are no specific MR findings that can accurately distinguish a plexiform neurofibroma from MPNST. 18F-fluorodeoxyglucose (^{18}F-FDG) positron emission tomography/computed tomography (PET/CT) is currently the modality of choice for detection of MPNST in patients with neurofibromatosis type I. Using a maximum standardized uptake value (SUV) above 3.5, the sensitivity and specificity of ^{18}F-FDG PET/CT have been reported to be 100% and 67%, respectively.

Primitive neuroectodermal tumors will be discussed in this portion of the chapter because they are considered to represent different stages of neuroectodermal differentiation. The tumors are composed of small round blue cells and also go by the names of Askin tumor, Ewing sarcoma, or Ewing sarcoma family of tumors. Although the Ewing sarcoma family of tumors is most often osseous lesions, they can also present as soft tissue tumors of muscle, subcutaneous tissue, and

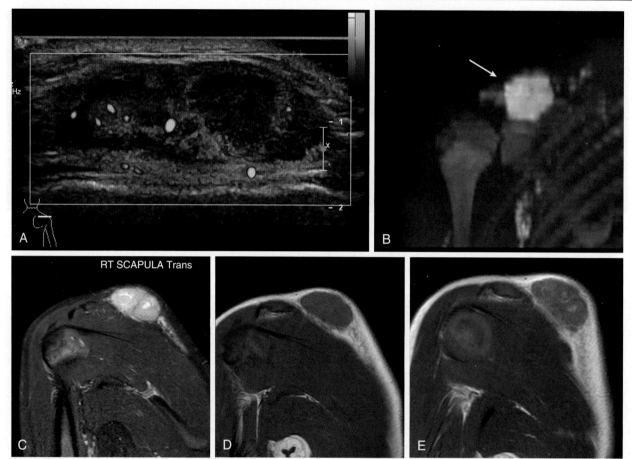

Fig. 16.13 Eleven-year-old boy presents with growing mass of right scapula. Ultrasound (A) demonstrates a well-circumscribed hypoechoic heterogeneous lesion with internal vascularity. Diffusion-weighted coronal reformatted maximum intensity image (B) demonstrates restricted diffusion throughout the mass (*arrow*). Coronal T2-weighted (C) and T1-weighted precontrast (D) and postcontrast (E) images demonstrate T2 prolongation throughout the lesion with heterogeneous enhancement. Biopsy was consistent with extraosseous Ewing tumor/Primitive neuroectodermal tumor.

the retroperitoneum. They are typically histologically indistinguishable from each other and share immuno-histochemical staining characteristics. The lesions are usually large at presentation (>5 cm).

The tumors may appear as a well-circumscribed soft tissue mass on plain film and CT. Thirty percent of lesions will have calcifications. US usually shows a hypoechoic heterogeneous well-defined mass with vascularity on color Doppler. MRI is nonspecific but usually shows a well-defined mass with T1 signal isointense to muscle with heterogeneous signal, and hyperintense signal on T2-weighted images is seen on almost all cases. The lesion typically enhances heterogeneously (Fig. 16.13). A pseudocapsule may be present in about a third of the cases, and internal fluid levels have also been described.

■ Skin and Subcutaneous Fat

Is There a History of Trauma?

This information can be a commonly overlooked aspect during the clinical interview but can be a key piece of information to formulating your differential diagnosis.

Subcutaneous fat necrosis may be accompanied by a history of trauma. Usually this is a nonlacerating, compressive-type trauma that leads to a "fat fracture." In neonates, hypothermia and hypoxia may also play a role in the development of fat necrosis. Due to accompanying hemorrhage and fibrosis, fat necrosis presents as a firm, mobile, well-defined, nontender mass on physical examination. Subcutaneous fat necrosis occurs over bony prominences that are more predisposed to trauma (e.g., shoulders, back, buttocks, thighs, and cheeks). These lesions are usually self-limited and may resolve, leaving focal atrophy of the subcutaneous tissues. On US, fat necrosis appears as a subcutaneous focal echogenic mass that will become heterogeneous before resolution. On MRI, fat necrosis appears as a linear pattern of abnormal signal intensity (low on T1-weighted images and either high or low on T2-weighted images) confined to the subcutaneous tissues (Fig. 16.14).

Hematoma is an entity worth keeping in the differential when a history of trauma is involved. Further imaging is normally not required but may sometimes be indicated if the patient is symptomatic or if there is not a known or clear history of trauma. Imaging of a hematoma with MRI will show a soft tissue mass with variable signal intensity depending on the age of the

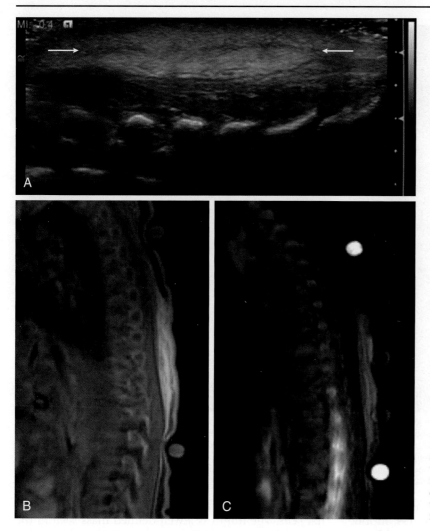

Fig. 16.14 Two-week-old with palpable back mass. Ultrasound image (A) shows an echogenic mass (*arrows*). Sagittal T2-weighted image (B) shows subcutaneous linear hyperintensity. Postcontrast T1-weighted image (C) shows linear enhancement. Follow-up ultrasound 2 months later shows complete resolution of the mass. Findings were felt to be related to subcutaneous fat necrosis of the newborn.

blood. T1 shortening of the methemoglobin and the T2 shortening of hemosiderin with characteristic signal loss or blooming with gradient-echo sequences is helpful for recognition of a hematoma.

Does It Contain Fat?

Adipocytic masses make up 6% of soft tissue tumors in children. Lipomas are benign masses that make up 66% of adipocytic tumors. They are categorized as superficial or deep, in respect to the superficial fascia, or as intermuscular or intramuscular masses. Superficial lipomas rarely grow larger than 5 cm in diameter and are typically diagnosed clinically without the use of imaging. Deep lipomas are most often intramuscular and have the potential to grow larger than superficial lipomas. Ultrasound may be helpful for superficial lipomas when the diagnosis is in question and will show a well-defined mass isoechoic to adjacent subcutaneous fat. Hypoechoic bands perpendicular to ultrasound beam are seen through the lesion. The masses are completely made up of fat; therefore MRI is sensitive and appears as homogeneous high-intensity signal on T1- and T2-weighted imaging and completely saturates out on fat-saturated sequences (Fig. 16.15).

Lipoblastoma is a benign neoplasm as well that originates from embryonal fat tissue and makes up to 30% of adipocytic masses in children. Lesions are diagnosed in the first 3 years of life, rapidly grow through early childhood, and have the potential to invade adjacent structures. Lipoblastoma has two subtypes: lipoblastoma proper and lipoblastomatosis. Lipoblastoma proper is encapsulated and more superficial, whereas lipoblastomatosis is not encapsulated and can invade nearby muscles. T1- and T2-weighted images reveal lobulated masses that have high signal intensity with signal loss on the fat-saturated sequences. These lesions can have thick septa and may have a heterogeneous appearance (Fig. 16.16), making it difficult to differentiate it from a liposarcoma.

Liposarcomas are malignant masses classified by the World Health Organization into five subtypes: well differentiated, dedifferentiated, myxoid, pleomorphic, and mixed. Although extremely rare in children, myxoid liposarcoma is the most common one in pediatrics, occurring in the second decade of life and often affecting the lower extremities, the thigh, or popliteal fossa regions in particular. Images are usually more heterogeneous than lipomas because there is less fatty tissue, and myxoid liposarcomas reveal a cystic appearance.

Hamartoma or fibrous hamartoma of infancy is a rapidly growing solitary benign lesion that most often

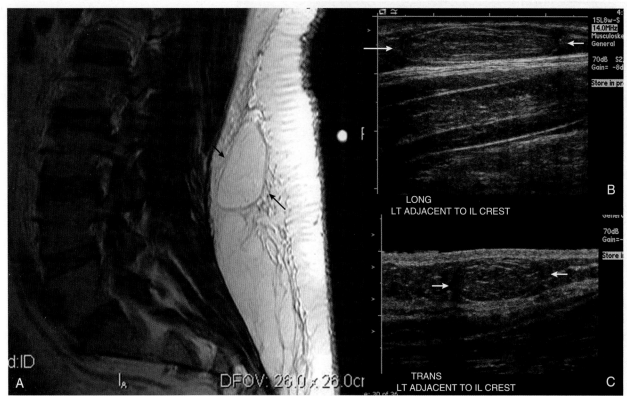

Fig. 16.15 Seventeen-year-old girl with posterior back mass demonstrates a well-encapsulated simple-appearing lipoma (*arrows*) on sagittal T2-weighted sequence (A) that completely saturated out on the fat-saturated sequences consistent with lipoma. A 13-year-old girl with a left posterior flank soft tissue mass present for years had a longitudinal and transverse ultrasound (B, C) that demonstrates a smooth oval well-defined lesion in the subcutaneous fat isoechoic to adjacent fat and with no suspicious imaging appearance consistent with lipoma.

occurs in the first year of life. The tumor is rare, most common in boys, and manifests as a painless, mobile mass often found in the axilla, upper trunk, and inguinal region. A minority of cases are present at birth. It is predominately composed of mature fat but also contains trabeculae of fibrocollagenous tissue and areas of primitive mesenchyme. Ultrasound typically shows a heterogeneously hyperechoic mass that is hypovascular to surrounding tissues on color Doppler ultrasound. The hyperechoic mass can have characteristic serpiginous hypoechoic bands representing the fibrocollagenous trabeculae (Fig. 16.17). MR reveals a fat-containing mass, apparent on T1-weighted imaging with and without fat suppression, or on in- and out-of-phase imaging. Foci of fibrous tissue, hypointense on T1- and T2-weighted imaging, may also serve as a clue to the diagnosis.

Is It a High-Flow Vascular Lesion?

Vascular lesions are classified as either neoplasms or malformations. Malformations are subdivided depending on the vessel type, such as arterial, venous, lymphatic, capillary, or mixed. High-flow lesions include neoplasms and arterial malformations; low-flow lesions include venous, lymphatic, capillary, and mixed malformations.

IH is the most common tumor of infancy. It is a mesenchymal tumor composed of arterial vascular channels that are lined by a single layer of endothelial cells. The tumor is a well-defined mass seen in the skin, subcutaneous fat, mucous membranes, airway, and parotid gland. If the lesion is superficial, it usually appears cherry red, but if the lesion is located in deeper tissues (deep dermis, subcutis, or muscle), it can have a blue hue. IH appears shortly after birth, after which it goes through a phase of rapid proliferation, peaking by 1 year of life. Pyogenic granuloma may mimic IH in appearance but clinically presents after 6 months of age. By the age of 3 to 5 years, IH regresses completely or leaves a small fibrous scar. Some complications associated with IHs are high-output congestive heart failure, hypothyroidism, and hemorrhage.

Ultrasound imaging of an IH will show a heterogeneous well-defined mass, with avid vascularity on color Doppler imaging and low-resistance arterial waveforms with spectral Doppler waveform analysis (Fig. 16.18). MRI of an IH will reveal a lobulated T1-hypointense, T2-hyperintense mass with flow voids (Fig. 16.19). Time-resolved MRA technique can be used to detect early arterial feeders and their point of origin. Similar findings can also be obtained with digital subtraction angiography, but this is usually reserved for the few situations when embolization is considered.

Rapidly involuting congenital hemangioma (RICH) and noninvoluting congenital hemangioma are lesions that undergo the rapid proliferation phase in utero, are fully formed at birth, and either rapidly involute or

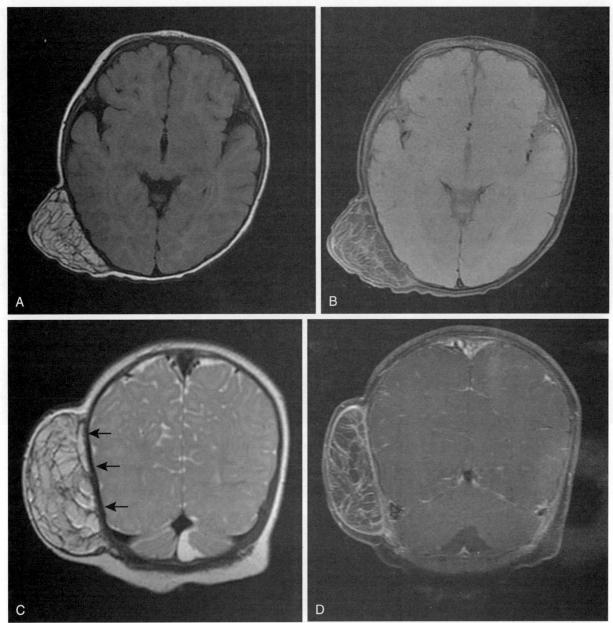

Fig. 16.16 Twenty-month-old boy with enlarging soft tissue mass and magnetic resonance imaging T1-weighted sequence without and with fat saturation (A, B) shows the lobulated mass with internal septa and significant internal fat that saturates out. The coronal T2-weighted sequence (C) demonstrates the adjacent subtle bony flattening of calvarium, and the coronal postcontrast T1-weighted fat-saturated image (D) demonstrates the enhancement of the capsule and internal septa. Histology was consistent with the preprocedure diagnosis of lipoblastoma.

persist into adulthood. On ultrasound, RICH appears as a hypoechoic lesion, sometimes with partial central necrosis. Foci of calcification and hemorrhage may also be seen in RICH. Feeding vessels, larger than those in IH, may be seen. Noninvoluting congenital hemangioma is similar to IH in imaging appearance (Fig. 16.20). Because there is significant overlap in the imaging appearances between congenital and IHs, imaging must be correlated with clinical history to make the correct diagnosis.

KHE is a locally aggressive vascular neoplastic lesion that is associated with the Kasabach-Merritt phenomenon, resulting in platelet sequestration and thrombocytopenia. Ultrasound usually demonstrates a hypervascular mass with ill-defined margins. MRI findings include an ill-defined T1-hypointense and T2-hyperintense mass with stellate borders, subcutaneous reticular pattern, and overlying skin thickening. Careful attention should be given to adjacent lymphatic channels and lymph nodes because these lesions will spread with contiguous tumor thrombus extending through dilated lymphatic channels (Fig. 16.21). Although KHE can regress over time much like IH, treatments for KHE are aggressive because of the possible lethal complications of thrombocytopenia. Treatments entail systemic therapies, with sirolimus

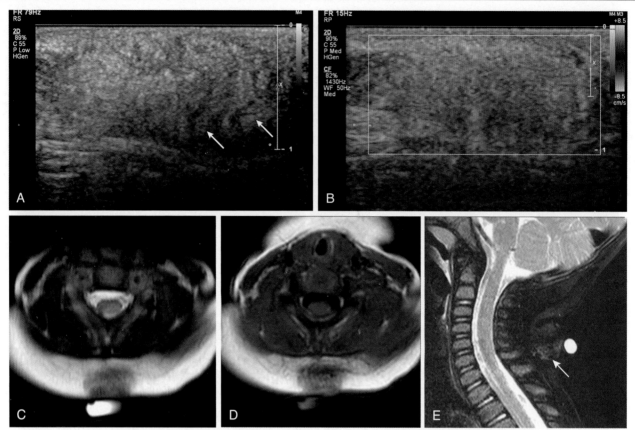

Fig. 16.17 Fourteen-month-old baby boy with congenital neck mass that has been growing since birth, with ultrasound (A) showing a heterogeneously hyperechoic lesion with serpiginous hypoechoic linear structures (*arrows*) and color Doppler showing no significant flow (B). Magnetic resonance imaging axial T2-wieghted sequence (C) demonstrated low signal, and axial T1-weighted images (D) also demonstrated low signal with sagittal T2-weighted fat-saturated sequence (E) showing focal internal fat saturating out (*arrow*) consistent with internal fat content. Biopsy showed fibrous hamartoma of infancy.

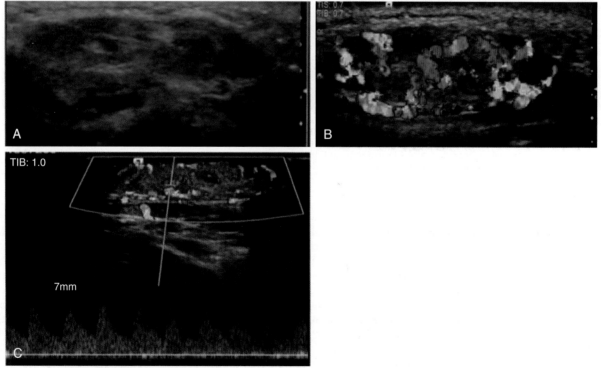

Fig. 16.18 Three-month-old baby with a palpable left chest wall mass. Grayscale ultrasound imaging (A) shows a well-circumscribed heterogenous-appearing mass. Color Doppler imaging (B) and spectral Doppler waveform analysis (C) show avid vascularity with low-resistance arterial waveforms. The imaging findings when interpreted in the context of the clinical history were consistent with infantile hemangioma.

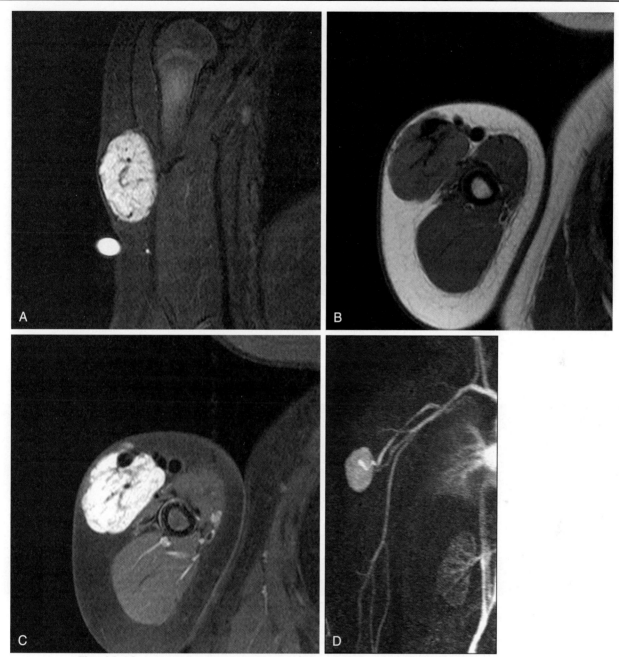

Fig. 16.19 A 9-month-old baby with an enlarging right upper extremity mass. Coronal STIR image (A) shows a lobulated hyperintense mass with flow voids. Axial precontrast (B) and postcontrast (C) T1-weighted images show a homogeneously enhancing mass. Time-resolved contrast-enhanced magnetic imaging angiography (D) shows the lesion is supplied by the brachial artery.

now becoming the first-line therapy with oral administration and vincristine being another known effective therapy.

AVMs are congenital high-flow abnormal connections between arteries and veins, with the absence of a capillary bed. Arteriovenous fistulas differ from AVMs in that they involve only a single connection between an artery and a vein typically. AVMs tend to become symptomatic during puberty as a result of changes in hormones or during episodes of infection, trauma, or thrombosis. Clinically, they can present as warm pulsatile masses with a thrill on the head, neck, trunk, or extremities. Both conditions have the potential to cause high-output heart failure. AVM differs from IH on imaging by the presence of a tangle of vessels in place of a parenchymal mass. The tangles are visible on T1- and T2-weighted imaging as flow voids and are discussed further in Chapter 15.

Is It a Slow-Flow Vascular Lesion?

Venous malformations are low-flow lesions and are the most common vascular malformation. For additional

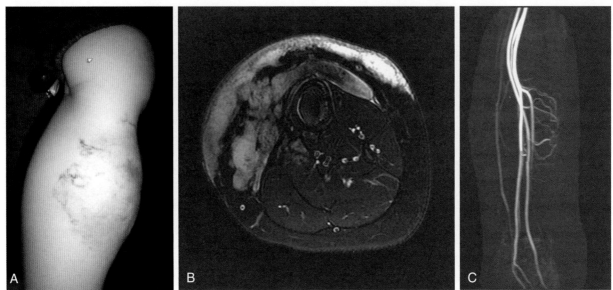

Fig. 16.20 Three-year-old boy with history of slowly growing warm vascular lesion of the left leg with dilated cutaneous vessels (A) and axial T2 fat-saturated sequence (B) demonstrated lobulated homogeneous T2 prolongation with superficial and deep components. The magnetic resonance angiogram (C) demonstrates multiple arterial feeding vessels from the posterior tibial and peroneal arteries on lateral projection. Biopsy findings were consistent with noninvoluting congenital hemangioma.

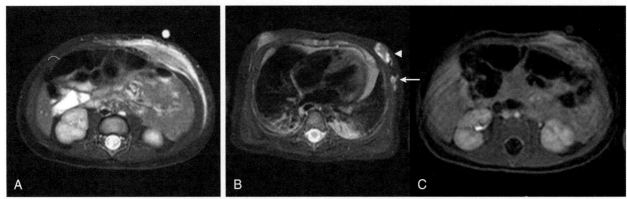

Fig. 16.21 Two-month-old with rapidly growing left abdominal mass with pigmented dark red skin and enlarged blood vessels. Axial T2-weighted fat-saturated images at the level of the tumor (A) and at the level of the breast buds (B) demonstrate an infiltrative mass invading the abdominal musculature with serpiginous T2 signal in the subcutaneous fat and tubular T2 prolongation tracking along the left chest (*arrow*) consistent with lymphatic extension with nodular increased signal within the left breast bud (*arrowhead*). Postgadolinium images on T1-weighted fat-saturated images demonstrate heterogeneous enhancement of the mass (C). Imaging and clinical findings are consistent with that of a kaposiform hemangioendothelioma.

discussion on venous malformation, see section on "Are There Calcifications?" and Chapter 15.

Lymphatic malformations are classified as either microcystic or macrocystic. Microcystic malformations are those that contain numerous septations, whereas macrocystic malformations contain only a few. The majority of malformations are mixed containing both microcystic and macrocystic regions. They can occur anywhere on the body. Ultrasound imaging of a lymphatic malformation typically reveals a multiseptated cystic mass, sometimes with fluid–fluid levels secondary to hemorrhage or infection. Color Doppler images shows septal vascularity but no internal vascularity. On MRI, lymphatic malformations are usually T2-hyperintense lesions with variable T1 signal intensity, owing to the presence of hemorrhage or proteinaceous contents within the malformation (Fig. 16.22). Treatment includes image-guided sclerotherapy, medical treatment with the mammalian target of rapamycin (mTOR) inhibitors, or surgical resection. A much more detailed discussion on this heterogeneous group of lesions can be found in Chapter 15.

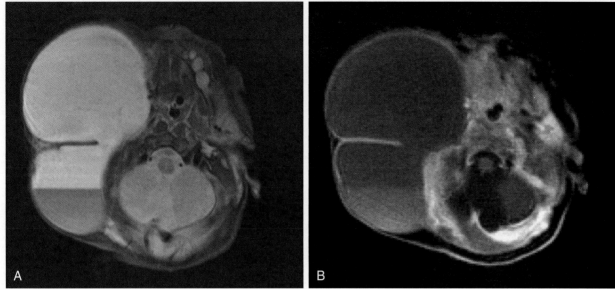

Fig. 16.22 Two-day-old baby with a prenatal history of the right neck mass. Axial T2-weighted image (A) shows a predominately hyperintense lesion, with a fluid–fluid level. Axial postcontrast gradient recalled-echo imaging (B) shows a fluid–fluid level with dependent T1 hyperintensity, secondary to hemorrhage. Imaging findings are typical of a macrocystic lymphatic malformation.

■ Summary

Soft tissue masses are often characterized by imaging. When presenting as a palpable mass, ultrasound may help characterize as cystic or solid and determine whether additional MRI may be necessary. Radiographs may occasionally be helpful, particularly for the presence of calcifications or adjacent osseous changes. MRI has excellent soft tissue mass characterization, however, may necessitate contrast as well as sedation/anesthesia. Consideration for imaging necessity and optimal initial imaging modality can guide correct diagnosis and appropriate therapy.

Bibliography

Behr, G. G., & Johnson, C. (2013). Vascular anomalies: Hemangiomas and beyond-part 1, fast-flow lesions. *American Journal of Roentgenology, 200*(2), 414–422.

Behr, G. G., & Johnson, C. (2013). Vascular anomalies: Hemangiomas and beyond-part 2, slow-flow lesions. *American Journal of Roentgenology, 200*(2), 423–436.

Biesecker, L. (2006). The challenges of Proteus syndrome: Diagnosis and management. *Eur J Hum Genetics, 14*(11), 1151–1157.

Blacksin, M., Ha, D., Hameed, M., & Aisner, S. (2006). Superficial soft-tissue masses of the extremities. *RadioGraphics, 26*(5), 1289–1304.

Chew, F. S., & Roberts, C. C. (2007). *Musculoskeletal imaging: A Teaching file* (2nd ed.). Philadelphia: Lippincott Williams & Wilkins.

Creeley, C. E., & Olney, J. W. (2010). The young: Neuroapoptosis induced by anesthetics and what to do about it. *Anesthesia & Analgesia, 110*(2), 442–448.

Dahnert, W. (2007). *Radiology review manual* (6th ed.). Philadelphia: Lippincott Williams & Wilkins.

Donnelly, L. F. (2005). *Diagnostic imaging: Pediatrics* (1st ed.). Salt Lake City, UT: Amirsys.

Dubois, J., & Alison, M. (2010). Vascular anomalies: What a radiologist needs to know. *Pediatric Radiology, 40*(6), 895–905.

Glatz, A. C., Patel, A., Zhu, X., et al. (2014). Patient radiation exposure in a modern, large-volume, pediatric cardiac catheterization laboratory. *Pediatric Cardiology, 35*(5), 870–878.

Glennie, D., Connolly, B. L., & Gordon, C. (2008). Entrance skin dose measured with MOSFETs in children undergoing interventional radiology procedures. *Pediatric Radiology, 38*(11), 1180–1187.

Greene, A. K., Karnes, J., Padua, H. M., Schmidt, B. A., Kasser, J. R., & Labow, B. I. (2009). Diffuse lipofibromatosis of the lower extremity masquerading as a vascular anomaly. *Annals of Plastic Surgery, 62*(6), 703–706.

Hammill, A., Wentzel, M. S., Gupta, A., et al. (2011). Sirolimus for the treatment of complicated vascular anomalies in children. *Pediatric Blood & Cancer, 57*(6), 1018–1024. doi:10.1002/pbc.23124. In press.Imperial, R., & Helwig, B. (1967). Verrucous hemangioma. A clinicopathologic study of 21 cases. *Archives of Dermatology, 96,* 247–253.

Knuuti, J., Saraste, A., Kallio, M., & Minn, H. (2013). Is cardiac magnetic resonance imaging causing DNA damage? *European Heart Journal, 34*(30), 2337–2339.

Kondrachuk, O., Yalynska, T., Tammo, R., & Lee, E. Y. (2012). Multidetector computed tomography evaluation of congenital mediastinal vascular anomalies in children. *Seminars in Roentgenology, 47*(2), 127–134.

Laffan, E. E., Ngan, B. Y., & Navarro, O. M. (2009). Pediatric soft-tissue tumors and pseudotumors: MR imaging features with pathologic correlation: Part 2. Tumors of fibroblastic/myofibroblastic, so-called fibrohistiocytic, muscular, lymphomatous, neurogenic, hair matrix, and uncertain origin. *RadioGraphics, 29*(4), e36.

Merrell, S. C., Rahbar, R., Alomari, A. I., et al. (2010). Infantile myofibroma or lymphatic malformation: Differential diagnosis of neonatal cystic cervicofacial lesions. *Journal of Craniofacial Surgery, 21*(2), 422–426.

Milla, S. S., & Bixby, S. D. (2010). *The Teaching files: Pediatric* (1st ed.). Philadelphia: Saunders Elsevier.

Moukaddam, H., Pollak, J., & Haims, A. H. (2009). MRI characteristics and classification of peripheral vascular malformations and tumors. *Skeletal Radiology, 38*(6), 535–547.

Nagarajan, K., & Banushree, C. (2015). Usefulness of MRI in delineation of dermal and subcutaneous verrucous hemangioma. *Indian Journal of Dermatology, 60*(5), 525.

Navarro, O., Laffan, E., & Ngan, B. (2009). Pediatric soft-tissue tumors and pseudo-tumors: MR imaging features with pathologic correlation. *RadioGraphics, 29*(3), 887–906.

Pavithra, S., Mallya, H., Kini, H., & Pai, G. S. (2011). Verrucous hemangioma or angiokeratoma? A missed diagnosis. *Indian Journal of Dermatology, 56*(5), 599–600.

Stoller, D. W. (2007). *Magnetic resonance imaging in Orthopedics and Sports medicine* (3rd ed.). Baltimore: Lippincott Williams & Wilkins.

Tennant, L. B., Mulliken, J. B., Perez-Atayde, A. R., & Kozakewich, H. P. (2006). Verrucous hemangioma revisited. *Pediatric Dermatology, 23*(3), 208–215.

Vogel, A. M., Alesbury, J. M., Burrows, P. E., & Fishman, S. J. (2006). Vascular anomalies of the female external genitalia. *Journal of Pediatric Surgery, 41*(5), 993–999.

Waner, M., North, P. E., Scherer, K. A., Frieden, I. J., Waner, A., & Mihm, M. C., Jr. (2003). The nonrandom distribution of facial hemangiomas. *Archives of Dermatology, 139*(7), 869–875.

CHAPTER 17
MSK Trauma

Azam Eghbal

CHAPTER OUTLINE

Common Musculoskeletal Trauma Imaging Techniques, 346
  Plain Radiographs, 346
  Ultrasound, 346
  Computed Tomography, 346
  Magnetic Resonance Imaging, 346
Pediatric Bone Anatomy, 346
Particularly Pediatric Fractures, 347
  Plastic Deformation, 347

  Buckle, 347
  Greenstick Fracture, 348
  Complete Fracture, 348
  Physeal Fractures, 348
Pearls and Pitfalls, 349
  How Can We Tell Abusive Fractures From Accidental Injury?, 349
  Normal Variants Not to Be Confused for Fracture, 350
Summary, 350

Whether the history is motor vehicle accident, fall from monkey bars, or sports-related injury, musculoskeletal trauma is one of the most common reasons for emergency department visits. Knowledge of the developing bone anatomy and specific pediatric fractures leads to appropriate diagnosis and treatment.

■ Common Musculoskeletal Trauma Imaging Techniques

Plain Radiographs

Multiorthogonal radiographs of the bones are a mainstay of trauma evaluation and are often the first line of evaluation.

Ultrasound

Ultrasound is often used in infants specifically for evaluation of cartilaginous portions of the bones. It is also used to assess for joint effusions, soft tissue lesions, or foreign body detection.

Computed Tomography

Complex fractures may necessitate additional evaluation by computed tomography (CT) to confirm/assess epiphyseal separation, comminution with fragments in the joint space, or the extent of fracture displacement or

to determine for possible need of open reduction internal fixation. Contrast is occasionally used for evaluation of vascular injuries.

Magnetic Resonance Imaging

Magnetic resonance imaging (MRI) is an excellent modality for evaluation of soft tissue and osseous injuries or bone marrow edema or to detect avascular necrosis. Contrast is typically not necessary unless infection or neoplasm is considered.

■ Pediatric Bone Anatomy

The most important differences between evaluating pediatric and adult bones are the anatomy of the developing bone, including the presence of growth plates, apophyses, and ossification centers.

Approximately 15% of extremity fractures in children involve disruptions of the growth plate, which is two to five times weaker than any other structure in the pediatric skeleton. In addition, the pediatric bone has greater porosity than mature adult bone, explaining unique pediatric fractures: plastic deformation, buckle, and greenstick fractures. Its greater porosity is secondary to its increased vascularity, which decreased with increasing age.

Long bones anatomy in pediatric patients include (Fig. 17.1):

Epiphysis: This is located at the end of the bone between the physis and the joint space.

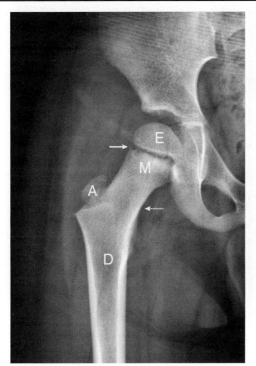

Fig. 17.1 Normal anteroposterior radiograph of the hip in a 6-year-old boy. *A,* Apophysis; *D,* diaphysis; *E,* epiphysis; *M,* metaphysis. *Arrow* indicates physis; *dotted arrow* indicates metadiaphysis.

TABLE 17.1   PELVIS APOPHYSES AND THEIR TENDINOUS ATTACHMENTS

Apophysis		Tendon
Anterior superior iliac spine	→	Sartorius
Anterior inferior iliac spine	→	Rectus femoris
Lesser trochanter	→	Iliopsoas
Greater trochanter	→	Gluteus medius
Ischial apophysis	→	Hamstring
Iliac crest	→	Abdominal wall muscles

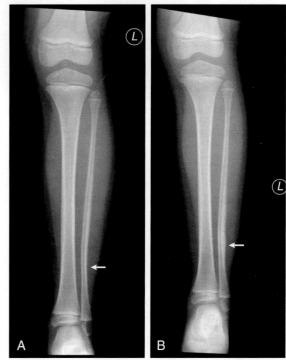

Fig. 17.2 Plastic deformation of the distal fibular diaphysis in a 6-year-old girl. (A) Anteroposterior radiograph of the left tibia and fibula shows medial apex bowing of the distal fibular diaphysis (*arrow*). (B) Subsequent radiograph 3 weeks later shows periosteal reaction along the distal fibular diaphysis (*arrow*) consistent with healing.

Physis (growth plate): The primary physis is made of hyaline cartilage and is responsible for the longitudinal growth via endochondral ossification. The newest bone forms on the metaphyseal side of the physis.

Metaphysis: This is a flared, highly vascularized segment of bone between the diaphysis and physis. It is made of immature bone. Its thinner cortex relative to the diaphysis is in part owed to its greater vascularity.

Metadiaphysis: A segment of bone between the diaphysis and metaphysis, where there is a transition in cortical thickness from the diaphyseal thicker cortex and the thinner metaphyseal cortex, increasing its susceptibility to fracture.

Diaphysis: The shaft between the proximal and distal metaphysis. The diaphysis has a thicker cortex than the metaphysis.

Apophysis: Bone that arises from a separate ossification than the parent bone and eventually fuses with the parent bone. It does not contribute to longitudinal growth and often has a tendinous attachment (Table 17.1).

■ Particularly Pediatric Fractures

Plastic Deformation

This fracture is caused by compressive trauma severe enough to deform a bone without a radiographically evident fracture. Plastic deformation is most often seen in the radius, ulna, and fibula. Although a fracture line is not visible, subsequent radiographs may show periosteal reaction as a result of fracture healing. Due to disruption of the "ring" in the forearm or distal lower extremity, an additional fracture may be present in the companion bone (Fig. 17.2).

Buckle

A buckle fracture is an incomplete fracture at the junction of the metaphysis and diaphysis on the compressive side of the bone resulting in a focal bulge on radiographs (Fig. 17.3). There is no discrete fracture

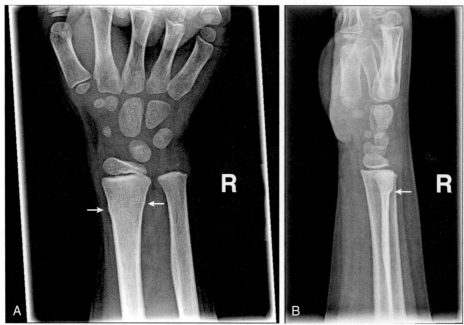

Fig. 17.3 *Buckle fracture of the right radius in a 7-year-old.* (A) Anteroposterior radiograph of the right wrist shows an undulating contour of the distal radial metadiaphysis, consistent with buckle fracture. (B) Lateral radiograph of the right wrist shows an undulating contour of the dorsal cortex of the radial metadiaphysis.

line, and the bulge does not extend along the circumference of the bone. These fractures are commonly seen in the distal radius and ulna, secondary to a fall on an outstretched hand.

Greenstick Fracture

A greenstick fracture is an incomplete cortical disruption along the tension side of bone, with a plastic deformation on the compressive side, usually occurring at the metadiaphysis (Fig. 17.4).

Complete Fracture

A complete fracture is one that propagates through the bone resulting in a circumferential disruption of the cortex.

Physeal Fractures

The Salter-Harris classification is the most commonly used classification system to describe fractures involving the physis (Fig. 17.5) (Table 17.2). Approximately 90% of growth plate fractures can be classified as Salter-Harris I–IV on plain radiograph. The other 10% of fractures may require either additional views or advanced

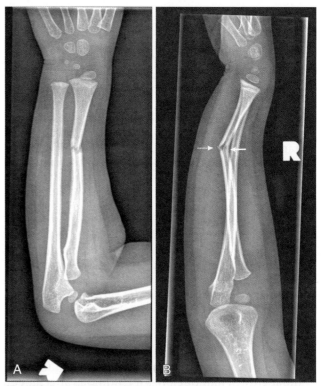

Fig. 17.4 *Greenstick fracture of the distal radial diaphysis in a 4-year-old girl.* Anteroposterior (A) and lateral (B) radiographs show a cortical disruption along the tension side of the bone (*dotted arrow*). The compression side of the bone (*arrow*) is intact, with volar bowing.

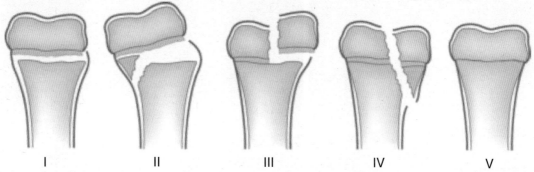

I   II   III   IV   V

Fig. 17.5 *Salter-Harris classification of fractures. (Reproduced with permission from Mettler, F. A. [2019] Essentials of radiology [pp. 199–290, Fig. 8.81]. Elsevier.)*

TABLE 17.2 SALTER-HARRIS-CLASSIFICATION OF FRATURES

Salter-Harris type I

6% of all growth plate fractures
Transverse fracture through the physis separating epiphysis from metaphysis
Can be radiographically occult
More common in young children and children
Ultrasound is useful adjunct tool in the setting of the proximal or distal humeral epiphyseal separation, when the cartilaginous epiphysis is not yet ossified (see Fig. 17.5)

Salter-Harris type II

Accounts for 75% of all physeal injuries
Transverse fracture through the physis accompanied by a vertical or oblique fracture through the metaphysis often making a triangular metaphyseal fragment of varying size (Fig. 17.6)

Salter-Harris type III

8% of physeal injuries
Transverse fracture through the growth plate accompanied by a vertical or oblique fracture through the epiphysis typically reaching the articular surface (Fig. 17.7)
Usually occurs in older children when growth plate closure starts
Because of intraarticular extension, arthritis may be a complication of Salter-Harris type III fractures

Salter-Harris type IV

10% of physeal fractures
Vertical or oblique fracture through metaphysis, physis, epiphysis, and articular cartilage (Fig. 17.8)
The triplane fracture is a unique pediatric fracture
Complications include growth arrest, limb-length discrepancy, and angular deformities (Fig. 17.9)

Salter-Harris type V

Compression fracture or crushing injury of the growth plate
Radiographically occult
Existence has been questioned

imaging for diagnosis. Although the majority of growth plate injuries heal without complication, limb length discrepancies or angular deformities are often the result of trauma to the physis, causing injury to the physis itself or disruption of the epiphyseal or metaphyseal blood supply and subsequent growth arrest and physeal bar development.

Other unique and common fractures in young children include the toddler's fracture and the trampoline, or type II toddler's fracture, and in older children include pelvic apophyseal avulsion fractures. For a full discussion, see Chapter 10. Pediatric elbow fractures are discussed in Chapter 13.

■ Pearls and Pitfalls

How Can We Tell Abusive Fractures From Accidental Injury?

The age of a patient, mechanism of trauma, underlying mineralization, presence of healing, or additional fractures are all important factors to consider in the determination if there should be concern raised for abuse. For a detailed discussion on nonaccidental trauma, see Chapter 21.

One of the most important concepts in evaluation of pediatric fractures is the correlation between the fracture pattern and the clinical history given by caregivers. There are chapters in this book dedicated to abusive skeletal trauma (see Chapter 21) and central nervous system injuries (see Chapter 20). Attention to those chapters is tantamount to understand fractures that have high specificity for child abuse, such as posterior rib fractures, and fractures that can be seen in both abuse and accidental trauma, such as clavicle fractures. Clavicle fractures are common accidental injuries and can also been seen from birth trauma. As with all fractures, the age of a patient, mechanism of trauma, underlying mineralization, and presence of healing or additional fractures are all important factors to consider in the determination whether there should be concern raised for abuse.

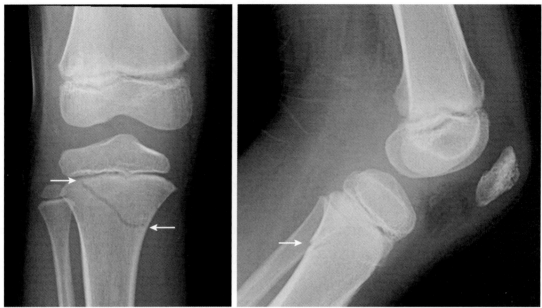

Fig. 17.6 Salter-Harris type II fracture of the proximal tibia in a 6-year-old girl. Anteroposterior and lateral radiographs of the knee show an oblique lucency (*arrows*) in the proximal tibial metaphysis extending to the physis consistent with a Salter-Harris type II fracture.

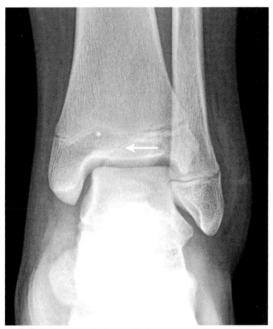

Fig. 17.7 Salter-Harris type III fracture of the distal tibia in a 14-year-old boy. Anteroposterior view of the ankle shows an obliquely oriented lucency through the distal tibial epiphysis. This fracture of the anterolateral distal tibial epiphysis is also called a juvenile Tillaux fracture. The fracture occurs at the time of physeal closure, which begins in the anteromedial physis (*asterisk*), referred to as "Kump's bump." The lateral physis closes after the medial physis, making it more prone to fracture.

Normal Variants Not to Be Confused for Fracture

There are many anatomical variants in the developing skeleton that can mimic traumatic injury. Although a few common variants are included in Figs. 17.10 and 17.11, the reader is directed to a more comprehensive

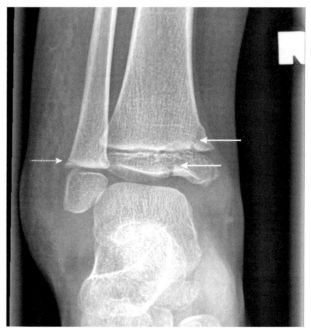

Fig. 17.8 Salter-Harris type IV fracture of the distal tibia in a 5-year-old girl. Anteroposterior view of the right ankle shows an irregular lucency through the distal tibial metaphysis extending through the physis and epiphysis (*arrows*). There is no offset at the articular surface. Also note the Salter-Harris type II fracture of the distal fibula (*dotted arrow*).

text, *Atlas of Normal Roentgen Variants That May Simulate Disease* by Keats (2003).

■ Summary

Familiarity with pediatric musculoskeletal anatomy and unique pediatric fractures is necessary for accurate interpretation.

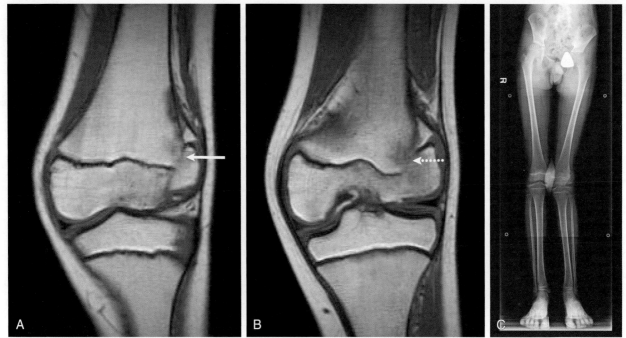

Fig. 17.9 *Salter-Harris type IV fracture of the distal femur in an 11-year-old boy.* Coronal T1-weighted image through the left knee (A) show a T1 hypointense line (*arrow*) in the lateral aspect of the distal femur, traversing the metaphysis, physis, and epiphysis consistent with Salter-Harris type IV fracture. There is proximal displacement of the fracture fragment with loss of articular congruence. Subsequent MRI (B) shows premature physeal fusion (*dotted arrow*). A standing anteroposterior radiograph of the lower extremities (C) shows resultant left genu valgum.

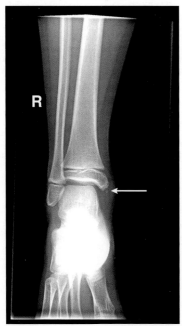

Fig. 17.10 *Medial malleolar secondary ossification center in an 8-year-old girl.* Anteroposterior radiograph of the right ankle showing a small ossific density inferior to the medial malleolus (*arrow*) consistent with a secondary ossification center. This variant of ossification typically appears between age 6 and 9 years in girls and 8 and 9 years in boys.

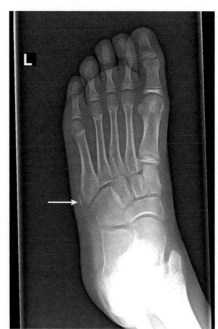

Fig. 17.11 *Base of fifth metatarsal apophysis in a 10-year-old girl.* Oblique radiograph of the left foot showing the apophysis of the base of the fifth metatarsal (*arrow*). This typically ossifies at age 10 years in girls and age 12 years in boys, with fusion in the following 2 to 4 years.

Bibliography

Alison, M., Azoulay, R., Tilea, B., Sekkal, A., Presedo, A., & Sebag, G. (2009). Imaging strategies in paediatric musculoskeletal trauma. *Pediatric Radiology*, *39*(Suppl. 3), S414–S421.

Appelboam, A., Reuben, A. D., Benger, J. R., et al. (2008). Elbow extension test to rule out elbow fracture: Multicentre, prospective validation and observational study of diagnostic accuracy in adults and children. *BMJ*, *337*, a2428.

Boutis, K., Komar, L., Jaramillo, D., et al. (2001). Sensitivity of a clinical examination to predict need for radiography in children with ankle injuries: A prospective study. *Lancet*, *358*, 2118–2121.

Brown, S. D., Kasser, J. R., Zurakowski, D., et al. (2004). Analysis of 51 tibial triplane fractures using CT with multiplanar reconstruction. *American Journal of Roentgenology*, *183*, 1489–1495.

Buhs, C., Cullen, M., Klein, M., et al. (2000). The pediatric trauma C-spine: Is the 'odontoid' view necessary? *Journal of Pediatric Surgery*, *35*, 994–997.

Bulloch, B., Neto, G., Plint, A., et al. (2003). Validation of the ottawa knee rule in children: A multicenter study. *Annals of Emergency Medicine*, *42*, 48–55.

Busch, M. T. (1990). Meniscal injuries in children and adolescents. *Clinics in Sports Medicine*, *9*, 661–680.

Chapman, V., Grottkau, B., Albright, M., et al. (2006). MDCT of the elbow in pediatric patients with posttraumatic elbow effusions. *American Journal of Roentgenology*, *187*, 812–817.

Connolly, S. A., Connolly, L. P., & Jaramillo, D. (2001). Imaging of sports injuries in children and adolescents. *Radiol Clin North Am*, *39*, 773–790.

Ducou Le Pointe, H., & Sirinelli, D. (2005). Limb emergencies in children. *Journal de Radiologie*, *86*, 251–252.

Egloff, A. M., Kadom, N., Vezina, G., et al. (2008). Pediatric cervical spine trauma imaging: A practical approach. *Pediatric Radiology*, *39*(Suppl. 3), S414–S421.

Fayad, L. M., Johnson, P., & Fishman, E. K. (2005). Multidetector CT of musculoskeletal disease in the pediatric patient: Principles, techniques, and clinical applications. *RadioGraphics*, *25*, 603–618.

Flynn, J. M., Wong, K. L., Yeh, G. L., et al. (2002). Displaced fractures of the hip in children. Management by early operation and immobilization in a hip spica cast. *J Bone Joint Surg Br*, *84*, 108–112.

Frank, J. B., Lim, C. K., Flynn, J. M., et al. (2002). The efficacy of magnetic resonance imaging in pediatric cervical spine clearance. *Spine*, *27*, 1176–1179.

Hernandez, J. A., Chupik, C., & Swischuk, L. E. (2004). Cervical spine trauma in children under 5 years: Productivity of CT. *Emergency Radiology*, *10*, 176–178.

Jacoby, S. M., Herman, M. J., Morrison, W. B., et al. (2007). Pediatric elbow trauma: An orthopaedic perspective on the importance of radiographic interpretation. *Semin Musculoskelet Radiol*, *11*, 48–56.

Jaffe, D. M., Binns, H., Radkowski, M. A., et al. (1987). Developing a clinical algorithm for early management of cervical spine injury in child trauma victims. *Annals of Emergency Medicine*, *16*, 270–276.

Jaramillo, D., & Laor, T. (2008). Pediatric musculoskeletal MRI: Basic principles to optimize success. *Pediatric Radiology*, *38*, 379–391.

Jaramillo, D., & Shapiro, F. (1998). Musculoskeletal trauma in children. *Magn Reson Imaging Clin N Am*, *6*, 521–536.

Johnson, K. J., Haigh, S. F., & Symonds, K. E. (2000). MRI in the management of scaphoid fractures in skeletally immature patients. *Pediatric Radiology*, *30*, 685–688.

Keats, T. E. (2003). Atlas of normal roentgen variants that may simulate disease (7th ed.). Mosby.

Khanna, G., & El-Khoury, G. Y. (2007). Imaging of cervical spine injuries of childhood. *Skeletal Radiology*, *36*, 477–494.

Launay, F., Barrau, K., Petit, P., et al. (2008). Ankle injuries without fracture in children. Prospective study with magnetic resonance in 116 patients. *Rev Chir Orthop Reparatrice Appar Mot*, *94*, 427–433.

Lee, S. L., Sena, M., Greenholz, S. K., et al. (2003). A multidisciplinary approach to the development of a cervical spine clearance protocol: Process, rationale, and initial results. *Journal of Pediatric Surgery*, *38*, 358–362 discussion 358–362.

Lennon, R. I., Riyat, M. S., Hilliam, R., et al. (2007). Can a normal range of elbow movement predict a normal elbow x ray? *Emergency Medicine Journal*, *24*, 86–88.

Major, N. M., & Crawford, S. T. (2002). Elbow effusions in trauma in adults and children: Is there an occult fracture? *American Journal of Roentgenology*, *178*, 413–418.

Mellado, J. M., Ramos, A., Salvado, E., et al. (2002). Avulsion fractures and chronic avulsion injuries of the knee: Role of MR imaging. *European Radiology*, *12*, 2463–2473.

Merrow, A. C., Reiter, M. P., Zbojniewicz, A. M., & Laor, T. (2014). Avulsion fractures of the pediatric knee. *Pediatric Radiology*, *44*(11), 1436–1445.

Myers, A., Canty, K., & Nelson, T. (2005). Are the Ottawa ankle rules helpful in ruling out the need for x ray examination in children? *Archives of Disease in Childhood*, *90*, 1309–1311.

Petit, P., Panuel, M., Faure, F., et al. (1996). Acute fracture of the distal tibial physis: Role of gradient-echo MR imaging versus plain film examination. *American Journal of Roentgenology*, *166*, 1203–1206.

Petit, P., Sapin, C., Henry, G., et al. (2001). Rate of abnormal osteoarticular radiographic findings in pediatric patients. *American Journal of Roentgenology*, *176*, 987–990.

Reed, M. H. (2008). Imaging utilization commentary: A radiology perspective. *Pediatric Radiology*, *38*(Suppl. 4), S660–S663.

Rossi, F., & Dragoni, S. (2001). Acute avulsion fractures of the pelvis in adolescent competitive athletes: Prevalence, location and sports distribution of 203 cases collected. *Skeletal Radiology*, *30*, 127–131.

Salamipour, H., Jimenez, R. M., Brec, S. L., et al. (2005). Multidetector row CT in pediatric musculoskeletal imaging. *Pediatric Radiology*, *35*, 555–564.

Simanovsky, N., Hiller, N., Leibner, E., et al. (2005). Sonographic detection of radiographically occult fractures in paediatric ankle injuries. *Pediatric Radiology*, *35*, 1062–1065.

Skaggs, D. L., & Mirzayan, R. (1999). The posterior fat pad sign in association with occult fracture of the elbow in children. *J Bone Joint Surg Am*, *81*, 1429–1433.

Smart, P. J., Hardy, P. J., Buckley, D. M., et al. (2003). Cervical spine injuries to children under 11: Should we use radiography more selectively in their initial assessment? *Emergency Medicine Journal*, *20*, 225–227.

Stevens, M. A., El-Khoury, G. Y., Kathol, M. H., et al. (1999). Imaging features of avulsion injuries. *RadioGraphics*, *19*, 655–672.

Swischuk, L. E., John, S. D., & Hendrick, E. P. (2000). Is the open-mouth odontoid view necessary in children under 5 years? *Pediatric Radiology*, *30*, 186–189.

Vialle, R., Pannier, S., Odent, T., et al. (2004). Imaging of traumatic dislocation of the hip in childhood. *Pediatric Radiology*, *34*, 970–979.

Viccellio, P., Simon, H., Pressman, B. D., et al. (2001). A prospective multicenter study of cervical spine injury in children. *Pediatrics*, *108*, E20.

Zaidi, A., Babyn, P., Astori, I., et al. (2006). MRI of traumatic patellar dislocation in children. *Pediatric Radiology*, *36*, 1163–1170.

Zuazo, I., Bonnefoy, O., Tauzin, C., et al. (2008). Acute elbow trauma in children: Role of ultrasonography. *Pediatric Radiology*, *38*, 982–988.

General

SECTION 3

General

CHAPTER 18

Imaging of the Neonate: Preterm Infant

Smyrna Tuburan

CHAPTER OUTLINE

Is This Neonate Preterm?, 355
Lines and Tubes in the Neonatal Intensive Care Unit, 355
   Umbilical Venous Catheter, 355
   Umbilical Arterial Catheter, 355
Chest, 356
   How to Approach Lung Opacities in the Preterm Infant?, 356
   Respiratory Distress Syndrome, 357
   Air Leak Complications in Respiratory Distress Syndrome, 357

Neonatal Chronic Lung Disease, 358
Patent Ductus Arteriosus, 359
Gastrointestinal, 359
   What to Look Out for in a Preterm Infant Abdominal Radiograph?, 359
   Necrotizing Enterocolitis, 359
Brain, 361
   Head Ultrasound Technique, 361
   What to Look for in a Preterm Head Ultrasound?, 361
   Germinal Matrix Hemorrhage, 361
Summary, 367

Preterm birth is birth before 37 weeks' gestational age. The incidence of preterm birth is approximately 1 in 10 births in the United States. The imaging of a preterm infant is not uncommon, and especially in the neonatal period, the radiologist plays a crucial role in the diagnosis of common complications related to preterm birth. Through a system-based approach, this chapter will review key imaging diagnoses commonly seen in the preterm infant.

■ Is This Neonate Preterm?

When evaluating any neonatal radiograph, a helpful initial step is to determine whether the neonate is preterm. Signs of prematurity include overall reduction in subcutaneous fat and lack of humeral head ossification. Humeral head ossification is almost never present before 38 weeks' gestational age.

■ Lines and Tubes in the Neonatal Intensive Care Unit

Umbilical Venous Catheter

Umbilical venous catheters (UVCs) are used in critically ill neonates for venous access for administra-

tion of intravenous fluids, parenteral nutrition, blood products, and medical medications, because peripheral and conventional central venous catheters are difficult to place. The typical course of the UVC is from the umbilical vein superiorly into the left portal vein, after which it courses through the ductus venosus into the inferior vena cava. The ideal positioning of the UVC is at the inferior vena cava–right atrial junction (Fig. 18.1).

Because of lack of imaging guidance during UVC placement, misplacement is not uncommon (Fig. 18.2). Complications of UVC misplacement include hepatic hematoma and necrosis in the setting of an intrahepatic placement of a UVC (Fig. 18.3), right or left atrial perforation, or umbilical vein perforation resulting in extravasation or hemoperitoneum (Fig. 18.4). Thrombosis in the inferior vena cava may occur even in an appropriately positioned UVC.

Umbilical Arterial Catheter

Umbilical arterial catheters (UACs) are used in neonates for blood pressure monitoring, blood sampling, and infusion of fluids and medications. The course of the UAC is from one of the two umbilical arteries inferiorly into the right or left internal iliac artery, after which it ascends through the common iliac artery into the aorta. A

UAC may be positioned with the tip between T6 and T9 (high UAC) or L3 and L5 (low UAC) to avoid the major aortic branches vessels (see Fig. 18.1). Complications of UACs include aortic thrombus, embolic events, and renal artery thrombus, which can result in hypertension or renal infarction.

■ Chest

How to Approach Lung Opacities in the Preterm Infant?

In the immediate neonatal period, particularly on the initial chest radiograph, surfactant deficiency syndrome is the most common diagnosis. Other diagnoses and superimposed conditions, such as infection, pulmonary edema, masses, and congenital anomalies, may

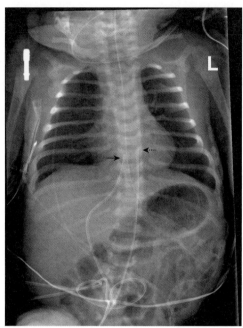

Fig. 18.1 Appropriate positioning of an umbilical venous and umbilical arterial catheter. Anteroposterior radiograph of the chest and abdomen shows the umbilical venous catheter *(arrow)* at the junction of the inferior vena cava and right atrium, and the umbilical arterial catheter *(dotted arrow)* at the T6/7 disc space.

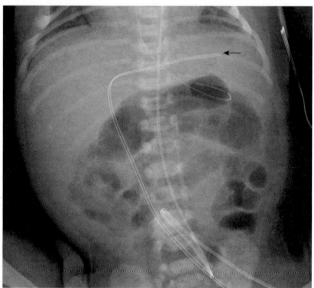

Fig. 18.2 Umbilical venous catheter malposition. Anteroposterior radiograph of the abdomen shows an umbilical venous catheter in the left portal vein.

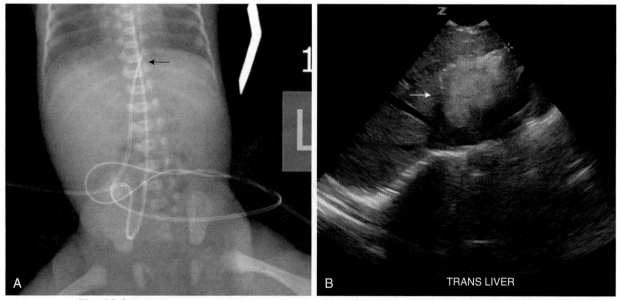

Fig. 18.3 Umbilical venous catheter malposition. Anteroposterior radiograph of the abdomen (A) showing an umbilical venous catheter projecting over the liver *(arrow)*. Transverse grayscale ultrasound image of the liver (B) performed for abnormal liver function tests shows an echogenic mass *(arrow)* in the left lobe of the liver, representing a region of hepatic necrosis after total parenteral nutrition infusion through the malpositioned umbilical venous catheter.

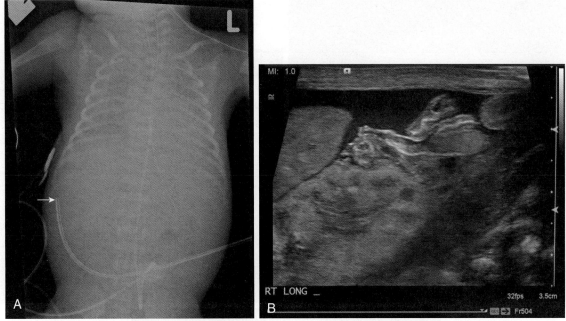

Fig. 18.4 Umbilical venous catheter malposition. Anteroposterior radiograph of the chest and abdomen (A) after emergent line placement in the delivery room showing an umbilical venous catheter coursing toward the right flank *(arrow)*, concerning for intraperitoneal placement. Longitudinal grayscale ultrasound image of the abdomen (B) after infusion of fluid through the umbilical venous catheter intraperitoneal free fluid.

also be present in preterm infants (see discussion in Chapter 19).

Respiratory Distress Syndrome

Respiratory distress syndrome (RDS) is the leading cause of death in babies who are born prematurely. RDS develops in approximately 10% of premature babies in the United States each year. RDS, now also known as surfactant deficiency syndrome, is the clinical manifestation of surfactant deficiency. Surfactant, a lipoprotein, synthesized by type II alveolar cells, lowers alveolar surface tension, thereby preventing alveolar collapse. Differentiation of type II alveolar cells occurs during the canalicular phase of lung development (18–28 weeks gestational age), after which surfactant is produced. Surfactant production increases with increasing gestational age. Alveolar development begins at 32 weeks gestational age and continues postnatally to 18 months of life.

Lack of sufficient surfactant in preterm infants results in increased surface tension within alveoli, and alveolar and acinar collapse. This radiographically manifests as low lung volumes, with granular opacification, and air bronchograms. The granular opacification that is typical of surfactant deficiency is secondary to collapse of alveoli with persistent aeration of the bronchioles and interstitial fluid secondary to capillary leakage. Radiographic findings are present shortly after birth and may progress in the first 24 hours of life (Fig. 18.5).

The treatment of RDS involves prenatal administration of corticosteroids, respiratory support (continuous positive airway pressure and high-frequency oscillatory ventilation), and exogenous surfactant administration. Exogenous surfactant administration can result in symmetrical or asymmetrical improvement in lung aeration,

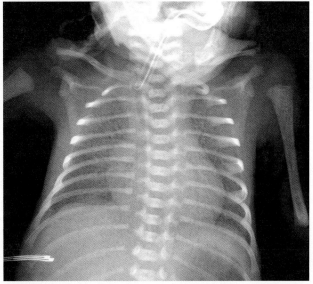

Fig. 18.5 Surfactant deficiency. Anteroposterior radiograph of the chest in a 29-week gestational age neonate shows bilateral diffuse granular opacities, typical of surfactant deficiency.

possibly secondary to heterogenous exogenous surfactant distribution. A known complication of exogenous surfactant administration is pulmonary hemorrhage, which clinically manifests as respiratory decompensation after a period of clinical improvement. Radiographs will demonstrate new dense airspace consolidation (Fig. 18.6).

Air Leak Complications in Respiratory Distress Syndrome

Air leak phenomena may develop in patients with RDS secondary to barotrauma and airway overdistension. It

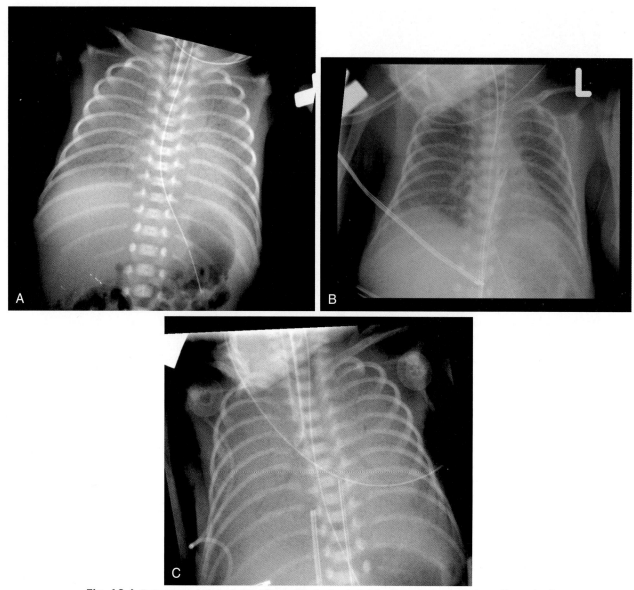

Fig. 18.6 Pulmonary hemorrhage after surfactant administration. Anteroposterior radiograph of the chest in a 26-week gestational age neonate at postnatal day 1 (A) showing bilateral diffuse granular opacities with multifocal atelectasis. A radiograph of the chest was obtained on day 2 after surfactant administration (B) showing improved aeration of the lungs likely caused by resolving atelectasis. After an abrupt period of desaturation, an anteroposterior radiograph of the chest obtained on postnatal day 3 (C) shows diffuse airspace opacification of the lungs, concerning for pulmonary hemorrhage. Bright red blood was suctioned from the endotracheal tube.

may occur in ventilated and nonventilated neonates. Air leak phenomena include pulmonary interstitial emphysema (PIE), pneumothorax, pneumomediastinum, and, rarely, pneumopericardium. PIE is the result of rupture at the bronchoalveolar junction, with subsequent tracking of air into the peribronchial and perivascular spaces. It may be focal or diffuse, and bilateral or unilateral. Radiographically, it manifests as branching lucencies, often cystic, along the expected course of the bronchovascular bundles (Fig. 18.7). PIE detection is important as a warning sign for other air leak complications. Pneumothoraces, pneumomediastinum, and pneumatoceles may also occur as a sequela of barotrauma in patients with RDS, with or without PIE (Figs. 18.8–18.10).

Neonatal Chronic Lung Disease

Neonatal chronic lung disease (CLD) is a common chronic pulmonary disease of infancy and is related to arrested lung development. Pathologically, CLD represents alveolar simplification and fibrosis. Radiographically, CLD manifests as coarsened interstitial markings with or without intervening cystic lucencies, as well as hyperinflation with regional air trapping and atelectasis (Fig. 18.11).

Long-term sequelae of BPD include hyperactive airways and increased susceptibility to lower airway infections.

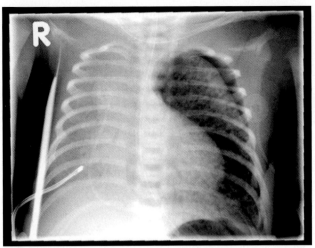

Fig. 18.7 Pulmonary interstitial emphysema. Anteroposterior radiograph of the chest in a 32-week gestational age neonate showing branching lucencies throughout the left lung consistent with pulmonary interstitial emphysema. There is an associated left pneumothorax.

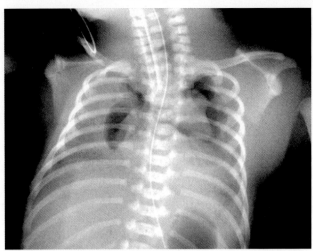

Fig. 18.9 Pneumomediastinum. Anteroposterior radiograph of the chest in a 28-week gestation age neonate showing two large lucencies over the mediastinum, superimposed on the thymus, consistent with pneumomediastinum. There is diffuse opacification of the lungs, thought to represent atelectasis in the setting of surfactant deficiency.

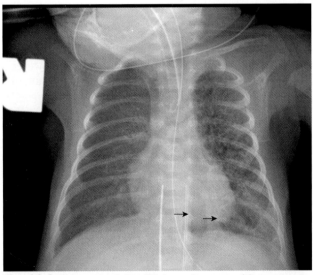

Fig. 18.8 Pulmonary interstitial emphysema with pneumatocele. Anteroposterior radiograph of the chest in a 30-week gestation age neonate showing branching left perihilar lucencies consistent with pulmonary interstitial emphysema. There are two larger ovoid lucencies *(arrows)* in the left lung base consistent with pneumatoceles.

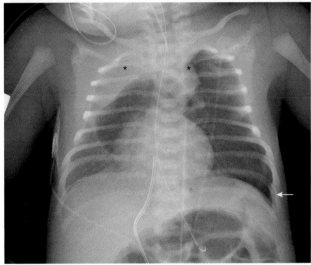

Fig. 18.10 Pneumomediastinum and pneumothorax. Anteroposterior radiograph of the chest in a 34-week gestational age neonate shows a large lucency over the mediastinum with superior displacement of both thymic lobes *(asterisk)* consistent with pneumomediastinum. There is also a left basilar pneumothorax *(arrow)* with increased lucency in the left costophrenic angle and a deep sulcus. Granular opacification in both lungs is consistent with surfactant deficiency.

Patent Ductus Arteriosus

The ductus arteriosus is patent at birth and closes within 3 days in term infants. In preterm infants, closure may happen as late as postnatal day 7. Moreover, because of the hypoxia associated with RDS, the ductus arteriosus may remain open. Normal shunting of blood flow across the patent ductus arteriosus is bidirectional. As pulmonary arterial pressure decreases in the first few days of life, left-to-right shunting increases, resulting in pulmonary venous congestion and pulmonary edema. Radiographic findings of a patent ductus arteriosus may include increasing heart size and increasing prominence of the central pulmonary vasculature (Fig. 18.12).

■ Gastrointestinal

What to Look Out for in a Preterm Infant Abdominal Radiograph?

Necrotizing Enterocolitis

Necrotizing enterocolitis (NEC) is the most common gastrointestinal condition in premature neonates. The exact cause of NEC is unknown, and it is theorized to have a multifactorial etiology, including a combination of ischemic and infectious etiologies superimposed on immature immunity. It is associated with significant mortality, ranging between 20% and 40%, which is even higher in very low-birth-weight infants, who are also at greater risk for NEC. It most often occurs in the first few days of life but can occur up to 3 weeks after birth or even later in some infants. The most common location of affected bowel is the terminal ileum; however, any part of the large or small bowel can be affected. It is also worth noting that NEC can occur in term infants, in particular those with underlying congenital heart disease.

Clinical signs and symptoms often overlap with that of neonatal sepsis and include tachypnea, tachycardia, and blood pressure lability, with abdominal distension, erythematous abdominal wall, feeding intolerance, and bloody stools. As such, abdominal radiographs and occasionally ultrasound play an important role in the

diagnosis of NEC. In addition, the radiologist plays a particularly important role at the time of diagnosis because radiological findings may precede the clinical signs. Medical NEC without imaging evidence of bowel perforation is treated with supportive care, which includes bowel rest, serial radiographs, and antibiotic therapy. NEC with perforation is treated with surgical resection of the perforated and necrotic bowel.

A range of radiographic findings are seen in NEC (Box 18.1). Radiographic findings suggestive of NEC

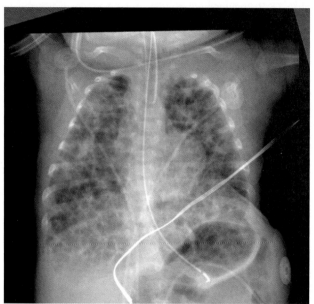

Fig. 18.11 Chronic lung disease of prematurity. Anteroposterior radiograph of the chest in a 3-month-old former 26-week gestational age infant showing markedly hyperinflated lungs with rounded lucencies throughout the lung parenchyma representing chronic lung disease of prematurity.

BOX 18-1　Necrotizing Enterocolitis Radiographic Findings

Suggestive

Focal or asymmetrical dilation of bowel (especially within the right lower quadrant)

Featureless "unfolded" bowel loops

Separation of bowel loops

Fixed bowel gas pattern over serial films

Diagnostic

Pneumatosis
- Bubble-like (submucosal) or curvilinear (serosal) lucencies
- Mimics fecal material or meconium; however, fecal material is uncommon in sick premature or nonfed infants in the intensive care unit

Portal venous gas
- Branching lucencies overlying the liver
- More peripheral extension than biliary gas

Pneumoperitoneum
- Triangles of anterior lucency (cross-table lateral radiograph)
- Lucency adjacent to liver (left lateral decubitus radiograph)
- Overall increased lucency (supine radiographs)
- Air on both sides of bowel wall (Rigler sign)
- Outline of falciform ligament (football sign)

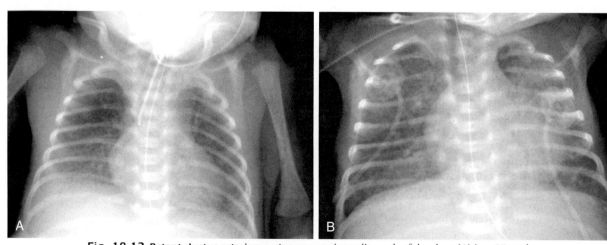

Fig. 18.12 Patent ductus arteriosus. Anteroposterior radiograph of the chest (A) in a 25-week gestational age infant on postnatal day 2 showing granular opacification of lungs representing surfactant deficiency. A follow-up radiograph (B) 10 days later shows increasing conspicuity of the perihilar vasculature with a slight increasing size of the cardiac silhouette. An echocardiogram showed a moderate-size patent ductus arteriosus with left-to-right shunting.

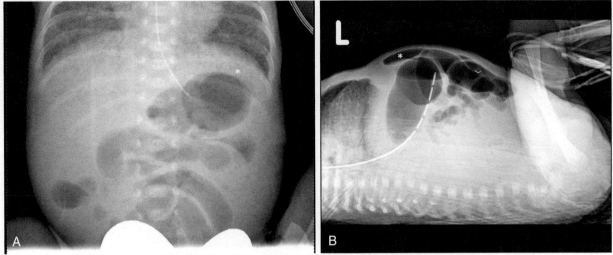

Fig. 18.13 Necrotizing enterocolitis. Anteroposterior radiograph of the abdomen (A) in a 15-day-old former 24-week gestational age neonate with abdominal distension shows dilated tubular loops of bowel in the lower abdomen with separation of bowel loops concerning for necrotizing enterocolitis. Cross-table lateral radiograph of the abdomen (B) obtained 2 days later shows pneumoperitoneum *(asterisk)*.

include asymmetrical and/or fixed dilatation of bowel and separation of bowel (Figs. 18.13 and 18.14). Hallmarks of NEC include pneumatosis, portal venous gas, and pneumoperitoneum (Figs. 18.15–18.17). If NEC is suspected clinically, or if there is concern on supine abdominal radiographs, additional cross-table lateral or left lateral decubitus radiographs should be obtained. The only radiographic finding seen in NEC that is considered an absolute indication for surgery is pneumoperitoneum.

The use of ultrasound can be helpful in cases of NEC when the radiograph demonstrates abdominal distension but a gasless abdomen. Ultrasound can detect early perforation by demonstrating complex fluid and portal venous gas in patients with suspected NEC in whom free air is not detected on abdominal radiography. Ultrasound may be able to demonstrate intramural gas and free intraperitoneal air (Fig. 18.18). Additional findings on ultrasound associated with NEC include thickened bowel loops with increased or absent color Doppler flow suggestive of inflamed or infarcted bowel.

A well-known complication of NEC is intestinal stricture, secondary to postinflammatory collagen deposition and fibrosis. Intestinal strictures develop in approximately 40% of infants with a history of NEC, typically within 3 months after the acute phase of NEC. Strictures are more common in the patients with surgically treated NEC. Patients may present with feeding intolerance, bowel obstruction, perforation, and sepsis. Strictures are most often in the colon but also can be present in the small bowel. The diagnosis can be made by contrast enema or small bowel follow-though.

■ Brain

Magnetic resonance imaging (MRI) is an excellent imaging modality for infant brain imaging, but it may be challenging or impossible to acquire in the critically ill infant. Head ultrasound is performed without sedation and can be performed portably in the neonatal intensive care unit (NICU), obviating the need to transport critically ill neonates. It is an excellent screening tool to look for hemorrhage and hydrocephalus. Although it is not as sensitive for detecting ischemia as MRI, ischemia and white matter injury can be identified if careful attention is made to subtle features.

Head Ultrasound Technique

Sonography of the neonatal brain is done primarily through the anterior fontanelle as a window. Both coronal plane and sagittal plane imaging are performed (Figs. 18.19 and 18.20). In addition, mastoid views obtained are helpful to evaluate the cerebellum often in axial and coronal planes (Fig. 18.21). Cerebellar injury is not uncommon in premature infants, and mastoid views have become more commonly performed in the evaluation of premature newborns in the NICU. Cine images and still images are obtained during cranial sonography using a dedicated neonatal head probe and high-resolution linear images for determination of near-field structures, such as extraaxial spaces and superior sagittal sinus patency.

What to Look for in a Preterm Head Ultrasound?

Germinal Matrix Hemorrhage
The germinal matrix is the site of future neuronal and glial cells and is located in the subependymal region. In the setting of poor cerebrovascular autoregulation during fetal/prenatal periods of physiological instability, the thin-walled vasculature of the germinal ma-

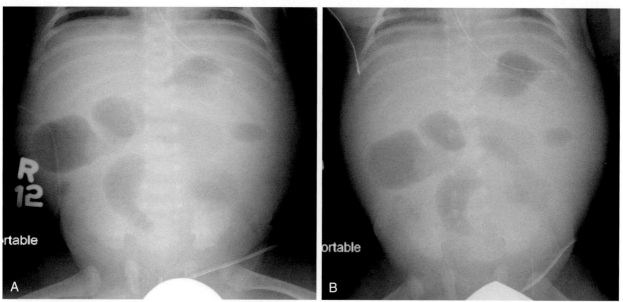

Fig. 18.14 Necrotizing enterocolitis. Two anteroposterior radiographs of the abdomen in a preterm infant obtained within 2 days of each other show dilated bowel in fixed pattern.

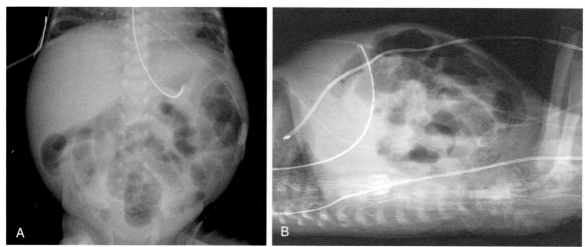

Fig. 18.15 Necrotizing enterocolitis. Anteroposterior radiograph of the abdomen (A) in a 2-month-old former 27-week gestational age infant with increasing abdominal distension shows bubbly lucencies in the left upper and lower quadrants and pelvis consistent with pneumatosis. Branching lucencies over the liver are consistent with portal venous gas. A subsequent cross-table lateral radiograph (B) obtained 4 hours later shows persistent pneumoperitoneum and portal venous gas without evidence of pneumoperitoneum.

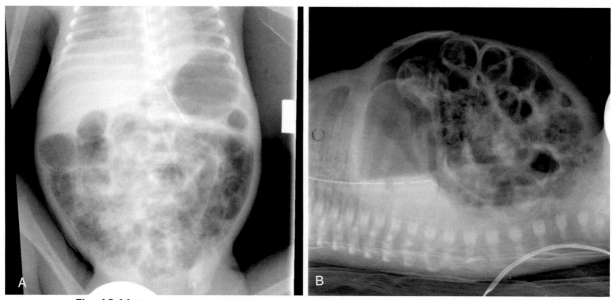

Fig. 18.16 Necrotizing enterocolitis. Anteroposterior radiograph of the abdomen (A) in a 13-day-old former 28-week gestational neonate shows diffuse pneumatosis. A cross-table lateral radiograph (B) obtained 1 hour later shows pneumoperitoneum.

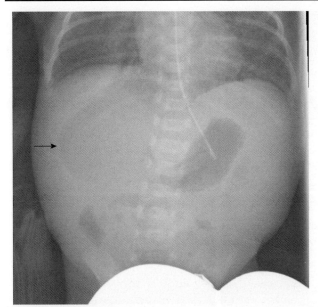

Fig. 18.17 Necrotizing enterocolitis. Anteroposterior radiograph of the abdomen in a 6-day-old former 24-week gestational age neonate showing a large lucency *(arrow)* over the liver, consistent with pneumoperitoneum.

trix may rupture, resulting in hemorrhage. Risk factors for germinal matrix hemorrhage (GMH) are extreme low birth weight (<1500 g) and extreme prematurity (<28 weeks). Hemorrhage most often occurs at the caudothalamic groove and can be confined to the subependymal region, grade I (Fig. 18.22), or extend into the lateral ventricles leading to intraventricular hemorrhage, grades II and III (Figs. 18.23 and 18.24). The difference between grade II and III is whether there is no dilation of the lateral ventricles at time of diagnosis (grade II) or whether there is significant volume and dilatation of the lateral ventricles at the time of diagnosis (grade III). Periventricular white matter parenchymal hemorrhagic infarction (grade IV) is thought to be due to mass effect from GMH at the caudothalamic groove, causing a venous ischemia of the parenchyma (Fig. 18.25). The GMH grading system corresponds to worsening prognosis with increased grade, with general good outcomes with grades I and II (Box 18.2).

Typically, acute GMH will have an echogenic homogeneous appearance. As the hemorrhage ages, it becomes more heterogeneous. The location at the

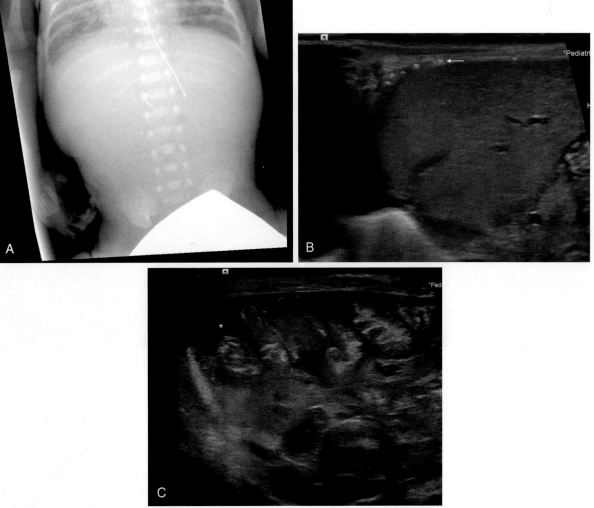

Fig. 18.18 Necrotizing enterocolitis. Anteroposterior radiograph of the abdomen (A) in an 8-day-old former 24-week gestational age neonate with increasing abdominal distension showing a nearly completely gasless abdomen. Grayscale ultrasound image of the liver (B) shows comet-tail artifact *(arrow)* along the anterior hepatic surface consistent with pneumoperitoneum. Grayscale ultrasound image through the right lower quadrant (C) shows complex fluid *(asterisk)*. These findings are highly suggestive of bowel perforation in the setting of necrotizing enterocolitis.

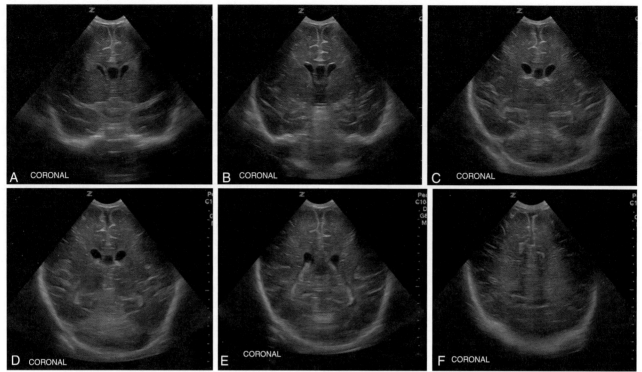

Fig. 18.19 Normal coronal ultrasound images through the brain obtained at (A) frontal horns of the lateral ventricles, (B) foramen of Monroe, (C) posterior aspect of the third ventricle, (D) quadrigeminal plate cistern, (E) trigones of the lateral ventricles, and (F) parietooccipital cortex.

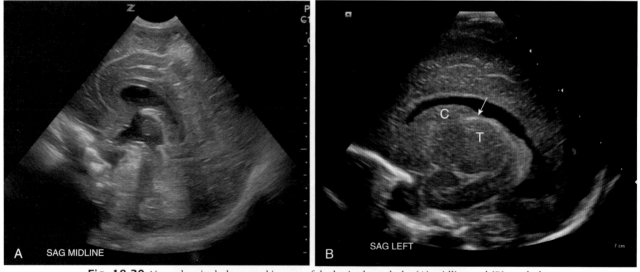

Fig. 18.20 Normal sagittal ultrasound images of the brain through the (A) midline and (B) caudothalamic groove *(arrow)* located between the head of the caudate nucleus *(C)* and the thalamus *(T)*.

caudothalamic groove makes grade I GMH relatively straightforward; however, grade II hemorrhage can occasionally be difficult, because the intraventricular choroid plexus is echogenic as well. Often, grade II hemorrhage will layer posteriorly in the occipital horn, which can be a helpful location to pay particular attention on the sagittal view. Asymmetrical lobulation of the choroid plexus can also suggest a grade II hemorrhage. Grade III hemorrhage is easy to diagnose given the large amount of echogenic material distending the ventricle. Parenchymal injury also has an echogenic appearance initially, and the echogenicity of the choroid plexus can be used as an internal "control," because the white matter is not typically as echogenic as the choroid plexus. Also, symmetry is helpful to diagnose abnormal echogenicity from grade IV injury.

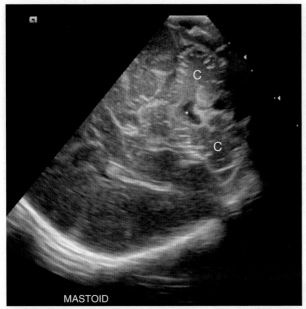

Fig.18.21 Mastoid ultrasound view showing the cerebellar hemispheres *(C)* and fourth ventricle *(*)*.

In addition, grade IV parenchymal hemorrhagic infarction is typically seen ipsilaterally after large grade I or grade III GMH, so attention on follow-up examinations is paramount.

Posthemorrhagic hydrocephalus can occur after intraventricular hemorrhage and is thought to occur as a result of impaired resorption of the cerebrospinal fluid. Serial ultrasounds looking for enlarging ventricular size are routine in follow-up for intraventricular hemorrhage. Some institutions use Doppler evaluation (resistive index) of the anterior cerebral artery as a marker for increased intracranial pressure. Lumbar punctures to draw off cerebrospinal fluid can temporize enlarging ventricles; however, neurosurgical placement of a ventricular shunt may be necessary if hydrocephalus continues to worsen.

White matter injury can be seen in premature infants, particularly the high-risk infants. Many use the term *periventricular leukoencephalopathy* given the typical location of the white matter injury. On ultrasound, periventricular leukoencephalopathy can start as increased echogenicity. Cystic change can be seen over time in

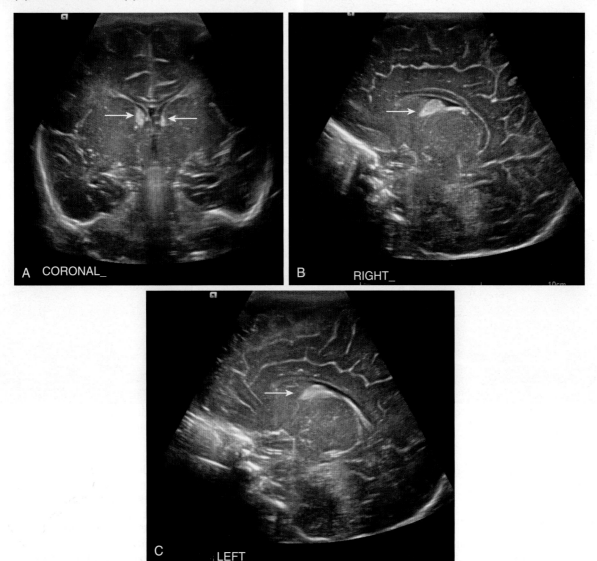

Fig. 18.22 Grade I germinal matrix hemorrhages. Coronal (A) and parasagittal ultrasound images through the right (B) and left (C) through the brain in an 11-week-old former 26-week gestational age neonate, showing echogenic foci in caudothalamic grooves bilaterally *(arrows)* consistent with bilateral grade I germinal matrix hemorrhages.

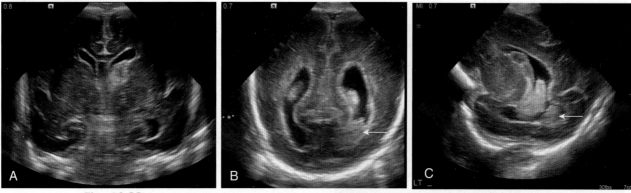

Fig. 18.23 Left grade II germinal matrix hemorrhage. Coronal (A, B) and sagittal images (C) through the brain in a 4-week-old former 23-week gestational age neonate show a predominantly echogenic focus in the left caudothalamic groove with an additional echogenic focus in the occipital horn of the left lateral ventricle *(arrows)* consistent with blood products and a grade II germinal matrix hemorrhage.

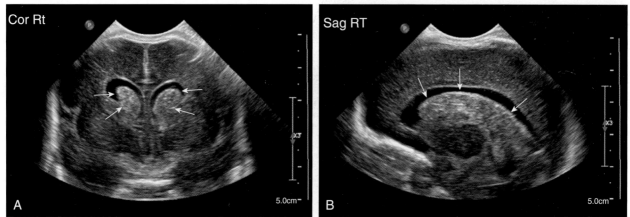

Fig. 18.24 Bilateral grade III germinal matrix hemorrhages. Coronal (A) and sagittal (B) ultrasound images of the brain in a 7-day-old former 26-week gestational age neonate with bilateral echogenic intraventricular hemorrhage *(arrows)* and mild-to-moderate enlargement of the lateral ventricles.

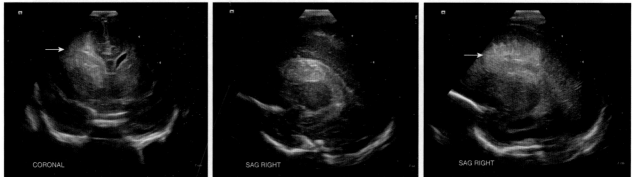

Fig. 18.25 Right grade IV germinal matrix hemorrhage. Coronal (A) and sagittal (B, C) ultrasound images in a 3-day-old former 27-week gestational age neonate showing blood filling the lateral ventricle with hemorrhage in the right periventricular white matter *(arrows)*.

BOX 18-2   Germinal Matrix Hemorrhage Grading System

Grade I   Confined to the caudothalamic groove
Grade II   Intraventricular hemorrhage without expansion/dilation of ventricles
Grade III   Intraventricular hemorrhage with expansion of ventricles
Grade IV   Periventricular parenchymal hemorrhagic infarction

more severe cases but is less frequently seen in recent years because of improvements and innovations in perinatal care of NICU infants. Subtle microcystic changes may be difficult to detect on ultrasound and even on neonatal MRI but may be detected later in the child's life after developmental delays are noted and subsequent MRI demonstrates white matter volume loss and gliosis.

■ Summary

The imaging of a preterm infant is not uncommon, and this chapter reviewed key imaging diagnoses that are unique to the preterm infant population. Keen knowledge to the imaging characteristics is important for prompt reporting to the pediatrician, because these diagnoses pose significant morbidity and mortality, and at times the radiographic findings can precede clinical symptoms.

Bibliography

Davidson, L. M., & Berkelhamer, S. K. (2017). Bronchopulmonary dysplasia: Chronic lung disease of infancy and long-term pulmonary outcomes. *Journal of Clinical Medicine, 6*(1), 4.

Knell, J., Han, S. M., Jaksic, T., & Modi, B. P. (2019). Current status of necrotizing enterocolitis. *Current Problems in Surgery, 56*(1), 11–38.

Liszewski, M. C., Stanescu, A. L., Phillips, G. S., & Lee, E. Y. (2017). Respiratory distress in neonates: Underlying causes and current imaging assessment. *Radiologic Clinics of North America, 55*(4), 629–644.

Luo, J., Luo, Y., Zeng, H., Reis, C., & Chen, S. (2019). Research advances of germinal matrix hemorrhage: An update review. *Cellular and Molecular Neurobiology, 39*(1), 1–10.

Maller, V. V., & Cohen, H. L. (2019). Neonatal head ultrasound: A review and update—Part 1: Techniques and evaluation of the premature neonate. *Ultrasound Quarterly, 35*(3), 202–211.

Taylor, G. A., Phillips, M. D., Ichord, R. N., Carson, B. S., Gates, J. A., & James, C. S. (1994). Intracranial compliance in infants: Evaluation with Doppler US. *Radiology, 191*(3), 787–791.

CHAPTER 19

Imaging of the Neonate: Term Infant

Gerald G. Behr

CHAPTER OUTLINE

Thorax, 368
How Do I Know If My Radiograph Is Technically
    Adequate for Diagnosis?, 368
    Collimation, 369
    Projection/Angulation, 369
    Positioning, 369
    Respiration, 369
    Exposure, 371
Is That Normal?, 371
    Humeral Ossification Centers, 372
    Broken Clavicle, 372
    Tracheal Buckling, 372
Troubleshooting a Narrowed-Appearing Airway, 372
Heart and Mediastinum: Is It Enlarged? Or Is It All
    Thymus?, 374
Pitfalls in Imaging Lungs: Normal Findings, 376
Approach to Pulmonary Vascularity, 377
Diffuse Granular Hazy Appearance: What Should I
    Be Thinking Of?, 378
Reticular Pattern: What Should I Be Thinking Of?, 378
    Entities Relating to Altered Fluid Dynamics, 378
    Entities Related to Infection, 379
    Meconium Aspiration Syndrome, 380

Interstitial Lung Disease, 380
Congenitally Hyperlucent Lung:
    Differential?, 381
Asymmetrical Smaller Lung: What Should I Be
    Thinking Of?, 382
    When There Is Pulmonary Artery Abnormality, 383
    When There Is Pulmonary Venous
        Abnormality, 384
Characteristic-Appearing Neonatal Lesions of the
    Lung, 385
    Congenital Pulmonary Airway
        Malformation, 385
    Bronchopulmonary Sequestration, 386
    Congenital Diaphragmatic Hernia, 387
    Esophageal Atresia With or Without
        Tracheoesophageal Fistula, 388
Abdomen, 390
Obstructed Bowel, 390
Pitfalls of Plain Film, 391
Highly Specific Findings on the Abdominal
    Radiograph, 392
Postnatal Workup of a Prenatally Diagnosed
    Abdominal Cyst, 393
Summary, 394

Encountering a neonatal imaging study may be an unsettling experience to radiologists who do not interpret them routinely. Normal structures often appear different from those of the adult or older child. Moreover, many differential diagnoses and disease processes are unique to the term neonate. In reality, however, there are a limited number of likely diagnoses that need to be considered for each imaging finding compared with the typically broader differential diagnosis that is generated for imaging findings in the adult or even older child. The accompanying medical history is brief. Finally, many disease states that affect the term neonate are based on altered anatomy that are amenable to detection on prenatal imaging. Because prenatal sonography is now commonplace, many diagnoses are no longer first made by postpartum imaging.

The goal of this chapter is to outline an approach to imaging the term neonate. It is broadly divided into two sections: the thorax and the abdomen. Discussion of disease entities and processes is organized around common imaging appearances. There is an emphasis on prob-

lem solving, both technical and interpretive. For further details regarding the relevant embryology, pathophysiology, and clinical aspects of term neonatal conditions, the reader is referred to several excellent articles and texts found in the Bibliography. A working knowledge of common findings encountered on neonatal imaging studies is essential to: (1) differentiate normal from abnormal; (2) accurately detect abnormalities; and (3) offer a concise differential or, when possible, a specific diagnosis.

■ Thorax

How Do I Know If My Radiograph Is Technically Adequate for Diagnosis?

The answer to this question depends in large part on what the clinical question is. Although every attempt

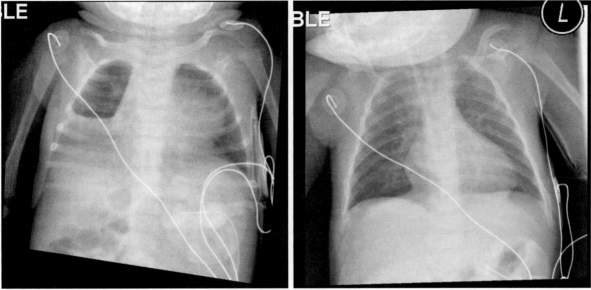

Fig. 19.1 Effects of apical lordotic technique. There is an uplifted cardiac apex, exaggerated horizontal ribs, anterior ribs projecting above their posterior segments, elevated diaphragms with loss of their sharp margins (A). Findings are resolved on repeat follow-up chest x-ray hours later (B).

should be made to acquire technically optimal images, poor technique should not blindly be used as "cover" to avoid interpreting aspects of the film that do carry diagnostic information.

In assessing technical adequacy, several observations should be made; these are discussed in the following subsections.

Collimation

Overcollimation is readily evident. Pertinent anatomy is excluded from the image. Conversely, undercollimation exposes extraneous anatomy to unnecessary ionizing radiation. In addition, the wider field of view increases scatter, decreasing image sharpness. In film/screen radiography, as well as in fluoroscopy, inclusion of very dense or very lucent regions (such as empty space outside the patient) increases the dynamic range, which falsely alters exposure parameters.

Projection/Angulation

It is simplest to image the newborn while supine, in anteroposterior (AP) projection. Fortunately, due to the geometry and small size of the infant thorax, there is no significant degradation of image quality or altered appearance of the mediastinum compared with the posteroanterior (PA) projection. As such, the AP projection is acceptable and widely used in the newborn and infant.

More problematic, however is unintended relative cranial angulation of the radiograph tube in relation to the chest, resulting in a lordotic projection (Fig. 19.1). Due to the conical shape of the chest, a lordotic view often results when the baby lies flat. The effect is exaggerated when the arms are held back in extension and the midtorso is arched. To remedy this, a foam pad with a 15-degree incline (higher end toward the head) may be placed under the thorax. Alternatively, the tube may be angled slightly caudally. The appearance of lordotic positioning can be further exacerbated by a low centered

beam, such as when acquiring a chest and abdomen on one cassette ("babygram"). In this instance the chest portion of the image is exposed by a more divergent beam. Ideally, the radiograph beam for a chest radiograph should be centered at the nipple line. The consequences of lordotic technique are outlined in Table 19.1.

Positioning

A well-positioned patient is judged on a frontal radiograph by assessing the medial heads of the clavicle. The sternoclavicular junction should be an equal distance between left and right. In addition, the rib lengths should be symmetrical. When these findings are not met, the patient is rotated about the vertical axis. Spurious relative hyperlucency of one hemithorax is most commonly a result of simple patient rotation. Rotation-related changes in projection of mediastinal structures are particularly pronounced in children, largely because of the thymus. As a relatively bulky anterior chest structure, a small degree of patient rotation results in substantial differences in its projection (Fig. 19.2). Indeed, this phenomenon can lead to a spurious impression of cardiomegaly or even upper lobe consolidation. Rotation uncovers the hilus of the side opposite the direction of rotation, resulting in accentuation of these structures (most typically on the left). With rotation, individual sternal ossification segments can appear as lung nodules or even as rib calluses (Fig. 19.3).

Respiration

In contrast with adults or older children, neonates and young children are imaged while freely breathing. Thus exposure time must be kept to a minimum to avoid motion blur. Just as important, though, is the phase of respiration that the image is acquired in. This is, of course, most challenging in a neonate because the normal neonatal respiratory rate is 20 to 60 breaths/min. Ideally, the image is acquired near peak inspiration. Attempted imaging during peak inspiration requires carefully observing the rise and fall of the chest and abdomen to synchronize the exposure at or close to peak inspiration. As a rule of thumb, on the frontal projection, six anterior ribs should be seen above the diaphragm (Fig. 19.4). In infants, counting anterior ribs is more reliable due to the more anterior dome of the diagram. Better yet is an overall assessment, including the degree of flattening of the diaphragm because other vari-

ables such as parallax as a result of positioning, will vary where the rib crosses the diaphragm.

Spurious findings commonly present because of inadvertent exposure during expiration are outlined in Table 19.2. When carefully examined, the findings could be suggested to be due to technique, although differentiation from true pathology may be tricky. For example, the hazy increased density seen on an expiratory film may not seem to be made up from acinar infiltrates, nor does it appear as a result of reticular densities. Rather, there is a generalized haze and a crowded appearance to the hilar vessels. It may be erroneous, however, to confidently ascribe such findings to technique. This is even more challenging in neonates where there is much overlap already between different patterns of disease on the chest radiograph. Most importantly, true findings may be missed entirely on an expiratory film. For example, focal lung disease may be "hidden" by a high diaphragm or may be rendered inconspicuous by the already generally increased lung density that decreases contrast in the image.

TABLE 19.1   Effects of Lordotic Projection on the Newborn Chest Radiograph

The cardiac apex appears "uplifted," simulating the appearance of right ventricular hypertrophy.

The anterior aspect of the first two or three ribs is projected at or above the remainder of the rib.

The clavicle is projected high above the lung apices.

Accentuation of bronchovascular markings and illusory airspace disease is most notable at the lung bases.

There may be loss of the sharp diaphragm as the diaphragm is now imaged more en face.

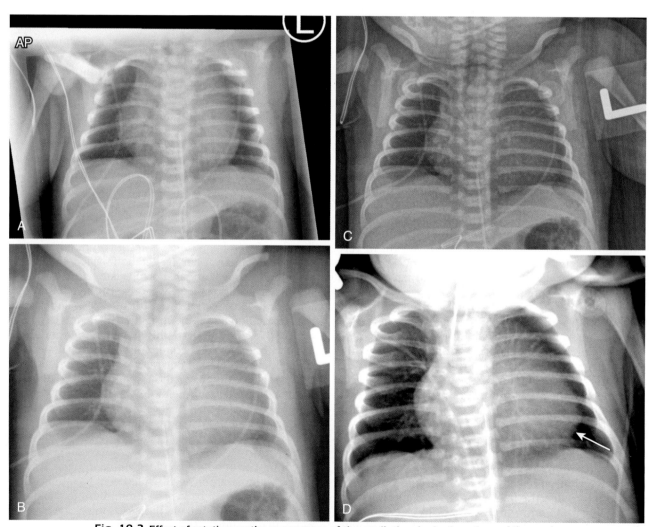

Fig. 19.2 Effect of rotation on the appearance of the cardiothymic shadow. Image (A) was taken 1 hour before image (B). The patient is rotated only slightly more leftward in (B) than in (A). This small difference is enough for the anteriorly positioned thymus to obscure much of the left lung, casting over it a "haze." However, lung markings are seen through this tissue. Image (C) is reprocessed from (B) using edge enhancement technique. The vessels are sharper and more apparent in this image, and the lungs are seen to be clear. The thymic notch (*arrow*) is seen in (D).

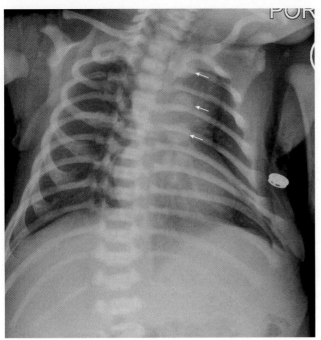

Fig. 19.3 Sternal ossification centers. Rotated chest radiograph obtained in a 6-week-old boy. Note the sternal ossification centers mimicking rib callus (*arrows*).

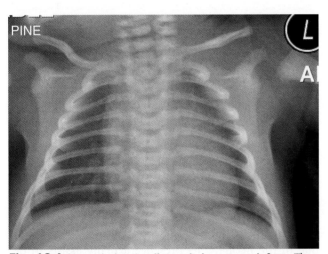

Fig. 19.4 Normal chest radiograph in a term infant. There is mild asymmetry in the position of the clavicles. The remainder demonstrates proper technique with six anterior ribs. Note that the humeral ossification centers are not yet visualized.

TABLE 19.2   Spurious Findings on an Expiratory Chest Radiograph

Cardiomegaly
Pulmonary edema
Overcirculation
Multifocal pneumonia
Illusory posterior mediastinal soft tissue

Exposure

Arguably, in the digital era, exposure factors have become less crucial to set with the same degree of precision as in the past. This is due to the much wider latitude digital radiography affords because it can record a far wider dynamic range than can film/screen. Still, setting proper exposure parameters is important for several reasons. First, the dynamic range is impressive but not infinite. At the extremes of density (such as dense, overlapping osseous structures and aerated lung), there still can be loss of detail that is not recoverable by adjusting the window and level settings on the display monitor (Fig. 19.5). In addition, regardless of overall exposure, the inherent contrast is still affected by exposure parameters such as kilovoltage peak (kVp). Importantly, an *underexposed* film can usually be brought back to the "correct" contrast on the display panel; however, the resulting increased noise in the film from quantum mottle renders a suboptimal image. This underexposure then imparts a "grainy" or hazy appearance to the image. When interpreting such a film, examining the soft tissues for these effects will help the reader differentiate this phenomenon from true lung pathology.

Within a large range of exposure values, *overexposure* in digital radiography may not compromise overall image quality. Because it is not visually readily evident, this actually creates a problem as there is no longer a feedback to the technologist to keep the dose in check. Whenever there is a quality issue, the dose can easily be raised to compensate for another deficiency. It is said that the exposure and final image product have been "decoupled." This results in ever-increasing radiation doses, known as "dose creep," and is something that both the technologist and radiologist should be aware of to adhere to the as low as reasonably achievable (ALARA) principle.

In addition to underexposure, the final image is affected by postprocessing techniques, such as use of an unsharp mask filter, or edge enhancement or changes in the gradient shift (see Fig. 19.2C). This can adjust the conspicuity of fine linear structures, including catheters, fissures, and the vascular markings. A detailed discussion of this, as well as other postprocessing techniques, is beyond the scope of this book.

Visualization of the lower vertebral endplates and pedicles through the mediastinal structures on a frontal radiograph suggests proper exposure. In addition, vascular markings should be easily seen in the central two-thirds of the lungs.

Is That Normal?

For the thoracic cage, the cliché "children are not just small adults" is as true in neonatal chest radiology as it is in much of pediatric medicine. To those unaccustomed to interpreting pediatric chest images, the appearance of the pediatric chest can be strange. Moreover, as discussed earlier, its appearance can change from one study to the next because small differences in patient and radiograph tube positioning can have a dramatic effect on the radiograph appearance. The normal full-term newborn thorax has a "lamp-shade" appearance on the frontal view. The ribs are relatively horizontal in configuration and develop the downsloping appearance later on in infancy. The bones can appear relatively dense (neonatal sclerosis). Exaggeration

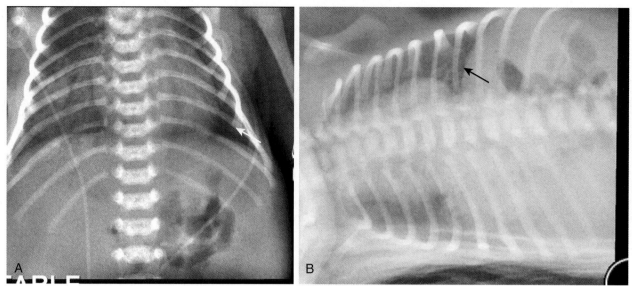

Fig. 19.5 Spurious pneumothorax. Frontal chest radiograph (A) obtained on the first day of life from a term newborn boy reveals absent lung markings at the left lung base (*arrow*) that was still not seen with window/leveling at the workstation. This is probably on technical grounds because sharp, conspicuous lung markings are present on the right lateral decubitus obtained minutes later (B). Presumably, this is from overexposure. With digital acquisition, "burned-out" areas are rare, except for the extremes of radiographic density and exposure.

of the horizontal configuration and upsloping of the first two or three anterior ribs may indicate inadvertent lordotic positioning.

Congenital masses of the chest wall are rare. Mesenchymal hamartoma of the chest wall is a benign rib mass with an ominous appearance on chest radiograph that shows relatively characteristic mass effect, rib erosion, calcification, and soft tissue (Fig. 19.6A). Magnetic resonance imaging (MRI) shows heterogenous signal because the histology consists of prominent cartilaginous tissue with hemorrhagic cysts (see Fig. 19.6C). Either partial or complete resection is recommended because there may be respiratory compromise and because there are case reports of malignant congenital tumors of the chest wall.

Humeral Ossification Centers
Presence of the proximal humeral ossification centers strongly suggests that the newborn is greater than 38 weeks of gestation (Fig. 19.7). The converse, however, is not true. That is, the humeral ossification centers are not always present yet in the full-term infant (see Fig. 19.4). Moreover, the appearance of the proximal humeral ossification centers, as well as the coracoid ossification center, is variably delayed in different populations.

Broken Clavicle
At delivery, occasionally a clavicle fracture may occur. Radiographs are often obtained to document and confirm the fracture (Fig. 19.8A). Not all broken-appearing clavicles are fractured. When the ends appear rounded and corticated, the possibility of a congenital pseudoarthrosis of the clavicle should be raised (see Fig. 19.8B). Similar to clavicular birth fractures, these may present with soft

tissue swelling and, occasionally, reduced movement of the arm. It is most often seen on the right side.

The appearance of pseudoarthrosis is distinct from the appearance of the clavicle in patients with cleidocranial dysostosis. Cleidocranial dysostosis is a disorder that affects intramembranous ossification and, to a lesser extent, endochondral ossification. As such, patients with cleidocranial dysostosis will present with hypoplastic or aplastic clavicles (see Fig. 19.8C). Common coexisting radiographic abnormalities include wormian bones and absence of ossification of the symphysis pubis (see Fig. 19.8D).

Tracheal Buckling
Not only is lateral and anterior tracheal buckling normal in the neonate, its presence actually assists in determining the side of the aortic arch. The typical convex rightward buckle of the trachea is consistent with a normal left-sided aortic arch. A leftward buckle is expected with a right-sided aortic arch. The buckling is more pronounced during expiration or with the head turned. It can give the false impression of a mass on the frontal view or prevertebral soft tissue thickening on the lateral view. If there is any uncertainty, repeating the radiograph with attention to head positioning and respiratory phase may confirm the buckling to have been only transient.

Troubleshooting a Narrowed-Appearing Airway

The newborn trachea often has a narrowed appearance. It is said that there can be up to 50% narrowing of the trachea between inspiration and expiration in

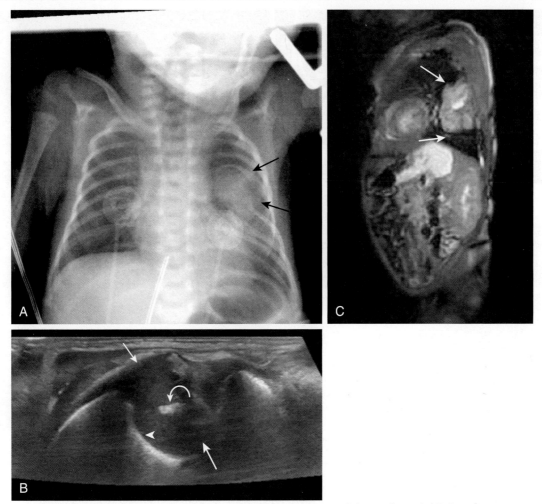

Fig. 19.6 Mesenchymal hamartoma of the chest wall. Frontal chest radiograph (A) demonstrates a large rounded density (*arrows*) projected over the left hemithorax. There is destruction, thinning, and splaying of the posterior ribs. Ultrasound (B) reveals a hypoechoic mass suggestive of cartilage (*arrow*) with small calcification (*curved arrow*). The mass displaces the lung inward (*ar*). Sagittal fluid-sensitive gradient echo magnetic resonance imaging (C) reveals a heterogeneous high signal mass (*arrows*) arising from the pleura or rib posteriorly. The higher signal is suggestive of cartilage; however, it is not specific. This child underwent surgical resection of the mass.

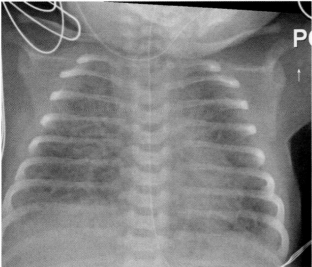

Fig. 19.7 Humeral ossification in term neonate with meconium aspiration syndrome. Frontal chest radiograph in a term infant shows course, reticular opacities diffusely throughout the lungs. The lungs are hyperinflated. Note the secondary ossification center of the left humeral head (*arrow*).

adults and children. In newborns, however, the airway narrowing in asymptomatic patients during the expiratory phase can be even more profound. Nonetheless, an AP and lateral study of the airway during fluoroscopy may be of benefit in selected patients who have clinical evidence of stridor. Unfortunately, the fluoroscopic findings of the normal overlap with those of tracheomalacia. However, the following generalizations may be helpful: (1) a focal expiratory collapse of the trachea is not normal and can suggest a vascular ring, (2) collapse of the trachea in the context of stridor suggests tracheomalacia, (3) a normal study does not exclude bronchomalacia, and (4) laryngomalacia is actually the most common cause of infantile stridor and will not be evident on routine radiological airway studies.

Multidetector computed tomography (CT) is more reliable than fluoroscopy. On CT, the caliber of the subglottic trachea may be used as an internal reference because it does not contain tracheal cartilage. Three-dimensional reconstructions of the airway are invaluable. More recently, some centers have been using real-time

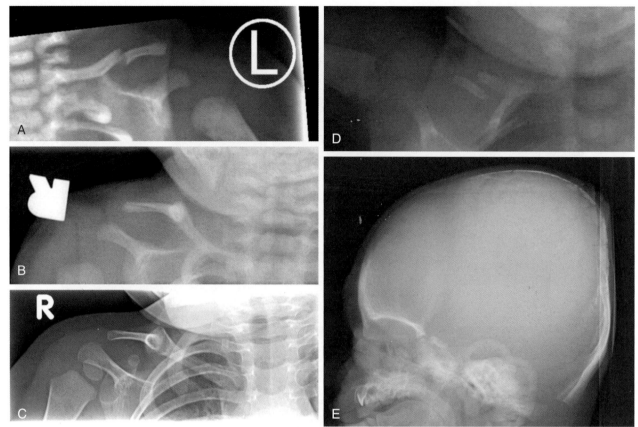

Fig. 19.8 *Spectrum of neonatal clavicle abnormalities.* Anteroposterior (AP) radiograph of the clavicle (A) showing a vertically oriented clavicle through the left midclavicle secondary to birth trauma. AP radiograph of the right clavicle in a neonate (B) showing a defect in the midclavicle with round and corticated margins along the defect consistent with a congenital pseudoarthrosis. A follow-up AP radiograph of the right clavicle (C) 2 years later shows that the defect is unchanged in appearance. AP radiograph of the right clavicle in a neonate (D) shows hypoplasia of the clavicle, consistent with cleidocranial dysostosis. Lateral skull radiograph (E) in the same patient shows wormian bone.

multidetector CT evaluation of the airway played back as cine clips, which is advantageous when the finding is transient. Most infants will instead undergo direct visualization under bronchoscopy for definitive diagnosis.

Tracheomalacia is divided into primary and secondary types. Primary tracheomalacia can occur in premature infants or in several systemic cartilaginous disorders, such as relapsing polychondritis and Larsen syndrome. Secondary tracheomalacia occurs in patients with tracheoesophageal fistula (TEF) (commonly), extrinsic vascular compression, and mediastinal soft tissue masses.

Tracheal stenosis is distinct from tracheomalacia and is differentiated by tracheal narrowing throughout the respiratory cycle and biphasic stridor. Long-segment tracheal stenosis is nearly synonymous with complete tracheal rings, an anatomic anomaly where the rings are less pliable because they lack the normal posterior membranous portion. A low position of the carina with horizontally positioned mainstem bronchus strongly suggests the condition (Fig. 19.9A). The trachea may appear consistently narrow on each chest radiograph. Although direct bronchoscopic visualization is diagnostic, a profoundly narrowed lumen may not allow passage of the bronchoscope to the most distal narrowed segment, which may include the bronchi.

In such case, CT scan may be obtained to detect bronchial involvement, which can establish surgical correctability. Approximately one-third of patients with tracheal stenosis/complete tracheal rings also have an aberrant left pulmonary artery arising from the right main pulmonary artery (type 2 pulmonary sling) (see Fig. 19.9B).

Short-segment stenosis (fewer than five rings involved) may be surgically corrected with resection and primary end-to-end anastomosis. Increasingly used techniques for the longer stenotic segments include the "slide tracheoplasty" and the use of tracheal stents.

Heart and Mediastinum: Is It Enlarged? Or Is It All Thymus?

The variability in the size and orientation of the thymus from one patient to the next and even from one radiograph to the next in the same patient renders cardiothoracic ratios limited in the full-term newborn, particularly when the image is acquired in expiration. A rule of thumb is that the transverse cardiothoracic ratio should be less than 60%. An attempt should still

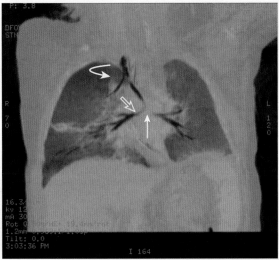
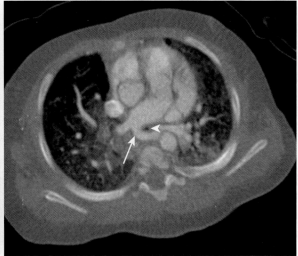

Fig. 19.9 Type 2 pulmonary sling with long-segment tracheal stenosis. Coronal chest computed tomographic (CT) reconstruction (A) showing a narrow trachea with a very low, T-shaped carina (*arrow*). There is an additional bronchus (*curved arrow*) arising from the trachea proximally on the right supplying the right upper lobe and bridging right bronchus (*open arrow*) supplying the right middle and lower lobes. Axial contrast-enhanced CT scan of the chest (B) shows the left pulmonary origin from the right pulmonary artery (*arrow*). Note the narrowed airway (*ar*).

be made to assess overall heart size and shape on the frontal radiograph, but the practice is a subjective one. The lateral view allows an unobstructed view of the posterior border, which should not extend to the spine.

There are several additional structures that may be normally seen on a neonatal chest radiograph that would be considered abnormal in an older child or adult. This includes occasional visualization of the right edge of the left atrium on the AP view, which projects to the right of the spine, near the upper heart border. Another finding considered normal is the "ductus bump." This typically represents the partially patent or closing ductus as the pulmonary pressures fall below left heart pressure.

One should attempt to assess the inferior margin of the thymus, particularly on the left. The extent of the cardiomediastinal silhouette that extends below this point provides an unobstructed view of a segment of heart border. This margin is often demarcated by a focal "notch" (see Fig. 19.2D). Cardiac border can often be differentiated from thymus by the presence of the so-called "thymic wave". This describes subtle undulation of the soft tissue border caused by the impression from the anterior ribs on the soft thymic gland. When the thymic gland is small, such as in the stressed state of an ill infant, or entirely absent, such as in DiGeorge syndrome, the cardiac contours and central vessels are better visualized. Further details regarding findings in congenital heart disease are covered in Chapter 3.

On a lateral view, obscuration of the retrosternal clear space in an infant is a normal finding because of the anterior mediastinal position of the thymus.

At times, the thymus can appear so large and irregular as to suggest the presence of a mass or vascular anomaly of the great vessels (Fig. 19.10). For example, a bulky thymic shadow can mimic the superior mediastinal fullness seen in supracardiac anomalous

pulmonary venous return or mimic the appearance of a soft tissue mass. If there are any red flags, such as mass effect on an adjacent structure (such as the airway), bone changes, or calcification, further investigation by cross-sectional imaging is mandatory. In the absence of such findings but still with a concern for a mediastinal abnormality, there are several approaches for further workup. First, review of any available prenatal imaging may prove helpful. Second, if it is believed that the image in question was captured in expiration, simply repeating the radiograph may be all that is required.

If uncertainty persists, fluoroscopy of the chest can show the expected change of size and shape of a normal thymus with respiration. Ultrasound is a more direct method for visualizing the thymus. This thymus appears as hypoechoic soft tissue with numerous foci of hyperechoic reflections creating a speckled or "starry sky" pattern (see Fig. 19.10D). Its margins will be seen to alter with respiration. The posterior extent of the thymus should be imaged to where it interfaces with lung. On a neonate, this is a relatively short distance. In addition, the sternum offers a better acoustic window in the neonate because of nonossified cartilage. As a result, even the posterior extent of the gland is readily visualized by ultrasound. Common variants include thymic extension behind the superior vena cava or superior extension into the neck, and ectopic locations in the anterior mediastinum and neck—all readily identifiable by ultrasound (see Fig. 19.10).

MRI, because of its exquisite soft tissue contrast, can confidently confirm the presence of a uniform thymus and exclude a pathological mass. However, because of its higher cost, less availability, risk for sedation (when needed), and potential artifacts, it can be reserved for cases that are unclear by ultrasound alone. For further discussion and additional images of the thymus, please see Chapters 1 and 2.

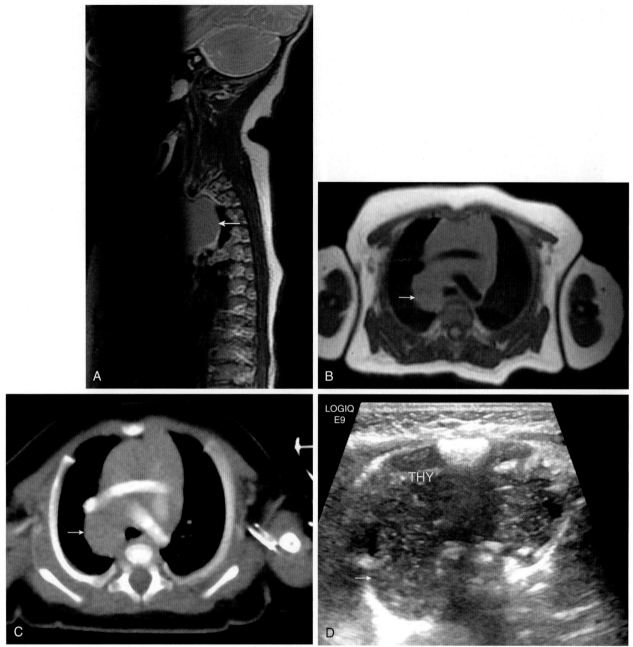

Fig. 19.10 Two-month-old boy who underwent spinal magnetic resonance imaging because of clinical signs of tethered cord. Sagittal T2-weighted sequence through the spine shows a posterior mediastinal mass (A). Thymic tissue was suspected. A saturation band obscures the mediastinum. Axial T1-weighted image (B) and subsequent axial chest computed tomography with intravenous contrast (C) demonstrate that this mass (*arrow*) is isointense and isodense to thymus. Transverse grayscale ultrasound image (D) at the same level shows the posterior mediastinal mass (*arrow*) isoechoic to the thymus (*THY; asterisk*), displaying its characteristic speckled appearance. It is ideal to avoid CT scan to confirm prominent thymic tissue.

Pitfalls in Imaging Lungs: Normal Findings

Several accessory fissures may be visible on a chest radiograph. A fissure is a visceral pleural-lined cleft extending into the lung to varying depths and is often incomplete. The azygos fissure and accessory inferior pulmonary fissure are common examples. The latter is typically seen vertically at the right base, separating the medial basal segment from the remaining right lower lobe basilar segments. The major fissure is typically not apparent on a frontal chest radiograph; however, with slight rotation, it may become visible (Fig. 19.11). Its appearance is most often seen in infants with cardiomegaly, probably because of resulting slight rotation of the right lower lobe. These fissures may be confused with atelectasis, scarring, a skin fold, or the pleural line of a pneumothorax.

A retrosternal triangular density seen inferiorly on some lateral chest radiographs is thought to reflect a

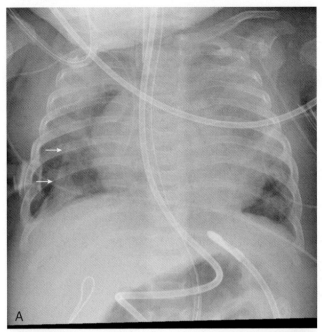

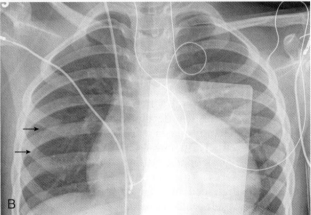

Fig. 19.11 Oblique fissure. Frontal chest radiograph (A) demonstrates an oblique fissure that is thought to be due to slight rotation of the lower lobe, often seen in patients with congenital heart disease. Frontal chest radiograph (B) in another with patient with a ventricular septal defect and heart block demonstrates a similar oblique fissure (*arrows*) that could be misconstrued as the pleural reflection of a pneumothorax.

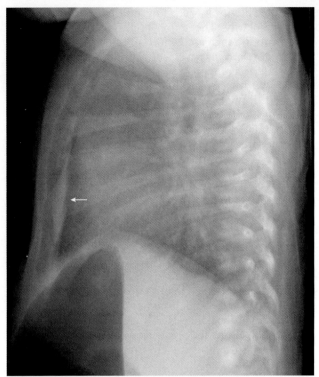

Fig. 19.12 Normal retrosternal density on a lateral chest radiograph in a 6-day-old boy (*arrow*).

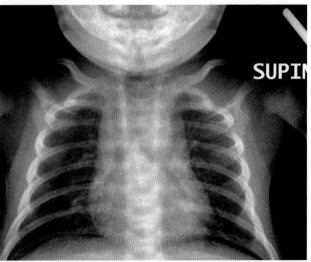

Fig. 19.13 Suprasternal fossa. Chest radiograph from a term 4-day-old boy demonstrates U-shaped lucency around the upper trachea of the neck and thoracic inlet. This is a normal finding related to the suprasternal fossa.

normal mediastinal soft tissue interface that extends more anteriorly than the left lung (Fig. 19.12).

The appearance of an ovoid vertically oriented lucency in newborns, mimicking the dilated esophagus of esophageal atresia (EA), is not uncommon (Fig. 19.13). This lucency is caused by the suprasternal fossa, a depression on the skin between the sternal heads of the sternocleidomastoid muscle and should not be confused with a dilated esophagus or trachea. It is more common in the setting of respiratory distress due to recruitment of these accessory muscles of respiration.

Approach to Pulmonary Vascularity

The newborn lungs often appear slightly more hyperlucent on radiograph than that of the older child. This is both due to the smaller-caliber vessels and the geometry of the newborn chest. Indeed, one of the most difficult aspects of pediatric chest radiograph interpretation is evaluation of the pulmonary vasculature. Simply stated, this is an assessment of vascular "plethora" versus decreased pulmonary vasculature. In practice, the findings are often subjective and may be influenced by variations in radiographic technique. A study by Tumkosit et al. (2012), using cardiac catheterization as the gold standard, did show reasonably good accuracy when the reader interprets shunt vascularity on frontal chest radiographs in children. The same study, however, showed poorer sensitivity in detecting mildly *decreased* pulmonary vascularity. The term "plethoric" vasculature reflects both the increased width of the vessel and the impression of "too *many* vessels." For the size of the vessel, it is useful to compare a vessel on end with an adjacent bronchiole, if seen. Another technique is to compare the diameter of the trachea to the right descending pulmonary artery, which should nearly equal in caliber.

This increased vascularity should not be confused with the physiology of venous hypertension, as seen with left-sided obstructive cardiac lesions or obstructed pulmonary venous return. Such findings appear more typical of interstitial edema, such as "fuzzy" margins of vessels and central hazy densities. In practice, this pattern may be identical to that of retained fetal fluid, and there is an overlap in appearance with other entities, including neonatal pneumonia. Even differentiating edema from shunt vascularity on many chest films can be challenging and, sometimes, an impossible task. In fact, with enough overcirculation, edema will result.

For the first several hours to days of life, pulmonary vascular resistance is still elevated. As such, most intracardiac shunt lesions will not be apparent on the neonatal chest radiograph. To make matters more complex, persistent fetal hypertension (also known as persistent pulmonary hypertension of the newborn) can persist beyond the newborn period, either because of lung hypoxia, acidemia, structural heart disease, or as an idiopathic condition. Its physiological hallmark is persistence of the fetal right-to-left shunting, which typically renders the vascular pattern on the chest radiograph either normal or decreased. The degree of hypoxemia in the newborn with this condition may be profound, but the lungs appear clear. When underlying structural heart disease needs to be excluded as a cause, it is usually accomplished with cardiac echo and is at this point beyond the capability of the chest radiograph. A more detailed discussion of the differential diagnosis of congenital heart disease can be found in Chapter 3.

General appearances and patterns of the abnormal lung parenchyma are described in the following section.

Diffuse Granular Hazy Appearance: What Should I Be Thinking Of?

A newborn lung with a ground-glass, granular, hazy pattern, with or without air bronchograms, typically evokes the diagnosis of respiratory distress syndrome of the premature infant due to surfactant deficiency, which is covered in detail in Chapter 18. Surfactant deficiency in the full-term or near-full-term infant is uncommon but can occur in the setting of gestational diabetes. Less common still are genetic disorders of surfactant causing congenital deficiency irrespective of the gestational age (Fig. 19.14).

More recently, a new classification of childhood interstitial lung disease (ChILD) has been established. Several of these appear as a diffuse hazy parenchymal opacification. These rare entities should be considered in a full-term newborn with persistent respiratory distress and may be deteriorating both clinically and radiographically. Entities with the appearance of diffuse hazy

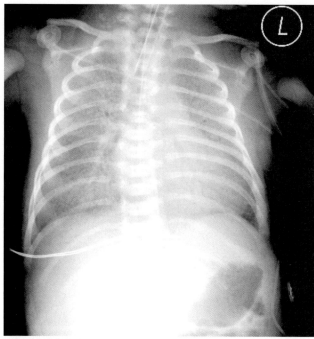

Fig. 19.14 Full-term infant with surfactant deficiency. Single anteroposterior view of the chest in this near-term (almost 37-week) baby girl with a mutation in *ABCA3* shows diffuse granular, hazy opacification of the lungs from surfactant deficiency. The phenotype of a defect in this gene manifests as surfactant deficiency. The appearance never improved.

opacities include several genetic deficiencies of surfactant and several diffuse developmental disorders (e.g., alveolar capillary dysplasia with misalignment of the pulmonary veins.) On chest CT, these often demonstrate ground-glass opacification with thickening of the interlobular septa. This "crazy-paving" appearance is identical to that seen in neonatal pulmonary alveolar proteinosis, which is also considered in the spectrum of ChILD (for further discussion of ChILD, see the section entitled "Interstitial Lung Disease" below).

Group B *Streptococcus* pneumonia may present as a granular hazy opacification on the chest radiograph mimicking respiratory distress syndrome related to surfactant deficiency; however, it is more likely to be accompanied by pleural fluid.

A mimicker of primary lung disease is that of pulmonary edema caused by left-sided obstructive congenital heart disease. A left-to-right shunt resulting in high-output cardiac failure could also present with hazy opacification of the lungs but would not manifest at birth because of the elevated pulmonary pressures. A left-to-right shunt, such as a patent ductus arteriosus, may be suggested if this finding develops *after* several days to weeks of life.

Reticular Pattern: What Should I Be Thinking Of?

Entities Relating to Altered Fluid Dynamics
When the newborn lung parenchyma is primarily characterized by prominent reticular densities, several entities

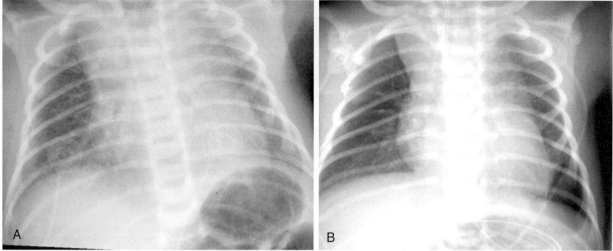

Fig. 19.15 Transient tachypnea of the newborn. Anteroposterior radiograph of the chest (A) shows prominent, reticular opacities throughout the lungs at birth. A follow-up chest radiograph (B) obtained 24 hours later shows near-complete resolution of the reticular opacities. There is still residual right basilar retained fluid that subsequently cleared.

should be considered, the most common of which is transient tachypnea of the newborn (TTN). In TTN, there is usually accompanying hyperinflation of the lungs and often a small pleural effusion with thickening of the fissures. The effusion and thickening may be most conspicuous along the minor fissure because of its orientation. The findings may be asymmetrical, often with a right-sided predominance. These radiographic findings are due to engorged lymphatic and venous channels caused by the delayed clearance of fetal lung fluid, most commonly seen after cesarean section, in children who are small for dates or those who have undergone a precipitous delivery. The natural history is that of rapid resolution, usually within 1 or 2 days (Fig. 19.15). Ultimately, because of overlap in appearance with other entities, a confident diagnosis can be made only after observing the rapid clearance of the chest radiograph and/or rapid improvement in the child's condition. The physiology of TTN of engorged pulmonary lymphatics and venous channels is similar to that of left-sided cardiac or pulmonary venous obstructive lesions. Not surprisingly, then, the findings of TTN can appear identical to cardiac or vascular causes of interstitial edema. In fact, finding a normal heart size on the chest radiograph does not exclude congenital heart disease. Total anomalous pulmonary venous return with obstruction is the prototypical example. These children, however, are usually far less clinically stable than those with TTN.

In a similar fashion, lung fluid drainage may be obstructed because of an abnormality of the lymphatic vessels themselves. Lymphangiectasia is defined as a pathological dilation of lymphatic channels and can occur as a result of a disturbance in lymph drainage related to congenital heart disease or may occur after surgery, radiation therapy, infection, or trauma. Primary lymphangiectasia, when presenting during the newborn period, is often more diffuse and carries a poor prognosis. Associated syndromes include Noonan, Turner, Ehlers-Danlos, and Ullrich-Turner syndromes. The appearance

is often indistinguishable from that of TTN; however, there is no improvement over time. If the primary lymphatic disorder is more generalized, such as in primary lymphatic disorder or lymphangiomatosis, there may be additional clues; in addition to recurrent chylous effusions, there may be chylopericardium and ascites because it may involve the viscera as well. There may be larger lymphatic collections, such as macrocystic lymphatic malformations that appear as variably sized fluid collections on ultrasound and MRI, often with fluid–fluid levels. Bone involvement is common and may be seen on the radiographs as lytic areas in the affected skeletal structures. Although often diagnostic, some refrain from biopsy of lung or bone because of the risk for furthering a chylothorax from lymph leakage at the incision site. If available, magnetic resonance lymphangiogram or lymph angioscintigraphy can be performed.

Entities Related to Infection

Pneumonia is seen in less than 1% of all live births. Its primary risk factor is premature rupture of membranes. The isolated lobar consolidative pattern of bacterial pneumonia seen in older children and adults is uncommon in the neonate. The radiographic appearance of neonatal pneumonias is diverse, and it can be difficult to distinguish pneumonia from other common parenchymal abnormalities such as TTN. Neonatal pneumonias may be suggested by ill-defined, patchy airspace opacities, often with accompanying perihilar reticular densities, or there may be coarse, irregularly distributed reticular markings. There is often an accompanying pleural effusion. Occasionally the lungs may even appear radiographically normal. Despite the general nonspecificity of findings of neonatal pneumonia, the published work has revealed several unique findings that, when present, may suggest one entity over another. Neonatal pneumonias are discussed as a group in this section because all *could* (and the majority *do*) demonstrate the interstitial/reticular pattern on chest radiograph.

TABLE 19.3   ChILD in Early Infancy

ALVEOLAR GROWTH ABNORMALITIES[a]	DIFFUSE DEVELOPMENTAL DISORDERS	GENETIC SURFACTANT DYSFUNCTION	SPECIFIC ENTITIES OF UNCLEAR CAUSE
Pulmonary hypoplasia	Acinar dysplasia	*ABCA3* gene defect	Neuroendocrine cell hyperplasia of infancy[b]
Chronic disease related to prematurity (bronchopulmonary dysplasia)	Congenital alveolar dysplasia	*SPB* gene defect	Pulmonary interstitial glycogenosis
Associated with congenital heart disease	Alveolar capillary dysplasia with misaligned pulmonary veins	*SPC* gene defect	
Several genetic disorders		*TTF-1* gene defect	

[a]Most common.
[b]Imaging findings are relatively more specific.

Group B streptococcus is the most common cause of neonatal pneumonia and is acquired in utero or during labor and delivery. As stated previously, its radiographic appearance can mimic surfactant deficiency. Group B streptococcus, like most neonatal pneumonias, is more likely to have pleural effusions, in contradistinction to surfactant deficiency. Similar to other neonatal pneumonias, it may also manifest as course reticular markings or patchy airspace opacities.

Chlamydia trachomatis is also contracted during passage through the infected birth canal and may cause neonatal conjunctivitis. Although the chest radiograph findings that are primarily reticular opacities are not unique, the pneumonia does not present until 2 to 12 weeks postnatally. Pleural effusions are uncommon.

TORCH infections (toxoplasmosis, other, rubella, cytomegalovirus [CMV], herpes) are rare. Pneumonia as a result of a TORCH infection is even more rare. For example, many newborns are exposed to CMV, with only 1% demonstrating a serological response. Among these few, only 10% show systemic signs, such as intrauterine growth retardation, hepatosplenomegaly, thrombocytopenia, or intracranial calcifications. Only 1% acquire CMV pneumonia, described as a diffuse reticulonodular pattern.

Neonatal herpes pneumonia is estimated to be seen in 1/7000 live births and is acquired transplacentally or transvaginally when the mother is actively shedding the virus. Radiographic findings include initial perihilar reticular opacities that worsen to become more diffuse alveolar opacities over time.

Syphilitic pneumonia (also known as "pneumonia alba") occurs in 5% to 25% of newborns with congenital syphilis. The unique clue on a chest radiograph is identifying the associated periosteal reaction of the long bones. Reportedly, the infiltrates in the lungs are more confluent and commonly diffuse.

Meconium Aspiration Syndrome

Meconium staining of amniotic fluid is common, occurring in 10% to 15% of live births. Meconium aspiration *syndrome* is present only when there is neonatal respiratory distress, meconium staining, characteristic chest radiograph findings, and no other explanation for the respiratory symptoms. It is a disease of term and postterm neonates and, when severe, is often managed successfully with inhaled nitric oxide or extracorporeal membrane oxygenation therapy. The outcome is related more to the associated pulmonary hypertension than to the amount of meconium. In line with this thinking, the apparent severity of the findings on chest radiograph correlate poorly with the clinical status and the eventual outcome.

The findings of meconium aspiration fall into the interstitial category. More specifically, the reticular markings are often coarse and patchy (see Fig. 19.7). There is usually accompanying hyperinflation. The tenacious meconium entrapped in the airway can cause areas of segmental atelectasis or air trapping. Pneumothoraces can be a complication seen after meconium aspiration. The meconium is caustic to the lung parenchyma, causing a chemical pneumonitis. The lung parenchyma can be susceptible to superimposed gram-negative pneumonia, complicating both the clinical and the radiographic picture.

Interstitial Lung Disease

The term *interstitial lung disease* (ILD), when referring to infants and children, refers to a heterogeneous group of parenchymal lung disorders that represent developmental, genetic, inflammatory, infectious, and reactive disorders. They are not all "interstitial" in the way we are accustomed to thinking of ILD in adults, and "diffuse lung disease" may be a better term. The new classification system is the result of a large collaborative effort of the Children's Interstitial Lung Disease (ChILD) Research Cooperative. The categories that are relevant in early infancy with several examples are listed in Table 19.3. Entities that manifest in the newborn and encompass a reticular appearance will be described in this section. The categories of surfactant deficiencies and the diffuse developmental disorders do not appear "interstitial" and were briefly described earlier in the Diffuse Granular Hazy Appearance: What Should I Be Thinking Of? section.

The most common form of the ChILD classification is that of alveolar growth abnormalities. These share a common histopathology. There is attenuated alveolarization, often described as "lobular simplification" with few large alveoli with decreased vascularity. This is similar to emphysema, both histologically and radiographically, although the pathogenesis is different. The

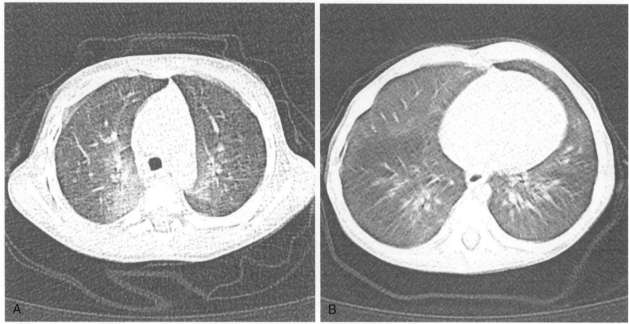

Fig. 19.16 Neuroendocrine hyperplasia of infancy (NEHI) in an infant with tachypnea. Axial computed tomography scan of the chest shows (A) perihilar and (B) right middle lobe and lingular ground-glass opacification, as can be seen in NEHI.

alveolar growth abnormalities may begin prenatally or postnatally. Pulmonary hypoplasia from in utero thoracic space compromise and bronchopulmonary dysplasia are the best known prenatal and postnatal examples of alveolar growth abnormalities, respectively. Alveolar growth abnormalities are also seen in association with congenital heart disease, genetic disorders, trisomy 21, or as an idiopathic condition of term infants.

Chest radiograph findings range from near-normal to thick, irregular reticular opacities and heterogeneously aerated lungs. Somewhat more specific and suggestive findings include cyst or cyst-like lucencies. CT findings have been described as pulmonary lobules of various shapes, sizes, and attenuations with interlobular septal thickening, ground-glass opacification, and cyst-like areas of hyperlucency. Often, subpleural linear opacities are present. Subpleural cysts may be present, particularly in children with trisomy 21.

Pulmonary interstitial glycogenosis, previously referred to as infantile cellular interstitial pneumonitis, is a disorder of unknown etiology. Its histological hallmark is interstitial infiltration by immature mesenchymal cells with increased glycogen that stain positive for vimentin. Pulmonary interstitial glycogenosis has not been observed in infants older than 10 months of age. Findings reported on chest radiograph include hyperinflation and interstitial opacities and on chest CT include interstitial thickening, architectural distortion and ground-glass opacities. Because imaging findings overlap with other interstitial processes such as alveolar growth abnormality, imaging cannot provide a definitive diagnosis. These patients are managed with corticosteroid therapy.

Neuroendocrine cell hyperplasia of infancy (NEHI), formerly known as persistent tachypnea of infancy, is another disorder of unknown etiology. Histologically, NEHI demonstrates numerous pulmonary neuroendocrine cells. During fetal lung development, these cells facilitate oxygen sensing. They normally diminish after the neonatal period. CT findings in NEHI carry a higher specificity for its diagnosis, which is in contrast with several other entities described in this section. NEHI should be suggested when there is mosaic attenuation on chest CT with distribution of ground-glass opacification predominantly affecting the right middle lobe, lingula, and paramediastinal region (Fig. 19.16). Interlobular septal thickening, bronchial wall thickening, and cysts are conspicuously absent. Treatment is supportive care, including oxygen supplementation. Bronchodilators and steroid therapy have not been shown to be effective.

Congenitally Hyperlucent Lung: Differential?

First and foremost, the most common cause of a hyperlucent thorax is patient rotation. This is usually apparent by looking for the symmetry of the ribs and medial clavicles.

On a supine chest radiograph, an anteriorly positioned pneumothorax can appear as a diffuse hyperlucency over the affected hemithorax. Often, there is a medial lucency, accentuating the mediastinal margin (Fig. 19.17). In confusing cases, decubitus films with the normal side down will confirm or refute the findings (see Fig. 19.5).

A large pneumomediastinum may be confused with the medial lucency of a pneumothorax. In this case, assessment of the thymus is helpful because mediastinal air will "lift" the thymus off the heart as the air insinuates between the thymus and pericardium (Fig. 19.18). A decubitus view is helpful to differentiate between the two. The lucency moves antidependently and away from the mediastinum with a pneumothorax. As in older children and adults, visualization of a pleural line without

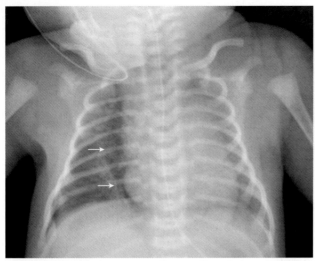

Fig. 19.17 Anterior pneumothorax. Frontal chest radiograph shows diffuse hyperlucency of the right lung with a more conspicuous lucency (*arrow*) adjacent to the right heart border and mediastinum, consistent with anterior pneumothorax.

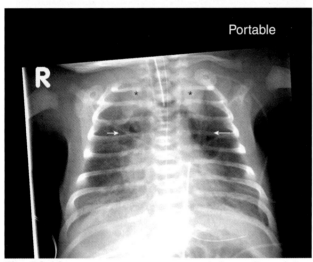

Fig. 19.18 Pneumomediastinum. Frontal chest radiograph in a newborn demonstrates a large ovoid lucency (*arrows*) projecting over the mediastinum uplifting the thymus.

further peripheral lung markings is diagnostic of a pneumothorax. This is not the most common appearance in a supine neonate.

Congenital lobar overinflation (CLO) is now considered an entity in the spectrum of bronchopulmonary malformations (BPMs) according to the Langston classification system. The other entities include congenital pulmonary airway malformation (CPAM), pulmonary sequestration, bronchial atresia, and bronchogenic cysts (the latter two are often incidental findings, less commonly discovered during prenatal imaging). Others have expanded the proposed BPM spectrum to include pulmonary vascular abnormalities such as AVM, pulmonary sling, and scimitar syndrome. Due to the changing and controversial classification schema, the practical radiologist would do well to adhere to a detailed description of the imaging findings. This is particularly useful when describing hybrid lesions that have features of two or more entities.

In its classic form, CLO is characterized by progressive lobar hyperexpansion, secondary to intrinsic bronchial cartilage hypoplasia or extrinsic compression. Hyperinflation of the affected lobe is due to a ball-valve mechanism, allowing air entry during inspiration but little or no air egress during expiration. The typical radiographic and CT appearance is hyperlucency of the affected lobe, which may displace the diaphragm inferiorly, shift mediastinal structures, and compress adjacent lobes (Fig. 19.19A–B). The pulmonary vasculature will be attenuated. On occasion, it may mimic a tension pneumothorax. CLO is most commonly encountered in the left upper lobe and right middle lobe. In the immediate postnatal period, the affected lung may retain fetal lung fluid, giving rise to a hyperdense lobe on imaging (see Fig. 19.19C). The mass effect will still be present to provide a clue to the diagnosis. As the fluid clears, the diagnosis becomes evident on subsequent imaging (see Fig. 19.19D). Treatment is surgical resection.

Poland syndrome is the unilateral absence of the pectoralis major muscle and often the pectoralis minor muscle with thoracic wall and breast hypoplasia. It most often affects the right side. Hand and arm anomalies are common. The chest radiograph reveals relative hyperlucency of the affected side as a result of decreased chest wall soft tissues. Associated anomalies include Klippel-Feil syndrome, and the affected child may experience development of pectus excavatum.

Pulmonary sling is a congenital anatomic abnormality in which the left pulmonary artery arises from the right pulmonary artery. It courses superior to the right mainstem bronchus and between the trachea and the esophagus en route to the left pulmonary hilum. There are two types of pulmonary sling. A type 1 pulmonary sling can result in distal tracheal and right mainstem bronchus compression and tracheobronchomalacia, with resultant hyperinflation of the right lung. A tracheobronchial branching pattern may be normal, or it may be a tracheal bronchus. It can be treated by reimplantation of the left pulmonary artery. A type 2 pulmonary sling cannot be treated reimplantation alone, because it is characterized by a low T-shaped carina, often with associated long-segment trachea stenosis with complete cartilaginous tracheal rings. The tracheobronchial branching pattern is abnormal, with a bridging bronchus arising from the left main stem bronchus to supply either part or all of the right lung (see Fig. 19.9). Additional cardiovascular anomalies may be present, including atrial and ventricular septal defects.

Asymmetrical Smaller Lung: What Should I Be Thinking Of?

Often a unilaterally small lung is readily evident from the chest radiograph. On other occasions, the findings are more subtle. Mediastinal shift (including cardiac dextroposition), elevated diaphragm, and closely spaced ribs are helpful clues. Associated hyperlucency, as may be seen in some of the alveolar development abnormalities, and certainly Swyer-James syndrome, as seen later in childhood, are *not* the typical imaging findings in most of the congenital hypoplastic lung entities. In fact, as detailed later, many of the anomalies feature *increased*

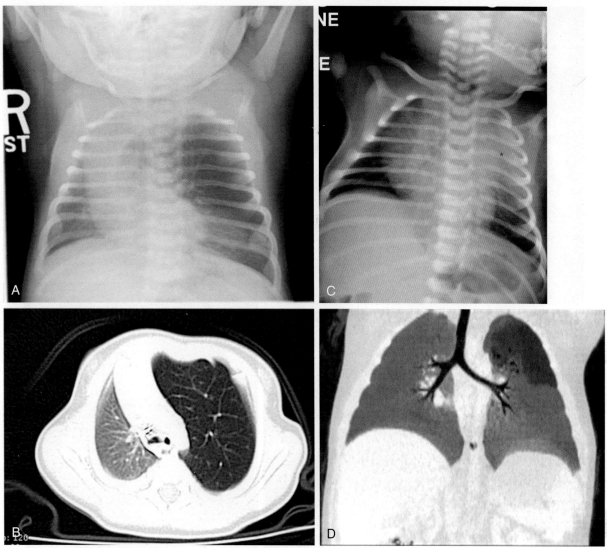

Fig. 19.19 Congenital lobar overinflation (CLO). Anteroposterior (AP) radiographs of the chest (A) in a 1-month-old boy show the typical presentation of CLO with hyperinflation and hyperlucency of the left upper lobe with mediastinal shift and a depressed left hemidiaphragm. Axial computed tomography scan (B) reveals hyperlucency with decreased vascularity in the left upper lobe. AP radiograph of the chest in a 1-day-old infant (C) shows increased density in the left upper lung (*red asterisk*). Minimum intensity projection coronal reconstruction from a thoracic CT scan in the same patient 1 week later (D) demonstrates a hyperlucent left upper lobe with clearance of the previously seen retained fluid consistent with CLO.

opacification of the affected lung with increased radiographic translucency of the contralateral lung.

When There Is Pulmonary Artery Abnormality

Underdevelopment of a lung is generally categorized into: (1) lung hypoplasia, (2) lung aplasia, and (3) lung agenesis. In pulmonary hypoplasia the affected lung is smaller due to decreased number and size of bronchopulmonary segments. The ipsilateral pulmonary artery is hypoplastic. Pulmonary hypoplasia can be primary or secondary. Pure primary pulmonary hypoplasia does occur but is rare. If there is no identifiable cause, pulmonary hypoplasia is classified as primary. Most cases of pulmonary hypoplasia are secondary and are the result of a maternal or fetal abnormality, such as oligohydramnios or congenital diaphragmatic hernia (CDH).

In those cases, there is pathological and radiographic overlap with the alveolar growth abnormalities. Pulmonary *aplasia* represents complete absence of the lung, with only a rudimentary, blind-ending mainstem bronchus. Pulmonary *agenesis* refers to complete absence of the lung, including the bronchus. The pulmonary artery on the affected side is absent in both entities. Patients with such entities are often asymptomatic or present with varying degrees of respiratory distress later in life.

Patients with such forms of underdevelopment of the lung may not be encountered in the neonate unless prenatally diagnosed or mildly symptomatic. The mediastinum is shifted to the affected side. The *contralateral* lung is hyperlucent and often herniates across the midline, which is seen as a hyperlucency anteriorly on the lateral view on a chest radiograph and is well depicted on a chest CT scan. The *ipsilateral* (hypoplastic side) lung

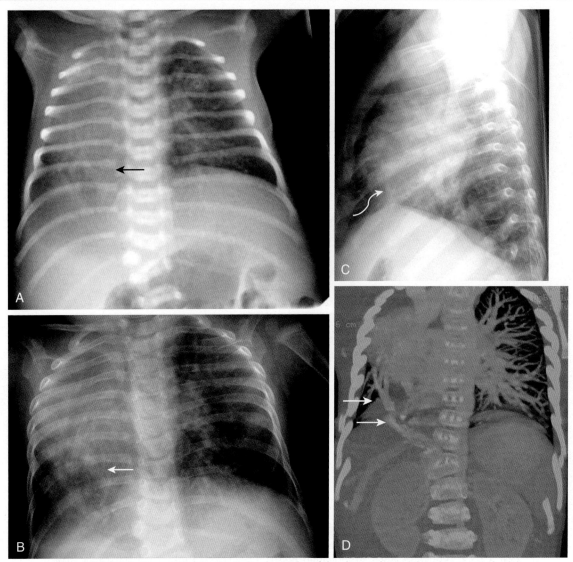

Fig. 19.20 Scimitar syndrome. Frontal radiographs of the chest at birth (A) and at 8 months (B) show the anomalous vein (*arrows*) and hypoplastic right lung. Lateral radiograph of the chest (C) reveals retrosternal lucency with a more posterior dense band (*curved arrow*), which is not the anomalous vein itself but rather an effect of the smaller right lung. Maximum intensity projection image in the coronal plane from a computed tomography (CT) angiogram (D) at 6 months of age reveals the anomalous vein (*arrows*) draining toward the inferior vena cava (not shown). The interruption of the scimitar vein is due to motion artifact. Note the right hemivertebra on the frontal radiographs and chest CT.

is usually opacified to varying degrees depending on degree of hypoplasia and shift of mediastinal contents. CT scan can distinguish agenesis, aplasia, and hypoplasia by identifying the presence of a bronchial stump in aplasia or the hypoplastic bronchial tree in lung hypoplasia.

Proximal interruption of the pulmonary artery is a special subcategory of lung hypoplasia. The vascular supply of the affected lung is supplied from the ductus arteriosus, which communicates directly with the otherwise "interrupted" hilar pulmonary artery. The affected lung is on the contralateral side to the aortic arch. As the ductus closes, lung perfusion of the affected lung (usually right lung) becomes reliant on collateral systemic vessels. Some patients may present later in childhood with recurrent pneumonias, pulmonary hypertension, or hemoptysis. Still, many are asymptomatic. The radiological findings are similar to those of the

other underdeveloped lung syndromes related to abnormal pulmonary artery supply except that in proximal interruption of the pulmonary artery, rib notching and pleural thickening may be present, both as a result of systemic collateral arterial supply.

When There Is Pulmonary Venous Abnormality

Hypogenetic lung syndrome (also known as scimitar syndrome) refers to lung hypoplasia with associated anomalous venous drainage to the right heart via the inferior vena cava, portal vein, hepatic vein, azygos vein, coronary sinus, or directly into the right atrium. It is a form of partial anomalous pulmonary venous return. The classic appearance is that of a smaller right lung with a dense, vertically oriented curvilinear structure (the "scimitar," or Turkish sword) seen at the right lung base medially on the frontal view (Fig. 19.20A–B). On the lateral view, a dense retrosternal band has been described (see Fig. 19.20C). This is not the anomalous vein but rather a lung–soft tissue interface created because of the smaller affected lung. The vascular and pulmonary lobar anatomy is better depicted with chest CT scan with administration of intravenous contrast material. Absence of the ipsilateral inferior pulmonary vein on CT scan supports the diagnosis of hypogenetic lung syndrome.

Characteristic-Appearing Neonatal Lesions of the Lung

Characteristic neonatal lesions of the lung are often diagnosed during prenatal life. They include congenital lobar emphysema, bronchial atresia, bronchopulmonary foregut malformations, CPAMs, bronchopulmonary

sequestrations (BPSs), and hybrid lesions composed of cystic pulmonary airway malformations and BPSs.

Congenital Pulmonary Airway Malformation

Congenital Pulmonary Airway Malformation or CPAM is characterized by overexpression of bronchial structures with deficient cartilage and focally underdeveloped alveoli. It is considered to be a form of BPM. They range from one or several large cysts with intervening septa to numerous tiny cysts to an increasingly solid appearance on both chest radiograph and chest CT scan (Fig. 19.21). Assigning nomenclature to a CPAM based on its varying appearances is fraught with controversy because the underlying pathogenesis is incompletely understood. In its pure form, arterial supply and venous drainage of a CPAM are from the pulmonary artery and vein, respectively. Given there may be components of a BPS (hybrid lesion), a detailed de-

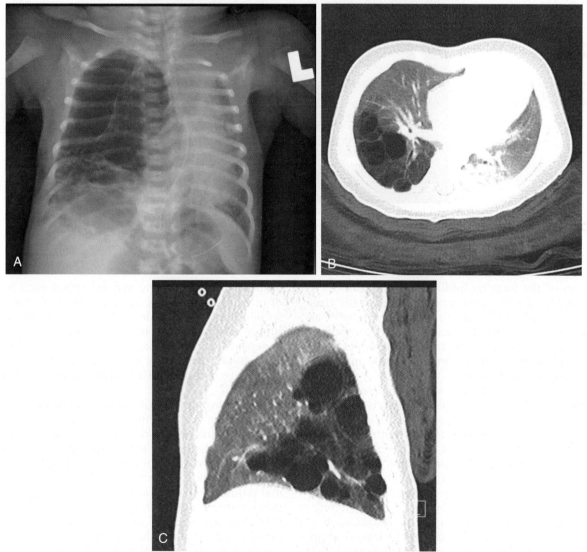

Fig. 19.21 Congenital pulmonary airway malformation (CPAM). Frontal radiograph of the chest in a newborn infant (A) shows a large cystic lesion occupying the right lung with mass effect on the mediastinum. This patient has a prenatal diagnosis of right lower lobe CPAM. Axial (B) and sagittal (C) images from computed tomography of the chest in a different patient showing a cystic lesion in the right lower lobe consistent with CPAM.

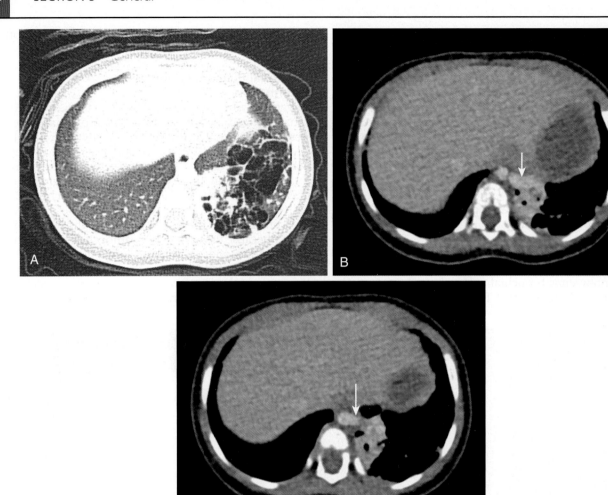

Fig. 19.22 **Hybrid lesion.** Axial image of the chest in lung windows from a computed tomography angiogram (A) shows a mixed solid and cyst lesion in the left lower lobe. Axial images in mediastinal windows (B, C) show a large artery (*arrows*) arising from the descending thoracic aorta supplies the left lower lobe lesion, consistent with a hybrid lesion, composed of congenital pulmonary airway malformation and bronchopulmonary sequestration.

scription of the imaging findings is important. CT is best completed with intravenous contrast of the chest with angiography technique to define any systemic arteries that would suggest a sequestration component (Fig. 19.22). Imaging should include the upper abdomen, because the systemic arterial supply may arise from the abdominal aorta.

Symptomatic CPAMs are surgically resected. The management of an asymptomatic CPAM is controversial. Asymptomatic CPAMs have often been resected because of their overlapping imaging features with pleuropulmonary blastoma type I (PPB). Feinberg et al., 2016 advocate for expectant management for those with asymptomatic lesions with a high likelihood of CPAM based on clinical and imaging features, including prenatal detection, systemic feeding vessel, and hyperinflation. Imaging features that suggest high likelihood of PPB include multilobar lesion or bilateral lesions, mediastinal shift, and the presence of a complex cyst. PPB is also more likely to develop a pneumothorax.

Bronchopulmonary Sequestration
A BPS is a congenital lung malformation of nonfunctioning lung parenchyma without a communicating

bronchus, although there may be pathological features of other malformations, such as bronchial atresia and sequestration. BPS is defined by its systemic arterial supply classically from the aorta, which may be readily depicted on CT angiography (Fig. 19.23A). Similar to other BPMs, the masses are often identified prenatally but may be occult on the initial postnatal neonatal chest radiograph.

Twenty-five percent of sequestrations are extralobar. An extralobar BPS is defined by having its own pleural investment and venous drainage to a systemic vein (see Fig. 19.23B). Extralobar BPS appears as a solid or microcystic mass and occasionally is infradiaphragmatic. In contrast, intralobar sequestrations occur within a normal pulmonary lobe, and its venous drainage is via the pulmonary venous system (Fig. 19.24). Intralobar BPS may demonstrate aeration on CT, presumably because of collateral air drift, although this appearance is not common in the neonatal period. It may be difficult to distinguish a BPS from a more solid CPAM. Indeed, there may be elements of both, indicating the presence of a hybrid lesion.

Treatment of intralobar BPS is most often surgical resection. The management of extralobar BPS, however,

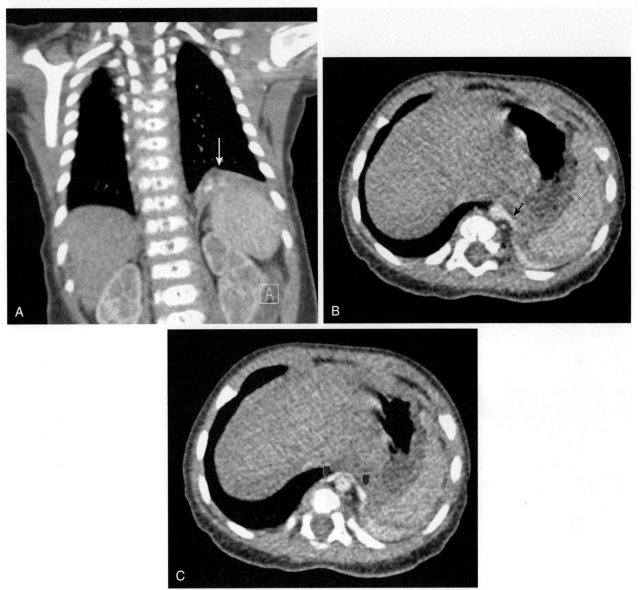

Fig. 19.23 Extralobar bronchopulmonary sequestration (BPS). Coronal reconstruction of the chest from a computed tomography angiogram (CTA) (A) shows a mass (*arrow*) abutting the left hemidiaphragm. Axial images through the chest from a CTA (B, C) show that the lesion has systemic arterial supply from the aorta (*arrow*) and systemic venous drainage in the azygous system (*ars*) consistent with an extralobar BPS.

is more controversial. Arterial embolization of the feeding vessel has been advocated in selected cases.

Congenital Diaphragmatic Hernia
CDH occurs through a diaphragmatic developmental defect, through which abdominal structures may herniate. Although there is the rare exception, left-sided hernias represent a posterior diaphragmatic defect known as the Bochdalek hernia, and right-sided CDHs tend to be due to anterior defect known as the Morgagni hernia. In the rare pentalogy of Cantrell, a midline defect is believed to be due to a defect in the septum transversum. Ectopic cordis, omphalocele, pericardial defects, and sternal clefts are then associated.

Most often, the chest radiograph findings are straightforward with stomach and/or numerous bowel loops in the thorax with mass effect manifested as contralateral shift of the mediastinal structures (Fig. 19.25A). There

may be a paucity or complete absence of abdominal bowel gas. If there is a nasogastric tube, it is commonly seen reentering the chest. Occasionally the appearance can mimic the cysts in CPAM. In this rare instance, a follow-up chest radiograph usually reveals a change in the intrathoracic bowel gas pattern, allowing more confident diagnosis of a CDH. Conversely, if the intrathoracic bowel loops are fluid filled, the appearance can be that of a mass such as a BPS. Again, follow-up chest radiograph may be valuable. The intrathoracic position of an nasogastric tube often offers the definitive clue (see Fig. 19.25B–C). Upper GI contrast studies to assess the position of the stomach and bowel loops are rarely necessary in the preoperative setting. If this were to be performed, midgut malrotation of the bowel is to be expected because it is often associated.

Prognosis of CDH relates to the degree of pulmonary hypoplasia, which can be assessed on prenatal imaging.

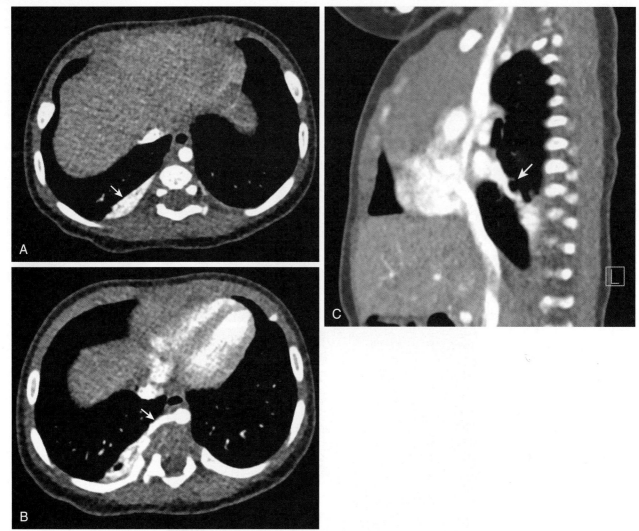

Fig. 19.24 Intralobar bronchopulmonary sequestration (BPS). (A) Axial image of the chest from a computed tomography angiogram (CTA) (A) shows a hyperdense lesion in the right lower lobe. (B) Axial image of the chest from a CTA shows a large artery arising from the descending aorta (*arrow*) supplying the right lower lobe hyperdense lesion. Sagittal reformatted image of the chest (C) shows that the lesion has systemic venous draining in the right inferior pulmonary vein (*arrow*), consistent with an intralobar BPS.

Most patients have prenatal imaging and diagnosis at time of delivery (see Chapter 23).

Esophageal Atresia With or Without Tracheoesophageal Fistula

There are two major subgroups of EA: those who have EA with a distal TEF and those who do not have the TEF. Typically patients with EA without TEF are detected on prenatal ultrasound because of the lack of fluid in the stomach. In contradistinction, EA with TEF may not be detected on prenatal ultrasound because the TEF will allow fluid from the trachea to enter the distal esophageal pouch and pass into the stomach. Because prenatal sonography always looks for fluid in the stomach, the TEF may allow the EA to go undetected until the baby is born. Occasionally a prenatal sonogram may detect a dilated proximal esophageal pouch in the setting of a normal fluid-filled stomach, and this may allow prenatal detection of a patient with EA-TEF. This diagnosis is often confirmed by fetal MRI.

TABLE 19.4   Neonatal bowel obstruction

HIGH BOWEL OBSTRUCTION	LOW BOWEL OBSTRUCTION
Antral web or atresia	Ileal atesia
Pyloric web or atresia	Meconium ileus
Duodenal stenosos or atresia	Functional immaturity of bowel[a]
Jejunal atresia	Hirschsprung disease
Multiple intestinal atresia syndrome	Colonic atesia
Malrotation with midgut volvulus	Anorectal malformation/ Imperforate anus

[a]Previously known as small left colon syndrome or meconium plug syndrome.
Please see chapter 4 for a more detailed discussion on neonatal bowel obstruction.

Initial diagnosis may be made when the child is unable to tolerate feeds, and an enteric tube is seen coiling in or unable to be passed through the proximal esophagus (Fig. 19.26). When an initial chest radiograph shows an enteric tube in the proximal esophagus, a few pertinent points should be addressed in the report: Is there distal bowel gas (in stomach/small bowel), is cardiac silhouette normal, is aortic arch and descending aorta appropriate, and are any vertebral anomalies present? These are specifically referring to the VACTERL/VATER association of vertebral, anal, cardiac, tracheoesophageal, renal, and limb abnormalities.

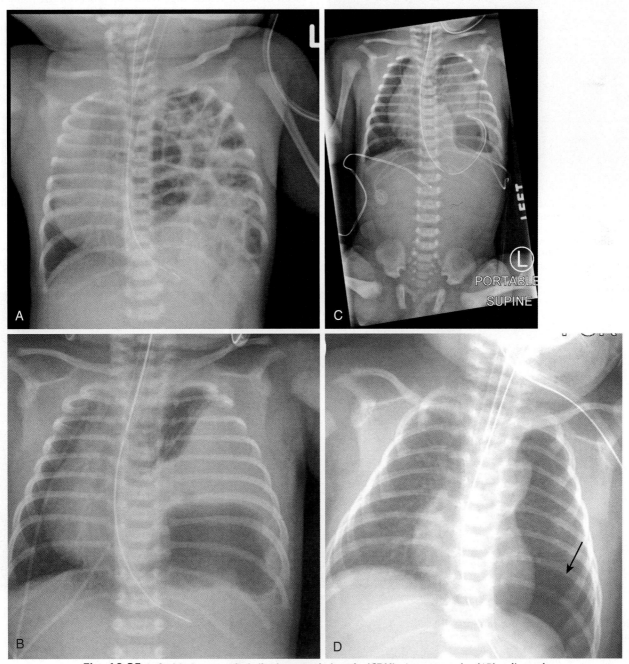

Fig. 19.25 Left-sided congenital diaphragmatic hernia (CDH). Anteroposterior (AP) radiograph of the chest in a newborn (A) showing the typical appearance of a CDH with multiple air-filled loops of bowel throughout the left hemithorax. AP radiograph of the chest (B) in a different newborn with CDH. The mediastinum is shifted rightward. There is hyperlucency at the left lower lung through which lung markings are seen and a large triangular density in the left mid to upper lung. Findings are highly suggestive of left-sided CDH. A follow-up radiograph (C) was obtained after the nasogastric tube was then advanced, clearly defining the intrathoracic position of the stomach. Note the absence of abdominal bowel gas. The dense, atelectatic hypoplastic left lung is now partially aerated. AP radiograph of the chest (D) after CDH repair (C). There is left-sided *ex vacuo* pneumothorax (*arrow*). This is an expected postoperative finding and only rarely requires evacuation.

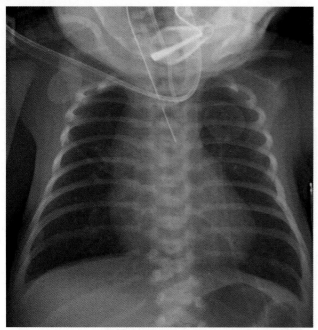

Fig. 19.26 Portable supine radiograph in a baby with intolerance of feeds. Two enteric tubes are seen, both terminating in the upper esophagus consistent with esophageal atresia. Gas is seen in the stomach, demonstrating a patent distal tracheoesophageal fistula. Also noted on the examination are vertebral segmentation anomalies.

■ Abdomen

Obstructed Bowel

Diagnosis of bowel obstruction in the neonatal setting is categorically different from both the adult and child. Instead of small versus large bowel obstruction, the primary point of imaging triage in the neonate is "high" versus "low" obstruction (Table 19.4). The rationale is based both on the unique set of differential diagnosis in this age group and the intrinsic limitations of imaging the bowel at this age.

Haustral folds are incompletely developed in the neonate. With the exception of the rectum, it is difficult, if not impossible, to reliably distinguish small from large bowel on an abdominal plain film of the newborn, even by position (Figs. 19.27A and 19.28A). Instead, one distinguishes between high and low obstruction. In general, the more loops of bowel distention, the more distal the obstruction. If there are "few loops" of distended bowel without distal bowel gas, then a high obstruction is diagnosed. If there are multiple air-distended bowel loops (usually more than four), a lower obstruction is diagnosed.

If there is a low obstruction, a water-soluble contrast enema under fluoroscopy is imperative to further narrow the differential, which still includes both surgi-

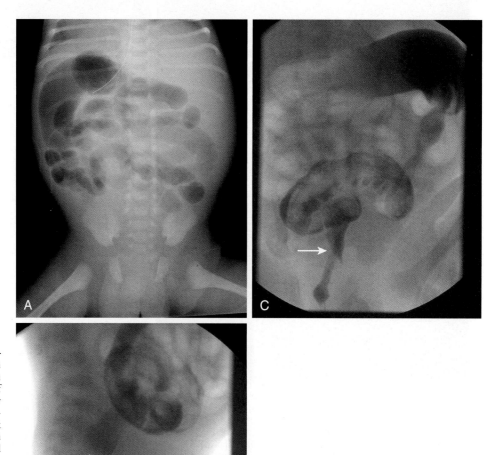

Fig. 19.27 Hirschsprung disease. Prone abdominal radiograph (A) obtained at birth in this term neonate shows multiple loops of dilated bowel consistent with a low obstruction. Attempt at further refining the differential with respect to the site of obstruction on plain radiograph is fruitless. On the third day of life, a contrast enema (B, C) was performed using iothalamate meglumine revealing a transition point in the upper rectum (*arrows*). The diagnosis of Hirschsprung disease was confirmed by biopsy.

cally and medically managed entities (Figs. 19.27B–C and 19.28B). High osmolar agents such as diatrizoate meglumine (Gastrografin) should be avoided in favor of agents that are closer to physiological osmolality, such as iothalamate meglumine (Cysto-Conray).

Pitfalls of Plain Film

There are few pitfalls of the abdominal plain film of the neonate besides those already mentioned. Among these few include a radiograph of the abdomen taken immediately after delivery. At this time, air may not have had enough time to transit to the alimentary canal. With bowel gas seen only proximally, especially with excessive air swallowing, the image may give the false impression of a high bowel obstruction. Conversely, with enough aerophagia, particularly in the setting of continuous positive airway pressure therapy, the entire bowel may reveal gaseous distention,

mimicking a low bowel obstruction. A true bowel obstruction usually demonstrates more distention. Here, the clinical history and physical examination are important in determining whether to pursue a contrast enema.

The level of obstruction is dictated only by the most *proximal* point of obstruction. Although a high bowel obstruction does not require a contrast enema (nor would it aid in its diagnosis), a contrast enema may be requested to detect more *distal* atresias. For example, a microcolon in the setting of a high obstruction on plain film would suggest both proximal and distal sites of atresia. Such information may be helpful to the individual surgeon.

A high bowel obstruction with specifically two dilated loops of bowel in the absence of further distal air is termed the "double bubble" sign, and it suggests duodenal atresia (Fig. 19.29). Extrinsic compression, such as Ladd bands, midgut volvulus, or preduodenal portal vein, can on rare occasion mimic this appearance

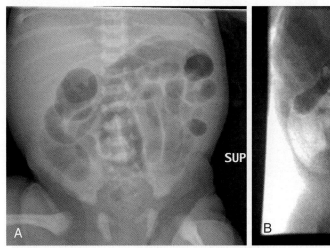

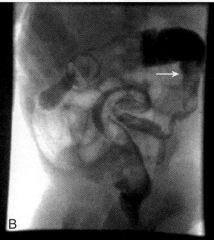

Fig. 19.28 **Functional immaturity of the colon.** Frontal supine abdominal radiograph (A) in this term baby boy on the first day of life reveals multiple dilated loops of bowel consistent with a low obstruction. A contrast enema performed the same day shows a transition point at the splenic flexure (*arrow*). Note the lucent linear filling defect in the sigmoid colon as a result of a meconium "plug" (*curved arrow*) in (B). Also note the more normal-caliber rectum in comparison with that in Fig. 19.28.

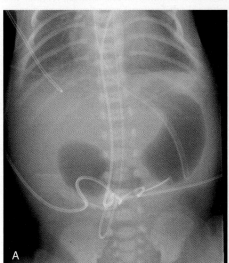

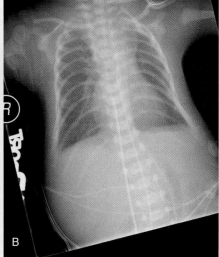

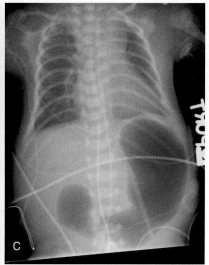

Fig. 19.29 Duodenal atresia, transient appearance: three frontal radiographs including the abdomen on this newborn boy with trisomy 21 taken several hours apart. The initial image (A) shows the classic findings of a dilated stomach and proximal duodenum (double bubble), diagnostic of duodenal atresia. After suction decompression via the nasogastric catheter, the diagnosis cannot be made (B) without seeing the initial image. The final image (C) represents reintroduction of gas into this high obstruction.

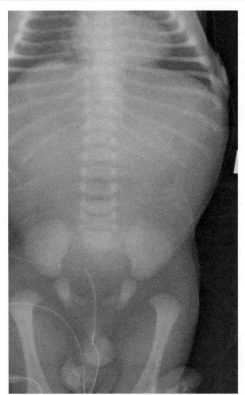

Fig. 19.30 Meconium peritonitis. Abdominal radiograph in the newborn showing plaque-like calcification in the peritoneum on the right and ill-defined rounded densities reflecting calcification on the left. Also note the calcification in the right hemiscrotum.

and will have distal bowel gas. There is typically only limited distention of the proximal duodenum with greater gastric distention in an acute obstruction, such as volvulus, as opposed to a chronic obstruction, such as duodenal atresia, where both structures are markedly dilated, yielding a true double bubble. Occasionally the two "bubbles" do not appear distended enough to confidently make the diagnosis of duodenal obstruction (often because of decompression from vomiting or nasogastric tube), or there is uncertainty regarding the presence of any distal bowel gas. Instead of using positive contrast material, gentle insufflation of air via a nasogastric tube, either under fluoroscopy or followed with an abdominal radiograph, may allow confident diagnosis.

A single dilated loop of bowel in the absence of further bowel gas is seen with neonatal gastric outlet obstruction, either from antral web or pyloric atresia. The latter is strongly associated with epidermolysis bullosa, aplasia cutis congenital, and multiple intestinal atresia.

Highly Specific Findings on the Abdominal Radiograph

Peritoneal calcification is readily evident on the radiograph, and its presence is due to a sterile, meconium peritonitis from in utero bowel perforation (Fig. 19.30). If mass effect is seen, a meconium pseudocyst may be present, which can be confirmed by ultra-

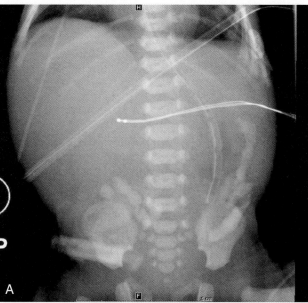

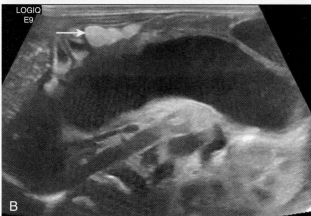

Fig. 19.31 Syndrome of multiple intestinal atresias with intraluminal calcification. Anteroposterior radiograph of the abdomen (A) in a neonate. The gas in the stomach is the only bowel gas present on the film. Dense material conforms to bowel lumen in an appearance suggesting previous administration of oral contrast, yet none was given. There is no peritoneal calcification. Grayscale ultrasound image of the abdomen (B) shows echogenic intraluminal material (*arrow*) corresponding to the high density on x-ray.

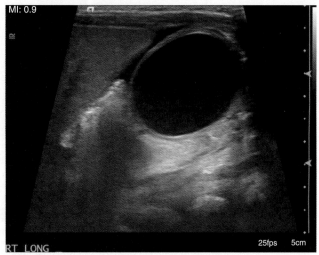

Fig. 19.32 Enteric duplication cyst. Abdominal ultrasound on this newborn girl reveals a cystic structure with internal debris demonstrating a layered wall (B), the so-called gut signature. This enteric duplication cyst was resected.

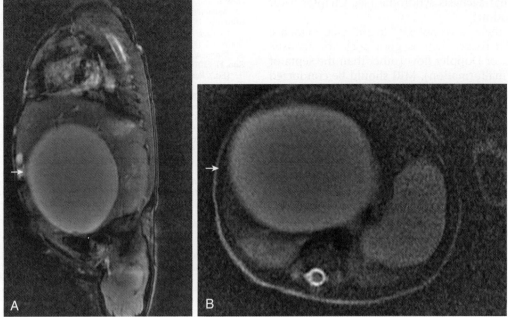

Fig. 19.33 Choledochal cyst. Single-shot fast spin echo sagittal (A) and axial (B) MRI sequence reveals a very large T2 hyperintense cyst (*arrow*) in the right upper quadrant on this 7-day-old boy.

sound. In the presence of a patent process vaginalis in males, intrascrotal, extratesticular calcifications may be observed.

Peritoneal calcifications should be differentiated from intraluminal calcium. Neonatal intraluminal calcification scattered throughout the bowel with a very high obstruction strongly suggest multiple intestinal atresias, a rare genetic disorder characterized by innumerable bowel atresia extending from stomach to distal colon (Fig. 19.31). Associations include biliary dilation and immunodeficiency. Intraluminal calcium may also be seen with stool admixed with alkaline urine, such as in anorectal malformation with a genitourinary fistula.

Postnatal Workup of a Prenatally Diagnosed Abdominal Cyst

If available, prenatal imaging or reports should be reviewed that may direct the postnatal imaging. Most often, the workup begins with a targeted ultrasound. Abdominal radiograph may be obtained if there is concern for bowel obstruction or to detect peritoneal calcification if a meconium pseudocyst is considered.

In females, large ovarian cysts are common due to maternal hormonal stimulation. If the relationship between the cyst and an ovary is not clearly established, a several-week follow-up ultrasound may reveal a decrease in size. It should be remembered that neonatal ovaries are relatively higher in the pelvis and descend during puberty.

Duplication cysts of the bowel are characterized sonographically by a rounded fluid collection with visualization of distinct bowel wall layers, the so-called gut signature (Fig. 19.32). It has been suggested

that the specificity of the sign increases as the number of distinct bowel wall layers become visible. There are, in total, five bowel layers that can potentially be seen.

A detailed discussion of choledochal cysts is beyond the scope of this chapter. The diagnosis can be made when communication with the bile duct is demonstrated. The diagnosis may be *suggested* when a right upper quadrant cyst without "gut signature" is encountered. The cyst may be very large (Fig. 19.33). The presence of a gallbladder should be documented because a single large right upper quadrant cyst could also represent neonatal gallbladder hydrops. A HIDA (hepatobiliary iminodiacetic acid) scan offers more specificity. MRI with a hepatobiliary-specific contrast agent such as gadoxetic acid can, in principle, demonstrate communication with the biliary system; however, there is at this time a paucity of literature advocating its use in this age group.

An abdominal cyst anywhere in the abdomen could represent a lymphatic malformation, but typically it is multicystic. These often, but not always, demonstrate fluid–fluid levels and septa. They are avascular, but the intervening septa may demonstrate Doppler flow.

A midline cyst, closely applied to the anterior abdominal wall between the umbilicus and the bladder, may represent a urachal remnant. If it is above the umbilicus and demonstrates Doppler signal, it may signify an umbilical vein varix. These can also occur (although less commonly) more distally, toward the liver.

Occasionally a "cyst" may be from collected fluid/debris within an obstructed vagina and uterus. Adjacent abnormalities of the fallopian tube may increase complexity in appearance. Additional imaging of the kidneys can be performed to look for possible associated unilateral renal agenesis as in the obstructed hemivagina and ipsilateral renal agenesis syndrome (see Chapter 9 for further discussion).

Finally, if there is complexity to the cyst, evidence of fat or solid tissue, such as poor posterior acoustic enhancement or Doppler flow (other than the septa of a lymphatic malformation), MRI should be conducted to define its extent because the lesion may represent a neoplasm such as a teratoma.

■ Summary

In summary, this chapter details an approach to chest and abdominal imaging of the term neonate. It provides overview on imaging patterns that one may encounter when imaging a term infant while also highlighting normal chest and abdominal radiographic findings that one must be familiar with for accurate interpretation.

Bibliography

Alazraki, N. P., & Friedman, P. J. (1972). Posterior mediastinal" pseudo-mass" of the newborn. *American Journal of Roentgenology, 116*(3), 571–574.

Al-Salem, A. H. (2014). *An illustrated guide to pediatric surgery.* Springer International Publishing.

Arthur, R. (2001). The neonatal chest Radiograph. *Paediatric Respiratory Reviews, 2*(4), 311–323.

Arthur, R. (2003). Interpretation of the paediatric chest radiograph. *Current Paediatrics, 13*(6), 438–447.

Baert, A. L., & Donoghue, V. B. (2010). *Radiological imaging of the neonatal chest.* Springer.

Balsam, D., Berdon, W. E., & Baker, D. H. (1974). The scapula as a cause of a spurious posterior mediastinal mass on lateral chest films of infants. *Journal of Pediatric Surgery, 9*(4), 501–503.

Barker, P. M., Esther, C. R., Jr., Fordham, L. A., Maygarden, S. J., & Funkhouser, W. K. (2004). Primary pulmonary lymphangiectasia in infancy and childhood. *European Respiratory Journal, 24*(3), 413–419.

Baud, C., Couture, A., Baert, A. L., et al. (2008). *Gastrointestinal Tract sonography in Fetuses and children.* Springer.

Berdon, W. E., Baker, D. H., Wung, J. T., et al. (1984). Complete cartilage-ring tracheal stenosis associated with anomalous left pulmonary artery: The ring-sling complex. *Radiology, 152*(1), 57–64.

Buonomo, C. (1997). Neonatal gastrointestinal emergencies. *Radiologic Clinics of North America, 35*(4), 845–864.

Cheng, G., Soboleski, D., Daneman, A., Poenaru, D., & Hurlbut, D. (2005). Sonographic pitfalls in the diagnosis of enteric duplication cysts. *American Journal of Roentgenology, 184*(2), 521–525.

Coley, B. D. (2013). *Caffey's pediatric diagnostic imaging, 2-Volume set: Expert Consult – Online and Print.* Elsevier: Health Sciences Division.

Coussement, A. M., & Gooding, C. A. (1973). Objective radiographic assessment of pulmonary vascularity in children 1. *Radiology, 109*(3), 649–654.

Davis, L. A. (1960). The vertical fissure line. *American Journal of Roentgenology, Radium Therapy & Nuclear Medicine, 84,* 451–453.

Dohlemann, C., Mantel, K., Vogl, T. J., et al. (1995). Pulmonary sling: Morphological findings. Pre- and postoperative course. *European Journal of Pediatrics, 154*(1), 2–14.

Eklöf, O., & Törngren, A. (1971). Pleural fluid in healthy children. *Acta Radiologica: Diagnosis, 11*(3), 346–349.

Enriquez, G., Garcia-Pena, P., & Lucaya, J. (2009). Pitfalls in chest imaging. *Pediatric Radiology, 39*(Suppl. 3), 356–368.

Esther, C. R., Jr., & Barker, P. M. (2004). Pulmonary lymphangiectasia: Diagnosis and clinical course. *Pediatric Pulmonology, 38*(4), 308–313.

Farrell, P. M. (2013). *Neonatal respiratory distress.* Elsevier Science.

Feinberg, A., Hall, N. J., Williams, G. M., et al. (2016). Can congenital pulmonary airway malformation be distinguished from Type I pleuropulmonary blastoma based on clinical and radiological features? *Journal of Pediatric Surgery, 51*(1), 33–37. https://doi.org/10.1016/j.jpedsurg.2015.10.019.

Fernandez, I., Patey, N., Marchand, V., et al. (2014). Multiple intestinal atresia with combined immune deficiency related to TTC7A defect is a multiorgan pathology: Study of a French-Canadian-based cohort. *Medicine, 93*(29), e327.

Fokin, A. A., & Robicsek, F. (2002). Poland's syndrome revisited. *The Annals of Thoracic Surgery, 74*(6), 2218–2225.

Gibson, G. J. (1996). Pulmonary hyperinflation a clinical overview. *European Respiratory Journal, 9,* 2640–2649.

Gilmartin, D. (1979). The serratus anterior muscle on chest radiographs. *Radiology, 131*(3), 629–635.

Godwin, J. D., & Tarver, R. D. (1985). Accessory fissures of the lung. *American Journal of Roentgenology, 144*(1), 39–47.

Goo, H. (2014). CT findings of congenital lung malformations. In I. O. Kim (Ed.), *Radiology illustrated: Pediatric radiology* (pp. 363–380). Springer Berlin Heidelberg.

Goo, H. W., Kim, H. J., Song, K. S., et al. (2001). Using edge enhancement to identify subtle findings on soft-copy neonatal chest radiographs. *American Journal of Roentgenology, 177*(2), 437–440.

Gupta, S. S., Singh, O., Sharma, S. S., & Mathur, R. K. (2010). Congenital fibrosarcoma of the chest wall: Report of a case. *Journal of Cutaneous and Aesthetic Surgery, 3*(3), 177–180.

Hedlund, G. L., & Kirks, D. R. (1990). Emergency radiology of the pediatric chest. *Current Problems in Diagnostic Radiology, 19*(4), 137–164.

Hernandez, R., Kuhns, L. R., & Holt, J. F. (1978). The suprasternal fossa on chest radiographs in newborns. *American Journal of Roentgenology, 130*(4), 745–746.

Herrmann, T. L., Fauber, T. L., Gill, J., et al. (2012). Best practices in digital radiography. *Radiologic Technology, 84*(1), 83–89.

Hertz, D. E. (2005). *Care of the newborn: A handbook for primary care.* Lippincott Williams & Wilkins.

Keats, T. E., & Anderson, M. W. (2013). *Atlas of normal roentgen variants that may simulate disease* (9th ed.). Philadelphia: Elsevier/Saunders.

Kesavan, A. (2013). *IAP textbook of pediatric radiology.* Jaypee Medical Limited.

Kohda, E., Tsutsumi, Y., Nagamoto, M., et al. (2007). Revisit image control for pediatric chest radiography. *Radiation Medicine, 25*(2), 60–64.

Langen, H. J., Kohlhauser-Vollmuth, C., Sengenberger, C., Bielmeier, J., Jocher, R., & Eschmann, M. (2014). Performing chest radiographs at inspiration in uncooperative children: The effect of exercises with a training program for radiology technicians. *Radiology Research and Practice, 2014,* 312846.

Langston, C. (2003). New concepts in the pathology of congenital lung malformations. *Seminars in Pediatric Surgery, 12*(1), 17–37.

Lanschot, J. J. B. V. (2005). *Integrated medical and surgical gastroenterology.* Thieme.

Leonidas, J. C., Berdon, W. E., Baker, D. H., & Santulli, T. V. (1970). Meconium ileus and its complications: A reappraisal of Plain film roentgen diagnostic criteria. *American Journal of Roentgenology, 108*(3), 598–609.

Mann, G. S., Blair, J. C., & Garden, A. S. (2012). *Imaging of Gynecological disorders in infants and children.* Springer.

Manning, P. B., Rutter, M. J., & Border, W. L. (2008). Slide tracheoplasty in infants and children: Risk factors for prolonged postoperative ventilatory support. *The Annals of Thoracic Surgery, 85*(4), 1187–1191;discussion 1191–1192.

Mata, J. M., Cáceres, J., Lucaya, J., & García-Conesa, J. A. (1990). CT of congenital malformations of the lung. *RadioGraphics, 10*(4), 651–674.

Moir, C. R., & Johnson, C. H. (2008). Poland's syndrome. *Seminars in Pediatric Surgery, 17*(3), 161–166.

Nason, L. K., Walker, C. M., McNeeley, M. F., Burivong, W., Fligner, C. L., & Godwin, J. D. (2012). Imaging of the diaphragm: Anatomy and function. *RadioGraphics, 32*(2), E51–E70.

Newman, B. (1999). Imaging of medical disease of the newborn lung. *Radiologic Clinics of North America, 37*(6), 1049–1065.

Newman, B. (2006). Congenital bronchopulmonary foregut malformations: Concepts and controversies. *Pediatric Radiology, 36*(8), 773–791.

Odita, J. C., Ugbodaga, C. I., Omene, J. A., & Okolo, A. A. (1983). Humeral head and coracoid ossification in Nigerian newborn infants. *Pediatric Radiology, 13*(5), 276–278.

Reid, J., Lee, E., Paladin, A., Carrico, C., & Davros, W. (2013). *Pediatric radiology.* USA: Oxford University Press.

Starc, M. T., Berdon, W. E., & Starc, T. J. (2014). Undiagnosed primary tracheal stenosis in tetralogy of Fallot: Complete rings with a low carina. *Pediatric Radiology, 44*(3), 362–363.

Sung, T. H., Man, E. M., Chan, A. T., & Lee, W. K. (2013). Congenital pseudarthrosis of the clavicle: A rare and challenging diagnosis. *Hong Kong Medical Journal, 19*(3), 265–267.

Swarnam, K., Soraisham, A. S., & Sivanandan, S. (2012). Advances in the management of meconium aspiration syndrome. *International Journal of Pediatrics, 359571* 2012.

Swischuk, L. E. (1997). *Imaging of the newborn, infant, and young child* (4th ed.). Williams & Wilkins.

Swischuk, L. E. (2000). *Emergency imaging of the acutely ill or injured child.* Lippincott Williams & Wilkins.

Tamrazi, A., & Vasanawala, S. S. (2011). Functional hepatobiliary MR imaging in children. *Pediatric Radiology, 41*(10), 1250–1258.

Traubici, J. (2001). The double bubble sign. *Radiology, 220*(2), 463–464.

Tumkosit, M., Yingyong, N., Mahayosnond, A., Choo, K., & Goo, H. (2012). Accuracy of chest radiography for evaluating significantly abnormal pulmonary vascularity in children with congenital heart disease. *Int J Cardiovasc Imaging, 28*(1), 69–75.

Whalen, J. P., Meyers, M. A., Oliphant, M., Caragol, W. J., & Evans, J. A. (1973). The retrosternal line. A new sign of an anterior mediastinal mass. *American*

Journal of Roentgenology, Radium Therapy & Nuclear Medicine, 117(4), 861–872.

Whitley, A. S., & Clark, K. C. (2005). *Clark's positioning in radiography* (12th ed.). Hodder Arnold.

Wiswell, T. E., Tuggle, J. M., & Turner, B. S. (1990). Meconium aspiration syndrome: Have we made a difference? *Pediatrics, 85*(5), 715–721.

Witte, C. L., Witte, M. H., Unger, E. C., et al. (2000). Advances in imaging of lymph flow disorders. *RadioGraphics, 20*(6), 1697–1719.

Wittenborg, M., Gyepes, M., & Crocker, D. (1967). Tracheal dynamics in infants with respiratory distress, stridor, and collapsing trachea 1. *Radiology, 88*(4), 653–662.

Yoo, S. J., & MacDonald, C. (2011). *Chest radiographic interpretation in pediatric cardiac patients.* Thieme.

Zylak, C., Littleton, J., & Durizch, M. (1988). Illusory consolidation of the left lower lobe: A pitfall of portable radiography. *Radiology, 167*(3), 653–655.

CHAPTER 20
Abusive Head and Spinal Trauma

Victoria Michelle Silvera

CHAPTER OUTLINE

Abusive Head Trauma, 396
    Demographics, Clinical Presentation, and
       Outcomes, 396
    Imaging of AHT, 398
    Skull Fractures, 399
    Subdural and Epidural Hematomas, 399
    Subarachnoid and Intraventricular Hemorrhage, 404
    Parenchymal Brain Injury, 404
    Retinal Hemorrhages, 406

    skull fractures, 406
    Imaging Strategies in the Evaluation of AHT, 407
Abusive Spine Trauma, 410
    Demographics, Clinical Presentation, and
       Outcomes, 410
    Imaging of Abusive Spine Trauma, 411
    Spinal Cord and Soft Tissue Injury, 413
    Subdural and Epidural Hematomas, 413
    Differential Diagnosis, 413
    Imaging Strategies of Abusive Spine Trauma, 413
Summary, 414

This chapter will review the basics of abusive head and spinal trauma, focus on common questions that arise when interpreting imaging studies of children with inflicted injuries of the central nervous system, and discuss the pros and cons of various imaging approaches. This chapter is written in a question-and-answer format.

■ Abusive Head Trauma

Demographics, Clinical Presentation, and Outcomes

What Is Abusive Head Trauma?
Various definitions of abusive head trauma (AHT) are found in the medical literature. The Centers for Disease Control and Prevention defines AHT as injury to the skull or intracranial contents of an infant or young child (<5 years of age) due to inflicted blunt impact and/or violent shaking.

How Common Is AHT?
The incidence of AHT in the United States is estimated at approximately 25-40 cases per 100,000 children younger than 1 year of age. The incidence of AHT then decreases over the next four years of life.

What Are the Classic Features of AHT?
Intracranial subdural hematomas (SDHs), retinal hemorrhages (RHs), and encephalopathy are the classic features of AHT. These findings are often observed in the absence of external signs of injury.

Which Signs and Symptoms May Be Observed in a Child with AHT?
Signs and symptoms that may be observed in a child with AHT include a decreased level of consciousness, such as irritablility or lethargy, recurrent vomiting (especially in the absence of fever or diarrhea), respiratory difficulties, seizures, and facial and scalp bruising and/or swelling. In a severe case of AHT, a child may present in a coma with respiratory difficulties or cardiopulmonary arrest.

Are There Certain "Red Flags" That Should Alert the Clinician to the Possibility of Abuse in a Child With Neurological Deficits?
Causes for concern include unexplained injuries (such as scalp swelling; bruising of the face, ears, neck, and torso, burns, and frenulum tears), inconsistencies or changes in the history provided by the caretaker, and unexplained delays in seeking medical care for an injured child. In addition, the mechanism of injury provided by the caretaker should adequately explain the pattern of injuries observed on the clinical and imaging examinations.

What Other Causes of Traumatic Head Injury Are There in Very Young Children Other Than Abuse?
Head injury can also be caused by accidental trauma, trauma related to recent birth, and trauma arising from

neglectful or inadequate supervision. The CDC does not include head injury arising from gunshot wounds, stab wounds, or penetrating trauma in the definition of AHT.

What Are the Proposed Mechanisms of Injury in Cases of AHT?

Mechanisms of injury include: (1) impulsive loading arising from rigorous and repetitive shaking of a child that may or may not terminate with blunt impact; (2) impact loading from blunt force (e.g., a child is thrown, dropped, punched, or hit in the head or the head is manually compressed; and (3) strangulation or suffocation. More than one mechanism may be contributory. Knowledge of these mechanisms of injury is derived from witnessed accounts of traumatic events and admissions by caretakers and is inferred based on known injury patterns with well-described causal accidental mechanisms.

Are There Certain Triggers That May Contribute to a Caretaker Intentionally Injuring a Child?

Commonly described triggers that can lead to a caretaker injuring a child are frustration and stress, which can occur or intensify when a child cries or has been crying for a period of time. Because a child will often stop crying when the brain is injured, the act of shaking may be reinforced.

Is There a Specific Age Range or Type of Child That Is at Increased Risk for AHT?

Most cases of AHT occur within the first year of life, with a peak incidence observed at approximately 10 to 13 weeks of age and then decrease in incidence thereafter. Children at greater risk for being abused are those with perinatal complications, those born prematurely or with major birth defects, "colicky" infants, and male infants. Additional risk factors include young parents, unstable family situations, families living at or below the poverty level, and caretakers with tendencies toward aggressive behavior and those with poor coping mechanisms regarding stress and impulse control. Substance abuse often plays a role in AHT. Despite these risk factors, abuse happens in families of all demographics, race, and economic circumstances.

When AHT Is Missed by a Healthcare Professional, What Are the Most Common Alternatively Entertained Diagnoses?

Accidental head trauma, viral gastroenteritis, influenza, and sepsis, amongst others.

How Often Is AHT Misdiagnosed by Healthcare Professionals?

In an important study by Jenny C. et al. (1999) the authors found that the diagnosis of AHT was not recognized in approximately one third of children with abusive head injuries who were seen by a physician. Approximately one third of those children sustained additional injuries after the missed diagnosis.

How Is the Nature of Injury Established in Cases of Suspected AHT?

Most commonly, a child with AHT is carefully examined and evaluated by a multidisciplinary team of professionals that work together in a coordinated and collaborative manner to determine whether abusive injury has occured. Occasionally the abuse is witnessed or the caretaker responsible for the inflicted injuries confesses to injuring the child. More commonly, however, the caretaker is not truthful about the inciting event. Evaluation of the cause of injury typically involves gathering information from the caretaker, family members, first responders, emergency department (ED) physicians, pediatricians, neurologists, ophthalmologists, neurosurgeons, radiologists, social workers, nurses, psychologists, psychiatrists, and law enforcement officers as appropriate and analyzing data provided by the physical examination, laboratory tests, imaging studies, and the scene investigation.

What Is the Composition of a Multidisciplinary Child Protection Team?

Depending on resources and geography, hospitals may have a multidisciplinary child protection team (CPT). CPTs typically consist of pediatricians whose clinical focus is child abuse (one or more of these pediatricians may be board-certified in the subspecialty of Child Abuse Pediatrics), social workers, nurses, psychologists, psychiatrists, and occasionally, attorneys. Team compositions may vary.

What Is the Role of the Radiologist in Evaluating Children With Suspected AHT?

The radiologist plays a critical role in the assessment of a child with head injury who may have been abused. First, the radiologist must attempt to determine whether the imaging abnormalities have been caused by trauma or by a medical condition or by both. A child with a medical condition may also have been abused and in fact, children with medical conditions are at greater risk for being abused than otherwise healthy children. Second, if it appears that the head findings are traumatic in nature, the radiologist should search for additional imaging abnormalities that may support or exclude abuse as the basis of the imaging abnormalities.

Based on the imaging abnormalities, it is helpful for the radiologist to provide recommendations for supplemental and/or follow-up imaging examinations that may further clarify and characterize the nature of the imaging findings. For example, if a radiologist identifies a SDH, on a head CT that is not explained by the medical condition of the child or by the history provided by the caretaker, the radiologist should discuss with the careteam whether obtaining a brain MRI as a next step would be helpful.

It is often informative for a radiologist to perform a comprehensive review of all imaging studies obtained during a care episode of a child being assessed for abuse to assess the evolution of imaging abnormalties on serial studies which often results in increased insight into the character of findings.

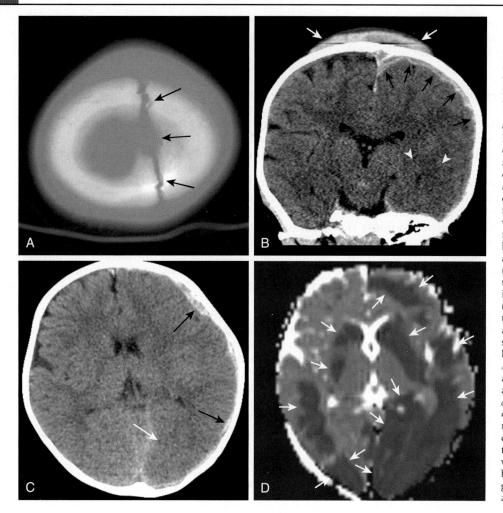

Fig. 20.1 Abusive head trauma (AHT). A 16-month-old girl with AHT. By report the infant fell from the couch and landed on the top of her head, then went into a "faint" and started seizing. Further examination revealed a tongue laceration, bilateral retinal hemorrhages, elevated transaminases, and a duodenal hematoma. The child was brain dead on day 2 of admission. (A) Axial head computed tomography (CT) image shows a fracture through the sagittal suture with diastasis. (B) Coronal reformatted image from the noncontrast head CT shows a heterogeneous-appearing thin subdural hematoma (SDH) over the left cerebral hemisphere with extension along the falx into the interhemispheric fissure (*black arrows*). A large scalp hematoma overlies the diastatic fracture at the vertex (*white arrows*). Note subtle parenchymal injury of the left temporal lobe (*arrowheads*). (C) Axial noncontrast head CT shows a thin, extensive, heterogeneous-appearing SDH on the left (*black arrows*). Ischemic injury is observed of the left occipital lobe (*white arrow*). (D) Axial apparent difusion coefficient (ADC) image shows extensive hypoxic ischemic injury involving multiple areas of the brain bilaterally, including the basal ganglia (*arrows*) not in a distribution of a vascular territory.

What Are the Potential Clinical Outcomes for Children With AHT?

An estimated 18 to 25% of children with AHT may not survive the traumatic incident, and it is estimated that 50% to 80% of survivors suffer significant long-term morbidity. Neurological outcomes include delayed psychomotor development, behavioral disorders, learning and language/speech difficulties, hemi- and quadriparesis, epilepsy, visual impairment, severe physical and mental disabilities and a persistant vegetative state.

Imaging of AHT

Are There Imaging Patterns That Are Considered Particularly Suggestive of AHT?

Imaging abnormalities vary based on the severity of the head injury. Findings include unilateral or bilateral SDHs, typically thin and extensive and located over the convexities and/or within the interhemispheric fissure, unilateral or bilateral parenchymal brain injury, typically hypoxic ischemic in nature, and retinal hemorrhages, which can be unilateral or bilat-

eral (Fig. 20.1). Bridging vein injury with partial or complete disruption of the bridging vein and cortical vein thrombosis may be apparent. A thin but extensive SDH with midline shift that is disproportionately greater than the width of the SDH (reflecting additional mass effect from ipsilateral brain swelling/injury) is particularly suggestive of AHT (Fig. 20.2) and warrants further investigation for possible abuse. An unexplained intracranial SDH as an isolated imaging finding is nonspecific, but raises the possibility of AHT. The medical team will attempt to determine the underlying cause of the SDH (e.g., abusive injury, accidental trauma, benign enlargement of the subarachnoid space [BESS], coagulopathy, metabolic disorder and other conditions) and assess the child for signs of possible inflicted injury.

Skull fractures are present in approximately 25% of cases of AHT and provide evidence of impact/impulse injury. The incidence of skull fractures in AHT is greater in autopsy series and lower in children with AHT without neurological deficits. As approximately 75% of children with AHT will *NOT* have a skull fracture, identification of an occult skeletal fracture on a SS provides additional data supporting a history of trauma.

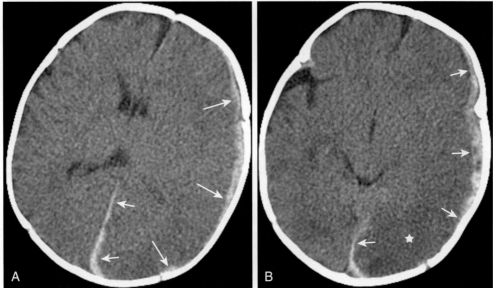

Fig. 20.2 Disproportionate midline shift. Two-month-old girl presented for progressive irritability, apnea, and seizures in the emergency department. This child had been seen before admission by the pediatrician for unexplained bruising and a subconjunctival hemorrhage. On this admission the child had bruising of the extremities and buttocks, bilateral retinal hemorrhages, and a skeletal survey showing fractures. (A, B) Thin, heterogeneous-appearing left-sided subdural hematoma (SDH) overlying the left cerebral hemisphere and extending along the interhemispheric fissure posteriorly (*arrows*). The degree of rightward midline shift is greater than the radial thickness of the SDH, which indicates left cerebral hemisphere swelling from parenchymal injury. The presence of hypoxic ischemic injury is supported by the loss of the gray white matter differentiation, most apparent in the left occipital region (*star*) and brain swelling.

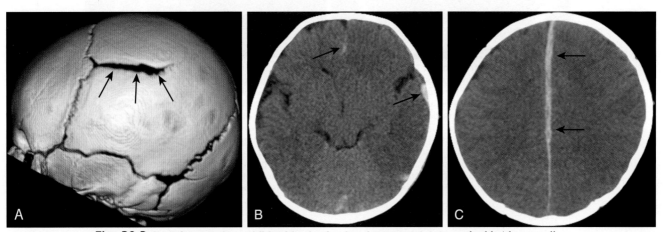

Fig. 20.3 Skull fracture in a child with abusive head trauma. A 2.5-month-old girl reportedly dragged out of her chair by an older sibling. The child presented to the emergency department with lethargy and vomiting and developed seizures. Further evaluation revealed no retinal hemorrhages and a positive skeletal survey. (A) Computed tomography (CT) three-dimensional model of the skull shows a diastatic parietal fracture (*arrows*). (B) Axial noncontrast head CT shows thin subdural hematomas (SDHs) along the interhemispheric fissure and left middle cranial fossa (*arrows*). (C) Axial noncontrast head CT reveals a thin SDH along the falx (*arrows*). The infant had been seen 6 weeks before this admission for biparietal skull fractures after reportedly falling from a bed.

Skull Fractures

What Is the Most Common Type of Skull Fracture in AHT?

linear parietal skull fracture is the most common type of skull fracture seen in AHT (Fig. 20.3). However, it is also the most common type of skull fracture observed in cases of accidental head trauma. Complex skull fractures (e.g., depressed, comminuted, diastatic, multiple,

bilateral, and suture-crossing) without appropriate history are more suggestive of abusive injury (Fig. 20.4).

Subdural and Epidural Hematomas

Please note that in this chapter a "subdural" hematoma/collection is referred to as blood and/or fluid located between the dura and the arachnoid membrane. On

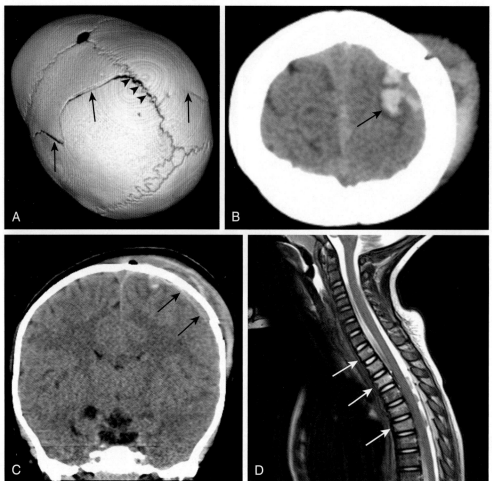

Fig. 20.4 *Skull fracture.* A 20-month-old girl with head trauma. Initially somnolent after a reported unwitnessed fall from a couch onto the hardwood floor. (A) The computed tomography (CT) three-dimensional model of the skull shows an irregularly configured crossover fracture at the vertex involving both parietal bones (*arrows*) and extending through the diastatic sagittal suture at the vertex (*arrowheads*). (B) The hemorrhagic contusion of the left frontal lobe was well seen on axial imaging, but not the adjacent extraaxial hematoma. (C) The coronal reformatted noncontrast head CT image depicts the left frontal extraaxial hematoma clearly. (D) Sagittal T2-weighted image of the upper spine shows multiple thoracic vertebral body compression fractures (*arrows*). The injury pattern was suggestive of a fall from a significant height with axial loading and was not consistent with the history provided by the caretaker. The skeletal survey showed no additional fractures. On further questioning the caretaker acknowledged the child had fallen from a second-story window while the caretaker was taking a nap.

histologic examination these hematomas/collections are identified within the dura, within a cleavage plane in the dural border cell layer.

What Causes Subdural Hematomas in Children With AHT?

The most widely cited cause of SDHs in children with AHT is partial or complete tearing of bridging veins at the vertex. In AHT secondary to acceleration and deceleration forces, bridging veins are subjected to tension and stretching, which in turn can lead to tearing of a bridging vein and bleeding into the subdural and subarachnoid spaces (Fig. 20.5). Occasionally a torn bridging vein with contracted clot at the point of disruption is observed on axial and/or coronal MRI as a discontinuous vein with an ovoid-, tadpole-, or comma-shaped configuration at the point of injury (Fig. 20.6). There

have been other alternative proposed theories for causes of subdural hemorrhage in AHT which have not been supported in the peer review literature.

What Is the Typical Appearance of a Subdural Hematoma in a Child With AHT?

In children with AHT, SDHs are usually thin, unilateral or bilateral, heterogeneous in attenuation, and located over the convexities and/or within the interhemispheric fissure (see Figs. 20.1–20.3 and 20.6). SDHs may also be observed within the posterior fossa along the squamosal portions of the occipital bones and along the clivus (retroclival) (see Fig. 20.5). Posterior fossa SDHs are often small, best appreciated on MRI, and are easily overlooked on CT, especially as CT images may be hampered by streak artifact and volume averaging between subdural blood and the occipital bones. A SDH may contain

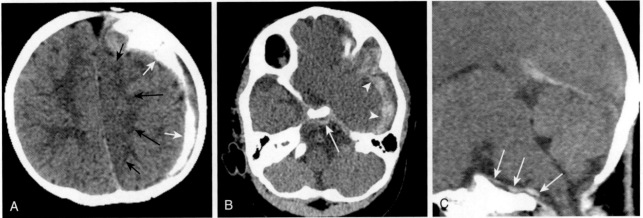

Fig. 20.5 Mixed-density subdural hematoma (SDH) from an avulsed bridging vein. Six-month-old boy found unresponsive and cyanotic in his crib, vomited once, and started seizing in the emergency department. The child had been seen twice by his pediatrician for cryptic bruising of the face, buttock, and arm. Negative workup for blood disorder. (A) Axial noncontrast head computed tomography (CT) image shows a left-sided heterogeneous-appearing SDH (*arrows*). The black arrows indicate parenchymal brain injury with loss of the gray-white matter distinction. The SDH was surgically evacuated. At surgery, a left hemispheric acute-on-chronic SDH was found with a large, avulsed, copiously bleeding bridging vein as well as ischemic brain tissue. The child did not survive. (B) Axial noncontrast head CT image shows a heterogeneous-appearing SDH in the left middle cranial fossa (*arrowheads*) and a retroclival hematoma (*arrow*) along the clivus. (C) The sagittal reformatted noncontrast head CT image shows the retroclival hematoma more clearly (*arrows*).

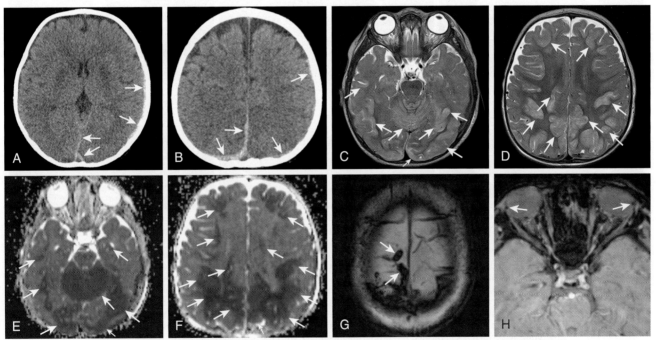

Fig. 20.6 Hypoxic ischemic injury (HII) and injured bridging veins. Fourteen-month-old girl who presented with vomiting and lethargy. Additional evaluation revealed bruising of the face, lip, jaw, and arms; a forehead contusion; bilateral retinal hemorrhages; and a negative skeletal survey. (A, B) Axial non-contrast head computed tomography images show thin, extensive subdural hematomas (*arrows*) along the falx, left frontoparietal region, and both parietal regions. Bilateral parenchymal injury is also evident as loss of gray white matter differentiation. (C, D) Axial T2-weighted images show extensive, patchy, bilateral parenchymal edema involving cortex and white matter and cerebellar injury (*arrows*). (E, F) ADC maps show that the areas of cerebral edema correspond to areas of restricted diffusion indicative of HII. (G) Axial susceptibility weighted imaging (SWI) at the vertex shows marked signal blooming of thrombosed injured or ruptured bridging veins (*arrows*). (H) Axial SWI image through the orbits shows bilateral peripheral retinal hemorrhages (*arrows*).

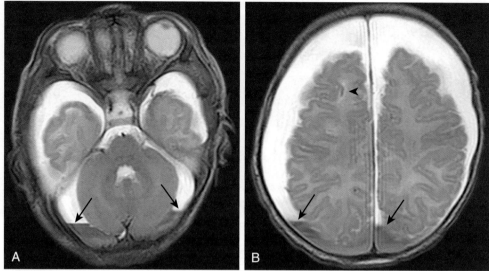

Fig. 20.7 Subdural hematomas (SDHs) with fluid–fluid levels. Three-month-old boy with upper respiratory symptoms, fever, congestion, and a prolonged seizure. The patient was evaluated for similar symptoms 2 weeks before admission. Further examination revealed hemiparesis, a crossover parietal skull fracture, hypoxic ischemic injury, no retinal hemorrhages, and a skeletal survey with fractures. (A) Axial T2-weighted image of the posterior fossa shows a large SDH with fluid–fluid levels (*arrows*). (B) Axial T2-weighted image of the supratentorial compartment shows bilateral, large SDHs with fluid–fluid levels overlying the entirety of the cerebral hemispheres. Sediment is dark (*arrows*) in signal and supernatant is bright. Note a small blood-filled cerebral contusional cleft (*arrowhead*).

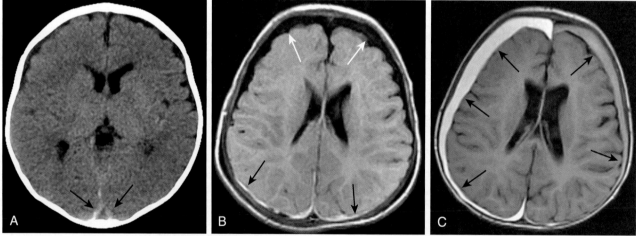

Fig. 20.8 Evolution of subdural hematomas. Three-month-old girl with bradycardia and bradypnea found unresponsive and limp by father. Further examination revealed a forehead contusion, body bruising, no retinal hemorrhages, and a skeletal survey with fractures. (A) The axial noncontrast head computed tomography (CT) image on day 1 shows thin, bilateral, high-attenuation subdural collections in the parietooccipital regions (*arrows*). Note the normal-appearing subarachnoid space in the frontal regions anteriorly. (B) Axial fluid-attenuated inversion recovery (FLAIR) magnetic resonance (MR) image on day 2 shows increase in the size of the bilateral subdural collections with fluid–fluid levels. Sediment layers dependently and posteriorly and is bright (*black arrows*), and the supernatant is distributed nondependently in the frontal regions (*white arrows*). (C) Axial FLAIR MR image on day 9 shows interval mixing of the hemorrhagic contents within the subdural space. Note the subdural collections are of different signal intensities but of the same age, which is established by comparing this image with the admission head CT.

a fluid–fluid level (Figs. 20.7–20.9), which reflects the separation of blood components within the collection; sediment layers dependently and supernatant layers in a non dependent fashion. Fluid–fluid levels within SDHs are also observed in cases of accidental head trauma. Typically, fluid–fluid levels resolve on follow-up imaging due to mixing and redistribution of blood products within the subdural space (see Fig. 20.8).

How Do Hematohygromas Form?

The most widely held theory on the etiology of hematohygromas in children with AHT is that the trauma causes a tear or rent in the arachnoid membrane that allows cerebrospinal fluid (CSF) to flow from the subarachnoid space into the subdural space. If the subdural space also contains blood, a hematohygroma is formed. If blood is not present within the subdural space, a hy-

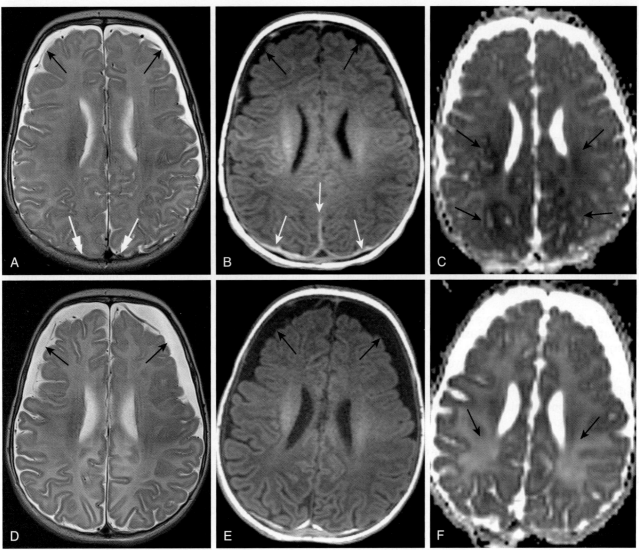

Fig. 20.9 Subdural hematohygromas. A 2.5-month-old boy found by his father to be grunting and shaking after waking from his nap. The infant was admitted for presumed sepsis and lethargy, and developed seizures on hospital admission. Additional examinations revealed bilateral retinal hemorrhages and a positive skeletal survey. (A–C) Performed 3 days after the onset of symptoms. (A, B) Axial T2- and T1-weighted images show small bilateral subdural collections that overlie the cerebral hemispheres and contain blood–fluid levels with sediment layering dependently (*white arrows*) and supernatant (*black arrows*) in a nondependent location. (C) The axial ADC map shows restricted diffusion in the posterior centrum semiovale and parietal lobes (*arrows*) bilaterally. (D–F) Follow-up magnetic resonance imaging 10 days after onset of symptoms. (D, E) Axial T2- and T1-weighted images show interval increase in the size of the subdural collections (*black arrows*), which could be explained by leakage/accumulation of CSF in the subdural space or ongoing bleeding. Sediment layers dependently (*white arrows*) and supernatant nondependently (*black arrows*). (F) Axial ADC map shows the diffusion to be mildly facilitated (*arrows*).

groma is formed. Additional theories posit that subdural hematohygromas arise from SDHs that accumulate CSF either through diffusion or effusion of CSF from the subarachnoid space into the subdural space, or that fluid accumulates within the subdural space from surrounding vessels. A hematohygroma may be indistinguishable from a hygroma based on the variable proportions of blood relative to CSF/fluid within the subdural space (Fig. 20.10). Along these lines, a hematohygroma that contains a low concentration of CSF/fluid resembles a SDH. Serial imaging of children with AHT in the first week to week and a half after the onset of symptoms may show an increase in the size of a subdural

collection (see Figs. 20.8 and 20.9), which can be caused by ongoing bleeding and/or influx or accumulation of CSF/fluid in the subdural space.

What Are the Causes of Heterogeneous-Appearing Subdural Hematomas on CT in Children With AHT?

In adults, a heterogeneous-appearing SDH on head CT often represents acute-on-chronic hemorrhage within the subdural space. In children with AHT there are three main reasons why a subdural collection may be heterogeneous-appearing. First, unclotted blood (which is intermediate or low in attenuation on CT) may be mixed with clotted blood (which is high in attenuation on CT) within the subdural space. This can occur in children who are acutely imaged, in cases with active, ongoing bleeding in the subdural space and in children with a coagulopathy. Second, the subdural fluid may represent a mixture of blood with CSF/fluid (i.e., a hematohygroma). Third, there is acute or subacute hemorrhage into a preexistent SDH (i.e., acute-on-chronic hemorrhage).

What Does a Membrane Within a Subdural Hematoma Signify?

As subdural hematomas evolve, vascularized membranes can form. The earliest time point at which a subdural membrane may be visualized on MRI has not been systematically studied in children. The earliest time point at which a subdural membrane has been observed in a histopathological study (thus not on a gross macroscopic level) of adults and children is 5 days. Care must be taken not to mistake a crossing bridging vein within the subdural space for a membrane.

Should I Attempt to Date a Subdural Hematoma in My Report Based on Imaging Characteristics?

It is preferable to use descriptive terminology in the radiology report when describing subdural collections and to refrain from using terms such as "acute," "chronic," or "acute-on-chronic" that suggest the age of the collection (see Fig. 20.10).

Why Does the Clinician Want to Know the Age of an Imaging Abnormality in Cases of Abuse?

If the age of a traumatic lesion, such as a SDH, can be determined by imaging, then the time frame during which the injury occurred can be established. This may help determine which caretaker(s) was/were in the presence of the child when the child was injured.

How Common Are Subdural Hematomas After Birth, and How Long Are They Evident on Imaging?

The reported prevalence of birth-related SDHs varies in the literature based on the sensitivity of the imaging modality used (i.e., ultrasound, CT, or MRI) to detect the SDHs; parturitional SDHs are estimated to occur in 15% to 63% of uncomplicated deliveries. Most parturitional SDHs resolve by 4 weeks, and in one study (Rooks VJ et al), all SDHs resolved by 3 months. SDHs related to birth are usually small and located posteriorly within the intracranial space in the region of the tentorium.

What Do Enlarged Low-Density Extraaxial Spaces in the Frontal Region on Imaging Represent in Infants?

Enlarged bifrontal extraaxial spaces can represent one of the following: (1) benign enlargement of the subarachnoid space; (2) chronic SDHs; and (3) acute, subacute, or chronic subdural hygromas or hematohygromas. In children with benign enlargement of the subarachnoid spaces, subarachnoid vessels will course through the subarachnoid space toward the dura in an undisturbed manner. When an enlarged extraaxial space represents a subdural collection, the subarachnoid membrane and the vessels within the subarachnoid space will be displaced toward the surface of the brain and a crowded apparance of the subarachnoid vessels is observed.

Are Retroclival Subdural or Epidural Collections Commonly Seen in Cases of AHT?

Retroclival collections are seen in up to one-third of cases of AHT depending on the resolution of the imaging and the imaging planes and sequences used. Most of these extraaxial collections are subdural in location (see Fig. 20.5) with small retroclival epidural hematomas (EDHs) uncommonly seen. Retroclival subdural collections can be caused by: (1) bleeding from dural injury; (2) a traumatic tear in the clival arachnoid membrane resulting in flow or effusion of CSF/fluid into the subdural space; or (3) redistribution of subdural blood/fluid from subdural collections along the occipital squama or supratentorial space. More than one cause may be contributory. A retroclival EDH may be caused by dural bleeding or disruption of local vasculature (e.g., the basilar plexus or meningohypophyseal trunk) and is likely related to hyperflexion and hyperextension injury of the craniocervical junction (CCJ). EDHs are observed at autopsy in children with fatal AHT.

Are Convexity Epidural Hematomas Common in Cases of AHT?

Convexity EDHs can be seen in cases of AHT, but they are not common. EDHs are usually associated with skull fractures and are much more commonly observed in children with accidental head trauma.

Subarachnoid and Intraventricular Hemorrhage

Is Subarachnoid or Intraventricular Hemorrhage Common in AHT?

A small volume of subarachnoid blood is commonly observed on imaging in cases of AHT and is almost always present in fatal cases of AHT at autopsy. Subarachnoid blood likely originates from torn bridging veins or from focal contusion or laceration of intracranial blood vessels. Subarachnoid blood is also commonly seen in accidental head trauma. Intraventricular hemorrhage (IVH) may accompany other intracranial trauma-related findings in children with AHT. Isolated IVH is uncommon.

Parenchymal Brain Injury

Which Types of Parenchymal Injury Are Seen in AHT?

The most common types of parenchymal brain injury seen in children with AHT are HII (Figs. 20.1, 20.6, and 20.9), traumatic axonal injury (particularly at the cervicomedullary junction), hemorrhagic and nonhemorrhagic contusional injuries (Fig. 20.11), and cerebral contusional tears, also known as white matter lacerations (Figs. 20.7 and 20.12) (see later discussion). Various combinations of parenchymal injury may be present concurrently. Diffuse axonal injury is considered uncommon.

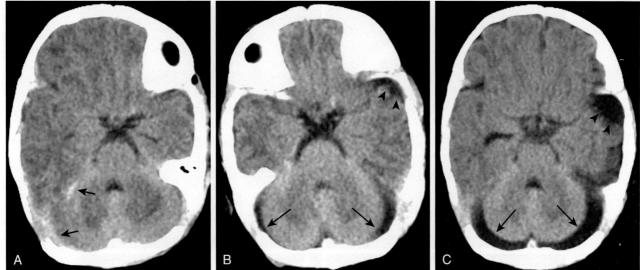

Fig. 20.10 Growing hematohygromas. Twenty-four-day-old girl with poor feeding, seizures 2 hours before presentation, and vomiting on the way to the emergency department. The father had dropped the baby several days before admission while feeding the baby and by report the baby was fine at the time. Further imaging revealed a parietal skull fracture, unilateral retinal hemorrhages, body bruising, a hard palate ulceration, and a positive skeletal survey. (A) Axial noncontrast head computed tomography (CT) performed on day 1 shows acute high-attenuation subdural blood along the right tentorial leaflet and over the cerebellum (*arrows*). Note the normal appearance of the left middle cranial fossa initially. (B) Noncontrast head CT on day 3 shows further enlargement of the posterior fossa subdural collection, which is now low in attenuation and consistent with a hematohygroma. Note the development of an acute low-density hygroma in the left middle cranial fossa (*arrowheads*). (C) The noncontrast head CT on day 10 shows further enlargement of the posterior fossa hematohygromas and left middle cranial fossa hygroma anterior to the left temporal lobe.

What Is the Imaging Appearance of HII in Children With AHT?

In cases of abuse, areas of HII are often patchy in appearance and scattered within the brain parenchyma in a nonarterial distribution (the distribution of injury does not adhere to an arterial territory). Injury may be located in the cortex, cerebral white matter, basal ganglia, cerebellum, and brainstem. A bilateral distribution of HII is more common than unilateral injury (Fig. 20.13). Parenchymal swelling and mass effect are variably present, and children may present with prominent bilateral cerebral swelling, unilateral cerebral swelling with midline shift (see Figs. 20.2 and 20.13), or mild or inapparent brain swelling (see Fig. 20.9). Evidence of HII can be seen on head CT shortly after the traumatic event.

In cases of unilateral HII (see Fig. 20.13), the SDH typically overlies the affected cerebral hemisphere. Unilateral HII in AHT can be mistaken for acute disseminated encephalomyelitis (ADEM), meningoencephalitis, and stroke, among others.

Regarding Parenchymal Hemorrhages, Is There a Distinctive Appearance in Children With AHT?

In AHT, parenchymal hemorrhages are usually small and scattered, but are occasionally more prominent in size in children with parenchymal contusions deep to a skull fracture.

Are Parenchymal Contusions Observed in AHT?

Parenchymal contusions are occasionally observed in AHT, in particular deep to impact injury (see Fig. 20.11).

What Are Cerebral Contusional Tears?

Cerebral contusional tears, also known as white matter lacerations, are rare parenchymal lesions usually observed in children ≤5 months of age with AHT. In the absence of appropriate history, cerebral contusional tears are considered very suggestive of abuse. These tears are sharply marginated clefts that extend in a radial manner through the cerebral white matter to the cortex. Occasionally, a cleft is oriented to the surface of the brain and runs parallel to the cortical margin. The clefts usually contain a small volume of contracted clot or a fluid–fluid level (see Fig. 20.12). The margin of the cleft may or may not show restricted diffusion. On head CT, cerebral contusional tears may be difficult to detect or distinguish from nonmyelinated white matter, especially if the hemorrhagic content is small or not apparent. Cerebral contusional clefts are often readily identified on MRI and ultrasonography. Cerebral contusional clefts have also been reported in the context of birth injury.

What Type of Posterior Fossa Abnormalities Are Seen on Imaging in AHT?

Cerebellar injury is seen in children with more severe patterns of AHT and may be apparent as cerebellar edema or HII. Brainstem injury involving the cervicomedullary junction is identified at autopsy in cases of AHT. Injury of the respiratory centers in the brainstem has been raised as a potential cause of the respiratory difficulties and apneic episodes observed in children with AHT. Posterior fossa SDHs are common in children with AHT, are often small, and are best appreciated on MRI.

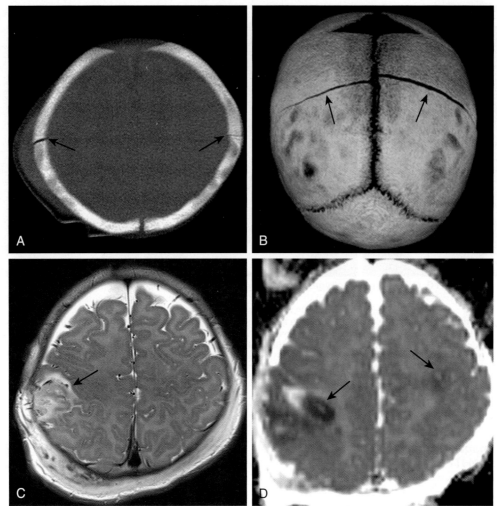

Fig. 20.11 Parenchymal contusion. Three-month-old boy status post fall from father's arms onto a wood floor, striking his head. The infant showed subclinical seizures in the hospital diagnosed by EEG. No retinal hemorrhages were seen but fractures were seen on a skeletal survey. (A) Axial noncontrast head computed tomography (CT) shows biparietal linear fractures (*arrows*) and a large right-sided scalp hematoma. (B) Noncontrast CT three-dimensional model of the skull better demonstrates the crossover fracture (*arrows*). (C) Axial T2-weighted image of the brain shows a right frontoparietal parenchymal contusion (*arrow*) deep to the right parietal fracture. (D) Axial ADC map shows restricted diffusion within the right frontal region of contused brain, as well as a contralateral area of parenchymal contusion (*arrows*) deep to the left-sided skull fracture. The head injury pattern suggests blunt force trauma, and the pattern is compatible with the provided history of a fall onto the head, which may have been accidental, neglectful, or intentionally inflicted. The multiple additional unexplained fractures supported abuse.

Retinal Hemorrhages

How Common Are Retinal Hemorrhages in Children With AHT, and Can They Be Detected on Imaging?

RHs are identified on fundoscopic examination in approximately 75% to 80% (range 50%–100% based on published series) of cases with AHT as opposed to approximately 20% of cases of accidental trauma. Children with AHT are more likely to have RHs that are too numerous to count, multilayered (i.e., intraretinal, preretinal, and subretinal), diffuse (i.e., covering a large area of the retina), and extend to the periphery of the retina. RHs are not generally appreciated on head CT and can be observed on MRI as small rounded or linear foci of T2 shortening and/or susceptibility (see Fig. 20.6). Traumatic retinoschisis (splitting of all retinal

layers), a severe form of retinal injury, manifests as linear, wavy-appearing folds along the posterior margin of the globe (Fig. 20.14).

Skull Fractures

Differential Diagnosis

WHICH MEDICAL CONDITIONS CAUSE PARENCHYMAL INJURY PATTERNS SIMILAR TO THOSE SEEN IN AHT?

Various conditions can mimic parenchymal brain injury patterns seen in AHT, including accidental trauma, infarcts from vascular disease, metabolic diseases (e.g., glutaric aciduria type I, Menkes disease), and infectious and postinfectious conditions (e.g., encephalitis

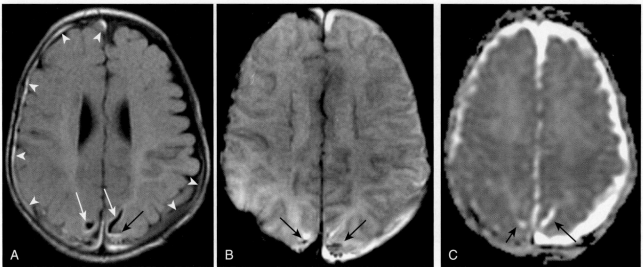

Fig. 20.12 Cerebral contusional tears. Same patient as in Fig. 20.10A. (A) Axial FLAIR image shows biparietal cerebral contusional tears (*white arrows*) with a subtle blood–fluid level on the left (*black arrow*). Arrowheads mark the bilateral subdural hematomas of different signal intensities. (B) Axial gradient echo sequence shows blood layering within both clefts. (C) Axial ADC map shows no definite restricted diffusion along the margins of the clefts.

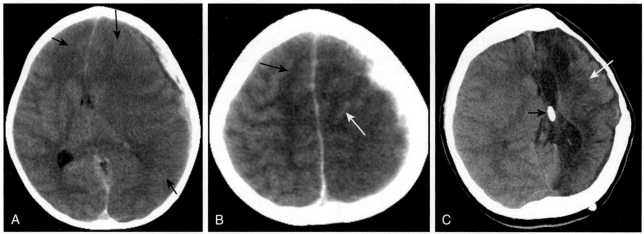

Fig. 20.13 Unilateral hypoxic ischemic injury (HII). Twenty-seven-month-old girl found unresponsive in the care of her mother's boyfriend. The child also had multiple bruises, bilateral retinal hemorrhages, and fractures on skeletal survey. (A) Axial noncontrast head computed tomography (CT) shows a thin mixed attenuation left-sided subdural collection (*white arrow*) with excessive rightward midline shift. Early left-sided brain injury is shown (*long black arrow*). The right frontal anterior cerebral artery (ACA) territory infarct is a secondary finding caused by subfalcine herniation (*short black arrow*). (B) Axial noncontrast head CT shows scant subarachnoid hemorrhage (*white arrow*) and the right-sided ACA territory infarct (*black arrow*). (C) Axial noncontrast head CT at follow-up shows extensive cystic encephalomalacia and atrophy of the left cerebral hemisphere (*white arrow*). The patient is shunted (*black arrow*).

and ADEM). Brain injury from suffocation or strangulation may appear similar to imaging abnormalities related to aspiration and cardiorespiratory arrest (e.g., apparent life-threatening event and sudden infant death syndrome).

WHICH MEDICAL CONDITIONS CAN CAUSE INTRACRANIAL SDHS?

Medical conditions that can cause intracranial SDHs include coagulopathies (such as hemophilia, vitamin K deficiency), hematological disorders (e.g., leukemia), cerebrovascular anomalies, metabolic conditions (e.g., glutaric aciduria type I, Menkes disease), intracranial hypotension, and surgical interventions such as ventricular shunting, among others.

Imaging Strategies in the Evaluation of AHT

If AHT Is Suspected in a Child, What Is My First-Line Imaging Study of Choice?

The American College of Radiology and the American Academy of Pediatrics recommend a noncontrast head CT in the initial assessment of suspected AHT. CT is superior to MRI and ultrasonography in identifying intracranial hemorrhage and skull fractures. In addition, CT is widely available, rapid, and allows for prompt triage of an injured child. In an asymptomatic or non-acute case of suspected child abuse, imaging evaluation of the head with a brain MRI instead of a head CT can be considered. This approach spares the child

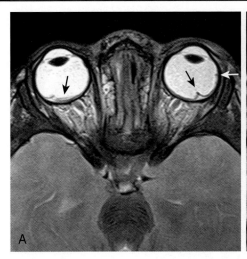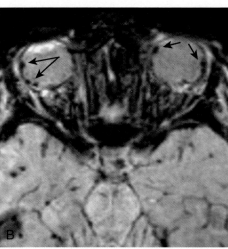

Fig. 20.14 Retinoschisis. Six-month-old girl with cardiac arrest while in the care of the babysitter. Cardiopulmonary resuscitation was performed for approximately 40 min before restoration of circulation. Head imaging showed diffuse cerebral edema, subdural hematomas, and retinal hemorrhages, and the skeletal survey was positive. Fundoscopic examination performed on the same day as the magnetic resonance imaging showed bilateral retinoschisis. (A) Axial T2-weighted image shows linear irregularities along the posterior aspects of the globes. (B) Axial SWI image shows rounded and linear foci of susceptibility artifact along the margins of the globes extending to the periphery of the retina.

the potentially harmful effects of ionizing radiation associated with CT. The downside of evaluating a child with possible AHT with MRI only is that nondisplaced and some displaced skull fractures, important pieces of diagnostic information, may not be appreciated (Fig. 20.15). It is estimated that approximately one-third of neurologically asymptomatic children with AHT will have evidence of intracranial injury (SDH, EDH, or cerebral edema) on CT and/or MRI, and almost half of these children will also have a clinically unsuspected skull fracture. In infants and young children with head imaging findings that raise the possibility of AHT, a SS is indicated.

Are Computed Tomography Sagittal and Coronal Reformatted Images Helpful in Cases of AHT?

Coronal reformatted head CT images aid in detecting linear, nondisplaced skull fractures oriented in the plane of section (Fig. 20.16) and increase the sensitivity for identifying small SDHs, EDHs and subarachnoid blood at the vertex (see Figs. 20.1 and 20.4), along the floor of the middle cranial fossae and along the tentorial leaflets. Coronal reformatted images also help distinguish superior sagittal sinus thrombosis from subarachnoid or subdural blood adjacent to the sinus. Sagittal reformatted images facilitate detection of subdural and epidural collections along the clivus (see Fig. 20.5) and CCJ.

Is a Computed Tomography Three-Dimensional Bone Model of the Skull Helpful in Cases of Head Trauma?

A three-dimensional (3D) bone model of the infant skull helps the radiologist differentiate sutures, synchondroses (cartilaginous joints present early in life, in a predictable location, and symmetrical in appearance), and anatomic suture variants from skull fractures. A 3D bone model is particularly useful when assessing the occipital region. At birth the occipital bone is composed of seven bony plates that are joined by synchondroses. A synchondrosis in this region can be mistaken for a skull fracture and, similarly, a bone fracture can be mistaken

for a synchondrosis (Fig. 20.17). A fracture through a suture or synchondrosis may be apparent on an axial head CT image as a widened suture or synchondrosis, but this abnormality can be difficult to appreciate in the axial plane and is more readily detected on a 3D bone model of the skull (see Fig. 20.4). Further, a 3D bone model depicts a skull fracture in a manner that is easily recognized and comprehended by laypeople involved in the care of the child (see Figs. 20.3, 20.4, 20.11, 20.15, and 20.17).

It is reasonable to consider generating 3D bone models fo the skull and sagittal and coronal reformatted images on all head CTs in children ≤1 year of age, regardless of the clinical indication. In the absence of a history of trauma, a subtle, linear, nondisplaced fracture may be overlooked. Occasionally the unexpected detection of a skull fracture on head CT is the first instance in which the radiologist is alerted to the possibility of abuse as a potential cause of a child's neurological deficits.

In Cases of Suspected AHT, Should I Recommend Brain Magnetic Resonance Imaging to Follow Computed Tomography of the Head?

Head CT and brain MRI are complementary in assessing children with AHT. The benefits of head CT are: (1) clear and unambiguous identification of acute intracranial blood, (2) more accurate information in regard to the age of blood (e.g., hyperdense blood indicates recent hemorrhage: hours to days old), (3) higher sensitivity for the detection of skull fractures, and (4) the ability to generate a 3D bone model of the skull. MRI offers advantages over head CT, including: (1) increased sensitivity in detecting and characterizing brain injury, such as HII and parenchymal contusions, including cerebral contusional tears; (2) improved ability to estimate the age of parenchymal injury with diffusion-weighted imaging; (3) increased sensitivity for posterior fossa injuries; (4) increased ability to detect membranes within SDHs and injured bridging veins; (5) improved ability to identify RHs; and (6) improved ability to provide prognostic information.

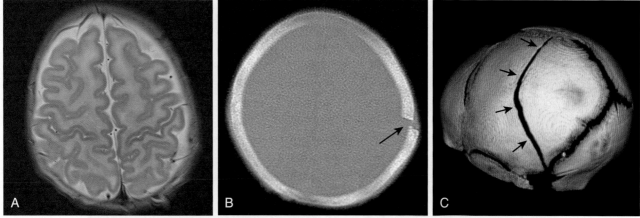

Fig. 20.15 Computed tomography (CT) versus magnetic resonance imaging for the evaluation of skull fracture. Six-week-old ex-34-week premature infant presents to the emergency department (ED) with new-onset seizure. The infant was seen 1 week earlier in the ED for a skull fracture after a fall from the bed onto a carpeted floor. (A) The diastatic left parietal skull is difficult to perceive on the axial T2-weighted image. (B) The axial noncontrast head CT image clearly shows the diastatic left parietal bone fracture at the same level. (C) The three-dimensional model of the skull depicts the vertically oriented diastatic parietal bone fracture clearly.

Fig. 20.16 In-plane skull fracture. Eighth-month-old girl who fell off of a 4-foot-high bed. The child presented to the emergency department with lethargy. (A) Axial noncontrast head computed tomography (CT) image shows right parietal scalp swelling but the right parietal skull fracture, which was oriented in a plane parallel to the angle of the gantry, could not be appreciated. (B) Coronal reformatted noncontrast head CT image clearly shows the nondisplaced linear fracture of the right parietal bone.

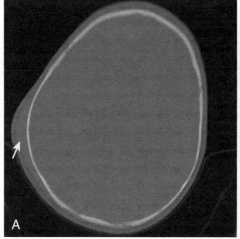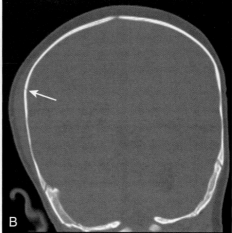

Should I Administer Gadolinium in Cases of Suspected AHT?

The American College of Radiology does not recommend administering gadolinium in cases of suspected AHT. Occasionally, however, the radiologist will have a postcontrast brain MRI available for review, for instance, in a patient with AHT initially suspected of having meningitis or sepsis. If a SDH is present on a contrast-enhanced MRI, an enhancing subdural membrane may be detected.

Is There a Role for Head Ultrasonography in Children With AHT?

Although head CT and MRI are recommended when assessing children with suspected AHT, ultrasound can be used as an adjunct to these imaging modalities and can detect some SDHs, parenchymal abnormalities (e.g., cerebral contusional tears), mass effect, hydrocephalus, superior sagittal sinus thrombosis, and arterial vasospasm. Ultrasound also has clear benefits: it

requires no sedation, can be performed bedside, and, as such, is useful in children ≤6 months of age, particularly in critically ill infants in the intensive care unit who are too unstable for transfer to radiology. Ultrasound is also helpful in the nonacute setting to distinguish a SDH from benign enlargement of the subarachnoid space. Head ultrasound is not usually sensitive for thin convexity and interhemispheric SDHs, which are common findings in AHT and many other intracranial injuries.

Should I Recommend Follow-Up Head Imaging in a Child With Suspected AHT?

More than one head imaging study in the acute phase of a child's hospital admission can be very helpful in gaining a more complete understanding of an intracranial abnormality. If an imaging abnormality evolves in a short period of time, this observation can provide the radiologist with additional insight into the age and nature of a traumatic injury (see Figs. 20.8–20.10). The full

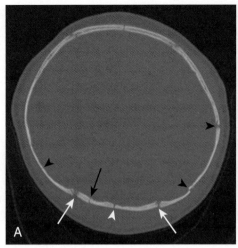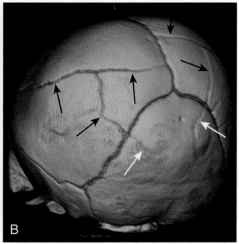

Fig. 20.17 Complex skull fracture. Seven-month-old girl with a prior history of a buttock burn of unknown cause and a fall from her bouncy chair 4 months before admission. The child presented to the emergency department with a change in mental status and a swollen head. She had no retinal hemorrhages and a negative skeletal survey. ^{18}F bone scan showed increased uptake of spinous processes of the lumbar spine, and magnetic resonance imaging showed corresponding bone marrow edema and edema within adjacent paraspinal soft tissues (not shown). (A) Axial noncontrast head computed tomography (CT) image of the skull shows a linear right occipital bone fracture (*black arrow*), which is difficult to distinguish from the lambdoid sutures (*white arrows*) and the midline occipital fissure (*white arrowhead*), a normal anatomic variant. Additional parietal fractures are observed (*black arrowheads*). (B) The three-dimensional model of the head CT allows easier differentiation of occipital fractures (*white arrows*) and parietal fractures (*black arrows*) from calvarial sutures.

extent of damage to the brain is best assessed by MRI at approximately 3 months after hospital discharge.

■ Abusive Spine Trauma

Demographics, Clinical Presentation, and Outcomes

Are Spinal Fractures Common in Cases of Abuse?

Spinal fractures are not common in cases of child abuse. The estimated prevalence of abusive spinal fractures derived from radiographic data is ≤3%, but it is substantially higher (up to approximately 10%) in children with a positive SS. These numbers, however, likely underestimate the true prevalence of spinal fractures in abused children because of the limited sensitivity of radiographs in detecting nondisplaced spinal fractures, minor compression fractures, fractures obscured by summation of anatomic structures, and fractures/injury involving the cartilaginous synchondroses and physes of the developing spine. In practice, clinically occult spinal fractures are occasionally identified in children with negative SSs undergong spine MRI for assessment of other injuries such as spinal ligamentous injury, spinal cord contusion, and intraspinal hematoma, on sagittal reformatted CT images of the chest, abdomen and pelvis obtained for evaluation of visceral injury.

Because of a more systematic approach to spine dissection at autopsy in recent years, as well as the increased use of postmortem imaging, postmortem examinations are showing an increased incidence of spinal injury in abused children.

Why Are Spinal Injuries Often Clinically Silent in Abused Children?

Spinal fractures, subluxations, ligamentous injuries, and spinal cord contusions may go undetected in abused children, as these children are often very young, preverbal, and incapable of vocalizing areas of pain. Moreover, it is challenging for a clinician to perform a detailed neurological examination in a very young child. Because abusive spinal injuries are strongly associated with head trauma, the injured child may be obtunded; also, in cases involving multitrauma, medical attention may be diverted elsewhere to more obvious injuries. In the intensive care unit setting a child may be sedated and intubated with peripheral lines and catheters inserted into the arms, which are secured by arm boards; movement of the extremities may therefore be limited, and spinal cord injury may not be apparent. Because spinal injuries are often clinically occult, it behooves the radiologist to diligently scrutinize imaging studies in search of spinal injury that may have gone undetected on the clinical examination.

What Are the Mechanisms of Injury in Abusive Spinal Trauma?

Mechanisms of injury in abusive spinal trauma include shaking of a child that is held by the torso resulting in hyperflexion and hyperextension of the spine; holding of the child's head and/or neck and swinging or shaking the child's body; intentional, manual, forceful hyperflexion or hyperextension of the spine; throwing the child resulting in impact and loading injury of the spine (with or without a rotational component on impact); and forceful downward placement of a child into a sitting position onto a firm surface such as a dressing table. Knowledge of these mechanisms of injury stems from witnessed accounts of injury, admissions by caretakers, and injury patterns with well-described causal accidental mechanisms.

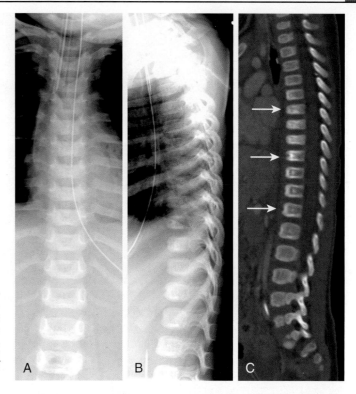

Fig. 20.18 Thoracic vertebral body compression fractures. One-year-old girl with a change in mental status. (A, B) Anteroposterior and lateral radiographic views of the thoracic spine from the skeletal survey. (C) The sagittal reformatted image from the computed tomography examination of the chest, abdomen, and pelvis better depicts the multilevel thoracic vertebral body compression fractures. Note the anterior notched appearance of the compressed vertebral bodies (*white arrows*).

What Are the Clinical Outcomes for Children With Abusive Spinal Injury?

No large systematic studies have examined the clinical outcomes of children who have suffered abusive spinal injury. Data derived from studies of children with accidental spinal injuries similar to children with abusive spinal injury suggest that outcomes vary from little or no long-term morbidity in children with simple compression fractures to significant morbidity or mortality in children with spinal cord contusions and transections and significant dislocations. Unrecognized ongoing spinal instability caused by spinal injury can result in ongoing back pain, spinal deformity, and myelopathy.

Imaging of Abusive Spine Trauma

Which Types of Spinal Injury Are Encountered in Cases of Abuse?

In cases of abuse, spinal fractures, subluxations and dislocations, fracture/separations of synchondroses, physes and apophyses, ligamentous and paraspinal soft tissue injury, spinal cord contusions, cord infarct and transections, spinal cord nerve root injuries and avulsions, and spinal SDHs and EDHs may be encountered.

SPINAL FRACTURES AND FRACTURE-SUBLUXATIONS

WHAT IS THE MOST COMMON TYPE OF SPINAL FRACTURE IN CASES OF ABUSE?. In cases of abuse the most common type of spinal fracture is a simple compression fracture and the most common location is the thoracic spine (Fig. 20.18). The next most common location for a spinal fracture is the lumbar spine

(in particular the upper lumbar spine in conjunction with lower thoracic spine injuries), followed by the sacral spine and the cervical spine. These compression fractures may be multiple and contiguous. However, noncontiguous spinal fractures are also observed. Therefore the entire spinal column should be carefully scrutinized for fracture.

Two main types of spinal compression fractures are seen in cases of abuse: (1) compression fractures of the vertebral body resulting in loss of vertebral body height (these can be symmetric or asymmetric; see Fig. 20.4); and (2) compression fractures of the anterior and superior end plate resulting in a notched, irregular appearance of the affected vertebral body margin (see Fig. 20.18) or a displaced, discrete bone fragment. These types of compression fracture may be single or multiple.

What Other Types of Spinal Fractures Should I Be Looking For?

An unusual but severe type of spinal injury that can be seen in an abused child is a spinal fracture-subluxation. This injury may be clinically occult, give rise to sensory and/or motor deficits with bowel and/or bladder incontinence, or become clinically apparent as a spinal deformity. These fracture-subluxations are typically unstable injuries and occur most commonly at the thoracolumbar junction with two main injury patterns noted: (1) fractures that involve the neurocentral synchondrosis and end plate physes with displacement of the ossified vertebral body centrum either anteriorly or posteriorly (Fig. 20.19); and (2) facet and posterior ligamentous injury with vertebral subluxation, which may or may not be accompanied by vertebral body, facet, and spinous process fractures and end plate physeal injury. Fractures through neurocentral synchondroses and growth plates

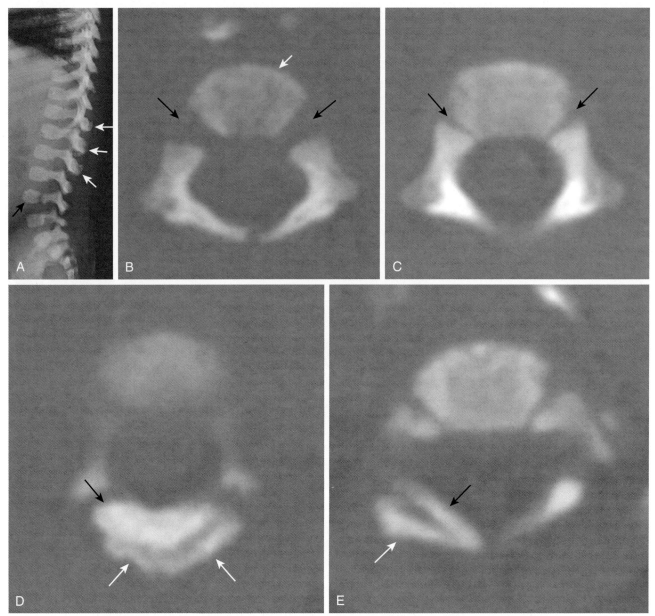

Fig. 20.19 Fracture dislocation, spinous process injury, and myositis ossificans. One-year-old boy admitted with hemorrhagic shock. Computed tomography (CT) scan revealed retroperitoneal and extraperitoneal hemorrhage and a fracture-dislocation of the lumbar spine. The child had been seen previously for a suspected humeral fracture. The skeletal survey revealed additional fractures. The child was neurologically intact. (A) Lateral radiograph of the spine reveals a fracture dislocation (*black arrow*). Healing spinous process fractures of the lower thoracic and upper lumbar spine (*white arrows*) are present. (B) Axial noncontrast CT of the lumbar fracture shows fractures and diastasis of both neurocentral synchondroses (*black arrows*) with anterior dislocation of the vertebral body ossification center (*white arrow*). (C) Axial noncontrast CT of a normal lumbar vertebral body for comparison shows normal-appearing neurocentral synchondroses (*arrows*). (D, E) Axial noncontrast CT shows myositis ossificans (*white arrows*) along the lamina of lower lumbar vertebrae (*black arrows*), providing evidence of prior injury. (Courtesy Timothy Higgins, MD)

without displacement are radiographically occult on SSs and CT. Subtle signs of spinal injury on radiographs include widening of the interpediculate distance, narrowing or widening of the disc space, and subtle loss of the normal spinal alignment. Periosteal thickening can indicate a healing spine fracture.

Less common types of abusive spinal fractures include pedicle fractures (Fig. 20.20), hangman-type fractures, Chance fractures, diastases of the vertebral body and intervertebral disks, and avulsion fractures of the spinous processes.

Are Spinous Process Fractures Detectable on the Skeletal Survey?

Occasionally, spinous process fractures are identified on the SS (see Fig. 20.19). Typically, these fractures are located in the middle and lower thoracic and upper lumbar regions. These injuries are caused by spinal hyperflexion resulting in avulsion of bone and/or the cartilaginous apophyses of the spinous processes where the interspinous and supraspinous ligaments attach. Spinous process fractures either occur in isolation or are associated with vertebral body compression fractures, fracture disloca-

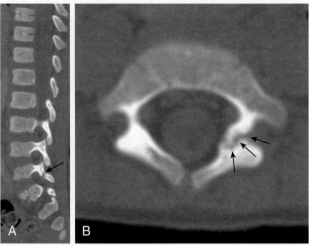

Fig. 20.20 Traumatic spondylolysis. Thirty-two-month-old girl not moving the right extremity after a fall from the couch. Additional imaging showed severe abusive head trauma and thoracic compression fractures (not shown). (A) Sagittal computed tomography (CT) reformat of the lumbar spine shows a chronic-appearing unilateral L5 spondylolysis. (B) Axial noncontrast CT shows the unilateral left L5 pars defect (also see Fig. 20.22).

tions, and paraspinal soft tissue injury. Spinous process fractures can be solitary or multiple, and may be apparent on radiographs if the avulsed bony spinous tip is displaced. On follow-up radiography, a spinous process injury may become apparent if there is new callus formation or ossification of fracture fragments. If the avulsion injury involves only the cartilaginous apophysis of the spinous process, then the injury will be radiographically occult, but it may be detected on MRI or bone scintigraphy.

Spinal Cord and Soft Tissue Injury

What Types of Spinal Cord Injury Are Found in Cases of Abuse?
Cord contusions, lacerations, and transections have been described in postmortem studies of fatal cases of abuse in addition to brainstem injuries, cervical nerve root avulsions, and dorsal root ganglion hemorrhage. Clinical evidence of cord injury in abused children is reported in large clinical series examining children with spinal injury and SCIWORA (spinal cord injury without radiographic abnormality).

Are Soft Tissue and Ligamentous Injuries of the Spine Common in Abused Children?
Injury of the cervical ligamentous complex (Fig. 20.21) is detected in as many as three-quarters of children with AHT when dedicated MRI of the neck is performed. The location of the cervical soft tissue injury supports a hyperflexion/hyperextension injury mechanism of the neck. In addition, cervical ligamentous injury is significantly associated with intracranial HII and extraaxial hemorrhage within the posterior fossa.

What Is the Significance of Myositis Ossificans in Children With Abusive Spine Trauma?
Edema and hemorrhage can be found within the paraspinal musculature of children with abusive spinal injury.

These injuries often resolve without appreciable residua. However, dystrophic calcification, termed *myositis ossificans*, may form in the process of healing. Myositis ossificans is indicative of a prior episode of soft tissue injury that has had sufficient time to calcify (see Fig. 20.19). Occasionally, myositis ossificans is quite large and can be mistaken for a paraspinal tumor, such as a neuroblastoma or ganglioglioma.

Subdural and Epidural Hematomas

ARE SPINAL SUBDURAL AND EPIDURAL HEMATOMAS COMMON IN CASES OF ABUSE?. Spinal SDHs are quite common in children with AHT. These intraspinal hematomas are usually clinically occult and are estimated to occur in more than 60% of children with AHT. In the absence of focal spinal injury, it is likely that these SDHs represent runoff of blood from intracranial SDHs. In children with accidental head injury, spinal SDHs are considered uncommon.

Small spinal EDHs are occasionally observed on MRI and at autopsy. In the thoracic and lumbar regions, these hematomas are usually associated with spinal fractures and localized injury. Small EDHs at the CCJ are usually encountered without a CCJ fracture and are likely related to hyperflexion/hyperextension injury.

Differential Diagnosis

WHICH ALTERNATIVE DIAGNOSES SHOULD I ENTERTAIN WHEN ASSESSING SPINAL FRACTURES IN CASES OF CHILD ABUSE?. The main alternative diagnostic considerations include accidental trauma, normal variants, congenital bony anomalies (e.g., congenital absence of the pedicles, which can simulate a traumatic spondylolysis), congenital spinal kyphosis, bone dysplasias, genetic conditions (e.g., osteogenesis imperfecta), metabolic bone diseases (e.g., Menkes disease), and prior discitis/osteomyelitis.

Imaging Strategies of Abusive Spine Trauma

The first-line imaging modality of choice to screen for occult spinal injury in a potentially abused child is radiography (as part of the SS). CT, MRI, radionuclide bone scintigraphy (technetium 99m-methyl diphospohonate/Tc-99m MDP) and fluorodeoxyglucose/FDG positron emission tomography/ PET scan (^{18}F-NaF) are generally used for problem solving when equivocal findings are observed on the SS, but they are also known to reveal additional, unsuspected spinal injuries. Follow-up SSs are recommended for children with equivocal findings on the initial SS and for those in whom abuse is strongly suspected and the initial SS is negative. Follow-up SSs performed after a short time interval (≥14 days) have been shown to increase the number of identified skeletal fractures by approximately 8% to 25%, in addition to confirming and further characterizing previously suspected fractures.

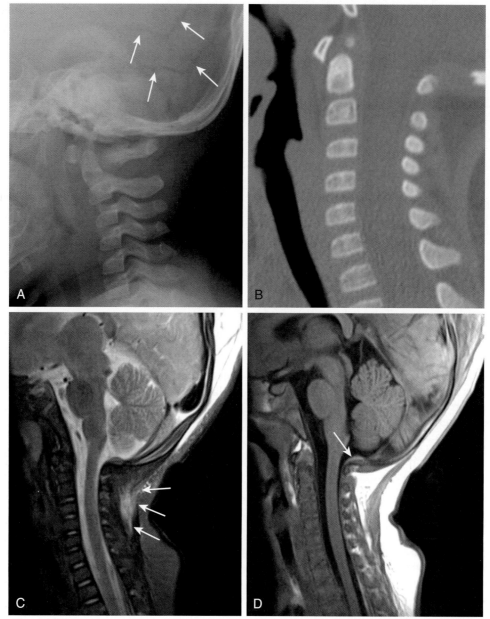

Fig. 20.21 Cervical soft tissue injury. Seven-month-old girl with a change in mental status and scalp swelling. The child had been seen previously for falls and a buttock burn of unknown cause. Additional imaging showed skull fractures and subdural hematomas (SDHs), no retinal hemorrhages, and a negative skeletal survey. ^{18}F bone scan showed increased tracer uptake at L1 and L5 and spinous processes, and magnetic resonance imaging showed marrow edema and paraspinal soft tissue edema at L1 (not shown). (A) Lateral radiograph shows bilateral skull fractures. (B) Sagittal noncontrast computed tomography reformat of the cervical spine was normal. (C) Sagittal T2-weighted image reveals deep cervical soft tissue edema (*arrows*) consistent with soft tissue injury. (D) Sagittal T1-weighted imaging shows a small posterior fossa SDH at the opisthion (*arrow*).

In children with evidence for AHT on head CT and/or brain MRI, additional MRI of the cervical spine should be considered to assess for cervical spine injury, in particular ligamentous injury. Conversely, imaging of the head should be considered in an abused child with a spinal fracture is identified (given the significant correlation between spinal fractures and intracranial injury). Extending spinal imaging beyond the cervical region to include the thoracic and lumbar spine may also identify clinically occult spinal SDHs, bone, and soft tissue inju-

ries. Spinal ultrasound in the youngest of patients may also detect spinal SDHs (Fig. 20.22).

■ Summary

Careful imaging evaluation of a child with abusive head and/or spinal injuries is important for the purposes of diagnosis and treatment, and facilitates the child's discharge from medical care to a safe environment. Many

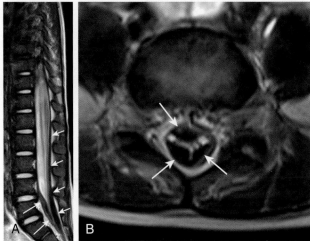

Fig. 20.22 *Spinal subdural hematomas (SDHs).* Same case as in Fig. 20.20. (A) Sagittal T2-weighted image of the lumbar spine shows spinal subdural hematomas (*arrows*), which are dark in signal. (B) Axial T2-weighted image shows that the SDHs are circumferential (*arrows*) and dark in signal.

mulate a safe discharge plan. Finally, it is not uncommon for the radiologist to be the first healthcare provider to recognize a clinically occult traumatic lesion in an abused child who is undergoing diagnostic imaging for nonspecific symptoms. By identifying and fully characterizing abusive head and spinal injuries, the radiologist is in a position to substantially affect the lives of infants and young children at risk.

victims of AHT do not survive, and those who do may suffer significant physical and mental disabilities. The role of the radiologist in the care of these vulnerable children is crucial: first in considering the possibility of abuse as the basis for the imaging and clinical abnormalities; second, in detecting and characterizing the injuries, which are often clinically occult, so that the child may receive appropriate medical treatment; and third, overseeing the appropriate imaging workup and carefully analyzing the imaging studies so that trauma, as the basis of the imaging abnormalities, is either supported or excluded, which in turn allows the care team to for-

Bibliography

Barber, I., Perez-Rossello, J. M., Wilson, C. R., Silvera, M. V., & Kleinman, P. K. (2013). Prevalence and relevance of pediatric spinal fractures in suspected child abuse. *Pediatric Radiology, 43*(11), 1507–1515.

Choudhary, A. K., Servaes, S., Slovis, T. L., Palusci, V. J., Hedlund, G. L., & Narang, S. K. (2018). Consensus statement on abusive head trauma in infants and young children. *Pediatric Radiology, 48*(8), 1048–1065.

Choudhary, A. K., Servaes, S., & Slovis, T. L. (2018). Consensus statement on abusive head trauma in infants and young children. *Pediatrics, 142*, 1048–1065.

Hymel, K. P., Rumack, C. M., Hay, T. C., Strain, J. D., & Jenny, C. (1997). Comparison of intracranial computed tomographic (CT) findings in pediatric abusive and accidental head trauma. *Pediatric Radiology, 27*(9), 743–747.

Jenny, C. (2014). Alternate theories of causation in abusive head trauma: What the science tells us. *Pediatric Radiology, 44*(Suppl. 4), S543–S547.

Jenny, C., Hymel, K. P., Ritzen, A., Reinert, S. E., & Hay, T. C. (1999). Analysis of missed cases of abusive head trauma. *Journal of the American Medical Association, 281*(7), 621–626.

O'Brien, W. T., Sr, Caré, M. M., & Leach, J. L. (2018). Pediatric emergencies: Imaging of pediatric head trauma. *Seminars In Ultrasound CT and MR, 39*(5), 495–514.

Orman, G., Wagner, M. W., Seeburg, D., Zamora, C. A., Oshmyansky, A., & Tekes, A. (2015). Pediatric skull fracture diagnosis: Should 3D CT reconstructions be added as routine imaging? *Journal of Neurosurgery: Pediatrics, 16*(4), 426–431.

Orru, E., Huisman, T. A. G. M., & Izbudak, I. (2018). Prevalence, patterns, and clinical relevance of hypoxic-ischemic injuries in children exposed to abusive head trauma. *Journal of Neuroimaging, 28*(6), 608–614.

Prabhu, S. P., Newton, A. W., Perez-Rossello, J. M., & Kleinman, P. K. (2013). Three-dimensional skull models as a problem-solving tool in suspected child abuse. *Pediatric Radiology, 43*(5), 575–581.

CHAPTER 21

Child Abuse (Radiology)

Alexis B.R. Maddocks, Mesha L.D. Martinez, William P. McCullough, and Sabah Servaes

CHAPTER OUTLINE

Background, 416
Fractures Associated With Child Abuse and Fracture
    Dating, 416
Soft Tissue Injuries in Child Abuse, 418
    American College of Radiology Criteria, 421
Differential Diagnosis of Skeletal Injuries, 422
    Accidental Injuries, 422
    Normal Variants, 422

Birth Trauma, 422
Cardiopulmonary Resuscitation, 423
Rickets, 424
Osteogenesis Imperfecta, 424
Scurvy, 424
Copper Deficiency, 425
Infections, 425
Periostitis and Child Abuse, 425
    Periostitis Differential Diagnoses, 426
Summary, 427

■ Background

Among the first to identify issues related to child abuse, Dr. John Caffey studied and published results in 1946 detailing multiple unexplained long-bone fractures of apparent traumatic origin in infants with chronic subdural hematomas. His work is cited in the landmark 1962 article, "The Battered-Child Syndrome," by Dr. C. Henry Kempe et al. Kempe and colleagues (1962) stated that "the physician's duty and responsibility to the child requires a full evaluation of the problem and a guarantee that the expected repetition of trauma will not be permitted to occur." Within several years of the publication of Kempe et al.'s article, every state in the United States mandated that medical professionals report all suspected cases of child abuse. In 1974, the Child Abuse Prevention and Treatment Act (CAPTA) was signed into law.

CAPTA has been amended several times, most recently by the CAPTA Reauthorization Act of 2019. CAPTA defines child abuse and neglect as "any recent act or failure to act on the part of a parent or caretaker which results in death, serious physical or emotional harm, sexual abuse or exploitation; or an act or failure to act, which presents an imminent risk of serious harm." Child maltreatment encompasses neglect, physical abuse, emotional abuse, and sexual abuse.

In 2019, an estimated 1840 children died as the result of abuse and neglect in the United States. Based on this estimate and population data, the national rate of child fatalities due to abuse and neglect was 2.5 deaths per 100,000 children. The youngest children are at greatest risk: 7% of all child maltreatment fatalities involved children younger than 3 years.

Based on US Child Protective Services (CPS) data, there were 674,000 victims of child abuse and neglect in 2017, equating to a rate of 9 victims per 1000 children in the US population. This number includes only those cases reported to and substantiated by CPS. Many additional cases go unreported. Children in their first year of life are at greatest risk, with a rate of victimization of 25.3 per 1000 children. Of reported cases of child maltreatment, 74.5% involved cases of neglect. Child physical abuse accounted for 18.3% of reports.

A majority of child physical abuse involves cutaneous injuries that never come to imaging. These injuries include bruises, bite marks, and burns. There are patterns of cutaneous injuries, which pediatricians and emergency medicine providers are trained to recognize as suggestive of physical abuse. Abusive head trauma, thoracic and abdominal organ injury, and orthopedic injuries with their associated soft tissue injuries are in the realm of imaging evaluation of child maltreatment. Imaging plays an important role in the diagnosis and follow-up care of these injuries, and it is our duty and responsibility to assist in diagnosing child physical abuse. In a battered child, a missed fracture or an injury misclassified as accidental exposes a child to further abuse and potentially death. This chapter details thoracic, abdominal, and orthopedic injuries of physical abuse. Abusive head trauma is addressed in Chapter 20.

■ Fractures Associated With Child Abuse and Fracture Dating

Any fracture can be the result of abuse, but some fractures are found almost exclusively in abused children.

416

These fractures are known to have a higher specificity for abuse than others and when seen by the radiologist should raise higher suspicion for child abuse in infants and toddlers (Table 21.1). The classic metaphyseal lesion (CML) is the most specific type of fracture one can see with child abuse up to the age of 1 year. This injury is caused by shearing, traction, or twisting (Fig. 21.1). Rib fractures (specifically posterior) have high specificity for child abuse, especially in infants (Fig. 21.2). Other highly specific types of injury that are less commonly seen are scapular fractures, spinous process fractures, and sternal fractures.

Multiple fractures or fractures of different ages are moderately specific for child abuse. Other fractures that have moderate specificity include epiphyseal separations, vertebral body fractures, digital fractures in infants, and complex skull fractures. In these cases the radiologist should always take into account the clinical situation and the patient's age when considering whether to raise concern for child abuse. One example of inappropriate history may be a clinical history that is not commensurate with the patient's developmental stage, such as a 1-month-old who rolled off of a changing table and presents with multiple injuries.

Although common, the fractures with low specificity for child abuse include long-bone fractures, linear skull fractures, clavicle fractures, and isolated subperiosteal new bone formation; however, keep in mind that abused children may have any or all of these fractures. The femur, humerus, and tibia are the most commonly injured long bones in child abuse. Again, the child's age is important in determining whether to raise concern for child abuse. For example, a femoral fracture in a nonambulatory child is more suspicious for abuse than in a child who is ambulatory, where the fracture is more likely to be accidental. Fractures of the humeral shaft in a child younger than 18 months is suspicious for child abuse compared with a supracondylar fracture in an ambulatory child. Linear skull fractures are usually not inflicted as opposed to complex or bilateral skull fractures that are more commonly associated with child abuse.

TABLE 21.1   Specificity of Fractures for Nonaccidental Trauma

SPECIFICITY	FRACTURE
High	Classic metaphyseal lesion (CML)
	Rib fractures
	Scapular fractures
	Sternal fractures
	Spinous process fractures
Moderate	Multiple fractures
	Fractures of different ages
	Epiphyseal separation
	Digital fractures
	Complex skull fractures
	Vertebral body fractures/subluxations
Low	Long-bone fractures
	Clavicle fractures
	Linear skull fractures

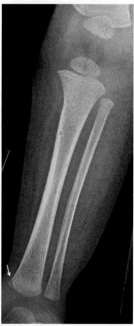

Fig. 21.1 AP radiograph of the tibia in a 5-month-old girl demonstrating a classic metaphyseal lesion along the medial aspect of the distal tibia (*arrow*).

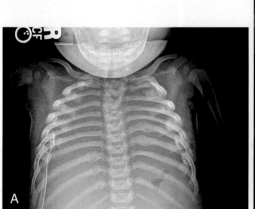
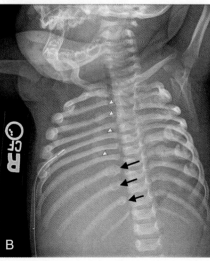

Fig. 21.2 Frontal view of the chest (A) in a 4-month-old girl demonstrates multiple lateral and posterior rib fractures. Postmortem oblique view of the ribs (B) demonstrates the appearance of sternal ossification centers (*arrowheads*), which can mimic callous formation from healing rib fractures (*arrows*) on oblique radiographs.

The important thing to remember is that although some fractures may be more specific for child abuse, we must always think about the possibility of child abuse, especially in children younger than 2 years.

Dating the age of fractures is a common request to the radiologist, and care should be used when attempting to determine the approximate age of fractures. There are phases of fracture healing that can be identified on plain radiographs. These include soft tissue swelling, periosteal reaction, soft callus, hard callus, bridging, and remodeling (Fig. 21.3). Even with these stages of fracture healing, it is still difficult to date a fracture exactly, although the fractures can be lumped into relatively broad time frames. Soft tissue swelling is most associated with acute fractures that are less than 1 week old. Periosteal reaction and soft callus with increasing hard callus and bridging are associated with recent fractures that are 8 to 35 days old. Old fractures (>36 days old) show a combination of periosteal reaction, hard callus, bridging, and remodeling. The more important task for the radiologist may be to determine whether fractures are of different ages rather than to specifically date the fractures. Multiple fractures of different ages indicate a pattern of repetitive trauma that places the child at greater risk for additional injuries and possibly even death.

■ Soft Tissue Injuries in Child Abuse

There are no specific imaging characteristics of soft tissue injury caused by child abuse. Unlike musculoskeletal and neurological findings pathognomonic for child abuse, traumatic radiographic findings of the soft tissues caused by motor vehicle accident or from a child falling on handlebars while bicycling can be identical to intentional injury by a parent, caregiver, or sibling. In addition, children can present with a combination of soft tissue injuries secondary to accidental and nonaccidental mechanisms, confusing the picture. Due to these facts, combined with the knowledge that the radiologist may be the first physician exposed to soft tissue injury caused by child abuse and that we are mandated reporters for intentional trauma, extensive research has been done to help educate radiologists in findings of accidental versus nonaccidental trauma.

Infants less than 1 year of age have the greatest incidence of soft tissue injury caused by child abuse. If a child is younger than 5 years with traumatic soft tissue injury and if the mechanism of injury given by the parent/caregiver does not match the diagnostic findings, abuse must be considered. Research has found accidental trauma causing soft tissue injuries is most often found in older children 7.6 to 10.3 years old. Child abuse that causes soft tissue injuries occurs in younger children, with the average age being 2.5 to 3.7 years. The most common soft tissue injuries associated with child abuse are liver injury, hollow visceral injury (predominately involving the distal duodenum and proximal jejunum), and pancreatic injury. In those scenarios, if there is no reported history of motor vehicle accident, fall onto handle bars while biking, or appropriate high-force blunt trauma history, child abuse should be considered. Suspicious histories that would not be concordant with those injuries include "falling out of bed" or rolling onto a sleeping infant.

As stated, most common injuries are to the liver, duodenum/proximal jejunum, and pancreas (Figs. 21.4–21.7). These injuries are due to lack of coverage by the ribs and fixation of these structures in the epigastric region of the abdomen (e.g., the ligament of Treitz fixates the proximal jejunum). Liver injury associated with child abuse more commonly involves the left lobe than accidental injury; however, abusive or accidental injury can occur in either left or right hepatic lobes. Children who are younger than 5 years and who present with a duodenal injury are most likely to have sustained that injury from abuse with complete transection/perforation being

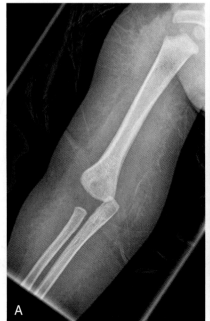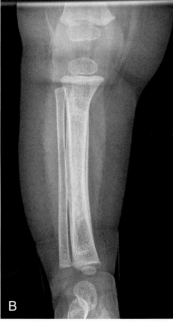

Fig. 21.3 Injuries of different ages in a 10-month-old. AP view of the humerus and elbow (A) demonstrates mild subperiosteal bone formation, as well as significant soft tissue swelling and malalignment of the elbow related to acute epiphyseal separation. AP view of the tibia (B) demonstrtes thick periosteal reaction along both medial and lateral aspects of the tibial shaft consistent with a healing fracture.

rare and duodenal hematomas causing proximal partial obstruction being the most common presentation (see Fig. 21.7). Bowel transections, unless caused by seat belt or bike handlebar injuries, are considered abusive in etiology unless proven otherwise. One-third of pancreatic injuries are nonaccidental, and some researchers claim that if the injury was not caused by motor vehicle accident or bicycle handle bar, then again the etiology is considered to be abuse unless proven otherwise.

Hypoperfusion complex, an entity associated with intracranial injury and severe neurological impairment and/or severe bleeding, can be a consequence of nonaccidental trauma (Fig. 21.8). In hypoperfusion complex, also known as shock abdomen, imaging findings are secondary to severe hypovolemia. Computed tomography (CT) findings include abnormal intense enhancement of the bowel wall, adrenal glands, kidneys, liver, and/or pancreas; decreased caliber of the inferior vena cava and aorta; bowel thickening; and/or dilatation. CT findings may precede clinical ones, making familiarity with this entity critical because the radiologist may be the first person to become aware of a child's tenuous volume status.

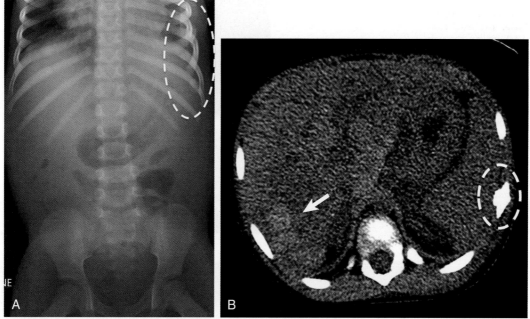

Fig. 21.4 A 4-year-old with abdominal pain. AP radiograph of the abdomen (A) demonstrates left-sided healing rib fractures (*circle*). Noncontrast axial CT image through the abdomen (B) demonstrates a right hepatic hematoma (*arrow*) and one of the healing rib fractures (*circle*). Skeletal survey subsequently performed on the patient's asymptomatic sibling (not shown) also showed healing rib fractures.

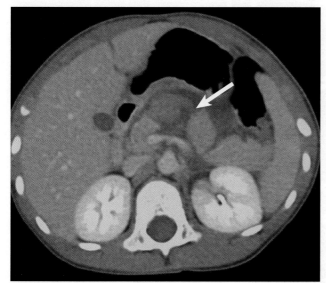

Fig. 21.5 A 4-year-old with abdominal pain and no reported history of trauma. Axial contrast-enhanced CT image through the abdomen shows pancreatic transection (*arrow*) with decreased enhancement in a portion of the pancreas and surrounding peripancreatic edema.

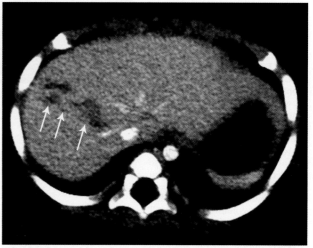

Fig. 21.6 A 5-month-old with multiple fractures (not shown) and elevated liver enzymes. Although suspected abuse patients may have benign abdominal examinations, referring clinicians will often perform laboratory tests to determine whether they need to do abdominal imaging. Axial contrast-enhanced CT image through the abdomen shows a grade III liver laceration in the right hepatic lobe (*arrows*), explaining the abnormal liver function tests in this patient.

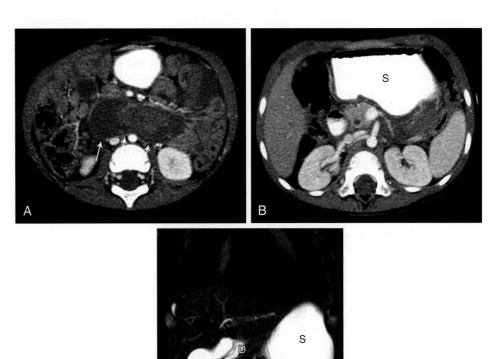

Fig. 21.7 Duodenal hematomas from abuse. Two axial contrast-enhanced CT images through the abdomen (A,B) shows a large duodenal hematoma (*arrows*) causing partial obstruction and distention of the proximal duodenum and stomach (*S*) containing oral contrast (B). Coronal T2-weighted MR image (C) throuugh the abdomen in another patient presenting with sudden-onset bilious emesis shows a submucosal fluid collection (*arrows*) found to a be a duodenal hematoma at surgery. The proximal duodenum (*D*) and stomach (*S*) are distended with fluid. There were multiple metaphyseal fractures on skeletal survey (not shown).

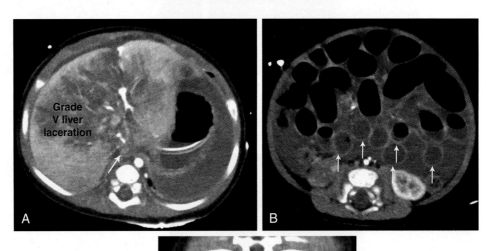

Fig. 21.8 Hypoperfusion complex, also known as shock syndrome. A 3-month-old, with known history of neonatal abstinence syndrome, found unresponsive by a parent and presented in cardiac arrest. Axial contrast-enhanced image through the abdomen (A) shows extensive liver injury. Also note decreased caliber of the inferior vena cava (*arrow*) and large amount of fluid in the left abdomen. Additional axial contast-enhanced CT scan image through the abdomen (B) shows multiple dilated loops of bowel throughout the abdomen with mucosal enhancement (*arrows*) and decreased caliber of aorta. Coronal reformatted contrast-enhanced CT image through the abdomen (C) shows hyperenhancement of the left adrenal gland and left kidney (*arrows*) and decreased contralateral renal/adrenal enhancement. There were posterior right rib fractures (not shown).

Rarer injuries, involving other organs, have been reported in the literature and include pharyngeal injuries and esophageal rupture (i.e., forced feeding or entry of foreign bodies), lung laceration/contusions associated with rib fractures (although these are uncommon findings in child abuse in comparison with accidental trauma because of the different mechanism causing the rib fractures), chylothorax (associated with multiple bone fractures), cardiac lacerations, commotio cordis, chylous ascites, portal venous gas, aortic pseudoaneurysms, adrenal injury (usually right-sided and accompanied by ipsilateral rib fractures and/or visceral injuries), and stomach, colon, and bladder rupture.

Infants, children, and adolescents who present late after sustaining nonaccidental type injuries can present with pseudocysts of the pancreas secondary to prior pancreatic contusion or partial tear, multiple osteolytic lesions in various bones caused by prior pancreatic injury and fat embolism, or focal posttraumatic bowel strictures, again typically seen involving the junction of the duodenum and jejunum, secondary to healed partial mural bowel tears.

Contrast-enhanced CT of the abdomen and pelvis is the gold standard whenever soft tissue injury caused by child abuse is suspected. No oral contrast is needed in the emergent setting, and a routine single-phase abdomen and pelvis protocol will suffice. The alliance for radiation safety for pediatric imaging dictates a low-dose radiation protocol for all pediatric patients. If a delayed phase must be acquired to rule out injury to the renal collecting system, consideration to decrease radiation is recommended. Focused assessment with sonography is not recommended because of its limited sensitivity of 50%. Although focused assessment with sonography is easily performed and widely available, positive findings require CT for further investigation to exclude more subtle injuries, while negative findings do not rule out injury. A routine complete abdominal ultrasound is suggested in patients younger than 2 years who are suspected of being abused but with low probability of internal soft tissue injury. For equivocal findings of bowel injury on CT or ultrasound, upper gastrointestinal series can help exclude intramural hematomas involving bowel caused by partial thickness tears and subserosal bleeding. Radiographs, often obtained on initial assessment, are often used to assess for free air or bowel obstruction (the latter can be associated with duodenal or other intramural hematoma of bowel). However, it is important to remember that free air from perforation of retroperitoneal structures (e.g., duodenum) may not show up on radiographs. Significant traumatic injury (i.e., multivisceral) without appropriate history should heighten the radiologist's suspicion.

American College of Radiology Criteria

The American College of Radiology Appropriateness Criteria are helpful in guiding clinicians and radiologists as to what imaging tests are appropriate given the history and physical examination. Sometimes the diagnosis of child abuse is clear based on the history and physical examination. In these cases, imaging may be used for documentation and for legal purposes. However, some cases are less straightforward, and imaging can be used

for detection of injuries. Radiologists must always consider the possibility of metabolic and genetic conditions when interpreting these studies, as described later in this chapter, although children with metabolic and genetic conditions are not exempt from abuse.

A radiographic skeletal survey is the first imaging test ordered for detection of fractures in a child younger than 2 years where there is a suspicion of possible child abuse. The skeletal survey should include frontal and lateral views of the skull, lateral views of the cervical and thoracolumbar spine, and single frontal views of all of the long bones separately using high-resolution including single frontal images of the hands and feet as well as single views of the chest and abdomen. Combining body parts on one image is not acceptable, as the large field of view and lack of attention/centering on each bone may reduce sensitivity. Oblique views of the ribs are also helpful in diagnosing rib fractures that are a strong indication of child abuse (see Fig. 21.2B). Skeletal surveys are less commonly performed in children older than 2 years; however, they are performed when the clinical findings suggest abuse or when there is a need to document the presence or absence of skeletal injuries. Skeletal survey should be performed in any child who has unexplained head or abdominal injuries that are suspicious for child abuse. Siblings of abused children are also at risk and should also be worked up for abusive injury.

Repeat skeletal surveys may be obtained 2 weeks after the initial survey in cases where the first skeletal survey was equivocal, abnormal, or in cases where abuse is still suspected based on the clinical assessment despite a normal initial skeletal survey. These repeat surveys often detect additional new or healing fractures, as well as confirm fractures of differing ages. The follow-up studies contain all of the same radiographic views as the initial study, omitting repeat imaging of the skull, pelvis, and spine (if no prior injury was seen in those areas) to reduce radiation exposure. Bone scintigraphy can be used (albeit rarely) as a complementary examination in cases where the skeletal survey is negative but clinical suspicion remains high. One may also consider the use of whole-body or focused MRI with Short Tau Inversion Recovery (STIR) imaging to identify injuries related to child abuse, for example, in the case of epiphyseal separation (Fig. 21.9). The usefulness of this technique needs to be weighed against the risks of sedation in the infants and toddlers who are the most at risk for child abuse. Ultrasound may also be a helpful technique, especially in young children where epiphyseal separation is suspected.

If the skeletal survey reveals multiple fractures or rib fractures in a child younger than 2 years or if the child is younger than 6 months, a CT of the brain without contrast should be obtained regardless of neurological symptoms because these patients may have abusive head trauma without clinical symptomatology.

In a child with suspected visceral or vascular injuries to the chest, abdomen, or pelvis secondary to child abuse regardless of age, a CT scan with IV contrast is highly recommended. This allows the radiologist to evaluate for vascular and solid organ injuries. It also allows for better visualization of fractures (particularly rib fractures) compared with the plain radiographs.

■ Differential Diagnosis of Skeletal Injuries

The differential diagnosis for skeletal injuries that result from physical abuse is broad and includes accidental injuries, birth trauma, normal variants, metabolic diseases of bone, skeletal dysplasia, and infection. A brief discussion of the more important differential considerations follows.

Accidental Injuries

Fractures are common injuries of childhood. As detailed earlier, certain fractures and fracture patterns are highly suggestive of physical abuse. Pediatric fractures that are not highly specific for abuse may be either accidental or the result of child maltreatment. It is incumbent on

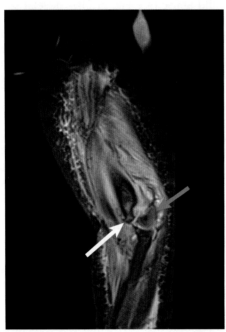

Fig. 21.9 Sagittal Short Tau Inversion Recovery (STIR) magnetic resonance image demonstrating physeal separation injury at the distal humerus in a 10-month-old boy. The nonossified capitellum (*red arrow*) is separated from the distal humeral metaphysis (*white arrow*) but remains aligned with the proximal radius.

the clinicians caring for children with fractures to ensure that the history of trauma and mechanism of injury adequately explain every fracture. This is of particular importance in infants and toddlers. The younger a patient with a fracture is, the more likely that fracture is the result of child maltreatment. In one study of children hospitalized with fractures, nearly 25% of the fractures in children younger than 12 months were attributed to abuse (Fig. 21.10).

Normal Variants

The CML is characteristic of child abuse. There are normal variants of the developing metaphysis, however, that can be confused with the CML. Kleinman et al. (1991) detailed four specific variants of the infant metaphysis in their 1991 paper. A metaphyseal beak is a medial projection off of the proximal humerus and tibia, and bilateral in 77% of cases in the Kleinman series (Fig. 21.11A). The authors describe the metaphyseal step-off as an acute angulation of nearly 90 degrees at the extreme edge of the metaphysis (see Fig. 21.11B). This finding was bilateral in 41% of patients in their series. The metaphyseal spur is a longitudinal projection, extending beyond the margin of the metaphysis, contiguous with the cortex of the metaphysis. The proximal tibial cortical irregularity, seen only at the medial aspect of the proximal tibial metaphysis, has the appearance of focal periosteal new bone formation. The spur and proximal tibial metaphyseal irregularity were bilateral in 25% of the Kleinman series (see Fig. 21.11).

Birth Trauma

Birth-related fractures are common, with the clavicle most frequently injured. These injuries occur in infants delivered both vaginally and via caesarian section. Long-bone fractures, classically associated with vaginal delivery of breech presentation, are now seen with increasing frequency in caesarian breech deliveries because planned caesarian delivery has been shown to reduce perinatal and infant mortality in breech pregnancies, and this method of delivery is now preferred in those

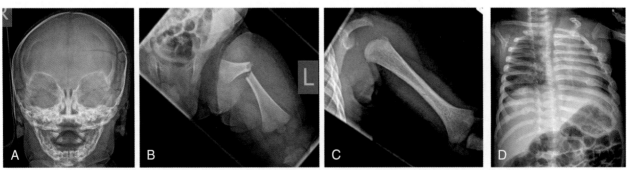

Fig. 21.10 Abusive fractures in three infants. AP radiograph of the skull (A) in a 7-month-old showing a left parietal skull fracture. Frog leg radiograph of the left femur (B) in the same patient demonstrates a transverse, angulated fracture of the proximal femur. (C) AP view of the left humerus (C) in a 2-month-old showing a left proximal humeral metaphyseal corner fracture. Oblique rib radiograph (D) in a 5-month-old showing multiple posterior and lateral rib fractures. All of these fractures were from abuse.

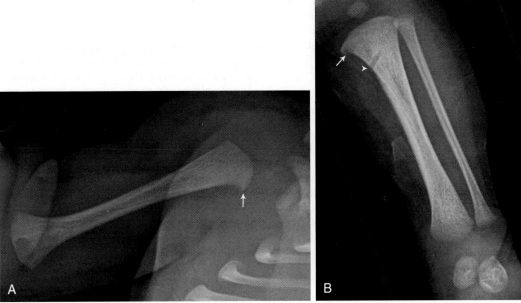

Fig. 21.11 Normal variants. A 3-week-old infant presented to an outside pediatrician in respiratory distress that progressed to respiratory failure and cardiac arrest. The infant was resuscitated in the field. AP radiograph of the right humerus (A) shows a proximal humerus metaphyseal beak (*arrow*). AP radiograph of the left tibia (B) shows a proximal tibial metaphyseal step-off (*arrow*). Note the needle tract from an intraosseous needle in the proximal left tibia (arrowhead).

cases (Fig. 21.12). Fractures secondary to caesarian delivery are, however, still uncommon. In one series, only two fractures were identified in 425 infants after difficult caesarian delivery for breech presentation. Posterior rib fractures have been described in birth-related trauma of very large infants after difficult vaginal deliveries. O'Connell and Donoghue (2007) described three neonates who were found to have CMLs after routine uncomplicated caesarian delivery. Birth-related spine, skull, mandibular, and epiphyseal injuries have also been reported. When discovered before discharge after delivery, these injuries are easily associated with birth trauma. Discovery of these injuries later in the neonatal period becomes more complicated, but in many cases a history of difficult delivery can help distinguish birth trauma from child maltreatment.

Cardiopulmonary Resuscitation

In a review published in 2006, Maguire et al. found that rib fractures associated with cardiopulmonary resuscitation (CPR) were rare and, when present, involved the anterior ribs. In 2000, the American Heart Association changed the recommended technique in two-rescuer newborn and infant CPR from a two-finger technique to a two-thumb technique with the hands encircling the chest. All but one of the studies included in the Maguire analysis were performed before 2000. In a large postmortem cohort, Reyes et al. (2011) found CPR-related anterior and lateral rib fractures in 3.3% of patients, many of which were not evident on postmortem radiographs. They found no posterior rib fractures. The rate of CPR-related rib fractures significantly increased from 1.2% before to 7.9% after their hospital

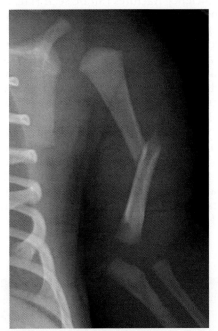

Fig. 21.12 Birth trauma. AP radiograph of the left humerus showing a displaced, angulated left humerus fracture in term newborn delivered by an elective repeat caesarian section.

adopted the encircling hands two-thumb technique. There is one report in the literature of posterior rib fractures in four infants who received CPR before death. A recently published study was designed to identify CPR-related rib fractures in infants who received CPR after the CPR guidelines were changed. This study reviewed all radiographs performed in 80 infants who received CPR. A total of 546 radiographs were reviewed, averaging seven radiographs per infant. In 39 patients (49%), at least one radiograph performed at least 10 days after CPR was available for review. No rib fractures were identified. These studies show that rib fractures related to CPR are uncommon and usually anterior and lateral. Posterior rib fractures remain highly suggestive of physical abuse.

Rickets

Rickets is a clinical disease of impaired ossification and mineralization of growth plates in children. In most cases, rickets is caused by vitamin D deficiency. Vitamin D can be absorbed from the diet or synthesized in the skin. Dark-complexion, breast-fed infants/children are at greatest risk. Breast milk contains only 20% to 30% of the concentration of maternal vitamin D, and dark-complected children require 5 to 10 times more sun exposure than fairer-skinned children for equivalent vitamin D production. Radiographic findings of rickets include widening of the growth plate, reduced mineralization of the zone of provisional calcification, fraying of the metaphyses, and metaphyseal cupping (Fig. 21.13). In the diaphysis, subperiosteal resorption, cortical thinning, intracortical tunneling, endosteal resorption, periosteal new bone formation, bowing, and insufficiency fractures can be seen (Fig. 21.14). In evaluating fractures in infants and children with rickets, one must consider that children with rickets can be subject to physical abuse (Fig. 21.15). Any fracture in a nonambulatory infant must be suspect, and there should always be remembrance that children with rickets could also be victims of abuse. In one study of 45 infants and toddlers with rickets, fractures were identified in 17.5% and were seen only in those who were ambulatory. These fractures did not resemble those highly suggestive of physical abuse, and fractures were observed only in those patients with severe rickets and obvious rachitic changes on radiography. Many diseases that result in impaired calcium or phosphorus homeostasis can cause bone disease similar to rickets (Fig. 21.16).

Osteogenesis Imperfecta

Osteogenesis imperfecta (OI) is a heterogeneous group of connective tissue diseases characterized by increased bone fragility, blue sclera, and joint hyperlaxity. The prevalence of OI is 1 in 12,000 to 15,000 children. Ninety percent of cases are autosomal dominant, although many present as new mutations in children with no family history of the disease. There are multiple types of autosomal dominant OI ranging in severity for the mild, nondeforming Sillence type I disease to the lethal Sillence type II disease seen in infants who are born with multiple fractures. Rib fractures can be seen in the more severe forms of OI. Classic metaphyseal lesions have never been described in OI. OI can, however, present in infancy with unexplained long-bone fractures in nonambulatory infants (Fig. 21.17). The diagnosis of OI is often suggested by a family history of fractures or clinical findings, such as blue sclera. When such history and physical findings are absent, these infants are likely to be evaluated for nonaccidental trauma. Genetic testing can help confirm the diagnosis but requires genetic sequencing of peripheral blood or cultured fibroblasts and can be complicated because more than 1500 dominant mutations have been identified to date. Bone biopsy can also be helpful in making the diagnosis in difficult cases.

Scurvy

Scurvy is caused by deficiency of vitamin C, which is important in collagen production. Scurvy is a rare disease today, but it can result in metaphyseal corner fractures similar to the CML. Additional radiographic

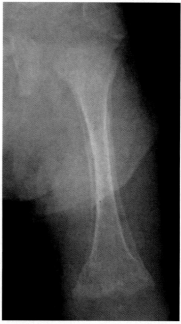

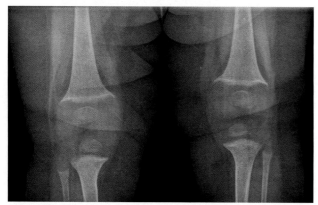

Fig. 21.13 Rickets metaphyseal findings. AP radiographs of both knees in a 9-month-old with rickets shows widening of the growth plate, reduced mineralization of the zone of provisional calcification, metaphyseal fraying, and metaphyseal cupping.

Fig. 21.14 Rickets diaphyseal findings. AP radiograph of the left femur demonstrating osteopenia, cortical thinning, and periosteal new bone formation in a 4-month-old with severe rickets.

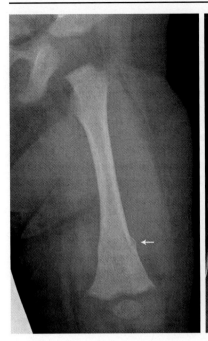
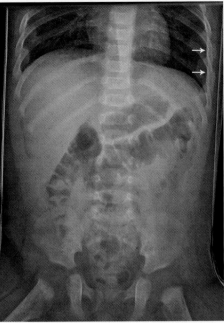

Fig. 21.15 Rickets with fractures. (A) Healing. This 9-month-old sustained a femur fracture when her 2-year-old sister attempted to pull her out of her crib, through the bars. AP radiograph of the left femur (A) shows a distal left femoral metadiaphysis buckle fracture (*arrow*). There is lack of ossification of the proximal femoral epiphyses, which are normally beginning ossification by 6 months. Subtle findings of decreased bone density should be identified. AP radiograph of the abdomen (B) shows healing lateral left sixth and seventh ribs fracture with callus.

findings in scurvy include ground-glass appearance of the long bones caused by trabecular atrophy, periosteal elevations secondary to subperiosteal hemorrhages (Fig. 21.18), dense zones of provisional calcification, and metaphyseal lucent lines. Clinically these patients have anemia, bleeding, and bruising. Widely distributed osseous changes and a dietary history revealing a restrictive diet should facilitate the correct diagnosis, distinguishing scurvy from child maltreatment.

Copper Deficiency

Copper is important in the development of cartilage. Copper deficiency is rare but can be complicated by fractures. Radiological findings in copper deficiency include metaphyseal cupping and fraying, metaphyseal spurs, osteopenia, and subperiosteal new bone formation. Menkes disease is a rare X-linked recessive disorder of copper metabolism, usually diagnosed clinically in infants. Classic radiographic findings include metaphyseal fractures, long-bone diaphyseal fractures, and lambdoid intersutural bones (wormian bones). Like scurvy, copper deficiency results in widespread osseous abnormalities distinguishing these diseases from child abuse.

Infections

Osteomyelitis preferentially involves the metaphyses resulting in mixed sclerotic and lytic lesions potentially resembling CMLs (Fig. 21.19). Radiographic findings in congenital syphilis include the classic Wimberger sign of bony destruction affecting the medial metaphysis of the tibia, metaphyseal destructive lesions involving other bones, and periosteal reaction affecting the diaphyses of long bones.

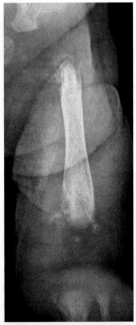

Fig. 21.16 Metaphysis changes in familial hypocalciuric hypercalcemia. AP radiograph of the left femur demonstrating demineralization with subperiosteal bone resorption, coarsened trabecular pattern, and poor ossification with islands of unossified cartilage in a 1-week-old with familial hypocalciuric hypercalcemia.

■ Periostitis and Child Abuse

Periostitis (inflammation of the periosteum of bone) leads to new bone formation or periosteal reaction that can be observed on radiographs, CT, and MRI and may be a subtle to obvious indicator of child abuse. Periosteal reaction associated with pathognomonic fractures of child abuse or involving multiple fractured bones with varying ages of healing should indicate to the radiologist that the source of injury is nonaccidental.

However, periostitis/periosteal bone formation alone is not pathognomonic for child abuse, and in cases where no obvious fracture is seen, knowing the patient's demographics and clinical history and through pattern recognition, one can deduce what the cause may be.

Periostitis Differential Diagnoses

There are three main categories of periosteal reaction without associated fracture: (1) diffuse/near diffuse (Fig. 21.20), (2) focal (Fig. 21.21), and (3) multifocal (Fig. 21.22).

For periosteal reaction involving most or all visualized bones, systemic processes must be considered.

In the newborn infant, diagnostic considerations include physiological periosteal bone formation (~6 weeks to 6 months) and iatrogenic causes (e.g., administration of prostaglandin in infants with congenital heart disease~ whose survival is dependent on the ductus arteriosus staying open). In older infants and children, differential diagnoses include rickets, a neoplastic process (leukemia and metastatic neuroblastoma), and rare disorders such as vitamin C deficiency (scurvy), copper deficiency (Menkes kinky hair syndrome), iatrogenic (interleukin-11), hypervitaminosis A and D, Caffey disease, and congenital syphilis.

Focal periosteal reaction involving a single bone without a visualized fracture can be a manifestation of a healing occult fracture, osteomyelitis, primary

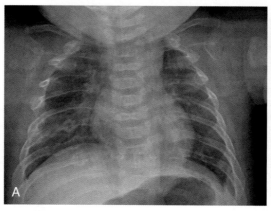
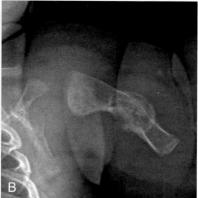

Fig. 21.17 Osteogenesis imperfecta. AP radiograph of the chest (A) showing multiple right posterior rib fractures in a 3-month-old infant with osteogenesis imperfecta. AP radiograph of the left humerus (B) showing a healing mid-humeral fracture in the same patient at 4 months of age. Note diffusely demineralized bones.

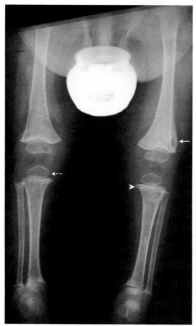

Fig. 21.18 Subperiosteal hemorrhage (*white arrow* seen best at the left distal femoral metaphysis) and dense zones of provisional calcification (*arrowhead*) seen best at left proximal tibial metaphysis in this child with scurvy.

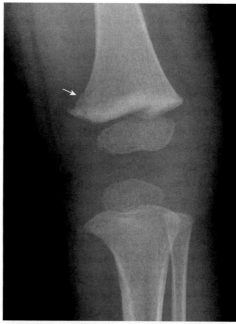

Fig. 21.19 Osteomyelitis. AP radiograph of the knee showing a lucency involving the medial distal femoral metaphysis (*arrow*) in a 19-month-old with osteomyelitis, which could easily be mistaken for a fracture.

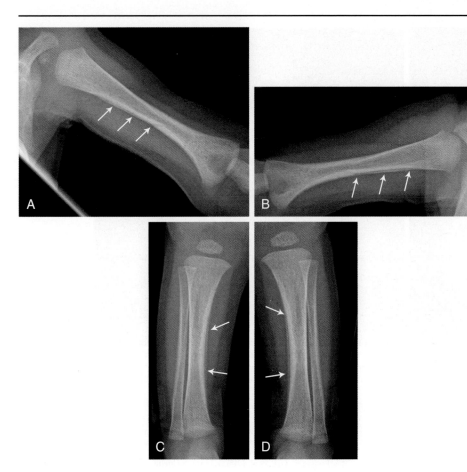

Fig. 21.20 Diffuse/near-diffuse periosteal reaction pattern, typically reflecting a systemic process. AP view of the humeri (A, B) and AP view of the tibiae (C, D) in a 1-month old with diffuse thin periosteal bone formation, nearly symmetrical, along the bilateral humeri and tibias (*arrows*) and noted to involve all long bones on postmortem skeletal survey to rule out nonaccidental trauma. No acute or healing fractures were found.

bone lesion, or focal bone involvement of systemic disease.

For multifocal pattern without fracture(s), focal areas of periosteal reaction involving multiple bones, differential diagnosis includes multisite disease processes, including infectious osteomyelitis, chronic noninfectious osteomyelitis, leukemic osseous involvement, and metastatic neuroblastoma.

All in all, periosteal reaction as the only finding has low specificity for predicting child abuse.

■ Summary

Child abuse is an important topic that all radiologists and pediatric caregivers should be acutely aware of. Abusive injury should always be considered when looking at fractures or soft tissue injuries where the clinical history does not match the visualized injury/injuries. Radiologists should know the fractures that are highly specific for child abuse and raise awareness to the referring clinician when necessary. The appropriate performance of these radiological examinations and documentation of any suspicious findings are important in protecting these children, as well as for any possible future legal proceedings. Awareness of the differential diagnoses for abusive trauma is also important, to raise concern for alternative diagnoses when appropriate.

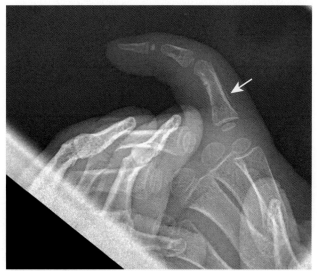

Fig. 21.21 Focal periosteal reaction, often representing a subacute distinct process causing inflammatory, reparative process, such as a fracture, an infection, or a focal site of systemic disease. Lateral radiograph of the fifth digit in a 3-year-old with pain and swelling of the fifth digit demonstrates periosteal reaction (*arrow*) in a patient with focal osteomyelitis.

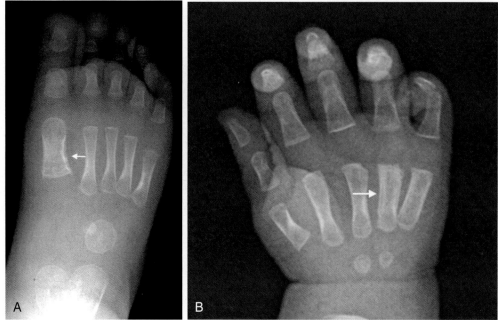

Fig. 21.22 Multifocal areas of periosteal reaction involving multiple bones. A 2-month-old presenting with right foot and hand swelling. AP radiograph of the right foot (A) showing periosteal reaction involving the first metatarsal. AP radiograph of the right hand (B) showing periosteal reaction involving the fourth metacarpal. This patient was diagnosed with multfocal infectious osteomyelitis in the setting of chronic granulomatous disease.

Bibliography

Adams, P. C., et al. (1974). Kinky hair syndrome: Serial study of radiological findings with emphasis on the similarity to the battered child syndrome 1. *Radiology, 112*(2), 401–407.

Amador, E., et al. (2010). Long-term skeletal findings in Menkes disease. *Pediatric Radiology, 40*(8), 1426–1429.

American Heart Association in collaboration with the International Liaison Committee on Resuscitation (AHA). (2000). Guidelines 2000 for cardiopulmonary resuscitation and emergency cardiovascular care. Part 11: Neonatal resuscitation. *Circulation, 102*, 343–357.

Armangil, D., et al. (2009). Early congenital syphilis with isolated bone involvement: A case report. *Turkish Journal of Pediatrics, 51*(2), 169–171.

Clouse, J. R., & Lantz, P. E. (2008). Posterior rib fractures in infants associated with cardiopulmonary resuscitation. In *American Academy of Forensic Science (Ed.), Proceedings of the American Academy of Forensic Science 60th annual meeting* (pp. 254–255).

Darling, S. E., et al. (2014). Frequency of intrathoracic injuries in children younger than 3 years with rib fractures. *Pediatric Radiology, 44*(10), 1230–1236.

Hilmes, M. A., et al. (2011). CT identification of abdominal injuries in abused pre-school-age children. *Pediatric Radiology, 41*(5), 643–651.

Kempe, C. H., Silverman, F. N., Steele, B. F., et al. (1962). The battered-child syndrome. *Journal of the American Medical Association, 181*(1), 17–24.

Kleinman, P. K., Belanger, P. L., Karellas, A., & Spevak, M. R. (1991). Normal metaphyseal radiologic variants not to be confused with findings of infant abuse. *American Journal of Roentgenology, 156*(4), 781–783.

Kwon, D. S., et al. (2002). Physiologic subperiosteal new bone formation: Prevalence, distribution, and thickness in neonates and infants. *American Journal of Roentgenology, 179*(4), 985–988.

Lonergan, G. J., et al. (2003). From the archives of the AFIP: Child abuse: Radiologic-pathologic correlation 1. *RadioGraphics, 23*(4), 811–845.

Maguire, S. A., et al. (2013). A systematic review of abusive visceral injuries in childhood—their range and recognition. *Child Abuse & Neglect, 37*(7), 430–445.

Nimkin, K., et al. (1994). Adrenal hemorrhage in abused children: Imaging and postmortem findings. *American Journal of Roentgenology, 162*(3), 661–663.

O'Connell, A., & Donoghue, V. B. (2007). Can classic metaphyseal lesions follow uncomplicated caesarean section? *Pediatric Radiology, 37*(5), 488–491.

Offiah, A., et al. (2009). Skeletal imaging of child abuse (non-accidental injury). *Pediatric Radiology, 39*(5), 461–470.

Raissaki, M., et al. (2011). Abdominal imaging in child abuse. *Pediatric Radiology, 41*(1), 4–16.

Reyes, J. A., Somers, G. R., Taylor, G. P., & Chiasson, D. A. (2011). Increased incidence of CPR-related rib fractures in infants—is it related to changes in CPR technique? *Resuscitation, 82*(5), 545–548.

Servaes, S., & Haller, J. O. (2003). Characteristic pancreatic injuries secondary to child abuse. *Emergency Radiology, 10*(2), 90–93.

Sheybani, E. F., et al. (2014). Pediatric nonaccidental abdominal trauma: What the radiologist should know. *RadioGraphics, 34*(1), 139–153.

Soundappan, S. V. S., Albert, H., Lam, & Daniel, T. C. (2006). Traumatic adrenal haemorrhage in children. *ANZ Journal of Surgery, 76*(8), 729–731.

CHAPTER 22

Dose Optimization and Risk Management in Pediatric CT

Robert D. MacDougall, Matthew M. Jones, Shreya Mozer, and Michael J. Callahan

CHAPTER OUTLINE

Basics of Radiobiology and Risks of Ionizing Radiation, 430
How Does Radiation Damage the Cell?, 430
Why Is Radiation a Greater Concern in Children Than in Adults?, 430
What Evidence Is There to Support Carcinogenic Effects Associated With Ionizing Radiation?, 430
Fundamentals of CT Dosimetry, 431
What Is the Radiation Dose for a CT Scan?, 431
CT Dose Index, 431
Dose Length Product, 432
Size-Specific Dose Estimate, 432
Effective Dose, 433
Dose and Image Quality Targets, 433
What Is an Appropriate CT Dose?, 433
CT Protocol Design, 434
How Can I Create Pediatric CT Protocols?, 434
Advanced Topics, 436
What Is Tube Current (mA) and Rotation Time (mS), and How Do They Affect Patient Dose?, 436
What Is Kilovolt Peak, and How Does It Affect the Patient Dose?, 436
What Are Acceptable Kilovoltage Ranges for Imaging of Children?, 437
What Is Pitch, and How Does It Affect the Patient Dose?, 437
What Are the Advantages of Higher Pitch?, 437
Automatic Exposure Control, 438
What Is Iterative Reconstruction, and How Does It Compare With Filtered Backprojection?, 438
Communicating Risk, 439
How Should I Communicate the Risk and Benefits to a Parent or Patient?, 439
What Challenges Will I Face in Discussing Radiation Risks With Patients?, 439
How Should I Discuss Dose?, 439
How Should I Discuss Risk?, 440
Summary, 440

The radiologist's most obvious "product" is the interpretation rendered for an imaging study. Although this visible document is a key component of the radiologist's job, it is only one of many responsibilities under the modern radiologist's purview. Many radiologists also oversee departmental practice functions, including, but not limited to, licensing and certification requirements, regulatory compliance, quality improvement, patient and staff safety, equipment purchasing and maintenance, patient scheduling, technologist training, study optimization, communication of results, and billing. Foremost among these responsibilities is ensuring patient safety. Since the early 2010s, regulatory agencies and national societies have placed a new focus on a poorly understood but critical component of patient safety: radiation dose awareness and optimization.

Radiation biology, or radiobiology, is a field that examines the interaction of ionizing radiation on living things down to their DNA. It is constantly evolving and continues to offer new perspectives into the effects of radiation within living cells. The study of past radiation events can offer insight into the long-term carcinogenic risks of ionizing radiation. However, to achieve these goals, a study population must be extremely large to offer an accurate risk estimate because of a multitude of uncontrolled geographical and environmental variables, in addition to the challenges posed by a very small absolute cancer risk at low levels of radiation.

The most widely cited estimates of cancer risk come from long-term studies of atomic bomb survivors. These data have been parsed in numerous ways, most visibly in the Biological Effects of Ionizing Radiation (BEIR) VII report (2006). More recent retrospective cohort studies in patients actually exposed to medical radiation have supported the conclusion that medical radiation is indeed a risk factor for secondary malignancies, although the methods used in these studies are controversial. For example, in a *Lancet* article published by Pearce et al. in 2012, the authors note an increased risk for brain cancer and leukemia for children undergoing head computed tomography (CT). However, the estimated radiation doses in this study were taken from national surveys and not from individual patients. Second, because the absolute risk for development of these cancers is extremely small to begin with, any increase (albeit small and uncertain) will result in a relatively large excess risk.

As a matter of practicality, most radiologists and medical physicists have come to accept a linear no-threshold (LNT) model for radiation dose and stochastic effects, such as the development of secondary malignancies. Although some may argue with to what degree the effects exist, there is near-universal agreement that the prudent approach is to reduce radiation dose when possible, particularly in children.

It is important to understand that there are many limitations to our current understanding of risk associated with medical imaging. If an "estimate" of radiation risk is discussed in such a way that causes alarm to a patient or parent, this creates a real risk if that clinically indicated examination is then delayed or refused. It is imperative to explain the medical need for the examination, along with the speculative and unknown risk for ionizing radiation.

Because of the rapidly dividing nature of children's cells and their proportionally longer life span, a child's risk for secondary malignancy is thought to be even greater than adults. Although the risks remain small overall, they must be constantly and meticulously weighed against the diagnostic yield of imaging studies that do, and do not, require the use of ionizing radiation. When the risks are gauged and justify a radiation-based imaging study, the radiologist must remember the ethical imperative codified in the Hippocratic Oath to "first, do no harm." That is, the radiologist in collaboration with a technologist and medical physicist must optimize the ordered imaging study such that the lowest radiation dose possible is used to answer the clinical question. This is especially true in children. This mantra is championed by the *Image Gently®* campaign, founded by the American College of Radiology, the Society for Pediatric Radiology, the American Association of Physicists in Medicine, and the American Society of Radiologic Technologists. The Image Gently campaign has succeeded in raising awareness in the radiology community of the potential risks of ionizing radiation. In this chapter, we will offer an overview of basic principles related to CT and radiation risk, along with practical steps that the radiologist can use to improve the safety and consistency of medical imaging.

■ Basics of Radiobiology and Risks of Ionizing Radiation

How Does Radiation Damage the Cell?

Radiation damage occurs at a cellular level. At energies in the diagnostic range (10–150 keV), radiation interacts with matter in two fundamental ways: via Compton scatter and the photoelectric effect. In both cases the result is the production of a free electron. Although injury to cellular components may occur by direct injury from the incident photon/electron, the vast majority of the initial energy will be conferred to other electrons via an exponential cascade of ionization and excitation; hence

the phrase *ionizing* radiation. The end result of this cascade is the disruption of ionic bonds and the formation of free radicals, which are the dominant mechanism by which cellular components are ultimately damaged. The most important cellular component damaged in this fashion is DNA, which is required for the replication and survival of the cell and, if damaged, can lead to genetic mutations. Cells can repair DNA damage, but only to a certain point—at a certain threshold level, damage may be irreversible. Deterministic (nonstochastic) effects such as radiation burns and skin necrosis occur when a sufficient dose has been delivered to result in cell death. Stochastic (or probabilistic) effects such as induction of malignancy occur when DNA damage is sufficiently severe to alter tumor suppressor pathways, but not so severe as to result in immediate cell death.

Why Is Radiation a Greater Concern in Children Than in Adults?

DNA is more likely to become damaged when it is in an unwound state, which occurs before, during, and immediately after cell division. Therefore, as the frequency and duration of cell division increases, so does the possibility of DNA damage. In addition, the frequency by which a mutation will be expressed is directly related to cellular activity and cell division. As a result, more rapidly dividing cells have a higher probability of expressing and replicating DNA errors than a dormant cell.

These factors help explain why rapidly dividing cells are more susceptible to radiation damage than other cells. The most susceptible cell lines include lymphocytes and hematopoietic stem cells, because of their high rate of division. Similarly, cells in a child's body generally divide more rapidly than those in an adult, as a consequence of normal growth and development. For this reason, it is estimated that children may be at least two times more sensitive than adults to the effects of ionizing radiation. With decreasing age, the degree of radiosensitivity is thought to increase.

In addition to a greater degree of radiosensitivity, children are also more vulnerable due to a proportionately longer life span and longer lag time during which mutations can manifest. Even if the biological sensitivity of a neonate and a 90-year-old were exactly the same, the radiation damage sustained by the neonate would have a much longer period to manifest, compared with the relatively shorter expected life span of the 90-year-old.

For the reasons outlined earlier, we must take radiation safety seriously in children and strive to keep exposures as low as reasonably achievable (ALARA) when using ionizing radiation.

What Evidence Is There to Support Carcinogenic Effects Associated With Ionizing Radiation?

The most widely studied radiation-exposed population is the survivors of the atomic bombs detonated over Japan to end World War II. This effort has been termed the

Life Span Study. This study is the major source of data with respect to radiation-induced solid malignancies and leukemia. The most comprehensive report summarizing the characteristics of this cohort is the BEIR VII report. This report was published by the National Academy of Sciences, the National Academy of Engineering, the Institute of Medicine, and the National Research Council. Notably, this committee-based study sought to quantify risk estimates of radiation exposure in the medical range, which represents the "low-level" range.

Needless to say, this is an extremely challenging task. The first requirement of the BEIR studies, as with any other studies looking retrospectively at the consequences of radiation exposure, is an estimate of the initial dose received above background radiation. Since 1957, dose estimates have been produced by a joint Japanese–United States organization called the Radiation Effects Research Foundation in an attempt to quantify survivors' doses at the time of detonation. These models became increasingly more complex, using real data from exposed materials within the atomic bomb radius in combination with survivor descriptions of their specific locations and relative adjacent shielding (or lack thereof) at the time of exposure. The BEIR VII report improved on prior studies by using the most accurate, computer-aided dose estimates to date. BEIR VII also used interim published data of radiation-exposed nuclear workers and even some early studies of patients exposed to radiation in the medical setting.

In summary, BEIR VII concluded that the stochastic effects of radiation (such as development of a secondary malignancy) are best represented by a LNT model. That is, even at very small doses, an increased risk is conferred. The BEIR VII report also presents a methodology for calculating lifetime attributable risk from data in tables 12D-1 and 12D-2. These tables present values for cancer incidence and mortality per 100,000 persons exposed to 100 mGy and at various ages of exposure. It should be noted that these tables have been used to create sensationalistic numbers of potential cancer deaths by dividing an "average" or "typical" dose absorbed for a CT study by 100 mGy and multiplying the result by the number of patients undergoing CT studies, divided by 100,000 persons. The result is a speculative number predicting future cancer risk. This calculation is inappropriate for two reasons. First, effective dose (E dose), as defined by the International Commission on Radiological Protection, is not intended as an epidemiological tool for risk assessment. This is discussed further in the upcoming section. Second, the LNT model is a "preferred" model, but a large degree of uncertainty is present at doses less than 100 mSv, with error bars that include *zero* excess risk. To date, there has been no direct evidence of increased cancer risk to patients exposed to a level less than 100 mSv.

In direct response to media reports in the popular press regarding the risks of radiation, the American Association of Physicists in Medicine (AAPM, 2011) released a public position statement that contains the following statement: "Risks of medical imaging at E doses below 50 mSv for single procedures or 100 mSv for multiple procedures over short periods of time are too low to be detectable and may be nonexistent. Predictions of hypothetical cancer incidence and deaths in patient populations exposed to such low doses are highly speculative and should be discouraged."

■ Fundamentals of CT Dosimetry

What Is the Radiation Dose for a CT Scan?

Before we can answer this common question, we need to understand the terminology used to describe radiation dose in CT. Typically when a patient, parent, or clinician asks, "How much radiation is used for a CT study?" they are indirectly asking, "What is the risk incurred by the patient by undergoing this study?" Approaches to answering this question are provided in the Communicating Risks section at the end of this chapter. In this section, we lay the groundwork by defining the various metrics used to describe radiation dose in CT examinations.

The term *radiation dose* in the context of CT can be split into three categories:
1. the radiation output of the CT scanner, quantified by the Computed Tomography Dose Index (CTDI; mGy) and the dose length product (DLP; mGy∗cm);
2. the radiation absorbed by the patient, quantified by absorbed organ dose (mGy) and E dose (mSv); and
3. carcinogenic risk to the patient, typically estimated in terms of lifetime attributable risk from the BEIR report VII or calculated as an equivalent surrogate examination (i.e., number of chest radiographs).

The absolute and relative risks to the patient are the most difficult questions to answer, because insufficient data exist at the low dose levels of radiation used in diagnostic CT to allow us to accurately predict cancer risk with any degree of certainty. The definitions of each quantity mentioned earlier are explained later.

CT Dose Index

It is instructive for any radiologist to review the definition of $CTDI_{VOL}$, the most widely used descriptor of "dose." This value and the DLP are exported by the scanner via a Radiation Dose Structured Report (RDSR) on modern scanners that can be included in the patient's medical record. It is also available in the form of a secondary capture dose screen, typically viewable on a PACS (picture archiving and communication system) workstation. $CTDI_{VOL}$ is also measured on an annual basis for typical examinations (e.g., pediatric head, pediatric abdomen, adult head, and adult abdomen) by a Qualified Medical Physicist (QMP) as part of compliance testing and American College of Radiology accreditation requirements.

$CTDI_{VOL}$ is a calculated value based on a measured quantity, termed $CTDI_{100}$. The quantity $CTDI_{100}$ is the dose measured by placing a 100-mm ionization chamber in the peripheral and central holes of a standard 16- or 32-cm CTDI phantom during one axial rotation (Fig. 22.1).

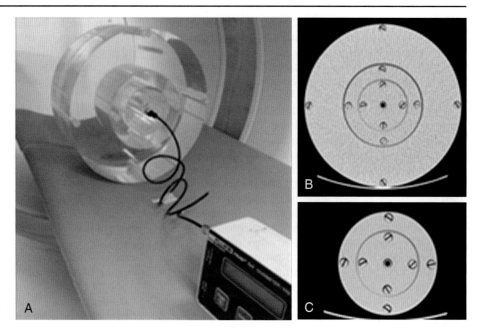

Fig. 22.1 (A–C) Computed Tomography Dose Index (*CTDI*) phantoms. *DLP*, Dose length product.

Dose report				
Series	Type	Scan range (mm)	CTDIvol (mGy)	DLP (mGy-cm)	Phantom cm
1	Scout	-	-	-	-
2	Helical	S22.750-1457.250	5.36	268.80	Body 32
			Total exam DLP:	268.80	

Fig. 22.2 Secondary capture dose screen: sample screen.

The quantity $CTDI_w$ (CTDI weighted) is calculated from measurements of $CTDI_{100}$ at the periphery and center to estimate the average dose across the radial cross section:

$$CTDI_w = \frac{2}{3}CTDI_{100}^{periphery} + \frac{1}{3}CTDI_{100}^{center}$$

The quantity $CTDI_{VOL}$ includes the effect of pitch and is calculated by the following equation:

$$CTDI_{vol} = CTDI_w / pitch$$

Pitch will be discussed further in the Advanced Topics section. Historically, the 16-cm CTDI phantom was intended to represent the approximate size of an adult head or pediatric abdomen, while the 32-cm CTDI phantom was intended to represent an adult abdomen. However, the use of these phantom sizes is not consistent across CT manufacturers. For example, Siemens calculates CTDI using the 32-cm phantom for all body protocols and the 16-cm phantom for all head protocols, while GE uses the 32-cm phantom only for adult body protocols and the 16-cm phantom for pediatric body and all head protocols. The $CTDI_{VOL}$ value should always be displayed with the size of the CTDI phantom (16 or 32 cm) used for the calculation and is available on the dose capture screen as shown in Fig. 22.2. Using identical scanning techniques, the $CTDI_{VOL}$ measured with the 16-cm phantom will be approximately twice as high compared with the $CTDI_{VOL}$ measured with the 32-cm phantom, with some deviation from this rule at lower kilovoltage (kV) (80 and 100) where the ratio is slightly greater than 2. $CTDI_{VOL}$ is typically used as the metric for protocol design and optimization because it eliminates the variable of scan length (unlike DLP), which can vary significantly with patient height.

Dose Length Product

The DLP is the product of $CTDI_{VOL}$ and scan length (in units of mGy*cm). It describes the CT scanner's radiation output to the CTDI phantom along the entire scan length:

$$DLP = CTDI_{vol} * \text{Scan Length}$$

DLP also includes overscanning that occurs in helical scanning protocols. Overscanning is required in helical scanning to obtain sufficient projection data to reconstruct images at the beginning and end of the scan range. The actual irradiated length can be obtained by calculating the DLP/$CTDI_{VOL}$ ratio. As such, DLP is the most comprehensive value for total radiation output of the scanner. DLP is typically used to estimate E dose by using DLP-ED conversion factors with units mSv/mGy*cm. This will be discussed further in the Effective Dose section.

Size-Specific Dose Estimate

The size-specific dose estimate (SSDE) is a quantity derived from $CTDI_{VOL}$ to estimate the absorbed dose to the patient instead of a standard plastic cylinder. SSDE was developed by the American Association of Physicists in Medicine (AAPM) Task Group (TG) 204. The TG report published conversion factors that could be used to calculate SSDE from CTDI by measuring the patient anteroposterior (AP) and/or lateral dimensions. The TG 204 conversion factors applied only to body parts of solid soft tissue. To account for body parts with heterogeneous density (e.g., thorax), TG 204 was supplemented with TG 220, which defines water equivalent diameter as the standard for estimating patient size. In theory, each z-axis position along the scan length has an associated SSDE. In an effort to simplify the calculation of a single SSDE, it has been shown that using the scan-average output (i.e., $CTDI_{VOL}$ from the dose report) and measuring water equivalent diameter at the center of the scan range results in acceptable error.

Effective Dose

The quantity E dose was developed by the International Commission on Radiological Protection (ICRP) as a method of accounting for the different radiosensitivities of organs. By weighting absorbed dose with the biological sensitivity of the exposed organ, it is possible to calculate an equivalent "whole-body" dose, that is, a uniform whole-body exposure that carries the same carcinogenic risk. Although E dose was originally intended to regulate occupational exposures, it has become a standard value for reporting patient dose with an implication of being a measure of patient risk, although this is incorrect. The potential for misuse of E dose was recognized and made explicit in Executive Summary item (k) of ICRP Report 103 https://www.icrp.org/docs/ICRP_Publication_103-Annals_of_the_ICRP_37(2-4)-Free_extract.pdf:

The collective E Dose quantity is an instrument for optimization, for comparing radiological technologies and protection procedures predominantly in the context of occupational exposure. Collective E Dose is not intended for a tool for epidemiological risk assessment and it is inappropriate to use it in risk projections. The aggregation of very low individual doses over extended time periods is inappropriate, and in particular the calculation of the number of cancer deaths based on collective E Doses from trivial individual doses should be avoided.

Despite these warnings, lay media and peer-reviewed scientific journals have used estimates of E dose, multiplied by risk coefficients taken from BEIR tables 12D-1 and 12D-2 to create sensationalistic numbers of future cancers as a result of medical imaging. These inappropriate uses of E dose and associated risk pose a different risk to the patient who may avoid a necessary study as a result of fear of a perceived risk for cancer.

E dose is difficult to calculate with a high degree of precision because accurate organ doses are typically unknown. To allow for quicker E dose estimates, DLP-to-E dose conversion factors have been developed for different body sizes and beam energies, most recently by Deak et al. (2010) E dose estimates using conversion factors provide a mechanism for comparison of dose across different modalities and body parts, and they can be used as an optimization tool but should stop short of being used to calculate risk.

■ Dose and Image Quality Targets

What Is an Appropriate CT Dose?

There are several approaches to determining appropriate dose levels for pediatric CT examinations. In an optimized scenario, tube output (i.e., CTDI) should be tailored to patient size, anatomical region, and clinical indication. As an example, the dose required for an initial head CT is typically much higher than a follow-up abdomen CT. The Image Gently campaign website contains practical information for designing size-specific protocols. The AAPM CT Protocol working group also routinely publishes CT Protocol Guidelines that can be used in conjunction with the Image Gently website.

The task of designing optimized dose levels for an individual practice necessarily involves an empirical component. This could take the form of gradually optimizing dose levels over time or using physics and phantom testing before scanning patients in an effort to achieve a previously derived image quality target. Although this may seem like a daunting task, numerous resources can be used as a starting point. The Quality Improvement Registry for CT Scans in Children is a consortium of six pediatric hospitals that contribute data to the American College of Radiology (ACR) Dose Index Registry (DIR). These data were used to develop pediatric abdominal diagnostic reference ranges (DRRs) for various clinical indications. The DRRs defined 25th, 50th, and 75th percentile ranges for various sizes. Doses less than the 25th percentile are at risk for being nondiagnostic, while doses greater than the 75th percentile might be unnecessarily high. Based on these DRRs, Image Gently published size-based "dose reduction factors" with the 50th percentile values serving as the basis for the "aggressive" dose reduction factors. The Image Gently approach will be discussed later in the CT Protocol Design section.

Another consideration for optimizing dose and image quality, in addition to tailoring dose to patient size and anatomic region, is the scan indication. Even when patient size and anatomy are similar, doses should also be tailored to achieve a level of image quality necessary to answer the clinical question while following the ALARA principle. A CT examination performed for suspected appendicitis may not require the same level of image quality (i.e., noise reduction) as a first-pass CT examination for suspected cancer. In 2011, Boston Children's Hospital implemented an indication-based "dose class" system for pediatric abdominal imaging that was designed to reduce the overall radiation burden for our pediatric population without sacrificing diagnostic confidence. This tiered approach to CT radiation dosing for pediatric abdominal imaging is one method to performing indication-based CT imaging. We prescribe relatively higher doses with less inherent image noise for staging abdominal oncological studies and trauma imaging (dose class 1), lower doses for suspected appendicitis or certain follow-up oncology studies (dose class 2), and even lower doses for suspected renal stones (dose class 3). Our belief is that certain diagnostic tasks require lower levels of quantum mottle (dose class 1 studies), and certain diagnostic tasks can be performed in the setting of a relatively higher level of quantum mottle at a substantially lower dose (dose class 3). In theory, many dose classes are possible, but as a matter of practicality, our institution uses three dose classes for body CT imaging (Fig. 22.3).

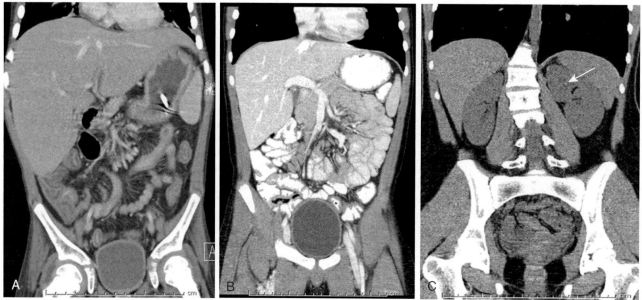

Fig. 22.3 (A–C) Abdominal dose class system example using filter backprojection.

CT Protocol Design

How Can I Create Pediatric CT Protocols?

The most basic approach to designing size-specific protocols is to scale tube current (mA) with patient size. Other factors that could be used to achieve further dose reductions (e.g., iterative reconstruction [IR], low kV) will be discussed in the Advanced Topics section.

In 2014, the Image Gently campaign published a document titled "Image Gently® Development of Pediatric CT Protocols 2014" https://radiologiadetrinchera.files.wordpress.com/2018/01/ig-ct-protocols-111714.pdf that serves as an excellent starting point for designing CT protocols for pediatric patients. Suggested "dose reduction factors" allow the user to calculate appropriate dose levels in terms of CTDI or SSDE for different patient size categories, using an appropriate adult dose level as a reference. The AAPM CT Protocol Guidelines (https://www.aapm.org/pubs/CTProtocols/) provide a great reference for appropriate dose levels and allow the radiologists to compare a hospital's adult doses with vetted benchmarks. Once the adult dose level is established, the pediatric dose can be determined for a range of patient sizes based on "limited," "moderate," or "aggressive" reduction factors. For institutions just beginning the process of optimization or those with a small pediatric patient population, it might be wise to begin with the "limited" dose conversion factors and gradually move to "moderate" or "aggressive," if acceptable. Tables for pediatric abdominal, thoracic, and head CT examinations are provided. The abdominal CT table is provided as an example (Table 22.1).

We will illustrate an example of how to create a CT protocol for patients with lateral dimensions of 16 cm. First, an adult reference dose should be established. If we assume the adult reference SSDE of 23 mGy is acceptable and uses 200 mAs (milliampere-seconds), we can use the "moderate mAs reduction factor" to multiply the adult mAs value of 200 mAs × 0.62 (reduction factors) = 124 mAs. Designing a protocol with 124 mAs and leaving all other technical parameters untouched will result in SSDE = 20 mGy for patients with lateral dimensions of approximately 16 cm. Alternatively, a more conservative or more aggressive reduction factor can be selected depending on the noise tolerance of the interpreting radiologist. A reasonable number of patient size categories should be used. Typically, seven is sufficient to provide size-based protocols without being too onerous for the technologists. It should be noted that this approach applies to fixed-mA protocols. Automatic exposure control (AEC) protocols can also be used to modulate the tube current based on the attenuation of the patient. AEC will be discussed in the Advanced Topics section.

Using the Image Gently approach, pediatric CT protocols can be designed for all patient sizes by reducing the tube mAs. In the earlier example, lateral dimension was used to measure patient size because this value can easily be measured using electronic calipers on a posteroanterior "localizer" image. The workflow in our institution for pelvis and abdomen studies begins with the acquisition of a posteroanterior localizer to measure the lateral dimension at the level of the iliac crest (Fig. 22.4). Different anatomic landmarks must be identified for each examination type.

In the previous section, we discuss modulating mA, which is linear with tube output and "dose," as a means of creating size-specific protocols. However, dose (i.e., SSDE) is only a surrogate for image noise. Although commonly used interchangeably with the term *image quality*, image noise is only one factor that affects overall quality. Other factors include image contrast, noise texture (i.e., the size or granularity of image noise), and artifacts. Noise *texture* and artifacts will be discussed in the Advanced Topics section. Later, another surrogate for overall image quality, the contrast-to-noise ratio (CNR), is discussed as an alternative to dose as an optimization tool.

Using the ACR CT phantom, the CNR can be easily measured following the standard test instructions on the ACR website. If size-based protocols have been

TABLE 22.1   Dose Conversion Table for Pediatric Abdominal Computed Tomography Provided by Image Gently

Fixed parameters: KVP = 120; MA = 200; TIME (S) = 1; Pitch during measured CTDIVOL = 1.0; Pitch during clinical examination = 1.0; Adult SSDE = 23

ABDOMEN/PELVIS AP THICKNESS (CM)	ABDOMEN/PELVIS LAT THICKNESS (CM)	ABDOMEN/PELVIS EFFECTIVE DIAMETER (CM)	MASS (KG)	AGE	LIMITED MAS REDUCTION FACTOR	MODERATE MAS REDUCTION FACTOR	AGGRESSIVE MAS REDUCTION FACTOR	LIMITED MAS SSDE (MGY)	MODERATE MAS SSDE (MGY)	AGGRESSIVE MAS SSDE (MGY)	LIMITED NB = ADULT SSDE ESTIMATED MAS	MODERATE NB = 0.75 * ADULT SSDE ESTIMATED MAS	AGGRESSIVE NB = 0.5 * ADULT SSDE ESTIMATED MAS
10	14	11 8	4	Newborn	0.52	0.39	0.25	23	17	11	104	77	50
11	16	13.3	10	1 y	0.55	0.42	0.29	23	18	12	110	64	59
14	20	16.7	18	5 y	0.62	0.50	0.39	23	19	15	123	100	78
16	25	20.0	33	10 y	0.70	0.62	0.53	23	20	18	140	123	106
19	29	23.5	54	15 y	0.80	0.74	0.68	23	21	20	160	148	137
22	32	26.5	65	20 y	0.89	0.86	0.83	23	22	22	179	172	165
25	35	29.6	75	Medium adult	1.00	1.00	1.00	23	23	23	200	200	200
31	41	35.7	110	Large adult	1.21	1.28	135	23	25	27	242	256	270

AP, Anteroposterior; CTDI, Computed Tomography Dose Index; LAT, lateral; NB, Newborn; SSDE, size-specific dose estimate.

developed for a single scanner in a department and are judged to be acceptable, the CNR can be measured for each of these size-based protocols and compared. Protocols can then be developed for a "nonoptimized" scanner by adjusting the kV and mA such that the measured CNR matches that of the optimized scanner for each protocol. In this way, image quality is matched across all scanners accounting for different kV, slice thickness, and image reconstruction as opposed to simply dose, which is a surrogate for image noise.

■ Advanced Topics

What Is Tube Current (mA) and Rotation Time (mS), and How Do They Affect Patient Dose?

Tube current (mA) and rotation time (mS) determine the tube current–time product, referred to as "mAs."

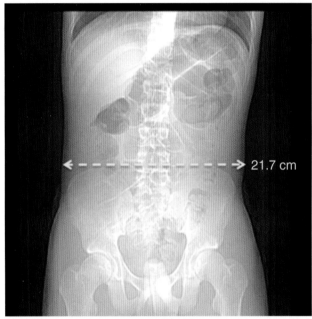

Fig. 22.4 Lateral measurement of the iliac crest on a posteroanterior localizer image.

Generally speaking, the quality of CT images improves by increasing the number of x-rays used to form the image. This can be accomplished by increasing the mA and/or rotation time. Typically, we attempt to reduce the rotation time in pediatric CT imaging to reduce motion artifacts, except in cases that require very high in-plane resolution (e.g., temporal bone imaging). In such cases, it may be necessary to use a longer rotation time to achieve sufficient projection data to prevent compromise of image resolution. The effect of rotation time on resolution can be tested by a QMP to provide guidance on rotation time for certain examination types. When the rotation time is decreased, the tube current should be increased to maintain sufficient mAs and an acceptable level of image noise. The tube current determines the number or the quantity of electrons that bombard the x-ray tube target and produce x-rays. When all other parameters are held constant, an image becomes less noisy when a greater number of x-rays are used. However, this also results in higher radiation dose. The tube current (mA) and patient dose are directly related, such that doubling the tube current roughly doubles all radiation dose metrics (CTDI, SSDE, and E dose). The mA and dose are inversely proportional to quantum mottle or noise, all other factors being equal, as demonstrated in Fig. 22.5.

What Is Kilovolt Peak, and How Does It Affect the Patient Dose?

The kV reflects the energy (voltage) applied between the anode and cathode in the x-ray tube and determines the maximum (peak) amount of energy that can be transferred to an individual photon (termed *kilovolt peak* [kVp]). The x-ray beam contains all energies up to the maximum defined by the kVp. Higher kV results in higher-energy photons, or x-ray beams that are more penetrating. If the mAs is held constant, increasing the kV will decrease the quantum mottle as more photons reach the detector. This will also increase the patient dose as a result of more ionizing events per interaction with matter and reduce image contrast because of a smaller difference in attenuation between biological materials at higher energies. The relationship between kV and patient dose is more complex than mA or mAs,

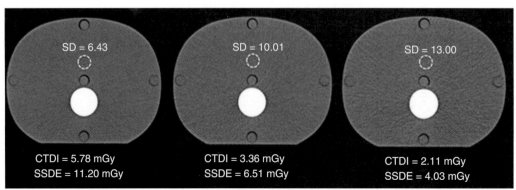

Fig. 22.5 Variation in image noise at three dose levels. *CTDI*, Computed Tomography Dose Index; *SSDE*, size-specific dose estimate.

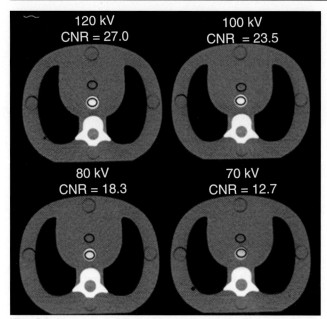

Fig. 22.6 Variation in contrast-to-noise ratio (*CNR*) at different kV levels.

with increasing kV resulting in exponential increases in patient dose. For instance, an increase of 20 kVp will increase patient dose by approximately 35% to 40%.

Increasing mAs while decreasing the kV can help lower the radiation dose while simultaneously improving image contrast, particularly when imaging with intravenous contrast media. The dose differential can be calculated by comparing CTDI of low and high kV techniques. Studies performed with intravenous contrast generally benefit from a lower kV because the k-edge of iodine provides better subject contrast at lower kV values (Fig. 22.6). As a result, more noise can be tolerated while still maintaining the CNR. It is important to note that at very high levels of image noise, improved contrast does not improve image quality because structures are no longer visible above the image noise.

One potential downfall of decreased tube voltage is the change in E dose. Lower-energy photons from lower kV values are less penetrating and are more likely to be absorbed. This can result in higher exposures to peripheral tissues, such as glandular breast tissue, orbits, and red bone marrow in the spine, all of which are considered to be relatively radiosensitive. This is why it is recommended to use only low kV techniques on small patients with low to moderate mAs settings. Using very high mAs values to compensate for increased absorption in large patients could result in high absorbed doses to sensitive organs.

The importance of CT dose optimization is not just to adjust parameters to reduce radiation but to ensure that the quality of the study is not compromised. Otherwise, regardless of dose, the study may be significantly limited or nondiagnostic. It is especially important to keep a kV of 120 in patients with larger diameters or girth for most CT scanners. However, in younger patients, especially infants, the kV values may need to be higher than suggested by size alone to account for relative paucity

of fat between organs, necessitating less image noise. In older children or those with more girth the presence of intraabdominal fat would allow for greater quantum mottle.

What Are Acceptable Kilovoltage Ranges for Imaging of Children?

Prior studies have provided rough guidelines for kV ranges while imaging children. Although the indication and presence of contrast affect decisions, recent literature supports 70 to 80 kV when performing contrast-enhanced studies in smaller children. In larger patients in studies performed without intravenous contrast, values as high as 120 kVp may be necessary for accurate delineation of soft tissues. Tube voltage values of 100 kVp are probably adequate for medium-size older children for most clinical indications, although when certain anatomic areas are being scanned, the tube voltage may be lowered. For instance, there is inherently more contrast between aerated lung and adjacent mediastinum than the soft tissues crowded within the abdomen, allowing for lower tube voltage settings.

What Is Pitch, and How Does It Affect the Patient Dose?

Pitch is the ratio of the distance traveled by the CT table in one 360-degree tube rotation and the distance of the collimated x-ray field at isocenter in the z direction. Three different pitch values are illustrated in Fig. 22.7.

A higher pitch means faster table motion and shorter period of irradiation to the patient, and thus lower dose if all other factors are unchanged. The dose is therefore inversely proportional to pitch when mA and rotation time are held constant. However, mA and rotation time can be increased or decreased to maintain the same patient dose (by matching scanner $CTDI_{VOL}$) as pitch is increased or decreased. Therefore pitch should be modified primarily to change scan speed and not to decrease patient dose, which can be accomplished separately by adjusting the mA. Caution should be exercised when increasing pitch to ensure the scanner is able to achieve the desired level of image noise. The advent of multidetector CT scanners allows implementation of higher pitch values without significant image degradation. Currently, most multidetector CT studies can be performed at pitch values greater than 1 to mitigate motion artifacts.

What Are the Advantages of Higher Pitch?

Higher pitch results in faster data acquisition, which translates into fewer motion artifacts. As mentioned earlier, it is our opinion that increasing pitch should not be the primary means to reduce dose, because this can be achieved more simply by adjusting mA. Most pediatric imaging uses pitch values greater than 1.0. When

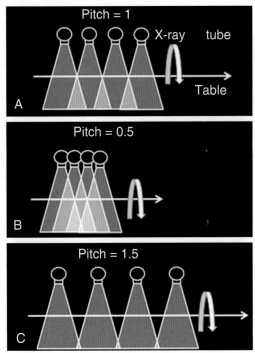

Fig. 22.7 Illustration of pitch (A–C).

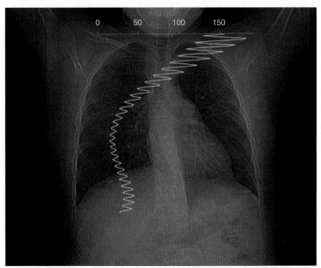

Fig. 22.8 mA trace overlayed on localizer image.

pitch values are less than 1, this results in overlapping irradiation of anatomy in the z direction (see Fig. 22.7). Although this increases patient dose, pitch values less than 1 may be necessary for certain indications, such as cardiac studies, and may be advantageous when high-detail imaging is required for certain musculoskeletal applications.

■ Automatic Exposure Control

AEC in the context of CT imaging refers to tube current modulation. When AEC is used in a CT protocol, a desired noise level is defined by user input within the protocol (e.g., GE "Noise Index" or Siemens "Quality Reference mAs"). Based on this value, tube current is varied by the CT scanner to achieve the desired noise level along the entire scan length. The mA used by the scanner is based on attenuation along the z-axis. The nominal result is a study of uniform quality with acceptable quantum mottle regardless of varying patient thickness in the included scan range. The human body is not a perfect cylinder, and some parts of the body are thicker or more attenuating than others. Without AEC, tube current is a constant value irrespective of body area being imaged or the rotational projection of the beam. In the absence of AEC and low mAs, there is inhomogeneous noise distribution and image degradation through thicker body parts, such as the shoulders or the pelvis. At higher mAs values the absence of AEC unnecessarily exposes thinner or less attenuating body parts, such as the lungs, to higher radiation doses.

There are two components to tube current modulation: longitudinal modulation and angular modulation. Longitudinal modulation refers to modulation along

the z-axis and is determined based on attenuation calculated from the localizer image. Angular modulation is determined by assuming an elliptical patient shape or "on the fly" during a scan based on the previous rotation and is designed to account for the differences in patient shape in the AP and lateral directions. An example of an mA trace for a chest–abdomen examination is shown in Fig. 22.8.

■ What Is Iterative Reconstruction, and How Does It Compare With Filtered Backprojection?

The CT gantry is mounted with detector arrays and a collimated x-ray source that rotates around the patient. At each angular position of the x-ray tube, incident x-rays are altered by attenuation characteristics of the tissues encountered. This creates a projection at each angular position of the x-ray tube. These projectional data form a sinogram, or a two-dimensional array. In filtered backprojection, all projections are *equally* weighted. This helps to reduce some of the image noise. With IR, there are additional statistical and geometric models that weigh the data *individually* and perform several passes over the raw data to create a more accurate noise model. These multiple passes reduce image noise, which is the main advantage of IR.

In general, dose reduction of approximately 20% to 40% can be achieved when using IR without degrading image quality (Fig. 22.9). With newer "model-based" IR techniques, CT radiation dose reduction can range anywhere from 40% to 80% compared with FBP. The drawback, however, is that IR necessitates higher computer processing speeds, and high levels of IR may produce images with a somewhat artificial or "plastic" appearance. The reason for this plastic appearance is that IR minimizes the noise *power* but also changes the noise *texture*, typically resulting in a lower-frequency (i.e., smoother) noise pattern. This is often perceived as "artificial" and undesirable.

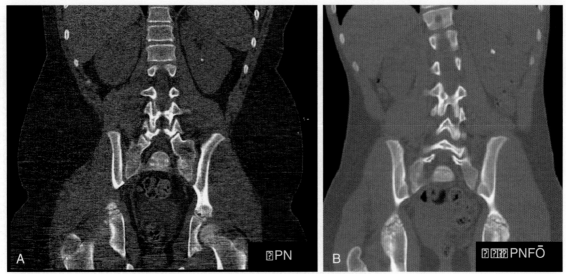

Fig. 22.9 (A, B) Effect of iterative reconstruction on image quality.

■ Communicating Risk

How Should I Communicate the Risk and Benefits to a Parent or Patient?

In this era of heighted public awareness, the lay press has hyperbolized a few incidences of overirradiated imaging errors and amplified the public's fear of radiation. These events tend to exaggerate and erroneously present diagnostic imaging as deterministic and tumor inducing. As imaging professionals, it is our obligation to reassure patients and their families of the real, tangible, sometimes lifesaving benefits of diagnostic imaging from the more elusive potential radiation risks. Although most people within the field of radiology would agree that quantifying and assessing risk is complex, many, if not all, would also agree that the benefits of CT scans, when indicated and properly performed, significantly outweigh these theoretical risks.

How do we convey this message when the discussion of individual risk is so abstract? Although the task of communicating risk remains challenging, we owe it to the patient to at least have a discussion. The initial discussion should involve the ordering clinician who is familiar with the patient's history and physical examination. Based on this information, the radiologist should actively guide the choice of imaging study for the indication and then accordingly, with the help of a QMP, adjust CT parameters to minimize the radiation dose, while still preserving image quality.

What Challenges Will I Face in Discussing Radiation Risks With Patients?

Radiologists face a number of significant challenges when discussing radiation dose with patients, particularly in the pediatric setting. Medical testing of a child is an inherently emotional experience for any parent, which can have a significant effect on their cognitive processing and retention of information. Therefore it is critical for the radiologist to be as clear and concise as possible when discussing the indication and expected benefit of the imaging study to the parent of a pediatric patient.

Although the patients or parents often develop a rapport with their primary physician, the radiologist is typically a new, unknown face and may be mistaken for a technologist in certain circumstances. Although challenging for many reasons, it is important for the radiologist to rapidly establish trust with the patient and their family, and to make it clear they are working together with the patient's other clinical providers to arrive at the correct diagnosis as accurately, rapidly, and safely as possible.

After establishing oneself as an important member of the clinical team, the radiologist should attempt to assess the baseline level of knowledge and anxiety that a patient or parent may have regarding the examination. Asking open-ended questions such as "What is your understanding of the test that has been ordered for your child?" or encouraging questions such as "explain to me your concerns or ask any questions you might have?" may help start a fruitful conversation. Once these basic details are established, the radiologist can then tailor the conversation appropriately. As an example, a parent with an engineering or physics degree may have different expectations of your conversation than a parent without a scientific background. Similarly, a parent who has lost a previous child or has themselves had an unwanted diagnosis may carry additional anxiety that must be acknowledged and addressed appropriately.

How Should I Discuss Dose?

After gaining some understanding of the parents' or patient's concerns, an initial discussion of dose can be introduced. Because the general population has little

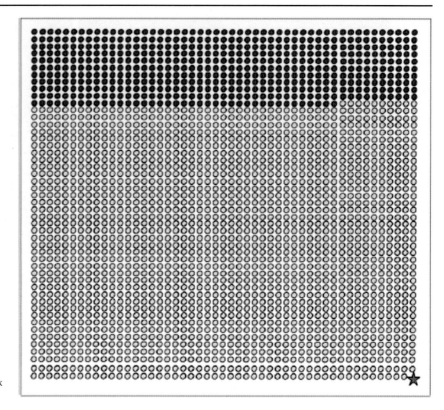

Fig. 22.10 Demonstration of 1 in 2500 risk in comparison with 550 in 2500.

familiarity with the medical and physics jargon surrounding dose estimates and dose risks, comparisons with real-life examples can facilitate an understanding of dose estimates. Visual aids comparing the dose expected from a given study with the natural background radiation received over a single day or year can be helpful; most parents do not realize that we are exposed to radiation all the time. Although not totally analogous (and somewhat controversial), comparison with radiation exposure on routine airline flights (e.g., from New York to Seattle) may also be helpful. Of course, it is important to remember and to remind parents that all dose estimates are truly estimates.

How Should I Discuss Risk?

Once dose has been discussed, one must address the more challenging topic of risk. As described earlier in this chapter, the risks of radiation-induced malignancy are thought to be real by most radiologists and medical physicists; however, quantifying a risk estimate for a single patient undergoing a single radiation-utilizing examination is an extremely difficult task.

Perhaps as a consequence of our evolution occurring before the development of complex mathematics, humans find it extremely difficult to think about and assess risk in a quantitative fashion. Psychologists have extensively studied this phenomenon. Most laypeople do not have a strong grasp of statistical modeling, and even most physicians are unlikely to know the difference between stochastic and deterministic effects of radiation. Therefore the simplest approach is favored.

There are several approaches to discussing risk. A numerical or statistical approach can be used to compare the risks for death from malignancy from an imaging examination with the risks of death from everyday activities like traveling cross-country by automobile.

For some individuals a graphical representation of the risk may be more understandable (Fig. 22.10).

Again, it cannot be overemphasized that these risk estimates are truly *estimates* and that they are *stochastic*, not deterministic. Above all, the radiologist must emphasize the medical benefits of accurate diagnosis when discussing risk.

The Image Gently campaign has several downloadable patient-oriented pamphlets on the Image Gently website https://www.imagegently.org/, which are a useful resource for a pediatric imaging waiting room. These pamphlets, written at a grade school level, are meant to provide a broad introduction to the ideas of radiation, dose, and risk. They discuss the basics of medical radiation and the innumerable benefits of using imaging studies to arrive at the correct diagnosis.

■ Summary

Understanding principles of radiation sensitivity, utilizing doses as low as reasonably achievable, and being able to communicate risks and benefits of studies are important aspects to the practice of Pediatric Radiology. This chapter explains these issues as well as guides readers in creation of pediatric CT protocols and evaluation of their radiation doses.

Bibliography

AAPM. (2011). AAPM position statement on radiation risks from medical imaging procedures. Available at http://www.aapm.org/org/policies/details.asp?id=318&type=PP¤t=true.

BEIR VII Phase 2. (2006). Health risks from exposure to low levels of ionizing radiation. Committee to Assess Health Risks from Exposure to Low Levels of Ionizing Radiation. The National Academies Press, Washington, DC. Available at: http://www.nap.edu/reportbrief/11340rb.pdf.

Deak, P. D., Smal, Y., & Kalender, W. A. (2010). Multisection CT protocols: Sex- and age-specific conversion factors used to determine effective dose from dose-length product. *Radiology, 257*(1), 158–166.

https://radiologiadetrinchera.files.wordpress.com/2018/01/ig-ct-protocols-111714.pdf.

www.icrp.org/docs/ICRP_Publication_103-Annals_of_the_ICRP_37(2-4)-Free_extract.pdf.

https://www.imagegently.org/.

Pearce, M. S., Salotti, J. A., Little, M. P., McHugh, K., Lee, C., Kim, K. P., Howe, N. L., Ronckers, C. M., Rajaraman, P., Craft, A. W., Parker, L., & de González, A. B. (2012). Radiation exposure from CT scans in childhood and subsequent risk of leukaemia and brain tumours: a retrospective cohort study. *The Lancet, 380*(9840), 499–505. https://doi.org/10.1016/S0140-6736(12)60815-0.

Fetal

CHAPTER 23
Fetal Body MRI

Dorothy Bulas and Matthew Jason Winfeld

CHAPTER OUTLINE

Why Fetal Body Magnetic Resonance Imaging?, 445
When Should Fetal Magnetic Resonance Imaging Be Performed?, 446
How Is Fetal Magnetic Resonance Imaging Performed?, 446
How Should the Patient Be Prepared?, 446
What Is the Fetal Magnetic Resonance Imaging Protocol?, 446
Should Intravenous Contrast Be Given for Fetal Magnetic Resonance Imaging?, 447
Approach to Interpretation, 447
What Maternal Structures Should Be Assessed?, 447
What Is the Fetal Situs?, 448
Fetal Face and Neck, 448
What Is the Normal Appearance of the Fetal Face and Neck?, 448
What Can Fetal Magnetic Resonance Imaging Add to the Diagnosis of Cleft Lip and/or Palate?, 449
What Can Fetal Magnetic Resonance Imaging Add to the Diagnosis of Micrognathia?, 450
What Neoplasms and Masslike Malformations Can Be Found in the Face and Neck?, 450
Fetal Thorax, 451
What Does the Normal Fetal Thorax Look Like on Magnetic Resonance Imaging?, 451
What Is the Significance of Diffuse T2 Hyperintensity in the Lungs?, 451
What Is the Significance of Focal Signal Abnormalities in the Lungs?, 452
What Might Be the Significance of Pleural Effusions?, 453
If a Congenital Diaphragmatic Hernia Is Present, What Should Be Evaluated?, 454
Can Magnetic Resonance Imaging Help Determine Whether the Fetal Thorax Is Small?, 457
What Might It Mean If the Heart Is Abnormally Positioned?, 457
Can Esophageal Atresia Be Diagnosed by Fetal Magnetic Resonance Imaging?, 457
Fetal Abdomen and Pelvis, 458
What Do the Normal Gastrointestinal System Structures Look Like by Fetal Magnetic Resonance Imaging?, 458
What Do the Normal Genitourinary System Structures Look Like?, 458
What Is the Differential Diagnosis for a Suprarenal Mass?, 458
An Upper Abdominal Cystic Mass Is Present, What Might This Be? 458
Can Distal Bowel Obstruction Be Diagnosed Prenatally?, 460
What Is the Spectrum of Abdominal Wall Abnormalities, and What Should Be Reported?, 460
What Do Large Kidneys Signify?, 462
What Is the Best Approach for the Evaluation of Hydronephrosis?, 463
What Might a Cystic Mass in the Lower Abdomen or Pelvis Be?, 465
What Is the Differential Diagnosis for a Presacral Mass?, 467
What Other Visceral Abdominopelvic Neoplasms May Present in Fetal Life?, 469
Fetal Musculoskeletal System, 469
Is Magnetic Resonance Imaging Useful in Evaluating the Fetal Musculoskeletal System?, 469
Is There a Role for Magnetic Resonance Imaging in the Evaluation of Skeletal Dysplasias?, 469
How Might Magnetic Resonance Imaging Aid the Assessment of Fetal Clubfoot?, 469
What Soft Tissue Tumors May Be Encountered in the Musculoskeletal System?, 469
Multifetal Gestations, 470
What Is the Role of Magnetic Resonance Imaging in Multifetal Gestations?, 470
Summary, 470

■ Why Fetal Body Magnetic Resonance Imaging?

Imaging is an essential component of the evaluation and care of the developing fetus. Ultrasound remains the core screening modality because of its availability, safety profile, and low cost. Standard of care includes a complete anatomy scan during the second trimester to assess for appropriate development. When anomalies are identified, ultrasound is critical in the assessment of fetal well-being, including interval growth, Doppler parameters, and cardiac function.

Magnetic resonance imaging (MRI) has become an important complementary modality in fetal assessment. Its large field of view and exquisite contrast and spatial resolution make it an invaluable tool in the further assessment of abnormalities. Fetal MRI has thus far been proven safe, with limited animal and human studies available that have demonstrated no firm evidence that embryos are sensitive to magnetic fields encountered from magnetic resonance systems.

■ When Should Fetal Magnetic Resonance Imaging Be Performed?

When an anomaly is identified by ultrasound, fetal MRI may provide useful additional information that will help guide pregnancy management and counseling. MRI is avoided in the first trimester because of the small size of the fetus and degraded resolution as a result of movement. Determining the optimal time to scan requires a balance between the need to identify abnormalities as early as possible and the desire to obtain images of the highest quality and resolution, which would come later in pregnancy with a larger fetus whose movement is more restricted. MRI can be performed as early as 17 to 18 weeks of gestation for counseling and prenatal management. Late third-trimester studies can be useful in planning delivery and perinatal management (Levine, 2013).

The American College of Radiology and Society for Pediatric Radiology have developed guidelines for the use of fetal MRI. These indications are summarized in Table 23.1.

TABLE 23.1 Body Indications for Fetal Magnetic Resonance Imaging

Face/Neck	Cystic and solid masses
	Masses that cause airway obstruction
Thorax	Masses
	Volumetric analysis of lung
Abdomen/Pelvis	Abdominopelvic cysts
	Complex genitourinary anomalies, such as cloacal malformations
	Complex renal anomalies
	Complex bowel anomalies
Multifetal gestations	Complications of monochorionic pregnancies
Miscellaneous	Consider magnetic resonance imaging when assessment of fetus by ultrasound is limited by oligohydramnios or maternal obesity

Adapted from *ACR–SPR Practice Parameter for the Safe and Optimal Performance of Fetal Magnetic Resonance Imaging (MRI)*. American College of Radiology. https://www.acr.org/-/media~/ACR/Files/Practice-Parameters/mr-fetal.pdf Revised 2020 (Resolution 45) (ACR–SPR)

■ How Is Fetal Magnetic Resonance Imaging Performed?

How Should the Patient Be Prepared?

In contradistinction to the screening obstetric ultrasound, which many prospective mothers look forward to as they get a first look at their fetus, fetal MRI can be a source of great stress to a family because they are typically performed to further evaluate a known or potential abnormality. Of ultimate importance to the success of the examination is the comfort and cooperation of the patient.

The American College of Radiology does not recommend written consent from patients for fetal MRI. Nonetheless, it is important to discuss with the family potential risks and benefits. To date, there is no conclusive medical evidence that MRI at 1.5T causes either short- or long-term negative effects on the fetus. It should be acknowledged, however, that MRI effects at 3T or greater are being investigated at the time of this chapter's writing (Bulas and Egloff, 2013).

As with all MRI examinations, patients need to be carefully screened for metal on or in their bodies. Some centers recommend not having the mother eat immediately before the MRI in an attempt to decrease fetal motion. However, no studies have conclusively showed that this measure actually improves image quality. Patients should also be encouraged to empty their bladders before scanning to improve comfort and image quality.

MRI can be an uncomfortable examination for any patient. Care should be taken to determine whether the patient would be more comfortable on her back or side to improve her ability to lie still. Sufficient pillows should be provided to support the patient in whichever position is deemed most comfortable. Earplugs and/or headphones should be provided to distract patients from the excessive noise generated by the magnetic resonance gradients. It may be helpful to have a partner in the room with the mother to decrease anxiety.

What Is the Fetal Magnetic Resonance Imaging Protocol?

The entire fetus, as well as large field-of-view images that include the uterus, cervix, and placenta, should be evaluated in every fetal MRI study (Bahado-Singh and Goncalves, 2013). Nonetheless, imaging protocols should be tailored to the clinical indication for the study. In case the mother cannot complete the examination because of discomfort, the earliest sequences obtained should help address the specific diagnostic question being asked.

The examination should begin with a standard three-plane localizer. Initial large field-of-view sequences of the maternal pelvis provide a global view of the uterus, placenta, and cervix and help delineate the position of the fetus relative to maternal anatomy. More directed sequences can then be acquired of specific fetal anatomy. As the fetus moves throughout the examination, subsequent sequences can be planned on the basis of earlier ones. Ideally, three planes of both the fetal brain and body should be obtained.

In the case of multiple gestations, after initial large field-of-view sequences, each fetus should be imaged separately. Distinguishing twins for purposes of imaging presents an additional challenge, and using labeling defined by ultrasound is helpful.

Single-shot techniques, which are spin-echo acquisitions in which the entirety of k-space is filled during one excitation, are the workhorses in fetal imaging because they are fast, thus limiting the deleterious effects of motion while providing excellent contrast resolution. Steady-state free precession images offer good contrast resolution with flowing blood demonstrating hyperintense signal. These display a ratio of T2/T1 contrast, thus accentuating fluid-sensitive signal, and may be performed as cine acquisitions to assess fetal movement. T1-weighted sequences are also of use, particularly to evaluate the meconium content of the bowel, subacute blood, and fat, which are hyperintense on these acquisitions. Echoplanar imaging can better delineate the fetal skeleton, providing excellent contrast between cartilage (bright) and bone (dark). Diffusion-weighted imaging can be useful in brain and renal imaging.

Should Intravenous Contrast Be Given for Fetal Magnetic Resonance Imaging?

Intravenous contrast is not recommended for fetal MRI. The gadolinium remains within the amniotic fluid for prolonged periods. If required for maternal or placental indications, the recommendation is to deliver the fetus as quickly as possible after contrast administration in the third trimester.

■ Approach to Interpretation

What Maternal Structures Should Be Assessed?
Large field-of-view images should include the mother's abdomen and pelvis. The maternal kidneys often demonstrate some degree of collecting system dilatation

because of ureteral compression by the gravid uterus, particularly late in pregnancy (Fig. 23.1). Any maternal abnormalities should be described if identified.

MRI also provides a global view of the pregnant uterus. The integrity of the cervix should be evaluated and cervical length measured in the sagittal plane. Any anomalies of the uterus, such as septate or bicornuate morphology, should be described, as should the size and location of fibroids (Fig. 23.2).

It is also important to evaluate the thickness and position of the placenta and the cord insertion. The normal placenta is discoid in configuration and homogeneously T2 hyperintense early in pregnancy, measuring 2 to 4 cm in maximal thickness, but becomes increasingly heterogeneous and lobulated later in gestation (Allen and Leyendecker, 2013). An abnormally thin placenta may indicate vascular compromise, whereas an abnormally thick placenta could be an associated finding of fetal hydrops, infection, aneuploidy, or anemia. A low-lying placenta or placenta previa, in which the placenta covers the internal cervical os, must be reported (Fig. 23.3).

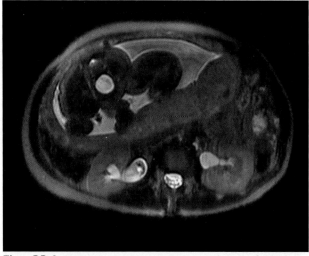

Fig. 23.1 Maternal hydronephrosis. Axial large field-of-view T2-weighted image of a 36-year-old pregnant woman demonstrates bilateral hydronephrosis, a common finding in the later stages of pregnancy.

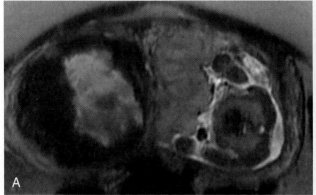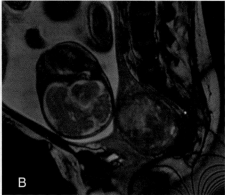

Fig. 23.2 Fibroids. (A) Axial large field-of-view T2-weighted image of a 42-year-old woman demonstrates a large fibroid with central necrosis along the right uterine wall. (B) Sagittal large field-of-view steady-state free precession image of a 35-year-old woman demonstrates a heterogeneous well-circumscribed cervical mass consistent with a fibroid.

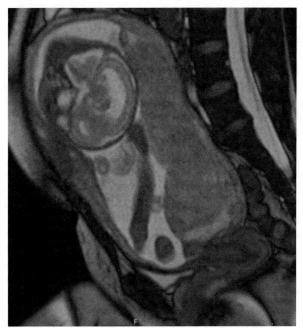

Fig. 23.3 Placenta previa. Sagittal steady-state free precession image of a uterus demonstrates the internal cervical os covered by the inferior margin of the placenta consistent with placenta previa.

MRI also may provide useful assessment of abnormal placentation, which is suggested by the presence of T2 dark intraplacental bands, increased placental vascularity, and focal bulging with interruption of the smooth uterine contour.

What Is the Fetal Situs?

Determining situs requires a three-dimensional understanding of fetal anatomy relative to that of the mother. Simply observing that the stomach has the same laterality as the heart is not sufficient for accurate assessment of situs because situs inversus totalis may occur; a specific "left" and "right" side of the fetus must be defined. Two simple questions need be answered to confidently determine situs:

1. Is the fetus cephalic or breech?
2. Is the fetus facing the mother's front, back, left side, or right side?

The easiest scenario to conceptualize is the front-facing breech fetus, because this position is identical to that of the mother. In this case, the fetus's left is the mother's left. A rear-facing cephalic fetus will also have the same left-right orientation as the mother. The front-facing cephalic fetus and the rear-facing breech fetus will have opposite left-right assignments relative to the mother.

If the fetus is facing the mother's left or right, the side of the fetus closest to the mother's spine will match the facing side if breech but be opposite if cephalic. For example, a breech fetus facing right will have its right side posterior relative to the mother. The same fetal left/right designation would be inferred in a cephalic fetus facing left. Some common scenarios are summarized in Table 23.2.

Once the left/right designation has been determined, the laterality of several anatomic structures should be sought. Among the structures to note are the heart, stomach, and liver.

TABLE 23.2   Defining Fetal Situs

FETAL LIE	FETUS IS FACING THE MOTHER'S...	FETAL LEFT IS MOTHER'S...
Cephalic	Front	Right
Cephalic	Back	Left
Breech	Front	Left
Breech	Back	Right
Cephalic	Left	Front
Cephalic	Right	Back
Breech	Left	Back
Breech	Right	Front

With regard to the heart, efforts should also be made to determine the side on which the apex lies; the apex pointing leftward defines levocardia, whereas the apex pointing rightward signifies dextrocardia. A right-sided heart with apex pointing left is not dextrocardia but rather levocardia with dextroposition.

Normal anatomic positioning of abdominal structures is known as situs solitus, and the presence of dextrocardia in this setting portends a high association with congenital heart disease (>95%). Abdominal situs inversus describes the scenario in which anatomic structures are reversed in orientation but otherwise maintain normal anatomic structure and relationships. Levocardia in this setting guarantees congenital heart malformation, whereas dextrocardia with abdominal situs inversus portends a slightly higher incidence of congenital heart disease than the general population (3%–5%). Any situs that is not solitus or inversus is classified as situs ambiguous, or heterotaxy, in which the anatomic relationships of major organs are altered. In the case of left isomerism, multiple spleens may be present. In fetuses with right isomerism, there may be no spleen (Lapierre et al., 2010). The liver is midline in either case (Fig. 23.4A–C).

Multiple other anomalies that have a high association with heterotaxy should also be sought, including intestinal malrotation, gallbladder absence, inferior vena cava interruption with azygous continuation (see Fig. 23.4D), and anomalous pulmonary venous return. Fetal echocardiogram should be performed because of the high risk for complex congenital heart disease.

Fetal Face and Neck

What Is the Normal Appearance of the Fetal Face and Neck?

A top-down approach may be used to survey the normal fetal face and neck. Both globes should be present, equal in size, and normally seated in the orbits (Fig. 23.5A). Asymmetry in globe size may indicate a genetic or chromosomal abnormality that can have important prognostic implications. Proptosis could signal the presence of an intraorbital abnormality or craniosynostosis. The interocular diameter should be roughly

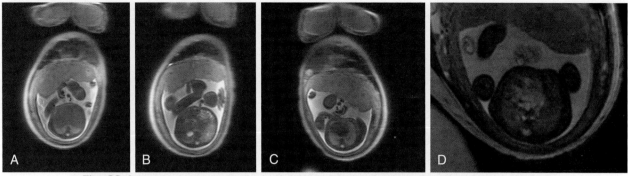

Fig. 23.4 Heterotaxy, 26-week fetus. Axial T2-weighted images demonstrate (A) midline liver, (B) right-sided stomach and left-sided fluid-filled small bowel loops, and (C) dextrocardia. (D) Axial steady-state free precession image demonstrating two prominent posterior vessels, the normal aorta to the left and enlarged azygous vein on the right, indicative of azygous continuation of an interrupted inferior vena cava.

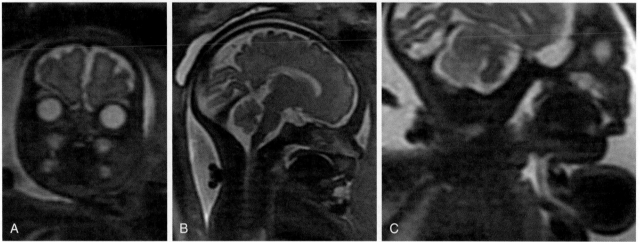

Fig. 23.5 Normal fetal face and neck, 32-week fetus. (A) Coronal T2-weighted image demonstrates symmetrical globes within normal-size orbits. (B) Sagittal paramidline T2-weighted image demonstrates a normal-size tongue within the oral cavity. (C) Sagittal paramidline T2-weighted images demonstrate fluid signal intensity within a normal-size upper pharynx.

equal to orbital width; hypotelorism and hypertelorism can both indicate chromosomal abnormalities or syndromic conditions of the fetus.

The maxilla, mandible, lip, and palate should be symmetrical and intact (Mirsky et al., 2012). Abnormally small mandible, or micrognathia, is a finding associated with a plethora of syndromes, best noted on sagittal images. Nasal bone hypoplasia is better assessed with ultrasound. The tongue should not protrude beyond the confines of the oral cavity (Fig. 23.5B); macroglossia can impede the airway postnatally and has syndromic associations, such as with Beckwith-Wiedemann syndrome (BWS).

The fetal airway is well delineated by MRI. Although the fetus does not require pharyngeal patency for growth and survival, because it draws oxygen from the maternofetal circulation, any airway impedance will have serious implications at delivery. The airway should be uniformly T2 hyperintense because of the presence of amniotic fluid (Fig. 23.5C). Any narrowing or frank obstruction of the pharynx must be identified.

What Can Fetal Magnetic Resonance Imaging Add to the Diagnosis of Cleft Lip and/or Palate?

Cleft lip and/or palate are relatively common and typically treatable craniofacial defects. Ultrasound is a reliable tool in the evaluation of cleft lip and primary palate, although sonographic evaluation of the fetal face can be somewhat limited depending on maternal body habitus and the lie of the fetal head at the time of scanning. MRI is better in assessing the secondary palate, which forms the majority of the hard palate (Arangio et al., 2013).

In up to 11% of cases, there is an association between cleft lip and/or palate and chromosomal abnormalities. MRI is particularly useful for complex clefts and central clefts, which have a high incidence of associated central nervous system anomalies. This association increases in frequency as the size and extent of the cleft increases. The two most important features of cleft lip and palate for defining the surgical approach are the laterality and anteroposterior extents of the defect(s), which have been shown to be more precisely assessed by MRI (Fig. 23.6).

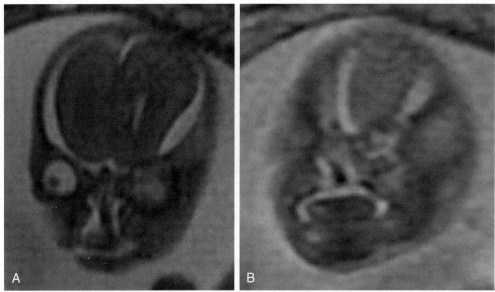

Fig. 23.6 Cleft lip and/or palate, 29-week fetus. (A) Coronal steady-state free precession image demonstrates bilateral cleft lip and palate. (B) Coronal T2-weighted image further posterior helps to evaluate the extent of the cleft palate.

What Can Fetal Magnetic Resonance Imaging Add to the Diagnosis of Micrognathia?

Micrognathia may be missed in the second trimester because rapid mandibular growth occurs later in gestation. Research by (Nemec et al., 2015) proposed quantitative parameters to assess micrognathia, including measurement of the inferior facial angle (IFA) and jaw index. The IFA is drawn on a midline sagittal image of the face with a line through the nasal root perpendicular to the plane of section and another parallel to the outer surface of the mandible. An IFA less than 50 degrees is concerning for micrognathia (Fig. 23.7A–B). The jaw index is the mandibular anteroposterior diameter normalized to biparietal diameter, which helps eliminate some of the effects of gestational age. A jaw index of less than the fifth percentile for gestational age suggests micrognathia. These calculations can be made with ultrasound, but MRI may provide greater accuracy.

Once the diagnosis of micrognathia has been made, there is a strong association with chromosomal abnormalities, necessitating comprehensive assessment of the fetal body for anomalies (Fig. 23.7C–D). Furthermore, true micrognathia may be associated with a small oral cavity, leading to posterior displacement of the tongue, potentially compromising airway integrity and affecting delivery planning.

What Neoplasms and Masslike Malformations Can Be Found in the Face and Neck?

Several masses can develop in the fetal face and neck. These can be cystic and/or solid. The most critical feature of the mass is its location in relation to the airway. Regardless of the cause of the mass, airway obstruction can lead to rapid decompensation in the delivery room. Various fetal and early perinatal interventions are available but require advance planning, including ex utero intrapartum treatment, in which a surgical airway is established with the fetus outside of the uterus but with maintenance of maternofetal circulation as the source of oxygen for the baby.

The majority of fetal neck masses are one of four entities: lymphatic malformation, teratoma, congenital hemangioma, and goiter. Lymphatic malformations result from failure of connection between the lymphatic and venous systems, resulting in isolated collections of lymph. In the neck, they tend to be posterior or posterolateral T2-hyperintense multiseptate masses that insinuate among normal structures and involve multiple anatomic spaces (Fig. 23.8). Fluid–fluid levels are not uncommon and are the result of internal hemorrhage. Cervical teratomas have a variable imaging appearance because of their composition of tissues from multiple germ cell layers. They may contain solid and cystic components, and calcifications are nearly pathognomonic, although not well seen by MRI (Fig. 23.9). Hemangiomas are vascular tumors that typically contain prominent vascular flow voids and are T2 hyperintense. Follow-up postnatal imaging may demonstrate decreased size if the lesion is of the rapidly involuting variety versus the noninvoluting hemangioma, which will not regress spontaneously after birth (Fig. 23.10). Fetal goiter may result from maternal thyroid dysfunction, such as autoimmune thyroid diseases in which thyroid-stimulating antibodies can cross to the fetal circulation and stimulate the fetal thyroid gland. Imaging appearance is unique, as the homogeneously T1-hyperintense bilobed thyroid gland is significantly enlarged (Fig. 23.11).

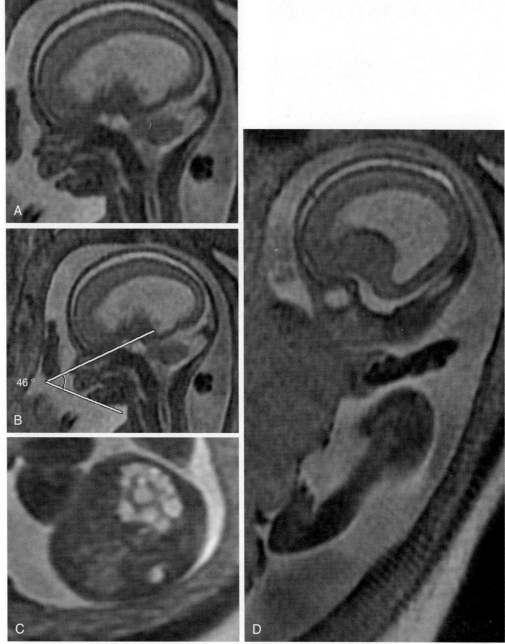

Fig. 23.7 Micrognathia, 21-week fetus. (A) Midline sagittal T2-weighted image shows micrognathia, confirmed by measurement of the inferior facial angle in (B) of 46 degrees. This fetus had additional abnormalities, including (C) multicystic dysplastic kidney and (D) abnormal flexed positioning of the right forearm and wrist.

Fetal Thorax

What Does the Normal Fetal Thorax Look Like on Magnetic Resonance Imaging?

A central-to-peripheral approach is recommended for comprehensive evaluation of the fetal thorax. The intrathoracic trachea should be patent and filled with fluid, similar to the upper airway in the neck. The heart should be located in the midline with leftward-pointing apex. The lungs should be relatively symmetrical in size, homogeneous in signal intensity, and slightly hyperintense on T2-weighted images be-

cause of the presence of amniotic fluid in the lungs (Fig. 23.12). A fluid-filled esophagus is typically not seen; if the proximal esophagus is particularly conspicuous, tracheoesophageal fistula should be considered. In some cases the great vessel branching pattern can be assessed.

What Is the Significance of Diffuse T2 Hyperintensity in the Lungs?

Diffuse hyperintense T2 signal throughout the lung parenchyma may be secondary to impedance of the outflow of amniotic fluid from the lungs (Table 23.3). This

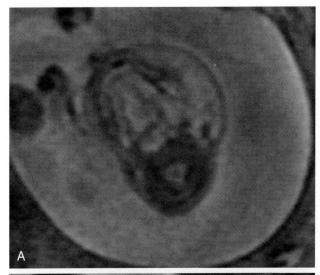

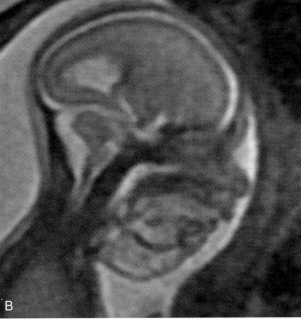

Fig. 23.8 Lymphatic malformation, 22-week fetus. (A, B) Axial (A) and sagittal (B) T2-weighted images demonstrate a hyperintense lower facial mass with multiple internal septations characteristic of a lymphatic malformation.

can be caused by tracheal obstruction. Cervical masses that compress the pharynx and thoracic masses, native to either the lung or mediastinum, also can cause airway compression with similar fluid retention in the lungs. At times, amniotic fluid can dilate the more distal airways. Unrecognized and untreated, high airway obstruction has a mortality rate of 80% to 100%. An obstructed airway as a result of intrinsic atresia or stenosis is known as congenital high airway obstruction syndrome. The most severe airway obstruction should be managed perinatally with the ex utero intrapartum treatment procedure.

Other causes of diffusely heterogeneous lung signal include primary and secondary lymphangiectasia. Primary lymphangiectasia is due to obstruction of the pulmonary lymphatics, whereas secondary lymphangi-

ectasia is the sequela of cardiac dysfunction related to congenital heart disease (Fig. 23.13).

What Is the Significance of Focal Signal Abnormalities in the Lungs?

Focal signal abnormality in the lungs is most likely to be a manifestation of an intrinsic lung mass from a developmental malformation (Barth, 2012). The signal characteristics, location of a lesion, and presence or absence of systemic feeding vessels will suggest its pathology (see Table 23.3).

Congenital pulmonary adenomatoid malformation (CPAM), formerly known as congenital cystic adenomatoid malformation, results from early airway maldevelopment and can have a variable appearance from primarily cystic to primarily solid (Fig. 23.14). These are the most common lung lesions discovered prenatally. Because they take the place of normal lung and cause mass effect that impedes development of normal lung, large size and bilateral involvement can be indicators of poor prognosis. The contribution of fetal MRI is to quantify lesion size and assess the amount of residual normal lung tissue. An important measure is the CPAM volume ratio, the volume of the mass divided by head circumference. CPAM volume is calculated by multiplying its length, width, and height by 0.52. Ratios less than 1.6 have a more favorable prognosis.

Pleuropulmonary blastoma, a rare malignant neoplasm, may have a similar imaging appearance to CPAM. Nonetheless, pleuropulmonary blastoma tends to grow throughout pregnancy, whereas CPAM has the tendency to decrease in size in the third trimester.

Pulmonary sequestration is a solid developmental lesion with a systemic arterial blood supply. Ultrasound may be able to demonstrate the arterial feeder using Doppler techniques (Fig. 23.15). MRI can assess overall size, location, and at times demonstrates the feeding vessel. Sequestrations may be intralobar or extralobar; extralobar lesions have separate pleural coverings, whereas intralobar lesions do not (Pacharn et al., 2013). A lesion may have pathological and imaging features of both CPAM and sequestration with mixed cystic and solid components and a systemic feeding vessel, known as a hybrid lesion.

Congenital lobar overinflation (CLO) is caused by intrinsically weak or absent bronchial wall cartilage or extrinsic compression of a lobar bronchus resulting in a one-way valve that allows amniotic fluid in but not out. The classic lesion usually involves the left upper lobe, right middle lobe, and right upper lobe, with lower lobe involvement being relatively rare. Nevertheless, a second subtype of CLO has been recognized, characterized by segmental or lobar hyperinflation and highly associated with bronchial atresia, more prevalent in the lower lobes. This subtype is now the most common form discovered on prenatal imaging. MRI will demonstrate a homogeneously T2-hyperintense hyperexpanded pulmonary lobe with normal distribution of pulmonary vessels (Fig. 23.16).

Another abnormality that manifests as focal lung signal abnormality is bronchial atresia. The airway immediately proximal to the atretic segment can fill with fluid,

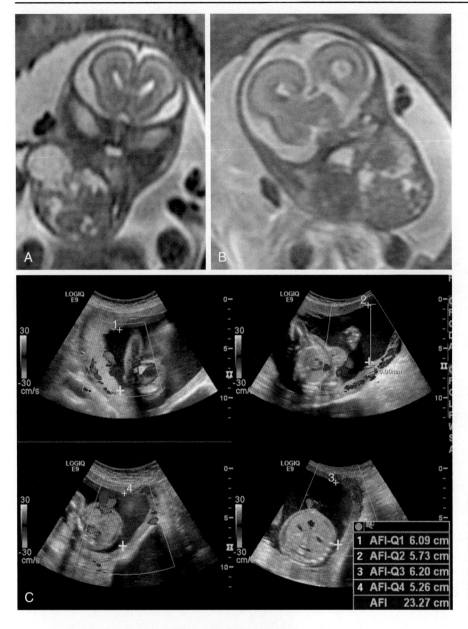

Fig. 23.9 Cervical teratoma, 20-week fetus. (A) Coronal T2-weighted image showing a large heterogeneous mass in the right neck region. (B) Slightly more posterior T2-weighted image demonstrates significant narrowing of the upper airway by the mass. (C) Sonographic images show an elevated amniotic fluid index likely caused by impairment of fetal swallowing from the mass.

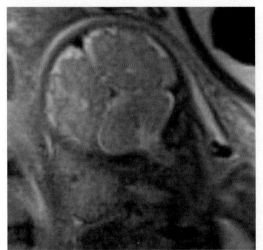

Fig. 23.10 Congenital hemangioma. A coronal T2-weighted image of a fetus demonstrates a T2-hyperintense mass with small hypointense flow voids.

demonstrating hyperintense signal on T2-weighted images. Bronchogenic cysts may arise in the lung parenchyma and account for focal signal abnormality. T1 images may be helpful because these tend to contain proteinaceous fluid and can be both T2 and T1 hyperintense. Bronchogenic cysts more commonly arise in the mediastinum, particularly subcarinal (Fig. 23.17).

MRI is particularly useful in differentiating lung masses from congenital diaphragmatic hernia (CDH). CDH contents are heterogeneous due to the presence of bowel and liver in the chest and will cause significant mass effect proportional to size. These will be discussed in a subsequent section.

What Might Be the Significance of Pleural Effusions?

Pleural effusions may be detected prenatally with varied etiologies (Yinon et al., 2008). First, it should be determined whether the pleural effusion is a manifestation of hydrops fetalis, a serious complication of many fetal anomalies; one may look for fluid in other fetal body compartments, such as abdominal ascites, skin thickening, and polyhydramnios. Hydrops can be a manifestation of genetic syndromes or chromosomal abnormalities, such as Down syndrome, Turner syndrome, or Noonan syndrome. A lung mass may also be the cause of pleural effusion; in these cases, focal pulmonary parenchymal signal abnormality will also be present. Pulmonary lymphangiectasia, which manifests as diffuse lung signal abnormality, can also present with pleural effusions because of the backflow of lymphatic drain-

age. Cardiac causes should be sought, because of increased right heart pressures and fluid leakage, and fetal echocardiography may be indicated.

If a Congenital Diaphragmatic Hernia Is Present, What Should Be Evaluated?

MRI has become a useful adjunct in the prenatal evaluation of CDH (Fig. 23.18A). Although ultrasound can make the diagnosis, the excellent contrast resolution of MRI allows for the accurate determination of many findings that may affect prognosis, prenatal interventions, and postnatal management (Mehollin-Ray et al., 2012) (Box 23.1).

WHERE IS THE LIVER?

If the liver is "up," within the thorax as part of the herniated abdominal contents, the prognosis for the fetus is worse. Furthermore, a greater volume of herniated liver portends a poorer prognosis. Various methods have been proposed for quantifying liver volumes within a hernia.

IS A HERNIA SAC PRESENT?

A hernia sac would be composed of peritoneum and/or parietal pleural and would manifest as a thin hypointense line surrounding herniated abdominal contents on fluid-sensitive sequences. Its presence has been associated with a better prognosis.

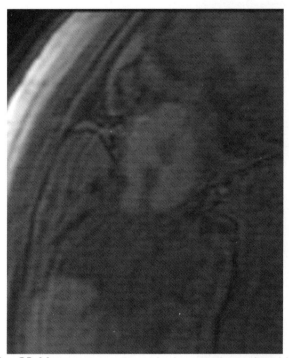

Fig. 23.11 Fetal goiter. T1-weighted images show enlarged bilobed mass extending from neck into upper chest representing enlarged thyroid. Ex utero intrapartum treatment procedure was performed.

TABLE 23.3   Differential Diagnosis for Fetal Lung Signal Abnormalities

DIFFUSE	FOCAL
Airway compression by mass	Congenital pulmonary airway malformation
Congenital high airway obstruction syndrome	Pulmonary sequestration
Pulmonary lymphangiectasia	Congenital lobar overinflation
	Bronchial atresia
	Bronchogenic cyst
	Congenital diaphragmatic hernia

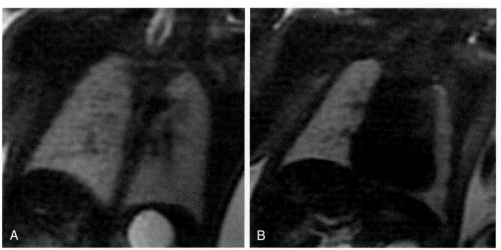

Fig. 23.12 Normal fetal thorax, 32-week fetus. (A) Coronal T2-weighted image demonstrates homogeneous signal intensity throughout both lungs, which are roughly equal in size. (B) Anterior coronal T2-weighted image further anterior showing the heart in the left chest with apex pointing to the left.

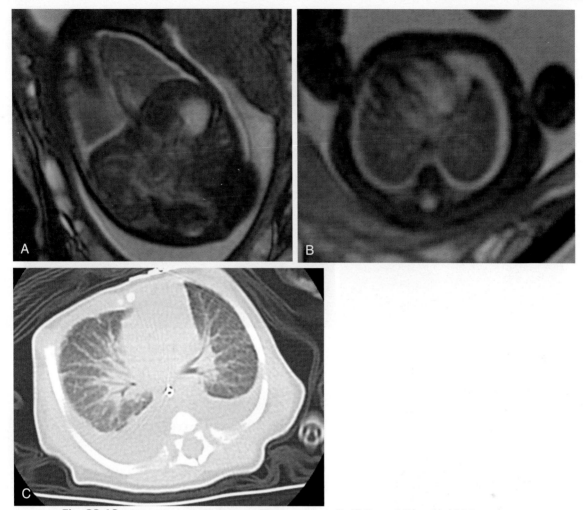

Fig. 23.13 Primary lymphangiectasia, 28-week fetus. (A, B) Coronal (A) and axial (B) steady-state free precession images demonstrate enlarged hyperintense lungs and bilateral pleural effusions characteristic of primary lymphangiectasia. (C) Postnatal axial computed tomography image demonstrates bilateral pleural effusions and interlobular septal thickening.

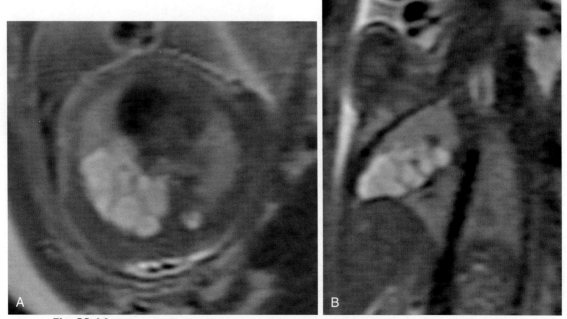

Fig. 23.14 Congenital pulmonary airway malformation (CPAM), 23-week fetus. (A, B) Axial (A) and coronal (B) T2-weighted images show a multicystic lesion in the right lung consistent with a CPAM.

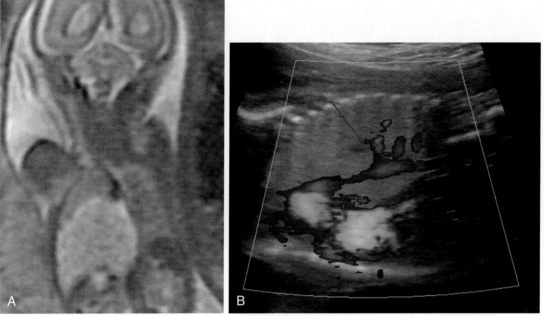

Fig. 23.15 Intralobar pulmonary sequestration, 26-week fetus. (A) Coronal T2-weighted image demonstrates an expansile hyperintense mass in the lower right hemithorax. (B) Ultrasound image with Doppler shows feeding arteries arising from the thoracic aorta.

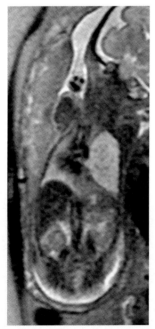

Fig. 23.16 Congenital lobar overinflation (CLO), 25-week fetus. Coronal T2-weighted image shows hyperintense expansion of the left upper lobe compatible with CLO. Note the normal distribution of hypointense vessels throughout the lesion.

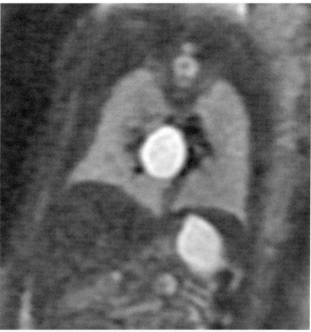

Fig. 23.17 Bronchogenic cyst, 27-week fetus. Coronal T2-weighted image demonstrates a simple cystic lesion in the subcarinal region consistent with a bronchogenic cyst.

WHAT ARE THE FETAL LUNG VOLUMES?

The severity of pulmonary hypoplasia is a useful prognostic indicator in fetuses with CDH. With abdominal contents herniated into the chest, both ipsilateral and contralateral lung will not grow normally.

Several quantitative ultrasound measures are available, including the lung/head ratio, which has been used to help predict fetal outcome in CDH. Three-dimensional ultrasound has provided volumetric data regarding existing lung tissue. MRI has helped improve the specificity of lung volume measurements. Using T2-weighted images, regions of interest are drawn around the lungs, generating a lung area for each slice that has a known thickness based on the image acquisition parameters, generating a volume (see Fig. 23.18B). The volumes are then summed to give a total fetal lung volume (TFLV), which can be compared with the expected fetal lung volume (EFVL) for gestational age. Ratios of TFLV to EFVL of less than 0.25 to 0.35 are associated with a higher mortality.

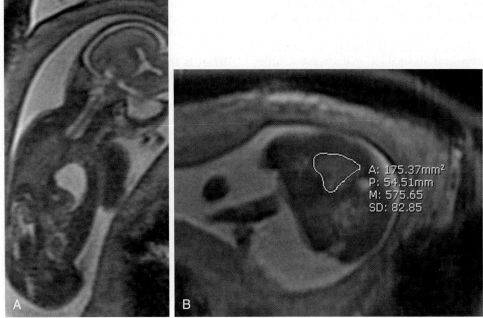

Fig. 23.18 Congenital diaphragmatic hernia (CDH), 20-week fetus. (A) Coronal T2-weighted image demonstrates the stomach and a portion of the left liver lobe herniating into the left hemithorax. (B) Axial T2-weighted image shows small bowel in the left hemithorax and a region of interest drawn around the normal right lung as part of volumetric analysis.

BOX 23.1 Congenital Diaphragmatic Hernia Checklist

Is the liver in the defect?
Is there a hernia sac?
What are the lung volumes?
Are there other congenital anomalies?

Another method of fetal lung volume quantification involves comparing the TFLV with the summed total thoracic volume less the mediastinal volume, termed the *expected lung volume*. This requires drawing three sets of regions of interest: lung, thorax, and mediastinum. If there are uncertainties regarding gestational age, this method may provide a viable alternative. A ratio of TFLV to expected lung volume of less than 0.15 is associated with a poorer prognosis.

ARE THERE OTHER ANOMALIES?

CDH can be associated with other anomalies that can affect prognosis and management. The most common associated abnormalities are cardiac, seen in approximately 35% of cases. Gastrointestinal and genitourinary anomalies are seen in approximately 10% of cases, including bowel atresias and lower urinary tract obstruction. There are syndromic associations, including Fryns syndrome, which can also present with nuchal thickening, pulmonary hypoplasia, and craniofacial abnormalities and has a poor prognosis.

Can Magnetic Resonance Imaging Help Determine Whether the Fetal Thorax Is Small?

Severe pulmonary hypoplasia of any etiology can have a poor prognosis. Causes of pulmonary hypoplasia can

be classified as intrathoracic or extrathoracic, of which CDH is considered an intrathoracic etiology. The previously described lung and mediastinal masses can also result in lung hypoplasia. Extrathoracic causes include oligohydramnios (as a result of urinary tract obstruction or prolonged rupture of membranes) or skeletal dysplasias (e.g., thanatophoric dysplasia or Jeune syndrome), which manifest with short ribs and a small thoracic cage; these are discussed further later in this chapter. Total lung volumes can be measured by MRI and compared with available normative data for gestational age. Fetal lung MRI volumetric measurements more than two standard deviations below the mean for gestational age may correlate with severe pulmonary hypoplasia.

What Might It Mean If the Heart Is Abnormally Positioned?

Once the fetus's left and right sides have been defined, correct cardiac position should be determined. There are three potential reasons the fetal cardiac axis is not oriented to the left: (1) there is an abnormality of situs, either situs inversus or heterotaxy; (2) there is an intrinsic abnormality of the heart; or (3) there is an abnormality in the fetal thorax causing the heart to shift. Any of the previously described thoracic lesions can cause mass effect, shifting the heart. Pulmonary agenesis, aplasia, or hypoplasia can cause the heart to deviate toward the absent or underdeveloped lung.

Can Esophageal Atresia Be Diagnosed by Fetal Magnetic Resonance Imaging?

Typically the normal esophagus is collapsed and not seen by ultrasound or MRI unless the fetus is imaged in the act of swallowing. Secondary findings, such as polyhydramnios and microgastria, can suggest the diagnosis of esophageal atresia. A dilated proximal esophageal pouch at times may be identified but typically is not a persistent finding (Fig. 23.19). Esophageal atresia should be considered if other anomalies of the VACTERL (vertebral anomalies, anal atresia, cardiac defects, tracheoesophageal fistula, esophageal atresia, renal and/or radial anomalies, and limb defects) association are present (Ethun et al., 2014).

Fetal Abdomen and Pelvis

What Do the Normal Gastrointestinal System Structures Look Like by Fetal Magnetic Resonance Imaging?

The liver should be visible predominantly in the right upper quadrant and will be of relatively homogeneous mild T1 hyperintensity and mild T2 hypointensity (Fig. 23.20A). The fetal gallbladder is usually identified during the second trimester as an ovoid T2-hyperintense/T1-hypointense structure (Fig. 23.20B). Later in gestational age, as the gallbladder improves in its ability to concentrate bile, it may become more T1 hyperintense and T2 hypointense, decreasing inherent contrast resolution with the adjacent liver. The gallbladder also becomes more efficient at contraction, and so may not be visible on all sequences later in gestation. The spleen is relatively T1 and T2 hypointense. The pancreas may be difficult to visualize particularly in second trimester studies and is relatively T2 hypointense and T1 hyperintense.

Fluid-filled stomach and small bowel are T2 hyperintense (see Fig. 23.20A). The small bowel should be predominantly left sided in the upper abdomen and more midline/right sided in the lower abdomen as the ileum approaches the cecum (Rubesova, 2012).

Meconium is high in signal intensity on T1-weighted images and low in signal intensity of T2-weighted sequences due to its proteinaceous contents; distal small bowel may also demonstrate similar signal intensity. Meconium signal should be present in the rectum by 20 weeks of gestation and geographically defined by being posterior to the bladder and extending approximately 1 cm below the bladder neck. As gestation progresses, more of the colon will fill with meconium in a retrograde fashion, with approximately half of all normal fetuses having a T1-hyperintense ascending colon by 31 weeks of gestation (see Fig. 23.21D–E) (Rubesova et al., 2009).

What Do the Normal Genitourinary System Structures Look Like?

The kidneys appear as relatively symmetrical intermediate signal intensity retroperitoneal structures with central T2-hyperintense fluid-filled pelvis (see Fig. 23.20C). Renal length in the craniocaudal dimension in millimeters is roughly equal to the gestational age in weeks. The adrenal glands are superior to the kidneys, best seen in the second trimester as T2-hypointense triangular structures. The ureters are typically not seen. The urinary bladder is a midline, fluid-filled pelvic structure with a thin wall (see Fig. 23.20A). The normal urethra should

not be visualized. The normal uterus and ovaries in the female fetus are very difficult to delineate. External genitalia should also be evaluated.

What Is the Differential Diagnosis for a Suprarenal Mass?

Suprarenal location of a mass portends a short differential diagnosis, which can be further narrowed by specific imaging findings (Box 23.2). First, determine whether the "suprarenal" mass is actually renal in origin. Potential renal etiologies include upper pole cystic dysplasia of a duplicated collecting system or urinoma as the result of urinary obstruction. These will appear hyperintense on T2-weighted images. Enteric duplication cysts may arise in the suprarenal region; ultrasound may demonstrate alternating bands of concentric echogenicity, although this is usually difficult to see prenatally.

Solid suprarenal masses include neuroblastoma or extralobar pulmonary sequestration, both of which will be relatively T2 hyperintense and T1 hypointense. Suprarenal neuroblastomas arise from the adrenal gland, so no normal adrenal gland will be noted adjacent to the mass. They are more commonly right sided (Fig. 23.21). Extralobar sequestrations are defined by a feeding vessel supplied by the systemic arterial system, which may manifest as an internal flow void on T2 images. They are more commonly found on the left. An additional consideration for a "solid" renal mass is adrenal hemorrhage. When the hemorrhage is subacute, the blood products may be high signal on T1-weighted images and low signal on T2-weighted images.

An adrenal "mass" that retains its adeniform shape may represent an enlarged adrenal gland (Maki et al., 2014). Among considerations for this finding are congenital adrenal hyperplasia and BWS. Congenital adrenal hyperplasia may present with ambiguous genitalia. In BWS, entities such as macroglossia and hemihypertrophy may also be seen.

An Upper Abdominal Cystic Mass Is Present, What Might This Be?

The first determination to make regarding a cystic upper abdominal lesion is whether this "mass" is, in fact, bowel, such as a dilated duodenum. A fluid-containing structure connecting with the stomach clinches the diagnosis of duodenal atresia, forming the classic "double bubble" (Fig. 23.22). Duodenal atresia is prevalent in trisomy 21, and thus other related abnormalities should be sought. The differential diagnosis includes duodenal stenosis or web, annular pancreas, preduodenal portal vein, and malrotation with Ladd bands. Distinguishing these entities prenatally is typically not possible, but all require surgery shortly after birth.

Other cystic upper abdominal masses include choledochal cysts and enteric duplication cysts. Choledochal cysts form as the result of cystic dilatation of a portion of the biliary tree. Enteric duplication cysts may arise anywhere along the gastrointestinal tract. Lymphatic malformations may also arise in the abdomen (Fig. 23.23).

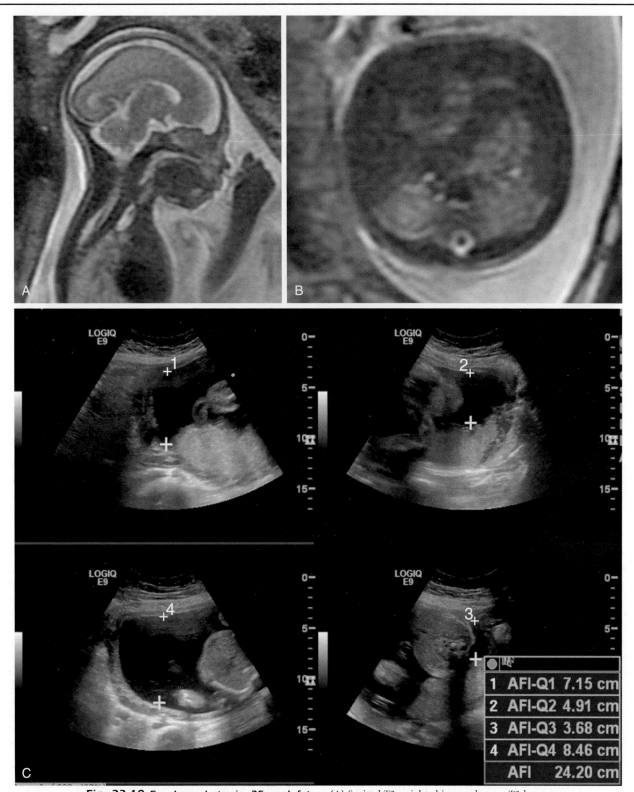

Fig. 23.19 Esophageal atresia, 25-week fetus. (A) Sagittal T2-weighted image shows a T2-hyperintense structure in the upper mediastinum compatible with an esophageal pouch. (B) Axial T2-weighted image in the upper abdominal region shows a collapsed stomach with no discernible fluid. (C) Ultrasound image demonstrates an elevated amniotic fluid index, the result of impaired swallowing caused by esophageal atresia.

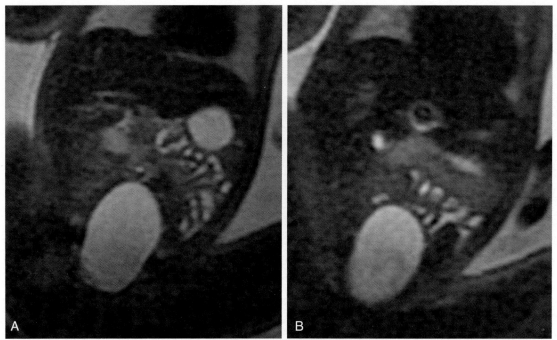

Fig. 23.20 Normal fetal abdomen and pelvis, 32-week fetus. (A) Coronal T2-weighted image demonstrates a hypointense liver in the right upper quadrant, a fluid-filled stomach in the left upper quadrant, and multiple nondilated small bowel loops in the left hemiabdomen. (B) Coronal T2-weighted image slightly more anterior to (A) shows a small round T2-hyperintense structure in the right upper quadrant consistent with the gallbladder.

Can Distal Bowel Obstruction Be Diagnosed Prenatally?

Fetal small bowel loops are considered dilated when they measure more than 7 mm in diameter. Fetal colonic loops are dilated when they measure more than 15 mm. With bowel obstruction, proximal bowel loops are dilated and distal bowel loops are decompressed beyond a transition zone. Jejunal atresia may present as a "triple bubble," with the three cystic upper abdominal "masses" representing the dilated stomach, duodenum, and proximal jejunum, respectively (Fig. 23.24). More distal small bowel obstructions may be a result of ileal atresia or meconium ileus. In these cases the colon may appear small with minimal meconium filling the distal loops because of the obstruction proximal to the ileocecal valve.

Very distal colonic obstruction, such as anal atresia or Hirschsprung disease, may not be identified on prenatal imaging (Alamo et al., 2013). A patent anal canal is functionally obstructed in the fetus, and so it may be difficult to distinguish between a normal anus, imperforate anus, and rectum devoid of ganglion cells. These diagnoses could be suggested if rectal meconium is not present or if the distal sigmoid is unusually prominent (Fig. 23.25). When there are additional findings of syndromic associations, such as VACTERL or OEIS (omphalocele, cloacal exstrophy, imperforate anus, and spinal dysraphism), the lack of distal meconium is more likely to suggest anal atresia. One very specific finding is the presence of calcifications within the bowel lumen as the result of admixture of urine and meconium related to a colovesical fistula (Capito et al., 2014). These may appear as discrete T2 hypointensities, and correlation with ultrasound may be helpful to better define these calcifications within a urine-filled colon.

What Is the Spectrum of Abdominal Wall Abnormalities, and What Should Be Reported?

Abdominal wall defects may be distinguished by location, relationship to the insertion of the umbilical cord, covering membrane, and nature of the herniated contents. The two most common ventral abdominal wall defects are omphalocele and gastroschisis. Omphaloceles are midline herniations of abdominal contents covered by peritoneum (Fig. 23.26). The umbilical cord inserts into the hernia. Gastroschisis is a paramidline defect through which primarily bowel herniates and is not covered by a membrane (Fig. 23.27). The umbilical cord inserts adjacent to the abdominal wall defect.

Omphaloceles have a higher association with aneuploidy and syndromes, making comprehensive assessment for other abnormalities critical in the assessment of outcome. Associations include BWS, Turner syndrome, and various aneuploidies, such as trisomy 18 and 21. There is a high risk for cardiac defects; thus, a fetal echocardiogram should be performed in these cases.

Gastroschisis is believed to result from a vascular insult later in gestation and thus is not associated with aneuploidy and other anomalies (Brugger and Prayer, 2011). It is more commonly found in younger mothers and tends to be sporadic.

A midline abdominal wall defect inferior to the umbilicus may be a manifestation of bladder exstrophy,

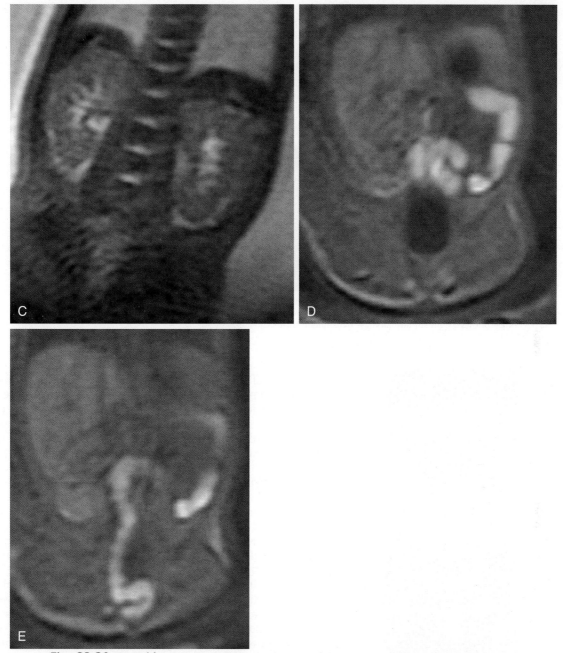

Fig. 23.20—cont'd (C) Coronal T2-weighted image of the retroperitoneum demonstrates normal kidneys that are symmetrical in size and homogeneous in parenchymal signal intensity with nondilated, fluid-filled pelvis. (D, E) Coronal T1-weighted images demonstrate hyperintense meconium signal throughout nondilated loops of the colon to the level of the rectum.

BOX 23.2   Differential Diagnosis for Fetal Supra-renal Lesions

Neuroblastoma
Extralobar pulmonary sequestration
Adrenal hemorrhage
Adrenal hyperplasia
Enteric duplication cyst
Renal upper pole cystic dysplasia (mimic)

which results from a defect in the cloacal membrane and subsequent eversion of bladder mucosa. A fluid-filled bladder will not be seen, and some tissue may be noted bulging below the cord insertion (Fig. 23.28). The kidneys are often normal, making the diagnosis difficult if the absent bladder is not noticed (Goldman et al., 2013).

Cloacal exstrophy is a rare and severe disorder affecting the infraumbilical mesoderm and both the

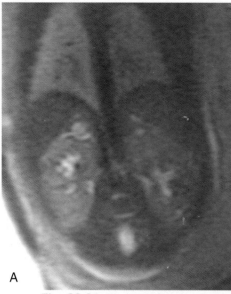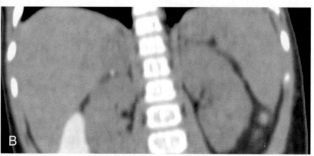

A
B

Fig. 23.21 Congenital neuroblastoma, 36-week fetus. (A) Coronal T2-weighted image demonstrates a solid right suprarenal mass. (B) Coronal computed tomography image of the child at 8 months of age shows a right suprarenal mass with calcifications.

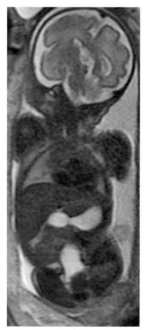

Fig. 23.22 Duodenal atresia, 30-week fetus. Coronal T2-weighted image demonstrates a "double bubble" consisting of a dilated stomach connected with a dilated proximal duodenum.

genitourinary and gastrointestinal tracts. Imaging findings include a lower anterior abdominal wall defect and absent fluid-filled bladder. MRI is particularly useful in demonstrating the lack of meconium signal in the rectosigmoid (Calvo-Garcia et al., 2013). The prolapsed blind-ending terminal ileum that herniates through the defect is difficult to see by both ultrasound and MRI. Normal external genitalia will not be seen. Cloacal exstrophy can be associated with anomalies of OEIS complex, which include omphalocele, imperforate anus, and spinal dysraphism (Fig. 23.29) (Winkler et al., 2012).

The most severe ventral wall defect, "limb-body wall complex," results from early failure of the major embryological folds to fuse. A majority of internal viscera projects outside of the fetal body. An unusually short umbilical cord is also seen. Major limb malformations, such as complete absence, and severe scoliosis may also result.

What Do Large Kidneys Signify?

When renal lengths measure more than two standard deviations above expected for gestational age, it must first be determined whether hydronephrosis is present; this is discussed in a subsequent section. A duplex collecting system can also result in a larger-than-expected kidney and may be a bilateral finding.

In the absence of hydronephrosis or duplex collecting systems, bilateral nephromegaly is most likely syndromic or genetic. Polycystic renal disease, both autosomal recessive and dominant forms, may present in fetal life as large kidneys with possibly some macrocysts (Chung et al., 2014). Autosomal recessive polycystic kidney disease may appear normal in the early second trimester and grow later in gestation. Because cysts are predominantly tiny, the kidneys typically manifest diffusely increased T2 signal with loss of corticomedullary differentiation (Fig. 23.30). Hepatic fibrosis is a rare manifestation of prenatal onset disease. Autosomal dominant polycystic kidney disease rarely presents prenatally, but when it does may have a similar appearance to autosomal recessive polycystic kidney disease. The characteristic large cysts seen postnatally and in adults are later findings. Close attention to family history should help clarify the diagnosis. Other rare genetic syndromes may also present as bilateral renal enlargement, such as Meckel-Gruber syndrome, and so a search for a posterior encephalocele and polydactyly is required. BWS may also present with large kidneys, which should otherwise be normal in signal intensity.

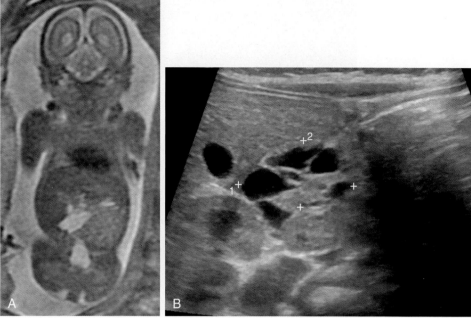

Fig. 23.23 Right upper quadrant lymphatic malformation, 23-week fetus. (A) Coronal T2-weighted image shows a cystic lesion in the right upper quadrant. The gallbladder and duodenum were identified separately. (B) Postnatal ultrasound image of the same lesion better demonstrates multiple septations.

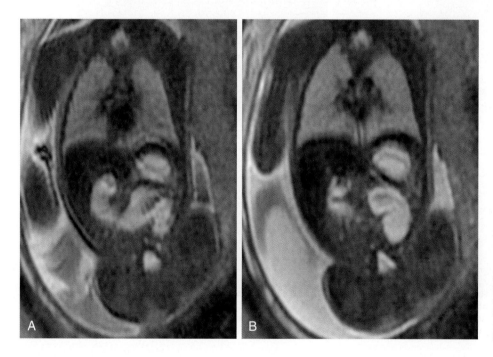

Fig. 23.24 Jejunal atresia, 28-week fetus. (A) Coronal T2-weighted image demonstrates a dilated fluid-filled stomach and duodenal sweep. (B) More anterior image shows a dilated proximal jejunum abruptly tapering.

What Is the Best Approach for the Evaluation of Hydronephrosis?

When hydronephrosis is believed to be present, it is important to first exclude multicystic dysplastic kidney (MCDK). The key is to assess the relationship between cysts; cysts that do not connect with the renal pelvis are more likely a manifestation of MCDK (Fig. 23.31). MCDK will typically involute postnatally. Bilateral MCDK is rare but when present is lethal. MRI, because of its ability to evaluate the fetus even with oligohydramnios, at times is superior to ultrasound in assessing the renal pathology in these fetuses.

Once hydronephrosis has been confirmed, the differential diagnosis will depend on three additional clinical and imaging features: fetal sex, involvement of the ureter(s) and bladder or not, and unilateral versus bilateral (Clayton and Brock, 2014) (Box 23.3).

WHAT IS THE SEX OF THE FETUS?

The differential diagnosis of hydronephrosis is more extensive in males. Two entities must be considered that would not be considerations in female fetuses: posterior urethral valves and prune belly syndrome. Posterior urethral valves occur at the prostatic urethra, causing

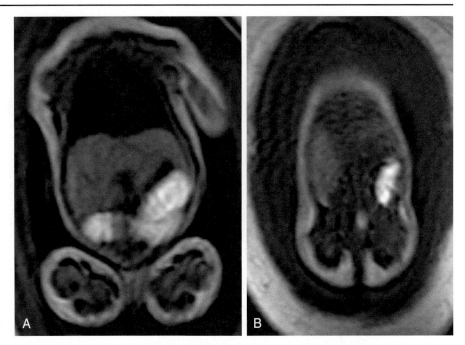

Fig. 23.25 Anal atresia, 31-week fetus. (A, B) Coronal T1-weighted images demonstrate hyperintense meconium within dilated loops of distal colon and no discernible meconium signal in the low posterior pelvis.

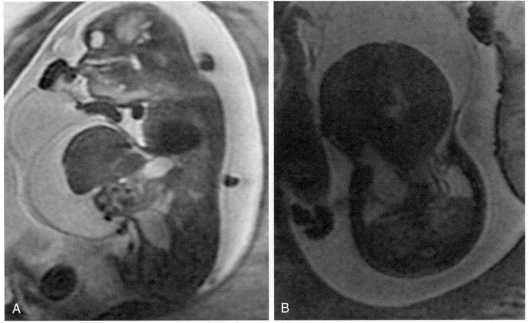

Fig. 23.26 Omphalocele, 32-week fetus. (A, B) Sagittal (A) and axial (B) T2-weighted images show a large midline abdominal wall defect with numerous bowel loops and liver extending beyond the confines of the body wall with a discrete covering membrane.

obstruction of the urinary system (Fig. 23.32). Prune belly syndrome involves replacement of smooth muscle of the urinary tract by connective tissue, making the system patulous. Both may manifest with bilateral hydroureteronephrosis and bladder enlargement. Prune belly syndrome is rarely seen in girls.

Megacystis-microcolon-intestinal hypoperistalsis syndrome is an autosomal recessive condition with a strong predilection for females. The genetic defect results in a smooth muscle myopathy. Imaging findings include enlargement of the bladder, urinary tracts, and small bowel.

If genitalia are truly ambiguous, cloacal malformation should be considered (see later).

ARE THE URETER(S) AND/OR BLADDER DILATED?

Further downstream dilatation of the urinary tract implies obstruction distal to the kidney. Bladder dilatation can be caused by obstruction at the urethral level, such as in posterior urethral valves, and can also be seen in prune belly syndrome and megacystis-microcolon-intestinal hypoperistalsis syndrome. Ureteral dilatation without bladder dilatation can be seen with

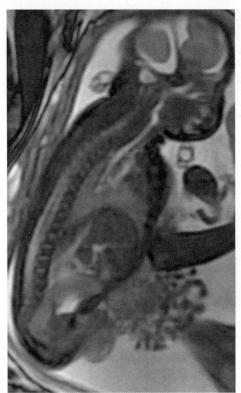

Fig. 23.27 Gastroschisis, 31-week fetus. Sagittal steady-state free precession image demonstrates bowel herniating through an anterior abdominal wall defect with no covering identified. The liver remains normally positioned.

ureterovesical junction obstruction, vesicoureteral reflux, and primary megaureter. If hydroureter is present, it is important to evaluate for a duplex collecting system. If the ureters are nondilated, hydronephrosis may be caused by ureteropelvic junction obstruction or vesicoureteral reflux.

IS THE HYDRONEPHROSIS UNILATERAL OR BILATERAL?

Entities that cause obstruction distal to the bladder level will most likely result in bilateral hydronephrosis. Outcome is more worrisome if both kidneys are obstructed. Any other entity causing hydronephrosis may be unilateral or bilateral.

In the setting of hydronephrosis, it is important to analyze the kidneys for the presence of macrocysts, which may indicate obstructive cystic dysplasia, a poor prognostic sign. Amniotic fluid levels must be followed. In severe urinary system obstruction, oligohydramnios may develop, which can lead to pulmonary hypoplasia.

What Might a Cystic Mass in the Lower Abdomen or Pelvis Be?

When a cystic mass is identified in the lower fetal abdomen or pelvis, knowing the sex of the fetus is important. If the fetus is female, the diagnosis is most commonly an ovarian cyst. If the cyst is in the pelvis in a female, vaginal and uterine anomalies should be considered as well.

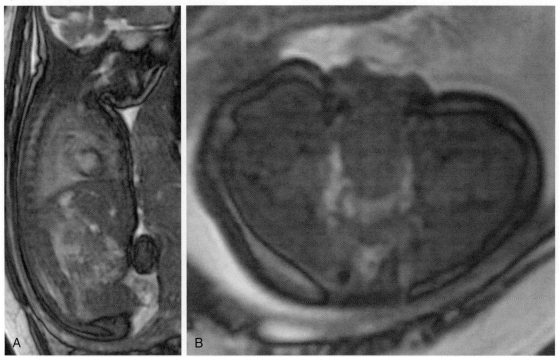

Fig. 23.28 Bladder exstrophy, 29-week fetus. (A, B) Sagittal (A) and axial (B) steady-state free precession images demonstrate an infraumbilical abdominal wall defect with herniating soft tissue and no normal bladder identified.

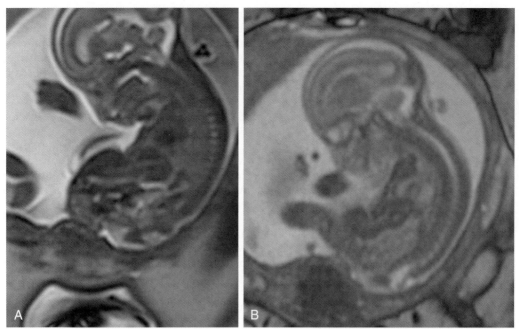

Fig. 23.29 OEIS (omphalocele, cloacal exstrophy, imperforate anus, and spinal dysraphism) complex, 18-week fetus. (A) Sagittal paramidline T2-weighted image demonstrates an omphalocele-containing bowel and more than half of the liver. (B) Sagittal midline T2-weighted image shows a low neural tube defect and absence of the urinary bladder. No meconium signal was seen in the expected region of the rectum, suggesting imperforate anus.

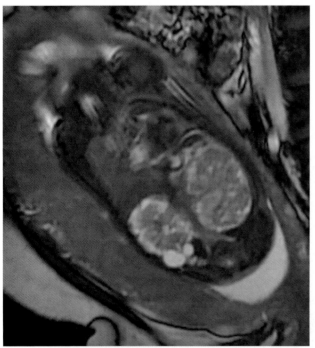

Fig. 23.30 Autosomal recessive polycystic kidney disease, 30-week fetus. Coronal steady-state free precession image demonstrates enlarged heterogeneous kidneys with a few macrocysts.

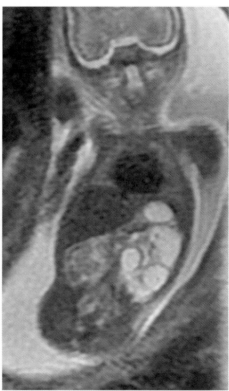

Fig. 23.31 Multicystic dysplastic kidney, 20-week fetus. Coronal T2-weighted image demonstrates multiple large discrete noncommunicating cysts in the left renal fossa with no discernible normal renal parenchyma.

Ovarian cysts typically manifest as thin-walled, round, T2 high signal abdominopelvic cysts. As ovarian cysts increase in size, they tend to move superiorly into the abdomen (Fig. 23.33). They are believed to arise as the result of stimulation by circulating maternal hormones. If homogeneous, they are simple cysts that involute after delivery. If complex, there may have been internal hemorrhage and possibly ovarian torsion.

If there is a partially T1-hyperintense cystic mass, diagnosis of meconium pseudocyst can be suggested, particularly if there is an abnormal appearance of the bowel.

A T2-hyperintense "mass" in the midline pelvis of a female fetus may be a hydrocolpos or hydrometrocolpos, the result of distal obstruction of the female genital tract. Hydrocolpos refers to dilatation of the vagina, and hydrometrocolpos involves the uterus as well. Potential causes include imperforate hymen, transverse vaginal septum, and vaginal stenosis. Often these are associated with renal anomalies, renal agenesis, or urogenital sinus anomaly.

A midline pelvic cystic "mass" may rarely signify a much more complex embryological disorder: cloacal

malformation. This entity is distinct from cloacal exstrophy, described earlier, because it does not involve a defect of the anterior abdominal wall. Rather, the urinary, genital, and gastrointestinal tracts join to form a common channel, the cloaca, which does not appropriately partition in utero. The "mass" is usually a complex hydrocolpos with a fluid–debris level. The bladder will be present but will connect with the cloaca. The urinary tracts are typically dilated. The distal hindgut may be dilated as it approaches the cloaca with loss of the normal expected hyperintense meconium signal on T1-weighted images. Oligohydramnios may develop, resulting in pulmonary hypoplasia. Genitalia are ambiguous.

The differential diagnoses for lower abdominopelvic cysts include lymphatic malformations and enteric duplication cysts. Lymphatic malformations are typically multiseptate and often are transspatial/multicompartmental. If they bleed, they may contain fluid–fluid levels. Enteric duplication cysts arise from the embryological foregut and can be found anywhere in the chest, abdomen, or pelvis.

What Is the Differential Diagnosis for a Presacral Mass?

The presacral region is the most common location of the most common fetal tumor, the teratoma (Kocaoglu and Frush, 2006). Teratomas are believed to arise from aberrantly located primordial germ cells that were not appropriately incorporated into the primitive sex cords to form the fetal gonads and subsequently did not degenerate. They contain derivatives of all three germ cell layers: ectoderm, mesoderm, and endoderm.

MRI will demonstrate a heterogeneous presacral mass, potentially with both solid and cystic components. They may also contain fat, which will be bright on T1-weighted images. Among the important observations to provide for prognosis are the relative

---

BOX 23.3 Causes of Fetal Hydronephrosis

Ureteropelvic junction obstruction
Vesicoureteral reflux
Ureterovesical junction obstruction
Posterior urethral valves
Prune belly syndrome
Megacystis-microcolon-intestinal hypoperistalsis syndrome
Cloacal malformation
Multicystic dysplastic kidney (mimic)

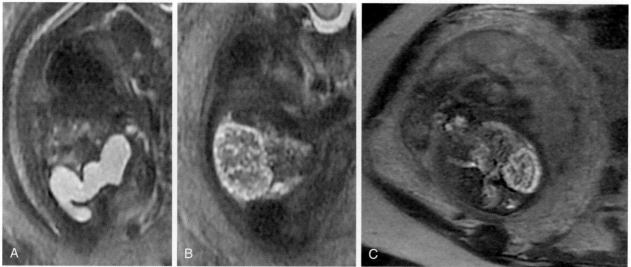

Fig. 23.32 Posterior urethral valves, 25-week fetus. (A) Sagittal T2-weighted paramidline image demonstrates dilatation of the left renal collecting system, urinary bladder, and proximal urethra in this male fetus. (B) Sagittal T2-weighted image shows numerous cysts throughout the left kidney consistent with obstructive cystic dysplasia. (C) Axial T2-weighted larger field-of-view image demonstrates virtually no amniotic fluid.

proportions of cystic and solid components, the relative proportions of internal and external components, and the presence of complicating factors, such as hydrops and polyhydramnios. Correlative ultrasound is important to assess vascularity. Teratomas with greater cystic components tend to have a better prognosis, presumably because solid components have the potential to be very vascular and cause a "steal" phenomenon, which

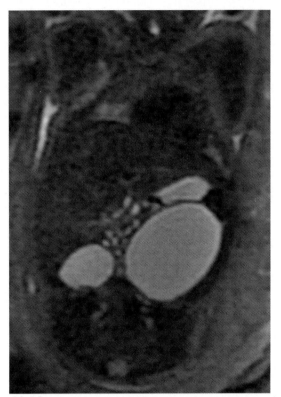

Fig. 23.33 Ovarian cysts, 33-week fetus. Coronal T2-weighted image demonstrates bilateral simple cysts in the midabdomen. Ovarian cysts move superiorly into the abdomen as they get larger.

can lead to heart failure. Hydrops would develop as a result. The proportion of internal and external components of the teratoma has greater implications postnatally, because a larger internal component portends a higher probability of malignant transformation. Total size is important to report but does not correlate well with prognosis. Very large tumors may, however, predispose to dystocia and make cesarian section a necessity for delivery (Fig. 23.34).

The primary differential diagnosis for a fetal presacral mass is an anterior myelomeningocele, which should also demonstrate intracranial findings of Chiari type II malformation. A potential imaging pitfall is intraspinal extension of a primarily cystic teratoma that may be mistaken for a myelomeningocele. These, however, would not demonstrate the posterior fossa findings characteristic of Chiari type II.

What Other Visceral Abdominopelvic Neoplasms May Present in Fetal Life?

IN THE LIVER
Fetal hepatic masses include infantile hepatic hemangioma (also known as infantile hemangioendothelioma), mesenchymal hamartoma, and hepatoblastoma. Infantile hepatic hemangiomas are typically hyperintense on T2-weighted images with vascular flow voids possibly seen in larger lesions (Fig. 23.35). They should be relatively hypointense to normal liver on T1-weighted sequences with possible areas of internal T1-hyperintense hemorrhage. They have the potential to cause significant arteriovenous shunting, which could lead to fetal heart failure and the development of hydrops. Mesenchymal hamartomas are predominantly cystic lesions that may also predispose to hydrops because of fluid shifts into the cystic component. Hepatoblastomas are malignant tumors that have a poor prognosis in the prenatal period. They are solid, heterogeneous masses with a pseudocapsule that gives the appearance of a well-demarcated lesion. They may contain calcifications and may bleed, leading to potentially serious complications (Woodward et al., 2005).

Fig. 23.34 Sacrococcygeal teratoma, 36-week fetus. (A, B) Axial (A) and sagittal (B) T2-weighted images demonstrate a predominantly cystic presacral mass with large external component.

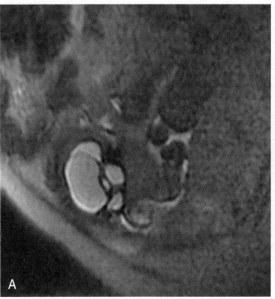

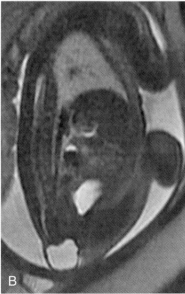

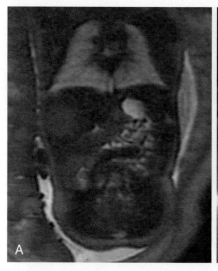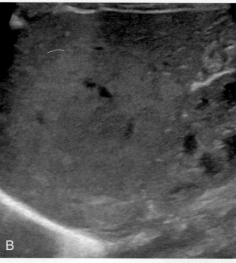

Fig. 23.35 *Infantile hepatic hemangioma, 37-week fetus.* (A) Coronal T2-weighted image demonstrates round T2-hyperintense signal in the right liver lobe. (B) Postnatal ultrasound image shows a circumscribed hepatic mass with prominent internal hypoechoic areas that proved to be blood vessels.

IN THE KIDNEY

The most common fetal renal mass is a mesoblastic nephroma, a usually benign hamartomatous lesion. They are commonly large, well-circumscribed, solid lesions that involve at least half of a kidney. Polyhydramnios is a frequent associated finding, although the etiology is not well understood.

Fetal Musculoskeletal System

Is Magnetic Resonance Imaging Useful in Evaluating the Fetal Musculoskeletal System?

Ultrasound remains the mainstay of fetal musculoskeletal system evaluation; however, MRI applications are continuing to grow. MRI is particularly helpful in providing large field-of-view looks at the fetal skeleton.

The fetal skeleton is not well imaged in the second trimester on conventional MRI sequences. Echoplanar imaging is useful in accentuating contrast between fetal bone and cartilage. Cartilage is hyperintense and bone is hypointense on this sequence. Muscle is of intermediate to low signal intensity on T1- and T2-weighted sequences.

On fetal MRI studies, the presence of each extremity and its components should be documented. Cine images will help establish fetal movement, an adjunct to ultrasound.

Is There a Role for Magnetic Resonance Imaging in the Evaluation of Skeletal Dysplasias?

Ultrasound remains the workhorse in the evaluation of skeletal dysplasias. MRI can be useful at times in identifying other anomalies that can pinpoint the diagnosis. It may also be helpful if ultrasound is limited, for example, in the setting of oligohydramnios. The use of MRI in skeletal dysplasia evaluation continues to be developed (Fig. 23.36). CT has also been used in cases of fetal skeletal dysplasia, with the understanding of radiation concerns.

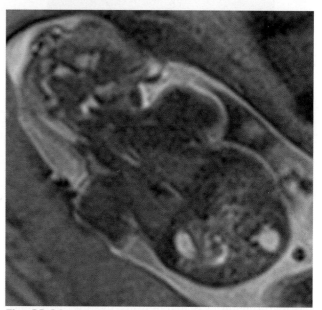

Fig. 23.36 *Thanatophoric dysplasia, 22-week fetus.* Coronal T2-weighted image demonstrates a small, narrow thorax in this fetus with a lethal skeletal dysplasia.

How Might Magnetic Resonance Imaging Aid the Assessment of Fetal Clubfoot?

Clubfoot, also known as talipes equinovarus, is an abnormality of foot alignment composed of hindfoot equinus, hindfoot varus, and forefoot varus. The diagnosis is typically made with ultrasound, although a study by (Nemec et al., 2012) demonstrated that MRI can aid in confirming equivocal ultrasound cases and can help identify concurrent abnormalities (Nemec et al., 2015) (Fig. 23.37). Clubfoot may be an isolated anomaly, but could also have associations with aneuploidy, brain and spine anomalies, and systemic musculoskeletal disorders.

What Soft Tissue Tumors May Be Encountered in the Musculoskeletal System?

A variety of benign and malignant soft tissue tumors may be seen in the musculoskeletal system of the fetus. Fibrous tumors are characteristically of homogeneous

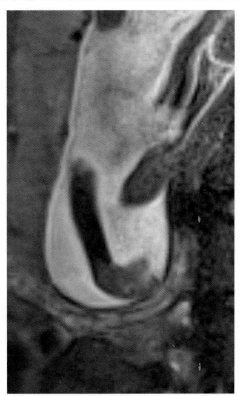

Fig. 23.37 Clubfoot, 20-week fetus. Coronal T2-weighted image demonstrates equinovarus positioning of the right foot. This fetus had other limb anomalies as well believed to be related to amniotic bands.

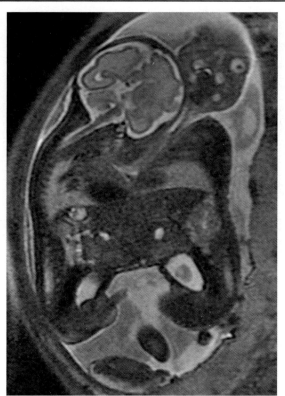

Fig. 23.38 Conjoined twins, 29-week fetuses. Sagittal T2-weighted image demonstrates conjoined twins sharing a liver. These twins were successfully separated postnatally.

low signal intensity on all sequences and may have an infiltrative appearance. Their malignant counterpart, fibrosarcoma, is more likely to be large and heterogeneous in signal intensity. Rhabdomyosarcomas may also appear heterogeneous and can arise almost anywhere in the musculoskeletal system, neck, face, and retroperitoneum. Vascular lesions include hemangiomas, lymphatic malformations, and hemangiopericytomas. Lymphatic malformations have been discussed previously. Hemangiomas are T2-hyperintense lesions that may contain flow voids, also discussed previously. Hemangiopericytomas arise from capillary mesenchymal cells called pericytes and tend to behave in a benign fashion in the fetus, as opposed to those that arise postnatally.

Multifetal Gestations

What Is the Role of Magnetic Resonance Imaging in Multifetal Gestations?
Specific indications for fetal MRI of multifetal gestations include assessment of monochorionic pregnancies at risk for twin–twin transfusion syndrome (Hu et al., 2006). MRI is also indicated for any reason applicable to a singleton pregnancy.

In twin–twin transfusion syndrome, arteriovenous anastomoses within the placenta result in shunting of blood from one fetus to another, resulting in asymmetrical fetal size and complications of hypovolemia in the donor twin and hypervolemia in the recipient twin. Among the available interventions is laser ablation of the culprit vessels. MRI may be indicated for procedural planning to help the fetal surgeon guide a safe and effective approach.

Co-twin demise in a monochorionic pregnancy may place the living twin at risk. The primary mechanism is infarction of major organs, possibly because of loss of circulatory equilibrium between the fetuses. MRI may be indicated to provide a better assessment of the living fetus for evidence of infarctions and to more accurately determine prognosis.

Fetal MRI is useful in the evaluation of conjoined twins for delivery and preoperative planning. With larger field-of-view images and superior anatomic information, MRI is useful to pediatric surgeons for planning interventions and counseling parents more effectively as to the risks of a separation operation (Fig. 23.38).

■ Summary

Fetal MRI has become an important prenatal diagnostic tool used in conjunction with and extension from fetal ultrasound. Additional information is gained for appropriate prognosis, delivery, and perinatal care. Understanding of fetal magnetic resonance techniques and images is relatable to pediatric imaging and the varied syndromic and congenital diagnoses seen in our field.

Bibliography

ACR–SPR Practice Parameter for the Safe and Optimal Performance of Fetal Magnetic Resonance Imaging (MRI). American College of Radiology. https://www.acr.org/-/media~/ACR/Files/Practice-Parameters/mr-fetal.pdf Revised 2020 (Resolution 45)

.Alamo, L., Meyrat, B. J., Meuwly, J. Y., et al. (2013). Anorectal malformations: Finding the pathway out of the labyrinth. *RadioGraphics, 33*(2), 491–512.

Allen, B. C., & Leyendecker, J. R. (2013). Placental evaluation with magnetic resonance. *Radiol Clin North Am, 51*(6), 955–966.

Arangio, P., Manganaro, L., Pacifici, A., et al. (2013). Importance of fetal MRI in evaluation of craniofacial deformities. *Journal of Craniofacial Surgery, 24*(3), 773–776.

Bahado-Singh, R. O., & Goncalves, L. F. (2013). Techniques, terminology, and indications for MRI in pregnancy. *Seminars in Perinatology, 37*(5), 334–339.

Barth, R. A. (2012). Imaging of fetal chest masses. *Pediatric Radiology, 42*(Suppl. 1), S62–S73.

Brugger, P. C., & Prayer, D. (2011). Development of gastroschisis as seen by magnetic resonance imaging. *Ultrasound in Obstetrics and Gynecology, 37*(4), 463–470.

Bulas, D., & Egloff, A. (2013). Benefits and risks of MRI in pregnancy. *Seminars in Perinatology, 37*(5), 301–304.

Calvo-Garcia, M. A., Kline-Fath, B. M., Rubio, E. I., et al. (2013). Fetal MRI of cloacal exstrophy. *Pediatric Radiology, 43*(5), 593–604.

Capito, C., Belarbi, N., Paye Jaouen, A., et al. (2014). Prenatal pelvic MRI: Additional clues for assessment of urogenital obstructive anomalies. *Journal of Pediatric Urology, 10*(1), 162–166.

Chung, E. M., Conran, R. M., Schroeder, J. W., et al. (2014). From the radiologic pathology archives: Pediatric polycystic kidney disease and other ciliopathies: Radiologic-pathologic correlation. *RadioGraphics, 34*(1), 155–178.

Clayton, D. B., & Brock, J. W., 3rd. (2014). Lower urinary tract obstruction in the fetus and neonate. *Clinics in Perinatology, 41*(3), 643–659.

Ethun, C. G., Fallon, S. C., Cassady, C. I., et al. (2014). Fetal MRI improves diagnostic accuracy in patients referred to a fetal center for suspected esophageal atresia. *Journal of Pediatric Surgery, 49*(5), 712–715.

Goldman, S., Szejnfeld, P. O., Rondon, A., et al. (2013). Prenatal diagnosis of bladder exstrophy by fetal MRI. *Journal of Pediatric Urology, 9*(1), 3–6.

Hu, L. S., Caire, J., & Twickler, D. M. (2006). MR findings of complicated multi-fetal gestations. *Pediatric Radiology, 36*(1), 76–81.

Kocaoglu, M., & Frush, D. P. (2006). Pediatric presacral masses. *RadioGraphics, 26*(3), 833–857.

Lapierre, C., Déry, J., Guérin, R., et al. (2010). Segmental approach to imaging of congenital heart disease. *RadioGraphics, 30*(2), 397–411.

Levine, D. (2013). Timing of MRI in pregnancy, repeat exams, access, and physician qualifications. *Seminars in Perinatology, 37*(5), 340–344.

Maki, E., Oh, K., Rogers, S., et al. (2014). Imaging and differential diagnosis of suprarenal masses in the fetus. *Journal of Ultrasound in Medicine, 33*(5), 895–904.

Mehollin-Ray, A. R., Cassady, C. I., Cass, D. L., et al. (2012). Fetal MR imaging of congenital diaphragmatic hernia. *RadioGraphics, 32*(4), 1067–1084.

Mirsky, D. M., Shekdar, K. V., & Bilaniuk, L. T. (2012). Fetal MRI: Head and neck. *Magn Reson Imaging Clin N Am, 20*(3), 605–618.

Nemec, U., Nemec, S. F., Brugger, P. C., et al. (2015). Normal mandibular growth and diagnosis of micrognathia at prenatal MRI. *Prenatal Diagnosis, 35*(2), 108–116.

Nemec, U., Nemec, S. F., Kasprian, G., et al. (2012). Clubfeet and associated abnormalities on fetal magnetic resonance imaging. *Prenatal Diagnosis, 32*(9), 822–828.

Pacharn, P., Kline-Fath, B., Calvo-Garcia, M., et al. (2013). Congenital lung lesions: Prenatal MRI and postnatal findings. *Pediatric Radiology, 43*(9), 1136–1143.

Rubesova, E. (2012). Fetal bowel anomalies—US and MR assessment. *Pediatric Radiology, 42*(Suppl. 1), S101–S106.

Rubesova, E., Vance, C. J., Ringertz, H. G., et al. (2009). Three-dimensional MRI volumetric measurements of the normal fetal colon. *American Journal of Roentgenology, 192*(3), 761–765.

Winkler, N. S., Kennedy, A. M., & Woodward, P. J. (2012). Cloacal malformation: Embryology, anatomy, and prenatal imaging features. *Journal of Ultrasound in Medicine, 31*(11), 1843–1855.

Woodward, P. J., Sohaey, R., Kennedy, A., et al. (2005). From the archives of the afip: A comprehensive review of fetal tumors with pathologic correlation. *RadioGraphics, 25*(1), 215–242.

Yinon, Y., Kelly, E., & Ryan, G. (2008). Fetal pleural effusions. *Best Practice & Research Clinical Obstetrics & Gynaecology, 22*(1), 77–96.

CHAPTER 24
Fetal CNS MRI

Nilesh K. Desai and Sarah Sarvis Milla

CHAPTER OUTLINE

Fetal Central Nervous System Magnetic Resonance Imaging Techniques, 473
At What Gestational Age Is Fetal Central Nervous System Magnetic Resonance Imaging Best Performed?, 473
What Are Common Indications for Fetal Central Nervous System Magnetic Resonance Imaging?, 473
What Protocol Should Be Used to Evaluate Fetal Central Nervous System Abnormalities?, 473

Fetal Central Nervous System: Normal Development, 473
What Is the Initial Approach to Evaluating the Fetal Brain on Magnetic Resonance Imaging?, 473

Ventriculomegaly, 475
What Is the Value of Fetal Magnetic Resonance Imaging in Evaluating Ventriculomegaly?, 475
How Do I Decide if the Ventriculomegaly Is Obstructive or Nonobstructive?, 475
Is the Corpus Callosum Normal?, 475
Are the Right and Left Cerebral Hemispheres and the Central Gray Matter Fully Divided?, 476
Is the Cavum Septum Pellucidum Present?, 478
Are There Small or Large Portions of the Lobar Cerebral Brain Parenchyma That Are Not Present?, 478
Are There Regions of Cortical Irregularity or Abnormal Layering and/or Dissimilarity to the Contralateral Side?, 479
Is One Ventricle Larger Than the Other?, 479
Are the Ventricle Margins Smooth and of Normal Signal Intensity?, 480
Is There a Solid and Cystic Intracranial Mass?, 481

Posterior Fossa, 481
Is There Cystic Enlargement of the Posterior Fossa?, 481
Does the Cystic Enlargement of the Posterior Fossa

Communicate With the Fourth Ventricle?, 482
Is There Elevation of the Torcular Herophili?, 482
Is the Vermis Normal?, 482
Are the Cerebellar Hemispheres Too Small?, 483
Are the Cerebellar Hemispheres Fused?, 483
Does the Brainstem Have a "Kinked" Appearance?, 484

Vascular, 484
Are There Abnormal Intracranial Flow Voids (e.g., Flow Voids That Are Too Large and/or Are Increased)?, 484
Is There a Vascular Nidus?, 484

Complication of Monochorionic Twin Pregnancy, 485
Are There Regions of Brain Destruction in a Monochorionic Pregnancy in the Living Fetus After One Fetus Dies?, 485

Head and Neck, 485
Is There a Midline Cystic Scalp Lesion?, 485
Is One or Both Globes Absent or Too Small?, 486
Is the Interocular or Binocular Distance Abnormal?, 486
Is There a Defect in the Upper Lip or Palate?, 486
Does the Mandible Appear Recessed or Too Small?, 487
Is a Cystic Head and Neck Mass Midline or off Midline?, 487
Does a Neck Mass Have Flow Voids?, 488
Are There Solid and Cystic Components?, 488

Spine, 488
Is There an Open Defect in the Lower Spine?, 488
Does the Spine Abruptly Stop Before the Coccyx?, 489
Is There a Segment of the Spine That Is Absent?, 489
Is There a Fluid-Filled Sac Anterior to the Sacrococcygeal Spine Separate From the Bladder?, 489

Summary, 489

Since first being performed in 1986, fetal MRI has rapidly become a standard of care for the secondary evaluation of fetal abnormalities involving the central nervous system (CNS) and thoracic and abdominopelvic cavities. Fetal MRI is most commonly performed for the evaluation of the fetal CNS when prenatal ultrasound demonstrates an abnormality. This chapter will provide an overview of fetal MRI by addressing foundations of fetal neuroimaging followed by a case-based approach to various disease entities of the brain and spine.

■ Fetal Central Nervous System Magnetic Resonance Imaging Techniques

At What Gestational Age Is Fetal Central Nervous System Magnetic Resonance Imaging Best Performed?

There are no known fetal contraindications to MRI at any gestational age. However, fetal CNS MRI before 20 weeks of gestation is of limited diagnostic value mainly because of the small size of the fetus and the noncompletion of organogenesis. Furthermore, fetal motion at such an early gestational age, even with single-shot techniques, makes imaging extremely difficult. Therefore, the majority of fetal CNS MRI is recommended at or after 20 weeks gestational age. Thereafter, fetal imaging should occur at a time point that not only best answers the question at hand but also provides information for management of the pregnancy. Most severe CNS malformations can be seen by 20 weeks of gestation. For these reasons, fetal CNS MRI commonly occurs between 20 and 24 weeks. It should be remembered, however, that there are diagnoses that may not be seen at such an early gestational age, including such things as cortical malformations that are focal or regional, gray matter heterotopia, subependymal nodules in tuberous sclerosis, and split cord malformations, among many others. Other times, it may be acceptable to both the patient and the ordering physician that fetal CNS MRI be performed late in the third trimester. For example, a fetus with mild ventriculomegaly for which expectant management is desired may be imaged late in the third trimester to then obviate the need for postnatal MRI. At other times, it may be critical for a fetus to be imaged late in the pregnancy just before delivery, for example, a fetus with a neck mass that warrants its evaluation with respect to the airway and for which an ex utero intrapartum treatment procedure is being contemplated. Other indications include maternal and/or fetal trauma, expected postnatal instability that would thwart a postnatal MRI and other expectant perinatal delivery management. Fetal MRI for CNS abnormality is usually not repeated during the pregnancy after the initial diagnostic fetal MRI, unless perinatal decisions would be affected, such as the one just described.

What Are Common Indications for Fetal Central Nervous System Magnetic Resonance Imaging?

The most common indication for fetal MRI is for the evaluation of cerebral ventriculomegaly. Under this premise, the primary clinical question is whether the ventriculomegaly is isolated (without identifiable cause or additional abnormalities) or nonisolated (with an underlying cause, such as aqueductal stenosis or additional abnormalities detected). Suspected corpus callosal abnormalities are a common indication, with the cavum septum pellucidum being an easily detected structure, and a marker of callosal development, on fetal ultrasound. Evaluation of the posterior fossa is also a common indication for fetal CNS imaging, which primarily involves evaluation of cerebellar development. Vascular abnormalities, including hemorrhage, malformations, and vascular insults, particularly as a complication of monochorionic twin pregnancies, are additional indications for fetal CNS evaluation. Fetal spine imaging typically serves to evaluate neural tube defects, scoliosis, and occasionally mass lesions, such as sacrococcygeal teratomas. Finally, evaluation of head and neck masses, especially their relation to the airway, encompass a small group of patients undergoing fetal imaging. An important point to make is that fetal MRI is indicated only when ultrasound adjunctive information is sought and when such information will have meaningful implications for patient care or counseling. Such implications include pregnancy management, mode or location of delivery, expected perinatal resuscitation needed (e.g., ex utero intrapartum treatment procedure), and parental education to include more accurate prognostication and to ultimately address parental anxiety.

What Protocol Should Be Used to Evaluate Fetal Central Nervous System Abnormalities?

The most important initial step in performing a successful fetal MRI after patient positioning is the ideal placement of the coil. The initial three-plane localizer should be used as a quick estimate of coil positioning with ideal placement resulting in clear visualization of the entirety of the gestational sac, preferably centered on the CNS structure in question. It is advisable that the radiologist be in a supervision position at the console or from the reading room as the technologist is performing the examination to evaluate the need for repeat sequences.

Standard protocols should exist for fetal imaging, including at least a body and CNS protocol. An example of a standard CNS protocol is listed in Table 24.1.

■ Fetal Central Nervous System: Normal Development

What Is the Initial Approach to Evaluating the Fetal Brain on Magnetic Resonance Imaging?

The initial approach to all fetal MRI is evaluation of the maternal anatomy, including evaluation of placenta location (and with twins, chorionicity and amnionicity), the subjective amount of amniotic fluid, the presence of a two- or three-vessel cord, gross evaluation of the cervix, and finally the evaluation of extrauterine pathology of the maternal pelvis and spine.

Next, attention to the fetal anatomy is warranted. Before evaluating the brain parenchyma, it is important to first determine situs. Although the initial temptation

TABLE 24.1   **Fetal Central Nervous System Imaging Protocol**

SEQUENCE	PLANE	TR (MS)	TE (MS)	VOXEL SIZE (MM)	COMMENT
Maternal gestational sac localizer	Axial, sagittal, coronal	6.7	2.95	1.8 × 1.8 × 7.0	Entire uterus/pelvis
T2 HASTE	Axial	700	133	1.0 × 1.0 × 7.0	Entire uterus/pelvis
T1 FLASH	Axial	125	1.86	1.3 × 1.3 × 7.0	Entire uterus/pelvis
Fetal TrueFISP localizer	Axial, sagittal, coronal	3.2	1.6	3.5 × 3.5 × 7.0	Entire fetus
Fetal brain localizer	Axial, sagittal, coronal	3.2	1.6	3.5 × 3.5 × 2.0	Fetal brain
T2 HASTE	Axial, sagittal, coronal	1000	133	1.0 × 1.0 × 3.0 or 1.0 × 1.0 × 2.0	Fetal brain
T1 FLASH	Axial	110	2.5	1.2 × 1.2 × 4.0	Fetal brain
DWI/ADC MAP	Axial	5500	129	2.0 × 2.0 × 4.0	Fetal brain
Spine localizer	Axial, sagittal, coronal	3.2	1.6	3.5 × 3.5 × 7.0	Fetal spine
T2 HASTE	Sagittal	1000	133	1.0 × 1.0 × 3.0	Fetal spine
TrueFISP	Sagittal	3.90	1.95	1.0 × 1.0 × 3.0	Fetal spine
T2 HASTE	Axial, coronal	1000	133	1.0 × 1.0 × 3.0	Fetal abdomen and thorax
T1 FLASH	Sagittal	3.9	1.95	1.3 × 1.3 × 5.0	Fetal abdomen and thorax

DWI, Diffusion-weighted imaging; *TE,* echo time; *TR,* repetition time.

is to identify the cardiac apex, the liver, and stomach to decide on brain sidedness, this should not be performed because a fetus may have situs inversus. Instead, it is best to determine by orienting to the fetus in three dimensions. By determining whether the fetus is breech or cephalic in presentation and on which side of the maternal pelvis the fetus lies, the radiologist can determine situs.

Evaluation of the brain then involves a thorough biometric evaluation of the fetal brain. Biometric evaluation includes measurement of the cerbral biparietal diameter (BPD), bone parietal diameter, frontooccipital diameter (FOD), corpus callosal length (AP length).

Additional biometrics that should be performed include the greatest transverse dimension of the cerebellum measured in the axial plane, the transverse cerebellar dimension (TCD). The cisterna magna (CM) should also be measured and should not exceed 10 mm. Measurements of the TCD and CM are shown in Figure 24.1. Other biometrics include cranial caudal and AP measurements of the vermis and pons. Nomograms for these measurements are readily available in definitive fetal textbooks. Beth Kline Fath et al. Fundamental and Advanced Fetal Imaging Ultrasound and MRI 2015).

And finally, the lateral ventricles are measured typically in the coronal plane at its maximal transverse width at the level of the atrium. Coronal measurements have been shown to be highly concordant with axial measurements of ultrasound. Lateral ventricles less than 10 mm are considered normal. Ventricles between 10 and 12 mm represent mild ventriculomegaly, between 12 and 15 mm moderate ventriculomegaly, and greater than 15 mm severe ventriculomegaly. Some authors simplify this scheme and classify mild ventriculomegaly as ventricles between 10 and 15 mm and severe ventriculomegaly as greater than 15 mm. The third and fourth

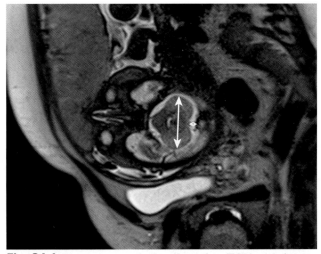

Fig. 24.1 Transverse cerebellar dimension (TCD) and cisterna magna (CM). The TCD is measured at the greatest transverse dimension of the cerebellum (*long arrow*). The CM is measured at midline (*short arrow*).

ventricles are not typically quantitatively measured, although both should be qualitatively assessed as being normal or enlarged.

The initial evaluation of the fetal brain is not complete until the gyral/sulcal pattern of the brain is evaluated and compared with expected for the given gestational age. Although a detailed discussion of normal gyration and sulcation as a function of gestational age is beyond the scope of this chapter, there exists multiple excellent atlases on normal fetal MRI brain anatomy. Both the experienced and inexperienced fetal imager benefit from comparative evaluation of case patients with reference images to ensure normal cortical development. Focal or regional cortical malformations remain among the most difficult diagnoses to make in utero, particularly until the mid- to late third trimester.

■ Ventriculomegaly

As previously noted, ventriculomegaly is the most common indication for fetal MRI. After deciding that ventriculomegaly is indeed present, the primary objective of the radiologist is to decide whether the ventriculomegaly is isolated, in that no other intracranial abnormalities are present, or nonisolated, in that causative or additional abnormalities are present. It is important to remember that the diagnosis of isolated ventriculomegaly on imaging is a diagnosis of exclusion. However, it does not imply that a causative factor is absent. It simply indicates that the cause is not identified on imaging. Of course a causative factor may become apparent later in pregnancy, postnatally, or even later in childhood. Table 24.2 lists common causes of nonisolated ventriculomegaly.

What Is the Value of Fetal Magnetic Resonance Imaging in Evaluating Ventriculomegaly?

Numerous studies have evaluated the ability of MRI to offer additional findings compared with ultrasound and, more importantly, offer additional findings that result in a change in management. Such a change in management often is a result of MRI to offer a more exact diagnosis than can be offered by ultrasound alone. For example, obstructive ventriculomegaly can be confirmed to be secondary to aqueductal stenosis or associated with a syndrome such as Walker-Warburg. These additional findings may change management, modify the mode or location of delivery, or alter the anticipatory perinatal care of the fetus, including neurosurgical intervention. Another important point is that even when MRI does not detect additional abnormalities, in many cases it affords confidence in the correct diagnosis initially made by ultrasound.

How Do I Decide if the Ventriculomegaly Is Obstructive or Nonobstructive?

Deciding whether ventriculomegaly is obstructive or nonobstructive is a logical initial step that helps hone the differential. First, evaluations of which ventricles are involved can be very helpful. The overwhelming majority of obstructive processes occur at the level of the posterior fossa beginning with the cerebral aqueduct. Therefore significant third ventricle dilatation is a strong clue that an obstructive process may be present. Then, attention should be placed on the subarachnoid spaces overlying the supratentorial convexities. Effacement of the cerebral convexities is a strong clue that an obstructive process is present. This often coexists with thinning of the cortical man-

TABLE 24.2   Causes of Nonisolated Ventriculomegaly

Congenital Malformation
- Chiari type II
- Dandy-Walker
- Aqueductal stenosis (congenital or acquired)
- Walker-Warburg
- Agenesis or hypogenesis of the corpus callosum
- Holoprosencephaly
- Schizencephaly
- Polymicrogyria syndromes

Destructive
- Hydranencephaly
- Stroke
- Intracranial hemorrhage
- Teratogens

tle and associated effacement of age-appropriate cerebral sulci, such as the sylvian fissure. And finally, the presence of macrocephaly can be another clue that an obstructive process is present (Fig. 24.2). Two important points should be made. Fetuses with Chiari type II malformation do not typically have macrocephaly in contradistinction to obstructive processes, such as aqueductal stenosis (see Fig. 24.2). Note the presence of CSF effacement in Chiari type II malformation due to intracranial hypotension. And finally, it is important to remember that although macrocephaly is often secondary to obstructive hydrocephalus, there are rare instances where megalencephaly, defined as enlargement of the brain parenchyma itself, is the primary cause of macrocephaly. Fetuses with megalencephaly may have diffuse supratentorial cortical dysplasia as can be seen with perisylvian syndromes. Ventriculomegaly may coexist with megalencephaly but may not be obstructive in origin.

Is the Corpus Callosum Normal?

Abnormalities of the corpus callosum are a common cause of ventriculomegaly and should be the initial evaluation in patients with nonobstructive ventriculomegaly. The corpus callosum is embryologically completely formed by 20 weeks of gestation and therefore is identifiable at the onset of when fetal MRI is typically offered. Evaluation of the corpus callous heavily relies on the multiplanar capabilities and superb resolution of MRI (Fig. 24.3). It cannot be stressed enough that proper evaluation of the corpus callosum must include thin-slice, preferably 2 mm skip 0 mm sagittal T2-weighted imaging, and that the sagittal sequence must be perfectly aligned. Also acceptable is 3-mm slice thickness, but one may still find some difficulty in visualizing the corpus callosum completely at early gestational ages. It is not uncommon that initial attempts at performing a sagittal sequence be plagued by mild obliquity because of constant or inconstant fetal motion. The technologist should make reasonable attempts to perform the perfect sagittal imaging and of course should recognize when such an image has been successfully obtained (see Fig. 24.3). Ideally the

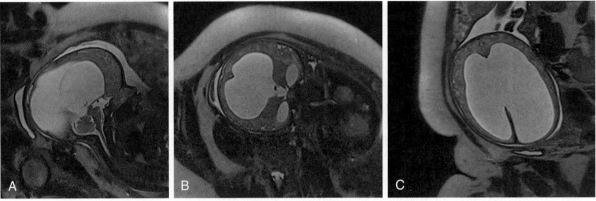

Fig. 24.2 Aqueductal stenosis. Multiorthogonal images (A-C) demonstrate severe supratentorial hydrocephalus characteristically sparing the fourth ventricle. Note the diffuse effacement of the subarachnoid space and the absence of the septum pellucidum from long-standing hydrocephalus. Cephalic biometrics revealed macrocephaly.

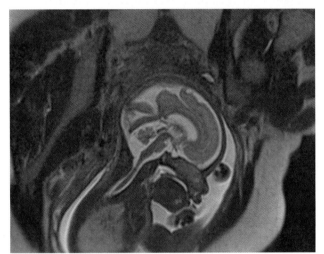

Fig. 24.3 Normal corpus callosum. The corpus callosum is embryologically complete by 20 weeks and thus is well seen with high-quality multiorthogonal imaging by this age.

corpus callosum should be imaged in its entirety, but as noted, even with perfect sagittal imaging this may be difficult. Identification of the C-shaped corpus callosum is necessary, including the splenium, to interpret as normal. Complete evaluation of the callosum also relies on visualizing the callosum on axial images and coronal images and identification of the cavum septum pellucidum. Coronal images show the cavum septum pellucidum and the commissural fibers of the corpus callosum especially well. If there is agenesis of the corpus callosum, Probst bundles and the characteristic "longhorn" dysmorphology of the lateral ventricles are well seen in the coronal plane. Axial images are also helpful in identifying the normal cavum septum pellucidum or colpocephaly or "teardrop" configuration of the posterior ventricles in agenesis or severe hypogenesis of the corpus callosum (Fig. 24.4). Mild hypogenesis of the corpus callosum, however, can be difficult to evaluate in some cases, but is especially difficult on axial and coronal images because of suboptimal evaluation of the polar segments of the corpus callosum. Corpus callosum biometry with normogram reference is thus especially important for all fetuses.

Notably, in rare instances, agenesis of the corpus callosum may coexist with interhemispheric cysts that either communicate or do not communicate with the lateral ventricles. In cases in which agenesis of the corpus callosum is associated with cysts that communicate with a ventricular system obstruction at the cerebral aqueduct is present. These cysts are diverticula of the ventricular system (see Fig. 24.4).

Finally, agenesis and hypogenesis of the corpus callosum can occur in isolation and nonisolation. Numerous syndromic and nonsyndromic diagnoses are associated with abnormalities of the corpus callosum.

Are the Right and Left Cerebral Hemispheres and the Central Gray Matter Fully Divided?

Holoprosencephaly is defined by a lack of complete division of the respective cerebral hemispheres of varying severity. The mildest form, referred to as lobar holoprosencephaly, has the most complete division from the contralateral hemisphere with only partial fusion at the level of the frontal lobes often with falcine hypoplasia. This is in contradistinction to the alobar subtype, where there is essential lack of differentiation between the right and left brain. Alobar holoprosencephaly is in fact the most common form of holoprosencephaly seen in the prenatal period. Such fetuses have a large "pancake"-shaped brain in the anterior cranial fossa with a large monoventricle and dorsal cyst. The corpus callosum and falx are absent, and the central gray matter and hypothalamus are fused (Fig. 24.5). Semilobar holoprosencephaly exists between the continuum of lobar and alobar holoprosencephaly. It should be noted that the distinction between the respective subtypes of holoprosencephaly is not concrete, and therefore the fetal imager should not be overly concerned with distinguishing a severe semilobar from alobar holoprosencephaly, for example. More importantly, the fetal imager should ensure high-quality 2- to 3-mm axial and coronal T2-weighted imaging to be able to assess for milder cases of holoprosencephaly. This includes close scrutiny for frontal lobe fusion in lobar holoprosencephaly and fusion of the superior frontal and parietal lobes in the

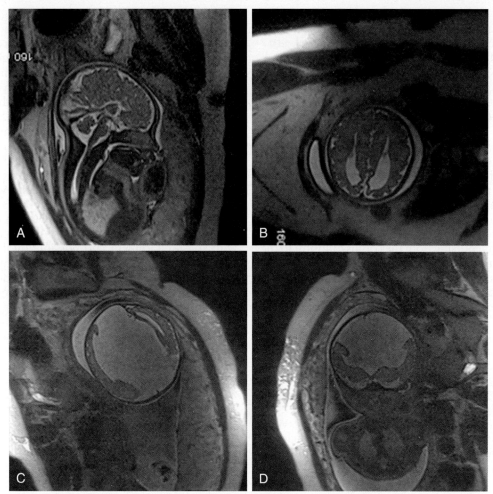

Fig. 24.4 Agenesis of the corpus callosum (ACC). Classic ACC with sulci radiating to the third ventricle (A). Note the colpocephalic configuration of the lateral ventricles (B). In some cases, ACC may be seen with interhemispheric cyst(s) (C, D). The cerebral hemispheres are splayed by the interhemispheric cyst, and the cyst is in communication with the lateral ventricles.

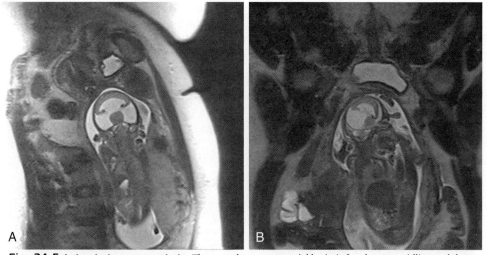

Fig. 24.5 Lobar holoprosencephaly. The pancake supratentorial brain is fused across midline and there is fusion of the thalami with a monoventricle (A). Sagittal image (B) demonstrates a dorsal cyst posteriorly.

middle interhemispheric variant of holoprosencephaly, also referred to as syntelencephaly. And finally, fusion of the diencephalon at the level of the thalamus may easily be missed without close scrutiny of this region. In isolated diencephalic fusion, ventriculomegaly may be seen. Agen-

esis of the corpus callosum and interhemispheric cysts may also be present. Scrutiny of this region is also important in evaluation of diencehalic mesencephalic junction dysplasia (Severino M, Righini A, Tortora D, Pinelli L, Parazzini C, Morana G, Accorsi P, Capra V, Paladini D,

Rossi A. MR Imaging Diagnosis of Diencephalic-Mesencephalic Junction Dysplasia in Fetuses with Developmental Ventriculomegaly. AJNR Am J Neuroradiol. 2017 Aug;38(8):1643-1646.   doi:10.3174/ajnr.A5245.   Epub 2017 Jun 8. PMID: 28596193; PMCID: PMC7960408.)

Is the Cavum Septum Pellucidum Present?

Identification of the cavum septum pellucidum is an extremely important exercise in evaluating the fetal brain. As with other parts of the fetal brain, high-quality, high-resolution fetal brain imaging is critical in identifying the cavum septum pellucidum and any associated abnormalities. It is best identified on coronal images as two separate thin leaflets coursing from the corpus callosum to the fornix partitioning the right from the left lateral ventricle.

Identification of a normal septum pellucidum is important because in greater than 95% of cases, absence of the septum pellucidum occurs as a nonisolated abnormality. Absence of the septum pellucidum is seen with callosal agenesis, with presence of the septum pellucidum arguing against callosal agenesis. Furthermore, absence of the cavum septum pellucidum may be seen with a variety of congenital abnormalities, including holoprosencephaly, septo-optic dysplasia, and bilateral schizencephaly, among many others.

One especially important note should be made. With chronic severe hydrocephalus the septum pellucidum may be absent. In such cases, however, the septum pellucidum is usually absent as a function of acquired fenestration with primary agenesis less common.

Are There Small or Large Portions of the Lobar Cerebral Brain Parenchyma That Are Not Present?

Porencephalic cysts or regions of porencephaly are areas of brain parenchyma that have undergone some form of injury. It is not uncommon for such regions of injury to be wedge shaped, and by definition such regions are isointense to cerebrospinal fluid (CSF) on all sequences. The cause of porencephalic cysts is thought to vascular in nature, posttraumatic or posthemorrhagic, or even secondary to infection. Notably, ischemia of varying severity and of various organs, including the brain, may occur in the living fetus after singular fetal demise in a monochorionic pregnancy (Fig. 24.6). The resulting injury to the remaining fetus may be life-threatening.

Regions of porencephaly and other diagnoses contained within this section differ significantly from a potential mimicker, an arachnoid cyst. Although both maintain CSF signal intensity on all sequences, an arachnoid cyst is a volume-positive lesion that results in regional mass effect on the adjacent brain parenchyma with sulcal effacement and possibly midline shift with larger cysts. Furthermore, there may be expansion of the regional cranial vault with thinning of the skull. These latter findings may be well seen with larger arachnoid cysts in the anterior middle cranial fossa, for example (Fig. 24.7).

Open lip schizencephaly can have a similar appearance as regions of porencephaly. The differentiating feature is that regions of porencephaly are lined by white matter as a function of their origin, whereas schizencephalic clefts are lined by dysplastic gray matter. Therefore one should evaluate for microlobulated T2 signal isointense to the germinal matrix or cortex lining the margins of a CSF cleft to clinch the diagnosis of schizencephaly. The presence of T2-hyperintense margins would support the diagnosis of porencephaly. Although such differentiation is fairly clear late in the third trimester, the differentiation may prove extremely difficult at earlier gestational ages, especially at 20 to 24 weeks of gestation. Closed lip schizencephaly will not present the aforementioned diagnostic challenge.

When regions of porencephaly are extremely severe, encompassing large symmetrical portions of the lobar cerebral hemispheres, in an anterior and middle cerebral artery distribution, the diagnosis of hydranencephaly

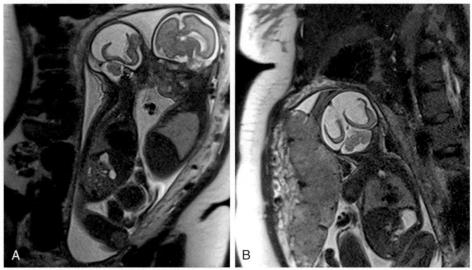

Fig. 24.6 Porencephaly. Multiplanar images (A-B) in a monochorionic pregnancy in which demise of fetus C resulted in multiple broad regions of bilateral porencephaly.

is made. Small tufts of parasagittal frontal lobe parenchyma may be present, but the posterior circulation, including the occipital lobes, thalami, cerebellar hemispheres, and brainstem, are entirely spared. The etiology is presumed to be the result of catastrophic compromise of the anterior circulation early in gestation. As with many other fetal diagnoses, high-quality imaging is necessary to exclude the possibility of severe hydrocephalus as would be diagnosed if a peripherally marginalized thinned cortical mantle was seen.

Are There Regions of Cortical Irregularity or Abnormal Layering and/or Dissimilarity to the Contralateral Side?

The radiological rule of finding symmetry between the cerebral hemispheres is extremely important in fetal imaging. The initial approach to a cortical malformation is to ensure an understanding of normal cortical lamination in the fetal brain, as well as normal gyration and sulcation for age. An aberration of cortical layering can be an important clue to the presence of a cortical

dysplasia (Fig. 24.8). Evaluation of the peripheral cortex for asymmetrical gyration or sulcation, whether it be undergyration or overgyration, should be honed in on. Micronodularity of the cortical surface, a subtle but still identifiable finding, is an additional finding that indicates cortical dysplasia. Such micronodularity may be the only clue of a cortical dysplasia in early gestational ages when little to no sulcation of the brain is yet present. Notably, subtle cortical dysplasia can be difficult to diagnosis in utero.

Is One Ventricle Larger Than the Other?

As was emphasized in the previous section, symmetry is a vital component of the evaluation of the fetal brain. After identifying a discrepancy in the size of the cerebral hemispheres, a decision should be made as to which hemisphere is indeed pathological. In deciding, an important clue is the size of the ventricle. Generally, if the larger ventricle coexists with the larger hemisphere, one should strongly suspect the presence of hemimegalencephaly. Hemimegalencephaly is defined as a diffusely

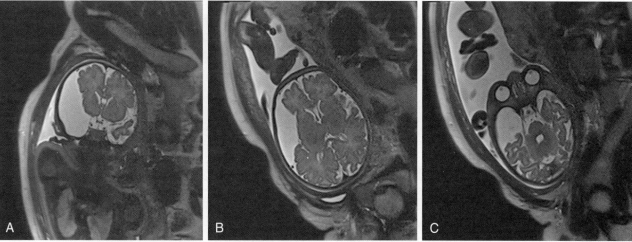

Fig. 24.7 Arachnoid cyst. Multiorthogonal images (A-C) demonstrate a large supratentorial arachnoid cyst extending from the anterior middle cranial fossa into the sylvian fissure. Note the expansion of middle cranial fossa indicating a long-standing benign lesion (C).

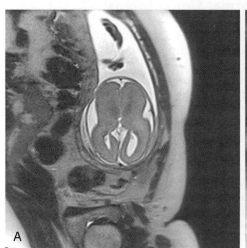
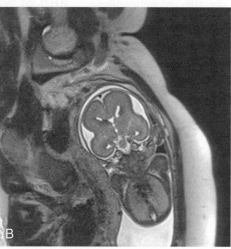

Fig. 24.8 Cortical dysplasia. Diffuse enlargement of the bilateral cerebral hemispheres with diffuse T2 shortening of the brain parenchyma and without normal lamination of the fetal brain (A-B). Megalencephaly syndrome was diagnosed based on this study with megalencephaly capillary malformation polymicrogyria syndrome diagnosed at birth. This neonate died in the perinatal period as a result of uncontrollable seizure and congenital heart disease.

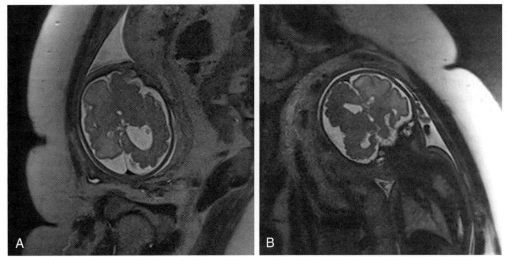

Fig. 24.9 Hemimegalencephaly. Classic overgrowth of one hemisphere, diffuse T2 shortening, and blurring of normal parenchymal lamination with ipsilateral ventriculomegaly (A-B).

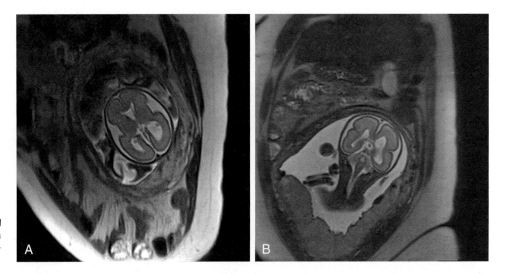

Fig. 24.10 *Unilateral isolated ventriculomegaly (A-B).* Such patients typically have an excellent prognosis.

dysplastic enlarged cerebral hemisphere. Unlike many other cortical dysplasias that occur more focally or regionally, because of the diffuse nature of the process and the usually dramatic overgrowth of the ipsilateral hemisphere, hemimegalencephaly can be detected at earlier gestational ages. Often the affected hemisphere will demonstrate diffuse T2 shortening and blurring of the usually seen parenchymal layers compared with the contralateral normal hemisphere (Fig. 24.9). Although it may occur in association with entities such as neurofibromatosis type I and hypomelanosis of Ito, it often occurs in isolation.

Unilateral ventriculomegaly may occur as a result of a variety of insults that mimic many of the same causes of bilateral ventriculomegaly. These include many of the diagnoses already mentioned but also include infection, vascular ischemic or hemorrhagic injury, and other congenital malformations including schizencephaly. Some of these affected fetuses may have chromosomal abnormalities.

As a diagnosis of exclusion, when no abnormality is identified of either cerebral hemisphere, the diag-nosis of isolated unilateral ventriculomegaly is given (Fig. 24.10).

Are the Ventricle Margins Smooth and of Normal Signal Intensity?

At all gestational ages, the contour of the ependymal margin of the lateral ventricles should be smooth. In addition, the germinal matrix should be seen as a smooth subependymal T2 hypointense band with restricted diffusion along the lateral aspect of the lateral ventricle margin centered often best seen at the caudothalamic groove (Fig. 24.11). Notably, the germinal matrix is a structure best seen between 8 and 28 weeks that completely involutes by 32 weeks of gestation. It is a highly metabolically active vascular site of neuronal and glial cell origin that eventually migrates to the developing cerebral cortex. And of course, it is the origin of prematurity-induced germinal matrix hemorrhage. Appreciating the normal anatomy of the germinal matrix is important to avoid interpreting its normal presence

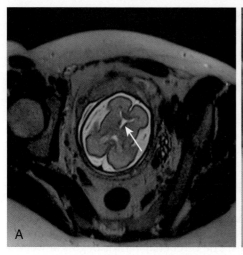 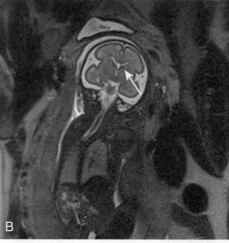

Fig. 24.11 Germinal matrix. The normal germinal matrix is a T2-hypointense band (*arrows in A-B*) that extends from the caudothalamic groove posteriorly along the ependymal margin of the lateral ventricle. The germinal matrix should not be mistaken for hemorrhage.

as representative of intraventricular hemorrhage. When such T2 shortening appears nodular, intraventricular hemorrhage should be considered. A susceptibility weighted, gradient-echo or echo planar sequence should be used to identify hemorrhage and distinguish between other causes of ependymal irregularity.

Additional differential considerations include tuberous sclerosis and gray matter heterotopia. Although both appear as nodular foci of T2 shortening, subependymal nodules demonstrate T1 shortening. The presence of classic extraventricular findings is paramount in clenching the diagnosis of tuberous sclerosis. Cortical tubers will appear as regions of cortical and subcortical T1 and T2 shortening on fetal MRI (Fig. 24.12). The presence of a cardiac rhabdomyoma, especially when multiple, will add a diagnostic clue to the presence of tuberous sclerosis. Subependymal giant cell astrocytomas are exceedingly rare in fetal and neonatal periods but have been reported.

Gray matter heterotopia may occur in isolation or may occur with other congenital malformations, such as polymicrogyria and schizencephaly, and as part of broader malformations, such as Dandy-Walker and Chiari type II. Notably, when gray matter heterotopia is confluent, one should consider the presence of X-linked inherited filamin A gene mutation. Such patients will nearly always be female and have coexisting congenital heart disease.

Is There a Solid and Cystic Intracranial Mass?

Congenital brain neoplasms are fortunately rare. Teratomas are the most common neonatal brain tumor and may present as small or grossly massive solid and cystic midline tumors. In contrast with older children for whom teratomas are most commonly seen infratentorially, prenatally diagnosed teratomas are typically supratentorial. The exact origin of these mass lesions is ultimately quite difficult. Fetal macrocephaly with rapid head size growth with or without hydrocephalus, replacement or displacement of normal brain parenchyma by the mass, and CNS dysfunction induced poly-

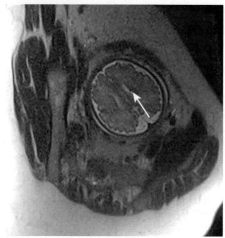

Fig. 24.12 Tuberous sclerosis (TS). Small subependymal nodule seen as a focus of T2 shortening along the ependymal surface.

hydramnios from impaired fetal swallowing. Additional differential considerations of solid and cystic congenital masses include primitive neuroectodermal tumor, glial neoplasms, ependymomas, craniopharyngiomas, and choroid plexus neoplasms.

■ Posterior Fossa

Is There Cystic Enlargement of the Posterior Fossa?

A common reason for fetal MRI is the presence of an enlarged CM. The CM is the fluid-filled space posterior to the cerebellum and vermis. On fetal MRI, the CM is measured per ultrasound convention at midline between the inner table of the squamosal occipital bone and the dorsal most margin of the vermis. It should measure no more than 10 mm. The role of the fetal imager asked to evaluate the cystic enlarged posterior fossa is to decide if the findings represent a normal variant or a truly abnormal state. The general differential diagnosis for cystic enlargement of the posterior fossa can be remembered by the acronym MADEC for mega CM, arachnoid cyst,

Dandy-Walker malformation, epidermoid cyst, and cerebellovermian hypoplasia.

Does the Cystic Enlargement of the Posterior Fossa Communicate With the Fourth Ventricle?

After the diagnosis of cystic enlargement of the posterior fossa is made, the next most important step that the fetal imager should decide is whether the fourth ventricle is in communication with the cystic enlargement of the posterior fossa. An arachnoid cyst, epidermoid cyst, and mega CM do not communicate with the fourth ventricle. An arachnoid cyst is a benign CSF-filled sac that is fully invested by arachnoid mater that follows CSF signal intensity on all pulse sequences, including diffusion-weighted imaging. It may be unilateral, bilateral (symmetrical or asymmetrical), and typically overlies the dorsal margin of the cerebellum and vermis. Regional mass effect and sulcal effacement can be helpful in favoring the presence of an arachnoid cyst over that of mega CM. Mega CM is simply representative of an enlarged subarachnoid space overlying the dorsal cerebellum and vermis and is therefore a diagnosis of exclusion that requires all the posterior fossa contents to be normal. An epidermoid cyst is also a congenital cyst lined by squamous epithelial cells but filled with cholesterol and keratinous debris that may mimic an arachnoid cyst on T1- and T2-weighted images. However, in contradistinction to arachnoid cysts, epidermoid cysts demonstrate restricted diffusion and incomplete suppression on T2 FLAIR sequences. Notable is that arachnoid and epidermoid cysts may occur anywhere in posterior fossa (and supratentorium), including the cerebellopontine angle and superior cerebellar cistern. In rare instances, such cysts may be transtentorial. An additional differential consideration for a transtentorial cystic structure includes a ventricular diverticulum (typically from the lateral ventricle) in which a portion of an obstructed lateral ventricle herniates into the posterior fossa. Such a finding is rare and would be found only with severe obstructive hydrocephalus.

Is There Elevation of the Torcular Herophili?

Elevation of the torcular herophili is a helpful clue into the potential diagnosis of a congenital malformation. It is classically seen and reported in the Dandy-Walker malformation and therefore should be a strong clue for the fetal imager to closely scrutinize the vermis when the posterior fossa demonstrates cystic enlargement (Fig. 24.13).

Is the Vermis Normal?

An intimate understanding of normal vermian anatomy is important in the evaluation of posterior fossa malformations. The cerebellar vermis begins at week 9 of gestation superiorly and continues inferiorly, closing by week 15. However, researchers have sonographically recorded that the posterior inferior vermis may remain patent as late as 17.5 weeks, and therefore the diagnosis of inferior vermian hypoplasia cannot reliably be made until week 18 of gestation at which time the vermis is developmentally complete. However, in a small case series by Limperopoulos et al. (2006), it was noted that of 19 fetuses who underwent prenatal MRI between 18 and 28 weeks, 6 of 19 were diagnosed with a normal postnatal MRI. This raises the issue that inferior vermian hypoplasia may in fact be overdiagnosed in the second trimester as a function of delayed normal variant closure of the vermis. Inherent to this issue is that given the exquisite detail of the vermis afforded by fetal MRI, the true normal imaging appearance of the vermis, including its embryological closure, is not completely understood. In real practice, therefore, the fetal imager should be cautious in dogmatically diagnosing inferior vermian hypoplasia except for more severe cases where the vermis is grossly hypoplastic. This is central to using the tegmentovermian angle (angle drawn along the dorsal margin of the brainstem and the ventral vermian surface that classically effaces by 17 weeks as a result of closure of the vermis) with caution.

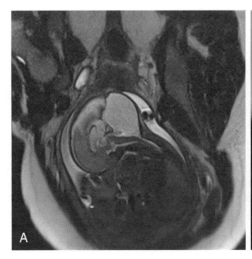
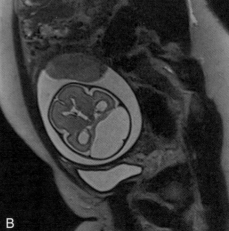

Fig. 24.13 Classic Dandy-Walker malformation. Cystic enlargement of the posterior fossa in communication with the fourth ventricle and near-complete vermian absence (A-B). Note severe elevation of the torcular herophili.

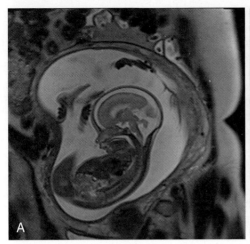
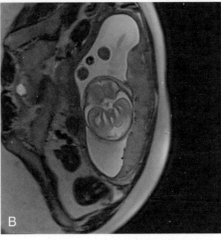

Fig. 24.14 Joubert syndrome. Sagittal image at midline (A) demonstrates a hypoplastic vermis. Axial image (B) demonstrates the "molar tooth" configuration at the level of the midbrain caused by lack of decussation of the superior cerebellar peduncles.

Abnormalities of vermian development may occur in isolation, referred to as inferior vermian hypoplasia. The term *Dandy-Walker variant* is not favored in the present terminology. When cystic enlargement of the posterior fossa in communication with the fourth ventricle coexists with torcular herophili elevation and vermian hypoplasia, the classical Dandy-Walker malformation is diagnosed. Another important diagnosis to consider when vermian hypoplasia is present is the "molar tooth-"like malformations, the prototype being Joubert syndrome. With high-quality imaging, the classic molar tooth appearance of the midbrain with thickening of the superior cerebellar peduncles secondary to lack of their decussation can be identified along with other findings, such as a narrow isthmus (pontine-mesencephalic junction) with a deep interpeduncular cistern (Fig. 24.14). Admittedly the diagnosis of the more subtle brainstem findings of Joubert syndrome may be quite difficult in early gestational ages.

Notably, normal measurements of the craniocaudal and AP of the vermis do exist and should be consulted for every fetal study. Furthermore, the fastigium of the fourth ventricle and primary fissure should be identifiable at all gestational ages. The absence of the fastigium, the dorsal apex of the fourth ventricle where the superior and inferior medullary velum meet, is a strong clue of an underlying cerebellovermian abnormality.

Are the Cerebellar Hemispheres Too Small?

Biometrics plays a crucial role in the evaluation of fetal anatomy. The normal range for the TCD measured in the axial plane at the greatest cerebellar width should be consulted as part of every fetal CNS survey. An abnormal TCD may be the first clue to a significant posterior fossa abnormality that may escape a qualitative survey. Cerebellar hypoplasia may accompany a wide variety of congenital malformations, including posterior fossa malformations, such as Dandy-Walker malformation and rhombencephalosynapsis, and genetic syndromes, such as Joubert. It may also be seen in fetuses with chromosomal abnormalities, including trisomies 13 and 18.

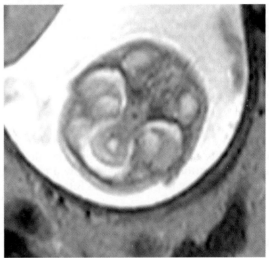

Fig. 24.15 Rhombencephalosynapsis. Abnormal fusion of the cerebellar hemispheres across the midline, without separation and normal vermis. Folia cross the entirety of the cerebellum in the transverse plane.

Furthermore, cerebellar volume loss may be seen as the result of an insult, such as from in utero infection, vascular injury, or exposure to teratogens.

Are the Cerebellar Hemispheres Fused?

After diagnosing an abnormally small cerebellum, one diagnosis that is worthy of special mention is rhombencephalosynapsis. Its special consideration is deserving because if the diagnosis is not purposefully considered, the study may be misinterpreted by the fetal imager. As has been thematic in this chapter, high-quality, high-resolution imaging is paramount. The diagnosis is made by identifying fusion of the cerebellar hemispheres. Typically the cerebellum will measure abnormally small with transversely oriented sulci across the entire cerebellum and lack of visualization of a normal-appearing vermis (Fig. 24.15). Other midline fusion abnormalities may coexist, such as aqueductal stenosis with obstructive hydrocephalus.

Does the Brainstem Have a "Kinked" Appearance?

On sagittal high-resolution imaging, the ultrastructure of the brainstem, including the mesencephalon, pons, and medulla, should be scrutinized. The brainstem should have a relatively straight noncontoured dorsal margin. There are rare instances of hindbrain–midbrain malformations that result in a distinctive abnormal contour to the brainstem referred to as brainstem "kinking" or a Z-shaped brainstem. Brainstem kinking occurs as a normal embryological phenomenon early in gestation with persistence indicative of a significant disturbance at approximately 7 weeks of gestation that effectively halts the brainstem into this configuration. When associated with cerebellar hypoplasia, obstructive hydrocephalus presumably as a result of tectal fusion, cobblestone lissencephaly, and retinal abnormalities, one should consider the merosin-positive cerebromuscular dysplasias, especially Walker-Warburg syndrome (Fig. 24.16). Of note is that cobblestone lissencephaly may be difficult to diagnose until late in gestation. Other diagnoses, such as lissencephaly syndromes with cerebellar hypoplasia and tectocerebellar dysraphism, may appear similar. Also, finally, at least some of these fetuses may have diagnoses that cannot be made in utero and/or are not yet realized by the literature.

The importance of closely evaluating the brainstem cannot be stressed enough because the presence of such an abnormality carries dramatic prognostic information for the fetus. Furthermore, it may imply a genetic process that might have implications for future pregnancies for the couple.

■ Vascular

Are There Abnormal Intracranial Flow Voids (e.g., Flow Voids That Are Too Large and/or Are Increased)?

On fetal MR, normal vascular flow voids of the anterior and posterior circulation are quite subtle, seen as wispy structures traversing the subarachnoid spaces. Therefore in the presence of an intracranial vascular malformation when numerous enlarged arterial and venous flow voids are found, the findings are typically quite striking. The presence of a high-output cardiac state is commonly the initial clue to an intracranial vascular abnormality. In addition, such lesions may first be seen as a result of ventriculomegaly and go on to initial identification by Doppler sonography.

Is There a Vascular Nidus?

Identifying abnormal multiple and enlarged flow voids is the initial step in identifying a vascular abnormality. After this, the most important step is to identify a nidus, defined as the central portion of an arteriovenous malformation (AVM) where the feeding arteries and draining veins communicate with an intervening capillary bed. Such a nidus will typically appear as a ball of tangled vessels. The presence of a nidus is a defining feature of an AVM. Although AVMs are congenital lesions, they are rarely diagnosed in the prenatal period because they do not usually result in high-output cardiac failure (because of the presence of an intervening capillary bed), nor do they cause hemorrhage. They are often not seen on routine prenatal sonography and thus do not usually present for fetal MRI.

Unlike in an AVM, an arteriovenous fistula (AVF) does not contain a nidus. Instead, there is direct communication of feeding arteries and draining veins without an intervening capillary bed. As such, when shunting of blood is severe enough, the fetus will present with high-output failure. As stated, a subcomponent of such patients will present with ventriculomegaly or the primary sonographic detection of the lesion as a result of large vascular flow voids. The vein of Galen AVF is a product of multiple AVFs between thalamoperforators, anterior cerebral and choroidal, and the embryologically persistent median prosencephalic vein of Markowski (Fig. 24.17). Two subtypes exist, including choroidal and mural subtypes, with the former accounting for up to 90% of vein of Galen AVFs. The choroidal subtype typically becomes symptomatic in the neonatal period with high-output failure

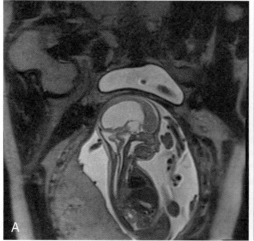 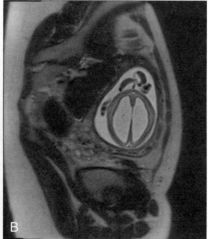

Fig. 24.16 Walker-Warburg syndrome. Sagittal image at midline (A) demonstrates classic imaging findings of brainstem "kinking." The vermis is also dysplastic. Severe supratentorial hydrocephalus is present (B) as a result of coexisting aqueductal obstruction, a common finding in such fetuses. On ultrasound, this entity is typically mistaken for isolated aqueductal stenosis.

because of a larger number of arteriovenous fistulous connections and therefore more shunting. The mural subtype, in contrast, has fewer albeit larger fistulous connections and therefore presents with seizures, hydrocephalus, or even hemorrhage later in childhood or adulthood (if not prenatally diagnosed). Although differentiating between the two subtypes on fetal MRI is less important, close evaluation of the brain parenchyma is important to assess for secondary brain injury due to chronic steal phenomenon and high venous pressures seen by the brain parenchyma. This is especially important postnatally before undergoing treatment because severe brain injury may mitigate against treatment. The treatment of these lesions is endovascular.

Although vein of Galen fistulas will be the most commonly encountered type of AVFs by fetal imagers, non-Galenic AVFs may also be seen in rare instances.

Dural venous sinus enlargement and partial thrombosis have been described on fetal MRI with a significantly expanded dural venous sinus, often involving the torcula, with internal abnormal T1 hyperintensity. Whether this is truly a dural venous sinus malformation versus simply prenatal venous sinus thrombosis is questioned, because many of these patients have resolution over time and have good outcomes postnatally.

■ Complication of Monochorionic Twin Pregnancy

Are There Regions of Brain Destruction in a Monochorionic Pregnancy in the Living Fetus After One Fetus Dies?

In rare instances, because of fetal demise in a monochorionic pregnancy, regions of parenchymal insult in the brain and solid visceral organs of the living fetus may occur. Such injury may result in adverse neurodevelopment or be so severe as to be lethal.

■ Head and Neck

Is There a Midline Cystic Scalp Lesion?

Cystic lesions of the midline scalp should be scrutinized carefully. The initial step in evaluating such lesions is to assess for whether the lesion is associated with a defect in the calvarium. When a defect in the calvarium is identified, the diagnosis of a cephalocele is made. A meningocele is a CSF-only-containing lesion, whereas an encephalocele is an open defect that also contains brain parenchyma. When such lesions are large, they are readily identifiable and easily diagnosed. However, such lesions may be missed when small and especially in the case of meningoceles when they are partially effaced against the uterine wall. Of note is that cephaloceles may occur as part of a broader set of abnormalities as in Meckel-Gruber syndrome or Walker-Warburg syndrome or occur in isolation. The treatment for these lesions includes surgical resection and closure. Postnatal MRI with MR venography and MR angiography are prerequisite to closure in most cases.

If the calvarium is closed, then the differential considerations broaden. A midline cystic lesion at the level of the parietal calvarium may represent an atretic parietal encephalocele, a type of cephalocele that has since lost its communication with the intracranial contents. Such lesions are termed *encephaloceles* even despite lack of intralesional brain on imaging because of the presence of glial cells at pathology. These lesions may

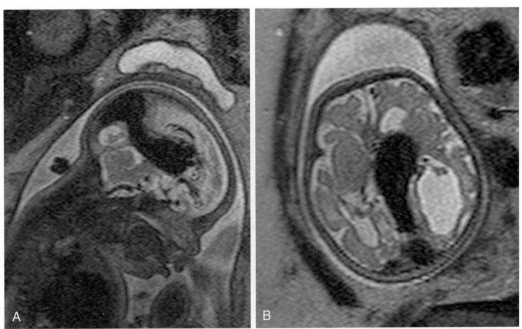

Fig. 24.17 Vein of Galen malformation (VOGM). Large VOGM (A-B) draining into the superior sagittal sinus via a persistent falcine sinus. Note the hypoplastic straight sinus. The left greater than right cerebral hemispheres demonstrate significant volume loss as a result of chronic venous hypertension, commonly referred to as "melting brain."

be associated with intracranial anomalies, including a persistent falcine sinus, split superior sagittal sinus, and even true abnormalities such as cerebral dysgenesis in rare cases. Additional differential considerations for midline cysts include dermoid and epidermoid cysts that may or may not communicate with the intracranial compartment.

Is One or Both Globes Absent or Too Small?

The fetal orbits are an important part of a relevant review of systems for all indications for fetal MRI, mainly because it is an organ that can be affected in a number of genetic and acquired abnormalities. Nomograms do exist for ocular diameter, binocular distance (BOD), and interocular distance (IOD) by sonography and by fetal MRI. Such measurements should be part of the normal fetal MRI evaluation of the head and neck. Microphthalmia is defined as an ocular distance in the less than 5th percentile. Anophthalmia refers to complete absence of the globe but with the presence of the eyelid, conjunctiva, and lacrimal apparatus (Fig. 24.18). Anophthalmia and microphthalmia may be seen with a variety of syndromic and genetic disorders, including trisomy 13, CHARGE syndrome, and Walker-Warburg syndrome, among others. In addition, acquired, secondary insults to the globe include congenital infections, such as TORCH (toxoplasmosis, other [e.g., syphilis, varicella, mumps, parvovirus, and HIV], rubella virus, cytomegalovirus, and herpes simplex) and toxic metabolic exposures, as can be seen with fetal alcohol syndrome and in utero retinoic acid exposure.

Is the Interocular or Binocular Distance Abnormal?

Hypertelorism refers to an abnormally increased IOD/BOD. Isolated hypertelorism occurs only very rarely. Rather, hypertelorism occurs in association with many other abnormalities, such as chromosomal abnormalities, and even from toxic exposure, such as from antiepileptic drugs. Furthermore, once the finding of hypertelorism is made, a disciplined effort to identify frontal skull base defects (anterior cephalocele) should ensue.

Hypotelorism refers to an abnormally decreased IOD/BOD. Rather than an isolated abnormality, it too is associated with aneuploidy and midline abnormalities, such as holoprosencephaly.

Is There a Defect in the Upper Lip or Palate?

Cleft lip and palate are the most common craniofacial abnormalities in the fetus with an incidence estimated at 1:700 to 1:1000. Eighty percent of cleft lip defects are associated with cleft palate. Cleft lip and palate may be seen in isolation or be seen with a variety of syndromes and aneuploidies, including trisomies 13 and 18, for example. They may also be the result of infection and teratogens. Cleft lips may be bilateral, unilateral or midline. Midline cleft lip may be especially associated with other abnormalities, including intracranial midline abnormalities. Cleft palate defects may involve the primary palate (anterior to the incisive foramen) and/or secondary palate (posterior to the incisive foramen). Again, high-quality imaging is paramount to evaluation for cleft lip and palate abnormalities. This includes performing perfect 2- to 3-mm coronal and sagittal imaging through the entirety of the face. As for the palate, it is important to identify the palate on more than one image to avoid overlooking an off-midline cleft defect. Although fetal MRI is generally more sensitive than 2D and 3D sonography, the generalized use of fetal MRI for suspected cleft defects is not cost-effective. Instead, fetal MRI should generally be reserved for evaluation of additional abnormalities when a midline cleft is present or when cleft defects are seen to occur with other sonographically

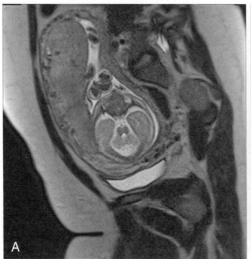 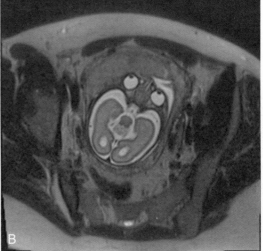

Fig. 24.18 Anophthalmia/Microphthalmia. Right anophthalmia and severe left microphthalmia (A). Normal globes (B).

confirmed abnormalities if management or counseling would vary with additional information.

Does the Mandible Appear Recessed or Too Small?

Micrognathia refers to an abnormally small mandible, whereas retrognathia reflects posterior displacement of the mandible. Agnathia refers to an absent mandible. It is not uncommon for micrognathia and retrognathia to occur together. Currently the diagnosis of retromicrognathia remains mostly qualitative on fetal MRI. In the sonographic literature, there are, however, quantitative measure to diagnose retromicrognathia that include the inferior facial angle, mandible/maxillary ratio, and the jaw index. Retromicrognathia results in a small oral cavity and may be associated with cleft palate and glossoptosis. Therefore such fetuses may be at risk for airway difficulty at the time of birth. Anticipatory delivery, including the use of ex utero intrapartum procedure, may be necessary. In all cases of retromicrognathia the role of the fetal imager is to evaluate the entirety of the airway to the tracheal bifurcation and to detail normal and abnormal segments to properly prepare the delivery team for potential resuscitative needs.

Is a Cystic Head and Neck Mass Midline or off Midline?

The initial approach to a cystic or cystic and solid mass neck mass is to decide whether the lesion is midline or off midline. A cystic lesion that is at midline that occurs at the skull base should suggest a cephalocele, dermoid, or epidermoid cyst. Notable is that nasal gliomas, heterotopic glial tissue that no longer communicates with the subarachnoid space, are not typically cystic in nature. For any midline facial mass, diffusion-weighted imaging and high-resolution (2–3 mm) sagittal imaging are critical. Sagittal imaging is most ideal to establish whether a skull base lesion maintains communication with the intracranial compartment. If the lesion occurs more inferiorly, at the level of the oral cavity, the differential considerations include lingual choristomas that are foregut duplication cysts, epidermoid and dermoid cysts, and lymphatic malformations. It can be difficult, if not impossible, to distinguish between these respective cysts except for the presence of restricted diffusion in epidermoid cysts. Midline cysts within the neck include thyroglossal duct cysts and epidermoid and dermoid cysts. Off-midline cysts in the head and neck include branchial cleft cysts and venolymphatic malformations (Fig. 24.19). Notably, teratomas may occur off midline or at midline in the head and neck (Fig. 24.20).

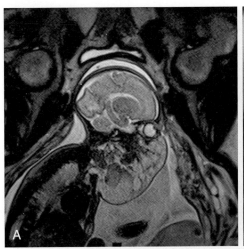
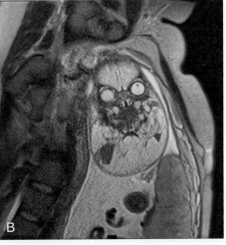

Fig. 24.19 Venolymphatic malformation. Extensive venolymphatic malformation of the face and neck (A-B) causing severe facial distortion. An ex utero intrapartum treatment procedure was performed at the time of delivery.

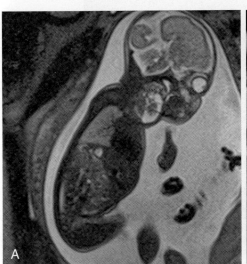
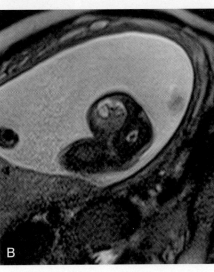

Fig. 24.20 Teratoma. Small, off-midline neck mass with solid and cystic components consistent with a teratoma (A-B). Note that the most important evaluation of fetuses with head and neck masses is to identify the relationship of the mass with regard to the airway.

Does a Neck Mass Have Flow Voids?

The presence of flow voids radiating to a T2-hyperintense mass strongly argues in favor of an infantile hemangioma. Infantile hemangiomas are the only neoplastic entity in the vascular malformations seen in childhood. Such lesions are typically unispatial and are typically off midline. When numerous, infantile hemangiomas may be associated with PHACES, a rare phakomatosis that may have coincident posterior fossa malformations, intracranial infantile hemangiomas, and intracranial and extracranial vascular anomalies.

Without the presence of a well-defined mass, stroma, the presence of numerous flow voids in the head and neck suggests the presence of an AVF or AVM.

Are There Solid and Cystic Components?

A mass lesion with solid and cystic components strongly argues in favor of teratoma (see Fig. 24.20). Teratomas may also have hemorrhagic components and calcification. After the sacrococcygeal region, the head and neck is the next most common location for teratomas to occur. They may occur anywhere in the head and neck, including the orbit, nasal cavity, oral cavity, and neck.

As with all the head and neck lesions that have been described within this section, it cannot be stressed enough that the primary goal of the fetal imager is to describe location, spatiality, and the degree and location of involvement of the airway so as to prepare for appropriate resuscitative measures. Deriving the primary or differential diagnosis is of secondary importance.

■ Spine

Is There an Open Defect in the Lower Spine?

A common indication for fetal MRI is for evaluation of the Chiari type II malformation. Patients who are being considered for in utero closure at select institutions are required to undergo fetal MRI before intervention. The Chiari type II malformation is defined by the presence of an open spinal dysraphism that typically occurs in the lumbosacral spine but may also extend as high as the thoracic spine. An open spinal dysraphism indicates that the neural placode is exposed to the amniotic environment by way of a large defect in the midline soft tissues and posterior spinal elements (Fig. 24.21). A protruding

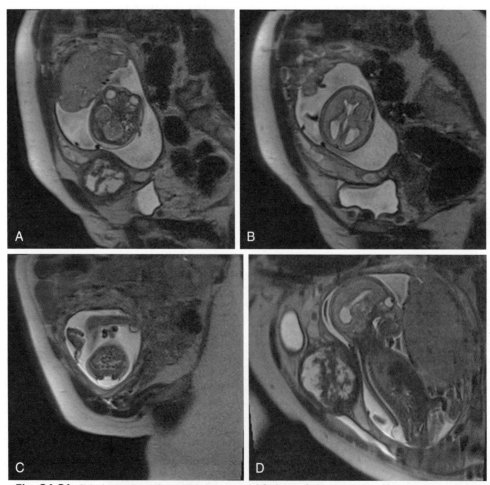

Fig. 24.21 Chiari type II malformation. Intracranial findings of Chiari type II malformation are present, including a small posterior fossa with crowding of its contents and partially effaced fourth ventricle with supratentorial hydrocephalus (A, B). Note that such fetuses are typically not macrocephalic. Myelomeningocele is present involving the lower lumbar, sacral, and coccygeal spine (C, D). Large uterine fibroid is present (A, C).

myelomeningocele sac is often evident, although when such a sac is absent the dysraphism is referred to as a myelocele. The cord is by definition tethered to the dorsal dural margin of the thecal sac at the inferior most intact posterior bony element. Of technical note is that it may be difficult to accurately determine the exact level that the spinal dysraphism begins by MRI. This is better determined by ultrasound.

The characteristic intracranial findings of Chiari type II malformation have been well documented and should be confirmed when an open spinal dysraphism is identified (see Fig. 24.21). The lack of the below intracranial findings of Chiari type II malformation negates the presence of an open spinal dysraphism and should prompt the fetal imager to reevaluate the spinal findings. An initial clue to the diagnosis is ventriculomegaly with diffuse subarachnoid space effacement without macrocephaly. Before 24 weeks, bilateral frontal bone scalloping, referred to as the "lemon sign," will be a characteristic finding. This sign will resolve typically by 24 weeks. Interdigitation of the cerebral gyri as a function of falcine hypoplasia may also be seen. In the posterior fossa, the fourth ventricle is effaced and the cerebellum wraps itself around the brainstem. The resulting configuration of the cerebellum is referred to as the "banana sign." Towering cerebellum, posterior beaking of the tectum, and petrous scalloping are additional findings that may be seen.

The presence of a closed spinal dysraphism, as in a meningocele, terminal myelocystocele, lipomyelomeningocele, and lipomyelocele, does not produce the characteristic intracranial findings in Chiari type II malformation.

Does the Spine Abruptly Stop Before the Coccyx?

Abrupt premature termination of the spine, including the thecal sac and spinal cord, is most consistent with caudal regression syndrome, a constellation of findings that is associated with maternal diabetes. Caudal regression syndrome is a complex closed spinal dysraphism that occurs as a fairly broad continuum from lower sacrococcygeal hypogenesis to hypogenesis involving all of the lumbosacrococcygeal spine. The conus medullaris may abruptly terminate having a blunted appearance without its typical conical tapering. Such an appearance of the conus may be seen even in milder forms of caudal regression. Cord tethering is also common. Anomalies of the gastrointestinal tract and genitourinary tract are common. Depending on the severity of the hypogenesis, patients will have a variable outcome with regard to lower-extremity function. In the most severe of cases, severely hypoplastic lower limbs may be present. Sphincter dysfunction is essentially universal.

Is There a Segment of the Spine That Is Absent?

In rare cases, a short segment of the spine may be hypoplastic or aplastic, a condition referred to as segmental spinal dysgenesis. Such segmental defects are most often seen in the thoracolumbar, lumbar, or lumbosacral spine. The spinal cord and thecal sac are markedly thinned at the level of the dysgenesis. Caudal to the segmental dysgenesis, the spine may be hypoplastic. Severe kyphoscoliosis is typically present.

Is There a Fluid-Filled Sac Anterior to the Sacrococcygeal Spine Separate From the Bladder?

As with the vertebral column, the thecal sac termination should be definitively localized. In an anterior sacral meningocele, hypogenesis of the sacrococcygeal spine is associated with a meningocele that herniates ventrally into the pelvis. The meningocele may be mistaken for the bladder. In addition, the anterior sacrum will be scalloped, and there may be a sickle-shaped scoliosis of the sacral spine. Cord tethering may be associated.

■ Summary

CNS indications are the most common indications for fetal imaging, with ventriculomegaly encompassing a majority of such studies. Ensuring high-quality, high-resolution imaging is paramount to procuring accurate diagnoses and thereby exacting prognostication and optimizing management options. A systematic, repetitive approach is best when interpreting imaging findings given the recurrence of common disease entities in the developing fetuses.

Bibliography

Arulkumaran, S., Skurr, B., Tong, H., Kek, L. P., Yeoh, K. H., & Ratnam, S. S. (1991). No evidence of hearing loss due to fetal acoustic stimulation test. *Obstetrics & Gynecology, 78*(2), 283–285.

Baker, P. N., Johnson, I. R., Harvey, P. R., Gowland, P. A., & Mansfield, P. (1994). A three-year follow-up of children imaged in utero with echo-planar magnetic resonance. *American Journal of Obstetrics and Gynecology, 170*(1 Pt 1), 32–33.

Bromley, B., Nadel, A. S., Pauker, S., Estroff, J. A., & Benacerraf, B. R. (1994). Closure of the cerebellar vermis: Evaluation with second trimester US. *Radiology, 193*(3), 761–763.

Burns, N. S., Iyer, R. S., Robinson, A. J., & Chapman, T. (2013). Diagnostic imaging of fetal and pediatric orbital abnormalities. *American Journal of Roentgenology, 201*(6), W797–W808.

Clements, H., Duncan, K. R., Fielding, K., Gowland, P. A., Johnson, I. R., & Baker, P. N. (2000). Infants exposed to MRI in utero have a normal paediatric assessment at 9 months of age. *British Journal of Radiology, 73*(866), 190–194.

Coakley, F. V., Glenn, O. A., Qayyum, A., Barkovich, A. J., Goldstein, R., & Filly, R. A. (2004). Fetal MRI: A developing technique for the developing patient. *American Journal of Roentgenology, 182*(1), 243–252.

De Santis, M., Straface, G., Cavaliere, A. F., Carducci, B., & Caruso, A. (2007). Gadolinium periconceptional exposure: Pregnancy and neonatal outcome. *Acta Obstetricia et Gynecologica Scandinavica, 86*(1), 99–101.

Expert Panel on MR Safety, Kanal, E., Barkovich, A. J., Bell, C., Borgstede, J. P., Bradley, W. G., Jr., et al. (2013). ACR guidance document on MR safe practices: 2013. *J Magn Reson Imaging, 37*(3), 501–530.

Fanou, E. M., Reeves, M. J., Howe, D. T., Joy, H., Morris, S., & Russell, S. (2013). In utero magnetic resonance imaging for diagnosis of dural venous sinus ectasia with thrombosis in the fetus. *Pediatric Radiology, 43*(12), 1591–1598.

Folkerth, R. D., McLaughlin, M. E., & Levine, D. (2001). Organizing posterior fossa hematomas simulating developmental cysts on prenatal imaging: Report of 3 cases. *Journal of Ultrasound in Medicine, 20*(11), 1233–1240.

Garel, C. (2006). New advances in fetal MR neuroimaging. *Pediatric Radiology, 36*(7), 621–625.

Glover, P., Hykin, J., Gowland, P., Wright, J., Johnson, I., & Mansfield, P. (1995). An assessment of the intrauterine sound intensity level during obstetric echo-planar magnetic resonance imaging. *British Journal of Radiology, 68*(814), 1090–1094.

Griffiths, P. D., Reeves, M. J., Morris, J. E., Mason, G., Russell, S. A., & Paley, M. N. (2010). A prospective study of fetuses with isolated ventriculomegaly investigated by antenatal sonography and in utero MR imaging. *AJNR American Journal of Neuroradiology, 31*(1), 106–111.

Hadlock, F. P., Deter, R. L., Harrist, R. B., & Park, S. K. (1982). Fetal head circumference: Relation to menstrual age. *American Journal of Roentgenology, 138*(4), 649–653.

Kanal, E. (1994). Pregnancy and the safety of magnetic resonance imaging. *Magnetic Resonance Imaging Clinics of North America, 2*(2), 309–317.

Kathary, N., Bulas, D. I., Newman, K. D., & Schonberg, R. L. (2001). MRI imaging of fetal neck masses with airway compromise: Utility in delivery planning. *Pediatric Radiology, 31*(10), 727–731.

Laing, F. C., Frates, M. C., Brown, D. L., Benson, C. B., Di Salvo, D. N., & Doubilet, P. M. (1994). Sonography of the fetal posterior fossa: False appearance of mega-cisterna magna and Dandy-Walker variant. *Radiology, 192*(1), 247–251.

Levine, D. (2001). Fetal magnetic resonance imaging. *Topics in Magnetic Resonance Imaging: TMRI, 12*(1), 1–2.

Levine, D., Barnes, P. D., Robertson, R. R., Wong, G., & Mehta, T. S. (2003). Fast MR imaging of fetal central nervous system abnormalities. *Radiology, 229*(1), 51–61.

Limperopoulos, C., Robertson, R. L., Estroff, J. A., Barnewolt, C., Levine, D., & Bassan, H. (2006). Diagnosis of inferior vermian hypoplasia by fetal magnetic resonance imaging: Potential pitfalls and neurodevelopmental outcome. *American Journal of Obstetrics and Gynecology, 194*(4), 1070–1076.

Liu, F., Zhang, Z., Lin, X., Teng, G., Meng, H., & Yu, T. (2011). Development of the human fetal cerebellum in the second trimester: A post mortem magnetic resonance imaging evaluation. *Journal of Anatomy, 219*(5), 582–588.

Mirsky, D. M., Shekdar, K. V., & Bilaniuk, L. T. (2012). Fetal MRI: Head and neck. *Magnetic Resonance Imaging Clinics of North America, 20*(3), 605–618.

Poretti, A., Boltshauser, E., & Doherty, D. (2014). Cerebellar hypoplasia: Differential diagnosis and diagnostic approach. *America Journal of Medical Genetics. Part C, Seminars in Medical Genetics, 166C*(2), 211–226.

Raybaud, C. A., Strother, C. M., & Hald, J. K. (1989). Aneurysms of the vein of Galen: Embryonic considerations and anatomical features relating to the pathogenesis of the malformation. *Neuroradiology, 31*(2), 109–128.

Robinson, A. J., Blaser, S., Toi, A., Chitayat, D., Pantazi, S., & Keating, S. (2008). MRI of the fetal eyes: Morphologic and biometric assessment for abnormal development with ultrasonographic and clinicopathologic correlation. *Pediatric Radiology, 38*(9), 971–981.

Rodegerdts, E. A., Gronewaller, E. F., Kehlbach, R., Roth, P., Wiskirchen, J., & Gebert, R. (2000). In vitro evaluation of teratogenic effects by time-varying MR gradient fields on fetal human fibroblasts. *Journal of Magnetic Resonance Imaging: JMRI, 12*(1), 150–156.

Rufener, S. L., Ibrahim, M., Raybaud, C. A., & Parmar, H. A. (2010). Congenital spine and spinal cord malformations-pictorial review. *American Journal of Roentgenology, 194*(Suppl. 3), S26–S37.

Sandow, B. A., Dory, C. E., Aguiar, M. A., & Abuhamad, A. Z. (2004). Best cases from the AFIP: Congenital intracranial teratoma. *RadioGraphics, 24*(4), 1165–1170.

Simon, E. M., Goldstein, R. B., Coakley, F. V., Filly, R. A., Broderick, K. C., & Musci, T. J. (2000). Fast MR imaging of fetal CNS anomalies in utero. *AJNR American Journal of Neuroradiology, 21*(9), 1688–1698.

Stroustrup Smith, A., Levine, D., Barnes, P. D., & Robertson, R. L. (2005). Magnetic resonance imaging of the kinked fetal brain stem: A sign of severe dysgenesis. *Journal of Ultrasound in Medicine, 24*(12), 1697–1709.

Vadeyar, S. H., Moore, R. J., Strachan, B. K., Gowland, P. A., Shakespeare, S. A., & James, D. K. (2000). Effect of fetal magnetic resonance imaging on fetal heart rate patterns. *American Journal of Obstetrics and Gynecology, 182*(3), 666–669.

Whitby, E. H., Variend, S., Rutter, S., Paley, M. N., Wilkinson, I. D., & Davies, N. P. (2004). Corroboration of in utero MRI using post-mortem MRI and autopsy in foetuses with CNS abnormalities. *Clinical Radiology, 59*(12), 1114–1120.

Wiskirchen, J., Groenewaeller, E. F., Kehlbach, R., Heinzelmann, F., Wittau, M., & Rodemann, H. P. (1999). Long-term effects of repetitive exposure to a static magnetic field (1.5 T) on proliferation of human fetal lung fibroblasts. *Magnetic Resonance in Medicine, 41*(3), 464–468.

Brain

CHAPTER 25
Pediatric Head CT

Jennifer A. Vaughn and Tina Young Poussaint

CHAPTER OUTLINE

Introduction, 493
Computed Tomography Techniques and Radiation
    Awareness, 493
Special Computed Tomography Examination
    Considerations, 494
Key Imaging Questions, 494
    Are the Vascular Structures Hyperdense?, 494
        Sinovenous Thrombosis, 494
        Acute Arterial Stroke, 496
    Is There Cerebral Edema?, 496

Is There Mass Effect/Midline Shift or Herniation?, 497
Are the Ventricles Too Big?, 498
Are the Cerebrospinal Fluid and Extraaxial Spaces
    Normal?, 499
Is There Intraparenchymal Hemorrhage?, 501
Are the Midline Structures Intact?, 502
Are There Intracranial Calcifications?, 502
Are There Foreign Bodies?, 505
Are There Any Abnormal Masses Associated With the
    Skull or Soft Tissues?, 505
Summary, 506

■ Introduction

Neuroradiological imaging of the pediatric patient has undergone tremendous change since the late 2000s. Although the use of magnetic resonance imaging (MRI) is on the rise, in part because of concerns over exposing children to medical radiation, there is still an important role for pediatric head computed tomography (CT), which provides fast imaging, often without the need for sedation. CT therefore remains an important tool for evaluating patients in the emergency department, especially in cases of acute trauma and critically ill inpatients who may be too unstable to undergo a lengthier MRI examination (Prabhu and Young-Poussaint, 2010). MRI also carries the additional risk of sedation and anesthesia for young children who have limited or no verbal skills and have difficulty remaining still in the magnetic resonance (MR) scanner long enough for the technologist to produce diagnostically useful images. At our institution, CT can be performed portably, making it an accessible test for children who cannot be transported to the radiology department. In addition, for patients who cannot undergo MRI secondary to implanted devices or external monitoring hardware, CT serves as the only available cross-sectional imaging modality.

The aim of this chapter is to provide an approach for interpreting pediatric head CT scans with a focus on recognizing intracranial structures in the developing brain while highlighting common disease entities seen in children. We will not, however, describe all potential neurological diseases of childhood that may be detected on head CT. As with the other chapters in this book, our goal is to present key findings that will enable the busy clinician to arrive at an appropriate or probable differential diagnosis by using a systematic approach to interpreting head CTs that will aid in clinical decision making.

■ Computed Tomography Techniques and Radiation Awareness

As CT use continues to grow among all age groups, the risks associated with exposure to ionizing radiation must be disclosed, as well as the fact that children experience disproportionate sensitivity to the effects of radiation. CT now accounts for the largest contribution to medical radiation dose in the United States. Children are at a greater risk for both short- and long-term effects of radiation, in part because their smaller bodies and organs are more susceptible to damage from higher doses and in part because their developing tissues and rapidly dividing cells are more radiosensitive than those of adults. These factors, combined with longer life expectancy, place children at higher risk for eventually developing cancers as a result of exposure to ionizing radiation, especially when CT must be repeated over months or years.

As a medical community, we can all play a role in minimizing radiation exposure through a variety of techniques. For example, shielding tissues outside of the imaging field can reduce the dose delivered to adjacent organs. Proper protocols should be selected for pediatric patients that take into account smaller body size with adjustments in the milliampere (mA) and peak kilovoltage (kVp). Protocols can also be further tailored depending on the clinical indication. Often a lower-dose scan can yield sufficient diagnostic information to answer a specific clinical question. At our institution, we select different scanning parameters for patients who are being followed for hydrocephalus where visualization of fine anatomic detail at the expense of a higher radiation dose does not add value to the clinical decision-making process (Pindrik et al., 2013; Rybka et al., 2007; Udayasankar et al., 2008). Single-phase contrast examinations should be part of the routine standard of care because additional information is rarely captured from the noncontrast or delayed phases to justify the added radiation dose. The scanning parameters for children must also be adjusted to image only the region of interest, with care taken to minimize imaging of any collateral tissues or organs.

With the promotion of the Image Gently campaign, numerous resources are now available to help guide the selection of appropriate CT parameters for clinical practice (Image Gently). At our institution, CT imaging protocols are continually reviewed by a team of radiologists, medical physicists, and radiology technologists to ensure scans are being optimized to achieve images of the highest diagnostic quality at the lowest possible levels of radiation exposure (The ALARA (as low as reasonably achievable) concept in pediatric CT: Intelligent dose reduction, 2002). The parameters selected for our head CT protocol are presented in Table 25.1. Modern multidetector scanners enable the acquisition of submillimeter (mm) thin-section images, which can then be reformatted into multiple viewing planes, but with no additional radiation dose delivered to the patient. Three-dimensional (3D) rotating models can also be generated from the axial data. These 3D models can both aid the radiologist in detecting pathology and provide surgeons and clinicians with a helpful visual aid for future disease management.

■ Special Computed Tomography Examination Considerations

As in adults, CT angiography (CTA) is also used for specific indications in the work-up of the pediatric patient. CTA is used to evaluate children with acute, nontraumatic parenchymal or subarachnoid hemorrhage; to evaluate for intracranial aneurysms, vascular malformations, or intracranial arterial dissections; or when concern exists for acute stroke where intravascular thrombolysis is being considered. At our institution, a single-phase, arterial-phase CT is performed that omits the noncontrast phase of the examination often performed in adult patients. CT venography is performed at some institutions for the evaluation of venous sinus thrombosis when MRI is either unavailable or contraindicated (Saposnik et al., 2011).

Occasionally contrast-enhanced CT may also be performed for the work-up of a mass, for assessing metastatic spread of disease, or for evaluating infectious processes. In pediatric patients with headache in the setting of sinusitis or mastoiditis, contrast-enhanced CT may be used to evaluate for intracranial complications. In most instances, MRI is preferred for these indications; however, as mentioned previously, in patients for whom MRI is not indicated, contrast-enhanced CT can play a vital role in reaching a diagnosis. Under these circumstances, the noncontrast portion of the examination is generally omitted because postprocessing techniques can evaluate cases where there is a question of enhancement in the presence of hemorrhage or mineralization.

■ Key Imaging Questions

In order to systematically approach pediatric head CTs we have organized this chapter around key imaging questions and finding encountered in clinical practice.

Are the Vascular Structures Hyperdense?

Sinovenous Thrombosis
The causes of cerebral sinovenous thrombosis differ significantly between children and adults. In children and young adults the causes include conditions that result in narrowing of the sinuses and invasion of the sinus walls and may predispose to stasis and coagulation. Trauma with skull fractures extending to the venous sinuses can cause occlusion or compression of the sinus, thereby altering flow and predisposing to thrombosis.

TABLE 25.1   Pediatric Head Computed Tomography Protocol

AGE	DISPLAY FIELD OF VIEW (DFOV) (cm)	KILOVOLTAGE (kVp)	MILLIAMPERE (mA)
Newborn to 6 months	20	120	155
7 months to 2 years	25	120	155
3 years to adult	25	120	215

- Orientation: head first
- Coverage: from base of skull to the vertex
- Scout 10 mA, 100 kVp
- Images are reconstructed in bone and soft tissue algorithms at 5.0 × 5.0 mm, as well as in bone algorithms at 0.625 × 0.625 mm
- Images are reformatted in bone and soft tissue windows in coronal and sagittal planes
- Three-dimensional rotating models of the calvarium are performed for all suspected cases of suspected nonaccidental trauma in patients younger than 1 year and for cases of suspected skull fracture, craniosynostosis, and other indications on request
- For ventricle check computed tomography, the mA is reduced to 95, 95, and 130 for the given age groups, respectively

Neoplastic and infectious processes may directly invade the sinus walls resulting in sinus occlusion secondary to the infiltrate and associated narrowing. In the pediatric population a prothrombotic state may be caused by inherited disorders of coagulation, dehydration, certain medications, and various systemic diseases, including malignancies, anemias, chronic renal disease, and autoimmune disorders, such as systemic lupus erythematous. In the neonate, additional maternal and obstetric factors predispose to sinovenous thrombosis, including maternal infection and diabetes, traumatic delivery, and placental abnormalities including abruption (Dlamini et al., 2010).

Familiarity with the cerebral venous anatomy is necessary to evaluate for cerebral sinovenous thrombosis. Cortical veins are superficially located along the brain surface and drain centrally to the dural venous sinuses. Deep cerebral veins, including the internal cerebral, medullary, and subependymal veins, drain blood from the deep brain structures to the vein of Galen, which, in turn, joins with the inferior sagittal sinus and together drain to the straight sinus. The major dural venous sinuses receiving blood from these superficial and deep systems include the torcula, sigmoid sinuses, transverse sinuses, and superior sagittal sinuses. The cavernous sinuses are also part of the deep venous system receiving blood from the ophthalmic veins and sphenoparietal sinuses. Each of these structures must be evaluated for abnormalities on CT. Thrombosis within any of these structures is collectively referred to as cerebral venous thrombosis.

Findings suggestive of sinovenous thrombosis on noncontrast head CT include increased attenuation and distension of the sinuses with possible extension of the hyperdensity into adjacent cortical veins known as the cord sign (Fig. 25.1A–C). Direct detection of the thrombus is seen in only approximately 20% of patients, however, so looking for secondary signs is important (Leach et al., 2006). In the presence of adjacent infection such as otomastoiditis or orbital cellulitis, there is also the possibility of spread to the adjacent venous structures. With fractures, it is important to evaluate for extension of the fracture to the sinus, as well as for osseous displacement into the sinus with resultant compression

and narrowing. Thrombosis can result in areas of parenchymal infarct and hemorrhage. Although infarcts typically present with loss of gray/white differentiation and edema, they do not characteristically correspond to a typical arterial distribution but may be associated with hemorrhage and proximal to the involved sinus or vein (Fig. 25.1B–D). When the thrombus involves the deep venous system, hyperdensity within the internal cerebral veins is usually seen. It is also important to look for subtle changes in low density in both thalami, specifically with blurring of the margins between the thalami and the internal capsule occurring secondary to venous congestion and edema.

Identifying sinovenous thrombosis is particularly challenging in the neonate where hemoconcentration results in diffuse, increased attenuation in the sinuses on unenhanced head CT, especially in contrast with the low-density, unmyelinated brain (Provenzale and Kranz, 2011). In hemoconcentration, all of the dural venous sinuses will have a homogeneously hyperdense appearance. Although secondary parenchymal signs or complications of thrombosis may suggest underlying hemoconcentration, it is also important to determine whether the sinuses just appear relatively hyperdense secondary to the presence of diffuse cerebral edema. An additional challenge in identifying hemoconcentration in the newborn is the presence of birth-related, extraaxial hemorrhage that is often present posteriorly and adjacent to the sinuses. Parturitional subdural hemorrhage is a very common finding in both vaginal and cesarean deliveries and is seen with increased frequency in vacuum- or forceps-assisted deliveries. Up to 46% of neonates have small, parturitional subdural hemorrhages, which can be both supratentorial and infratentorial in location, and may occur with concurrent subgaleal and cephalohematomas within the scalp. Establishing the location of hyperdensity is therefore critical because birth-related hemorrhages are most often subdural, and thus will be located deep to the dural venous sinuses and separated by the overlying dura. These small hemorrhages typically track along the subdural space at a distance from the dural sinuses, offering an additional clue as to their location.

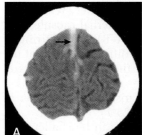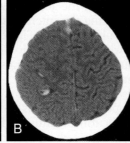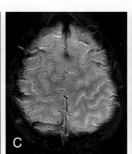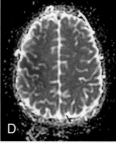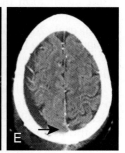

Fig. 25.1 *Sinovenous thrombosis.* (A) Sinovenous thrombosis and cord sign on computed tomography (CT). Axial CT image demonstrates hyperdensity within the superior sagittal sinus (*arrow*) and extending into cortical veins. (B) Sinovenous thrombosis with venous hemorrhage on CT. Axial CT image demonstrates hyperdensities in right frontal lobe with mild surrounding edema. (C) Superior sagittal sinus and cortical vein thrombosis on magnetic resonance. Axial susceptibility image demonstrates hypointensities within the superior sagittal sinus and cortical veins. (D) Venous infarct. Axial apparent diffusion coefficient map demonstrates restricted diffusion consistent with infarct in the right frontoparietal lobe. (E) Delta sign on CT venography. Axial CT image demonstrates central nonenhancement of the superior sagittal sinus (*arrow*).

Overall, noncontrast CT is insensitive for the diagnosis of sinovenous thrombosis, with positive results in only roughly 30% of cases, even when considering all of the findings. If there is high clinical suspicion, however, or if noncontrast CT shows any of the suggestive findings described earlier, further imaging with a contrast-enhanced CT venogram or MRI venogram is recommended. On contrast CT venography, the empty delta sign, which represents the nonenhancing thrombus surrounded by the enhancing dura, is generally noted (Fig. 25.1E) (Rodallec et al., 2006).

Acute Arterial Stroke

Although pediatric arterial stroke occurs only rarely in children, with an incidence of approximately 1.6 per 100,000 per year, it still represents a major public health burden because of the long-term morbidity associated with significant neurological deficits that typically result from this event. The incidence of arterial stroke is highest in children younger than 1 year. Unfortunately, the diagnosis is often delayed secondary to the absence of risk factors typically associated with adult stroke (e.g., clinical history of heart disease, hypertension, obesity, nicotine use) and variability of clinical presentation. The primary causes for stroke in children include cardiac shunts, sickle cell disease, and inherited coagulation disorders, which account for most of the underlying causes. In children with multiple strokes, occlusive vasculopathy including moyamoya disease, radiation therapy, trisomy 21, and neurofibromatosis type 1 should be considered as possible causes (Mallick et al., 2014).

The dense middle cerebral artery (MCA) sign refers to the hyperattenuating appearance of the M1 segment of the MCA secondary to thrombosis of the vessel. It is an important early indicator of ischemic stroke on unenhanced CT. Although this sign is very specific, it is insensitive and present in only 30% of patients with a proximal MCA occlusion (Petitti, 1998). Caution should be exercised when subjectively assessing the density of the MCA, however, because apparent, increased vessel attenuation can also be seen in cases of elevated hematocrit such as in polycythemia and in herpes encephalitis secondary to edema in the subjacent brain parenchyma. An absolute attenuation cutoff of 43 Hounsfield units and a ratio of the attenuation of the contralateral MCA above 1.2 have been shown to reliably exclude false-negative cases (Gadda et al., 2002; Koo et al., 2000). The hyperdense vessel sign can also be applied to the other intracranial vessels, including the carotid and basilar arteries (Fig. 25.2), although this is seen less commonly than in the MCA.

To achieve optimal therapeutic management, children with acute ischemic stroke must be identified as quickly as possible because thrombolysis and antithrombotic therapy are increasingly being used at pediatric stroke centers and are key to recovery and rehabilitation (Arnold et al., 2009). In addition to the hyperdense MCA sign, other signs seen in the setting of early acute MCA territory stroke include edema, loss of gray/white differentiation, and effacement of the sulci within the region supplied by the MCA, including the ipsilateral insula, frontal, temporal, and parietal lobes, as well as the deep gray structures.

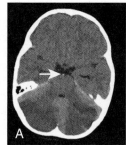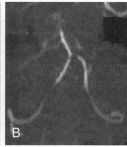

Fig. 25.2 Hyperdense artery sign. (A) Noncontrast head axial computed tomography image demonstrates hyperdense basilar artery (*arrow*) with ischemia in cerebellar hemispheres. (B) Magnetic resonance angiogram of the posterior circulation demonstrates absence of flow-related signal in distal basilar artery and posterior cerebral arteries secondary to thrombosis.

Is There Cerebral Edema?

Identifying the presence of edema in children is generally more challenging than in adults because the findings may appear more subtle and may be easily overlooked if the clinician is accustomed to interpreting adult head CTs. The normal pediatric brain has little space between the sulci and fissures, and ventricle size may be small. However, in the presence of edema, whether focal or diffuse, the brain volume enlarges compressing the cerebrospinal fluid (CSF) spaces. This loss of sulcation is frequently difficult to detect, so evaluating areas of the brain where sulci are normally seen (e.g., at the vertex) can be helpful (Fig. 25.3). Although the ventricles in pediatric patients are normally smaller than those of adults, they should be visible and fairly symmetrical in size. Any asymmetries of the ventricles suggesting ventricular effacement or a slitlike appearance can be found in the setting of edema. Similarly, the sylvian fissures and basilar cisterns should normally be visible and symmetrical in the normal pediatric brain. It is important therefore to visualize the suprasellar, quadrigeminal plate, and perimesencephalic cisterns for the presence of edema.

As edema progresses, there is loss of the gray/white differentiation (see Fig. 25.3A, C). In children, it is important to evaluate the deep gray structures and ensure that the basal ganglia and thalami can be seen as distinct from the adjacent white matter (WM) structures, including the internal and external capsules and periventricular WM (see Fig. 25.3A–B). Any blurring of the gray/white differentiation or diffuse haziness of the brain parenchyma should raise the possibility of cerebral edema.

Diffuse cerebral edema may arise from a number of causes in pediatric patients (Box 25.1).

The detection of diffuse edema can be challenging, however, because the brain may appear symmetrical. Important clues are blurring within the deep gray structures, effacement of the basilar cisterns, and nonvisualization of the sulci at the vertex. In addition, in the presence of diffuse cerebral edema, the cerebellum may appear hyperdense secondary to changes in low density within the edematous supratentorial brain known as the "white cerebellar" or "reversal" sign (Han et al., 1990).

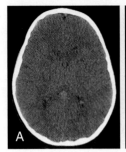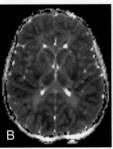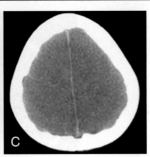

Fig. 25.3 Diffuse cerebral edema after cardiac arrest. (A) Noncontrast axial computed tomography (CT) image demonstrates low density within the basal ganglia and thalami with diffuse effacement of the cerebral sulci. (B) Axial magnetic resonance apparent diffusion coefficient map demonstrates restricted diffusion within the bilateral basal ganglia, thalami, and cerebral hemispheres consistent with infarct. (C) Axial CT image demonstrates diffuse cerebral edema with loss of the gray/white differentiation and effacement of the sulci at the vertex.

BOX 25.1   Causes of Diffuse Cerebral Edema

- Diabetic ketoacidosis
- Global anoxia: drowning/near drowning, arrest, hanging
- Hepatic or uremic encephalopathy
- Infection: sepsis, encephalomyelitis, meningitis
- Status epilepticus
- Trauma: diffuse axonal injury
- Toxin ingestion

BOX 25.2   Causes of Focal Cerebral Edema

- Stroke
- Posterior reversible encephalopathy syndrome
- Seizure
- Metabolic conditions presenting acutely
- Demyelinating disease: acute disseminated encephalomyelitis, multiple sclerosis
- Infection: cerebellitis, encephalitis, abscess
- Mass: neoplasm, arteriovenous malformation, cavernoma with hemorrhage

BOX 25.3   Herniation Patterns

- Subfalcine
- Uncal
- Descending transtentorial
- Ascending transtentorial
- Tonsillar

Focal edema in the pediatric patient is attributable to a variety of causes (Box 25.2). It may be easier to detect than the diffuse pattern, however, because asymmetry often exists in focal edema, with the contralateral side suggesting an abnormality. Certain diseases have a predilection for localizing to specific brain regions; thus familiarity with the common focal edema patterns is crucial to making a firm diagnosis. For example, herpes simplex encephalitis (HSE) should be considered when there is focal edema involving one or both medial temporal lobes, inferior frontal lobes, and/or insula, because this is a devastating, rapidly progressive, and potentially fatal infection. In the presence of edema involving the parietooccipital, watershed regions, cerebellum, and posterior frontal regions, especially in the clinical setting of hypertension or immunosuppressive drug use, a diagnosis of posterior reversible encephalopathy syndrome should be considered (McKinney et al., 2007; Shimizu et al., 2013). Edema confined to the cerebellum in a child may suggest cerebellitis. Cerebellitis can be seen with viral infections such as varicella zoster (after vaccinations) and in toxic encephalopathy in the setting of methadone overdose.

Is There Mass Effect/Midline Shift or Herniation?

Once edema is identified as focal or diffuse, determining the displacement and/or distortion of brain structures locally and remotely is crucial to understanding the extent of the condition. Moreover, identifying the presence or absence of mass effect plays a greater role in management decisions than determining the specific cause of the edema. In addition, the cause of the mass effect may not be readily apparent on unenhanced head CT, and any displacement of adjacent structures may be the only clue to the presence of underlying pathology.

The brain has inherent symmetry, which should be considered when evaluating for the presence of mass effect. It is important first to identify the midline and, second, to ensure that key midline structures, such as the anterior and posterior falx, septum pellucidum, and pineal gland, are in fact at midline. Although the lateral ventricles may be slightly asymmetrical, they should maintain a smooth contour, and neither side should be effaced, compressed, nor shifted.

In addition to midline shift, it is also important to identify and report any herniation patterns (Box 25.3) because specific types of herniations predispose the patient to additional complications secondary to the mass effect and may require immediate intervention. These herniation patterns are described later.

Subfalcine herniation, the most common type of herniation pattern, results when the paramedian frontal lobe, typically the cingulate gyrus, is displaced to the opposite side of the falx cerebri. To identify this, a line should be drawn from the anterior falx posteriorly to the posterior falx to assess whether the paramedian frontal lobe is deviated across this line (Fig. 25.4). As a result of subfalcine herniation, the anterior cerebral artery branches, which run within the interhemispheric fissure and cingulate sulci, can be compressed against, or be pulled under, the falx and secondarily occluded leading to infarcts within the anterior cerebral artery vascular territory. Also as a result of subfalcine herniation are trapping of the ventricles and hydrocephalus. As the frontal lobe and corpus callosum are pushed across to the opposite side, they may compress and obstruct

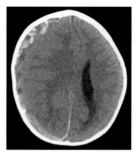

Fig. 25.4 Subfalcine herniation. Axial computed tomography image shows right subdural hemorrhage and right cerebral edema with resultant left to right subfalcine herniation and ventricular enlargement of the left lateral ventricle.

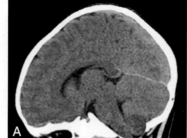
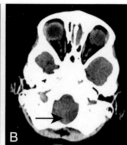

Fig. 25.5 Tonsillar herniation. (A) Sagittal computed tomography (CT) image demonstrates ischemia and edema in the cerebellar tonsils with herniation of the tonsils through the foramen magnum. (B) Axial CT image demonstrates crowding of the low-density tonsils (*arrow*) at the foramen magnum.

the contralateral foramen of Monro, resulting in contralateral hydrocephalus (see Fig. 25.4).

A second pattern of herniation requires identifying the uncus, the most medial part of the temporal lobe. Uncal herniation, a common type of descending transtentorial herniation, results when the uncus is displaced medially and inferiorly into the suprasellar cistern. As the herniation progresses, the hippocampus also herniates medially and effaces the quadrigeminal cistern. Eventually both uncus and hippocampus extend below the tentorial incisura, resulting in unilateral descending transtentorial herniation that compresses the midbrain. Uncal herniation may also compress the oculomotor nerve within the suprasellar cistern, resulting in pupillary dilation. It may also compress the ipsilateral posterior cerebral artery against the tentorium, giving rise to infarct in the posterior cerebral artery vascular territory.

With severe supratentorial mass effect, both medial temporal lobes may herniate medially and inferiorly push the midbrain and pons downward, reducing the angle between the midbrain and pons. When this occurs, it is termed *central* or *bilateral descending transtentorial herniation.*

When the mass effect occurs in the infratentorial brain, two types of herniation are seen. Typically the cerebellar tonsils will displace inferiorly through the foramen magnum, resulting in anterior displacement of the cervicomedullary junction and effacement of the fourth ventricle. This is most easily recognized on sagittal reformatted images. This type of herniation can occur with Chiari type I malformation acquired in patients with posterior fossa masses or posterior fossa edema (Fig. 25.5), or may present with intracranial hypotension. Less commonly, or when the mass effect is severe, the cerebellum can displace upward through the tentorium. This displacement in turn effaces the quadrigeminal plate cistern, compresses the tectum, and possibly obliterates the cerebral aqueduct, resulting in hydrocephalus. This type of herniation pattern is termed *ascending transtentorial herniation.*

Are the Ventricles Too Big?

Pediatric head CT imaging is often used to evaluate ventricular size to establish the presence of hydrocephalus.

Acute hydrocephalus can occur in a variety of clinical settings (e.g., obstructive and nonobstructive hydrocephalus), as well as in the presence of a malfunctioning ventricular shunt. When evaluating the ventricles, it is important to remember that the pediatric ventricles are normally small; however, all components of the lateral ventricles, as well as the third and fourth ventricles, should be visible in the healthy patient. Early signs of ventricular enlargement include dilation of the lateral ventricular temporal horns and rounding of the third ventricle, structures that are normally small and barely visible. Essential to assessing the third ventricle accurately is a sagittal reformatted image, which may depict the roof of the third ventricle and corpus callosum as superiorly bowed. It may also show the floor as inferiorly bowed, and the third ventricular recesses may be enlarged (Segev et al., 2001). The CSF spaces, including the sulci, fissures, and basilar cisterns, may become effaced or compressed. Low-attenuation change within the periventricular WM surrounding the ventricular margins may be seen, indicating transependymal edema or flow of CSF. However, it is important to distinguish any low-density periventricular change associated with edema from ependymitis granularis. Ependymitis granularis is a benign finding presenting as subtle, small regions of low attenuation within the WM, found anteriorly and laterally to the frontal horns and around the occipital horns of the ventricles. In the setting of transependymal edema, low-attenuation change will be lower in density and more pronounced in extent, that is, extending around the atria, bodies of the lateral ventricles, and around the temporal horns where changes related to ependymitis granularis should not be seen.

Determining the underlying cause for the hydrocephalus is critical to optimal disease management and clinical decision making. Acute hydrocephalus can be divided broadly into nonobstructive and obstructive types, with the latter being further divided into noncommunicating or communicating forms based on the cause of the obstruction (Rekate, 2009). In noncommunicating hydrocephalus, the cause of the obstruction may be readily apparent on head CT, for example, a mass in the posterior fossa, pineal, or tectal regions (Fig. 25.6), or a vascular malformation such as a vein of Galen malformation compressing sites where the CSF flow pathways are the narrowest. The sites typically prone to obstruction include the foramina of Monro, the cerebral aqueduct, and the fourth ventricle outlet foramina of Magendie and Luschka. In addition, many nonneoplastic causes can obstruct the ventricles at these same sites, for example, Chiari malformations (Fig. 25.7), arachnoid cysts (ACs), intraventricular adhesions and webs, and congenital stenoses. In cases of communicating hydrocephalus a number of diseases can result in poor extraventricular resorption of CSF by the arachnoid granulations, for example, subarachnoid hemorrhage, leptomeningeal tumor spread, leptomeningeal inflammation/infection from meningitis, and venous hypertension. Tumors of the choroid plexus may also lead to a nonobstructive hydrocephalus secondary to the overproduction of CSF.

The shunted patient represents a unique patient group frequently imaged to evaluate for signs of ventricular catheter malfunction. In these patients, ventricular size must be compared with the size recorded in any previous examinations. Knowing the "normal" baseline size of the ventricles in a particular shunted patient is critical because small changes in ventricle size from the initial baseline may indicate shunt malfunction. The entire visible course of any intraventricular catheter must also be traced. This should include both the intracranial portion and the component within the scalp and any visible extracranial course. On the scout image, catheter discontinuities or kinks are common sites of shunt fracture in the mobile neck. Fluid collections around the reservoir may indicate malfunction and should be routinely checked.

Evaluating the position of the tip of the catheter is also important because small changes in the location of the tip may indicate the catheter has migrated and may no longer be draining properly. Each portion of the ventricular system must be evaluated for any change in size because trapping of portions of the ventricles secondary to scarring and adhesions from repeated infections and hemorrhage may occur (Sivaganesan et al., 2012). Under these conditions a second catheter may be inserted to bypass these obstructions. Importantly, CT scans may demonstrate stable or even decreased ventricular size in patients experiencing shunt malfunction. A neurosurgical consult should be requested for patients with documented shunt malfunction regardless of imaging findings.

Finally, ventriculomegaly does not always indicate the presence of hydrocephalus. Many congenital syndromes present with ventriculomegaly, which is beyond the scope of this chapter. Additional abnormalities can alert to the likelihood that the ventricular enlargement is chronic. However, these children may also experience development of acute hydrocephalus in the presence of chronically enlarged ventricles; evaluating for specific signs of mass effect is therefore necessary. Ventriculomegaly is also seen in the presence of diseases resulting in cerebral volume loss, such as the end stage of many metabolic and neurodegenerative disorders, after prior hypoxic-ischemic injury and germinal matrix hemorrhage, and in chronic demyelinating diseases such as multiple sclerosis. With chronic ventriculomegaly resulting from congenital abnormalities and/or volume loss, there is often reduced volume of the periventricular WM, prominence of the CSF spaces, and enlargement of the extraaxial spaces. Although the lateral and third ventricles will be enlarged, there should be no evidence of transependymal edema, nor should the third ventricle demonstrate any bowing of the margins or widening of the ventricular recesses, as previously discussed. The temporal horns should also remain relatively preserved in size and should not demonstrate any rounding.

Are the Cerebrospinal Fluid and Extraaxial Spaces Normal?

Previously discussed conditions resulting in compression of the CSF and extraaxial spaces (e.g., cerebral edema and acute hydrocephalus) have been covered in this

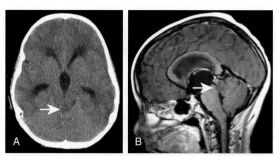

Fig. 25.6 Tectal glioma with obstructive hydrocephalus. (A) Axial computed tomography image shows a low-density mass within the tectum (*arrow*) with compression of the cerebral aqueduct and supratentorial hydrocephalus. (B) Sagittal postcontrast T1 magnetic resonance imaging shows nonenhancing tectal glioma (*arrow*) with obstructive hydrocephalus.

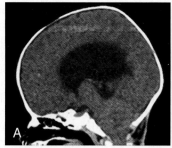
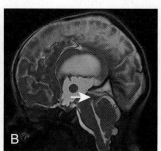
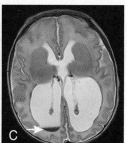

Fig. 25.7 Chiari type II with congenital obstructive hydrocephalus. (A) Sagittal noncontrast computed tomography image shows a small posterior fossa, inferior descent of the cerebellar tonsils through the foramen magnum, effacement of the fourth ventricle, and supratentorial hydrocephalus. (B) Sagittal T2 magnetic resonance (MR) image shows tectal beaking (*arrow*). (C) Axial T2 MR image demonstrates obstructive hydrocephalus with intraventricular hemorrhage (*arrow*) secondary to recent surgical repair of associated myelomeningocele.

chapter. However, several very common conditions in children may also result in enlarged extraaxial spaces, and the radiologist should be alert to these possible findings on head CT.

The term *extraaxial* is used to denote the space that is within the cranial vault but external to the brain parenchyma. Entities found within this region include masses, fluid collections, and cysts related to the pia, arachnoid, dura, and bridging vasculature. Although not the focus of this chapter, trauma, whether accidental or nonaccidental, may result in hyperdense, extraaxial collections classified as subarachnoid, subdural, and/or epidural determined by location. Importantly, as the hemorrhage ages, it progressively decreases in density and eventually may appear equal to or just slightly hyperdense to the surrounding CSF. It is crucial to detect any secondary signs of mass effect, but this is especially challenging because such signs are often subtle in appearance. Empyema, although also not the focus of this chapter, may present as a mildly hyperdense, extraaxial collection compared with the CSF that should be considered in the setting of complicated sinusitis. For further reading on the paranasal sinuses, please refer to Chapter 29.

In addition to conditions resulting in altered density within the extraaxial space, several conditions lead to enlarged, extraaxial, and CSF spaces of equal density to the CSF, including benign enlargement of the subarachnoid space (BESS), ACs, chronic subdural hematomas, and glutaric aciduria type 1.

In BESS, infants and very young children present with enlarged head circumference and have symmetrical enlargement of the bifrontal extraaxial spaces greater than 5 mm with equal density to the CSF and otherwise normal head CTs (Fig. 25.8A) The bridging veins may appear prominent, traversing the extraaxial spaces. These children are at increased risk for subdural hematomas in the setting of minor trauma secondary to stretching of these crossing veins (Fig. 25.8B). In BESS, however, there should be no mass effect from the enlarged extraaxial CSF spaces on the adjacent gyri as would be expected in cases of both chronic subdural hematomas and ACs, which typically have some mass effect on the brain. In the case of ACs, remodeling of the inner table of the overlying calvarium takes place. Furthermore, BESS is not associated with any parenchymal brain abnormality, nor is it associated with cerebral volume loss, and the ventricles are typically normal to very slightly enlarged in size.

This is in contrast with patients with glutaric aciduria type 1 who may have enlarged head circumference and expansion of subarachnoid spaces. Typically, however, enlargement is seen in the extraaxial spaces anterior to the temporal poles and in the Sylvian fissures. Glutaric aciduria type 1 is also characterized by a slow, progressive neurological deterioration with edema and subsequent atrophy of the basal ganglia (Fig. 25.9), additional features that enable the radiologist to distinguish it from BESS and middle cranial fossa ACs.

Posterior fossa CSF or extraaxial collections are also commonly noted on CT, the modality used most often for initial diagnosis, followed by MRI for definitive diagnosis. ACs, Dandy-Walker malformation, Blake

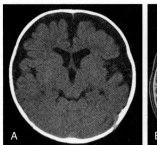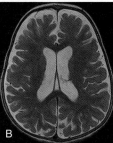

Fig. 25.8 Benign enlargement of subarachnoid spaces. (A) Axial computed tomography noncontrast image shows enlarged bifrontal cerebrospinal fluid (CSF) extraaxial spaces. (B) Axial T2 magnetic resonance image shows enlarged bifrontal CSF extraaxial spaces with prominent bridging vessels and mild ventriculomegaly for age.

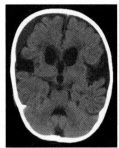

Fig. 25.9 Glutaric aciduria. Axial computed tomography noncontrast image demonstrates prominent cerebrospinal fluid spaces anterior to the temporal lobes and enlargement of the Sylvian fissures bilaterally with a small right subdural fluid collection and mild prominence of the cerebral sulci.

pouch cyst, and mega cisterna magna can all present with enlargement of the CSF spaces posterior to the cerebellum. In Dandy-Walker malformation, there will be partial or complete absence of the cerebellar vermis, elevation of the tentorium, and enlargement of the fourth ventricle (Fig. 25.10). In ACs and mega cisterna magna, these structures will be intact. The thin wall of the AC separates the CSF density posterior fossa structure from the rest of the subarachnoid space and distinguishes it from mega cisterna magna in which there is free communication of the enlarged CSF space. However, this thin wall is not easily seen on head CT.

Prominent intraaxial CSF spaces within the brain parenchyma can also be seen on CT with a limited differential diagnosis, including perivascular or Virchow-Robin spaces (PVSs) and hippocampal remnant cysts. PVSs are filled with interstitial fluid and surround penetrating vessels. They are typically found within the inferior basal ganglia, as well as within the subcortical and periventricular WM. Most are symmetrical, occur in clusters, and are several millimeters in size; however, they may enlarge under certain conditions, appearing as large, asymmetrical CSF-like lesions with mass effect. Patients with the mucopolysaccharidoses, including Sanfilippo, Hunter, and Hurler syndromes, as well as certain muscular dystrophies, can present with such enlarged, multiple PVSs (Fig. 25.11). Hippocampal remnant cysts are benign, small, CSF-like spaces similar in morphology to PVSs; however, they are found typically in a string along the medial temporal lobes, just medial

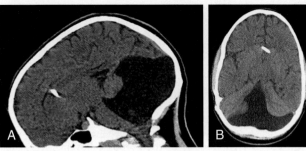

Fig. 25.10 Dandy-Walker malformation. (A) Sagittal computed tomography (CT) image shows a hypoplastic cerebellar vermis and enlarged posterior fossa cerebrospinal fluid (CSF) space that communicates with the fourth ventricle with elevation of the tentorium. There is a ventricular shunt in the frontal region. (B) Axial CT image shows a hypoplastic cerebellum with absent inferior vermis and an enlarged posterior fossa CSF space that communicates with the fourth ventricle.

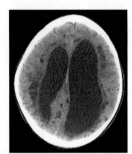

Fig. 25.11 Hunter syndrome. Axial computed tomography image shows enlarged perivascular spaces bilaterally with ventriculomegaly.

to the temporal horn of the lateral ventricle. Both entities are of no clinical significance and should not be mistaken for pathology.

Is There Intraparenchymal Hemorrhage?

Trauma, both accidental and nonaccidental, is a major cause of neurological morbidity and mortality in children, followed by spontaneous hemorrhage. Traumatic intraparenchymal hemorrhage in the form of contusion and diffuse axonal injury are not the focus of this chapter, however. For further reading on this topic, refer to Chapter 20. Additional causes for intraaxial hemorrhage in the pediatric age group include arteriovenous malformations (AVMs), arteriovenous fistulas, cavernous malformations, bleeding diatheses, certain infections including HSE, hemorrhagic masses, and rarely in children, aneurysms. In neonates, germinal matrix hemorrhage may be found in those born at less than 34 weeks of gestation and venous thrombosis with associated hemorrhage in those born at more than 34 weeks of gestation with the findings as described in the previous section. The age of the patient, presence of any underlying hematological disorder, location, and degree of any surrounding edema are important clues in distinguishing among these etiologies. The differential diagnosis and subsequent management strategy differ substantially between children and adults where hypertensive hemorrhage and hemorrhagic metastases account for a much larger percentage of intraparenchymal hemorrhages.

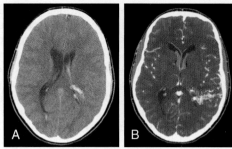

Fig. 25.12 Arteriovenous malformation rupture with intraventricular hemorrhage. (A) Axial computed tomography (CT) noncontrast image shows left periatrial hemorrhage extending into the left lateral ventricle with intraventricular hemorrhage within the left lateral ventricle and right occipital horn. (B) CT angiography shows a serpiginous tangle of vessels (*asterisk*) in the left periatrial white matter and left inferior parietal lobe without mass effect.

Cerebral vascular malformations are the most common cause for spontaneous intraparenchymal hemorrhage in children aged 1 to 18 years. The types of cerebral vascular malformation include parenchymal, dural, and mixed forms. AVMs tend to be solitary lesions with an incidence of approximately 1.34 per 100,000 person-years in the general population, although these individuals often remain asymptomatic. It is beyond the scope of this chapter to discuss the various types of AVM; however, they are classified by the Spetzler-Martin grading system based on their size, location, and venous drainage (Alexander & Spetzler, 2005). On unenhanced head CT, AVMs typically appear as a serpentine tangle of vessels with little intervening parenchyma. The enlarged draining veins and arteries may be visible as slightly hyperdense, tubular, vascular structures to the adjacent gliotic parenchyma, which may contain foci of dystrophic calcifications. The degree of mass effect and surrounding edema is typically minimal, if any, compared with a neoplastic mass of comparable size. In the setting of AVM rupture, hemorrhage may be seen within different compartments of the brain and associated vasogenic edema with mass effect (Fig. 25.12). Angiography remains the gold standard for diagnosing these lesions and also allows for treatment options in a subset of these patients.

Cavernous malformations (prior colloqual term also known as cavernomas) are commonly found within the subcortical WM, although they can be found in any region of the brain. It should be considered in the differential diagnosis for both single and multiple small foci of parenchymal hyperdensity, because multiple hereditary cavernoma syndromes do exist, although they are rarer than single lesions. When uncomplicated, cavernomas are typically asymptomatic and may not be detected on unenhanced CT. A small focus of hyperdensity or faint calcification not associated with any mass effect or surrounding edema may be seen. In the setting of hemorrhage, a larger, rounded region of parenchymal hemorrhage with surrounding vasogenic edema and mass effect may be observed. In these patients, MRI with susceptibility or gradient-echo imaging may aid in identifying classic features that characterize the lesions, additional cavernomas and associated developmental venous anomalies. Among the differential diagnoses for multiple spontaneous parenchymal hemorrhages are posterior reversible encephalopathy syndrome, septic emboli, vasculitis, and hematological disorders. In children, tumors are a rare cause of intraparenchymal hemorrhage. However, certain brain tumors have a predilection for hemorrhage and should be considered when a hemorrhage is seen in association with a large amount of mass effect and surrounding vasogenic edema. Metastasis, although accounting for a large percentage of tumoral hemorrhage in adults, is a rare cause of tumoral hemorrhage in children. High-grade, primary parenchymal tumors, including primitive neuroectodermal tumors (PNETs), glioblastomas, supratentorial ependymomas, atypical teratoid rhabdoid tumors, and choroid plexus carcinomas, should be considered among the differential diagnoses for a hemorrhagic neoplasm in children. As previously discussed, HSE can also cause a focal pattern of marked edema in association with parenchymal hemorrhage and should also be considered among the differential diagnoses.

Are the Midline Structures Intact?

It is important to determine whether the morphology of key midline structures is normal because many congenital brain malformations present with midline abnormalities. The first structures to locate and examine are the anterior and posterior falx cerebri. If the falx is absent, then the holoprosencephaly spectrum of disorders should be considered. Alobar holoprosencephaly is the most severe form presenting with no identifiable lobes, a single monoventricle that opens into a large dorsal midline cyst, a fused thalami, a variable amount of anteriorly fused cortex, and most telling, absent midline structures, including the falx and septum pellucidum. This disease can mimic hydranencephaly or severe hydrocephalus, which may also present in the neonate with a variable amount of thinned peripheral cortex; however, in both of these conditions, the falx cerebri should be present (Barkovich, 2005).

The corpus callosum should next be identified and determined to be present in its entirety and normal in morphology. Dysgenesis of the corpus callosum includes agenesis of the corpus callosum where the corpus callosum is absent, or hypogenesis, where the corpus callosum is incomplete (Fig. 25.13) (Barkovich and Kjos, 1988). Agenesis of the corpus callosum can be associated with aneuploidies, holoprosencephaly, Chiari type II malformation, Dandy-Walker spectrum, malformations of cortical development, midline facial anomalies, Aicardi syndrome, cephaloceles, intracranial lipomas, and interhemispheric cysts, among numerous other entities (Barkovich and Norman, 1988). Thus these patients should be referred for brain MRI because many of these conditions and associated congenital anomalies will be inconspicuous on head CT.

The corpus callosum consists of the genu, body, splenium, and rostrum. The corpus callosal development is a series of complex steps beyond the scope of this chapter; in general, however, it forms from an anterior to a posterior direction. The sagittal reformatted image is helpful for visualizing the corpus callosum, and all

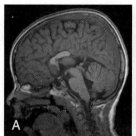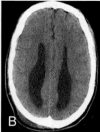

Fig. 25.13 Hypogenesis of the corpus callosum. (A) Sagittal T1 magnetic resonance image shows absence of the posterior body, isthmus, and splenium of the corpus callosum. (B) Axial computed tomography image shows colpocephaly with enlargement of the ventricle atria and teardrop configuration of parallel oriented ventricles.

portions are normally seen in this view. Normative values of callosal size and thickness are available in the literature and should be consulted for reference as the callosum thickens and elongates with age (Hetts et al., 2006). On imaging of callosal agenesis, a high third ventricle—a widened interhemispheric fissure characterized by widely spaced parallel lateral ventricles with enlarged occipital horns—gives rise to the teardrop configuration of the ventricles known as colpocephaly and Probst bundles. These structures are best seen on MR, which are WM bundles medial to the medial walls of the lateral ventricles and lateral to the cingulate gyri. Callosal anomalies in holoprosencephaly are atypical because the splenium may be present, or the body and splenium may be present with an absent genu. In the middle interhemispheric variant type of holoprosencephaly, the genu and splenium may be present with an absent body.

Moving inward, the septum pellucidi should be evaluated next. In neonates a cavum septum pellucidum is normally present with fusion of the anterior septal leaflets occurring in 85% of patients by approximately 3 months of age. Persistence beyond this age represents a normal anatomic variant. Similarly, cavum vergae reflects persistence of the CSF space between the splenium and the hippocampal commissure, often seen in association with cavum septum pellucidum as a common normal variant (Osborn, 2012). Absence of the septum is seen in patients with holoprosencephaly, as previously discussed, and in septo-optic dysplasias, as well as severe obstructive hydrocephalus. Septo-optic dysplasia can be thought of as the most minor variant within the holoprosencephaly spectrum and is characterized by absence of the septum, hypoplasia of the optic chiasm, and abnormalities in pituitary, most commonly pituitary hypoplasia. It may be associated with schizencephaly and numerous other congenital malformations (Fig. 25.14) (Raybaud, 2010). In longstanding, severe obstructive hydrocephalus, deficiencies of the septal leaflets secondary to elevated intraventricular pressure and postsurgical changes may be evident.

Are There Intracranial Calcifications?

Calcifications within the brain, extraaxial spaces, and ventricles can be seen in normal anatomic structures, as well as in a wide variety of diseases, including congenital

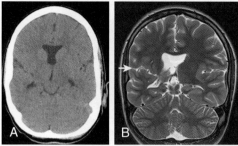

Fig. 25.14 *Septo-optic dysplasia and schizencephaly.* (A) Axial computed tomography image shows absence of the anterior septal leaflets. (B) Coronal T2 magnetic resonance image shows absence of the anterior septal leaflets and schizencephaly with a gray matter–lined cleft extending through the right temporal lobe to the margin of the right lateral ventricle (*arrow*).

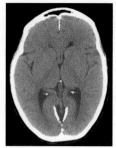

Fig. 25.15 Basal cell nevus syndrome with tentorial and falcine calcifications. Noncontrast axial computed tomography image shows calcifications along the tentorial leaflets and anterior and posterior falx.

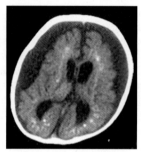

Fig. 25.16 *Congenital cytomegalovirus.* Axial computed tomography image shows bilateral periventricular calcifications with bilateral extracerebral cerebrospinal fluid density collections. There is ventriculomegaly and parenchymal volume loss.

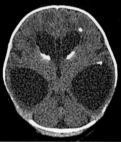

Fig. 25.17 *Congenital toxoplasmosis.* Axial computed tomography image shows bilateral periventricular calcifications and cystic encephalomalacia in the frontal lobes with ventriculomegaly.

diseases, vascular malformations, infectious and metabolic processes, toxic exposures, prior trauma, infarcts, or in association with certain tumors.

Normally calcified structures include the pineal gland, habenula, choroid plexus, and dura, which should not be mistaken for pathology, although evaluating the size and pattern of these calcifications is very important. The pineal gland, for example, is rarely calcified in children younger than 5 years. However, it undergoes an exponential increase in the incidence of calcification around the age of 15 such that by age 20, approximately 40% of patients have physiological calcification of the gland (Zimmerman and Bilaniuk, 1982). Calcifications within the pineal in children younger than 5 years and calcification at any age with associated enlargement of the gland greater than 1 cm should be regarded with suspicion because primary pineal tumors can present with calcific components. Calcifications are also commonly seen in the habenula in approximately 10% of pediatric patients. Calcifications within these paired structures located anterolaterally to the pineal gland along the medial thalamus bilaterally have been shown to correlate with the presence of pineal calcifications.

Similarly, choroid plexus calcification also increases in extent and incidence with age. Approximately 12% of patients younger than 10 years demonstrate normal physiological calcification, which progressively increases to 86% by the eighth decade of life (Whitehead et al., 2015). In children, however, calcification is normally confined to the glomus; calcifications within the choroid outside this location should raise suspicion for alternative diagnoses, such as prior infection or hemorrhage and tumors of the choroid plexus (Modic et al., 1980). Dural calcifications along the tentorium and falx, although common in adults, are rare in children, found in less than 1%. However, falx and tentorial calcifications can be seen with the basal cell nevus syndrome (Fig. 25.15) where associated calcification of the petroclinoid ligaments, odontogenic keratocysts of the maxilla and mandible, basal cell carcinomas, and medulloblastoma are typically detected. Dural calcifications are also more commonly seen after craniotomies.

Intrauterine infection with TORCH (toxoplasmosis, rubella, cytomegalovirus, herpesviruses, HIV) infections may also result in various intracranial calcifications. Cytomegalovirus is the most common congenital infection seen in developed countries. The timing of infection during gestation determines postnatal manifestations, with early gestational infection resulting in a more severe pattern, including periventricular calcifications and volume loss secondary to germinal zone necrosis (Fig. 25.16). Ventriculomegaly, microcephaly, cortical malformations (polymicrogyria and pachygyria), and sensorineural hearing loss are also common; however, these conditions remain difficult to appreciate on unenhanced head CT and should be further evaluated with MRI.

Congenital toxoplasmosis tends to cause a more diffuse pattern of calcification throughout the cortex and subcortical WM. Associated destruction of the parenchyma is not uncommon. In addition, these patients tend to present with macrocephaly, hydrocephalus, and rarely seen malformations of cortical development (Fig. 25.17).

In the differential diagnosis for periventricular calcification are the subependymal nodules seen in tuberous sclerosis, one of the neurocutaneous syndromes associated with cortical tubers, subependymal nodules, WM abnormalities, and subependymal giant cell astrocytomas within the brain. Subependymal nodules are found along the margins of the lateral ventricles, and although it is rare to have calcification within these nodules before 1 year of age, they progressively calcify over time so that eventually approximately 50% are calcified. Neonates with congenital HIV infection may also present with calcifications with a predilection in the bilateral basal ganglia and in the subcortical WM in association with marked cerebral volume loss. Neonates with herpes infection can also present with dystrophic calcifications and encephalomalacia within the brain parenchyma.

A variety of infections beyond the gestational/neonatal period can also produce calcifications with certain imaging patterns. Neurocysticercosis is caused by intracerebral infection with *Taenia solium* and is a common cause for seizures in children and young adults in endemic areas. The infection can be both intraaxial and extraaxial and progresses through four stages based on the viability of the parasite and the brain's response to its presence. The end stage of neurocysticercosis, in which the cysts are quiescent, may appear as numerous intracranial calcifications without any appreciable surrounding edema or mass effect with calcified cysts seen within the subarachnoid space, basilar cisterns, ventricles, as well as throughout the brain parenchyma. Contrast-enhanced MRI is useful for detection of active lesions.

Cerebral toxoplasmosis acquired postnatally causes multiple ring-enhancing lesions with surrounding edema in a central, predominant distribution. After treatment, there are diffuse scattered parenchymal calcifications. Tuberculosis remains endemic in many countries, and although central nervous system (CNS) infections, even among these patients, are rare, healed tuberculomas of the CNS may calcify and should be considered in patients presenting from developing nations and in immunocompromised individuals.

In adults, symmetrical calcification may be seen within the globus pallidus as an incidental finding; however, calcification in the basal ganglia in children should raise suspicion for conditions including infections previously discussed, metabolic syndromes including parathyroid diseases, inherited diseases, prior hypoxic injury, and toxic exposures, such as carbon monoxide, lead, and chemoradiation. Cockayne syndrome is a rare inherited dysmyelinating disease presenting with basal ganglia calcifications in addition to calcifications in the cerebellar dentate nuclei and cortical brain in association with atrophy (Fig. 25.18). Fahr disease is another neurological disorder that may present in childhood and is characterized by calcifications in these same brain regions. Typically, however, this disease remains asymptomatic until adulthood with additional calcifications seen in the thalami and subcortical WM. In patients treated with radiation and chemotherapy, calcifications occur within the basal ganglia and in other regions, including the cerebellar dentate and gray matter/WM junction secondary to mineralizing microangiopathy (Fig. 25.19).

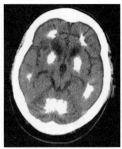

Fig. 25.18 Cockayne syndrome. Axial computed tomography image shows dense bilateral parenchymal, basal ganglia, and cerebellar calcifications involving lentiform nuclei, dentate, and subcortical white matter with parenchymal volume loss.

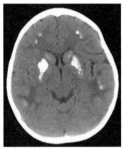

Fig. 25.19 Radiation therapy brain effects. Axial computed tomography image shows microangiopathy secondary to prior radiation with dense calcifications involving the basal ganglia and subcortical white matter.

Certain primary brain tumors in children have a tendency to calcify and should be included among the differential diagnoses when calcifications are seen in association with a mass. These include craniopharyngiomas, teratomas, intracranial lipomas, oligodendroglioma, PNETs, dysembryoplastic neuroepithelial tumor, gangliogliomas, and ependymomas.

Craniopharyngiomas are low-grade sellar and suprasellar neoplasms with an incidence in a bimodal distribution occurring in older children/teens and a second peak in adulthood. The childhood adamantinomatous subtype typically presents as a cystic mass with stippled and/or peripheral calcifications in more than 90% of patients, in contrast with the adult subtype in which calcification is rare and lesions are more solid (Fig. 25.20). Teratomas may also be present in the suprasellar region and contain calcification; in these cases, fat density in associated with a mixed cystic and solid mass. In addition, peripheral calcification in association with incidentally discovered intracranial lipomas may be seen. Within the supratentorial brain, oligodendroglioma and PNET in the differential for a partially calcified mass should be considered. Oligodendrogliomas are rare in children but commonly calcify. PNETs are more common in childhood and typically present as a large, heterogenous cellular mass with calcifications in approximately 70% of patients. Additional tumors, such as dysembryoplastic neuroepithelial tumors and gangliogliomas, may also occasionally demonstrate calcifications. Posterior fossa ependymomas can have scattered punctate calcifications.

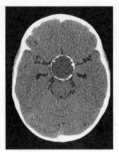

Fig. 25.20 Craniopharyngioma. Axial computed tomography image demonstrates round, marginated peripherally calcified suprasellar mass.

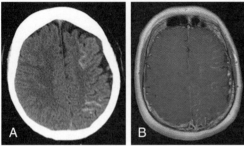

Fig. 25.21 Sturge-Weber syndrome. (A) Axial computed tomography image shows calcifications within the subcortical white matter of the left cerebral hemisphere with parenchymal volume loss. (B) Axial T1 postcontrast magnetic resonance imaging demonstrates left cerebral hemisphere leptomeningeal enhancement with thickening of the calvarium.

Finally, calcifications are also seen in association with several of the phakomatoses and neurocutaneous syndromes. As previously discussed, calcification is seen in tuberous sclerosis, both within the subependymal nodules along the ventricular margins and in association with subcortical and cerebral tubers as the child ages. Sturge-Weber syndrome, a disorder caused by a sporadic somatic mutation, is characterized by an angiomatosis involving the face, choroid of the eye, and the leptomeninges with a characteristic port wine stain involving the ipsilateral ophthalmic distribution of the trigeminal nerve. These children may have intractable seizures beginning in the first several years of life. Gyriform and subcortical calcification within the affected ipsilateral cerebral hemisphere (Fig. 25.21A) in association with atrophy and ipsilateral enlargement and enhancement of the leptomeninges (see Fig. 25.21B) and choroid plexus are also present. Calcifications in the brains of Sturge-Weber patients typically occur on the same side as the facial angioma and are likely caused by impaired venous drainage that results in chronic ischemia. Cortical calcifications can be bilateral in up to 20% of patients.

Are There Foreign Bodies?

Before assessing the normal intracranial structures with head CT, it is important to ascertain whether any foreign materials are present within the head, scalp, orbits, sinuses, or nasal cavity, including those purposely placed

in these areas by the child, parent, or surgeon or those that are involuntarily present. Specifically, metallic foreign bodies, such as surgical clips, coils, plates, screws, metallic facial jewelry, nails, and bullets, may result in streak artifact emanating from the object on CT. These metallic objects are important to report because many will preclude or require special consideration before obtaining an MRI study.

Occasionally wood is seen within the orbit or brain in the setting of a traumatic, penetrating injury. Because wooden objects will appear as air density on CT, a widening of the CT window level and width is often required to appreciate the full extent of the foreign body. Glass may be present in abrasions and lacerations involving the scalp and face. Remnants from shattered glass will be radiodense on CT but will not present with streak artifact, which helps in distinguishing glass from metal (Hunter and Taljanovic, 2003).

Finally, plastic catheters may be placed intentionally within the ventricles or subdural space for surgical drainage. In this situation, prior imaging studies should be viewed and compared with the most recent scans to determine whether any intentionally placed surgical materials have migrated, loosened, or fractured over time.

Are There Any Abnormal Masses Associated With the Skull or Soft Tissues?

Occasionally congenital, benign, and malignant masses within the scalp are incidental findings on head CTs obtained for other indications. Certain scalp masses should be further evaluated with CT to determine the pattern of any skull involvement. For additional reading on skull masses, please refer to Chapter 25.

In adults, sebaceous or trichilemmal cysts are commonly seen within the scalp, although these cysts are rare in children. Epidermoids and dermoids are more common causes of round, low- density, well-defined cystlike masses within the scalp in children. Dermoid cysts can be acquired or congenital. When congenital, they are often found in the midline and have a greater potential to extend through the skull intracranially (Sorenson et al., 2013). If there is a suspicion of a congenital dermoid cyst, the integrity of the adjacent bone should be assessed to look for sinus tracts or possible signs of erosion. MRI should be used to assess for intracranial extension. Hemangiomas and neurofibromas may present as well-defined scalp masses. However, these lesions are typically composed of soft tissue, are low in density, and do not extend into or erode the adjacent skull—features that should enable the radiologist to distinguish benign from malignant entities.

In children with Langerhans cell histiocytosis, a scalp mass is a characteristic finding. The skull is the most common site of involvement of eosinophilic granuloma, which presents as a well-defined, lytic lesion with a beveled edge. This type of lesion reflects the asymmetrical involvement of the inner and outer calvarial tables in association with an avidly enhancing soft tissue mass extending into the scalp. Occasionally the pattern of

Fig. 25.22 Sinus pericranii. (A) Axial contrast-enhanced computed tomography (CT) image shows vein coursing through a focal calvarial defect communicating with a well-defined enhancing scalp mass (*arrow*). (B) Sagittal contrast-enhanced CT image shows vein coursing through the calvarial defect communicates intracranially with the superior sagittal sinus. (C) Three-dimensional model from CT examination shows well-defined right parietal vascular scalp mass.

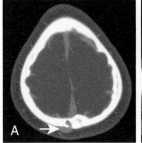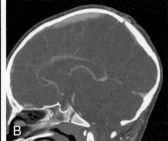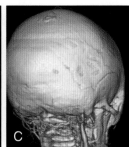

osseous involvement with eosinophilic granuloma will be more aggressive in appearance with irregular permeative lysis and differential considerations, such as osteomyelitis and metastasis from neuroblastoma (Pawar et al., 2011; Healy et al., 1981).

Several congenital conditions can cause protrusion of intracranial contents through the skull and into the scalp. These conditions present clinically as scalp masses unique to the pediatric population. Sinus pericranii is a venous anomaly presenting as an abnormal venous connection from the dural venous sinuses (typically the superior sagittal sinuses) to abnormal venous vasculature within the scalp. On CT, it presents as a mildly hyperdense scalp mass with thinning or scalloping of the adjacent calvarium secondary to pressure erosion and a focal defect traversing the inner and outer skull table, which transmits the connecting emissary vein to the dural sinus (Fig. 25.22) (Pavanello et al., 2015). MRI and MR venography should be used to delineate the venous connection and to identify any related vascular malformations and anomalies. Cephaloceles may also present as a scalp mass. These lesions vary in size and content that includes components of brain, CSF, meninges, and vessels. They are classified by their location and by the content of the CNS component protruding through the skull defect. Most of the lesions are at midline, with the occipital form being the most common type in the United States and the frontoethmoidal form being the most common type in Asia. They are seen in association with other congenital anomalies, although many cases are sporadic. The appearance on CT will vary based on their respective contents, with cranial meningoceles appearing as a fluid density sac and encephaloceles with various amounts of neural tissue of soft tissue density. CT is the optimal modality to define the extent of the osseous defect through which these lesions protrude, whereas MRI should be used to define the contents of the cephalocele and to identify additional intracranial anomalies.

■ Summary

CT is an important imaging tool for the management and diagnosis of numerous diseases of childhood that affect the brain. This chapter provides a broad overview of imaging patterns and key imaging questions that should be used in evaluating pediatric head CT, in narrowing differential diagnoses, and in guiding clinical management. An important role for CT brain imaging in pediatrics remains, particularly when radiation dose is taken into account, as well as the numerous clinical indications for which this modality is recommended or preferred.

Bibliography

Alexander, M. J., Spetzler, R. F., et al. (2005). Endovascular treatment of cerebral arteriovenous malformations in children. *Pediatric neurovascular disease: Surgical, endovascular and medical management* (pp. 167–175). New York: Thieme.

American College of Radiology (ACR). (2014). *ACR appropriateness criteria.* http://www.acr.org/Quality-Safety/Appropriateness-Criteria.

American College of Radiology (ACR). (2014). *Computed tomography accreditation.* http://www.acr.org/Quality-Safety/Accreditation/CT.

Arnold, M., Steinlin, M., Baumann, A., et al. (2009). Thrombolysis in childhood stroke: Report of 2 cases and review of the literature. *Stroke, 40*(3), 801–807.

Barkovich, A. J. (2005). *Pediatric neuroimaging* (4th ed.). Lippincott Williams & Wilkins.

Barkovich, A. J., & Kjos, B. O. (1988). Normal postnatal development of the corpus callosum as demonstrated by MR imaging. *AJNR. American Journal of Neuroradiology, 9*(3), 487–491.

Barkovich, A. J., & Norman, D. (1988). Anomalies of the corpus callosum: Correlation with further anomalies of the brain. *American Journal of Roentgenology, 151*(1), 171–179.

Dlamini, N., Billinghurst, L., & Kirkham, F. J. (2010). Cerebral venous sinus (sinovenous) thrombosis in children. *Neurosurgery clinics of North America, 21*(3), 511–527.

Gadda, D., Vannucchi, L., Niccolai, F., et al. (2002). CT in acute stroke: Improved detection of dense intracranial arteries by varying window parameters and performing a thin-slice helical scan. *AJNR. American Journal of Neuroradiology, 44*(11), 900–906.

Han, B. K., Towbin, R. B., De Courten-Myers, G., et al. (1990). Reversal sign on CT: Effect of anoxic/ischemic cerebral injury in children. *American Journal of Roentgenology, 154*(2), 361–368.

Healy, J. F., Marshall, W. H., Brahme, F. J., et al. (1981). CT of intracranial metastases with skull and scalp involvement. *AJNR. American Journal of Neuroradiology, 2*(4), 335–338.

Hetts, S. W., Sherr, E. H., Chao, S., et al. (2006). Anomalies of the corpus callosum: An MR analysis of the phenotypic spectrum of associated malformations. *American Journal of Roentgenology, 187*(5), 1343–1348.

Hunter, T. B., & Taljanovic, M. S. (2003). Foreign bodies. *RadioGraphics, 23*(3), 731–757.

Image gently. https://www.imagegently.org/. Accessed November 15, 2014.

Koo, C. K., Teasdale, E., & Muir, K. W. (2000). What constitutes a true hyperdense middle cerebral artery sign? *Cerebrovascular Diseases, 10*(6), 419–423.

Leach, J. L., Fortuna, R. B., Jones, B. V., et al. (2006). Imaging of cerebral venous thrombosis: Current techniques, spectrum of findings, and diagnostic pitfalls. *RadioGraphics, 26*(Suppl. 1), S19–S41; discussion S42-S13.

Mallick, A. A., Ganesan, V., Kirkham, F. J., et al. (2014). Childhood arterial ischaemic stroke incidence, presenting features, and risk factors: A prospective population-based study. *The Lancet Neurology, 13*(1), 35–43.

McKinney, A. M., Short, J., Truwit, C. L., et al. (2007). Posterior reversible encephalopathy syndrome: Incidence of atypical regions of involvement and imaging findings. *American Journal of Roentgenology, 189*(4), 904–912.

Modic, M. T., Weinstein, M. A., Rothner, A. D., et al. (1980). Calcification of the choroid plexus visualized by computed tomography. *Radiology, 135*(2), 369–372.

Osborn, A. G. (2012). *Osborn's brain imaging pathology and anatomy.* Lippincott Williams & Wilkins.

Pavanello, M., Melloni, I., Antichi, E., et al. (2015). Sinus pericranii: Diagnosis and management in 21 pediatric patients. *Journal of Neurosurgery: Pediatrics, 15*(1), 60–70.

Pawar, R. V., Hagiwara, M., Milla, S., et al. (2011). Eosinophilic granuloma presenting as post-traumatic scalp hematoma with epidural hemorrhage. A case report. *The Neuroradiology Journal, 24*(5), 767–771.

Petitti, N. (1998). The hyperdense middle cerebral artery sign. *Radiology*, *208*(3), 687–688.

Pindrik, J., Huisman, T. A., Mahesh, M., et al. (2013). Analysis of limited-sequence head computed tomography for children with shunted hydrocephalus: Potential to reduce diagnostic radiation exposure. *Journal of Neurosurgery: Pediatrics, 12*(5), 491–500.

Prabhu, S. P., & Young-Poussaint, T. (2010). Pediatric central nervous system emergencies. *Neuroimaging Clinics of North America, 20*(4), 663–683.

Provenzale, J. M., & Kranz, P. G. (2011). Dural sinus thrombosis: Sources of error in image interpretation. *American Journal of Roentgenology, 196*(1), 23–31.

Raybaud, C. (2010). The corpus callosum, the other great forebrain commissures, and the septum pellucidum: Anatomy, development, and malformation. *Neuroradiology, 52*(6), 447–477.

Rekate, H. L. (2009). A contemporary definition and classification of hydrocephalus. *Seminars in Pediatric Neurology, 16*(1), 9–15.

Rodallec, M. H., Krainik, A., Feydy, A., et al. (2006). Cerebral venous thrombosis and multidetector CT angiography: Tips and tricks. *RadioGraphics, 26*(Suppl. 1), S5–S18; discussion S42–S43.

Rybka, K., Staniszewska, A. M., & Bieganski, T. (2007). Low-dose protocol for head CT in monitoring hydrocephalus in children. *Medical Science Monitor, 13*(Suppl. 1), 147–151.

Saposnik, G., Barinagarrementeria, F., Brown, R. D., Jr., et al. (2011). Diagnosis and management of cerebral venous thrombosis: A statement for healthcare professionals from the American Heart Association/American Stroke Association. *Stroke, 42*(4), 1158–1192.

Segev, Y., Metser, U., Beni-Adani, L., et al. (2001). Morphometric study of the midsagittal MR imaging plane in cases of hydrocephalus and atrophy and in normal brains. *AJNR. American Journal of Neuroradiology, 22*(9), 1674–1679.

Shimizu, Y., Tha, K. K., Iguchi, A., et al. (2013). Isolated posterior fossa involvement in posterior reversible encephalopathy syndrome. *The Neuroradiology Journal, 26*(5), 514–519.

Sivaganesan, A., Krishnamurthy, R., Sahni, D., et al. (2012). Neuroimaging of ventriculoperitoneal shunt complications in children. *Pediatric Radiology, 42*(9), 1029–1046.

Sorenson, E. P., Powel, J. E., Rozzelle, C. J., et al. (2013). Scalp dermoids: A review of their anatomy, diagnosis, and treatment. *Child's Nervous System, 29*(3), 375–380.

The ALARA (as low as reasonably achievable) concept in pediatric CT (2002). Intelligent dose reduction. Multidisciplinary conference organized by the society for pediatric radiology, August 18–19, 2001. *Pediatric Radiology, 32*, 217–313.

Udayasankar, U. K., Braithwaite, K., Arvaniti, M., et al. (2008). Low-dose nonenhanced head CT protocol for follow-up evaluation of children with ventriculoperitoneal shunt: Reduction of radiation and effect on image quality. *AJNR. American Journal of Neuroradiology, 29*(4), 802–806.

Whitehead, M. T., Oh, C., Raju, A., et al. (2015). Physiologic pineal region, choroid plexus, and dural calcifications in the first decade of life. *AJNR. American Journal of Neuroradiology, 36*, 575–580.

Zimmerman, R. A., & Bilaniuk, L. T. (1982). Age-related incidence of pineal calcification detected by computed tomography. *Radiology, 142*(3), 659–662.

Head and Neck

CHAPTER 26

Approach to Lateral Neck Radiographs

Meryle J. Eklund

CHAPTER OUTLINE

Approach to the Lateral Neck Radiograph, 511
Technique, 511
How to Read the Lateral View, 511
    Tonsils and Adenoids, 512
    Epiglottis, 512
    Subglottic Airway, 512
    Prevertebral Soft Tissues, 513
    "Edge of Film" Findings, 513
Case Examples, 513
    Adenoid and Tonsillar Enlargement, 513

Retropharyngeal Abscess, 514
Epiglottitis, 514
Croup, 515
Bacterial Tracheitis, 515
Foreign Bodies, 516
Miscellaneous, 517
    Congenital Lesions, 517
    Neoplasm, 518
    Accidental and Iatrogenic Causes, 519
    Autoimmune Diseases, 519
Summary, 520

■ Approach to the Lateral Neck Radiograph

The lateral neck radiograph is a relatively inexpensive, readily available, and easy-to-perform examination that is very useful for the evaluation of suspected abnormalities in the upper aerodigestive tract. In the emergency setting the lateral neck radiograph is commonly obtained to evaluate for abnormalities causing acute respiratory distress or dysphagia. The examination also can be useful in the workup of chronic obstruction of the airway. The first portion of this chapter will outline the appropriate technique for acquiring the optimal lateral neck radiograph image and review pertinent anatomy. The common indications for obtaining the lateral neck radiograph will then be addressed, as well as the findings seen in some of the most common and most critical diagnoses encountered when this examination is ordered.

■ Technique

Before imaging the child, it is prudent for the radiologist to gather clinical data regarding the patient, if possible. This will facilitate the appropriate approach to imaging the patient in the safest manner, as well as help guide diagnosis. Important considerations include the onset and duration of symptoms, associated symptoms (e.g., fever, toxic appearance, or drooling), physical examination findings (e.g., stridor, barky cough, rales, rhonchi), and the known or suspected ingestion of a foreign body or caustic agent. For a patient in respiratory failure or impending respiratory failure, imaging should be deferred until an adequate airway is established.

When a child presents in acute respiratory distress, it is important to consider how positioning of the child can affect breathing, because maintaining the airway is of paramount concern. Given that the child's airway is incompletely developed and flexible compared with the adult, supine imaging can acutely worsen respiratory distress and result in complete respiratory obstruction. Thus the lateral radiograph is ideally obtained in an upright position.

To obtain maximal distention of the airway, the child is typically imaged with the neck extended and breath held in inspiration. Together, these techniques minimize prevertebral soft tissue redundancy and maximally distend the airway to better evaluate the anatomy (Fig. 26.1). When taking a breath in, the musculature of the upper airway contracts, which allows for increased air flow while maintaining or dilating the nasal, pharyngeal, and laryngeal airways. In the older child a command to take a deep breath is usually adequate. In the young child, timing the radiograph can be more difficult, often requiring more than one attempt. In addition, the prevertebral soft tissues in neonates, infants, and toddlers can be particularly difficult to efface even with optimal technique. If all else fails, airway fluoroscopy could be performed for real-time evaluation of the soft tissues of the neck.

■ How to Read the Lateral View

Evaluation of the lateral neck radiograph requires a good understanding of the relevant anatomy of the neck, and

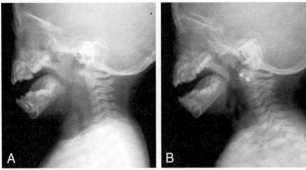

Fig. 26.1 Lateral radiographs of the neck taken minutes apart in a 2-year-old obtained in (A) expiration and slight flexion demonstrates thickened prevertebral soft tissues. Image obtained during inspiration in slight extension (B) shows resolution of prevertebral soft tissue thickening as a result of technical factors and patient's oropharyngeal phase.

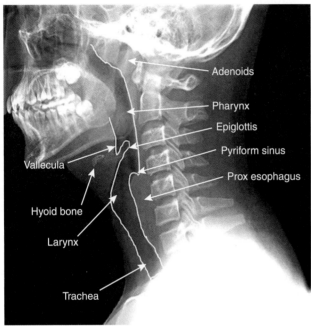

Fig. 26.2 Normal neck anatomy.

it is important for the radiologist to be familiar with the normal and abnormal appearance of the anatomical structures (Fig. 26.2). One approach is to evaluate the anatomy from the point of entrance of inspired air in the nasopharynx through the lower cervical trachea as it approaches the chest.

Tonsils and Adenoids

The adenoids, also known as the nasopharyngeal tonsils, are located superior to the palatine tonsils along the roof of the nasopharyngeal airway. As with other tonsillar tissues, the adenoids play a protective role against infectious disease in the upper airway. Adenoidal pathology predominantly relates to abnormally enlarged size, which can impinge on the nasopharyngeal airway and contribute to significant acute or chronic upper respiratory obstruction. Various methods for the radiographic evaluation of adenoidal enlargement have been pro-

posed in the literature. An easy and effective approach is to give a subjective assessment on the level of impingement on the nasopharyngeal airway (mild, moderate, or severe narrowing versus complete obstruction). One can also calculate the adenoidal/nasopharyngeal ratio, which provides a more objective description of nasopharyngeal impingement by way of measuring the adenoidal size (A) relative to the diameter of the nasopharynx (N) and reporting the A/N ratio. Distance "A" is measured from the margin of the basiocciput to the maximal convexity of the adenoid, while distance "N" represents the distance between the posterior superior margin of the hard palate and the anterior edge of the sphenobasioccipital synchondrosis. An A/N ratio greater than 0.8 indicates enlarged adenoids. Finally, a direct measurement of the diameter of the adenoids can also be reported. This is more difficult to interpret and generalize to all children, however, because the acquired measurement could have different implications based on the child's age and size.

Epiglottis

The epiglottis is a small, fibrocartilaginous flap of tissue that protects the airway from aspiration during swallowing by covering the trachea and facilitating the propulsion of an ingested bolus into the esophagus. It is located at the level of C3 and the hyoid bone. When normal in size, the epiglottis is a thin structure. An abnormally enlarged epiglottis has a thickened appearance and has been described as similar to the size and shape of a child's thumb. The aryepiglottic folds are the normally thin and delicate slips of tissue extending obliquely from the free edge of the epiglottis to the arytenoid cartilages. The laryngeal vestibule, or inlet of the larynx, is formed anteriorly by the epiglottis and posteriorly and laterally by the aryepiglottic folds and arytenoid cartilages. An infectious or inflammatory abnormality of the epiglottis causes airway obstruction not typically because of the enlargement of the epiglottis by itself, but because of the swelling of the surrounding soft tissues and obstruction of the laryngeal inlet.

Subglottic Airway

The subglottic airway extends from the true vocal cords to the lower margin of the cricoid cartilage. This region is vulnerable to significant pathological obstruction due to its small size and the relatively inflexible surrounding cricoid. Narrowing of the subglottic airway is an important indicator of even mild edema and inflammation associated with an acute infectious process. Although mild subglottic narrowing can sometimes be visualized on the lateral radiograph, findings are usually much more evident on the frontal view. Therefore in children who present with stridor or a barky cough, it is prudent to obtain a frontal view for optimal evaluation. In the normal anteroposterior appearance of the subglottic airway, there is shouldering of the subglottic trachea, with a nearly horizontal superior margin of the tracheal col-

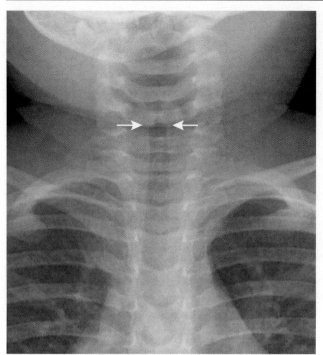

Fig. 26.3 Normal shouldering of the subglottic airway on a frontal view. Note the near-horizontal orientation of the superior margin of the subglottic tracheal column (*arrows*).

umn (Fig. 26.3). Symmetrical or asymmetrical narrowing, compression, or deviation of the tracheal column on the frontal view indicate significant pathology.

Prevertebral Soft Tissues

Evaluation of the prevertebral soft tissues can be one of the most important yet most frustrating components of interpretation of the lateral neck radiograph. This is particularly true in very young patients who have short necks, redundant soft tissues, and are unable to cooperate with instructions for respiration and positioning. Occasionally the presence of prevertebral soft tissue thickening remains unclear despite two or three attempts to acquire an adequate image. If the radiologist is not satisfied with the quality of examination achieved with static radiograph technique, further evaluation with dynamic fluoroscopic observation could quickly elucidate the upper airway anatomy and resolve any questions from the radiographic examination.

Determining the presence of prevertebral soft tissue thickening is critical in evaluation of potential retropharyngeal infection, trauma, or mass. Normal measurements of the prevertebral soft tissues vary considerably according to the cervical level and age of the patient. One simple technique is to compare the prevertebral soft tissue thickness with the anteroposterior dimension of the adjacent vertebral body, which adjusts for patient age and growth. The prevertebral soft tissues from C1 to C4 usually measure less than half the anteroposterior dimension of the adjacent vertebral body. In older children, because of increasing ossification of the adjacent vertebral bodies, the prevertebral soft tissues decrease in

relative thickness from C1 to C4. Below C4, up to one vertebral body width is considered normal, because of the esophageal soft tissues. These are general rules for a technically adequate radiograph. Close attention to imaging technique is important because lateral radiographs obtained in expiration and flexion can exaggerate prevertebral thickness. Repeat radiographs may be necessary. If there is persistent prominence of the soft tissues, retropharyngeal edema or abscess may be present, and computed tomography (CT) of the neck may be indicated (guided by history and level of clinical concern).

Secondary signs of infection or trauma are as important as, if not more important than, soft tissue swelling if present. Foci of gas (outside the esophagus) could indicate infection with gas-forming infectious agents or tracheal or esophageal perforation as a result of foreign body or trauma. Abnormal radiodensity may indicate ingested foreign body or calcification within a mass.

In general, paired calcified structures projecting in the soft tissues are likely normal. The hyoid bone ossifies progressively after birth at the level of C3. There may also be styloid processes extending caudally from the inferior surface of the temporal bones toward the hyoid and variable calcification of the stylohyoid ligaments. Although normal calcification of the thyroid, cricoid, and arytenoid cartilages occurs with age, these structures are generally noncalcified in childhood, with the exception of those seen in teens.

"Edge of Film" Findings

Although the majority of pathology in the neck will cause an alteration in the normal anatomy described earlier, one must scrutinize all structures included in the field of view. Occasionally, significant findings can be detected within the bones, sinuses, nasal cavity, or upper chest. Foreign bodies can be located anywhere along the aerodigestive tract, including the nasal cavity and thoracic inlet. Careful review of the osseous structures may reveal fracture, malalignment, or focal lesion that could point to trauma or neoplasm. Paranasal sinus opacification may indicate sinusitis or mass lesion.

■ Case Examples

Adenoid and Tonsillar Enlargement

Adenotonsillar hypertrophy results from growth of lymphoid tissue in Waldeyer ring in the nasopharyngeal region as a result of frequent infection and obstructive causes. The enlarged tonsillar tissue may cause respiratory compromise in the acute phase of infection, or on a chronic basis in the setting of obstructive sleep apnea. Other factors may also contribute to nasopharyngeal obstruction, such as craniofacial dysplasia, neuromuscular disorders, and palatal surgeries, so it is preferred to describe adenoidal size with respect to relative amount of impingement on the nasopharyngeal airway rather

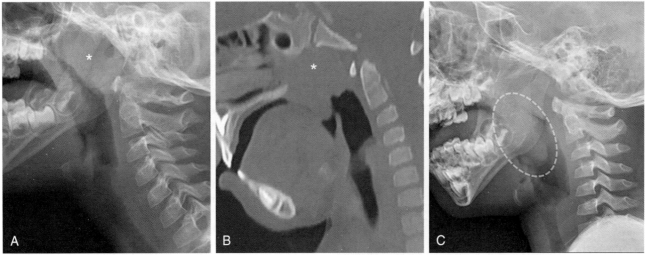

Fig. 26.4 Adenoid enlargement (*asterisk*) on lateral neck radiograph (A) and corresponding midline sagittal computed tomography image (B). Markedly enlarged palatine tonsils (*dashed ovals*) and adenoids in a different patient (C) with obstruction of the nasopharyngeal airway.

than a single measurement. As previously described, an A/N ratio greater than 0.8 indicates adenoidal enlargement with significant nasopharyngeal obstruction likely (Fig. 26.4).

Acute tonsillitis is accompanied by the clinical signs of fever, dysphagia, and odynophagia. Lymphadenopathy is often present, and occasionally the patient exhibits excessive drooling and altered voice quality. Airway compromise can result from enlargement of the tonsils themselves or from the formation of tonsillar or peritonsillar abscess or edema, which results in prevertebral soft tissue thickening. Retropharyngeal abscess is an important complication of tonsillitis and pharyngitis with potentially severe clinical implications, which will be discussed separately.

Obstructive sleep apnea consists of recurrent events of partial or complete airway obstruction during sleep, resulting in disrupted ventilation and sleep patterns. The point of obstruction is often in the nasopharynx or oropharynx, which again could be caused by adenotonsillar hypertrophy or other anatomical or neuromuscular abnormalities. Imaging plays an important role in determining the cause of obstruction, and early intervention is critical, because chronic obstructive sleep apnea has been linked to daytime hypersomnolence, behavior disorders, secondary enuresis, and failure to thrive. Delayed diagnosis can lead to more severe complications, such as cor pulmonale or neurological damage.

Retropharyngeal Abscess

Retropharyngeal abscess is most commonly diagnosed before 6 years of age, usually in association with upper respiratory tract infections and tonsillitis. Additional causative factors include injury from foreign body ingestion or iatrogenic injury (e.g., after traumatic intubation). Clinical symptoms include odynophagia, dysphagia, trismus, fever, drooling, and muffled voice.

Torticollis and displacement of the uvula may be present on physical examination. By radiography, prevertebral soft tissue swelling, loss of the cervical lordosis, and abnormal soft tissue gas are all indicators of retropharyngeal abscess. CT or MRI is necessary to confirm diagnosis and is helpful in identifying drainable fluid collections, providing more precise anatomical delineation and extent of infection, and evaluating for complications, such as vascular thrombosis (typically internal jugular thrombosis) or pseudoaneurysm (Fig. 26.5). The radiologist should also be aware of Grisel syndrome, a rare but severe complication of cervical infection where inflammation leads to cervical ligamentous laxity and atlantoaxial subluxation, with potential for development of permanent neurological sequelae.

Epiglottitis

Epiglottitis is a bacterial infection that historically was the most common cause of epiglottic enlargement in infants and children, with *Haemophilus influenza* the most frequent causative agent. The number of cases of bacterial epiglottitis decreased considerably after the institution of routine vaccination for *Haemophilus influenza* type B, and *Streptococcus* species is now the most common cause. The typical age group affected with epiglottitis is 3- to 6-year-olds. Children present with fever, respiratory distress, stridor, drooling, tachypnea, and trouble speaking, oftentimes after recent upper respiratory infection. They may lean forward to breathe and have respiratory retractions. It is critically important to ensure that the patient has an adequate, secured airway before bringing the child to the radiology suite if epiglottitis is suspected, because acute airway obstruction and respiratory failure are very possible consequences of this disease.

Imaging findings in epiglottitis include abnormal enlargement of the epiglottis and thickening of the

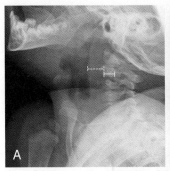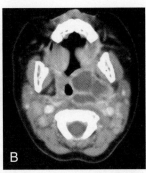

Fig. 26.5 Lateral radiograph of the neck in a 12-month-old with fever (A) demonstrates mild thickening of the prevertebral soft tissues (*dashed line*), greater than the width of the adjacent vertebral body (*solid line*). Subsequent neck computed tomography (B) shows abscess centered lateral to the airway with some retropharyngeal extension. Incision and drainage revealed methicillin-resistant *Staphylococcus aureus*.

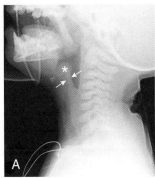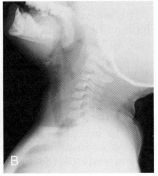

Fig. 26.6 Enlarged epiglottis (*asterisk*) with associated thickening of the aryepiglottic folds (*arrows*) in a young child with epiglottitis (A). Repeat lateral neck radiograph 5 months after treatment (B) shows resolution of epiglottic enlargement with normal, thin aryepiglottic folds measuring less than 5 mm.

aryepiglottic folds to greater than 5 mm (Fig. 26.6). This may be accompanied by loss of the normal cervical lordosis. As noted previously, it is the marked thickening of the aryepiglottic folds and arytenoid cartilage (which forms the lateral and posterior walls of the laryngeal vestibule) that results in acute airway obstruction, not enlargement of the epiglottis itself.

A few additional causes of epiglottic enlargement by radiography can be confused with epiglottitis. Omega epiglottis is a normal variant that leads to apparent epiglottic enlargement on the lateral neck radiograph, appearing almost identical to epiglottitis. This is due not to true epiglottic enlargement, but rather to elongation and lateral extension of the epiglottis with downward curving of the lateral flaps, which creates an omega shape (Ω). The distinguishing feature of omega epiglottis is the preservation of the normal thin and delicate appearance of the aryepiglottic folds, rather than the aryepiglottic fold thickening that is found in epiglottitis. Laryngoscopy may be necessary to diagnose omega epiglottis in indeterminate cases.

Vallecular cyst is a congenital lesion that can present with stridor in infancy. Superinfection of a vallecular cyst may also lead to acute respiratory distress in the older child. By radiography, a vallecular cyst usu-

ally presents as a bulging mass in the vallecular space. Demonstration of this finding can be difficult because of laxity and redundancy of the retropharyngeal soft tissues in the young child, sometimes requiring correlation with cross-sectional imaging or direct visualization with endoscopy. Resection or drainage is often required for treatment (Fig. 26.7).

Other considerations for an enlarged epiglottis and possible glottic obstruction include angioedema secondary to anaphylactoid reaction or complement deficiency, as well as diffuse involvement as part of a multispatial infection or inflammatory process. In addition, foreign bodies can become lodged in the vallecula and cause local inflammation with secondary enlargement of the epiglottis, or may become directly lodged in the laryngeal vestibule resulting in a very acute presentation. Patients with hemophilia may bleed in their mucous membranes, including the membranous covering of the epiglottis, causing radiographic enlargement of the epiglottis. Similarly, patients with Stevens-Johnson syndrome might have disease of the mucous membranes in the hypopharynx or larynx. Many of these conditions may be radiographically occult.

Croup

Croup, also known as acute laryngotracheitis, occurs most commonly in children ranging from 3 months to 3 years of age. It is usually caused by parainfluenza virus or respiratory syncytial virus and results in diffuse inflammation and edema of the larynx and trachea, but is worst in the subglottic region. Croup is characterized by a harsh, barky cough, and the diagnosis can be made clinically in most instances. Imaging is performed to rule out other causes of stridor that may mimic croup, including foreign body aspiration or ingestion, epiglottitis, or subglottic hemangioma. Croup is usually self-limited, and standard treatment consists of conservative measures, including nebulized racemic epinephrine and corticosteroids.

Typical findings include loss of the normal shouldering of the lateral walls of the subglottic trachea on the frontal view of the neck, which assumes a funnel-like or steeple-like configuration with tapering toward the glottis superiorly. The narrowing is seen 1 to 1.5 centimeters below the vocal cords as a result of subglottic swelling and varies little between inspiration and expiration. On the lateral view, mild subglottic narrowing is subtle, if present. The functional findings of an overdistended hypopharynx and proximal larynx are better indicators of subglottic obstruction on the lateral projection, caused by inflammatory edema and physiological response to airway resistance (Fig. 26.8).

Bacterial Tracheitis

Membranous croup, pseudomembranous croup, bacterial croup, purulent tracheobronchitis, membranous

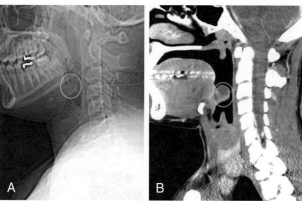

Fig. 26.7 Lateral scout (A) and sagittal (B) images from a neck computed tomography scans in a patient with superinfected congenital vallecular cyst (*circle*). Purulent material drained revealing methicillin-susceptible *Staphylococcus aureus*.

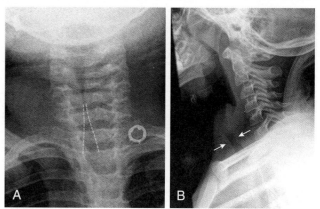

Fig. 26.8 Croup in a 6-year-old with smooth, symmetrical subglottic narrowing on the frontal view (*dashed lines*) (A) and mild subglottic narrowing (*arrows*) and distention of the hypopharynx on the lateral view (B).

laryngotracheobronchitis, and membranous tracheitis are all names that represent the same clinical entity as bacterial tracheitis, a disease characterized by a bacterial infection of the trachea with formation of thick mucopurulent exudates that obstruct the upper airway to variable degrees. Often, this is a secondary infection after an acute viral illness. Common bacterial agents include *Staphylococcus aureus*, group A *Streptococcus*, and *Moraxella catarrhalis*. The clinical course mimics that of viral croup, but the symptoms are nonresponsive to conventional therapy, and the patient may have high fever and a toxic appearance. The only definitive diagnosis is direct visualization of the trachea with endoscopy.

Imaging features may be very subtle and difficult to identify or radiographically occult. Some degree of subglottic narrowing is common. Diffuse haziness and irregularity of the anterior tracheal wall (the "candle dripping sign") is more specific but less frequent (Fig. 26.9). Abnormalities on the chest radiograph are frequently present, with 50% demonstrating evidence of pneumonia.

Foreign Bodies

The diagnosis of aspirated or ingested foreign body can be difficult without a witnessed event, yet delayed diagnosis can have grave consequences. Symptoms are nonspecific and can range from drooling to stridor to respiratory distress depending on the nature of the foreign body, its location, and time from aspiration or ingestion. Common sites of lodging of swallowed foreign bodies include the level at or just under the cricopharyngeal muscle as a result of weak peristalsis in that region (approximately C5–C6), as well as the thoracic inlet. If a foreign body is suspected, the included soft tissues should be closely scrutinized not only for detection of a radiopaque or radiolucent structure but also for the secondary signs of complication, such as swelling, mass effect on the airway, and the presence of soft tissue gas (Fig. 26.10).

The ingested button battery presents a particularly challenging scenario. Prompt medical attention and removal of the battery is of utmost concern because of the rapidity with which serious injury can be sustained. Severe tissue necrosis can occur within 2 hours of ingestion. Yet nonspecific symptoms and unwitnessed events can delay diagnosis considerably. Batteries measuring 20 mm or larger are more likely to become stuck, and removal should be pursued as soon as ingestion is confirmed. If batteries have already passed into the intestines, patients are typically monitored closely with reliable clinical follow-up.

There has been a dramatic increase in the number of serious injuries sustained from button battery ingestion, as use in small electronic devices and other household items has become more prevalent and more powerful. Radiographically, button batteries appear as a thin, round, metallic structure that typically demonstrates a radiodense double edge when viewed en face and a small step-off when viewed on the side (Fig. 26.11).

The radiologist should evaluate for soft tissue swelling and mass effect on the airway. Extensive edema and the presence of soft tissue gas indicate severe injury, and water-soluble esophagram should be considered to investigate the possibility of tracheoesophageal fistula, particularly if the smaller negative pole is forward facing against the posterior membranous trachea. Mucosal burns, mediastinitis, and even aortoesophageal fistula represent additional potential serious complications of ingestion.

Although the ingestion of coins is somewhat more innocuous, significant tissue injury can also occur when a coin becomes lodged in the esophagus. As with any foreign body ingestion, the soft tissues should be closely evaluated for the presence of swelling and gas, which indicate more serious tissue damage. If the coin demonstrates continuous antegrade motion through the gastrointestinal tract on serial radiographs, soft tissue injury is unlikely. Occasionally, coins can be mistaken for button batteries or other objects, particularly

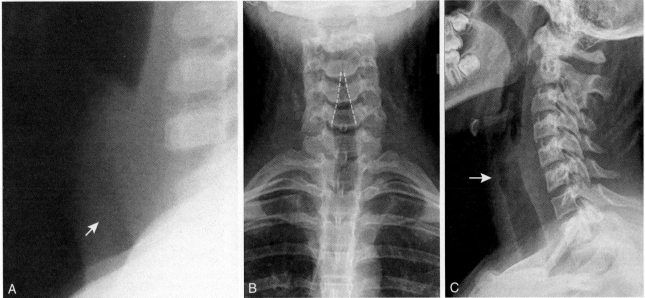

Fig. 26.9 Mild narrowing of the proximal trachea with irregularity of the anterior tracheal wall (*black arrow*) in a child with bacterial tracheitis (A). Marked subglottic narrowing (*dashed lines*) on the frontal view (B) and mild irregularity of the subglottic trachea (*white arrow*) on the lateral view (C) in a different 14-year-old patient with laryngotracheitis by laryngoscopy.

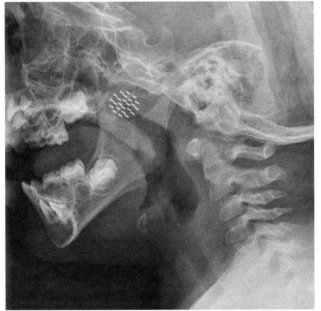

Fig. 26.10 Portion of a toothbrush lodged in the nasopharynx.

when two or more are ingested simultaneously and result in a stacked or double-edged appearance when viewed from the side.

Food products and bones may be difficult to identify by radiograph. Larger, dense bones can appear as radiopaque densities, but delicate fish bones may be impossible to visualize. Vegetative matter often appears radiolucent. As with any suspected foreign body, there should be careful evaluation for secondary signs of soft tissue injury, including the presence of prevertebral soft tissue swelling, soft tissue gas, or loss of the normal cer-

vical lordosis, regardless of whether a radiopaque foreign body is seen (Fig. 26.12).

Miscellaneous

Congenital Lesions

Many congenital masses can cause acute or chronic symptoms in the neck, as a result of primary mass effect or superinfection. The lateral neck radiograph can have a significant role in identifying these lesions, but a multimodality approach is often required. Thyroglossal duct cysts, branchial cleft cysts, and epiglottic cysts are examples of lesions that can all cause symptoms of mass effect in early childhood, but can also come to attention later on as a result of secondary infection. Being alert to the possibility of these lesions can expedite diagnosis and appropriate treatment in these patients, who often present with pain, dysphagia, or acute respiratory distress. Because discussion of each category of congenital lesion is beyond the scope of this chapter, please refer to Chapter 27 for a more comprehensive review.

Vascular anomalies comprise an additional class of lesions that are present at birth or shortly thereafter. Venous, lymphatic, or venolymphatic malformations tend to be multispatial and may cause respiratory obstruction at any level because of mass effect. Subglottic hemangioma is an example of a vascular neoplasm that has been associated with airway obstruction and respiratory distress, most commonly because of subglottic stenosis. Subglottic hemangiomas are often not visualized on radiography but can appear as a well-defined rounded or oval mass, often on the lateral or posterior wall of the subglottic trachea. The key to diagnosis is *asymmetrical* subglottic

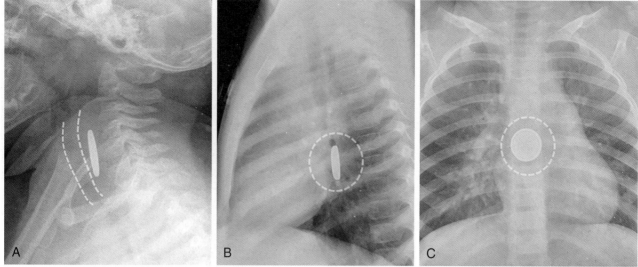

Fig. 26.11 Lateral radiograph of the neck (A) in a 1-year-old demonstrates a coin lodged in the distal cervical esophagus. Mild associated soft tissue swelling with slight anterior bowing of the trachea (*dashed lines*), but no significant narrowing of the airway. Foreign body in another patient demonstrates (B) beveled edge (*dashed circle*) on the lateral view and (C) concentric rings or "halo" appearance (*dashed circle*) on the frontal view.

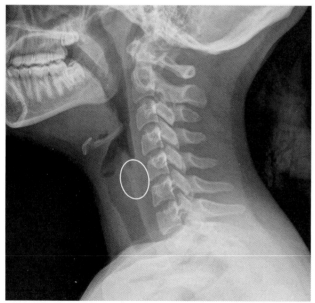

Fig. 26.12 Adolescent who swallowed a fishbone. A thin radiopaque linear density can be seen in the soft tissues anterior to the C5 vertebral body (*circle*). A small fishbone was retrieved endoscopically.

narrowing on the frontal view, which differentiates this lesion from other causes of subglottic narrowing, such as croup or bacterial tracheitis. Fifty percent of patients with subglottic hemangioma have cutaneous hemangiomas, which can be a good indicator of subglottic hemangioma if asymmetrical subglottic narrowing is present.

Other causes for neonatal stridor include laryngomalacia, tracheomalacia, tracheobronchomalacia, and congenital laryngeal or subglottic webs. Laryngomalacia, tracheomalacia, and tracheobronchomalacia are the result of immature cartilage and musculature of the airway, which allow the supralaryngeal, laryngeal, or tracheal structures to collapse during inspiration. These conditions are characterized by stridor in the first few weeks of life. Most commonly they are self-limiting and resolve by 1 year of age. Diagnosis with neck radiographs is extremely challenging and may be impossible depending on the level of obstruction and degree of inspiration or expiration at the time the radiograph was acquired. Laryngomalacia, tracheomalacia, and tracheobronchomalacia can be evaluated with airway fluoroscopy, which provides dynamic evaluation of the airway caliber in different phases of respiration. Oftentimes the definitive diagnosis is made with direct endoscopic visualization.

Neoplasm

Neoplasms can cause airway obstruction as a result of mass effect from the lesion or, in some cases of treated malignancy, from edema after radiation therapy. Rhabdomyosarcoma and neuroblastoma have relatively high incidence in the head and neck and can result in airway compromise. Metastatic disease to the cervical spine may result in extraosseous extension of soft tissue with mass effect on the airway (Fig. 26.13).

Antrochoanal polyp is an example of a benign neoplasm that may cause airway obstruction because of its growth into the nasopharynx from its origin in the maxillary sinus. Congenital or neonatal goiter can also result in respiratory distress secondary to mass effect on the trachea by the enlarged thyroid gland. Benign and malignant lymphadenopathy can likewise contribute to airway obstruction.

On the lateral neck radiograph, focal airway narrowing and soft tissue swelling or mass not otherwise explained by clinical presentation should be worked up for the possibility of underlying neoplasm.

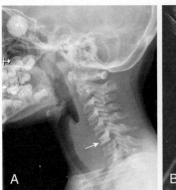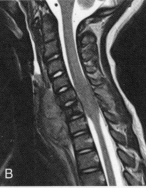

Fig. 26.13 A 6-year-old with a history of retinoblastoma and new right-sided weakness. Lateral neck radiograph (A) reveals sclerotic lesion in the C6 vertebra (*arrow*) with prevertebral soft tissue swelling. Note the prosthetic globe in the orbit (*asterisk*). Magnetic resonance imaging (B) demonstrates large metastatic mass centered at C5–C6 with extension into the epidural space, posterior elements, and prevertebral soft tissues.

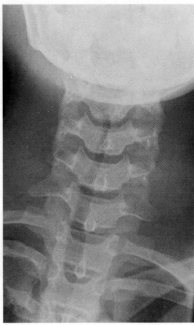

Fig. 26.14 Long-segment irregular subglottic stenosis caused by prior intubation.

Accidental and Iatrogenic Causes

Accidental caustic ingestion of strongly acidic or basic agents may cause mucosal injury in the oropharynx, hypopharynx, or esophagus, which in turn could cause edema and inflammatory changes in the epiglottis and surrounding structures. Thermal injury has similar effects. Inhalational injury of smoke or fumes from toxic substances may likewise cause swelling of the airway and result in respiratory distress or failure. Radiographic clues in the acute setting include thickening of the prevertebral soft tissues, enlargement of the epiglottis, thickening of the aryepiglottic folds, and narrowing of the subglottic airway. Often, the best clue to diagnosis is a thorough evaluation of available clinical information and situational evidence or a witnessed event of ingestion or inhalation of harmful substances. Respiratory symptoms can also occur in the chronic setting after accidental inhalation or ingestion as granulation tissue and scarring results in subglottic or upper tracheal stenosis.

One of the most common causes of iatrogenic respiratory distress is subglottic stenosis after intubation. The neck radiograph can be helpful in the initial identification of subglottic narrowing, but neck and chest CT is oftentimes performed for further delineation of anatomical location, features, and extent, and can also provide dynamic information about the degree of stenosis according to respiratory phase when images are acquired in inspiration and expiration (Fig. 26.14).

Another cause of postintubation subglottic narrowing is the formation of subglottic cysts, which are acquired mucosal retention cysts predominantly occurring after long-term intubation in the neonate. Subglottic cysts appear as asymmetrical foci of airway narrowing on the frontal or lateral neck radiograph, which can have a similar appearance to subglottic hemangioma. Definitive diagnosis is ultimately made by direct laryngoscopy.

Autoimmune Diseases

Autoimmune diseases affect the aerodigestive tract to varying degrees. Two autoimmune diseases, Wegener granulomatosis (a necrotizing vasculitis) and relapsing polychondritis (an inflammatory disorder of cartilage), have the highest incidence of upper airway involvement and can be seen in the pediatric population. Airway abnormalities and glomerulonephritis are the classic manifestations of Wegener granulomatosis, although other systems may be involved. Tracheal disease may be an isolated finding, but more commonly occurs in the setting of multisystem disease. Patients can present with dyspnea, hoarseness, or stridor. In the trachea, segmental, unifocal, or multifocal disease may be present, but there is usually focal involvement over a course of 2 to 4 cm. The subglottic trachea is most often affected, with smooth or nodular circumferential wall thickening. The posterior membranous trachea is always involved, which is a distinguishing feature from relapsing polychondritis.

Relapsing polychondritis is a rare autoimmune disease characterized by recurrent inflammation and destruction of cartilage. Common sites of involvement include the cartilaginous portions of the ears, nose, larynx and upper airway, tracheobronchial tree, eyes, and large joints. The respiratory tract is involved in about half of patients, and respiratory distress may occur because of central airway collapse relating to destruction and fibrosis of the laryngeal and tracheal cartilages or from narrowing of the peripheral airways. Once tracheal narrowing is identified on the neck radiograph, CT examination can be helpful to determine the exact anatomical extent of abnormality and evaluate for abnormal cartilaginous calcifications that can suggest the disease (Fig. 26.15).

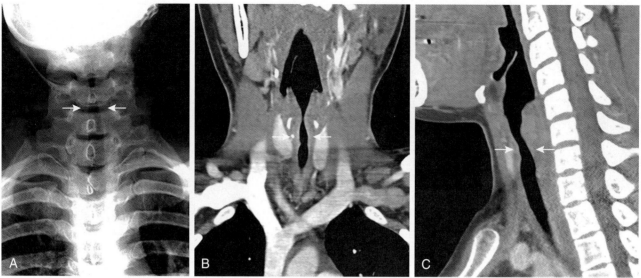

Fig. 26.15 Frontal radiograph (A) and coronal (B) and sagittal (C) computed tomography images of subglottic tracheal stenosis (*arrows*) in a 14-year-old female patient with relapsing polychondritis who presented with stridor.

■ Summary

Lateral neck radiographs can be challenging to optimize and interpret, particularly in young children. Understanding normal anatomy, recognizing pathology and distinguishing from suboptimal techniques are important to prevent unnecessary additional imaging. Evaluating for foreign bodies with rapid identification of ingested button batteries is necessary for emergent removal. This chapter elucidates many of the important and life threatening diagnoses.

Bibliography

Acar, M., Kankilic, E., Koksal, A., et al. (2014). Method of the diagnosis of adenoid hypertrophy for physicians: Adenoid-nasopharynx ratio. *Journal of Craniofacial Surgery, 25*(5), e438–e440.

Al-Mutairi, B., & Kirk, V. (2004). Bacterial tracheitis in children: Approach to diagnosis and treatment. *Paediatrics and Child Health, 9*(1), 25–30.

Anton-Pacheco, J. L., Villafuela, M., Martinez, A., et al. (2009). Congenital subglottic web: A rare cause of neonatal stridor. *Journal of Pediatric Surgery, 44*(1), e25–e27.

Berg, E., Naseri, I., & Sobol, S. E. (2008). The role of airway fluoroscopy in the evaluation of children with stridor. *Archives of Otolaryngology - Head and Neck Surgery, 134*(4), 415–418.

Breysem, L., Goosens, V., Vander Poorten, V., et al. (2009). Vallecular cyst as a cause of congenital stridor: Report of five patients. *Pediatric Radiology, 39*(8), 828–831.

Currarino, G., & Williams, B. (1982). Lateral inspiration and expiration radiographs of the neck in children with laryngotracheitis (croup). *Radiology, 145*(2), 365–366.

Faix, L. E., & Branstetter, B. F. (2005). 4th uncommon CT findings in relapsing polychondritis. *AJNR Am J Neuroradiol, 26*(8), 2134–2136.

Fujioka, M., Young, L. W., & Girdany, B. R. (1979). Radiographic evaluation of adenoidal size in children: Adenoidal-nasopharyngeal ratio. *American Journal of Roentgenology, 133*(3), 401–404.

Holinger, L. D., Toriumi, D. M., & Anandappa, E. C. (1988). Subglottic cysts and asymmetrical subglottic narrowing on neck radiograph. *Pediatric Radiology, 18*(4), 306–308.

Jatana, K. R., Litovitz, T., Reilly, J. S., et al. (2013). Pediatric button battery injuries: 2013 task force update. *International Journal of Pediatric Otorhinolaryngology, 77*(9), 1392–1399.

John, S. D., & Swischuk, L. E. (1992). Stridor and upper airway obstruction in infants and children. *RadioGraphics, 12*(4), 625–643 discussion 644.

John, S. D., Swischuk, L. E., Hayden, C. K., Jr., et al. (1994). Aryepiglottic fold width in patients with epiglottitis: Where should measurements be obtained? *Radiology, 190*(1), 123–125.

Karkos, P. D., Benton, J., Leong, S. C., et al. (2007). Grisel's syndrome in otolaryngology: A systematic review. *International Journal of Pediatric Otorhinolaryngology, 71*(12), 1823–1827.

Li, A. M., Wong, E., Kew, J., et al. (2002). Use of tonsil size in the evaluation of obstructive sleep apnoea. *Archives of Disease in Childhood, 87*(2), 156–159.

Martinez, F., Chung, J. H., Digumarthy, S. R., et al. (2012). Common and uncommon manifestations of wegener granulomatosis at chest CT: Radiologic-pathologic correlation. *RadioGraphics, 32*(1), 51–69.

McCook, T. A., & Kirks, D. R. (1982). Epiglottic enlargement in infants and children: Another radiologic look. *Pediatric Radiology, 12*(5), 227–234.

Salour, M. (2000). The steeple sign. *Radiology, 216*(2), 428–429.

Stoane, J. M., Haller, J. O., & Price, A. F. (1996). Neonatal goiter: Imaging findings in two children. *Pediatric Radiology, 26*(3), 20306.

Virk, J. S., Pang, J., Okhovat, S., et al. (2012). Analysing lateral soft tissue neck radiographs. *Emergency Radiology, 19*(3), 255–260.

CHAPTER 27
Pediatric Head and Neck Masses

Bradley S. Rostad, Adina L. Alazraki, and Erica L. Riedesel

CHAPTER OUTLINE

Part 1: Ocular and Orbital Masses (Box 1), 522
Ocular Masses, 522
  Is There a Mass Involving the Retina With Calcifications?, 522
  Is There a Mass Involving the Retina Without Calcifications?, 523
  Is the Mass Retrolental?, 524
  Does the Mass Involve the Iris?, 524
  Is the Vitreous Abnormal Without a Discrete Mass?, 524
  Is There Retinal Detachment?, 524
  Is There a Mass Involving the Optic Nerve?, 525
Extraocular Masses, 525
  Is the Mass Cystic and Unilocular?, 525
  Is There a Unilocular Cystic Lesion Near the Medial Canthus?, 526
  Is There a Unilocular Cystic Lesion That Is in Continuity With the Globe?, 526
  Is the Lesion Multicystic?, 527
  Is the Mass Solid and Hypervascular?, 527
Part 2: Sinonasal Masses (Box 2), 530
Nasofrontal Masses, 530
  Is the Mass Continuous With the Brain Through a Cranial Defect?, 531
  Is the Mass Discontinuous With Brain Tissue?, 531
  Is There a Persistent Sinus Tract or Inclusion Cyst?, 532
  Is the Mass Hypervascular?, 532
Sinus Masses, 532
  Is the Mass Polypoid and Protruding Into the Nasopharynx Without Aggressive Features?, 532
  Is There an Aggressive-Appearing Mass at the Roof of the Nasal Cavity?, 533
  Is the Mass Osseous Based, With a Mixed Lytic and Sclerotic Appearance?, 533
Nasopharynx Masses, 533
  Is There a Soft Tissue Mass With Aggressive Features?, 533
  Is the Patient Male With the Mass Centered on the Sphenopalatine Foramen?, 534
  Is There an Aggressive-Appearing Mass Involving the Lateral Nasopharyngeal Wall?, 535
Part 3: Oral Cavity, Floor of Mouth, and Mandibular Masses (Box 3), 535
Oral Cavity Masses, 535
  Is the Lesion Cystic and near the Vallecula?, 535

Floor of Mouth Masses, 536
  Is the Lesion Cystic and Midline?, 536
  Is the Lesion Cystic and Lateral to Midline?, 536
  Is There a Cystic Collection Associated With Dental Disease?, 536
Mandibular Masses, 537
  Is It an Aggressive-Appearing Lesion Centered on Bone?, 537
  Is It an Aggressive Soft Tissue Mass Involving Bone?, 537
  Is the Lesion Sclerotic and Well Circumscribed?, 537
  Is It a Lucent Lesion With Multifocal Mineralization?, 537
  Is the Lesion Cystic?, 538
  Is the Cyst Periapical?, 538
  Is the Cyst Expansile Without Erosion of Adjacent Teeth?, 538
  Is the Cyst Unilocular and Expansile With Erosion of Adjacent Teeth?, 538
  Is the Cyst Multilocular and Expansile With Erosion of Adjacent Teeth?, 538
  Does the Lesion Resemble Small, Malformed Teeth?, 538
  Is There an Expansile, Ground-Glass Appearance to the Mandible or Maxilla?, 538
  Is There Resorption of the Bone Around Multiple Teeth?, 538
Part 4: Neck Masses (Box 4), 538
Anterior Neck Masses, 538
  Is the Lesion Cystic?, 538
  Is the Cyst Midline?, 538
  Is the Cyst Lateral to Midline?, 539
Deep Neck Masses, 542
  Does It Involve the Sternocleidomastoid Muscle?, 542
  Is It Paraspinal, and Does It Contain Calcifications?, 542
  Does It Appear Locally Aggressive?, 543
  Does the Mass Contain Macroscopic Fat?, 544
  Is the Mass Well Circumscribed and Hypervascular?, 544
  Is the Lesion Multicystic and Transspatial?, 544
  Is There Expansion of the Nerve Roots?, 544
  Are There Rim-Enhancing Fluid Collections Involving the Tonsils?, 544
  Are There Rim-Enhancing Fluid Collections Involving the Retropharyngeal Space?, 545
Summary, 546

Evaluation of pediatric head and neck masses can be challenging because the anatomy is complex and the diseases that affect the head and neck are numerous. Grouping head and neck lesions into broad categories based on anatomic location and suspected type of lesion, whether it is solid or cystic, can greatly facilitate a practical approach to imaging.

For small, superficial lesions in the neck, ultrasound is an excellent initial step in imaging, particularly if the lesions are likely to be cystic. Cystic lesions in the neck may have a variable sonographic appearance. If the cysts contain simple fluid, they will appear anechoic and smooth walled. However, they may appear heterogeneous if they contain proteinaceous material or blood products. Checking to see if the debris in a cyst is mobile is helpful, because a cyst containing debris could be mistaken for a solid lesion. Increased through transmission is also a sonographic finding of cystic rather than solid contents. In addition, it is important to consider the effect that infection or inflammation may have on the imaging appearance of an otherwise asymptomatic cystic structure. Frequently, cystic lesions come to clinical attention when they become infected or are enlarged by internal hemorrhage. In these cases an otherwise simple-appearing cystic structure may contain debris and have a thickened and hypervascular wall.

If a lesion in the neck is suspected to extend into the upper mediastinum, deep structures of the neck, or the retropharyngeal space, or if the lesion is larger than can be practically imaged by the field of view of an ultrasound probe, magnetic resonance imaging (MRI) or computed tomography (CT) is the next step in imaging evaluation.

The choice between CT and MRI depends on many factors. CT is often more available than MRI and usually does not require sedation. For this reason, CT is often the preferred first imaging step beyond ultrasound for evaluation of head and neck lesions, particularly in emergent situations. CT may better demonstrate calcifications within a solid mass to help narrow a differential diagnosis. In addition, CT may provide more information regarding degree of osseous erosion by an aggressive mass. In contrast, MRI has superior soft tissue contrast and lacks ionizing radiation. MRI is the study of choice when imaging complex soft tissue structures, including orbital tumors, tumors of the oropharynx, and tumors of the nasofrontal region. For both CT and MRI, intravenous contrast significantly improves soft tissue visualization and is typically recommended for evaluation of head and neck masses.

Radiographs have limited value in the direct evaluation of head and neck masses. However, soft tissue radiographs of the neck are useful in evaluating the airway and are often ordered as the first line evaluation in a patient with difficulty breathing or abnormal upper airway sounds (Chapter 26, "Lateral Neck"). As with any imaging modality, safety is paramount. If a patient is having significant difficulty breathing, or if there is clinical suspicion of impending acute airway obstruction, it is important that this be addressed by emergency clinical personnel who should secure the airway before imaging is attempted.

■ Part 1: Ocular and Orbital Masses (Box 1)

Ocular Masses

The differential diagnosis for ocular masses in children includes retinoblastoma, persistent hyperplastic primary vitreous, Coats disease, medulloepithelioma, and *Toxocara* endophthalmitis. Although no imaging finding is pathognomonic, some imaging features are more suggestive of a specific diagnosis than others. Helpful imaging findings include the location of the abnormality (Fig. 27.1), presence of calcifications, microphthalmia, and laterality. Clinically relevant information includes recognizing whether the lesion is congenital or acquired, and if there is leukocoria on physical examination.

Is There a Mass Involving the Retina With Calcifications?

Retinoblastoma is the most common intraocular malignancy in childhood. On imaging, retinoblastoma usually appears as an intraocular mass involving the retina. Calcification is present in nearly all retinoblastomas and is considered a distinguishing feature of the disease. Although many chronic ocular processes may cause calcifications, and retinoblastoma may rarely present without calcifications, a mass involving the retina with calcifications is retinoblastoma until proved otherwise.

Retinoblastoma is not congenital but usually presents in the first few years of life. Symptoms include leukocoria (approximately half of children with leukocoria are diagnosed with retinoblastoma), squinting, and strabismus. Rarely retinoblastoma can present with extensive inflammation and be clinically mistaken for orbital cellulitis.

Retinoblastoma is caused by a defect in the *RB1* tumor suppressor gene on chromosome 13q14. Mutations in both alleles are necessary for tumor development. There are hereditary and nonhereditary forms of the disease.

BOX 27.1 Ocular and orbital masses	
Ocular Masses	**Orbital Masses**
■ Retinoblastoma	■ Dacryocystocele
■ Persistent hyperplastic primary vitreous	■ Dermoid
	■ Lymphatic malformation
■ Coats disease	■ Hemangioma
■ *Toxocara* endophthalmitis	■ Optic glioma
	■ Rhabdomyosarcoma
■ Medulloepithelioma	■ Neuroblastoma
■ Coloboma	

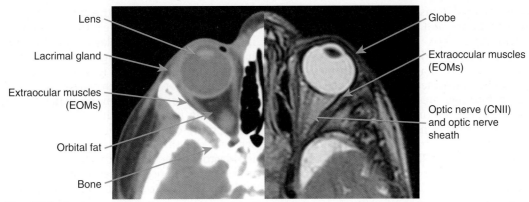

Fig. 27.1 Ocular and orbital anatomy on axial computed tomography and magnetic resonance imaging.

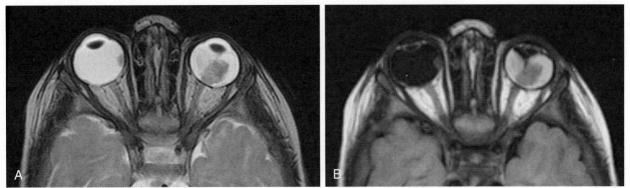

Fig. 27.2 **Bilateral retinoblastoma.** (A) Axial T2 weighted MRI of the orbits demonstrates bilateral hypointense intraorbital masses. (B) T1 image demonstrates the bilateral intraocular masses with retinal detachment of the left globe and associated T1 hyperintense proteinaceous fluid.

The nonhereditary form requires spontaneous mutations in both alleles. Those with hereditary retinoblastoma already have a mutation in one allele; the other mutation occurs spontaneously. The hereditary form is more likely to present earlier and to be bilateral. Patients with the hereditary form are also predisposed to development of primary synchronous intracranial tumors, usually seen in the midline in the suprasellar region or pineal region. When retinoblastoma is present in both globes and the suprasellar location, the presentation is described as "trilateral" retinoblastoma. These intracranial tumors are histologically identical to intraocular retinoblastoma. It is for this reason that dedicated MRI of the brain, as well as the orbits, should be obtained. In addition to intracranial tumors, patients with hereditary retinoblastoma have an increased risk for development of sarcomas elsewhere. This patient population is also particularly radiosensitive, and the risk for development of sarcomas is significantly increased if radiation therapy is used for treatment.

CT shows a hyperdense retinal mass with moderate enhancement and areas of necrosis and calcification. However, CT is no longer recommended for imaging in cases of known or suspected retinoblastoma. A combination of ocular ultrasound and MRI has been proved to be adequate for tumor characterization,

and this approach avoids ionizing radiation in this radiosensitive patient population.

On MRI, retinoblastoma is T1-hyperintense and T2-hypointense to the vitreous humor and demonstrates heterogenous enhancement (Fig. 27.2). It is important to assess the integrity of the sclera and to evaluate the optic nerve for invasion. Evaluation of the brain should also be made with special attention to the suprasellar and pineal regions, as well as assessment for leptomeningeal disease.

The main differential diagnostic considerations for retinoblastoma are other causes of childhood leukocoria, including persistent hyperplastic primary vitreous, Coats disease, *Toxocara* endophthalmitis, and retinopathy of prematurity. Rarely retinal astrocytoma and medulloepithelioma may be encountered.

Is There a Mass Involving the Retina Without Calcifications?

Toxocara endophthalmitis (ocular larva migrans) is a granulomatous response to infection of the vitreous or uvea of the eye by larva of the roundworm of the *Toxocara* genus. The normal hosts are dogs (*T. canis*) and cats (*T. cati*), and the eggs of the parasite are excreted in animal feces. Children can become infected after ingesting eggs from contaminated items or soil. The eggs hatch in the gastrointestinal tract, and the larvae can migrate to any organ, including the eye.

The disease is usually unilateral and can result in subretinal exudate and masslike granulomas. The most common clinical presentation is visual impairment. Imaging findings are nonspecific. On CT, it may be indistinguishable from Coats disease with vitreous hyperdensity and retinal detachment. Notably, there is no calcification, which helps to distinguish it from retinoblastoma. MRI may also demonstrate a granulomatous mass that enhances after contrast administration.

Is the Mass Retrolental?

Persistent hyperplastic primary vitreous (PHPV) is the second most common cause of pediatric leukocoria. It is congenital and is usually diagnosed in the early neonatal period. The disease is almost always unilateral, and the affected eye is usually microphthalmic. Bilateral cases of PHPV may be syndromic, such as Walker-Warburg syndrome. A mimic of bilateral PHPV may be bilateral retinal detachment from trauma or condition such as Norrie disease.

Pathologically, PHPV results from failure of the embryonic primary vitreous to completely regress. The result is a residual mass of retrolental fibrovascular tissue that proliferates. It may invade the lens or bleed, resulting in increased intraocular pressures (glaucoma). Half of cases also have a persistent hyaloid canal, which contains a persistent hyaloid artery extending from the optic disc to the posterior lens. The combined shape of the retrolental mass and contiguous hyaloid canal has been likened to a martini glass. Resulting tethering of the posterior retina at the optic disc may result in varying degrees of tenting or retinal detachment. On CT the retrolental tissue is hyperdense and enhances. The residual hyaloid canal may be seen. Unlike retinoblastoma, calcifications are absent. MRI shows similar findings with an enhancing retrolental mass (Fig. 27.3). Imaging findings may be complicated by the presence of intraocular hemorrhage or retinal detachment.

Does the Mass Involve the Iris?

Medulloepithelioma, a rare intraocular tumor, is a primitive neuroepithelial neoplasm. Both benign and malignant types exist. The average age at diagnosis is 5 years. Clinical findings include leukocoria, impaired vision, and pain. Most tumors originate in the ciliary body, but they can originate from the retina. CT demonstrates masses with irregular borders that can be located at the ciliary body or retina. Sometimes calcification can be seen, making this lesion difficult to distinguish from retinoblastoma when it involves the retina. On MRI the tumor is hyperintense to vitreous on T1-weighted imaging and hypointense to vitreous on T2-weighted imaging.

Is the Vitreous Abnormal Without a Discrete Mass?

Coats disease results from a congenital vascular malformation of the retina. The abnormal retinal blood vessels result in a breakdown of the blood–retina barrier. Over time this leads to the accumulation of large amounts of subretinal lipoproteins and blood products resulting in retinal detachment and vision loss. The process is commonly unilateral. Although it is congenital, it usually presents later at around 6 to 8 years of age. Symptoms include leukocoria, strabismus, glaucoma, and vision loss.

CT shows increased density in the subretinal fluid, which in some cases can be extensive enough to occupy the entire globe (Fig. 27.4). Unlike retinoblastoma, there are no calcifications. After contrast, there is enhancement of the retina, but not of the subretinal space. If the subretinal fluid collection is large enough, this results in a V shape of the retina, with the apex of the V at the optic disc, where the retina is tightly attached. On MRI the subretinal fluid is hyperintense on T1-and T2-weighted imaging because of its high lipid content. If there is hemorrhage or fibrosis, this may manifest as T2 heterogeneity. As on CT, after contrast the retina enhances, but the subretinal fluid does not.

Is There Retinal Detachment?

Retinal detachment can be a complication of retinoblastoma, PHPV, *Toxocara* endophthalmitis, Coats disease, and medulloepithelioma. It is a nonspecific finding, but if found, a careful search should be made for associated pathology.

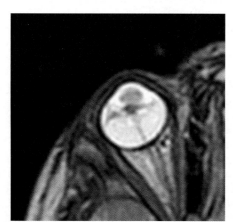

Fig. 27.3 Persistent hyperplastic primary vitreous (PHPV). Axial T2 magnetic resonance imaging shows triangular retrolental soft tissue mass with hyaloid remnant extending from lens to posterior pole of right globe.

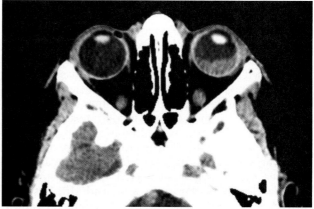

Fig. 27.4 Coats disease. Computed tomography shows posterior segment hyperdensity in the left globe representing subretinal exudate composed of proteinaceous fluid and blood product.

Is There a Mass Involving the Optic Nerve?

Optic nerve glioma is the primary consideration in an optic nerve mass or mass-like enlargement of the optic nerve in children. It can arise anywhere along the optic tracts, including the optic nerve, chiasm, and optic radiations. Histologically, optic nerve gliomas are identical to juvenile pilocytic astrocytomas. They are associated with neurofibromatosis type 1 (NF1) in half of cases, and bilateral optic nerve gliomas are diagnostic for NF1. Clinical findings include decreased vision and abnormal fundoscopic examination. On imaging the tumor most commonly presents as fusiform expansion of the optic nerve, but the mass can be eccentric. In some cases the optic nerve may be tortuous. A differential consideration for mild enlargement and enhancement may include optic neuritis, but optic nerve gliomas are typically much larger and indolent in symptom presentation.

On CT the optic nerve glioma is usually isodense to the extraocular muscles and may demonstrate variable enhancement. Calcifications are rare. On MRI the tumor is isointense or hypointense on T1-weighted imaging and hyperintense on T2-weighted imaging (Fig. 27.5). Enhancement is also variable. MRI with its superior soft tissue contrast is better able to demonstrate intracranial extension. Because the only practical imaging differential of an optic nerve glioma is a nerve sheath meningioma, which is rare in the pediatric population, the imaging findings of an optic nerve glioma by MRI are essentially pathognomonic. Fortunately, optic nerve gliomas typically have an indolent course and are therefore managed conservatively.

Extraocular Masses

Is the Mass Cystic and Unilocular?

Dermoid and epidermoid inclusion cysts are the most common benign extraocular orbital masses in children. They commonly occur in the upper outer orbit and may be located near to or involve cranial sutures. Clinically, they may present as facial asymmetry or become symptomatic when they are complicated by infection or cyst rupture.

Inclusion cysts are thought to originate from abnormal separation of the ectoderm from the mesoderm or aberrant in-folding of the ectoderm into the mesoderm during development and can occur anywhere throughout the head and neck. Although they are not neoplasms, they enlarge as the desquamated epithelium and/or sebum accumulates. The walls of epidermoid cysts consist only of squamous epithelium, but dermoid cysts contain dermal elements as well (hair follicles, sebaceous glands). Notably, rupture of inclusion cysts can cause an inflammatory reaction that may mimic orbital cellulitis. Imaging demonstrates well-circumscribed cystic lesions that may be adjacent to or within sutures. The adjacent bone may demonstrate remodeling, reflecting the slow growth of these lesions.

Imaging characteristics of dermoid and epidermoid cysts are similar regardless of location in the head and

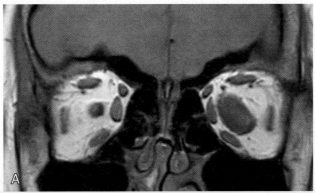

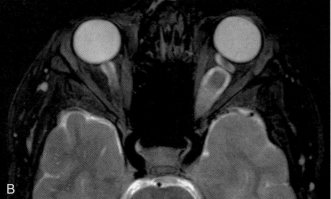
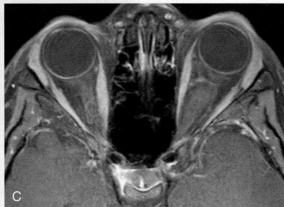

Fig. 27.5 Optic nerve glioma. (A) T1 coronal magnetic resonance imaging (MRI) demonstrates unilateral fusiform enlargement of the right intraorbital optic nerve. (B) T2 fat-saturated axial MRI shows tortuous and "kinked" appearance of the enlarged optic nerve with normal surrounding CSF within the optic nerve sheath. (C) No enhancement on postcontrast MRI.

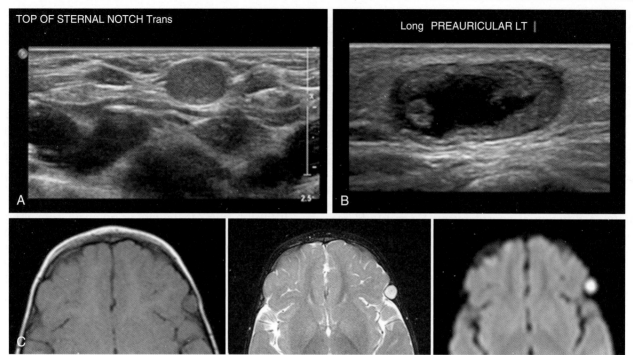

Fig. 27.6 Dermoid and epidermoid inclusion cysts. (A) Ultrasound with high-frequency transducer demonstrates well-circumscribed spherical mass which is "solid appearing," avascular, with posterior acoustic enhancement and edge shadowing in a dermoid cyst. (B) Epidermoid cyst with complex cystic appearance on ultrasound. On magnetic resonance imaging, dermoid/epidermoid cysts are typically (C) iso-intense on T1, (D) bright on T2 with (E) restricted diffusion on DWI.

neck (Fig. 27.6A–B). These developmental cysts are commonly seen at sutures with the most common location being near the zygomaticofrontal suture (level of lateral eyebrow). Orbital location of dermoid/epidermoid cysts is not uncommon given the multiple sutures. It can be difficult to differentiate dermoid cysts from epidermoid cysts so may be referenced as "dermoid/epidermoid" cysts. Ultrasound is the most appropriate initial imaging study for palpable masses in pediatric patients, and often provides a diagnosis given history, location, and sonographic appearance. On ultrasound, dermoid/epidermoid cysts will be seen as a well-circumscribed ovoid mass within the subcutaneous tissue, and occasionally seen scalloping subjacent bone or within the suture itself. Dermoid cysts may be "solid appearing" with mixed internal echogenic material. Posterior acoustic enhancement and edge shadowing are key imaging findings to confirm the cystic nature of these pseudosolid lesions. Epidermoid cysts may be more "cystic" appearing on ultrasound and may contain internal echogenic debris.

On CT, epidermoid cysts are well circumscribed and the density slightly greater than simple fluid, reflecting the proteinaceous contents of desquamated keratinized cells. However, dermoid cysts may demonstrate lipid material secreted from the sebaceous glands, and foci of calcification may also be seen. Keratin debris within dermoid cysts may float on top of the secreted lipid giving the appearance of a fluid–fluid level. If located within bone, both dermoid and epidermoid cysts will demonstrate a well-defined lucency with a rim of sclerosis and remodeling.

On MRI, epidermoid cysts may be bright on T2-weighted imaging, but their contents are distinguished from simple fluid-containing cysts because this signal will not suppress on fluid-attenuated inversion recovery imaging and will show diffusion restriction from the keratinized cellular debris within the cyst (see Fig. 27.6C). The lipid content of dermoid/epidermoid cysts can be isointense to mildly hyperintense on T1-weighted imaging and can show some suppression on fat-saturated sequences (suggesting dermoid).

Is There a Unilocular Cystic Lesion Near the Medial Canthus?

A dacryocystocele results from obstruction of the nasolacrimal duct. It appears as cystic dilation of the nasolacrimal duct, and may have inflammatory changes from superimposed infection causing an acute presentation (dacryocystitis). On CT and MRI a dacryocystocele appears as a thin-walled cystic lesion with fluid attenuation at the medial canthus of the eye (Fig. 27.7). The lacrimal duct may be seen as a tubular structure extending distally to the valve of Hasner at its communication to the inferior turbinate. These are treated conservatively with warm compresses and massage, and antibiotics if superinfected. Other approaches, such as probing the nasolacrimal duct or rarely more aggressive surgical procedures, are reserved for difficult cases.

Is There a Unilocular Cystic Lesion That Is in Continuity With the Globe?

Coloboma results from a failure of the embryonic choroidal fissure to close. It appears as an outpouching of the globe, is usually posterior, and may involve the optic disc. However, sometimes it can be so large that it looks

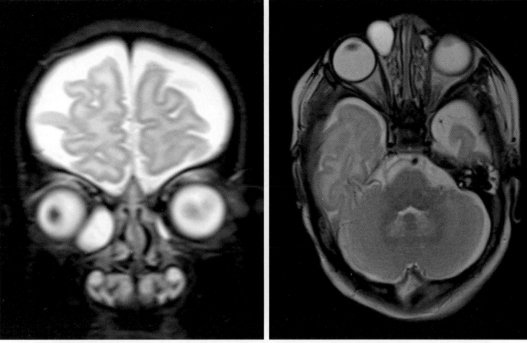

Fig. 27.7 Dacryocystocele. Magnetic resonance imaging demonstrates thin-walled, simple fluid-filled cystic lesion at the medial canthus of the eye.

like an extraocular orbital cystic lesion. Bilateral colobomas are associated with CHARGE syndrome (coloboma, heart anomaly, choanal atresia, growth retardation, genital and ear anomalies).

Is the Lesion Multicystic?

Venous and lymphatic malformations represent a spectrum of slow-flow vascular malformations. These lesions are transspatial, can involve any part of the orbit and adjacent face, and typically enlarge as the patient grows.

In the orbit, superficial lesions and the superficial components of large lesions are predominantly lymphatic, while deep lesions and the deep components of large lesions are predominately venous. Although these lesions are chronic, they often present acutely with proptosis from sudden expansion caused by internal hemorrhage or secondary infection.

MRI is preferred to evaluate the depth and extent of these lesions. Venous malformations are T1-hypointense, T2-hyperintense, and enhance after contrast. Lymphatic malformations are T1-hypointense and T2-hyperintense but do not enhance, although thin septa within the lesion may show linear enhancement (Fig. 27.8). Lymphatic malformations may show fluid–fluid levels from internal hemorrhage. Venous malformations may show fluid-fluid levels from extreme slow venous flow and separation of blood products. Venous malformations may also show filling defects related to clot or phleboliths.

Is the Mass Solid and Hypervascular?

Infantile hemangioma of the orbit is a benign neoplastic vascular lesion that is not congenital but develops shortly after birth, undergoes a period of rapid growth for several months (up to 1st year), and then slowly involutes over several years as it involutes into fibrous and fatty tissue.

The most common orbital location is the eyelid; however, these tumors can involve the orbit and retroorbital space. Deeper masses may present with proptosis and cause complications resulting in impaired vision.

For superficial lesions with characteristic physical examination findings and an appropriate clinical history, imaging may not be needed. However, ultrasound may be requested to support a clinical diagnosis. On ultrasound, hemangiomas appear as well-defined, homogenous masses with increased vascularity. Doppler evaluation will demonstrate low resistance arterial waveforms with relatively high velocities. If the lesion is suspected to involve deeper structures, or if the diagnosis is uncertain, MRI (preferred) or CT may be helpful.

Contrast enhanced CT demonstrates a lobular homogenous soft tissue mass without calcifications. If imaged in the proliferative phase, uniform avid-enhancement is seen with contrast administration. During the involuting phase, heterogeneity of the lesion may be seen due to the fibrous and fatty components. There may be remodeling of adjacent bone, but not aggressive bony changes (Fig. 27.9). On MRI an infantile hemangioma appears as a soft tissue mass, typically T1-isointense to muscle. On T2-weighted imaging, it is hyperintense to muscle and small arterial feeding vessels or flow voids are seen leading to and within the mass. Post contrast imaging during the proliferative phase demonstrates an avid enhancement beginning in the arterial phase with enhancement similar in signal to the aorta. During the involuting phase, heterogeneity can be seen. Asymptomatic lesions can be observed, and treatment with propranolol or surgery may be recommended for symptomatic lesions or lesions which could cause visual symptoms with lesion growth.

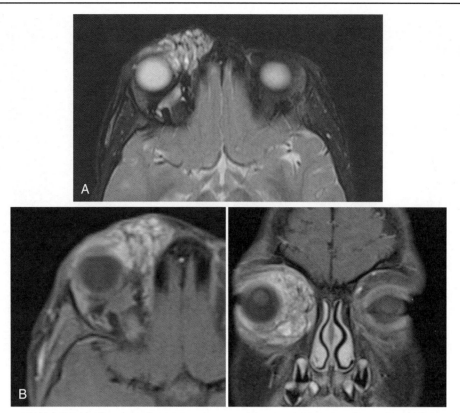

Fig. 27.8 Orbital microcystic lymphatic malformation. (A) T2 fat-supressed axial magnetic resonance imaging (MRI) demonstrates transspatial mass consisting of innumerable small (<2-mm) cysts in the medial right periorbital region and (B) septal enhancement on postcontrast axial and coronal MRI.

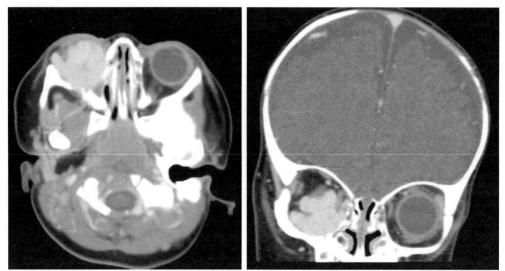

Fig. 27.9 Orbital hemangioma. Computed tomography with intravenous contrast demonstrates uniformly enhancing soft tissue retroorbital mass with remodeling of adjacent bone.

Does the Mass Appear Aggressive, Eroding Adjacent Bone?

IS THE MASS IN THE SUPERIOR ORBIT?

Rhabdomyosarcoma, although rare, is the most common extraocular orbital malignancy in children. It arises from pluripotent mesenchymal cells and can occur anywhere in the orbit, although it is most commonly found in the superior orbit. It is locally aggressive, invading adjacent structures. There are three types: alveolar, em-bryonal, and pleomorphic, with embryonal being the most common type in the orbit. Small tumors may appear well circumscribed and homogenous, but larger tumors may have ill-defined margins and demonstrate internal heterogeneity from cystic necrosis and hemorrhage. Although rare with orbital rhabdomyosarcoma, in advanced disease there may be metastatic lymphadenopathy and hematogenous metastases to the lungs and bones.

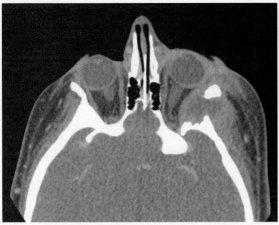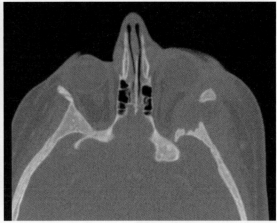

Fig. 27.10 Orbital Langerhans cell histiocytosis. Computed tomography demonstrates a soft tissue mass in the lateral orbit with diffuse, moderate enhancement and destructive osteolytic changes.

Both MRI and CT can be of value in imaging orbital rhabdomyosarcoma, however MRI is usually preferred. MRI is superior at demonstrating intracranial extension, while CT is superior in demonstrating osseous involvement. Additional imaging characteristics are described later in the Part 2: Sinonasal Masses.

IS THE MASS IN THE BONY ORBIT?

Langerhans cell histiocytosis (LCH) is a multisystem disease that has many clinical presentations. With orbital disease, patients most commonly present with proptosis. Additional symptoms include ptosis and palpebral or periorbital erythema. In the setting of orbital involvement, LCH is most commonly found in the lateral aspect of the frontal bone but can be found in other bones and extend into nearby soft tissues. Because they are locally aggressive, they need to be distinguished from other aggressive, potentially malignant lesions.

CT demonstrates a relatively homogenous soft tissue mass centered in and eroding the involved bone (Fig. 27.10) with well defined margins. The mass enhances homogeneously after contrast. On MRI, these lesions are T1-intermediate and T2-hyperintense. Like CT, on MRI they enhance after contrast.

The discovery of Langerhans cell histiocytosis of the orbit should initiate an evaluation for systemic disease. The treatment depends on the disease extent. Single lesions may heal spontaneously and are frequently observed after diagnostic biopsy, but multifocal disease may require a more aggressive approach with steroids and chemotherapy.

IS THE MASS CENTERED IN THE BONE OF THE LATERAL ORBITAL WALL WITH AN AGGRESSIVE PERIOSTEAL REACTION?

Neuroblastoma is the most common pediatric malignancy to metastasize to the orbit. The metastases typically involve the bones of the lateral orbital wall and orbital roof. Clinical findings usually consist of proptosis and periorbital ecchymosis.

CT demonstrates a soft tissue mass involving the bone with a permeative or erosive appearance (Fig. 27.11). There is typically an aggressive periosteal reaction with a "sunburst" pattern. The soft tissue component is typically hyperdense to muscle and may contain small calcifications and areas of cystic necrosis. The soft tissue component may extend into the lateral extraconal space, but only rarely does it involve the preseptal space. On MRI the soft tissue component is T1-hypointense to muscle, T2-hyperintense to muscle, and demonstrates heterogenous enhancement.

IS THERE A CLINICAL HISTORY OF LEUKEMIA?

Granulocytic sarcoma, formerly known as a chloroma, is a tumor of primitive granulocyte precursor cells that may be found in children with leukemia. Although rare, they are important to recognize because leukemia is the most common malignancy of childhood, and granulocytic sarcomas can be seen before presentation of systemic disease or be seen before diagnosis of relapse. Proptosis is the most common presentation, with tumors usually found along the lateral orbital wall. They may permeate through bone, although typically without eroding it, and extend into adjacent soft tissues. CT demonstrates a homogenous soft tissue mass with osseous and soft tissue involvement that enhances homogenously after contrast. On MRI, they are isointense to hypointense on T1-weighted imaging, heterogeneously slightly hyperintense on T2-weighted imaging, and enhance homogenously after contrast.

IS THERE AN EXPANSILE, GROUND-GLASS APPEARANCE TO THE BONY ORBIT?

Fibrous dysplasia is a developmental abnormality of the bones consisting of immature fibroosseous tissue that slowly grows over time. Most cases involve only one bone, but the disease can be polyostotic. Notably, polyostotic fibrous dysplasia is associated with McCune-Albright syndrome. When it involves the orbit, patients may present with facial deformity or visual impairment.

Classically, radiographs usually show a ground-glass matrix within a defined lesion centered in the medullary space with expansion and remodeling of the involved bone. There may be scattered areas of sclerosis. Similar to radiographs but with better anatomic detail, CT demon-

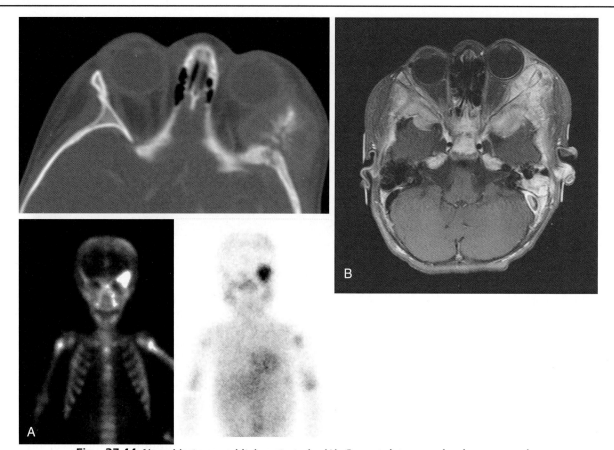

Fig. 27.11 Neuroblastoma orbital metastasis. (A) Computed tomography demonstrates lateral orbital soft tissue mass with aggressive "sunburst" periosteal reaction and uptake on both technetium-99m-methylene diphosphonate bone scan and iodine-123 MIBG scan. (B) Magnetic resonance imaging in a different patient with bilateral orbital metastases.

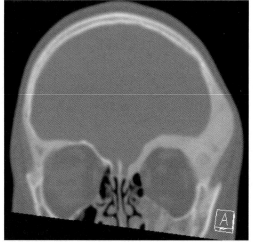

Fig. 27.12 Fibrous dysplasia. Computed tomography demonstrates classic "ground-glass" appearance of expanded bone around both orbits in this patient with McCune-Albright syndrome.

strates a predominantly ground-glass lesion with scattered areas of sclerosis (Fig. 27.12). MRI shows low to intermediate signal on T1 and variable signal on T2. Nuclear medicine bone scans show increased activity on all phases, and F-18 fluorodeoxyglucose-positron emission tomography/CT shows intense hypermetabolic activity.

■ Part 2: Sinonasal Masses (Box 2)

Nasofrontal Masses

When evaluating nasofrontal masses in children, the most important question to answer is whether there is intracranial involvement. However, before discussing the pathology that can occur in this area, a brief review of embryology of the nasofrontal region is helpful, particularly development of three transient nasofrontal structures: the fonticulus frontalis, the prenasal space, and the dural diverticulum that extends through the prenasal space.

BOX 27.2 Sinonasal masses		
Nasofrontal Masses	**Sinus Masses**	**Nasopharynx Masses**
▪ Encephalocele	▪ Sinonasal polyp	▪ Rhabdomyosarcoma
▪ Nasal glioma	▪ Esthesioneuroblastoma	▪ Juvenile nasopharyngeal angiofibroma
▪ Hemangioma	▪ Juvenile ossifying fibroma	▪ Nasopharyngeal carcinoma

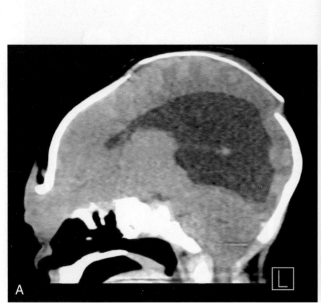
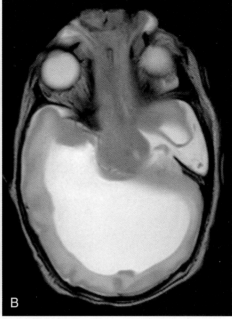

Fig. 27.13 Encephalocele. Large midline frontoethmoidal encephalocele on (A) computed tomography and (B) magnetic resonance imaging demonstrating protrusion of frontal meninges and brain tissue through midline bony defect at site of persistent embryological fonticulus frontalis.

The fonticulus frontalis is a transient anterior embryonic fontanelle located superior to the nasal bone that separates the nasal bone from the frontal bone. In normal embryonic development the fonticulus frontalis closes and becomes the nasofrontal suture. The prenasal space is inferior to the nasal bone and separates it from the cartilage of the nasal capsule. This cartilaginous nasal capsule is continuous with the cartilaginous skull base. Another transient structure, the dural diverticulum, extends through the prenasal space beneath the nasal bone but above the cartilage to contact the overlying skin. Eventually the diverticulum retracts from the skin and involutes, and the prenasal space closes. A small midline pit in the anterior cranial fossa known as the foramen cecum remains at the site of the previous prenasal space and contains the fibrous remnants of the dural diverticulum and occasionally an emissary vein. Failure of the fonticulus frontalis or prenasal space to close or persistence of the dural diverticulum can result in the various pathologies discussed later.

MRI is the study of choice for all of these anomalies. CT is of limited usefulness even for evaluation of the osseous portions of the cranium because the anterior skull base may not be completely ossified until 4 years of age.

Is the Mass Continuous With the Brain Through a Cranial Defect?

An encephalocele in the nasal region usually results from herniation of brain tissue through either a persistent fonticulus frontalis or prenasal space. Nasofrontal cephaloceles protrude through a persistent fonticulus frontalis, while nasoethmoidal cephaloceles protrude through a persistent prenasal space. Clinically, patients may present with a mass over the nasal bridge that enlarges when crying and hypertelorism. The mass may or may not be covered by skin. For the diagnosis of an encephalocele to be made, the extracranial mass and associated cerebral spinal fluid must be continuous with the intracranial brain and subarachnoid space, respectively. On MRI, herniated brain tissue present in the encephalocele should be similar in intensity with contiguous intracranial brain tissue however may be T2-hyperintense because of gliosis. Cerebrospinal fluid in an encephalocele will be T1-hypointense and T2-hyperintense. Like normal brain tissue, brain tissue in an encephalocele does not typically enhance. The cranial defect through which the encephalocele protrudes will often be wide with erosion of the anterior aspect of the crista galli (Fig. 27.13). Imaging is performed to evaluate the encephalocele, for potential presurgical planning, and to look for associated anomalies, including intracranial cysts, callosal agenesis, interhemispheric lipomas, and schizencephaly.

Is the Mass Discontinuous With Brain Tissue?

A nasal glial heterotopion or nasal cerebral heterotopion is brain tissue that herniates within the dural diverticulum in the prenasal space, then subsequently loses continuity with the intracranial brain. It is not a neoplasm, and so the term nasal glioma is not preferred. The sequestered brain tissue typically consists of dysplastic neuroglia and fibrovascular tissue. These lesions may be midline or just off midline.

Nasal glial heterotopia are classified as intranasal or extranasal. Intranasal heterotopia are found on the lateral wall or nasal septum of the nasal cavity and may present with nasal obstruction. Extranasal glial heterotopia are found on the bridge of the nose. Unlike an encephalocele, heterotopia typically will not enlarge with crying, but hypertelorism may be present. On MRI, they are typically isointense to brain matter

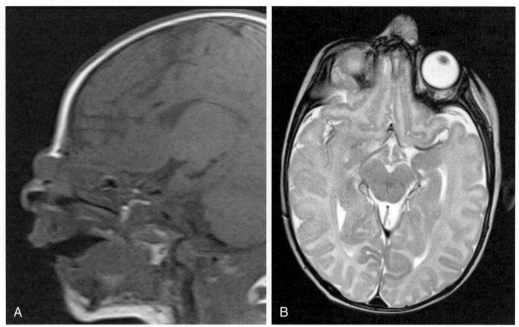

Fig. 27.14 Extranasal glial heterotopia. Heterotopic brain tissue at the nasal bridge isointense to the cerebral gray and white matter on A) Sagittal T1- and B) Axial T2-weighted magnetic resonance imaging.

on T1-weighted imaging and T2-weighted imaging (Fig. 27.14). A fibrous stalk may be seen attaching the nasal glioma to the brain. Nasal heterotopia do not enhance, but with intranasal heterotopia there may be enhancement of the adjacent compressed nasal mucosa.

Is There a Persistent Sinus Tract or Inclusion Cyst?

A persistent sinus tract may be found anywhere along the path between the foramen cecum at the anterior skull base to the bridge of the nose. It forms when the dural diverticulum, which protrudes through the embryonic prenasal space, fails to completely regress. If the tract is continuous from the skin to the meninges, there may be a history of recurrent meningitis from bacteria normally found on the skin surface. Sometimes a small pit with hairs or sebaceous secretions is visible on the bridge of the nose.

In addition to a persistent sinus tract, the dural diverticulum can fail to completely separate from its point of contact with the skin and, as it regresses back to the cranial vault, can contain a small amount of ectoderm, forming a dermoid or epidermoid inclusion cyst. Nasal dermoid and epidermoid cysts have similar imaging characteristics as these lesions found elsewhere in the body.

Is the Mass Hypervascular?

Infantile hemangiomas can occur anywhere in the head and neck, but infantile hemangiomas of the nasal bridge are significant because they must be distinguished from other nasal bridge masses, including encephalocele, nasal glioma, and nasal dermoid/epidermoid. These lesions can appear similar on clinical examination, so imaging is crucial to assist with diagnosis and to exclude

intracranial involvement of nasal bridge masses. Infantile hemangiomas are not congenital but arise shortly after birth, undergo rapid growth for about a year, and then slowly involute. Imaging characteristics are further characterized later in this chapter.

Sinus Masses

Is the Mass Polypoid and Protruding Into the Nasopharynx Without Aggressive Features?

Sinonasal polyps are benign mucosal lesions of the sinuses consisting of hyperplastic mucosal tissue. They form in response to chronic inflammation and can consist of both cystic and polypoid components, but the cystic component may be collapsed with opposed walls. The most common is the antrochoanal polyp, which originates in the maxillary sinus and grows along the path of least resistance into the nasopharynx, typically through the accessory ostium. These lesions grow slowly but can get very large and can present dramatically with acute airway obstruction. Other symptoms include chronic nasal obstruction and epistaxis.

Imaging demonstrates mass originating in the sinus and extending into the nasopharynx with enlargement of the ostium through which it protrudes. CT shows a uniformly low-density lesion with osseous remodeling of the involved ostium. On MRI the lesion is T1-hypointense, T2-hyperintense and demonstrates thin, peripheral enhancement after contrast (Fig. 27.15). Occasionally a more intense area of contrast can be seen from an angiomatous component, which is thought to develop from repeated infarction and revascularization of this elongated mass. Treatment is surgical.

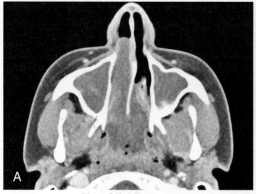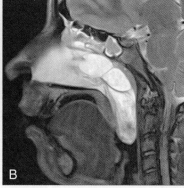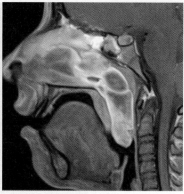

Fig. 27.15 Sinonasal polyp. (A) Contrast-enhanced computed tomography demonstrates a large hypodense, nonenhancing polypoid mass centered in the right nasal passage, obstructing the maxillary sinus ostia. (B) Polyp appears hyperintense on sagittal T2-weighted magnetic resonance imaging and extends into the nasopharynx and posterior pharynx with (C) peripheral enhancement on postcontrast T1-weighted images.

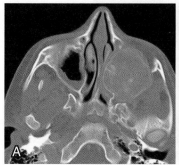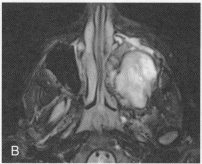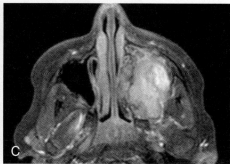

Fig. 27.16 Juvenile ossifying fibroma. (A) Expansile osseous mass in the left paranasal/maxillary region on computed tomography. (B) Soft tissue components are T2 hyperintense on magnetic resonance imaging and (C) enhancing.

Is There an Aggressive-Appearing Mass at the Roof of the Nasal Cavity?

Esthesioneuroblastoma is a rare malignancy located in the roof of the nasal cavity. It arises from olfactory neuroepithelium. A member of the primitive neuroectodermal tumor family, it could be considered an olfactory neuroblastoma. It is slow growing but locally aggressive and can erode through the cribriform plate with an intracranial component.

This tumor has a bimodal age distribution with peaks in the second and fifth to sixth decades of life. Symptoms include nasal obstruction, epistaxis, headache, and anosmia. If there is brain involvement, there may be neurological symptoms. Metastatic sites include cervical lymph nodes, the central nervous system, lung, liver, skin, eye, and bone.

Imaging demonstrates a highly vascular mass with areas of cystic necrosis. CT is helpful to assess osseous involvement. The tumor is isodense to hyperdense given the hypercellularity and enhances heterogenously after contrast. On MRI, it is T1-hypointense, T2-heterogenous, and has heterogenous enhancement.

Treatment includes surgery, chemotherapy, and radiation. This tumor has a tendency to recur and if successfully treated, long-term follow-up is needed. The differential includes other locally aggressive tumors, including Ewing sarcoma, rhabdomyosarcoma, and nasopharyngeal carcinoma.

Is the Mass Osseous Based, With a Mixed Lytic and Sclerotic Appearance?

Juvenile ossifying fibroma is a benign, slow-growing but locally aggressive osseous lesion that frequently originates in the facial bones of the paranasal sinuses. CT demonstrates an expansile osseous-based mass with lytic and sclerotic areas, surrounded by a thick rim of sclerosis that may be partially disrupted. The noncalcified portions of the tumor may have cystic components as well. On MRI the soft tissue component is T1-isointense, T2-hypointense and enhances after contrast (Fig. 27.16). As expected, the cystic portions are T2-hyperintense. The differential includes aneurysmal bone cyst and fibrous dysplasia. Treatment is surgical.

Nasopharynx Masses

Is There a Soft Tissue Mass With Aggressive Features?

Rhabdomyosarcoma is a malignant tumor that arises from pluripotent mesenchymal cells. Peak incidence is age 2 to 5 years and although this tumor can occur anywhere in the body, 40% of primary tumors involve the head and neck. It may be locally aggressive, invading adjacent structures. There are three types: alveolar, embryonal, and pleomorphic. Most of the disease presenting in children is of the embryonal and alveolar types.

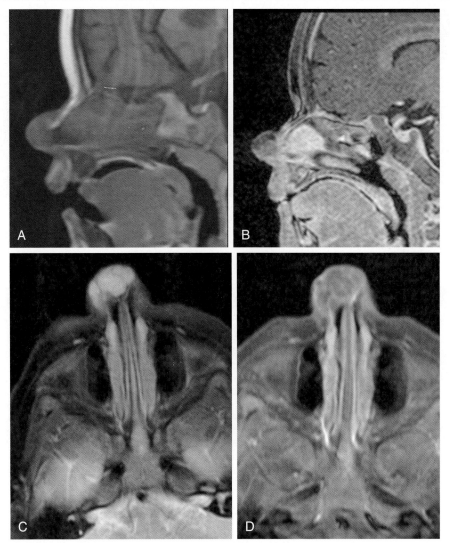

Fig. 27.17 Nasal rhabdomyosarcoma. On magnetic resonance imaging, sagittal T1 (A) and axial T2 (C) weighted images demontraste a soft tissue mass isointense to muscle on T1, slightly hyperintense on T2, with heterogeneous enhancement on postcontrast (B) sagittal and (D) axial imaging.

Locations of rhabdomyosarcoma in the head and neck are classified into parameningeal sites and nonparameningeal sites. The parameningeal sites include the nasopharynx, nasal cavity, paranasal sinuses, infratemporal fossa, pterygopalatine fossa, and middle ear area. Other locations in the head and neck are considered nonparameningeal. Prognosis is worse for parameningeal sites because these regions are anatomically complex and not easily visualized; thus disease is typically more advanced at presentation.

The tumors may have ill-defined margins and demonstrate internal heterogeneity from cystic necrosis and hemorrhage. On CT the tumor is isodense to muscle and may demonstrate enhancement. Erosion of adjacent bone is common. Although the tumor itself does not calcify, small calcifications may be seen in areas of osseous destruction. On MRI the tumor is usually isointense to muscle on T1-weighted imaging, slightly hyperintense to muscle on T2-weighted imaging, and enhances heterogeneously depending on the amount of cystic necrosis (Fig. 27.17).

Is the Patient Male With the Mass Centered on the Sphenopalatine Foramen?

Juvenile nasopharyngeal angiofibroma is a highly vascular lesion originating along the superior border of the sphenopalatine foramen. It is almost exclusively seen in males in the second decade of life. Although benign, this highly vascular lesion is locally aggressive, eroding bone and extending into adjacent anatomic spaces. These lesions bleed easily because their vessels are large and lack the elastic fibers found in normal vessels. The blood supply is typically from the ipsilateral internal maxillary artery.

Frequently, embolization is performed before surgery to avoid intraoperative blood loss. Although previously most surgeries were performed openly, now more endoscopic procedures are being done. Radiation therapy is pursued if the tumor is not amenable to complete surgical resection. Male predominance suggests a hormonal component, and these tumors are suspected to be androgen dependent; however, an effective hormonal therapy has not been found. Interestingly,

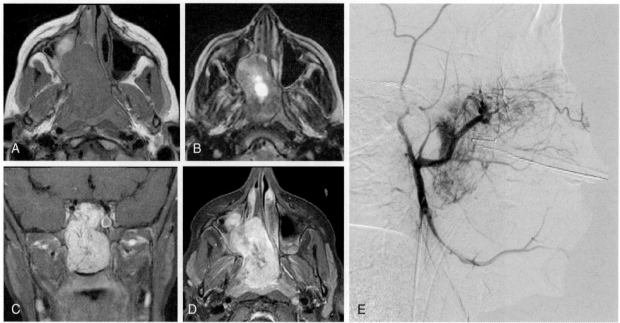

Fig. 27.18 Juvenile nasopharyngeal angiofibroma. Magnetic resonance imaging demonstrates a large nasopharyngeal mass centered in the sphenopalatine foramen that is isodense to muscle on (A) T1-weighted imaging has heterogeneous "salt-and-pepper" appearance on (B) T2 imaging with robust enhancement seen in coronal (C) and axial (D) imaging. (E) Selective angiogram of the ipsilateral external carotid artery demonstrates extensive contrast "blush" associated with hypervascular tumor.

some of these tumors may resolve spontaneously after adolescence.

On CT, juvenile nasopharyngeal angiofibroma appears as a soft tissue mass with marked enhancement. There may be erosion of the adjacent bone and anterior bowing of the posterior wall of the maxillary sinus. On MRI, these tumors are hypointense on T1-weighted imaging, heterogeneous intermediate signal intensity on T2-weighted imaging, and have large flow voids. As on CT, they avidly enhance after contrast (Fig. 27.18). The differential diagnosis includes nasopharyngeal carcinoma and rhabdomyosarcoma.

Is There an Aggressive-Appearing Mass Involving the Lateral Nasopharyngeal Wall?

Nasopharyngeal carcinoma is rare in children. Patients typically present late with advanced disease because of low clinical suspicion for carcinoma and because nasopharyngeal carcinoma is easily mistaken for benign adenoidal hypertrophy in its early stages.

Histologically, nasopharyngeal carcinoma in children differs from that seen in adults. In children the tumor consists of undifferentiated carcinoma or less commonly nonkeratinizing carcinoma, whereas in adults it is typically differentiated squamous cell carcinoma.

Although a definitive diagnosis can be made only by biopsy, suspicious imaging findings include asymmetrical adenoid enlargement, retropharyngeal lymphadenopathy, cervical lymphadenopathy, skull base erosion, unilateral mastoid opacification from eustachian tube obstruction, and widening of the petroclival fissure. With continued growth, the tumor may also involve the adjacent head and neck spaces, including the pterygopalatine fossa, masticator space, and parapharyngeal space. Cervical lymph node metastases are common, but distant metastases are possible.

CT may show a soft tissue mass in the nasopharynx with erosive changes of the adjacent bones. On MRI, it is isointense to hyperintense to muscle on T1-weighted imaging, hyperintense to muscle on T2-weighted imaging, and enhances homogenously. Treatment is with chemotherapy and radiation, with the role of surgery limited to biopsy. The differential diagnosis includes rhabdomyosarcoma, lymphoma, and juvenile nasopharyngeal angiofibroma.

■ Part 3: Oral Cavity, Floor of Mouth, and Mandibular Masses (Box 3)

Oral Cavity Masses

Is the Lesion Cystic and near the Vallecula?

A vallecular cyst is a rare benign cyst found in the region of the vallecula. It is thought to arise either from blockage of the submucosal glands or expansion of the laryngeal saccule. It is clinically significant because it can obstruct the airway and cause stridor. MRI may demonstrate a simple cyst with T1-hypointensity and T2-hyperintensity. Treatment is surgical marsupialization. The main differential diagnosis is a thyroglossal duct cyst at the base of the tongue.

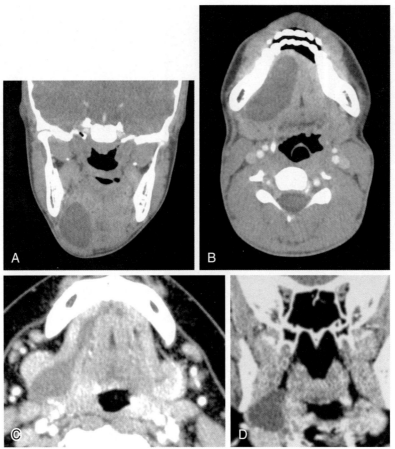

Fig. 27.19 Ranula. (A) Coronal and (B) axial Computed tomography (CT) with intravenous contrast demonstrates a low-density cyst localized to the sublingual space consistent with simple ranula. (C) Axial and (D) Coronal CT shows cystic mass in the right sublingual space extending posteriorly into the submandibular space consistent with diving ranula.

BOX 27.3 Oral cavity, floor of mouth and mandibular masses	
Oral Cavity and Floor of Mouth	**Mandibular Masses**
▪ Vallecular cyst	▪ Osteosarcoma
▪ Dermoid inclusion cyst	▪ Ewing sarcoma
▪ Ranula	▪ Osteoma
▪ Dental abscess	▪ Osteoblastoma
	▪ Dentigerous cyst
	▪ Keratocystic odontogenic tumor
	▪ Ameloblastoma
	▪ Fibroosseous dysplasia
	▪ Langerhans cell histiocytosis

Floor of Mouth Masses

Is the Lesion Cystic and Midline?

Dermoid inclusion cysts of the floor of the mouth are typically found in the midline. Their histopathology and imaging findings are similar to dermoid inclusion cysts found elsewhere. The primary differential diagnosis is an oral teratoma. Treatment is surgical removal.

Is the Lesion Cystic and Lateral to Midline?

Ranulas are benign cystic lesions associated with the sublingual gland. There are two types: simple and plunging (diving). The simple ranula is a retention cyst resulting from an obstructed sublingual gland. The simple ranula is located in the sublingual space, above the mylohyoid muscle. A plunging ranula forms when a simple ranula ruptures past the mylohyoid and extends into the submandibular space. Ranulas may present after becoming infected, so on imaging, superimposed inflammatory changes may be present. These lesions appear cystic on CT (Fig. 27.19). On MRI, they demonstrate simple fluid signal and are T1-hypointense and T2-hyperintense. Treatment is resection of the sublingual gland and associated cyst.

Is There a Cystic Collection Associated With Dental Disease?

Dental abscesses typically form when a periapical abscess ruptures through the mandibular cortex. It is more common to have cortical disruption on the lingual side of the mandible because the cortex of the mandible is thicker on the buccal side. Because of the location of the teeth roots in relation to the mylohyoid muscle, abscesses from dental disease of the second molar (or second and third molar in adults) are typically located in

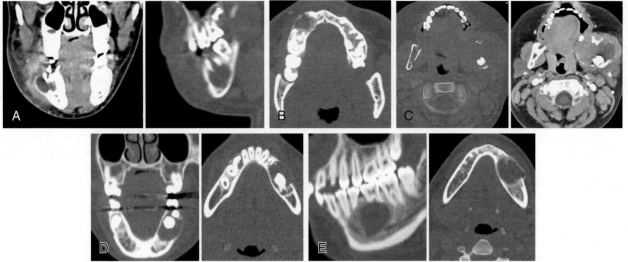

Fig. 27.20 Spectrum of mandibular lesions: (A) dental abscess, (B) osteosarcoma, (C) Ewing sarcoma, (D) dentigerous cyst, and (E) ameloblastoma.

the submandibular space, but abscesses resulting from more anterior teeth are located in the sublingual space. There may be associated osteomyelitis of the mandible.

On CT a soft tissue dental abscess appears as a rim-enhancing fluid collection adjacent to a focal defect in the mandible that usually is associated with a periapical lucency and dental disease of the involved tooth (Fig. 27.20A). CT findings of osteomyelitis of the jaw depend on chronicity but may include abnormal lucencies, areas of sclerosis, and periosteal reaction. The abscess will typically be adjacent to the mandible near a diseased tooth and demonstrate rim enhancement. On MRI the abscess will have variable T1 signal, increased T2 signal, and will enhance peripherally. Osteomyelitis of the jaw would manifest as decreased T1 marrow signal intensity.

Mandibular Masses

Primary lesions of the jaw are rare in children, but a wide variety of pathology can be seen. As with bones in other locations, nonodontogenic primary bone lesions, such as the simple bone cyst, aneurysmal bone cyst, giant cell tumor, chondrosarcoma, and osteosarcoma, can also present in the mandible, and their imaging findings are similar to that when present in other locations. A few primary bone tumors with special significance to the head and neck will be discussed here, along with some of the more frequent but nevertheless rare pediatric odontogenic lesions. Radiography and CT are the primary imaging modalities used to assess the mandible and maxilla.

Is It an Aggressive-Appearing Lesion Centered on Bone?

Osteosarcoma of the mandible, although rare, can occur (see Fig. 27.20B). Overall, osteosarcoma is the most common pediatric primary malignant bone tumor. Patients with primary osteosarcoma of the jaw tend to have a better prognosis than extremity osteosarcomas

because the risk for metastasis is lower. Notably, half of osteosarcomas in the head and neck are secondary and arise in sites of prior radiation therapy. In any aggressive pediatric bone lesion the possibility of osteosarcoma should be considered, particularly in the setting of prior radiation therapy.

Is It an Aggressive Soft Tissue Mass Involving Bone?

Although Ewing sarcoma, like osteosarcoma, rarely presents in the mandible, it is significant because it is the second most common primary malignant bone tumor in children. When it does present in the mandible, it typically involves the posterior ramus. On imaging, it appears as an aggressive soft tissue mass involving the bone with cortical destruction, osseous expansion, and may have a hair-on-end periosteal reaction (see Fig. 27.20C).

Is the Lesion Sclerotic and Well Circumscribed?

Osteomas are benign tumors of mature compact bone. When in the mandible, they are usually seen in the posterior body or condyle. They are sclerotic and well circumscribed. Although typically asymptomatic, they are significant because they are associated with Gardner syndrome (familial colorectal polyposis), which is highly associated with early colon cancer.

Is It a Lucent Lesion With Multifocal Mineralization?

An osteoblastoma is a benign tumor consisting of osteoid tissue. It can be painful and, unlike osteoid osteoma, a smaller lesion with similar histological features, the pain is not relieved by salicylates. Osteoblastomas typically occur in the posterior mandible. On imaging they may be confused with periapical or dental abscess, and careful clinical history taking to determine lack of prior dental caries in the affected region is helpful in making the diagnosis. These lesions are generally large (>1.5 cm) at detection, and CT imaging demonstrates a lucent lesion with associated bone expansion and multifocal mineralization.

Is the Lesion Cystic?
The differential diagnosis for a cystic lesion in the mandible includes a radicular cyst, dentigerous cyst, keratocystic odontogenic tumor, ameloblastoma, and giant cell granuloma. Although certain imaging features may be present as described later, for lesions other than an obvious radicular cyst, tissue sampling may be required for diagnosis.

Is the Cyst Periapical?
Radicular cysts are periapical cysts that develop from odontogenic infections that spread through root of the tooth. Unless acutely inflamed, they are usually asymptomatic. Periapical granulomas can also develop from severe odontogenic disease.

Is the Cyst Expansile Without Erosion of Adjacent Teeth?
Dentigerous cysts, also known as follicular cysts, are benign cysts that form around the crown of an unerupted molar. They attach at the tooth just below the crown, so that the crown of the involved tooth is within the cyst, but the root of the tooth is not. They can be expansile with remodeling of the mandible but are usually not erosive (see Fig. 27.20D). Multiple cysts are associated with mucopolysaccharidosis type 4 (Maroteaux-Lamy syndrome).

Is the Cyst Unilocular and Expansile With Erosion of Adjacent Teeth?
Keratocystic odontogenic tumor (previously called *odontogenic keratocyst*) is a benign but locally aggressive cystic tumor containing keratinaceous debris that originates from the dental lamina. It is expansile and may erode adjacent teeth. It is typically found in the posterior body and ascending ramus of the mandible. Recurrence after enucleation and curettage is common. They are associated with multiple syndromes, including basal cell nevus (Gorlin-Goltz), Ehlers-Danlos, and Noonan syndromes.

Is the Cyst Multilocular and Expansile With Erosion of Adjacent Teeth?
Ameloblastoma is a predominantly cystic tumor that originates from the odontogenic epithelium. It is typically an expansile unilocular or multilocular cystic lesion, although some lesions may have soft tissue components (see Fig. 27.20E). It is locally aggressive and can erode adjacent teeth and cortex. Recurrence after surgical resection is common. Rarely, these tumors may metastasize.

Does the Lesion Resemble Small, Malformed Teeth?
An odontoma is essentially a hamartoma of dental tissue, and it is the most common pediatric odontogenic tumor. These tumors typically consist of enamel and dentin. There are two types: compound and complex. Compound odontomas resemble small, malformed teeth, while complex odontomas appear as radiodense masses. Both have a lucent rim. They are typically asymptomatic.

Is There an Expansile, Ground-Glass Appearance to the Mandible or Maxilla?
Fibrous dysplasia is a developmental abnormality of the bones consisting of immature fibroosseous tissue that slowly grows over time. The lesions are expansile and have a ground-glass appearance on CT. As previously described, fibrous dysplasia may be associated with McCune-Albright syndrome and Jaffe-Lichtenstein syndrome.

Is There Resorption of the Bone Around Multiple Teeth?
Although rare, some infiltrative diseases such as Langerhans cell histiocytosis and a subtype of Burkitt lymphoma can involve the mandible and cause the resorption of bone. The imaging appearance of these entities can mimic periodontitis, which is unusual in the pediatric population.

■ Part 4: Neck Masses (Box 4)

Anterior Neck Masses

Is the Lesion Cystic?
Nonvascular cystic lesions in the pediatric neck include thyroglossal duct cysts, branchial apparatus cysts, thymic cysts, and foregut duplication cysts.

Is the Cyst Midline?
Thyroglossal duct cysts commonly present as small cysts in the midline or near the midline of the anterior neck. They are common and account for most of the congenital neck abnormalities in children.

A brief review of thyroid embryology is helpful in understanding formation of thyroglossal duct cysts. The thyroid primordium originates in the foramen cecum at the base of the tongue and descends along the anterior neck to its final infrahyoid position. The thyroglossal duct exists transiently along the path of the recently descended thyroid tissue and soon involutes, but remnants of this duct can develop into cysts. Consequently, thyroglossal duct cysts can be found anywhere near the midline from the foramen cecum to the thyroid gland, with an infrahyoid location most commonly seen.

BOX 27.4 Neck masses	
Cystic Masses	**Solid Masses**
■ Thyroglossal duct cyst	■ Ectopic thyroid
■ Branchial cleft cyst	■ Ectopic thymus
■ Thymic cyst	■ Lymphadenopathy
■ Foregut duplication cyst	■ Fibromatosis colli
■ Lymphatic (or venous) malformation	■ Teratoma
	■ Plexiform neurofibroma
■ Abscess	■ Hemangioma

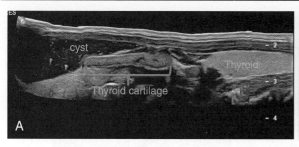
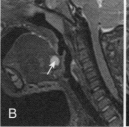
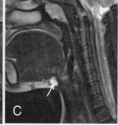
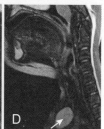

Suprahyoid~25%   Hyoid ~30%   Infrahyoid~45%

Fig. 27.21 Thyroglossal duct cyst. (A) Panoramic ultrasound image demonstrates infrahyoid cyst just above the thyroid cartilage. (B-D) Sagittal magnetic resonance imaging can identify thyroglossal duct cysts (arrows) along the midline from the foramen cecum base of tongue (B), anterior to the hyoid bone and (C) near the thyroid bed.

These lesions are easily imaged with ultrasound. Cyst fluid may be simple or proteinaceous (Fig. 27.21). Thyroglossal duct cysts usually come to clinical attention in the setting of acute infection, in which case surrounding inflammatory changes may be present.

Documentation of the relationship to the hyoid bone in the longitudinal plane is helpful for treatment planning. It is also important when assessing a potential thyroglossal duct cyst to document whether normal thyroid tissue is present. Treatment is surgical resection via the Sistrunk procedure in which the entire thyroglossal duct, including the middle of the hyoid bone, is resected. If the only thyroid tissue is ectopic tissue along the resected thyroglossal duct cyst, then the patient will become hypothyroid. Even asymptomatic thyroglossal duct cysts are resected if found because they have a 1% chance of harboring papillary thyroid cancer.

Is the Cyst Lateral to Midline?

The differential diagnosis for nonvascular cystic lesions off midline includes branchial apparatus cysts, thymic cysts, and foregut duplication cysts.

THE BRANCHIAL APPARATUS AND THEIR REMNANTS

A comprehensive description of the embryology of the branchial apparatus is beyond the scope of this text. However, a basic understanding of this topic facilitates the diagnosis of developmental abnormalities resulting in cervical cysts and tracts, and so will be briefly reviewed.

During the fourth week of embryonic development the branchial apparatus forms. It consists of multiple paired arches of tissue. Each arch consists of mesoderm, including an artery and a nerve. These arches are separated by external clefts lined by ectoderm and internal pouches lined by endoderm. From these arches, pouches, and clefts, several structures of the lower face and neck are formed. Only those parts of the branchial apparatus that result in clinically relevant cysts and tracts will be discussed here. In some cases the cysts can arise from arches, pouches, or clefts, so in those cases the term *branchial apparatus cyst*, rather than the traditional term branchial cleft cyst, will be used.

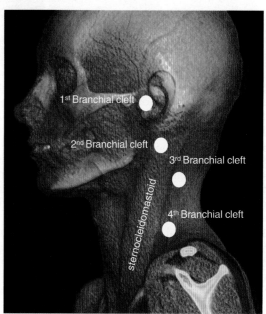

Fig. 27.22 Depiction of the primary anatomic location of branchial cleft cysts.

IS THE LESION NEAR THE EAR?

The first branchial apparatus cysts arise near the ear, either anterior or posterior to the pinna, or may arise near the parotid gland (Fig. 27.22).

Tracts may connect the cysts to either the skin surface or the external auditory canal. Although ultrasound can detect the cystic portions of this anomaly, tracts are better defined by MRI or contrast-enhanced CT.

IS THE LESION IN THE LATERAL NECK?

Second and third branchial apparatus cysts can arise in the lateral neck.

The second branchial apparatus cyst, which is the most common, may be found anywhere from the oropharyngeal tonsillar fossa to the supraclavicular region (Figs. 27.22 and 27.23). They have previously been classified into four different subtypes:

Type I: deep to the platysma, anterior to the sternocleidomastoid muscle

Type II: anterior to the sternocleidomastoid muscle, posterior to the submandibular gland, and lateral to the carotid sheath

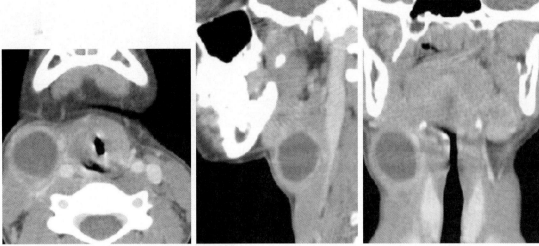

Fig. 27.23 *Second branchial cleft cyst.* Computed tomography shows a well-circumscribed peripherally enhancing cystic mass in the right neck anterior to and partially inseparable from the sternocleidomastoid muscle.

Type III: between the internal and external carotid arteries
Type IV: medial to the carotid sheath and adjacent to the pharyngeal wall

The most common type is type II. A type II second branchial apparatus cyst arises from the remnant of a transient structure called the *sinus of His*. It is interesting to note that although the sinus of His is predominantly formed from the second branchial cleft, it also contains components from the third and fourth branchial clefts as well.

The third branchial apparatus cyst is rare. It is usually found in the posterior triangle of the upper neck, deep to the sternocleidomastoid muscle and posterior to the carotid sheath. It can also be found in the anterior triangle of the lower neck anterior to the sternocleidomastoid muscle. This cyst and other remnants of the third and fourth branchial apparatus are typically found on the left side of the neck.

IS THE LESION CLOSELY ASSOCIATED WITH THE UPPER POLE OF THE THYROID GLAND?

Third and fourth branchial apparatus remnants are traditionally both thought to result in tracts in the neck that communicate with the pyriform sinus.

Practically, distinguishing between a third and fourth branchial requires determining the position of the tract to the superior laryngeal nerve. Third branchial apparatus tracts pass superior to the superior laryngeal nerve, whereas fourth branchial apparatus tracts pass inferior to it. This determination can only be made surgically. However, more recent research suggests that these tracts may not derive from the fourth branchial apparatus at all, and instead suggests that these tracts form from the thymopharyngeal duct of the third branchial apparatus. Regardless, because of the close proximity of these tracts to the superior pole of the thyroid gland, repeated infections of these tracts can result in repeated episodes of infectious thyroiditis or neck abscesses near the thyroid. If this remnant is suspected, direct visualization of the pyriform sinus for the tract opening should be performed via endoscopy for confirmation.

IS THE CYST NEAR THE LOWER NECK ON THE LEFT?

Thymic cysts, for unknown reasons, are usually left sided. As with most nonvascular cystic lesions of the neck, understanding the embryology is helpful. The thymus arises from the third branchial pouch near the angle of the mandible and descends into the mediastinum, where the right and left thymic primordium fuse. As the primordial thymic tissue descends, it leaves behind the thymopharyngeal duct. This duct normally involutes, but remnants can develop into cysts. These cysts parallel the course of the sternocleidomastoid muscle, just deep to it. They are usually closely related to the carotid sheath and may occur within the sheath or between the carotid artery and internal jugular vein. The cysts may extend to the level of the thymus and connect to it by a tract of tissue. The differential diagnosis for thymic cysts includes second and third branchial apparatus cysts. The diagnosis is confirmed by the presence of thymus tissue in the pathology specimen.

IS THE LESION ADJACENT TO A FOREGUT STRUCTURE?

Foregut duplication cysts develop from rests of foregut epithelium and can be found anywhere along the gastrointestinal tract. They are most commonly seen in the chest and abdomen but can occur in the head and neck.

Three criteria are required for diagnosis. The cyst must (1) be covered by smooth muscle, (2) contain foregut-derived epithelium, and (3) be attached to a normal derivative of the foregut. The pharynx, lower respiratory tract, esophagus, stomach, duodenum, and hepatobiliary system are all derived from the foregut, reflected in the cell types seen within foregut cysts, including squamous epithelium, gastric mucosa, and ciliated respiratory epithelium.

Imaging by ultrasound shows the cyst wall consists of an inner hyperechoic mucosal layer and an outer hypoechoic muscular layer. The cyst may be simple or contain layering debris. CT will demonstrate a cyst with variable density depending on cystic contents. On MRI, foregut duplications show variable T1 signal depending on cyst contents, are T2 hyperintense, and show thin enhancement of the cyst wall (Fig. 27.24).

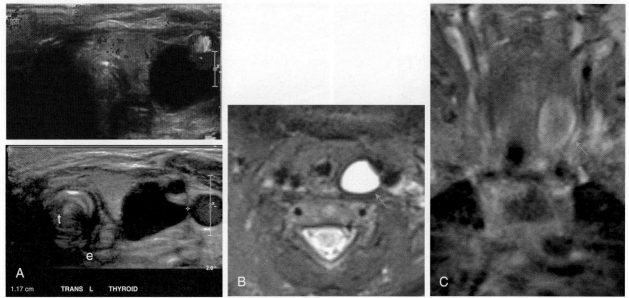

Fig. 27.24 Foregut duplication cyst. (A) Postnatal ultrasound evaluation of cystic neck mass initially identified on prenatal ultrasound demonstrates simple anechoic cyst at the level of the thyroid, immediately adjacent to the esophagus (*e*). The curvilinear echogenic structure to the right of the esophagus is a cartilagenous tracheal ring anterior to the air filled trachea (*t*). (B) On magnetic resonance imaging the cyst is T2 hyperintense with (C) thin enhancing rim after contrast administration.

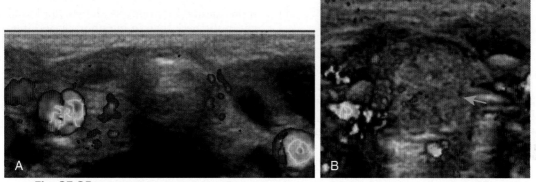

Fig. 27.25 Ectopic/lingual thyroid. Ultrasonography images (A) demonstrate an empty thyroid fossa with (B) thyroid tissue identified at the base of the tongue.

DOES IT INVOLVE THE THYROID?

Thyroid carcinoma is rare in children, but the possibility of thyroid cancer could be considered in any mass that involves the thyroid. The most common thyroid cancer in children is papillary thyroid carcinoma. Imaging findings that suggest papillary thyroid carcinoma include microcalcifications, heterogenous involvement of the gland, and cervical lymphadenopathy.

IS IT NEAR THE MIDLINE?

Ectopic thyroid tissue is most frequently found at the base of the tongue. Infrequently it will be found in the midline below the hyoid bone. Rarely ectopic thyroid tissue can be found in the lateral neck, mediastinum, and even abdomen. The imaging characteristics of ectopic thyroid tissue are identical to the normally located thyroid tissue (Fig. 27.25). It is important to realize that ectopic thyroid tissue is frequently the only thyroid tissue and if resected, the patient will become hypothyroid.

DOES IT HAVE A "STARRY SKY" APPEARANCE?

Ectopic thymus tissue, or cervical extension of the mediastinal thymus, can be present as a neck "mass." Apart from location, ectopic and orthotopic thymus have identical imaging characteristics. On ultrasound the thymus has a unique echogenic "starry sky" appearance on a homogenous background pattern. In infants the "starry sky" pattern may include linear and branching echogenic lines (Fig. 27.26). The dynamic component of the ultrasound examination is also helpful; thymic tissue will appear very soft and flexible and does not distort adjacent structures. As expected, on MRI, its signal characteristics are identical to mediastinal thymus.

ARE THERE ENLARGED LYMPH NODES?

Cervical lymphadenopathy is nonspecific and can be seen with infection, inflammation, or malignancy. Although by no means definitive, certain imaging features of cervical lymphadenopathy can provide a clue to the diagnosis.

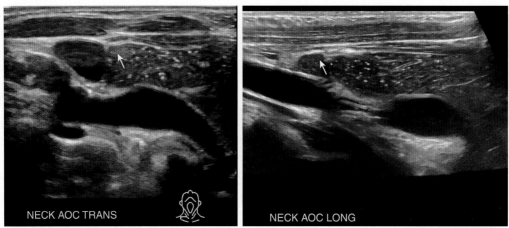

Fig. 27.26 Ectopic thymus. Ultrasound of the inferior right neck demonstrates cervical extension of thymic tissue above the level of the subclavian vein. Note the "starry sky" and "dot-dash" appearance of normal thymic tissue (arrows).

On ultrasound a normal lymph node is reniform in shape and has a well-defined border, a cortex that is hypoechoic to muscle, and a central echogenic hilum (Fig. 27.27A). Color Doppler imaging may show a hilar vessel with a few central branches. On CT, normal lymph nodes are hypodense to muscle and mildly enhance. On MRI, they are of intermediate T1 and intermediate to hyperintense T2 signal intensity.

DO THE LYMPH NODES HAVE PRESERVED ARCHITECTURE?

Infectious lymphadenitis is common in children and typically caused by viral or bacterial pathogens. On ultrasound, lymph nodes will be enlarged (measuring >1 cm in short-axis diameter) but have preserved reniform shape and internal architecture (see Fig. 27.27B). Some cases of infectious bacterial lymphadenitis progress to suppurative lymphadenitis where necrosis of the lymph node results in the development of phlegmon or abscess.

DO THE LYMPH NODES CONTAIN CALCIFICATIONS?

Atypical findings in infectious lymphadenitis include lymph node necrosis without significant adjacent inflammation and calcification. The differential for this atypical appearance includes atypical granulomatous infections, such as *Mycobacterium tuberculosis* or *Mycobacterium avium-intracellulare*, and malignancy. Calcifications also can be seen in treated lymphoma.

DO THE LYMPH NODES HAVE ABNORMAL ARCHITECTURE?

Lymphoma and metastatic disease should be considered if there is lymphadenopathy with abnormal nodal architecture, in the absence of infection or involving more. Ultrasound imaging features that suggest malignancy include round shape, distorted hilum, ill-defined borders, cystic necrosis, and abnormal capsular blood flow pattern (see Fig. 27.27C); however, tissue sampling is needed to make a definitive diagnosis.

Lymphoma is the most common solid extracranial malignancy in children, so it is an important diagnostic consideration in the setting of cervical lymphadenopathy. Lymphoma can be broadly categorized into two types: Hodgkin lymphoma and non-Hodgkin lymphoma.

Hodgkin lymphoma typically presents with nodal or splenic involvement and is more likely to affect adolescents. It commonly presents with cervical lymphadenopathy, although many patients also have mediastinal involvement. Less commonly, the disease presents in the axially or inguinal regions. Associated symptoms, such as weight loss, fever, and night sweats, may be present.

Non-Hodgkin lymphoma is typically extranodal and is more common in younger children. It is less likely to present in the neck than in intrathoracic and intraabdominal locations, but this disease can occur anywhere in the body. Cervical lymphadenopathy in the setting of non-Hodgkin lymphoma usually in an indication that the disease is widespread.

Deep Neck Masses

Does It Involve the Sternocleidomastoid Muscle?

Fibromatosis colli is a benign fibroblastic proliferation of the sternocleidomastoid muscle likely secondary to traumatic injury during late pregnancy or delivery.

Clinically, infants are usually healthy at birth but with time will present with a firm unilateral neck mass associated with torticollis, the head tilted and rotated toward the affected side and the chin tilted away.

The imaging study of choice for evaluation of suspected fibromatosis colli is ultrasound of the sternocleidomastoid muscles with comparison imaging of the contralateral side (Fig. 27.28). Images show fusiform enlargement of the involved muscle with variable echogenicity but without aggressive features. For most cases, treatment is physical therapy.

Is It Paraspinal, and Does It Contain Calcifications?

Neuroblastoma most commonly occurs in the abdomen, but it can originate anywhere along the sympathetic chain from the neck to the pelvis. When it originates from the sympathetic chain, it is seen as a paraspinal soft tissue mass that frequently involves the neural foramina.

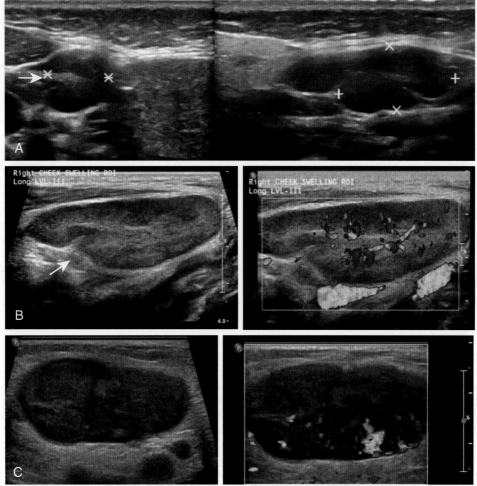

Fig. 27.27 Lymph nodes. (A) Ultrasound appearance of normal nodes with lobulated margins and a normal fatty hilum (*arrow*). (B) Reactive lymph node enlargement. Enlarged and echogenic nodes with maintained hilar anatomy. (C) An enlarged lymph node in a patient with lymphoma. Enlarged, infiltrated, hypoechoic nodes with loss of normal hilum.

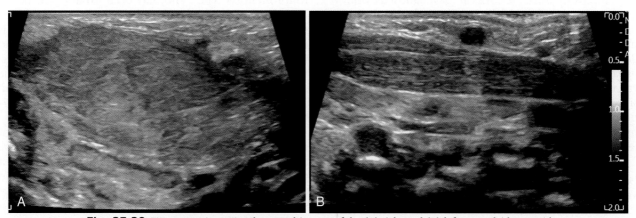

Fig. 27.28 Fibromatosis colli. Ultrasound images of the (A) right and (B) left sternocleidomastoid muscle in a 26-day-old infant with torticollis. The right side is diffusely and homogeneously enlarged and fusiform in shape.

On CT, neuroblastoma appears as a heterogenous soft tissue mass with sparse or heterogenous enhancement. It may contain areas of cystic necrosis and calcification. On MRI, it appears as a T1-hypointense, T2-hyperintense mass with variable heterogenous enhancement after contrast. Metastases may occur to lung, liver, and bone.

Does It Appear Locally Aggressive?

Langerhans cell histiocytosis is a multisystem disease that often mimics other inflammatory, infectious, and malignant processes. The majority of patients with Langerhans cell histiocytosis have head and neck involvement. In the neck, it most commonly presents with lymphadenopathy or skull lesions, although it can present as soft tissue masses as well. It appears locally aggressive with adjacent osseous destruction and can be difficult to differentiate from other aggressive soft tissue malignancies. On MRI the soft tissue component appears as T1-iso to hypointense, T2-hyperintense, and demonstrates marked enhancement after contrast administration. Ultimately biopsy is required for a definitive diagnosis.

Does the Mass Contain Macroscopic Fat?

Cervical teratoma, although rare, is the most common congenital mass of the head and neck. A teratoma is a congenital tumor that contains tissue from all three germ cell layers: ectoderm, mesoderm, and endoderm. It therefore typically has a heterogenous mixed cystic and solid appearance with variable enhancement and may contain fat and coarse calcifications. The CT and MRI appearances are consistent with areas of fat and calcium, and its soft tissue components may enhance. Although classically it presents as a large exophytic mass, it can also occur in the oropharynx or other compartments of the face, and is externally apparent only by mild mass effect.

Is the Mass Well Circumscribed and Hypervascular?

Hemangiomas are benign vascular tumors of early childhood. There are two main types: infantile hemangiomas, which are not present at birth but appear soon thereafter, and congenital hemangiomas, which are present at birth.

Infantile hemangiomas reach their maximum size at around 1 year of age and then slowly involute, becoming replaced by fat and fibrous tissue over a period of years. Congenital hemangiomas are of two types: rapidly involuting congenital hemangiomas, which involute by about a year of age, and noninvoluting congenital hemangiomas, which persist throughout life.

Imaging cannot adequately differentiate between these three types of hemangiomas, so clinical history is important. Superficial lesions can be diagnosed by physical examination, but if there is concern for involvement of deeper structures, particularly the orbit or airway, imaging is required. On ultrasonography the tumor will demonstrate a well-defined soft tissue mass of variable, usually increased, echogenicity with markedly increased vascularity. Doppler evaluation will demonstrate low-resistance arterial waveforms with relatively high velocities. On MRI, hemangiomas are robustly enhancing intermediate T1- and hyperintense T2- signal intensity lesions with large internal flow voids.

Is the Lesion Multicystic and Transspatial?

Venous and lymphatic malformations are slow-flow vascular malformations common in the head and neck. Although typically described as separate entities, they can be thought of as being on a spectrum, and each type of malformation frequently contains a small component of the other.

Venous malformations consist of dilated thin-walled venous channels that lack the smooth muscle of normal veins and typically appear on imaging as a network of torturous vessels with a transspatial distribution. Because they are malformations, they grow in proportion with the rest of the body. However, rapid enlarge-ment may occur in certain situations, such as trauma, infection, or hormonal changes associated with puberty. The slow flow through these lesions may lead to the development of phleboliths.

On ultrasound, venous malformations often appear as a heterogeneous, hypoechoic, "spongelike" soft tissue mass that is compressible. Doppler will typically demonstrate low-velocity internal venous flow; however, up to 15% of venous malformations will have no appreciable internal flow on ultrasound, and internal flow may be absent in the setting of thrombosis. Identification of phleboliths on ultrasound can help confirm diagnosis.

Because venous malformations may be very large, ultrasound may not be able to evaluate the full extent of these lesions. MRI is the study of choice to evaluate the depth and extent of tissue involvement. The venous channels are typically T1-hypointense, T2-hyperintense, and enhance after contrast.

Lymphatic malformations consist of dilated thin-walled lymphatic channels. Like venous malformations, they also frequently occur in the head and neck, are transspatial, and grow in proportion to the body. They may enlarge acutely if infected or from internal hemorrhage. Histologically, lymphatic malformations are categorized into two types based on the size of their channels, microcystic and macrocystic; however, lesions may be a combination of these two types. On MRI, microcystic lymphatic malformations appear as a lobulated mass composed of innumerable small (<2 mm) T1-hypointense, T2-hyperintense cysts with lacy septal enhancement. In contrast, the macrocystic type appears as a lobulated mass composed of large, thin-walled cysts (>2 mm) (Fig. 27.29). Fluid–fluid levels may be present if there has been intralesional hemorrhage.

Is There Expansion of the Nerve Roots?

Plexiform neurofibromas are pathognomonic for neurofibromatosis type I and may occur in any part of the body, including the head and neck. These are benign nerve sheath tumors composed mainly of Schwann cells that grow along nerves. They may become bulky, expand the neural foramen, and compress adjacent nerve roots. Sometimes they are invasive into adjacent soft tissue structures. On MRI, these tumors are T1-isointense and T2-hyperintense. They may have a central area of T2-hypointensity known as the "target sign" (Fig. 27.30).

In all plexiform neurofibromas, there is a risk for malignant degeneration to a malignant peripheral nerve sheath tumor. Clinical findings suspicious for a malignant peripheral nerve sheath tumor are rapid growth, pain, and neurological symptoms. Imaging findings include large size, cystic change, peripheral enhancement, and adjacent edema.

Are There Rim-Enhancing Fluid Collections Involving the Tonsils?

Tonsillar/peritonsillar abscesses are common in the pediatric population. On CT and MRI, they appear as rim-enhancing fluid collections involving the tonsil that do not extend beyond the superior pharyngeal constrictor muscle; however, they can rupture through and extend into the parapharyngeal and

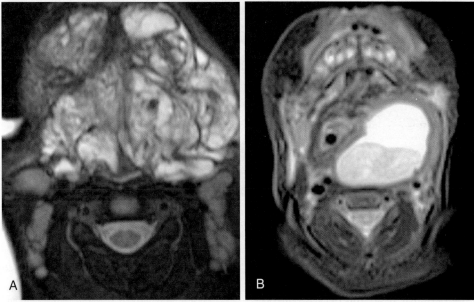

Fig. 27.29 Lymphatic malformation on magnetic resonance imaging. (A) Microcystic with numerous small cystic spaces in the floor of mouth. This mass extended into the retropharyngeal space and infratemporal fossa. (B) Macrocystic with large cystic structure in the retropharyngeal space. Note the fluid–fluid level suggesting internal hemorrhage.

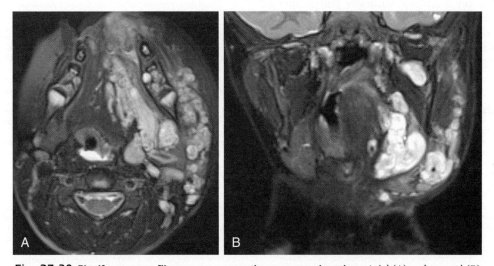

Fig. 27.30 Plexiform neurofibroma on magnetic resonance imaging. Axial (A) and coronal (B) fluid-sensitive images. Numerous hyperintense rounded "targetoid"-appearing structures with central hypointensity. They tend to follow a linear extension along nerve plexuses.

masticator spaces, causing deep neck abscesses, or into the retropharyngeal space, causing a retropharyngeal abscess.

Are There Rim-Enhancing Fluid Collections Involving the Retropharyngeal Space?

Retropharyngeal abscesses are common in children due to the frequency of upper respiratory tract infections seen in this age group. Frequently the primary physician will first order soft tissue radiographs of the airway to assess for retropharyngeal fullness. These radiographs should be obtained with the chin extended and in full inspiration because in expiration, redundant pharyngeal soft tissues can mimic retropharyngeal soft tissue fullness. If retropharyngeal fullness persists, CT of the neck with intravenous contrast should be obtained.

On CT, a retropharyngeal abscess presents as a rim-enhancing fluid collection posterior to the oropharynx between the superior pharyngeal constrictor muscles and the longus coli muscles (Fig. 27.31). It is important to determine the effect of the abscess on the airway and the full extent of the abscess, which can extend from the skull base to the superior mediastinum. It is also important to distinguish a retropharyngeal abscess from phlegmonous changes in a retropharyngeal lymph node, which is unlikely to be amenable to aspiration. Visualization of rim-enhancement is most helpful to differentiate. Occasionally in young children, there may not be robust inflammatory walling off of the abscess, limiting the enhancement.

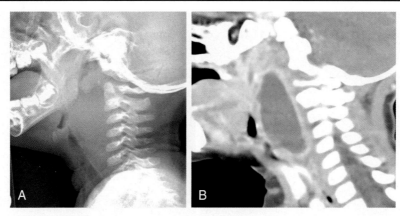

Fig. 27.31 Retropharyngeal abscess. (A) Lateral soft tissue neck radiograph demonstrates marked enlargement of the retropharyngeal soft tissues with mass effect on the cervical trachea. (B) Lateral intravenous contrast-enhanced computed tomography of the neck shows large rim-enhancing fluid collection in the retropharyngeal space.

■ Summary

The anatomy of the pediatric head and neck is complex, and the conditions that affect it are diverse-spanning from congenital anomalies to infections to neoplasm. However, a practical approach to imaging these lesions can be achieved by choosing an appropriate imaging modality based on anatomic location and suspected diagnosis. Although many lesions may require tissue sampling for diagnosis, often the combination of imaging features in correlation with location will help the radiologist suggest a specific diagnosis.

Bibliography

Abramson, S. J., & Price, A. P. (2008). Imaging of pediatric lymphomas. *Radiologic Clinics of North America, 46,* 313–338 ix.

Bak, M., & Wein, R. O. (2012). Esthesioneuroblastoma: A contemporary review of diagnosis and management. *Hematology/Oncology Clinics of North America, 26,* 1185–1207.

Balikci, H. H., Ozkul, M. H., Uvacin, O., et al. (2013). Antrochoanal polyposis: Analysis of 34 cases. *European Archives of Oto-Rhino-Laryngology, 270,* 1651–1654.

Barkovich, A. J., Vandermarck, P., Edwards, M. S., & Cogen, P. H. (1991). Congenital nasal masses: CT and MR imaging features in 16 cases. *AJNR. American Journal of Neuroradiology, 12,* 105–116.

Blount, A., Riley, K. O., & Woodworth, B. A. (2011). Juvenile nasopharyngeal angiofibroma. *Otolaryngologic Clinics of North America, 44,* 989–1004 ix.

Brennan, B. (2006). Nasopharyngeal carcinoma. *Orphanet Journal of Rare Diseases, 1,* 23.

Brennan, R. C., Wilson, M. W., Kaste, S., et al. (2012). US and MRI of pediatric ocular masses with histopathological correlation. *Pediatric Radiology, 42,* 738–749.

Breysem, L., Goosens, V., Vander Poorten, V., et al. (2009). Vallecular cyst as a cause of congenital stridor: Report of five patients. *Pediatric Radiology, 39,* 828–831.

Capps, E. F., Kinsella, J. J., Gupta, M., et al. (2010). Emergency imaging assessment of acute, nontraumatic conditions of the head and neck. *Radiographics, 30,* 1335–1352.

Chung, E. M., Murphey, M. D., Specht, C. S., et al. (2008). From the Archives of the AFIP. Pediatric orbit tumors and tumorlike lesions: Osseous lesions of the orbit. *Radiographics, 28,* 1193–1214.

Chung, E. M., Smirniotopoulos, J. G., Specht, C. S., et al. (2007). From the archives of the AFIP: Pediatric orbit tumors and tumorlike lesions: Nonosseous lesions of the extraocular orbit. *Radiographics, 27,* 1777–1799.

Chung, E. M., Specht, C. S., & Schroeder, J. W. (2007). From the archives of the AFIP: Pediatric orbit tumors and tumorlike lesions: Neuroepithelial lesions of the ocular globe and optic nerve. *Radiographics, 27,* 1159–1186.

de Graaf, P., Göricke, S., Rodjan, F., et al. (2012). Guidelines for imaging retinoblastoma: Imaging principles and MRI standardization. *Pediatric Radiology, 42,* 2–14.

De Vuysere, S., Hermans, R., & Marchal, G. (2001). Sinochoanal polyp and its variant, the angiomatous polyp: MRI findings. *European Radiology, 11,* 55–58.

Edwards, R. M., Chapman, T., Horn, D. L., et al. (2013). Imaging of pediatric floor of mouth lesions. *Pediatric Radiology, 43,* 523–535.

Flors, L., Leiva-Salinas, C., Maged, I. M., et al. (2011). MR imaging of soft-tissue vascular malformations: Diagnosis, classification, and therapy follow-up. *Radiographics, 31,* 1321–1340 discussion 1340–1341.

Freling, N. J. M., Merks, J. H. M., Saeed, P., et al. (2010). Imaging findings in craniofacial childhood rhabdomyosarcoma. *Pediatric Radiology, 40,* 1723–1738 quiz 1855.

Gaddikeri, S., Vattoth, S., Gaddikeri, R. S., et al. (2014). Congenital cystic neck masses: Embryology and imaging appearances, with clinicopathological correlation. *Current Problems in Diagnostic Radiology, 43,* 55–67.

Griauzde, J., & Srinivasan, A. (2015). Imaging of vascular lesions of the head and neck. *Radiologic Clinics of North America, 53,* 197–213.

Gujar, S. K., & Gandhi, D. (2011). Congenital malformations of the orbit. *Neuroimaging Clinics of North America, 21,* 585–602 viii.

Hedlund, G. (2006). Congenital frontonasal masses: Developmental anatomy, malformations, and MR imaging. *Pediatric Radiology, 36,* 647–662 quiz 726–727.

Hiorns, M. P., & Owens, C. M. (2001). Radiology of neuroblastoma in children. *European Radiology, 11,* 2071–2081.

Ho, M. L., Courtier, J., & Glastonbury, C. M. (2016). The ABCs (airway, blood vessels, and compartments) of pediatric neck infections and masses. *American Journal of Roentgenology, 206,* 963–972.

Hughes, D. C., Kaduthodil, M. J., Connolly, D. J. A., & Griffiths, P. D. (2010). Dimensions and ossification of the normal anterior cranial fossa in children. *AJNR. American Journal of Neuroradiology, 31,* 1268–1272.

Ibrahim, M., Hammoud, K., Maheshwari, M., & Pandya, A. (2011). Congenital cystic lesions of the head and neck. *Neuroimaging Clinics of North America, 21,* 621–639 viii.

James, S. H., Halliday, W. C., & Branson, H. M. (2010). Best cases from the AFIP: Trilateral retinoblastoma. *Radiographics, 30,* 833–837.

Joshi, M. J., Provenzano, M. J., Smith, R. J. H., et al. (2009). The rare third branchial cleft cyst. *AJNR. American Journal of Neuroradiology, 30,* 1804–1806.

Kadom, N., & Sze, R. W. (2010). Radiological reasoning: Pediatric midline nasofrontal mass. *American Journal of Roentgenology, 194,* WS10–WS13.

Kieran, S. M., Robson, C. D., Nosé, V., & Rahbar, R. (2010). Foregut duplication cysts in the head and neck: Presentation, diagnosis, and management. *Archives of Otolaryngology - Head and Neck Surgery, 136,* 778–782.

Kim, E. E., Valenzuela, R. F., Kumar, A. J., et al. (2000). Imaging and clinical spectrum of rhabdomyosarcoma in children. *Clinical Imaging, 24,* 257–262.

Koch, B. L. (2005). Cystic malformations of the neck in children. *Pediatric Radiology, 35,* 463–477.

Laffan, E. E., Ngan, B. Y., & Navarro, O. M. (2009). Pediatric soft-tissue tumors and pseudotumors: MR imaging features with pathologic correlation: Part 2. Tumors of fibroblastic/myofibroblastic, so-called fibrohistiocytic, muscular, lymphomatous, neurogenic, hair matrix, and uncertain origin. *Radiographics, 29,* e36.

LaPlante, J. K., Pierson, N. S., & Hedlund, G. L. (2015). Common pediatric head and neck congenital/developmental anomalies. *Radiologic Clinics of North America, 53,* 181–196.

Lewoczko, K. B., Rohman, G. T., LeSueur, J. R., et al. (2014). Head and neck manifestations of langerhan's cell histiocytosis in children: A 46-year experience. *International Journal of Pediatric Otorhinolaryngology, 78,* 1874–1876.

Lowe, L. H., Booth, T. N., Joglar, J. M., & Rollins, N. K. (2000). Midface anomalies in children. *Radiographics, 20,* 907–922.

Lowe, L. H., Marchant, T. C., Rivard, D. C., & Scherbel, A. J. (2012). Vascular malformations: Classification and terminology the radiologist needs to know. *Seminars in Roentgenology, 47,* 106–117.

Ludwig, B. J., Foster, B. R., Saito, N., et al. (2010). Diagnostic imaging in nontraumatic pediatric head and neck emergencies. *Radiographics, 30,* 781–799.

Ludwig, B. J., Wang, J., Nadgir, R. N., et al. (2012). Imaging of cervical lymphadenopathy in children and young adults. *American Journal of Roentgenology, 199,* 1105–1113.

Mautner, V. F., Hartmann, M., Kluwe, L., et al. (2006). MRI growth patterns of plexiform neurofibromas in patients with neurofibromatosis type 1. *Neuroradiology, 48,* 160–165.

Meesa, I. R., & Srinivasan, A. (2015). Imaging of the oral cavity. *Radiologic Clinics of North America, 53,* 99–114.

Murphey, M. D., Ruble, C. M., Tyszko, S. M., et al. (2009). From the archives of the AFIP: Musculoskeletal fibromatoses: Radiologic-pathologic correlation. *Radiographics, 29,* 2143–2173.

Nasseri, F., & Eftekhari, F. (2010). Clinical and radiologic review of the normal and abnormal thymus: Pearls and pitfalls. *Radiographics, 30,* 413–428.

Oomen, K. P. Q., Modi, V. K., & Maddalozzo, J. (2015). Thyroglossal duct cyst and ectopic thyroid: Surgical management. *Otolaryngologic Clinics of North America, 48,* 15–27.

Papaioannou, G., & McHugh, K. (2005). Neuroblastoma in childhood: Review and radiological findings. *Cancer Imaging, 5,* 116–127.

Paulino, A. C., & Okcu, M. F. (2008). Rhabdomyosarcoma. *Current Problems in Cancer, 32,* 7–34.

Peterson, C. M., Buckley, C., Holley, S., & Menias, C. O. (2012). Teratomas: A multimodality review. *Current Problems in Diagnostic Radiology, 41,* 210–219.

Pruna, X., Ibañez, J. M., Serres, X., et al. (2000). Antrochoanal polyps in children: CT findings and differential diagnosis. *European Radiology, 10,* 849–851.

Rauschecker, A. M., Patel, C. V., Yeom, K. W., et al. (2012). High-resolution MR imaging of the orbit in patients with retinoblastoma. *Radiographics, 32,* 1307–1326.

Reilly, B. K., Kim, A., Peña, M. T., et al. (2015). Rhabdomyosarcoma of the head and neck in children: Review and update. *International Journal of Pediatric Otorhinolaryngology, 79,* 1477–1483.

Restrepo, R., Oneto, J., Lopez, K., & Kukreja, K. (2009). Head and neck lymph nodes in children: The spectrum from normal to abnormal. *Pediatric Radiology, 39,* 836–846.

Restrepo, R., Palani, R., Cervantes, L. F., et al. (2011). Hemangiomas revisited: The useful, the unusual and the new. Part 1: Overview and clinical and imaging characteristics. *Pediatric Radiology, 41,* 895–904.

Richter, A., Mysore, K., Schady, D., & Chandy, B. (2016). Congenital hairy polyp of the oropharynx presenting as an esophageal mass in a neonate, a case report and literature review. *International Journal of Pediatric Otorhinolaryngology, 80,* 26–29.

Robson, C. D. (2010). Imaging of head and neck neoplasms in children. *Pediatric Radiology, 40,* 499–509.

Schmidt, S., Eich, G., Geoffray, A., et al. (2008). Extraosseous langerhans cell histiocytosis in children. *Radiographics, 28,* 707–726 quiz 910–911.

Stambuk, H. E., Patel, S. G., Mosier, K. M., et al. (2005). Nasopharyngeal carcinoma: Recognizing the radiographic features in children. *AJNR. American Journal of Neuroradiology, 26,* 1575–1579.

Sung, T. H. T., Sung, T., Man, E. M. W., et al. (2012). Paediatric thyroid carcinoma in disguise: Papillary thyroid carcinoma presenting with thyrotoxicosis and diffuse goiter. *Pediatric Radiology, 42,* 377–379.

Suzuki, J., Hashimoto, S., Watanabe, K., & Takahashi, K. (2011). Congenital vallecular cyst in an infant: Case report and review of 52 recent cases. *Journal of Laryngology & Otology, 125,* 1199–1203.

Thomas, B., Shroff, M., Forte, V., et al. (2010). Revisiting imaging features and the embryologic basis of third and fourth branchial anomalies. *AJNR. American Journal of Neuroradiology, 31,* 755–760.

Toma, P., Granata, C., Rossi, A., & Garaventa, A. (2007). Multimodality imaging of Hodgkin disease and non-Hodgkin lymphomas in children. *Radiographics, 27,* 1335–1354.

Wasa, J., Nishida, Y., Tsukushi, S., et al. (2010). MRI features in the differentiation of malignant peripheral nerve sheath tumors and neurofibromas. *American Journal of Roentgenology, 194,* 1568–1574.

Weissman, J. L., Tabor, E. K., & Curtin, H. D. (1991). Sphenochoanal polyps: Evaluation with CT and MR imaging. *Radiology, 178,* 145–148.

Wong, R. K., & VanderVeen, D. K. (2008). Presentation and management of congenital dacryocystocele. *Pediatrics, 122,* e1108–e1112.

Wu, J., Schulte, J., Yang, C., et al. (2016). Hairy polyp of the nasopharynx arising from the eustachian tube. *Head Neck Pathology, 10,* 213–216.

Yabuuchi, H., Fukuya, T., Murayama, S., et al. (2002). CT and MR features of nasopharyngeal carcinoma in children and young adults. *Clinical Radiology, 57,* 205–210.

Yu, T., Xu, Y. K., Li, L., et al. (2009). Esthesioneuroblastoma methods of intracranial extension: CT and MR imaging findings. *Neuroradiology, 51,* 841–850.

Zander, D. A., & Smoker, W. R. K. (2014). Imaging of ectopic thyroid tissue and thyroglossal duct cysts. *Radiographics, 34,* 37–50.

Spine

CHAPTER 28
Imaging of the Pediatric Cervical Spine

Diana P. Rodriguez

CHAPTER OUTLINE

Epidemiology, 551
  Mechanism of Trauma, 552
  Patterns of Cervical Spinal Injury, 552
Cervical Spine Developmental Anatomy and Normal Variants, 552
  Vertebral Body Shape Developmental Changes, 552
  Ossification Patterns of the Cervical Spine Vertebrae, 552
  Craniocervical Junction and Ligaments, 555
Clearance of the Cervical Spine, 556
Clinical Presentation of CSI, 559
Diagnostic Imaging of CSI, 559
  Plain Radiography, 559
  Computed Tomography, 561
  Magnetic Resonance Imaging, 562
Specific Cervical Spine Injuries, 562
  Atlantooccipital Dislocation or Craniocervical Dissociation, 562
  Imaging Evaluation, 562

Ligamentous Injury, 564
Atlantoaxial Rotary Subluxation, 565
  Imaging Evaluation, 565
  Plain Radiography, 565
C1 Vertebra Fractures, 568
C2 Vertebra Fractures, 570
  Hangman Fracture (Pars Interarticularis Fracture), 570
  Synchondrosal Fractures, 570
  Odontoid Fractures, 573
Subaxial C3–C7 Fractures, 573
Predisposing Conditions to Cervical Spine Injury, 574
  Down Syndrome, 574
  Os Odontoideum, 575
  Klippel-Feil Syndrome, 575
  Achondroplasia, 576
Summary, 576

The most common indication for pediatric cervical spine (C-spine) imaging is trauma. Although cervical spinal injuries are rare in children, the result can be devastating. The role of the radiologist is crucial in the early detection of cervical spinal injury (CSI) that may require immediate clinical attention. Imaging interpretation of the C-spine is particularly challenging and requires a thorough knowledge of its unique anatomic characteristics as the spine continues to develop and mature during childhood, reaching adult features at approximately 12 years of age. Knowledge of developmental changes allows differentiation of normal age-related anatomy from traumatic injury. Pediatric CSI results in extensive variability of injury patterns, closely related to age and mechanism of trauma. This chapter includes a review of the normal C-spine anatomy and common variants, a systematic approach for radiological interpretation, and illustrations of the most common traumatic injuries of the pediatric C-spine. The concept of "clearance" of the pediatric C-spine in the emergency department setting will also be discussed.

■ Epidemiology

Trauma leads as the most common cause of pediatric morbidity and mortality. Spinal injury occurs in 5% of trauma cases, and the region most frequently affected in children is the C-spine (60%–80% of cases). The incidence rate of CSI in pediatric blunt trauma is 1% to 1.5%, occurring more often in boys. CSI tends to increase with age and peaks at 9 to 12 years of age. Although CSI is rare, it can result in devastating outcomes, such as significant neurological injury or even death. The anatomy and biomechanics of the immature pediatric spine predispose to specific patterns of injury that are different from the adult spine. A study recently published by Leonard et al. (2011) evaluated a large, multicenter cohort of patients, including from 17 PECARN (Pediatric Emergency Care Applied Research Network) sites. This study retrospectively classified CSI in 540 patients and demonstrated that patterns of CSI with blunt trauma are closely related to *age* and *mechanism of trauma*, as has been also supported by other publications.

Mechanism of Trauma

Assessment by age subgroups shows that motor vehicle collision (MVC) and falls are the most common mechanisms of injury in both the youngest children (<2 years of age) and children aged 2 to 7 years. Pedestrian struck by motor vehicle is also a common mechanism in children aged 2 to 7 years. In the group ≥8 years of age, sports injuries and MVC are more frequent. CSI related to sports accounts for a quarter of ER visits of children. A multicenter retrospective case control study in children younger than 16 by Babcock et al. (2018) showed that football was the sport most frequently related to CSI, as well as diving, gymnastics/cheer, and hockey. CSI was also prevalent in unorganized activities such as trampolining, rough play or falls.

Patterns of Cervical Spinal Injury

Patterns of CSI are closely related to age and mechanism of trauma. Injuries from the atlantooccipital articulation to the C2 level, known as *axial injuries*, are more often seen in children ≤3 years of age. Factors that contribute to this pattern of injury include a large head relative to the C-spine with a fulcrum of motion at the C2/C3 level, underdeveloped neck musculature, lax ligamentous structures, vertebral body morphology, and the presence of vertebral synchondroses. Axial injuries include C1 and C2 fractures, as well as atlantooccipital dislocation (AOD) and atlantoaxial rotary subluxation (AARS). Increased morbidity and mortality is seen with AOD and may result in death. Cord injury is also more common in the young age group and can lead to severe neurological deficits. In children younger than 8 years, the bony spinal column allows significant stretching without tearing, while the spinal cord is much less stretchable and can result in shear injury.

Subaxial injuries, from the level of C3 to C7, occur more often in children older than 8 years and can frequently present with ligamentous injury and/or vertebral body fractures. At this age the fulcrum of motion is at the C5/C6 level, the neck muscles are more developed, and most of the vertebral synchondroses are fused. CSI in the teenager is similar to the adult.

Multilevel injuries are extremely rare in pediatric CSI. Injury to other organ systems is common in high-energy trauma and contributes to unfavorable outcome. Head trauma is the most common associated injury.

SCIWORA (spinal cord injury without radiographic abnormality) is a term that was first used by Pang and Wilberger (1982) to describe radiographically normal cases in patients with neurological abnormality. Historically, this term refers to spinal cord injury in the absence of findings on plain radiographs. However, with the advent of new imaging modalities to evaluate the spine, such as computed tomography (CT) and magnetic resonance imaging (MRI), this term has become confusing over time. Several authors have recently proposed the redefinition of this term, suggesting that "real-SCIWORA" should refer only to spinal cord injury with negative neuroimaging findings on all modalities, including plain radiographs, CT, and MRI. The incidence rate of SCIWORA in pediatric CSI ranges from 5% to 67%; this wide range may be in part related to differences in the use of this term among clinicians. The lack of MRI studies at the time of diagnosis may result in higher reports of SCIWORA by pediatricians and emergency department physicians, although it is often used less by neurosurgeons and orthopedic surgeons, who usually have magnetic resonance (MR) studies available at the time of diagnosis.

■ Cervical Spine Developmental Anatomy and Normal Variants

The radiologist must be aware of the normal developmental changes and anatomic variants of the pediatric C-spine on radiological studies to detect pathology and avoid misinterpretation. These include changes in vertebral morphology during the first decade of life, as well as the presence of synchondroses, apophyses, and secondary centers of ossification. Pitfalls may result from technically inadequate plain radiographs related to head positioning.

Vertebral Body Shape Developmental Changes

The shape of the vertebral bodies changes from birth until approximately the first decade of life. In infants, cervical vertebral bodies are oval shaped, whereas at around age 2 to 3 years, these appear relatively flattened. From 3 to 8 years of age, vertebral bodies demonstrate mild anterior wedging, especially C3 through C5, and should not be mistaken for compression fractures. At about 10 years of age, the cervical vertebrae acquire a more rectangular or square shape, similar to the adult spine. Other unique findings in the young child include shallow articular joints with slightly uncovered appearance of the facets and underdeveloped spinous processes with mild upward orientation (Figs. 28.1 and 28.2). Uncovertebral joints form during adolescence (see Fig. 28.2).

Ossification Patterns of the Cervical Spine Vertebrae

C1 (Atlas)

C1 is formed from three primary ossification centers (Box 28.1): the anterior arch and two neural (posterior) arches (Fig. 28.3). C1 is a ring structure and does not have a body. The anterior arch is mainly cartilaginous at birth, but some degree of ossification may be present in 20% of newborns. Otherwise, ossification of the anterior arch is expected to be visible at around 12 months of age but can be delayed until 24 months of age. The C1 anterior arch can also form from multiple ossification centers (2–4) in 25% of children. The most common variant is two ossification centers in 18% of the population (Fig. 28.4). Occasionally the anterior arch can be absent, and the neural arches may fuse anteriorly.

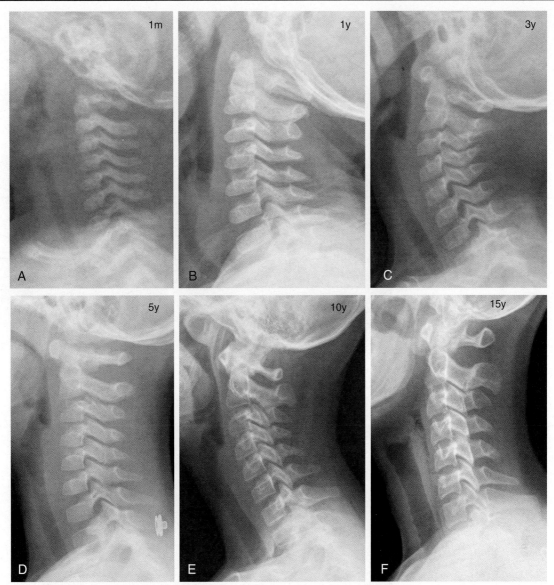

Fig. 28.1 Lateral radiographs of the cervical spine at (A) 1 month, (B) 1 year, (C) 3 years, (D) 5 years, (E) 10 years, and (F) 15 years of age. Vertebral body shape changes from oval shape in infancy, mild anterior wedge shape in the young child, and rectangular or square shape in the older child and adolescent. In the young child (A–C), there is uncovered appearance of the facets, overriding C1 on C2, and underdeveloped, upward orientation of the spinous processes. *m*, months; *y*, years.

The posterior arches begin to ossify in the seventh week of fetal life. The neurocentral synchondroses are between the anterior arch and posterior arches (see Fig. 28.3). A completely ossified anterior arch with fused neurocentral synchondroses usually occurs by 6 to 8 years of age. The posterior arches usually fuse by 3 to 5 years of age (see Fig. 28.3). Although rare, incomplete fusion of the posterior arches or a midline cleft may be seen in children ≤8 years of age. Another anatomic variant includes unilateral or bilateral paramedian clefts (see Fig. 28.4C).

C2 (Axis)

C2 is formed by four primary ossification centers that are present at birth: the body, two neural arches, and the odontoid process (Fig. 28.5). A single secondary ossification center, the os terminale (tip of the odon-

toid process), appears between 3 and 6 years of age (see Fig. 28.5C). C2 synchondroses can be seen until approximately 8 years of age and should not be mistaken for fractures. The subdental (odontocentral) synchondrosis (Figs. 28.6 and 28.7), located between the odontoid process and the body, begins to close around age 3 to 6 years of age and usually fuses around 11 to 12 years of age. Bilateral neurocentral synchondroses separate the body from each neural arch, while bilateral odontoneural synchondroses separate the odontoid process from each neural arch; these fuse between 3 and 6 years of age (see Figs. 28.6 and 28.7). The tip of the odontoid process (os terminale) fuses at approximately 12 years of age. Because the odontoid process forms from two ossification centers in utero, a vertical remnant synchondrosis can occasionally be seen. The posterior arches fuse around 2 to 3 years of age.

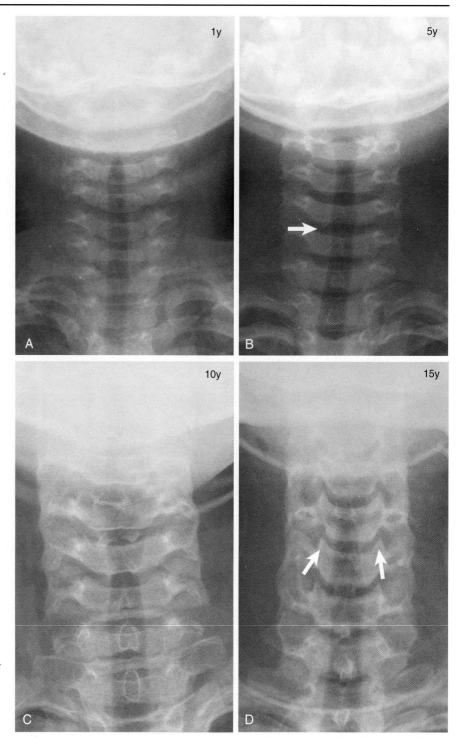

Fig. 28.2 Anteroposterior radiographs of the cervical spine at (A) 1, (B) 5, (C) 10, and (D) 15 years of age. Vertebral body joints are shallow in the young child (B) (*arrow*). There is development of the uncovertebral joints in the older child (*arrows*) (D).

C3–C7 Vertebrae

C3–C7 vertebrae each form from three ossification centers: the body and two neural arches. The neural arches fuse posteriorly at around 2 to 3 years of age, while the body and neural arches fuse between 3 and 6 years of age. C7 has the longest spinous process and C3 to C7 commonly have bifid spinous processes (Fig. 28.8).

Secondary ossification centers of C3–C7 include ring and spinous process apophyses. A ring apophysis is a wedge-shaped ossification center along the anterior and inferior aspect of the vertebral body and may be present at multiple levels. Ring apophyses ossify around 10 years of age and fuse between 18 and 25 years of age. The apophysis of the tip of the spinous process is seen more often at the C6 and C7 levels (Fig. 28.9).

Craniocervical Junction and Ligaments

The craniocervical junction (CCJ) is composed of the atlantooccipital and atlantoaxial joints, which are responsible for preserving stability, mobility, and rotation of the CCJ. The atlantooccipital joint allows for flexion and extension (F/E) movements and mainly depends on bony structures (the occipital condyles over the C1 sockets). The atlantoaxial joint allows for rotational movements and mostly depends on ligamentous structures. The major ligaments of the CCJ include the transverse ligament (major component of the cruciate ligament), alar ligaments, apical ligament, tectorial membrane (continuation of the posterior longitudinal ligament), anterior atlantooccipital (AAO) membrane and atlantoaxial ligament (continuation of the anterior longitudinal ligament), and posterior atlantooccipital (PAO) membrane (continuation of the ligamentum flavum) (Fig. 28.10).

Additional ligamentous complex of the posterior C-spine includes the ligamentum flavum and interspinous ligaments (continues cephalad as the ligamentum nuchae).

Transverse Ligament

The transverse ligament is the thickest and strongest of the CCJ and is a major component of the cruciform ligament, serving as the major stabilizing ligament of the atlantoaxial joint (Fig. 28.11). The superior and inferior limbs of the cruciform ligament are small and do not provide significant CCJ stability. The transverse ligament courses posterior to the odontoid process of C2 and attaches to each lateral tubercle of C1, keeping the odontoid process anteriorly against the posterior aspect of the anterior C1 arch. The spinal cord is located posterior to this ligament. The transverse ligament allows for atlantoaxial rotation up to approximately 47 degrees, whereas the alar ligaments limit excessive rotation. Rupture of the transverse ligament results in C1/C2 subluxation.

Alar Ligament

The alar ligament attaches to the odontoid process and skull base. This ligament limits excessive rotation and

---

BOX 28.1 Ossification and Fusion of the Cervical Vertebra Related to Age

C1

Anterior Arch
Ossification: present at birth (20%), visible by 12 months
Fusion: 6–8 years

Posterior Arch
Ossification: begins at seventh week of fetal life
Fusion: 3–5 years

C2

Body, Neural Arches, and Odontoid
Ossification: present at birth
Fusion
    Odontocentral synchondrosis: begins at 3–6 years, complete by 11–12 years
    Odontoneural and neurocentral synchondroses: 3–6 years
Posterior arches: 2–3 years

Os Terminale
Ossification: appears by 3–6 years
Fusion: 10–12 years

C3–C7

Body and Neural Arches
Ossification: present at birth
Fusion: neurocentral synchondroses: 2–3 years
Posterior arches: 3–6 years

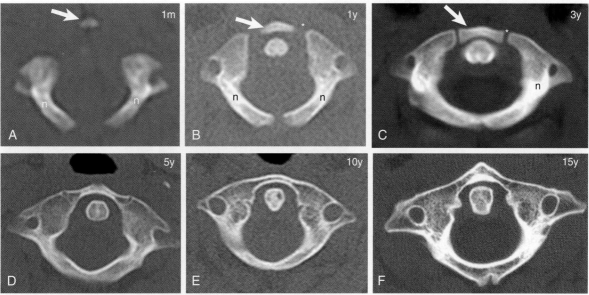

Fig. 28.3 C1 development. C1 forms from three ossification centers: anterior arch (*arrow*) and two neural arches (*n*). CT axial images at (A) 1 month, (B) 1 year, (C) 3 years, (D) 5 years, (E) 10 years, and (F) 15 years of age. Fusion of the neural arches posteriorly occurs by 3 to 5 years of age, while the anterior arch fuses by 6 to 8 years of age after closure of the neural-central synchondroses (*asterisks*).

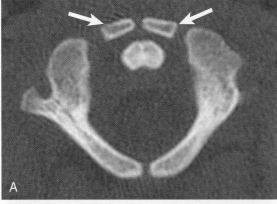
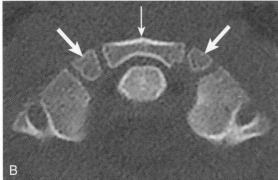
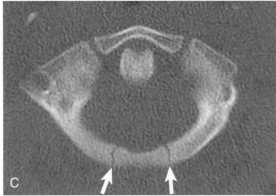

Fig. 28.4 A few examples of C1 anterior arch ossification variants. (A) Two ossification centers in a 1-year-old (*arrows*). (B) Three ossification centers in a 3-year-old (*arrows*). (C) Bilateral paramedian clefts in the posterior arch (*arrows*).

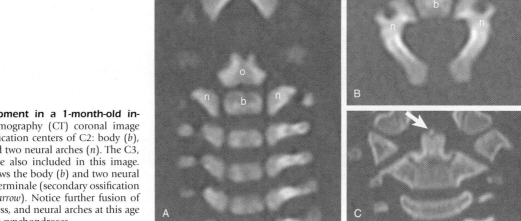

Fig. 28.5 C2 development in a 1-month-old infant. (A) Computed tomography (CT) coronal image shows four primary ossification centers of C2: body (*b*), odontoid process (*o*), and two neural arches (*n*). The C3, C4, and C5 vertebrae are also included in this image. (B) A CT axial image shows the body (*b*) and two neural arches (*n*) of C2. (C) Os terminale (secondary ossification center) in a 3-year-old (*arrow*). Notice further fusion of the body, odontoid process, and neural arches at this age with partial closure of the synchondroses.

lateral bending of the neck. It also stabilizes the atlanto-axial joint, preventing C1/C2 subluxation. The alar ligament may have a cranial caudal or horizontal orientation, and its shape is variable: tubular, round, elliptical, rectangular, or wing-shaped.

Apical Ligament
The apical ligament attaches to the tip of the odontoid process and basion and courses posterior to the alar ligament. Some have suggested the lack of function of this ligament. A study in cadavers demonstrated the absence of the apical ligament in 20% of specimens.

Tectorial Membrane
The tectorial membrane is a thin structure, formed by two to three layers that fuse at the posterior longitudinal ligament, and courses posterior to the cruciform ligament. The middle and thickest layer attaches from the clivus to the body of C2 (Fig. 28.11). Nerves and vessels are present between its layers. The tectorial membrane's function is controversial; some suggest it restricts flexion, whereas others consider it a CCJ stabilizer that resists extension.

Anterior Atlantooccipital Membranes
The AAO membrane is a continuation of the anterior longitudinal ligament and attaches to the anterior aspect of C1 and to the anterior rim of the foramen magnum (Fig. 28.10). This membrane courses posterior to the prevertebral neck muscles. The AAO membrane forms the anterior wall of the supraodontoid space, which contains fat and veins and the alar, apical, and Barkow ligaments.

Posterior Atlantooccipital Membrane
The PAO membrane attaches to the C1 posterior arch and to the posterior rim of the foramen magnum. The AAO and PAO membranes are considered stabilizers of the CCJ.

■ Clearance of the Cervical Spine

Suspected CSI in the setting of blunt trauma requires proper clinical evaluation in order to provide adequate management and prevent catastrophic outcomes such as

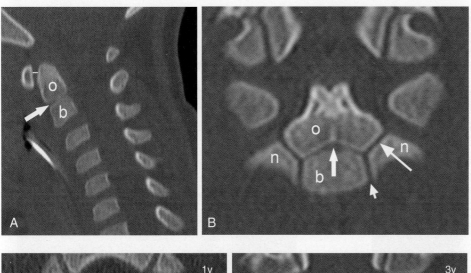

Fig. 28.6 C2 synchondroses in a 3-year-old. (A) Sagittal computed tomography (CT) image shows the subdental (odontocentral) synchondrosis (*arrow*) between the body (*b*) and the odontoid process (*o*). (B) Coronal CT image shows subdental (odontocentral) synchondrosis (*arrow*) between the body (*b*) and odontoid process (*o*), bilateral odontoneural synchondroses (*long thin arrow*), and bilateral neural-central synchondroses (*short arrow*).

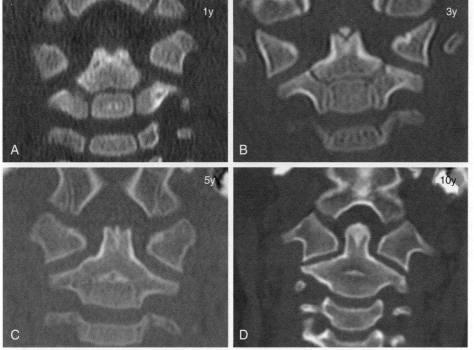

Fig. 28.7 Closure of C2 synchondroses. Coronal CT images at (A) 1, (B) 3, (C) 5, and (D) 10 years of age. The subdental synchondrosis begins to close by 3 to 6 years of age and fuses by 11 to 12 years of age. The tip of the odontoid process fuses at approximately 12 years of age.

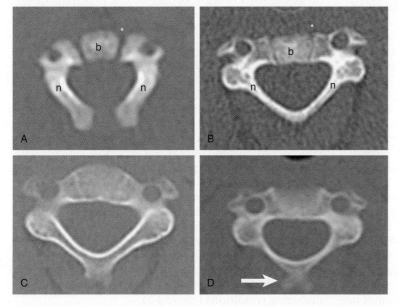

Fig. 28.8 C3–C7 development. The C3–C7 vertebral bodies form from three ossification centers: body (*b*) and two neural arches (*n*). Axial computed tomography images of C3 at (A) 1, (B) 5, (C) 10, and (D) 15 years of age. Neural arches fuse posteriorly by 2 to 3 years of age, while the body and neural arches (neural-central synchondroses; *asterisks*) fuse at between 3 and 6 years of age. Bifid spinous processes are common in these vertebrae (*long arrow*).

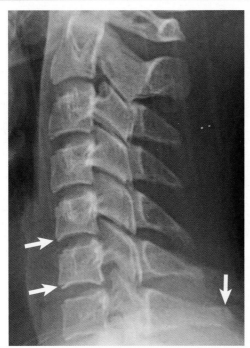

Fig. 28.9 Cervical spine apophyses. C7 has the longest spinous process; there is an apophysis at its tip (*vertical arrow*). Ring apophyses (*horizontal arrows*) are seen at the anterior aspect of the inferior end plates of C3–C7.

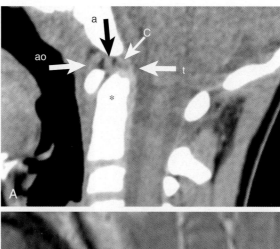

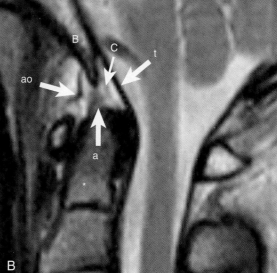

Fig. 28.10 Craniocervical junction ligaments. (A) Sagittal computed tomography image in soft tissue window shows the dense craniocervical junction (CCJ) ligaments. The anterior atlantooccipital ligament (*ao*) attaches from the anterior aspect of the C1 arch to the clivus and is a continuation of the anterior longitudinal ligament; the apical ligament (*a*) attaches from the tip of the odontoid process (*asterisk*) to the tip of the clivus or basion; cruciate ligament (*c*); the tectorial membrane (*t*) attaches from the posterior body of C2 to the dorsal surface of the clivus and is a continuation of the posterior longitudinal ligament. (B) Sagittal T2-weighted magnetic resonance image shows the hypointense CCJ ligaments. The anterior atlantooccipital ligament (*ao*), the apical ligament with a triangular configuration (*arrow*), the cruciate ligament (faintly seen, *c*), and the tectorial membrane (*t*). Basion (*B*).

death, quadriplegia or other serious neurologic sequelae. The purpose of a pediatric cervical spine protocol is to detect clinically significant CSI in children who have sustained blunt trauma, to identify all significant injuries, to decrease unnecessary radiation exposure, and permit the removal of a rigid cervical collar that is no longer necessary. *Pediatric clearance of the C-spine* is the process to evaluate clinically a child with suspected CSI (history and physical examination), who may require diagnostic imaging evaluation, in order to determine that CSI has not occurred. The clinical history should also include the mechanism of injury such as diving, axial load, "clothes-lining", or a high-risk motor vehicle collision. Cervical spine clearance is the responsibility of physicians with expertise in evaluating a child with suspected CSI; this includes ED physicians, general and trauma surgeons, neurosurgeons, and orthopedic surgeons. Less than 50% of level-I pediatric trauma centers, until recently, had a written protocol for c-spine clearance. The Pediatric Cervical Spine Clearance Working Group (PCSCWG), a subgroup of the Pediatric Cervical Spine Study Group, recognized the need for a consensus on comprehensive standardized guidelines for pediatric c-spine clearance. This multidisciplinary group of experts in pediatric c-spine clearance just recently developed an algorithm to guide institutional protocols for c-spine clearance (Herman et al., 2019). By consensus, this group created three pathways according to the Glasgow Coma Scale (GCS) score and its pediatric modification. Pathway 1: patient with a GCS score of 14 or 15; pathway 2: patient with a GSC score of ≤8, and pathway 3: patient with a GCS of 9 to 13. These pathways determine the imaging modality indicated. Most children that undergo blunt trauma have a GSC score of 14 or 15. If the children in this group cannot be

cleared clinically, conventional radiography is the next step recommended, which consists of a high-quality lateral radiograph. CT is indicated in children who have suffered blunt trauma and have a GCS score of ≤8. MRI is an excellent modality in all age groups, and indicated for the evaluation of CSI in the obtunded child when rapid neurologic recovery is not expected. Patients with GCS score of 9-13 require spinal immobilization and radiographic imaging. In this group, CT is done when radiographs are abnormal, or if an abnormal physical finding is detected. Children with congenital vertebral anomalies such as Klippel-Feil syndrome, spinal canal stenosis as seen in achondroplasia, os odontoideum and atlanto-axial instability in children with Down syndrome, are at increased risk for CSI. Further evaluation with CT or MRI is usually indicated in children with predisposing conditions (Box 28.2).

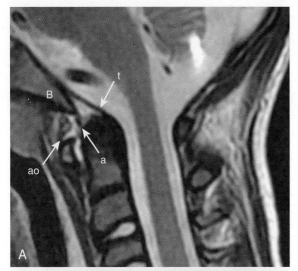

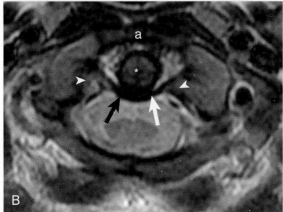

Fig. 28.11 Craniocervical junction ligaments. (A) Sagittal T2-weighted magnetic resonance (MR) image shows the anterior atlantooccipital ligament (*ao*), the apical ligament (*a*), and the tectorial membrane (*t*). The cruciate ligament is often not visible. (B) Axial T2-weighted MR image shows the transverse ligament (*arrows*), which courses posterior to the odontoid process (*asterisk*) and attaches to each lateral tubercle of C1 (*arrowheads*), keeping the odontoid process anteriorly against the posterior aspect of the anterior C1 arch (*a*).

BOX 28.2 Pediatric Cervical Spine Clearance: A Consensus Statement and Algorithm from the Pediatric Cervical Spine Clearance Working Group (Herman, MJ et al 2019)

Three pathways:
- Pathway 1: patient with a *GCS score of 14 or 15
- Pathway 2: patient with a GCS score of ≤ 8
- Pathway 3: patient with a GCS score of 9-13

* GCS = Glasgow Coma Scale

Children with congenital vertebral anomalies, such as Klippel-Feil syndrome (KFS), spinal canal stenosis as seen in achondroplasia, os odontoideum, and atlantoaxial instability (AAI) in children with Down syndrome, are at increased risk for CSI. Further evaluation with CT or MRI is indicated in patients with these predisposing conditions.

■ Clinical Presentation of CSI

Symptoms of CSI may include localized neck tenderness, muscle spasm, decreased range of neck motion, and torticollis. Spinal cord injury may manifest as sensory loss (paresthesias, dysesthesias, etc.) or motor loss (weakness), or even respiratory arrest when injury occurs at the C5 level or higher.

■ Diagnostic Imaging of CSI

The choice of imaging modality for evaluation of CSI depends on the patient's clinical status. Reducing radiation exposure in children should always be considered as well, given the potential risk for radiation-induced cancer, particularly thyroid cancer when imaging the C-spine. For instance, the estimated amount of ionizing radiation exposure is 30-fold higher for C-spine CT (approximate radiation dose: 6 mSv) versus plain radiography (approximate radiation dose: 0.2 mSv). The role and indication of plain radiographs, CT, and/or MRI in pediatric CSI will be subsequently reviewed.

Plain Radiography

Plain radiographs have high sensitivity in suspected pediatric CSI and are accepted as the imaging modality of choice in the initial evaluation of a child with a history of blunt trauma. For example, Nigrovic et al. (2012) reported a sensitivity of 90% (95% confidence interval [CI], 85%–94%) when using two or more radiographic views to detect CSI. In this study, radiographs in children with normal neurological examinations missed a small number of injuries; however, none required neurosurgical intervention. Furthermore, the Appropriateness Criteria of the American College of Radiology indicate radiography as the imaging method of choice for children younger than 16 years for evaluation of suspected CSI.

In the alert patient ≥5 years of age, with normal neurological examination, a three-view C-spine series (lateral, anteroposterior [AP] and open-mouth odontoid views) is recommended. In children younger than 5 years, only the lateral and AP views are done. The odontoid view is not indicated in this age group because of its technical difficulty and low yield. The lateral view is always obtained first while the patient is wearing a cervical collar. It is important to identify children at risk for CSI that will need further evaluation with CT and/or MRI to avoid missing clinically important injuries. In the critical patient a cross-table lateral film is done initially.

Flexion and Extension Lateral Views
F/E lateral views are not performed to clear the C-spine in the acute setting in children. These views are usually done on a follow-up visit in patients who report persistent cervical tenderness and have negative plain films or CT. F/E views are useful in detecting vertebral subluxation, which can be seen with ligamentous injury.

Technically adequate F/E views are defined as 30 degrees of change from neutral position and should include the C7-T1 junction. F/E views are accepted as standard for evaluation of ligamentous injury.

Normal Parameters of C-Spine Radiographs

LATERAL RADIOGRAPH

A technically adequate lateral radiograph includes the skull base through the C7-T1 disk space and should be obtained in neutral position. Loss of the cervical lordosis (straightening of the C-spine) is often a normal finding in children, usually as a result of mild head flexion. It is frequently seen in the child wearing a cervical collar or may be occasionally caused by muscle spasm.

Appropriate vertebral alignment should be assessed on the lateral radiograph (Fig. 28.12). Three curved lines demonstrate the alignment of the vertebral bodies and the spinal canal. Disruption of these lines may indicate subluxation in the presence of ligamentous injury or displaced fracture fragments. A fourth line can be drawn at the tips of the spinous process to also highlight any offset. The C1–C2 interspinous distance (measured from the inferior aspect of the C1 spinous process to the superior aspect of the C2 spinous process) should measure less than 12 mm. Increased interspinous distance suggests possible posterior ligamentous injury.

1. Anterior vertebral line: Demarcates the anterior margin of the vertebral bodies.
2. Posterior vertebral line: Demarcates the posterior margin of the vertebral bodies.
3. Spinolaminar or posterior cervical line (Swischuk line): This line demarcates the posterior margin of the spinal canal. The posterior cervical line is measured from the anterior aspect of the spinous process of C1 to the anterior aspect of the spinous process of C3. This line should overlap the anterior aspect of the spinous process of C2 or measure less than 2 mm from it (Fig. 28.13A). A distance of greater than 2 mm indicates true subluxation (see Fig. 28.13B).
4. Posterior spinous line: Follows the tip of the spinous processes.

PREVERTEBRAL SOFT TISSUES

Thickness of the prevertebral soft tissues should measure less than 6 mm at the retropharyngeal level and less than a cervical vertebral body width (approximately <14 mm) in the subglottic/retrotracheal level (see Fig. 28.12). Expiration and head flexion may result in apparent soft tissue thickening, which should resolve with adequate technique (inspiration and mild head extension).

ATLANTODENTAL INTERVAL

Atlantodental interval (ADI) is the distance between the posterior margin of the anterior arch of C1 and the anterior aspect of the odontoid. A normal ADI value is ≤5 mm in children and ≤3 mm in adults (Fig. 28.14). Increased ADI may indicate ligamentous injury or AAI, such as in children with Down syndrome.

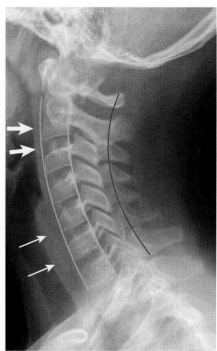

Fig. 28.12 Lateral radiograph of the C-spine. Cervical lines should be parallel and smooth and are useful in assessing vertebral alignment. Anterior vertebral line (green) along the anterior aspect of the vertebral bodies; posterior vertebral line (yellow) along the posterior aspect of the vertebral bodies, and spinolaminar line (red) or Swischuk posterior cervical line, which demarcate the posterior margin of the spinal canal. Prevertebral soft tissue thickness in the retropharyngeal level from C1 to C4 measures less than 5 mm (*short arrows*), while the thickness increases in the subglottic region at the C4 level (*thin arrows*), as a result of the presence of the esophagus, measuring usually less than a vertebral body width. In addition, the distance between the inferior spinous process of C1 to the superior spinous process of C2 is <12 mm.

C1 SPREAD OR PSEUDOSPREAD

On the odontoid view the distance between the odontoid process and the lateral masses of C1 should be symmetrical and measure less than 6 mm. Increased lateral spaces (>6 mm) with misalignment of the C1 lateral masses and C2 vertebral body indicate spread of the C1 lateral masses as a result of fracture. *Pseudospread* refers to increased distance between the dens and the lateral masses, but with preserved alignment of C1 and C2. This is a normal variant often seen in children younger than 4 years and may be asymmetrical with mild head rotation (Fig. 28.15).

PSEUDOSUBLUXATION

Mild physiological anterolisthesis (pseudosubluxation) of C2 on C3 and C3 on C4 is a common finding, especially in children younger than 8 years (see Fig. 28.13A). To exclude true subluxation, the posterior cervical line should be measured as described previously. A distance greater than 2 mm to the anterior margin of the C2 spinous process would indicate true subluxation, as seen with C2 fractures, which will be discussed later in this review (see Fig. 28.13B).

INTERSPINOUS DISTANCE

Interspinous distances should be symmetrical and less than <1.5 times greater than the space above and below.

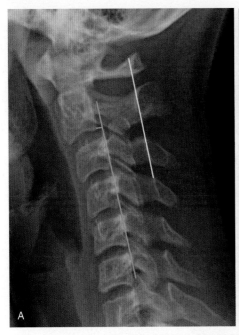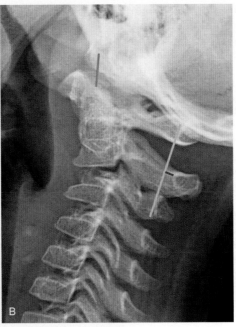

Fig. 28.13 Posterior cervical (Swischuk) or spinolaminar line. This line is useful to differentiate pseudosubluxation from true subluxation. Lateral radiographs show the posterior cervical line measured from the anterior aspect of the C1 spinous process to the anterior aspect of the C3 spinous process (A, *yellow line*; B, *orange line*). This line should overlap the anterior aspect of the spinous process of C2 or measure <2 mm from it. (A) There is minimal anterolisthesis of C2 on C3 (*light blue line*) with a normal posterior cervical line (*yellow line*), consistent with pseudosubluxation. (B) The posterior cervical line (*orange line*) shows a distance ≥2 mm to the sclerotic spinous process of C2, consistent with true subluxation in this child with a C2 fracture.

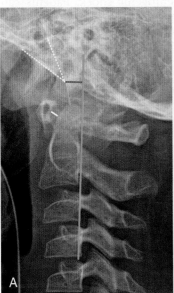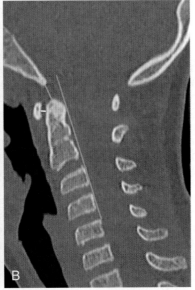

Fig. 28.14 Harris method combines basion–dens interval (BDI) and basion–axial interval (BAI). Lateral radiograph (A) and sagittal computed tomography (B) image show a normal BDI (*light blue line*) from the basion (tip of the clivus bone delineated by *dotted line* in A) to the tip of the odontoid (dens) and should measure ≤12 mm. BAI is the distance from the basion to a line traced along the posterior vertebral body cortex and should measure ≤12 mm (*red line*). (A, B) Normal atlantodental intervals that should measure less than 5 mm in children (*white lines*).

The C1/C2 interspinous distance is normally greater than those at other levels. The intervertebral disk spaces should be symmetrical.

Radiographic methods used to evaluate the CCJ will be reviewed in detail later with AOD.

Computed Tomography

Although CT is more sensitive than plain radiographs in the detection of CSI, it carries a higher radiation exposure. Given the low incidence of CSI in children (approximately 1%) and the high sensitivity of plain films (≥90%) in detecting CSI, CT should *not* be used in the initial evaluation of the child with low risk for CSI in blunt trauma. However, CT may be indicated in the child with neurological deficits or worsening clinical status, or in the critically injured child. Hannon et al. (2014)

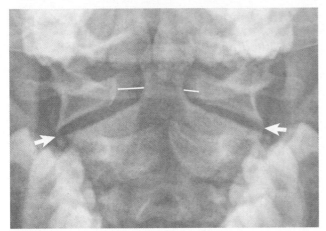

Fig. 28.15 Open-mouth odontoid view in a 10-year-old. There is mild asymmetry of the lateral spaces between the odontoid process and the lateral masses of C1 (*lines*), which is secondary to mild rotation. C1 lateral masses are well aligned with the body of C2 (*arrows*).

recently published a Clinical Decision Analysis in the evaluation of pediatric CSI with blunt trauma and concluded that clinical clearance and screening radiographs are the preferred strategies in the initial evaluation.

Conversely, CT is the initial C-spine screening test in adults with blunt trauma. CT is more sensitive and possibly more cost-effective in detecting injury in adults with moderate-to-high risk for CSI, and it was recently included in the guidelines of the Eastern Association for the Surgery of Trauma. For this reason a considerable number of children who are evaluated in general trauma centers where only adult protocols are in place often undergo screening with CT of the head and C-spine.

CT is the imaging modality of choice to evaluate osseous structures, including fracture details and alignment of the CCJ. Although normal CCJ ligaments can be seen on CT images in soft tissue algorithm (see Fig. 28.10A), this modality does not demonstrate well ligamentous injury. However, indirect signs of ligamentous injury, such as hematomas at the CCJ or along the clivus with elevation of the tectorial membrane, and prevertebral soft tissue edema can be detected with CT. CT has very low sensitivity in detecting spinal cord injury.

Magnetic Resonance Imaging

MRI is the imaging modality of choice in the evaluation of the cranial cervical junction and C-spine ligaments, intraspinal contents, bone marrow, and paraspinal soft tissues. Excellent definition of these structures is particularly achieved at high magnetic field strengths, such as 3T, allowing for better signal-to-noise ratio. Ligaments are composed of fibrous tissue and have low signal intensity on all MR sequences, including T1-weighted imaging, T2-weighted imaging (T2WI), and proton density. The AAO and PAO membranes, the tectorial membrane, and the apical ligament are better visualized on sagittal images, while the transverse is best seen on axial images. Coronal images can show the alar ligaments. MRI can well demonstrate the following findings: spinal cord abnormalities, such as focal edema, hemorrhage, myelomalacia, or cord compression; hematomas at the CCJ, along the clivus or in the spinal canal; and marrow edema associated with fractures, disk injury or herniation, and paraspinal soft tissue edema.

■ Specific Cervical Spine Injuries

Atlantooccipital Dislocation or Craniocervical Dissociation

Axial injuries of the C-spine occur more frequently in children younger than 8 years. AOD is more common in children younger than 2 years, while both AOD and AARS occur more often in children 2 to 7 years old.

AOD results from injury to the CCJ stabilizing ligaments, including the alar and tectorial membrane ligaments. Fractures are rarely present. See a detailed description of the CCJ ligaments earlier in this chapter.

Mechanisms of trauma include MVC (often an unrestrained passenger), falls from heights, motor vehicle to pedestrian accident, and head and neck blunt trauma. These mechanisms usually involve high-energy trauma with sudden acceleration-deceleration and hyperextension and/or hyperflexion of the head. Specific anatomic features of young children predispose to AOD, such as increased head size relative to the body, shallow occipital condyles, horizontally oriented atlanto-occipital joints, C2/C3 fulcrum of motion, vertebral body shape, and ligamentous laxity. AOD is an extremely unstable injury, traditionally known to result in death or persistent neurological deficit. However, survival rate in childhood has increased with time because of awareness of this entity and improved prehospital treatment of patients.

AOD is a difficult diagnosis that requires a high level of suspicion and is frequently associated with injury to other organs or systems, most often head injury. Clinical presentation of AOD is variable, ranging from a normal neurological examination to an unconscious patient with respiratory arrest. Spinal cord injury can manifest as motor or sensory deficits (weakness, quadriplegia), abnormal reflexes, or neurogenic shock. Patients can also present with lower cranial nerve (CN) involvement or cerebrovascular injury (vertebral or carotid artery dissection).

Traynelis et al. (1986) classified AOD in three groups in 1986: type I, anterior displacement of the occiput relative to the atlas; type II, distraction of the occiput from the atlas; and type III, posterior displacement of the occiput relative to the atlas. However, many authors now agree that given the hypermobility of these injuries, any of these categories may be artificially created by the patient's head positioning.

Horn et al. (2007) proposed a two-grade classification based on CT and MR findings that could help in determining treatment choice. Grade I represents normal CT findings with moderately abnormal MRI findings (edema in atlantooccipital joints or posterior ligaments). Grade II indicates at least one abnormal measurement on CT or definite abnormal MRI findings in the atlantooccipital joints and/or ligaments.

Imaging Evaluation

Plain Radiography and Computed Tomography

Multiple radiodiagnostic methods have been used over the years to detect AOD; however, no single method is ideal in determining ligamentous injury of the atlantooccipital and atlantoaxial articulations. Standard tests (i.e., Powers ratio, Harris method, Wackenheim line) rely on measurements using bony landmarks. These tests detect abnormal relationships that result from shifted bony structures on lateral plain radiographs or sagittal CT reformatted images. Therefore, if structures have reshifted back, these tests will be erroneously interpreted as normal, when in fact AOD is present. On plain radiographs, limitations include nonvisualization of the bony landmarks because of incompletely ossified or superimposed bony structures. Given that these

BOX 28.3   Imaging Methods for Evaluation of Atlantooccipital Dislocation in Children (Normal Measurements)

Condylar–C1 interval (CCI) on CT: *Most sensitive and specific method
Normal infants and young children: up to 4mm
Older teens and young adults: up to 2.5 mm

Harris Method
Basion–dens interval (BDI): children <12 mm and adults <10 mm
Basion–axial interval (BAI): children <12 mm in children and adults 12 to 4 mm
Powers ratio: BC/OA ≤ 0.9 (normal) and BC/OA ≥ 0.9 (AOD suspected)
Wackenheim line: normal—line along posterior clivus intersects posterior half to a third of the dens

are low-sensitivity tests, at least two methods should be used in conjunction to assess suspected AOD. Prevertebral soft tissue swelling is a frequent finding.

Standard methods (radiographs and CT):
1. *Harris method* (Box 28.3): This method combines the following two measurements:
   a. *Basion–dens interval (BDI):* Distance between the basion and tip of the dens. Normal BDI is less than 12 mm in children and less than 10 mm in adults (see Fig. 28.14).
   b. *Basion–axial interval (BAI):* Distance between a line traced along the posterior cortex of C2 body and the basion (tip of the clivus). Normal BAI is less than 12 mm in children, and 4 to 12 mm in adults (see Fig. 28.14).
2. *Powers ratio:* This includes measurements from the skull base to C1. This ratio is easy to measure on CT. Distance from basion (B) to midpoint anterior cortex of the C1 posterior arch (BC). Distance from the opisthion (O) to midpoint posterior cortex of the C1 anterior arch (OA). BC/OA ≤0.9 (normal) and BC/OA ≥0.9 (AOD suspected) (Fig. 28.16).
3. *Wackenheim line:* Line drawn along the posterior aspect of the clivus that should intersect the posterior half to third of the dens. Given that the odontoid tip is cartilaginous in young children, this line should be traced using soft tissue windows on CT to avoid pitfalls (Fig. 28.17).

Computed Tomography
Caution is required when using CT to assess AOD, because the CCJ may appear well aligned despite the presence of extensive ligamentous injury. Although fractures are rarely seen with AOD, these can be best evaluated with CT.

Condylar Gap Method or Condyle–C1 Interval
Occipital condyle- C1 interval (CCI), also known as the condylar gap method, is currently the preferred test to evaluate AOD. CCI is the only method that directly evaluates the atlanto-occipital joint structures, and can

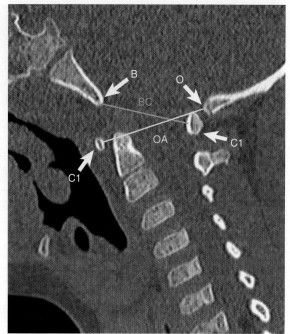

Fig. 28.16 Powers ratio. Sagittal computed tomography image of a 3-year-old in bone window shows normal Powers ratio. Line BC is measured from the basion (*B*) to the midpoint anterior cortex of the posterior C1 arch. Line OA is measured from the opisthion (*O*) to the midpoint cortex of the anterior C1 arch. BC/OA ≤ 0.9 (normal) and BC/OA ≥ 0.9 (suspect atlantooccipital dissociation).

assess coronal misalignment (Fig. 28.18). In 2007, Pang et al. (2007) published normal CCI values in children, and subsequently compared this method to other radiodiagnostic criteria and indicators. Pang's results showed that the CCI method had the highest diagnostic sensitivity and specificity for AOD. More recently, Smith et al. (2016) demonstrated CCI morphology and measurements change with development, and concluded CCI is largest from 2–4 years of age, and decreases through late childhood and adolescence. CCI is measured on reformatted coronal or sagittal CT images, perpendicular to the articular surfaces of the occipital condyle and lateral mass of C1 ccipital condyle notch (Fig. 28.18). Sagittal images are preferred to avoid including the occipital condyle notch. Coronal values are larger and more variable: medialmost coronal measurement is greater than the lateralmost measurement in the younger child. A normal CCI for infants and children less than 13 years is up to 4mm. In older teens and young adults, a CCI up to 2.5 mm is normal (Box 28.3). Figs. 28.19 and 28.20 show two different cases of AOD diagnosed with CT using the condylar gap method. On the first patient (4-year-old), both Power's ratio and Wackenheim line method, failed to show abnormality (Fig. 28.21).

Magnetic Resonance Imaging
MRI is the imaging modality of choice to assess for CCJ ligamentous injury. MR is indicated in patients with suspected CSI high-energy mechanism of injury or when the neurological examination is unreliable. MRI is useful to further evaluate abnormalities detected on CT or plain films (see Fig 28.20). MRI can also demonstrate spinal cord contusions or edema, spinal cord

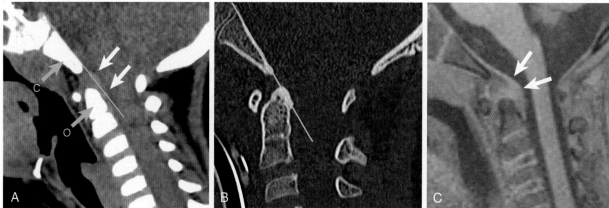

Fig. 28.17 Wackenheim line. Sagittal computed tomography (CT) image in soft tissue window in a 3-year-old (A) and sagittal CT image in a 9-year-old (B) show the Wackenheim line traced along the dorsal surface of the clivus (C), which should intersect the posterior third of the odontoid process (O). Notice that in (A) the odontoid is partially cartilaginous (*arrows*), while in (B), it is completely ossified. (C) Sagittal T1-weighted magnetic resonance image shows a normal craniocervical junction in a 3-year-old with a partially cartilaginous odontoid process (*arrows*) that is hyperintense compared with bone.

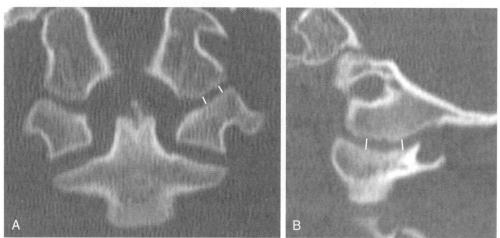

Fig. 28.18 Condylar gap method or condyle–C1 interval (CCI). Coronal computed tomography (CT) image (A) and sagittal CT image (B) in a 9-year-old show the gap between the occipital condyles and the articular surface of C1 (*lines*). Avoid occipital condyle notch (*arrow*). Normal measurement: up to 4 mm (infants and children less than 13 years), and up to 2.5 mm in older teens and young adults.

transection (see Fig. 28.22), marrow edema in fractures, CCJ or clival hematomas, perimedullary subarachnoid hemorrhage, and spinal subdural or epidural hematomas. Bright fluid on T2WI with fat saturation or short T1 inversion recovery images can be seen at the atlantoaxial joints in the presence of joint capsule injury (see Fig. 28.21E–F).

■ Ligamentous Injury

Injury of the *tectorial membrane* can be seen as an interruption of the T2-hypointense line or coiling of the ends of the disrupted membrane. The tectorial membrane may also appear intact, but lifted from the clivus and/or dens with associated blood or fluid between the membrane and these osseous structures (see Fig. 28.21C–D).

Injury to the *transverse ligament* presents as increased T2 signal at the site of insertion of the ligament and can be associated with small avulsion fractures of

the tubercles in the inner cortex of the anterior C1 arch. The atlantodens interval (>5 mm) may also be increased.

Injury to the *anterior and posterior atlantoaxial ligaments* presents with interruption or absence of these ligaments and associated blood and/or edema between the dens and the clivus. Soft tissue edema can be present in the C1/C2 prevertebral fascia and posterior soft tissues between C1 and C2 (see Fig. 28.21C–D).

Rupture of the *alar ligament* is difficult to assess and can show absence of the T2-hypointense band or "dot" with contralateral shift of the dens within the C1 ring.

Treatment for AOD consists of early occipitocervical stabilization, fixation, and fusion. There are several types of internal fixation from the occiput to C2. The technique of choice depends on the patient's age and anatomic variations, including placement of rib grafts alone in young children (<6 years), contoured loop technique (rodwire constructs) in children between 7 and 10 years, and rigid instrumentation in children older than 10 years (see Fig. 28.21G). Cervical traction

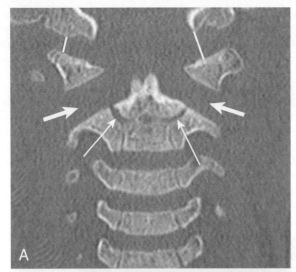

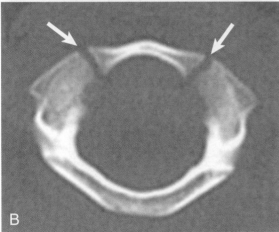

Fig. 28.19 Atlantooccipital dislocation. (A) Coronal computed tomography (CT) image in a 4-year-old shows abnormal CCI (*white lines*) measuring >4 mm, as well as increased C1/C2 joint spaces (*thick arrows*). There is a nondisplaced C2 fracture of the subdental and bilateral odontoneural synchondroses (*thin arrows*). (B) Axial CT image of C1 in the same patient shows mildly diastatic fractures through the neural-central synchondroses (*arrows*).

is avoided because of the associated risk for neurological deterioration. Hydrocephalus is the most common complication reported.

■ Atlantoaxial Rotary Subluxation

AARS is a rare condition of unknown incidence, consisting of an apparent fixed rotation of C1 on C2. Many terms have been used to refer to this condition, such as acute acquired torticollis, AARS, atlantoaxial rotary fixation, and atlantoaxial rotary dislocation. The variety of names, as commented in Neal and Mohamed's (2015) review article, likely represents a spectrum of the same condition rather than different etiologies or severities. The term AARS will be used in this review.

Previously mentioned anatomic characteristics of the pediatric C-spine allow for hypermobility, making the atlantoaxial region susceptible to instability and injury, which predisposes to AARS. The normal C-spine can rotate up to 180 degrees, and the atlantoaxial joint is responsible for up to 60% of this rotation. During neck rotation, C1 rotates first and then C2, resulting in a natural C1/C2 subluxation. This differs from AARS, where the facet of C1 is locked on the facet of C2, preventing its return to a normal position, as a result of muscle spasm or a mechanical block. The transverse ligament plays a key role in stabilizing the atlantoaxial complex, keeping the odontoid process against the anterior arch of C1. The alar ligaments also prevent excessive rotation and lateral bending.

The most common causes of AARS include traumatic and inflammatory etiologies. Minor trauma, such as blunt head trauma or falls, or manipulation of the C-spine during surgical procedures can result in AARS. In severe trauma, AARS can present in association with C-spine fractures. Head and neck inflammatory events, such as tonsillitis, retropharyngeal abscess, or upper respiratory infections, may also precede AARS. Inflammation of the joints and ligaments occur via lymphatic or venous spread. The term *Grisel syndrome*, described in 1930, refers to AARS related to inflammation. AARS has also been reported in patients with Down syndrome, congenital vertebral anomalies, rheumatoid arthritis, and tumors.

Clinically, AARS presents with torticollis, neck pain, and the typical "cock-robin" posture (face tilt and turn to the opposite side with some chin depression) (Fig. 28.23A). The definition of acute, subacute, and chronic AARS is difficult. A number of classifications based on the duration of symptoms have been published, without reaching a general consensus. For example, Beier et al. (2012) divided their population with AARS into three groups: acute group (symptom duration of <1 month), subacute group (symptom duration between 1 and 3 months), and chronic group (symptom duration of >3 months). In contrast, Neal and Mohamed (2015) classifies AARS into two groups: acute presentation (<2 weeks from onset of symptoms) and chronic presentation (>2 weeks from onset of symptoms). AARS also has been classified based on imaging findings, specifically using CT. Both the duration of symptoms and on occasion imaging findings will help in deciding treatment options.

Imaging Evaluation

AARS is considered primarily a clinical diagnosis made through careful history and physical examination. The role of imaging examinations is to exclude associated traumatic or inflammatory disorders and help in AARS classification.

Plain Radiography

The initial evaluation of AARS with plain radiographs can show underlying congenital abnormalities or traumatic osseous injury. However, plain radiographs are technically difficult in patients with significant head rotation because of torticollis (see Fig. 28.23A). The open-mouth view can demonstrate asymmetry of the spaces between the odontoid process and the lateral masses of C1, as a result of lateral displacement of the odontoid process. This view is not indicated in children younger than 5 years. The lateral radiograph, which is often nondiagnostic for AARS, may occasionally show anterior displacement of C1 with increased atlantodens interval (>5 mm) or C2/C3 subluxation.

Computed Tomography
CT with three-dimensional reconstructed images can nicely show rotation of C1 on C2 and anterior displacement of one of the lateral masses of C1 with posterior displacement of the contralateral mass (see Fig 28.23B-C).

In 1977, Fielding and Hawkins (1977) classified AARS into four types: type 1, the most common, consists of rotation of C1 on C2 without anterior or posterior displacement; type 2, consists of 3 to 5 mm anterior displacement of C1 on C2; type 3, consists of anterior displacement of C1 on C2 greater than 5 mm; and type 4, consists of posterior displacement of C1 on C2. CT should be used with caution, especially in patients with acute torticollis, given its risk for ionizing radiation without necessarily yielding additional substantial information. The use of dynamic CT is questioned, and new evidence demonstrates poor reliability and reproducibility of these examinations in the acute setting. It is not recommended by a number of authors in the evaluation of acute AARS.

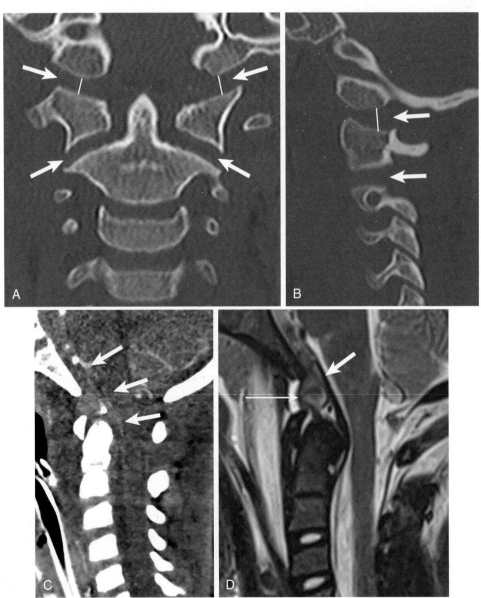

Fig. 28.20 Atlantooccipital dislocation (AOD)/ligamentous injury in a 7-year-old. (A) Coronal computed tomography (CT) image shows abnormal CCIs (*top arrows* and *lines*) and mildly increased C1/C2 joint spaces (*bottom arrows*). (B) Sagittal CT image shows increased CCI (*line and top arrow*) and increased C1/C2 joint space (*bottom arrow*). (C) Sagittal CT image in soft tissue window shows elevation of the tectorial membrane secondary to hematoma at the craniocervical junction (CCJ; *arrows*). The prepontine and premedullary spaces are effaced. (D) Sagittal T2-weighted magnetic resonance (MR) image shows ligamentous injury with discontinuity of the superior aspect of the tectorial membrane (*thick arrow*), CCJ hematoma (*thin arrow*), and discontinuity of the posterior atlantooccipital membrane (*short arrows*). (E) Coronal T2-weighted MR image shows increased occipital condyle–C1 joint spaces with presence of fluid (*arrows*). (F) Coronal T2-weighted MR image shows mildly increased C1/C2 joint spaces with fluid (*arrows*). (G) Lateral radiograph shows postoperative changes from occipital–cervical fusion.

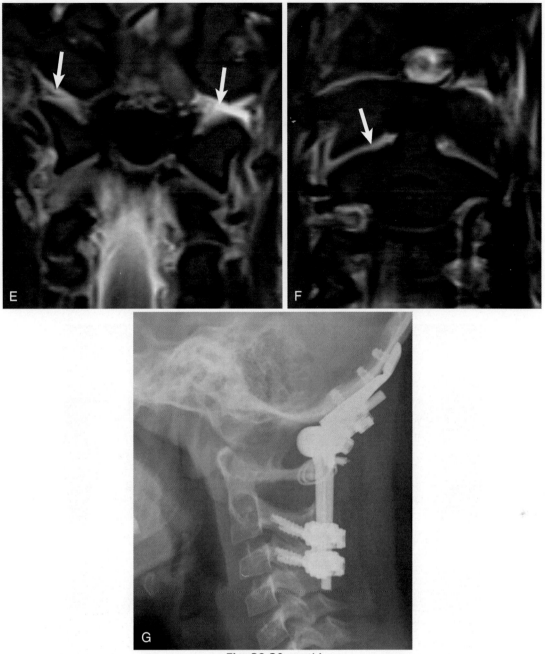

Fig. 28.20 cont'd

Magnetic Resonance Imaging

MRI is the imaging modality that provides the best anatomic detail of the ligaments, other soft tissue structures, and bone marrow. Short T1 inversion recovery and T2WI with fat suppression can nicely show bright fluid signal in any of these structures. Some structures that can be injured with AARS include the transverse, alar, and posterior longitudinal ligaments, as well as the C1/C2 joint capsules. These abnormalities are identified in the acute phase and resolve with time. MRI is also useful in detecting other underlying conditions, such as infection or tumor. The vertebral arteries, which are rarely affected in AARS, can be evaluated with time-of-flight MR angiography.

Treatment for AARS ranges from conservative measures to invasive surgical procedures and is determined by the patient's age, duration of symptoms, and underlying conditions. Acute cases of AARS can occasionally resolve spontaneously; however, realignment is often required. Options to reduce AARS include cervical collar, halter or skeletal traction, halo immobilization, or surgical fusion. Patients with acute AARS usually respond to conservative measures, although chronic cases and acute cases who do not respond positively to conservative treatment will occasionally require surgical intervention with posterior fixation.

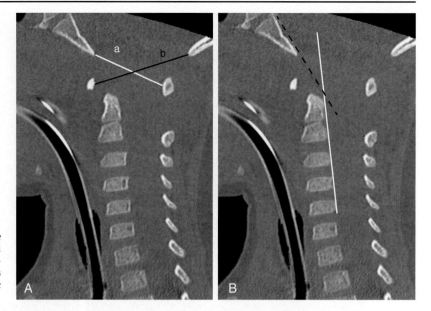

Fig. 28.21 Atlantooccipital dislocation in the same patient. Powers ratio (A) was normal and Wackenheim line (B) was borderline in this patient with a partially cartilaginous odontoid. This is an example of false-negative results using these methods.

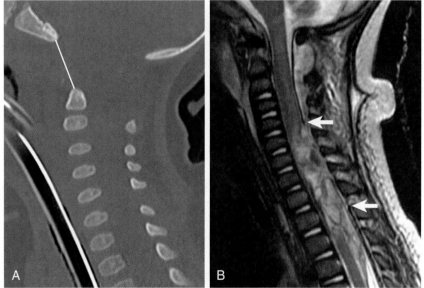

Fig. 28.22 Atlantooccipital dislocation (AOD) and spinal cord transection in a 12-month-old, status post motor vehicle accident, not moving lower extremities and left arm. (A) Sagittal computed tomography image shows AOD with abnormally increased Basion–dens interval (*white line*). Oval-shaped vertebral bodies are a normal finding at this age. (B) Sagittal T2-weighted magnetic resonance image shows complete disruption of the cord between C5 and the top of T3. The disrupted cord segment is encased in a large amorphus clot filling the gap (*arrows*) between the proximal and distal ends of the spinal cord.

■ C1 Vertebra Fractures

Fractures of the C1 vertebra (atlas) usually result from axial loading injury. However, the mechanism of trauma of C1 fractures differs in adults and children. In the adolescent and adult, C1 fractures tend to occur in high-energy trauma, such as motor vehicle accidents with high deceleration forces. In young children (<7 years of age), C1 fractures can result from minor forces, such as hitting the head against the bar at the top of a slide or from falling on the buttocks with inertial mass of the head.

Jefferson fracture refers to a fracture of the ring of C1 involving the anterior and posterior arches, caused by vertical forces transmitted through the occipital condyles to the lateral masses of C1 (Fig. 28.24). These fractures are more common in the adolescent and are considered unstable when osseous fragments are displaced and the transverse ligament is ruptured. On imaging, this fracture may present with spread of the lateral masses and abnormal alignment with the C2 body. The distance between the lateral C1 masses and the odontoid process is usually increased, measuring greater than 6 mm. This finding can be evaluated

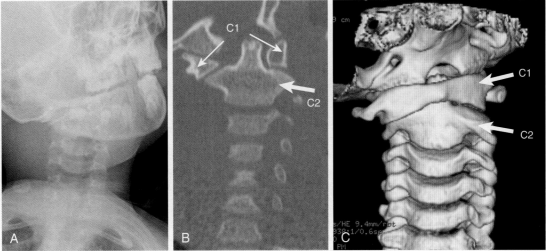

Fig. 28.23 Atlantoaxial rotary subluxation (AARS) in an 8-year-old boy status post motor vehicle accident 2 days prior now presenting with severe torticollis. (A) Anteroposterior radiograph shows typical "cock-robin" posture with face tilted and turned to the opposite side with some chin depression. (B) Coronal computed tomography (CT) image shows rotation of the lateral masses of C1 over C2 with asymmetrical lateral atlantodental spaces. (C) CT three-dimensional reconstructed image shows leftward rotation of C1 on C2.

on the open-mouth odontoid view. Pseudospread, a normal variant mentioned earlier, may mimic C1 fractures in children younger than 4 years. Other C1 fracture patterns include isolated fracture of the anterior arch, isolated fracture of the posterior arch, fracture of the transverse process, and isolated fracture of the lateral mass.

In the young child, synchondroses can be the site of fractures and may be subtle with only the presence of diastasis, which can be detected on CT or MR (see Fig. 28.19B). For this reason, open or diastatic sutures at an age when these should be already fused should raise concern for injury. Isolated fractures of C1 are difficult to diagnose, particularly in young children in whom plain radiographs of the C-spine are often normal, including normal prevertebral soft tissue thickness. Furthermore, the odontoid view is not indicated in children younger than 5 years. It is important for the radiologist to be familiar with the patterns of ossification of C1 to be able to differentiate normal anatomic variants from fractures. Variants include synchondroses between multiple ossification centers of the anterior arch, as well as clefts in the posterior arch (see Fig. 28.4). As a reminder, the anterior arch usually fuses by 3 to 5 years of age, and the posterior arch fuses completely by 6 to 8 years of age (see Fig. 28.3).

Clinically, young children present with neck pain, cervical muscle spasm, or torticollis, after blunt head trauma. These signs and symptoms should prompt further assessment with CT and/or MRI to evaluate for fractures and/or ligamentous injury. Atlantoaxial ligamentous injury, including rupture of the transverse ligament, is best evaluated with MRI.

Treatment of isolated, nondisplaced C1 fractures without ligamentous injury is usually conservative

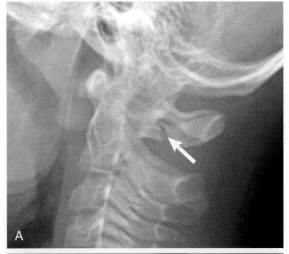
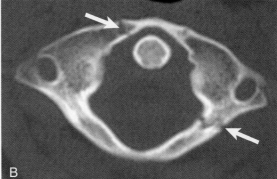

Fig. 28.24 C1 fractures in a 6-year-old, status post sledding accident. (A) Lateral radiograph shows a nondisplaced fracture of the posterior C1 arch. (B) Computed tomography axial image shows a nondisplaced linear fracture of the anterior arch through the right neural-central synchondrosis (*arrow*) and a nondisplaced linear fracture of the posterior arch on the left side (*arrow*).

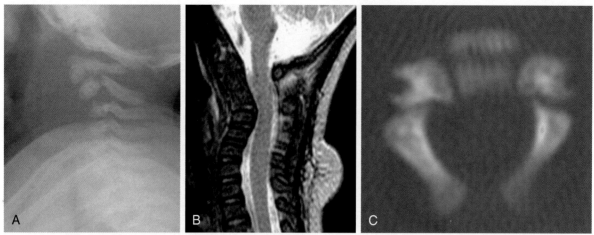

Fig. 28.25 C2 pars fracture in a 4-week-old infant. (A) Lateral radiograph shows linear fracture of the C2 pars interarticularis, with anterior tilt of the C2 body and odontoid process. C2/C3 intervertebral disk space is widened, and C1/C2 interspinous space is increased. There is moderate prevertebral soft tissue edema. (B) Sagittal T2-weighted magnetic resonance image shows focal kyphosis centered at C2/C3 resulting in mild spinal canal stenosis, but no cord compression. (C) Axial computed tomography image shows bilateral nondisplaced C2 pars fractures.

with immobilization, applying rigid neck orthosis for 8 to 12 weeks. At the end of treatment, flexion-extension radiographs are sometimes obtained to evaluate for residual AAI.

■ C2 Vertebra Fractures

Hangman Fracture (Pars Interarticularis Fracture)

Hangman fracture refers to bilateral fractures of the pars interarticularis. Although this type of fracture is more frequently seen in children older than 8 years, it may also present in children 2 to 8 years of age and rarely occurs in children younger than 2 years. C2 pars fractures result from hyperextension and axial loading. Mechanisms of injury include motor vehicle accidents, diving, and fall from elevations.

On radiography and CT, C2 pars fractures usually show anterior displacement and/or angulation of the odontoid process, as well as increased C1/C2 interspinous space, without or with anterior subluxation of C2 on C3 (Fig. 28.25). An abnormal posterior cervical line will help differentiate from C2/C3 pseudosubluxation. CT shows the coronal orientation of these pars fractures and best demonstrates details of atypical fractures. Again, MRI can best assess associated ligamentous injury or C2/C3 disk injury (see Fig. 28.25). Spinal fractures at other levels and vertebral artery dissection can also present with Hangman fracture.

Treatment is mostly conservative with halo immobilization; however, significantly displaced fractures and nonunion fractures may require surgical intervention.

Synchondrosal Fractures

Patterns of C2 fractures vary with age and mechanism of trauma. In the young child (<6 years of age), C2 is the vertebra most frequently injured due to its anatomic characteristics, in addition to the unique anatomy of the immature C-spine described earlier. Open or incompletely fused synchondroses are susceptible sites for fractures and can occur secondary to minor or severe head blunt trauma in association with excessive flexion-extension of the C-spine.

Mechanisms of injury include trampoline, sledding, and motor vehicle accidents. Complete and displaced fractures tend to be more frequent and usually occur with major trauma, whereas incomplete, nondisplaced synchondrosal fractures present more often with minor trauma. Rusin et al. (2015) recently proposed a classification of C2 synchondrosal fractures based on a spectrum of patterns. In this review the most common fracture pattern involved both odontoneural synchondroses, as well as the odontocentral synchondrosis, with varying degrees of anterior displacement or distraction (Figs. 28.26 and 28.27). Other patterns of displaced fractures include involvement of the bilateral neurocentral and odontoneural synchondroses with anterior displacement of the odontoneural segment, or fracture of the bilateral odontoneural and bilateral neurocentral synchondroses. Ligamentous injury is almost nearly present.

Findings on plain radiographs include displaced and angulated osseous fragments (i.e., odontoid fragment), increased interspinous C1/C2 distance, abnormal posterior cervical line, prevertebral soft tissue edema, and on occasion associated signs of AOD (see Figs. 28.26 and 28.27). Nondisplaced incomplete fractures are more often not visible on plain radiographs.

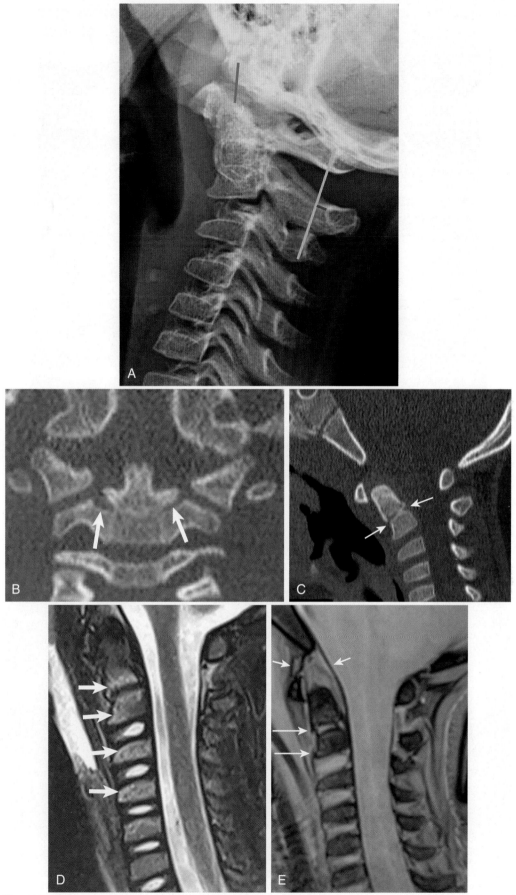

Fig. 28.26 C2 synchondrosis fracture in a 2-year-old after blunt facial trauma. (A) Lateral radiograph shows abnormal posterior cervical line indicating subluxation (*red line distance*). Basion–dens interval was normal (*blue line*). There is mild anterior tilt of the C2 body and increased C1/C2 interspinous space. (B) Coronal computed tomography (CT) image shows fracture of the bilateral odontoneural synchondroses (*arrows*). (C) Sagittal CT image shows fracture of the subdental synchondrosis. Condyle–C1 intervals and C1/C2 joints were normal. (D) Sagittal T2-weighted magnetic resonance (MR) image shows marrow edema of C2, C3, and C4 vertebral bodies with mild height loss, and (E) sagittal MERGE MR image shows discontinuity of the anterior longitudinal ligament at the C2 level (*long arrows*) and intact anterior atlantooccipital and tectorial membranes (*short arrows*). The patient received conservative treatment with halo orthosis immobilization.

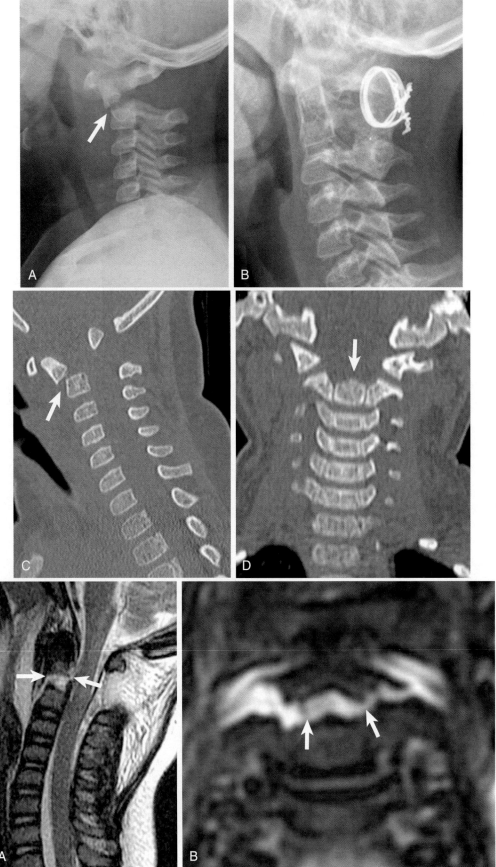

Fig. 28.27 C2 subdental fracture in a 20-month-old. (A) Lateral radiograph shows diastatic fracture of the subdental synchondrosis with anterior tilt and displacement of the odontoid and increased C1/C2 interspinous space. (B) Follow-up posttreatment (cerclage) lateral radiograph at 6 years of age demonstrates healing and normal alignment. (C) Sagittal computed tomography (CT) image shows anterior displacement and angulation of the odontoid process (*arrow*) and increased C1/C2 interspinous space. (D) Coronal CT image shows absent odontoid process (*arrow*), which is displaced anteriorly. Craniocervical junction and C1/C2 joints were preserved. (E) Sagittal T2-weighted magnetic resonance (MR) image shows diastatic subdental fracture and ligamentous injury with discontinuity of the anterior and posterior longitudinal ligaments at the C2 level (*arrows*). There is moderate prevertebral and suboccipital soft tissue edema. (F) Coronal T2-weighted MR image shows diastatic fracture through the subdental and bilateral odontoneural synchondroses (*arrows*).

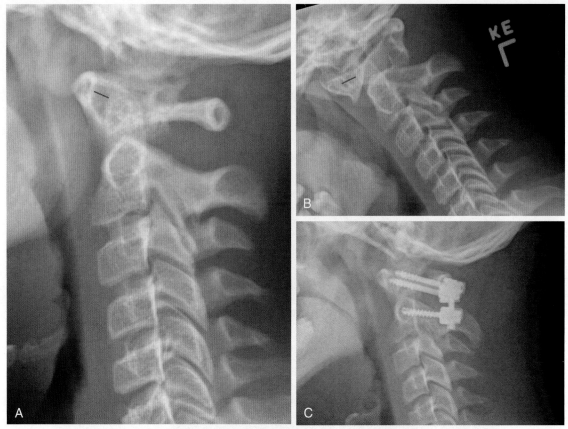

Fig. 28.28 Atlantoaxial instability in a 13-year-old boy with Down syndrome. (A) Lateral radiograph in neutral position shows increased atlantoaxial interval (AAI). (B) Lateral radiograph obtained with flexion shows further increase in AAI. (C) Postoperative lateral radiograph shows atlantoaxial posterior fusion with normal alignment.

Evaluation with cross-sectional imaging is mandatory. CT imaging with multiplanar and 3D reformatted images best demonstrates the fracture characteristics and can detect AOD. CT can also show prevertebral soft tissue edema and hematoma at the CCJ or along the clivus, lifting the tectorial membrane. MRI is indicated to evaluate ligamentous injury, cord contusion or compression, and associated AOD (see Figs. 28.26D–E and 28.27E–F).

Treatment mostly consists of reduction and halo stabilization, until fusion is achieved. However, surgical stabilization may be indicated to treat significantly displaced fractures (Fig. 28.27B).

Odontoid Fractures

The traditional classification of odontoid fractures was introduced by Anderson and D'Alonzo in the 1970s and includes three types of fractures that are usually seen in adults and children older than 10 years. Type I fracture consists of an avulsion fracture of the odontoid tip at the insertion of the alar ligament and is rare (1%–3%). Type II fractures occur at the base of the dens and are the most common pattern, with the highest incidence of nonunion. These are considered unstable and require immediate surgical stabilization. Type III fractures extend to the C2 vertebral body and are usually displaced. These are treated nonsurgically with halo immobilization.

■ Subaxial C3–C7 Fractures

Subaxial injuries, from C3 to C7, are more frequent in adolescents, followed by children 4 to 12 years of age, and they rarely occur in children younger than 4 years (see Fig. 28.26D). Mechanisms of trauma include motor vehicle accidents and sports injuries. In high-energy trauma, injury to multiple spinal levels and other organs is more common and can present with neurological deficits. In low-energy trauma, most often a single vertebral level is involved, typically C7 or C6, usually without ligamentous injury. Subaxial patterns of injury include ligamentous injury without fracture, multilevel vertebral body fractures other than burst, multilevel vertebral body burst fractures, single-level vertebral body compression fracture, single-level vertebral body burst fracture, other single-level vertebral body fractures with dislocation and/or disk injury, single-level teardrop fracture, single-level disk injury, and facet fractures.

Treatment is usually conservative with a collar; however, halo immobilization or surgical intervention may on occasion be indicated depending on degree of severity and instability.

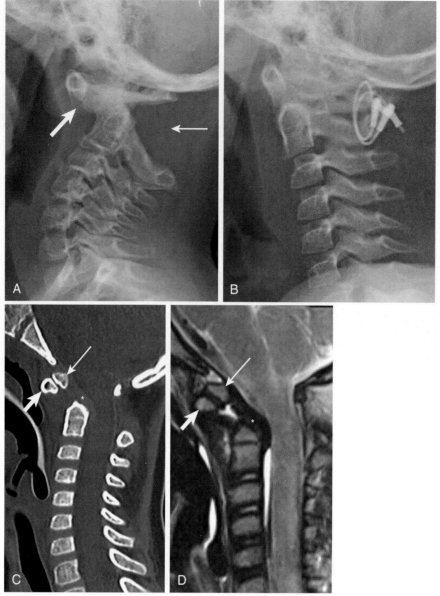

Fig. 28.29 Os odontoideum and atlantoaxial instability in a 3-year-old boy. (A) Lateral radiograph shows C1/C2 subluxation with markedly increased atlantoaxial interval (*white line*) and increased C1/C2 interspinous distance (*posterior arrow*). (B) One-month postoperative lateral radiograph, status post C1/C2 cerclage, shows normal alignment. Sagittal CT image (C) and sagittal T2-weighted magnetic resonance image (D) show an os odontoideum (*long arrow*) partially fused to the anterior of C1 (*short arrow*), as well as blunting of the odontoid process (*asterisk*). There is mild spinal canal stenosis at the C2 level. Craniocervical junction ligaments are intact.

■ Predisposing Conditions to Cervical Spine Injury

Children with underlying genetic conditions may have C-spine anomalies that predispose to CSI. These include disorders such as Down syndrome (trisomy 21), KFS, mucopolysaccharidosis, achondroplasia, and os odontoideum.

Down Syndrome

In children with Down syndrome, AAI is present in approximately 10% to 30% of cases and is most often asymptomatic. In addition to laxity of the transverse lig-

ament, abnormal development of bony structures can contribute to AAI, such as hypoplasia of the occipital bone condyles, assimilation of the atlas, hypoplasia and aplasia of the odontoid process, os odontoideum, and C1 hypoplasia (Fig. 28.28).

AAI is not a static condition; signs and symptoms may slowly progress over time, and complications of cord compression can occur suddenly. Therefore normal C-spine radiographs should not be used as predictors for the development of AAI. The American Academy of Pediatrics 2011 revision guidelines for the care of children with Down syndrome now emphasize family education and annual well-child visits, with a thorough and careful history and clinical examination to identify myelopathic signs and symptoms, as well

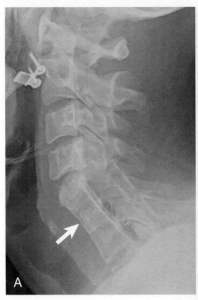
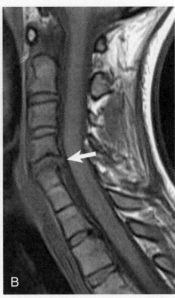

Fig. 28.30 Klippel-Feil syndrome in a 20-year-old woman. (A) Lateral radiograph shows fusion (nonsegmentation) of the C5, C6, and C7 vertebral bodies and posterior elements with "wasp-waist sign" of these vertebral bodies. (B) Sagittal T1-weighted magnetic resonance image shows C4/C5 disk herniation at the motion segment C4/C5, mildly impinging on the spinal cord (*arrow*).

as anticipatory guidance of AAI and protection of the C-spine. Screening with radiographs is no longer recommended in the asymptomatic child. Children with Down syndrome are cautioned to not participate in full-contact sports, such as football and soccer, and sports like gymnastics, wrestling, diving, or trampoline use.

Clinical symptoms that should prompt attention include development of neck pain, weakness, spasticity, changes in tone, gait difficulties, hyperreflexia, change in bowel or bladder function, or other myelopathic symptoms.

Evaluation of AAI with lateral radiographs in neutral and flexion position has traditionally consisted of measuring ADI (>5 mm) (see Fig. 28.28), the basilar-dental distance (>12 mm), and Powers ratio above 1.0. More recently, Nakamura et al. (2016) proposed evaluating two parameters in neutral position, including the inclination angle of C1 and the coefficient C1/SAC-C4. This avoids possible complications of cord compression with flexion. CT can further evaluate morphology of developmental bony abnormalities. MRI is helpful in evaluating cord compression and cord signal abnormalities consistent with myelomalacia. Treatment consists of posterior fixation (see Fig. 28.28C).

Os Odontoideum

Os odontoideum is an ossicle with smooth and well-corticated margins, separate from a hypoplastic or foreshortened odontoid. Etiology is congenital or traumatic, and it is thought to occur early in development. Os odontoideum can be located just posterior to a hypertrophied anterior C1 arch, or fused to the basion (tip of the clivus), and can result in variable degrees of AAI (Fig. 28.29). Conversely, an acute fracture at the dens base (type II) will show irregular, lucent contours. Os odontoideum is seen in 6% of children with Down syndrome.

Clinically, os odontoideum can be asymptomatic or may manifest with neurological symptoms from cord compression. Even with minor trauma, acute cord compression has been reported in children with os odontoideum.

Os odontoideum can be detected incidentally on radiographs for evaluation of C-spine trauma. CT provides excellent anatomic detail of the osseous structures (see Fig. 28.29C). MRI will demonstrate the degree of cord compression, as well as changes in the spinal cord, such as decreased caliber and hyperintense foci in the cord on T2WI, which may represent edema or myelomalacic changes (see Fig. 28.29D).

Treatment consists of fixation and fusion to prevent myelopathy and to avoid the risk for acute cord compression, which can occur even with minor trauma.

Klippel-Feil Syndrome

KFS is a congenital malformation of the C-spine due to failure of vertebral segmentation resulting in fusion of two or more vertebral bodies. This results in a short neck, with appearance of a low hairline at the back of the head and limited range of motion in the neck. Genetic mutations have been recently identified that could explain the pathogenesis. KFS can be associated with other spinal or cerebral anomalies, such as diastematomyelia, syringomyelia, agenesis of the corpus callosum, meningocele, cervical occult spina bifida, or spinal masses like dermoid cysts and lipomas. Other organ systems also can be affected. Children with KFS should avoid sports or activities that can injure the neck.

Imaging studies will show vertebral fusion with AP narrowing of the vertebral bodies (wasp-waist sign) (Fig. 28.30) and occasionally other findings, such as spina bifida, hemivertebra, scoliosis, and Sprengel deformity (congenital elevation of the scapula). CT and MR can assess for spinal canal stenosis. MRI can

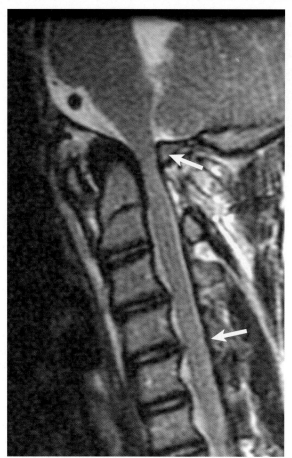

Fig. 28.31 Achondroplasia in a 9-year-old boy. Sagittal T2-weighted magnetic resonance image of the upper cervical spine shows stenosis of the foramen magnum with prominence of the opisthion (*top arrow*) and spinal canal stenosis throughout (*bottom arrow*).

demonstrate associated disk herniation at the motion segment (at the junction between the nonfused and fused segment), as well as cord compression (see Fig. 28.30B). Treatment for KFS is symptomatic and may require surgical intervention to correct instability.

Achondroplasia

Achondroplasia is an autosomal dominant dwarfism syndrome and the most common hereditary dysplasia, caused by mutations in the *FGFR3* gene. This leads to abnormal endochondral bone formation of the skull base that results in a shallow posterior fossa and abnormal shape and narrowing of the foramen magnum with occasional overgrowth of the opisthion. These bony abnormalities can cause cervicomedullary junction compression. Other osseous findings include stenosis of the jugular foramina and spinal canal stenosis secondary to short pedicles of the vertebral bodies (Fig. 28.31).

Myelopathy secondary to cervicomedullary compression can present clinically with clonus and hyperreflexia, hypotonia, sleep apnea, or even sudden death.

MRI can demonstrate the degree of cervicomedullary compression, spinal canal stenosis, and effacement of the subarachnoid spaces, as well as signal changes in the medulla and cervical spinal cord. Dynamic MRI in neutral, extension, and flexion positions and cerebrospinal fluid flow study can further assess the effects of cervicomedullary compression.

Treatment consists of foramen magnum decompression. In asymptomatic children, prophylactic decompression is strongly considered to avoid the risks of progressive apnea, sudden death, or neurological injury after trauma.

■ Summary

Imaging of the pediatric cervical spine can be challenging to interpret, given the varied appearances during different ages and the presence of synchondroses and apophyses. Attention to learning normal appearances, how to identify anatomic variants, and identifying preexisting conditions and diagnoses which may increase risk for injury. Fracture patterns and review of subluxations and instabilities are important to recognize given the significant neurologic sequelae that can occur if missed.

References

Adelgais, K. M., Browne, L., Holsti, M., Metzger, R. R., Murphy, S. C., & Dudley, N. (Feb 2014). Cervical spine computed tomography utilization in pediatric trauma patients. *Journal of Pediatric surgery*, 49(2), 333–337.

Ahmed, R., Traynelis, V. C., & Menezes, A. H. (Oct 2008). Fusions at the craniovertebral junction. *Child's Nervous System*, 24(10), 1209–1224 ChNS : official journal of the International Society for Pediatric Neurosurgery.

American College of Radiology (ACR). (2012). *Appropriateness criteria – Suspected Spine Trauma*. Available at: https://acsearch.acr.org/docs/69359/Narrative/.

Anderson, L. D., D'Alonzo, R. T. (1974). Fractures of the odontoid process of the axis. *Journal of Bone and Joint Surgery*, 56(8):1663–1674.

Astur, N., Klimo, P., Jr., Sawyer, J. R., Kelly, D. M., Muhlbauer, M. S., & Warner, W. C., Jr. (Dec 18 2013). Traumatic atlanto-occipital dislocation in children: Evaluation, treatment, and outcomes. *The Journal of Bone and Joint Surgery American*, 95(24), e194 volume, 191-198.

AuYong, N., & Piatt, J., Jr. (Jan 2009). Jefferson fractures of the immature spine. Report of 3 cases. *Journal of Neurosurgery: Pediatrics*, 3(1), 15–19.

Babcock, L., et al. (2018). Cervical spine injuries in children associated with sports and recreational activities. *Pediatric Emergency Care*, 34(10), 677–686.

Beier, A. D., Vachhrajani, S., Bayerl, S. H., Aguilar, C. Y., Lamberti-Pasculli, M., & Drake, J. M. (2012). Rotatory subluxation: Experience from the hospital for sick children. *Journal of Neurosurgery: Pediatrics*, 9(2), 144–148.

Bilston, L. E., & Brown, J. (Oct 1 2007). Pediatric spinal injury type and severity are age and mechanism dependent. *Spine*, 32(21), 2339–2347.

Easter, J. S., Barkin, R., Rosen, C. L., & Ban, K. (Aug 2011). Cervical spine injuries in children, part I: Mechanism of injury, clinical presentation, and imaging. *Journal of Emergency Medicine*, 41(2), 142–150.

Easter, J. S., Barkin, R., Rosen, C. L., & Ban, K. (Sep 2011). Cervical spine injuries in children, part II: Management and special considerations. *The Journal of Emergency Medicine*, 41(3), 252–256.

Fielding, J. W., & Hawkins, R. J. (1977). Atlanto-axial rotatory fixation. (Fixed rotatory subluxation of the atlanto-axial joint). *The Journal of Bone Joint Surgery*, 59(1), 37–44.

Hall, G. C., Kinsman, M. J., Nazar, R. G., et al. (Mar 18 2015). Atlanto-occipital dislocation. *World Journal of Orthopedics*, 6(2), 236–243.

Hannon, M., Mannix, R., Dorney, K., Mooney, D., & Hennelly, K. (Mar 2014). Pediatric cervical spine injury evaluation after blunt trauma: A clinical decision analysis. *Annals of Emergency Medicine*, 65(3), 239–247.

Herman, M. J., et al. (2019). Pediatric cervical spine clearance: A consensus statement and algorithm from the pediatric cervical spine clearance working group. *Journal of bone and joint surgery American volume*, 101(1), e1.

Hoffman, J. R., Mower, W. R., Wolfson, A. B., Todd, K. H., & Zucker, M. I. (Jul 13 2000). Validity of a set of clinical criteria to rule out injury to the cervical spine in patients with blunt trauma. National Emergency X-Radiography Utilization Study Group. *New England Journal of Medicine*, 343(2), 94–99.

Horn, E. M., Feiz-Erfan, I., Lekovic, G. P., Dickman, C. A., Sonntag, V. K. (2007). Survivors of occipitoatlantal dislocation injuries: Imaging and clinical correlates. *Journal of Neurosurgery Spine*, 6(2), 113–120.

Junewick, J. J. (May 2011). Pediatric craniocervical junction injuries. *AJR American Journal of Roentgenology*, 196(5), 1003–1010.

Junewick, J. J., Chin, M. S., Meesa, I. R., Ghori, S., Boynton, S. J., & Luttenton, C. R. (Nov 2011). Ossification patterns of the atlas vertebra. *AJR American Journal of Roentgenology*, 197(5), 1229–1234.

Karwacki, G. M., & Schneider, J. F. (Nov 2012). Normal ossification patterns of atlas and axis: A CT study. *AJNR American Journal of Neuroradiology*, 33(10), 1882–1887.

Knox, J. B., Schneider, J. E., Cage, J. M., Wimberly, R. L., & Riccio, A. I. (Oct-Nov 2014). Spine trauma in very young children: A retrospective study of 206 patients presenting to a level 1 pediatric trauma center. *Journal of Pediatric Orthopaedics*, 34(7), 698–702.

Leonard, J. C. (Oct 2013). Cervical spine injury. *Pediatric Clinics of North America*, 60(5), 1123–1137.

Leonard, J. C., et al. (2019). Cervical spine injury risk factors in children with blunt trauma. *Pediatrics*, 144(1).

Leonard, J. R., Jaffe, D. M., Kuppermann, N., Olsen, C. S., & Leonard, J. C. (May 2014). Cervical spine injury patterns in children. *Pediatrics*, 133(5), e1179–1188.

Leonard, J. C., Kuppermann, N., Olsen, C., et al. (Aug 2011). Factors associated with cervical spine injury in children after blunt trauma. *Annals of Emergency Medicine*, 58(2), 145–155.

McCracken, B., Klineberg, E., Pickard, B., & Wisner, D. H. (Jul 2013). Flexion and extension radiographic evaluation for the clearance of potential cervical spine injures in trauma patients. *European Spine Journal*, 22(7), 1467–1473 official publication of the European Spine Society, the European Spinal Deformity Society, and the European Section of the Cervical Spine Research Society.

Murphy, R. F., Davidson, A. R., Kelly, D. M., Warner, W. C., Jr., & Sawyer, J. R. (Mar 2015). Subaxial cervical spine injuries in children and adolescents. *Journal of Pediatric Orthopaedics*, 35(2), 136–139.

Nakamura, N., Inaba, Y., Aota, Y., et al. (2016). New radiological parameters for the assessment of atlantoaxial instability in children with down syndrome: The normal values and the risk of spinal cord injury. *Bone & Joint Journal*, 98-B(12), 1704–1710.

Neal, K. M., & Mohamed, A. S. (Jun 2015). Atlantoaxial rotatory subluxation in children. *Journal of the American Academy of Orthopaedic Surgeons*, 23(6), 382–392.

Nigrovic, L. E., Rogers, A. J., Adelgais, K. M., et al. (May 2012). Utility of plain radiographs in detecting traumatic injuries of the cervical spine in children. *Pediatric Emergency Care*, 28(5), 426–432.

O'Brien, W. T., Sr., Shen, P., & Lee, P. (2015). The dens: normal development, developmental variants and anomalies, and traumatic injuries. *Journal of Clinical Imaging Science*, 5, 38.

Pang, D., Nemzek, W. R., & Zovickian, J. (Nov 2007). Atlanto-occipital dislocation--part 2: The clinical use of (occipital) condyle-C1 interval, comparison with other diagnostic methods, and the manifestation, management, and outcome of atlanto-occipital dislocation in children. *Neurosurgery*, 61(5), 995–1015 discussion 1015.

Pang, D., Nemzek, W. R., & Zovickian, J. (2007). Atlanto-occipital dislocation: Part 1--normal occipital condyle-C1 interval in 89 children. *Neurosurgery*, 61(3), 514–521, discussion 521.

Pang, D. (1982). Spinal cord injury without radiographic abnormalities in children. *Journal of Neurosurgery*, 57(1), 114–129.

Patel, J. C., Tepas, J. J., 3rd, Mollitt, D. L., & Pieper, P. (Feb 2001). Pediatric cervical spine injuries: Defining the disease. *Journal of Pediatric Surgery*, 36(2), 373–376.

Rao, R. D., Tang, S., Lim, C., & Yoganandan, N. (Sep 4 2013). Developmental morphology and ossification patterns of the C1 vertebra. *Journal of Bone and Joint Surgery American*, 95(17), e1241–1247 volume.

Riascos, R., Bonfante, E., Cotes, C., Guirguis, M., Hakimelahi, R., & West, C. (Nov-Dec 2015). Imaging of atlanto-occipital and atlantoaxial traumatic injuries: What the radiologist needs to know. *RadioGraphics*, 35(7), 2121–2134 a review publication of the Radiological Society of North America, Inc.

Rusin, J. A., Ruess, L., & Daulton, R. S. (2015). New C2 synchondrosal fracture classification system. *Pediatric Radiology*, 45(6), 872–881.

Sierink, J. C., van Lieshout, W. A., Beenen, L. F., Schep, N. W., Vandertop, W. P., & Goslings, J. C. (Jun 2013). Systematic review of flexion/extension radiography of the cervical spine in trauma patients. *European Journal of Radiology*, 82(6), 974–981.

Smith, P., et al. (2016). Normal development and measurements of the occipital condyle-C1 interval in children and young adults. *AJNR American Journal of Neuroradiology*, 37(5), 952–957.

Sobolewski, B. A., Mittiga, M. R., & Reed, J. L. (Dec 2008). Atlantoaxial rotary subluxation after minor trauma. *Pediatric Emergency Care*, 24(12), 852–856.

Szwedowski, D., & Walecki, J. (2014). Spinal Cord Injury Without Radiographic Abnormality (SCIWORA) - clinical and radiological aspects. *Polish Journal of Radiology*, 79, 461–464 Polish Medical Society of Radiology.

Tat, S. T., Mejia, M. J., & Freishtat, R. J. (Dec 2014). Imaging, clearance, and controversies in pediatric cervical spine trauma. *Pediatric Emergency Care*, 30(12), 911–915 quiz 916-918.

Traynelis, V. C., Marano, G. D., Dunker, R. O., & Kaufman, H. H. (1986). Traumatic atlantooccipital dislocation: Case report. *Journal of Neurosurgery*, 65, 863–870.

Tubbs, R. S., Hallock, J. D., Radcliff, V., et al. (Jun 2011). Ligaments of the craniocervical junction. *Journal of Neurosurgery: Spine*, 14(6), 697–709.

Vassiou, K. (2012). Magnetic resonance imaging of the ligaments of the craniocervical region at 3Tesla magnetic resonance unit: Quantitative and qualitative assessment. *Journal of Biomedical Science and Engineering*, 5, 9.

Viccellio, P., Simon, H., Pressman, B. D., Shah, M. N., Mower, W. R., & Hoffman, J. R. (Aug 2001). A prospective multicenter study of cervical spine injury in children. *Pediatrics*, 108(2), E20.

Yucesoy, K., & Yuksel, K. Z. (May 2008). SCIWORA in MRI era. *Clinical Neurology and Neurosurgery*, 110(5), 429–433.

Zhang, Z., Wang, H., & Liu, C. (Jun 2015). Acute traumatic cervical cord injury in pediatric patients with os odontoideum: A series of 6 patients. *World Neurosurgery*, 83(6), 1180 e1181–1186.

CHAPTER 29
Neonatal Spine Imaging

Thierry A.G.M. Huisman and Sarah Sarvis Milla

CHAPTER OUTLINE

Neonate With a Sacral Dimple, 578
Neonate With a Non-Skin-Covered Bump/Lesion at the Back, 578
Neonate With a Skin-Covered Bump/Lesion at the Back, 579
Neonate With a Midline Fluid-Discharging Skin Pit, 581
Neonate With Hypoplastic Lower Extremities, 583
Neonate With a Congenital Caudal Tumor, 584
Neonate With a "Duplicated" or Widened Spinal Canal, 586
Neonate With a Focal Scoliosis or Hyperkyphosis, 588
Additional Rare Spinal Abnormalities, 589
Neonate With a Spinal Injury, 589
Neonate With Nonaccidental Spinal Injury, 590
Summary, 591

In the neonatal period the most frequently encountered spinal pathologies are of developmental nature. Spinal tumors or infections are exquisitely rare in neonates. Spinal trauma may occasionally be encountered and typically result from a complicated/traumatic delivery. This chapter will consequently focus on spinal malformations.

The development of the spinal canal and its contents is highly complex and involves multiple "programmed" anatomic and functional developmental and maturational processes. Malformations of the spinal canal and cord may be an isolated anomaly involving "only" the neuroaxis (brain and spinal cord/canal) or may be part of a complex syndrome or malformation (e.g., cloacal malformation). Next to the primary developmental etiology, the malformed spinal canal and cord may be secondarily injured because of prenatal, perinatal, or postnatal factors (e.g., long-standing exposure of the neural tissue to the amniotic fluid, mechanical injury during delivery, or postnatal infection). Detailed knowledge about normal neonatal spine imaging, as well as malformations, is essential to recognize malformations early (preferably prenatally) to counsel the parents during pregnancy, to plan possible intrauterine interventions, to make decisions about the mode of delivery, to optimize postnatal care, and to predict functional outcome.

In both the prenatal and postnatal period, ultrasound (US) and magnetic resonance imaging (MRI) give highly sensitive and specific information about the full extent and character of the spinal anomaly. Conventional radiography and computed tomography (CT) are rarely indicated and should be avoided to limit radiation exposure. In the following paragraphs the most common spinal malformations will be discussed based on their most apparent clinical findings.

■ Neonate With a Sacral Dimple

This is a common history seen in neonatal spinal sonography. Physical examination features that are more correlative with spinal abnormalities are dimple locations higher along the gluteal cleft or at lumbar level, larger or draining pits, and skin findings such as hairy patches and vascular anomalies. Sonography is an excellent initial evaluation for the spinal canal in the first few months of life because of the lack of ionizing radiation, relative ease of performing the examination, and presence of dorsal cartilage allowing sonographic window into the canal. Often, the sonographic findings are reassuring for normal spinal development. Features that are used to determine normal development are normal location of the conus medullaris at/above L2, normal appearance of a thin filum terminale, and normal pulsation of the cauda equina nerve roots. Pulsation of the conus can be documented with cine imaging or M-mode interrogation. The sonographic numbering of the vertebral bodies can be performed by counting caudal to cranial or by looking for the lumbosacral angle at L5-S1. Variants of normal that are frequently seen include a mildly prominent distal central canal (also known as ventricularis terminalis) and/or a filar cyst just below the conus.

■ Neonate With a Non-Skin-Covered Bump/Lesion at the Back

If there is no skin covering a spinal defect, the neural placode is exposed to the surface and is termed an *open neural tube defect*. If the neural placode is level with the adjacent skin, the lesion is classified as a myelocele (MC); if the neural placode is pushed outside of the hypoplastic/malformed osseous spinal canal, the neural placode appears raised in relation to the adjacent skin and will "pull out" the attached meninges, appearing as a bulging fluid-filled sac. Consequently, this lesion is classified as a myelomeningocele (MMC). Both lesions result from an incomplete or segmental defective closure of the neural tube in which the resultant neural placode did not detach from the adjacent surface ectoderm. The exposed surface of the neural placode should have become the inside of the neural tube, is consequently covered by ependyma, and leaks cerebrospinal fluid (CSF). The neural placode itself is believed to be less functional because of multiple complex primary and secondary processes, including the failure of closure itself with resulting deranged neuroarchitecture but also because of chronic injury as a result of the longlasting exposure of the neural tissue to the amniotic fluid. Adjacent bone, muscle, and skin are also deficient in various degrees of severity. These malformations most frequently occur at the lumbosacral levels; however, the thoracic or cervical spinal cord may also be involved.

Furthermore, nearly all neonates with an open spinal dysraphism will have an associated Chiari type II malformation. It is believed that the chronic leakage of CSF at the level of the spinal dysraphia during the early second trimester is causative for the occurrence of an associated Chiari type II malformation. In several fetal centers around the world, based on this hypothesis, open spinal dysraphias are closed during intrauterine life with the goal to limit the severity of the Chiari type II malformation and to reduce the degree of associated hydrocephalus and possible need for ventriculoperitoneal shunt.

Identification of an open spinal dysraphism is often done on prenatal imaging (US and MRI) (Figs. 29.1–29.3). A midline neural placode is seen either in level with the adjacent surface ectoderm (MC) or protruding like a bubble above the level of the surface ectoderm

(MMC). Nerve roots appear along the anterior surface of the neural placode and, depending on the degree of neural placode protrusion, will appear "stretched" in their course toward the neural foramina. In MMC malformations, various degrees of meningeal structures will be encountered herniating lateral to the neural placode. The spinal canal is usually widened with absent or hypoplastic lateral and dorsal musculoskeletal structures. Infrequently, the neural placode may protrude asymmetrically outside of the malformed spinal canal. In addition, various degrees of hydromyelia may be encountered in the intact spinal cord superior to the spinal dysraphia. Within the cranial vault the typical stigmata of a Chiari type II malformation are encountered. Prenatal US typically identifies the spinal dysraphism and Chiari type II malformation, and fetal MRI is typically used to increase the level of anatomic detail and should focus on evaluating additional malformations or complications (Fig. 29.4). Fetal MRI is especially helpful for the complete diagnostic workup of the Chiari II malformation (see Fig. 29.1). The associated findings often determine the long-term motor and neurocognitive outcome.

■ Neonate With a Skin-Covered Bump/Lesion at the Back

Skin-covered focal bumps/lumps along the midline of the neonatal back have a significantly better functional and neurocognitive prognosis than the non-skin-covered spinal dysraphias. In skin-covered dysraphias (closed neural tube defects) the neural placode is covered/protected by skin and subcutaneous tissue, limiting injury during intrauterine life. In addition, no leakage of CSF is observed; consequently, Chiari type II malformations are typically not seen. Depending on the degree of herniation of the neural placode outside of the malformed/hypoplastic osseous spinal canal and

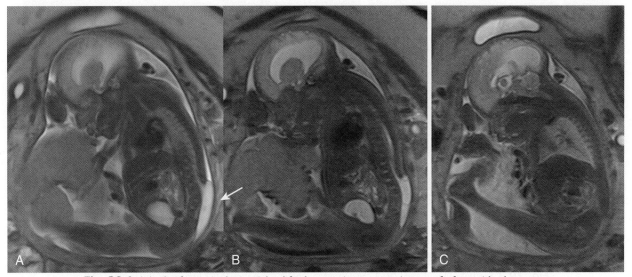

Fig. 29.1 (A) Ultrafast sagittal T2-weighted fetal magnetic resonance images of a fetus with a large non-skin-covered low thoracolumbar myelomeningocele (*arrow*). (B) The cystic dilatation of the spinal canal is seen with the neural placode herniating outside of the widened spinal canal. (C) In addition, a small posterior fossa is seen compatible with an associated Chiari type II malformation. The lower extremities are extended.

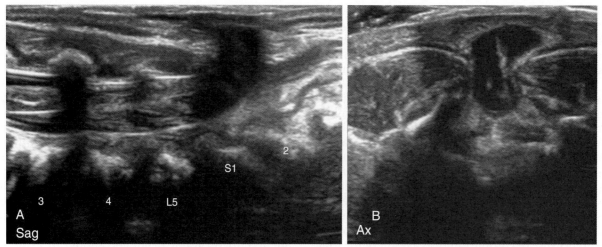

Fig. 29.2 Postnatal sagittal (A) and axial (B) ultrasound images of a neonate with a myelomeningocele. The cerebrospinal fluid-filled hypoechogenic myelomeningocele sac is identified with the neural placode on top of the myelomeningocele sac. The nerve roots are seen as linear hyperechogenic structures coursing through the widened spinal canal. A standoff pad is positioned on top of the neural placode to enhance the image quality, simulating superficial soft tissue.

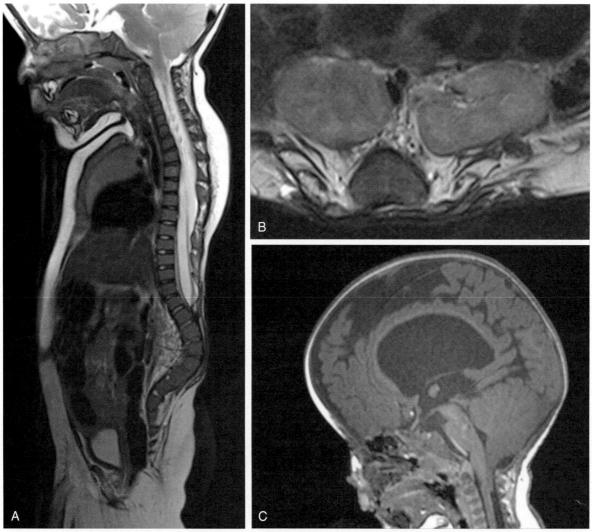

Fig. 29.3 Sagittal (A) and axial (B) T2-weighted magnetic resonance (MR) images of the spinal canal of a neonate with repaired thoracolumbar myelomeningocele. The spinal cord is hypoplastic/thinned, the dorsal soft tissue and bony elements are completely lacking at the level of the spinal dysraphia, the skin was closed surgically over the defect. No dorsal musculature is seen. The kidneys are partially malrotated and approach each other in the midline anterior to the vertebral body. The sagittal T1-weighted MR image of the brain (C) shows the classical stigmata of a Chiari type II malformation.

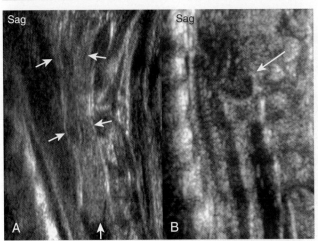

Fig. 29.4 (A,B) Sagittal (*Sag*) ultrasound images of the craniocervical junction of two neonates with classical Chiari type II malformation. The cerebellar tonsils are herniating dorsally to the kinked upper cervical spinal cord (*arrows*) as typically seen in the Chiari type II malformation. Significant crowding is noted of the foramen of magnum.

the size of the associated subcutaneous lipoma, these spinal dysraphias are categorized as myeloschisis with intradural lipoma, lipomyelocele (LMC), or lipomyelomeningoceles (LMMCs).

These skin-covered spinal dysraphias are believed to result from a premature dysjunction of the neural tube from the adjacent surface ectoderm before the neural tube has completely closed. The associated lipoma attached to the neural placode is believed to result from the interaction of adjacent mesodermal cells with the inner lining of the nonclosed neural tube during development, which induces the development of excessive amounts of fat. The resultant lipoma is consequently in close contact to the neural placode. Depending on the amount and extension of the fat, variant size lipomas occur that may be located exclusively intradural or may extend through the osseous defect into the subcutaneous region. On clinical inspection, significant lumps/bumps may be seen. Furthermore, cutaneous stigmata, including hairy tufts or focal skin discolorations, may be seen overlying the dysraphia. LMCs and LMMCs most frequently occur in the lumbar region.

Most children have a normal neurocognitive development but may require urological, orthopedic, and gastroenterological assistance. Their long-term morbidity consists mostly of neurogenic bladder dysfunction with possible renal damage if not treated appropriately.

Prenatal and postnatal neuroimaging (US and MRI) rely on the identification of the osseous defect with a fat-covered neural placode within the level or dorsally of the osseous defect (Figs. 29.5 and 29.6). Similar to the open spinal dysraphias, the closed malformations are classified depending on the amount of tissue that is protruding outside of the spinal canal. The spinal cord is often tethered. If no significant lipoma is present, the skin-covered spinal dysraphias may be easily missed by prenatal US. Fetal MR usually displays the skin-covered spinal dysraphia in better detail but may also occasionally fail to identify the anomaly. T1-weighted MR sequences may be helpful for identification of the

T1-hyperintense lipoma. Chiari type II malformations are exquisitely rare in skin-covered spinal dysraphia. The size of the lipoma can vary significantly and may pose a large cosmetic issue for the child, especially as the child grows older. Surgical reduction of the lipoma is frequently performed later in life. A precise identification of the interface between the lipoma and the neural placode is essential for guiding surgical correction. A large lipoma may exert massive mass effect on the neural placode, even resulting in partial rotation of the neural placode with asymmetric protrusion of meninges outside of the level of the spinal canal. Finally, evaluation for additional associated malformations is important, for example, urogenital or anorectal malformations.

■ Neonate With a Midline Fluid-Discharging Skin Pit

Dorsal dermal sinuses usually become apparent as a midline dimple or small pin point opening from which clear CSF may intermittently leak. In addition, a focal skin discoloration or hairy tuft may be seen in close proximity to the skin dimple. The CSF leakage is frequently missed by the parents because the neonatal diapers absorb the leaked CSF. Dorsal dermal sinuses consist of an epithelium-lined fistulous canal or tract extending from the neonatal back through the adjacent subcutaneous tissues, toward the spinal canal, where it courses through the dural sac to reach the adjacent spinal cord. In the majority of cases an associated intradural lipoma is noted that is adherent to the spinal cord. Based on their embryology the fistulous tract may extend into the central canal of the spinal cord. Dorsal dermal sinuses are believed to result from a focal or incomplete disjunction of the neuroectoderm from the surface ectoderm while the skin is closing dorsally to the neural tube. During embryological neural tube/spinal cord migration from the surface into the developing spinal canal, a persistent connection between ectoderm and neural tube can occur, resulting in a fistulous tract. Most dorsal dermal sinus lesions are in the lumbar region; however, thoracic and cervical cases have been described in the literature. They represent a port of entry for infections and meningitis and may result in a caudal syndrome with extensive inflammation of the cauda equina nerve roots.

Dorsal dermal sinuses may be recognized on prenatal US based on a cord tethering and/or by the simultaneous identification of the adjacent intradural, perimedullary lipoma. The fistulous tract is rarely seen on prenatal US. Prenatal MRI usually correctly characterizes the malformation. In contrast with an MMC, the spinal cord appears closed, no neural placode is noted, and most importantly the spinal cord below the lipoma is intact. No associated Chiari type II malformation is seen. A mild dilatation of the central canal may be seen. Furthermore, the tip of the spinal cord may be low ending. Postnatal US and in particular neonatal MRI easily identify the malformation (Fig. 29.7). The fistulous tract is well seen on thin-sliced, high-resolution T1- or T2-weighted images as a T1-hypointense, T2-hypointense, or hyperintense linear streak extending from the cutaneous dimple

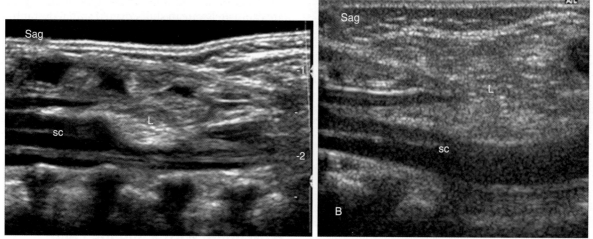

Fig. 29.5 Sagittal ultrasound images of two neonates (A,B) with large lumbar lipomyelomeningoceles. The spinal cord (sc) is tethered and the distal neural placode is covered by hyperechogenic lipoma (L) extending into the subcutaneous region.

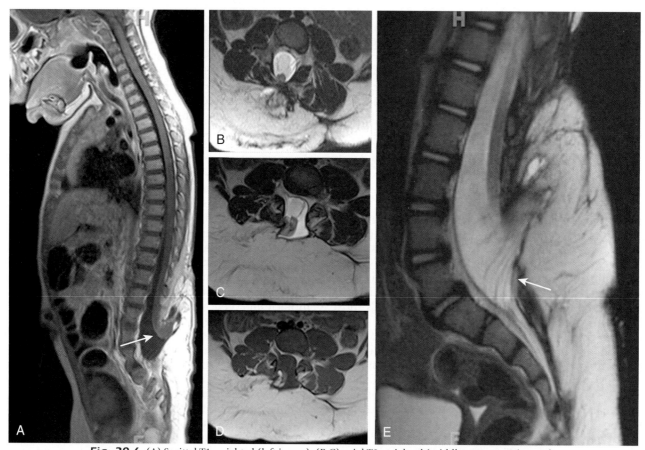

Fig. 29.6 (A) Sagittal T1-weighted (left image), (B,C) axial T2-weighted (middle, upper two images), (D) axial T1-weighted (middle, lower image), and (E) magnified sagittal T2-weighted (right image) magnetic resonance images of a neonate with a skin-covered lumbar lipomyelomeningocele. The neural placode is herniating outside of the widened spinal canal and is dorsally covered by a T2/T1-hyperintense lipoma that is extending from the subcutaneous region into the widened spinal canal. The neural placode is partially rotated. The anterior and posterior nerve roots are located along the anterior surface of the neural placode and are seen as thin, stretched nerves coursing through the cerebrospinal fluid-filled dural sack (*arrow*). The musculature is rather well developed; no Chiari type II malformation was seen.

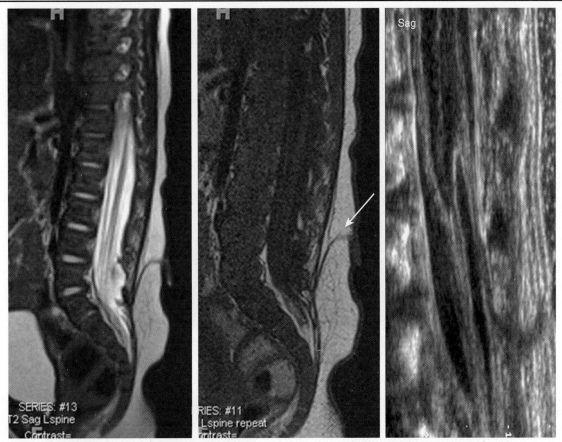

Fig. 29.7 Sagittal T2 (left), T1 (middle) magnetic resonance, and ultrasound (right) images of a neonate with a dorsal dermal sinus. The fistulous tract is seen extending from the skin through the subcutaneous tissue into the spinal canal. The fistulous tract is outlined by T1/T2-hyperintense fat. The lesion is equally well seen on ultrasound as a hypoechogenic tract.

toward the spinal cord. The tract is usually well seen on non-fat-saturated sequences because the adjacent subcutaneous fat renders a good lesion contrast. The tract is most frequently directing upward/cranially and will end in up to 50% of cases in an intradural lipoma, which is adherent to the involved segment of the spinal cord. On very thin sliced, heavily T2-weighted long-echo imaging the fistulous tract may be directly identified coursing between the nerve roots of the cauda equina. Contrast-enhanced sequences may be considered if inflammation is suspected. CT is rarely indicated.

Differential diagnosis includes a sacral dimple, which is known as a focal depression of the skin just above the neonatal buttocks. Sacral dimples are a common variant, occurring in up to 5% of the neonates. The lower the dimple, the less likely that is connected to the spinal canal/cord. If clear fluid can be discharged from the dimple, if a hairy tuft is associated, or if there are clinical features of lower extremity or bladder dysfunction, US or MRI should be considered to rule out a spinal malformation.

■ Neonate With Hypoplastic Lower Extremities

Lower-limb abnormalities in combination with a partial absence of the caudal spinal cord and matching vertebral osseous elements may be seen in the caudal regression syndrome. The syndrome is frequently associated with urogenital tract malformations, pulmonary hypoplasia (as a result of renal insufficiency), or imperforate anus or may be part of the omphalocele exstrophy imperforate anus syndrome, VACTERL association (vertebral anomalies, anal atresia, cardiac defects, tracheoesophageal fistula and/or esophageal atresia, renal and radial anomalies and limb defects), or Currarino triad.

The caudal regression syndrome is believed to result from an anomalous secondary neurulation and/or primary neurulation. The primary neurulation refers to the transformation of the surface ectoderm into neuroectoderm and subsequent neural groove and tube formation, which eventually becomes the upper nine-tenths of the final spinal cord. Secondary neurulation is responsible for the development of the lowest part of the spinal cord, including conus medullaris, cauda equina, and filum terminale. During secondary neurulation, multiple pluripotent cells gather along the inferior tip of the primary neural tube, coalesce, and form a central cavity, which eventually fuses with the distal tip of the primary neural tube. If the secondary neurulation is deficient, a caudal regression syndrome ensues.

Clinically the findings are usually straightforward with dysplastic lower limbs, distal leg atrophy, short intragluteal cleft, genital anomalies, anal atresia, and,

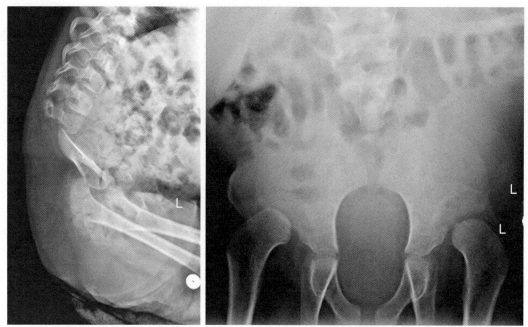

Fig. 29.8 Lateral and frontal radiography of a neonate with a severe caudal regression syndrome. The lower lumbar vertebral bodies, including sacrum, are lacking. The iliac wings are approaching each other in the midline. The hip joints are dysplastic.

in very severe cases, fusion of the lower extremities (sirenomelia). The renal abnormalities are easily identified by US examination and are likely linked to pulmonary hypoplasia. Maternal diabetes mellitus during pregnancy increases the risk for a caudal regression syndrome. On plain film imaging an agenesis of the coccyx/sacrum and/or absence of the lower vertebrae may be seen (Fig. 29.8).

High-resolution prenatal US and MRI are sensitive and specific for the detection of the caudal regression syndrome and match the postnatal US and/or MRI findings (Figs. 29.9–29.11). The most distal segments of the spinal cord and matching musculoskeletal elements are lacking. Typically the spinal cord terminates higher than usual with a club- or wedge-shaped inferior border. The sacrum and coccyx are not seen. Depending on the level of affection, additional lumbar or thoracic vertebral bodies may be lacking. The hips are frequently dislocated, and the musculature is typically highly hypoplastic. The brain is usually without pathology, and surviving children have normal cognitive functions. Caudal regression syndrome can be subclassified into two types depending on the location and shape of the distal spinal cord. In type I the distal cord ends high and abrupt (i.e., "blunted conus"); in type 2 the distal cord is low and tethered. LMMC and terminal myelocystocele are reported in 20% of cases.

■ Neonate With a Congenital Caudal Tumor

Congenital tumors within the sacrococcygeal region are most frequently sacrococcygeal teratomas. These "benign" tumors are believed to arise from the pluripotent cells of the caudal cell mass that is linked to the

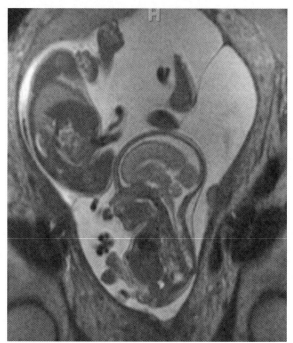

Fig. 29.9 Sagittal T2-weighted fetal magnetic resonance imaging of a twin pregnancy in which the lower twin presented with a severe caudal regression syndrome. The caudal part of the spinal canal is completely lacking, and the lower extremities were hypoplastic.

secondary neurulation. They consist of derivates from all three germ cell layers, including the ectoderm, mesoderm, and endoderm. Sacrococcygeal teratomas may be isolated, may be associated with additional anorectal anomalies, or may be seen as part of the Currarino triad.

The tumor is usually easily identified at birth as a large cystic and/or solid mass lesion in the region of the sacrum and coccyx. The anatomy of the pelvic floor

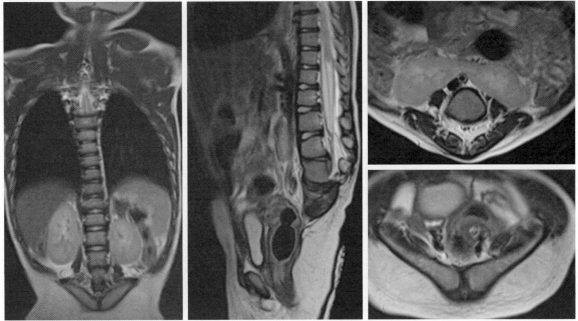

Fig. 29.10 Coronal, sagittal, and axial T2-weighted magnetic resonance images of a neonate with a severe caudal regression syndrome (same neonate as in Fig. 29.8). The lower vertebral bodies, including sacrum, are completely lacking; the caudal spinal cord, including conus medullaris, is absent; the inferior end of the spinal cord appears club or wedge shaped; and the kidneys and iliac wings are fused.

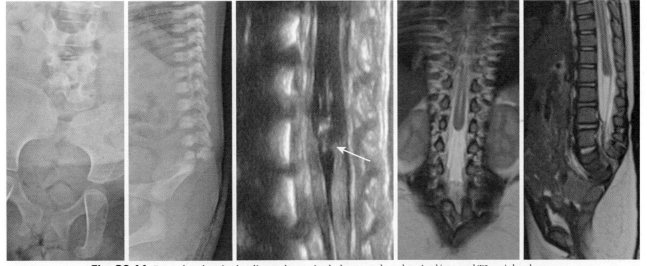

Fig. 29.11 Frontal and sagittal radiography, sagittal ultrasound, and sagittal/coronal T2-weighted magnetic resonance (MR) images of a neonate with caudal regression syndrome. The lower lumbar and sacral osseous elements are lacking; on ultrasound the spinal cord is malformed, wedge shaped, and ends too high in the spinal canal. The matching T2-weighted MR images confirm the caudal regression syndrome with blunt-ending spinal cord.

may be significantly distorted. Based on their location and extension, these tumors are classified in four types being purely or predominantly intrapelvic, extrapelvic, or combined intrapelvic and extrapelvic. Intraspinal extension is rarely present.

Prenatal diagnosis by US and MRI is essential for guiding delivery and determining the immediate perinatal and postnatal care. The lesion is easily identified on prenatal US; MRI may, however, give important additional anatomic information. In addition, fetal MRI may better evaluate the hemodynamic effect of the tumor on the fetus. Fetal hydrops, including ascites and pleural effusion, cardiomegaly, and obstruction of the kidneys are easily depicted. Moreover, fetal MRI also allows to exclude placental hydrops. Postnatal neuroimaging is typically performed for guidance of the surgical procedure (Fig. 29.12). Solid and cystic components may coexist, and calcifications and fat inclusions are easily identified. Surgical resection aims at complete resection of the teratoma, typically with resection of the coccyx and restoration of a functional pelvic anatomy.

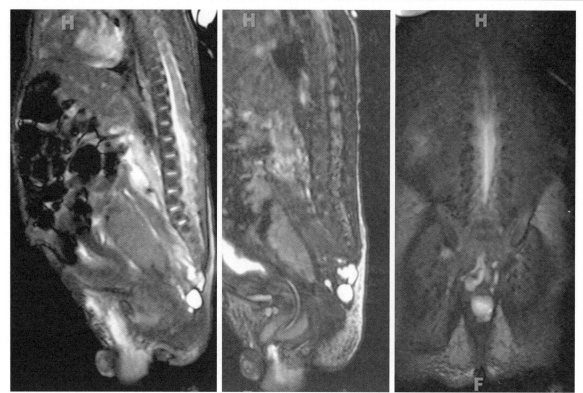

Fig. 29.12 Sagittal (left and middle) and coronal T2-weighted magnetic resonance images of a neonate with a multicystic sacrococcygeal teratoma inferior to the distal pole of the coccyx. No extrapelvic component is noted. The spinal cord is intact and unremarkable.

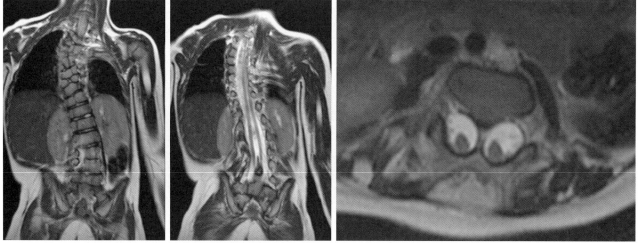

Fig. 29.13 Coronal (left and middle) and axial (right) T2-weighted magnetic resonance images of a child with a lumbar diastematomyelia. The spinal cord is split by a T2-hypointense bony spur; the two hemicords are located within a separate bony canal at the level of the bony spur. In addition, the spinal cord is tethered. Furthermore, multilevel segmentation/formation anomalies are seen of the thoracic vertebral bodies. Mild S-shaped thoracolumbar scoliosis.

■ Neonate With a "Duplicated" or Widened Spinal Canal

Focal hairy tufts, cutaneous birthmarks like hemangiomas, dorsally to the spine, focal scoliosis, or a widened spinal canal may suggest a split notochord syndrome or diastematomyelia. In diastematomyelia the spinal cord is divided in two hemicords, which can be separated by a membranous septum or a bony spur. Each hemicord has one ventral and one dorsal nerve root. The diastematomyelia is usually uni-focal but may be multifocal and is most commonly encountered at the lumbar or thoracic level. The spinal cord usually fuses superior or inferior to the diastematomyelia.

Diastematomyelia is believed to result from a duplication of the notochord secondary to an abnormally wide primitive streak. Because the notochord induces the transformation of the overlying surface ectoderm into neuroectoderm, two hemicords develop.

Prenatal and postnatal US and MRI imaging features are basically identical (Figs. 29.13–29.15).

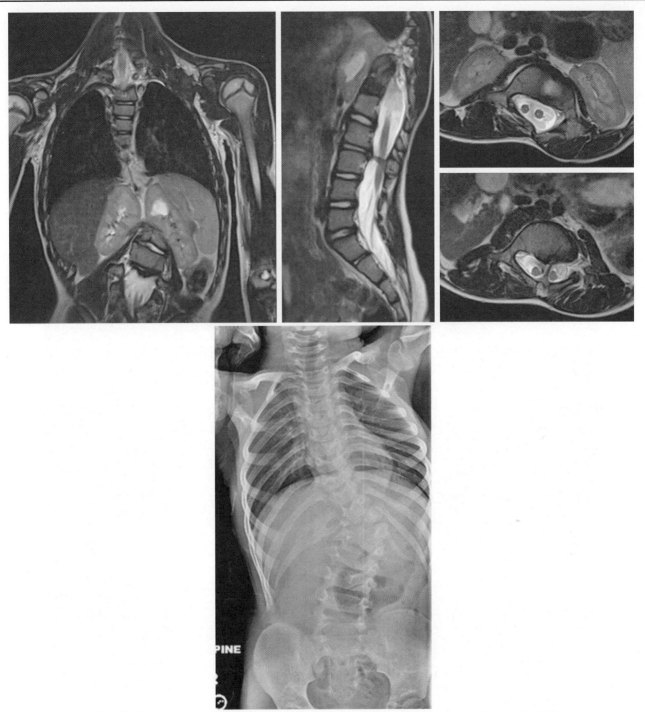

Fig. 29.14 (A) Coronal (left), sagittal (middle), and axial (right) magnetic resonance images of a child with a lumbar diastematomyelia. A tin bony spur is dividing the spinal canal in two compartments. The hemicords have a small T2-hyperinetnse central canal. Next to a levoscoliosis of the lumbar spine the kidneys are approaching each other in the midline. (B) Matching frontal radiography shows the segmentation/formation anomaly of the lower thoracic and upper lumbar vertebral bodies, as well as malformed ribs.

Typically a widened spinal canal is encountered with two hemicords outlined by T2-hyperintense CSF. Short-segment diastematomyelia may go undetected. Multiplanar MRI is essential to prevent misdiagnosis. The fibrous band or bony spur that divides the spinal canal into two separate compartments is typically well seen on axial or coronal imaging as a T2-hypointense band. Cord tethering is seen in the majority of patients with lumbar diastematomyelia. Additional spinal dysraphias may be encountered. Diastematomyelia can also occur in fetuses with an MMC. Furthermore, associated segmentation and formation anomalies of the osseous vertebral column are frequently seen. There is, however, no increased incidence of intracranial malformations with isolated diastematomyelia.

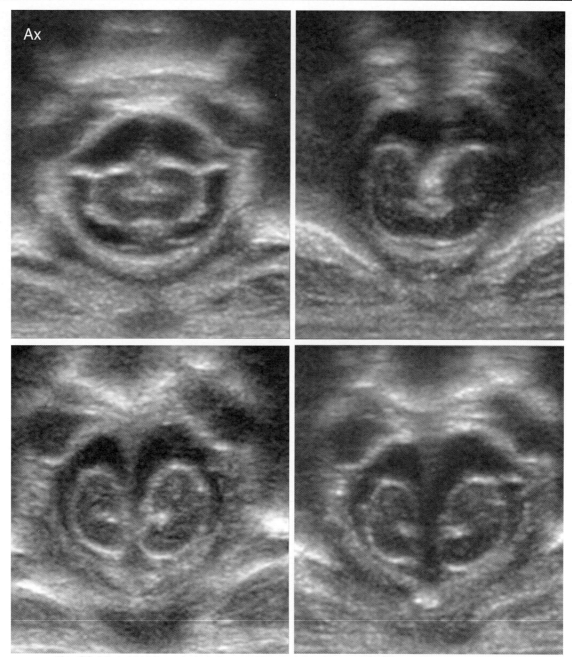

Fig. 29.15 Axial high-resolution ultrasound images of a neonate with a fibrous diastematomyelia. The two hemicords are easily identified covered by hyperechogenic pia mater. The central canal in each hemicord is also hyperechogenic.

■ Neonate With a Focal Scoliosis or Hyperkyphosis

Segmentation or formation anomalies result in a spectrum of vertebral anomalies, including, for example, hemivertebrae, butterfly vertebrae, or block (Fig. 29.16). "Isolated" focal segmentation and formation anomalies are usually recognized on prenatal MRI because of a focal scoliosis or kyphosis. If multiple segments are involved, the malformation is usually more complex and frequently part of well-defined disorders of the primary and secondary neurulation or notochordal development. These anomalies may also be encountered as part of various well-defined syndromes and associations, such as Klippel-Feil syndrome or VACTERL association.

These formation anomalies result from a segmental derangement of the developing musculoskeletal somites. During the development of the neural tube a somite plate develops on each side of the neural tube. This somite plate becomes segmented and by the end of the fifth week of gestation, 42 pairs of somites are noted

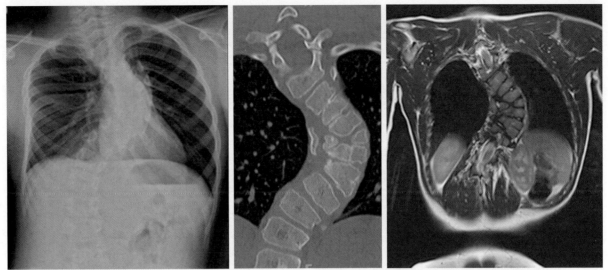

Fig. 29.16 Frontal radiography (left), coronal computed tomography (middle), and coronal T2-weighted magnetic resonance images in a child with multifocal segmentation/formation anomalies of the thoracic spine resulting in a significant scoliosis.

lateral to the neural tube. The somites subsequently develop a central cavity. The internal side gives rise to the sclerotome, which migrates and surrounds the notochord, eventually becoming the vertebral primordia. The caudal half of each sclerotome joins the superior half of the adjacent sclerotome resulting in the vertebral bodies. The lowest part of the cranial half of each sclerotome forms the intervertebral disk. The notochord regresses at the level of the vertebral bodies but persists at the level of the intervertebral disks to become the nucleus pulposus.

■ Additional Rare Spinal Abnormalities

Next to the previously described more common developmental anomalies of the neonatal spine, multiple well-defined rare anomalies may be encountered, which include, for example, the terminal myelocystocele (skin-covered neural tube defect with herniation of a focally expanded lumbosacral central canal outside of the widened/dysraphic spinal canal), neuroenteric fistula or cyst (midline cleft connecting the peritoneal cavity/bowel with the dorsal skin while crossing/dividing the spinal canal and cord), segmental spinal dysgenesis (focal agenesis/dysgenesis of the spinal cord and nerve roots), as well as multilevel anomalies that are less well understood. In these cases the radiologist should describe the anomaly in full detail in case of surgical intervention.

■ Neonate With a Spinal Injury

In neonates the stability of the pediatric spine relies predominantly on the cartilaginous spine and the relatively lax ligaments. In addition, the large head to body pro-

portion, weak neck musculature, shallow occipital condyles, horizontal orientation of the facet joints, small uncinate processes, immature uncovertebral joints, and increased elasticity of the posterior joint capsules make the neonatal craniocervical junction and upper cervical spine very vulnerable for injury.

Consequently, a traumatic vaginal delivery may result in injuries of the craniocervical junction. Next to ligamentous and cartilago-osseous lesions, the spinal cord may be injured ranging from smaller focal hemorrhages up to complete transections. In addition, nerve root avulsions and brachial plexus injuries may be seen.

US has little value in the sensitive diagnosis of these lesions. CT may show osseous injuries, fractures, and dislocations, but may underestimate the degree of ligamentous injury and/or spinal cord injury. MRI has proved to be the most sensitive imaging modality to evaluate the neonatal spinal column, canal, and cord (Fig. 29.17). T2-weighted MRI or short TI inversion recovery sequences may show an increased T2 signal of the injured ligaments, occasionally with T2-hyperintense edema of the injured ligaments. The high-resolution T2-weighted constructive interference in steady state (CISS) sequence may directly show the interruption/disruption of the injured ligaments. This MR sequence is especially helpful for the alar and apical ligaments, as well as the tectorial membrane. Retroclival hematomas may displace the tectorial membrane and extend into the epidural space of the upper spinal canal. Diffusion-weighted imaging may reveal injury to the spinal cord with high sensitivity and specificity.

Occipital osteodiastasis is a unique postnatal/neonatal finding characterized by a separation of the squamous and occipital bony plates as a result of an anterior displacement and upward rotation of the squamous portion of the occipital bone by suboccipital pressure. Occipital osteodiastasis typically occurs after breech

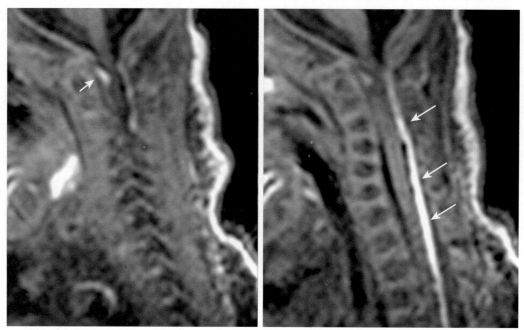

Fig. 29.17 Sagittal T1-weighted magnetic resonance images of a neonate with a traumatic vaginal delivery resulting in a T1-hyperinetsne epidural hematoma anterior and posterior to the cervical dural sack.

delivery and is associated with an increased risk for posterior fossa and intraspinal, subdural hematomas, as well as injury to the brainstem and cerebellum. Familiarity with the unique neonatal anatomy of the occipital bone enhances the detection rate. Sagittal images and a 3D reconstruction of the bony skull facilitate diagnosis. If CT identifies occipital osteodiastasis, MRI should be considered because of its higher sensitivity for soft tissue lesions in the posterior fossa and upper cervical spinal canal.

In neonates, it is of importance not to position the child in a supine position on a hard, flat board, because the prominent occipital protuberance increases a flexion at the craniocervical junction. This may aggravate compression of the spinal cord or lower brainstem, or increase a dislocation at the craniocervical junction.

Finally, in newborns, avulsion of the spinal nerve roots with formation of a pseudomeningocele or a direct injury/disruption of the brachial plexus may result from a traumatic delivery. In Erb palsy the upper motor neurons (C5/6) are involved, resulting in a lack of the Moro reflex, while in Klumpke palsy the lower motor neurons (C7/T1) are affected, resulting in the lack of the Moro and grasp reflexes. In addition, Horner syndrome may be present because of a simultaneous injury to the sympathetic fibers of T1. In addition, Horner sign may be present because of a simultaneous injury to the sympathetic fibers of T1. Isolated Klumpke palsy is extremely rare, and Klumpke palsy is almost always associated with Erb palsy as a complete plexus injury resulting in atonic "flail limb" and Horner sign. In most cases a spontaneous recovery is the rule. High-resolution heavily T2-weighted MRI and diffusion ten-

sor imaging may show a traumatic pseudomeningocele, as well as a disrupted nerve root.

■ Neonate With Nonaccidental Spinal Injury

Nonaccidental injury in the neonatal period most frequently results from vigorous shaking of the baby. Next to the typical diffuse shear injuries within the brain, which are possibly complicated by a hypoxic component as a result of chest compression while shaking or a cardiopulmonary arrest, injury may occur at the craniocervical junction. Thoracolumbar injury is typically seen in older infants (median age, 13.5 months) often with visible spinal deformity or focal neurological signs. Craniocervical or cervical spinal injuries are more common in younger infants (median age, 5 months) who present with impaired consciousness and respiratory distress. Typically, subdural and/or epidural hematomas are noted within this region; however, the intradural hemorrhage may redistribute throughout the entire spinal canal (Fig. 29.18). Cervical spine ligamentous injuries (predominantly involving the nuchal, atlanto-occipital, and atlantoaxial ligaments) are significantly more common in children with nonaccidental trauma compared with children with accidental trauma. If nonaccidental injury is suspected, it is mandatory to evaluate the entire spinal cord and canal for additional posttraumatic lesions, and a complete diagnostic work-up with skeletal survey, physical examination, and a psycho-social evaluation should be performed.

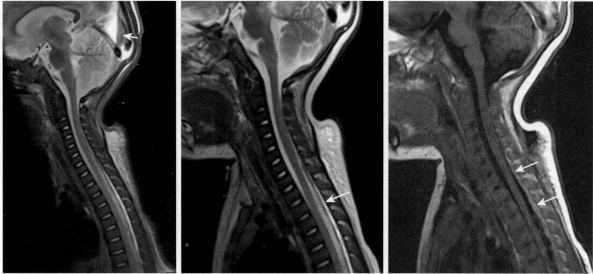

Fig. 29.18 Sagittal T2-weighted (left and middle) and T1-weighted magnetic resonance images of a 2-month-old newborn who suffered from proven nonaccidental injury. T2/T1-hyperintense blood is seen in the epidural space dorsally to the cervicothoracic spinal cord. In addition, sedimented blood products are noted superior to the cerebellar tentorium and in the posterior fossa.

■ Summary

A detailed understanding of the normal and abnormal development of the spinal canal and its contents is essential for the correct classification of most spinal malformations. In addition, clinical-radiological correlation will help narrow the differential diagnosis. Prenatal and postnatal US and MRI are the most valuable imaging modalities for the diagnostic workup. CT is rarely indicated and should be avoided whenever possible in the neonatal period.

Bibliography

Huisman, T. A. (2008). Fetal magnetic resonance imaging. *Seminars in Roentgenology, 43*(4), 314–336.

Huisman, T. A., Phelps, T., Bosemani, T., Tekes, A., & Poretti, A. (2015). Parturitional injury of the head and neck. *Journal of Neuroimaging, 25*(2), 151–166.

Huisman, T. A., Rossi, A., & Tortori-Donati, P. (2012). MR imaging of neonatal spine dysraphia: What to consider? *Magnetic Resonance Imaging Clinics of North America, 20*, 45–61.

Huisman, T. A., & Solopova, A. (2009). MR fetography using heavily T2-weighted sequences: Comparison of thin- and thick-slab acquisitions. *European Journal of Radiology, 71*(3), 557–563.

Huisman, T. A., Wagner, M. W., Bosemani, T., Tekes, A., & Poretti, A. (2015). Pediatric spinal trauma. *Journal of Neuroimaging, 25*(3), 337–353.

Koelble, N., Huisman, T. A., Stallmach, T., Meuli, M., Zen Ruffinen Imahorn, F., & Zimmermann, R. (2001). Prenatal diagnosis of a fetus with lumbar myelocystocele. *Ultrasound in Obstetrics and Gynecology, 18*(5), 536–539.

Tekes, A., Pinto, P. S., & Huisman, T. A. (2011). Birth-related injury to the head and cervical spine in neonates. *Magnetic Resonance Imaging Clinics of North America, 19*(4), 777–790.

Tortori-Donati, P., Rossi, A., Biancheri, R., & Cama, A. (2005). Congenital malformations of the spine and spinal cord. In P. Tortori-Donati (Ed.), *Pediatric neuroradiology head, neck, and spine* (pp. 1551–1608). Springer.

CHAPTER 30
Imaging of Back Pain

Diana P. Rodriguez

CHAPTER OUTLINE

Epidemiology, 592
Clinical Evaluation, 593
Imaging Evaluation, 593
Radiographs, 593
    Advanced Imaging: Computed Tomography, Magnetic Resonance Imaging, and Nuclear Medicine, 594
    Computed Tomography, 594
    Magnetic Resonance Imaging, 594
        Technetium-99m Bone Scan Whole Body With Single-Photon Emission Computed Tomography Spine, 594
    Spondylolysis and Spondylolisthesis, 594
    Disk Calcification, 595
    Scheuermann Disease/Kyphosis, 596
    Sacral Meningocele, 598
    Disk Degeneration and Herniation, 600
    Disk Cyst, 601

Infectious Disorders, 601
    Spondylodiskitis, 601
    Epidural Abscess, 602
    Chronic Recurrent Multifocal Osteomyelitis/Chronic Noninfectious Osteomyelitis, 603
Neoplastic Disorders, 604
Spinal Column Tumors, 604
    Langerhans Cell Histiocytosis, 604
    Aneurysmal Bone Cyst, 605
    Osteoid Osteoma, 606
    Osteoblastoma, 606
    Ewing Sarcoma, 607
    Lymphoma and Leukemia, 607
Intramedullary Tumors, 608
    Astrocytoma, 608
    Ependymoma, 609
Extramedullary Intradural Tumors, 611
    Schwannoma, 611
    Meningioma, 611
Summary, 612

Back pain is common in children and tends to increase with age, especially in the early teen years. Although back pain can be the presenting symptom of serious pathology, such as infection or neoplasm, recent studies have shown lower rates of identifiable disease in children with back pain. A nonpathological cause, such as mechanical low back pain, is frequently seen in children and responds to conservative treatment without requiring diagnostic imaging. A detailed clinical history and a thorough physical examination are critical to avoid unnecessary workups, and can identify patients with clinical red flags who will benefit from further radiographic or laboratory studies. Familiarity with common disorders that manifest with back pain in children, and the use of a systematic approach to choose the indicated imaging modality will lead to a correct diagnosis. This chapter will review the epidemiology, clinical evaluation, imaging workup, and radiological findings of common and a few rare disorders that cause back pain in children.

■ Epidemiology

There is wide variability in the reported prevalence of back pain in children, ranging from 12% to 50%. Difficulty in determining the prevalence of back pain in children includes several factors, such as differences among studies in defining "back pain" (some refer to back pain in general, while others refer exclusively to low back pain), variability in the time period assessed, sample size, and a small number of prospective studies on the epidemiology of back pain in children. Prevalence increases with age, and specifically low back pain shows a dramatic increase in the early teen years. Lifetime prevalence rate has been shown to increase from 12% at 11 years of age to 50% at 15 years of age. A 40.2% lifetime prevalence of back pain in children between 10 and 16 years of age has also been reported. Suggested risk factors include females, poor fitness in sedentary adolescents, and family history. The adolescent athlete can be considered a different subgroup in which low back pain more often results from acute injury or overuse injury.

Back pain in children is most often a symptom of a benign process, but it can also be the manifestation of a more serious pathology, including infectious/inflammatory, neoplastic, congenital, and traumatic etiologies (Table 30.1). Mechanical low back pain is common in children and refers to pain without an identifiable etiology on physical examination, radiographs, or advanced imaging evaluation. This condition responds to conservative treatment and usually does not require imaging evaluation.

TABLE 30.1   Etiology of Back Pain in Children and Adolescents

I. Traumatic	d. Giant cell tumor
A. Spondylolysis/spondylolisthesis	e. Chordoma
B. Vertebral column fractures	f. Osteogenic sarcoma
C. Disk herniation	g. Ewing sarcoma
D. Intraspinal hematoma	h. Osteochondroma
E. Spinal cord injury	i. Histiocytosis
II. Musculoskeletal	2. Secondary neoplasms
A. Scheuermann disease	a. Leukemia
B. Scoliosis	b. Lymphoma
C. Intervertebral disk degeneration	c. Neuroblastoma
D. Intervertebral disk herniation	d. Metastatic disease
E. Intervertebral disk calcification	B. Spinal cord
F. Nonspecific musculoskeletal back pain	1. Intramedullary
III. Infectious	a. Astrocytoma
A. Diskitis	b. Ependymoma
B. Vertebral osteomyelitis	c. Ganglioglioma
C. Epidural abscess	d. Gangliocytoma
D. Sacroiliac joint infection	2. Extradural tumors
E. Chronic recurrent multifocal osteomyelitis	a. Neuroblastoma
F. Nonspinal infection	b. Ganglioneuroblastoma
1. Pyelonephritis	c. Ganglioneuroma
2. Pneumonia	d. Lymphoma
3. Pelvic inflammatory disease	e. Peripheral primitive neuroectodermal tumor
4. Paraspinal muscle abscess	3. Intradural extramedullary
IV. Inflammatory	a. Schwannoma
A. Ankylosing spondylitis	b. Neurofibroma
B. Juvenile idiopathic arthritis	c. Meningioma
C. Arthritis	d. Cerebrospinal fluid dissemination of intracranial neoplasms
1. Psoriatic arthritis	VI. Congenital
2. Reactive arthritis	A. Syringomyelia
3. Inflammatory bowel disease–associated arthritis	B. Tethered cord syndrome
V. Neoplastic disorders	VII. Other
A. Spinal column	A. Sickle cell pain crisis
1. Primary neoplasms	B. Referred pain (e.g. Cholecystitis)
a. Osteoid osteoma	C. Chronic pain syndromes
b. Osteoblastoma	D. Osteoporosis
c. Aneurysmal bone cyst	

Modified from Rodriguez, D. P., & Poussaint, T. Y. (2010). Imaging of back pain in children. *AJNR American Journal of Neuroradiology, 31*(5), 787–802.

■ Clinical Evaluation

A detailed clinical history and a thorough physical examination are essential in identifying the source of back pain in children and determining whether further radiographic or laboratory studies are necessary. Children who have no significant physical findings, short duration of pain, and a history of minor injury can be treated conservatively without further work up. Pain should be characterized in terms of site, duration, frequency, mechanism of onset, time of onset (e.g., nighttime), acute or chronic nature, radiating pain, and association with recent-onset scoliosis. Pain associated with constitutional symptoms, such as fever, malaise, and night sweats, may suggest underlying infection or malignancy. Pain that improves with aspirin or nonsteroidal antiinflammatory drugs (NSAIDs) can be consistent with an osteoid osteoma. *Clinical red flags*, including constant pain, night pain, radicular pain, pain lasting longer than 4 weeks, and abnormal neurological examination should prompt further imaging evaluation. Laboratory tests are indicated in patients with suspicion for infection or systemic illness and must include inflammatory markers and a complete routine blood panel. If these tests are positive, imaging evaluation is indicated as well.

■ Imaging Evaluation

The American College of Radiology recently published an Appropriateness Criteria guideline for imaging evaluation of back pain in children (Booth et al., 2017). These guidelines and recommendations discuss the indications for imaging modalities according to different clinical variants. These variants include: (1) initial imaging evaluation in the child without clinical red flags; (2) initial imaging evaluation in the child with one or more clinical red flags: (3) child with negative radiographs and one or more clinical red flags; (4) child with positive radiographs and one or more clinical red flags; (5) child with chronic back pain associated with overuse (mechanical back pain); and (6) child with back pain associated with suspected inflammation, infection, or malignancy.

■ Radiographs

Radiographs of the entire spine are a good initial diagnostic tool for the evaluation of back pain in children and include anteroposterior and lateral views. Oblique views should not be obtained routinely in children, because these do not increase sensitivity while adding considerable radiation exposure. Radiographs are not necessary in children with short duration of symptoms that respond to conservative therapy. In 24% of cases, radiographic findings have been shown to lead to the diagnosis. Radiographs may detect bony lesions, such as vertebra plana, fractures, Scheuermann disease, spondylolysis, scoliosis, and expansile and destructive lesions like aneurysmal bone cysts (ABCs).

Advanced Imaging: Computed Tomography, Magnetic Resonance Imaging, and Nuclear Medicine

After radiographs, the best imaging technique for the evaluation of back pain in children is variable. The choice of computed tomography (CT), magnetic resonance imaging (MRI), or bone scintigraphy depends on the clinical presentation, suspected underlying pathology, and the child's age. Another important consideration when imaging children is the amount of radiation exposure with each technique. Ionizing radiation places children at risk for development of neoplasms and therefore should be kept to a minimum. Pediatric patients are more susceptible to the mutagenic effects of radiation, and their lifetime risk is greater because they have more years to live and therefore accumulate more radiation exposure throughout their life. The ALARA (As Low As Reasonably Achievable) principles must always be applied, and whenever possible, imaging modalities that do not use ionizing radiation, such as MRI, should be considered.

Computed Tomography

The use of CT in children should be limited because of its ionizing radiation, and when indicated, CT must be restricted to the smallest field of view possible. CT is considered the imaging technique of choice for characterizing fractures and bony lesions. Two-dimensional reformatted images and three-dimensional reconstruction models are useful in the preoperative evaluation of spinal trauma and scoliosis and for presurgical orthopedic planning.

Magnetic Resonance Imaging

MRI is the imaging technique of choice in diagnosing intraspinal or paraspinal pathology and is indicated in children with back pain and one or more clinical red flags. In patients with abnormal neurological findings, initial evaluation with MRI of the entire spine may be indicated. When there is suspicion of infection, inflammation, or neoplasm, precontrast and postcontrast MR sequences should be performed to assess patterns of enhancement. Generally, noncontrast MRI is done in the child with low back pain with suspected spondylolysis or disk pathology. The decision of using MRI must be weighed carefully against its relatively high cost and the need for sedation in younger children.

Technetium-99m Bone Scan Whole Body With Single-Photon Emission Computed Tomography Spine

Technetium-99m (^{99m}Tc) methylene diphosphonate bone scintigraphy with SPECT (single-photon emission computed tomography) is another tool in the imaging workup of back pain in children. It has high sensitivity in detecting spondylolysis and is superior to MRI in detecting active spondylolysis. Bone scans are particularly useful in identifying multifocal disease as well. However, bone scans expose patients to significantly more radiation than radiographs and CT. In particular, the urinary bladder is subjected to a large amount of radiation because the radioactive tracer is excreted through the urine and temporarily stored in the bladder before voiding. Coregistered CT is becoming a standard component of modern SPECT. Again, increased radiation exposure with this technique is a limiting factor for its use. Advantages of SPECT/CT over SPECT alone include improved anatomic localization of sites of abnormal uptake, identification of causes of abnormal uptake, and demonstration of bony abnormalities that do not show abnormal radiotracer uptake. Abnormalities of the posterior elements, including lumbar interspinous bursitis, spinous process avulsion, and facet hypertrophy can be better assessed with SPECT/CT.

Spondylolysis and Spondylolisthesis

Spondylolysis refers to a defect or fracture of the pars interarticularis, which is the weakest portion of the neural arch. The pars interarticularis is the bony segment formed by the junction of the vertebral pedicle, the superior and inferior articular processes, and the lamina. Although etiology remains unclear, risk factors include developmental defects and repetitive trauma from excessive hyperextension. A prevalence rate of 4.4% has been reported in children and 6% in the general population. The incidence of spondylolysis increases with the practice of sports such as gymnastics, soccer, volleyball, diving, and ballet. Bilateral involvement is more frequent than unilateral, and the most commonly affected vertebra is L5, followed by L4 and L3. Multilevel involvement can occur, and atypical involvement at a higher level, such as L2, tends to be more painful.

There is no general consensus for the imaging workup to evaluate suspected spondylolysis. However, evaluation typically begins with plain radiographs and can be further assessed with any of the following imaging modalities: MRI, CT, ^{99m}Tc bone scan whole body with SPECT spine, or SPECT/CT. Radiographs are considered a poor screening test with low sensitivity for spondylolysis in children; only two-view (anteroposterior and lateral) radiographs are recommended. It has been demonstrated that oblique views do not increase sensitivity and specificity, but rather add radiation exposure. A pars fracture can be seen as an oblique lucency at the base of the laminae on the lateral view (Fig. 30.1). Radiographs are useful for the evaluation of *spondylolisthesis*, defined as anterior slippage of a given vertebra over the one below it, in the presence of bilateral pars fractures. The degree

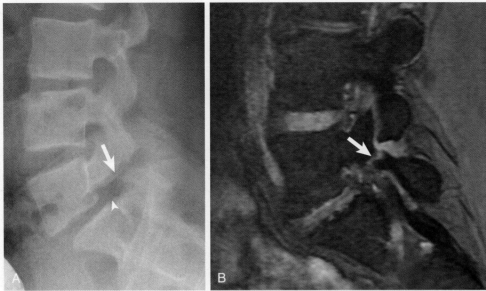

Fig. 30.1 (A) Lateral radiograph of the lumbosacral junction shows a diastatic L5 pars fracture (*arrow*) and grade 1 spondylolisthesis of L5 on S1 (*arrowhead*). (B) Sagittal gradient-echo magnetic resonance image shows a mildly diastatic chronic fracture (*arrow*).

of anterior vertebral displacement is graded as follows: grade 1, less than 25% displacement; grade 2, 25% to 50% displacement; grade 3, 50% to 75% displacement; and grade 4, 75% to 100% displacement. Grade 5 (spondyloptosis) refers to complete displacement of the vertebral body anteriorly (Fig. 30.1A).

MRI is currently a preferred imaging modality to diagnose spondylolysis due to the lack of radiation and its ability to assess soft tissue and bony structures. The following spectrum of abnormalities of the pars interarticularis can be demonstrated with MRI: focal marrow edema without a visible fracture consistent with stress reaction, incomplete or complete fractures with marrow edema (in the acute/subacute phase), or chronic (nonunion) fractures with no marrow edema. Paraspinal soft tissue edema can be seen occasionally in the acute setting. Incomplete fractures extend from inferior to superior. Marrow edema will show hypointense signal intensity on T1-weighted images (T1WIs), hyperintense signal on T2-weighted images (T2WIs) with fat saturation, or STIR (short-tau inversion recovery) pulse sequence. Sagittal multiple-echo recombined gradient-echo images are also recommended because they provide greater sensitivity for visualization of pars fractures (Fig. 30.1B). On axial images, pars fractures have a transverse orientation and should not be mistaken with the adjacent facet joints, which have an oblique orientation. The facet joints are seen one or two slices above and below the pars fractures (Fig. 30.2C,D).

Healing response of incomplete fractures is not well seen with MRI or CT; neither modality can assess whether an incomplete fracture is in an evolutionary or reparative phase. CT scans can best characterize the fracture and can show associated findings, such as bony fragmentation or surrounding sclerosis (Fig. 30.3).

SPECT bone scans are sensitive for detecting spondylolysis and reveal areas of bone turnover; findings are generally positive for a prolonged period (~6 weeks). Spondylolysis presents as increased radiotracer uptake in the posterior elements (pars interarticularis, lamina, or pedicle) (Fig. 30.4) (Booth et al., 2017). These findings may be consistent with stress reaction, stress fracture, or a symptomatic spondylolytic defect. Coregistered CT is now a standard component of modern SPECT systems. The advantages of SPECT/CT were mentioned earlier in this review.

The differential diagnosis of spondylolysis includes fractures of the vertebral pedicles, which are significantly less common, but can also show bilateral uptake in the posterior elements with SPECT. Fractures of the pedicle are most often unilateral but can be seen in association with contralateral spondylolysis. Bilateral pedicle fractures tend to occur in skeletally mature patients and are difficult to differentiate from pars fractures with SPECT. Coregistered CT can make this distinction as well as MRI (Fig. 30.5).

Nonsurgical treatment of spondylolysis includes restriction of activity that exacerbated symptoms, activity modification limited to specific forms of exercise (e.g., stationary biking and modified swimming), bracing, NSAIDs, and physical therapy.

Disk Calcification

Calcification of the intervertebral disk is a rare disorder in children of unknown etiology. Proposed causes include inflammation or infection (i.e., diskitis, osteomyelitis), trauma, or metabolic disorders (i.e., hyperparathyroidism). It also has been described in association with syndromes such as Morquio syndrome, I cell disease, and Patau syndrome. Disk calcification occurs more often in the cervical spine, followed by the thoracic and lumbar spine, and has a slight predilection for boys. This entity usually occurs during the first two decades of life and is self-limiting, with most symptoms resolving within 6 months. Disk calcification can completely resolve with time.

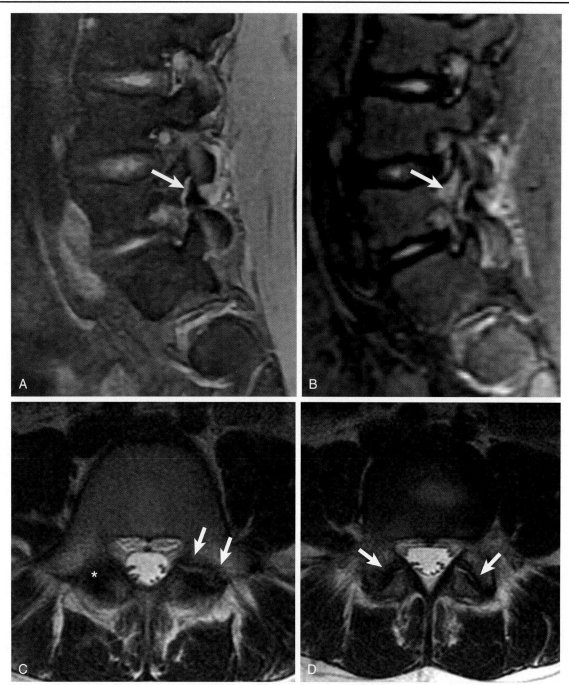

Fig. 30.2 Acute L5 spondylolysis in an 11-year-old. (A) Sagittal gradient-echo image of the lumbo-sacral junction shows a bright linear fracture of the left pars interarticularis (*arrow*). (B) Sagittal short-tau inversion recovery image at the same level shows marrow edema of the adjacent superior (*arrow*) and inferior articular processes. (C) Axial T2-weighted image shows horizontal orientation of the left linear pars interarticularis fracture (*arrows*) and sclerosis (low signal) of the right pars (*asterisk*). (D) Axial T2-weighted image caudal to the fracture shows bilateral facet joints with a normal oblique orientation (*arrows*).

Disk calcifications can be seen incidentally or can present with symptoms such as pain, stiffness, decreased range of motion, muscle spasm, tenderness, and torticollis. Fever and increased erythrocyte sedimentation rate (ESR) may also be present. Symptoms tend to be brief and rarely last for more than several weeks. Associated disk herniation may occur as well.

On radiographs and CT, disk calcification is seen as a round, oval, flattened, or fragmented calcification in the nucleus pulposus. On MRI the calcified disk will appear dark on T2WI and bright on T1WI. Associated

calcification of the posterior ligament can occur. MRI can best evaluate an associated disk herniation (Fig. 30.6).

Treatment is conservative; however, severe myelopathy or radiculopathy will require surgical intervention.

Scheuermann Disease/Kyphosis

Scheuermann disease is an osteochondrosis of the spine affecting the vertebral epiphyseal growth plates. This

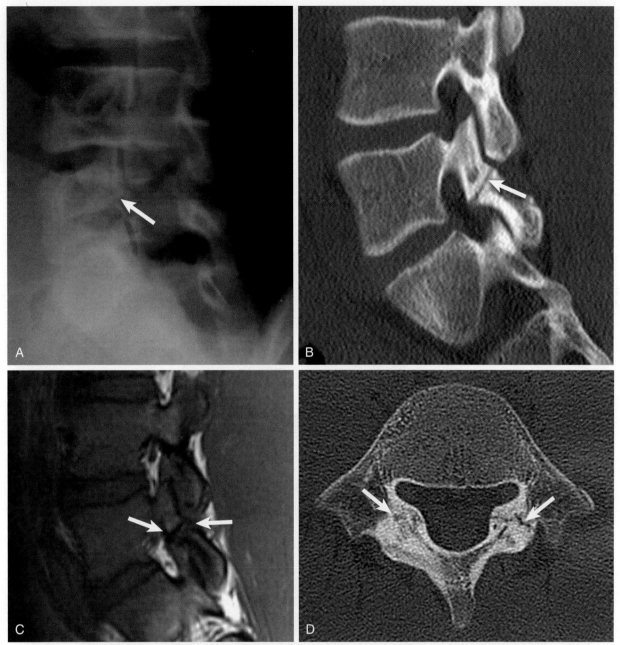

Fig. 30.3 Chronic bilateral L5 spondylolysis in a 16-year-old. (A) Oblique radiograph of the lumbosacral junction and (B) sagittal computed tomography (CT) image show a linear left pars interarticularis fracture (*arrow*). (C) Sagittal T1-weighted image shows the fracture (*arrows*); there was no marrow edema on T2-weighted images (not shown). (D) Axial CT image shows bilateral L5 pars fractures with moderate surrounding sclerosis (*arrows*).

condition is the most common cause of progressive thoracic or thoracolumbar angular hyperkyphosis in adolescents and is associated with back pain. Unlike postural kyphosis, this is a rigid deformity that does not correct when the patient is asked to stand straight. The radiological diagnosis consists of the following findings: anterior wedging of three or more contiguous vertebrae of 5 degrees or greater, resulting in a thoracic kyphosis greater than 35 degrees. Other associated findings include irregular end plates with Schmorl nodes, disk-height loss, and associated apophyseal ring fractures (Fig. 30.7).

Prevalence rates range from 0.4% to 10% depending on diagnostic inclusion criteria. Conflicting reports show

no consistent sex predilection in this disorder that occurs during the period of rapid bone growth between 12 and 15 years of age. Although pathogenesis remains unclear, genetic and mechanical factors likely are involved.

Clinical presentation consists of pain localized to the midscapular region at the level of the kyphotic deformity that usually intensifies gradually after activity, or after prolonged periods of sitting or standing, and improves with rest. The apex of the kyphotic deformity is more commonly localized to the T7-T9 vertebrae or at the thoracolumbar junction. Atypical Scheuermann kyphosis (lumbar type) is less common and occurs at the thoracolumbar junction with the apex between T10 and T12.

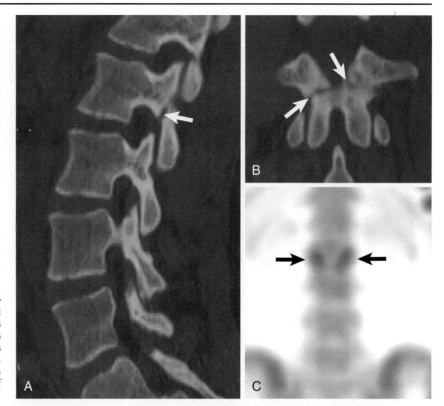

Fig. 30.4 Acute bilateral L2 spondylolysis in a 14-year-old. (A) Sagittal computed tomography (CT) image shows a linear L2 pars fracture (*arrow*). (B) Coronal CT image shows bilateral minimally displaced L2 pars fractures (*arrows*). (C) Technetium-99m methylene diphosphonate single-photon emission CT scan demonstrates increased uptake in the region of the bilateral L2 pars interarticularis (*arrows*).

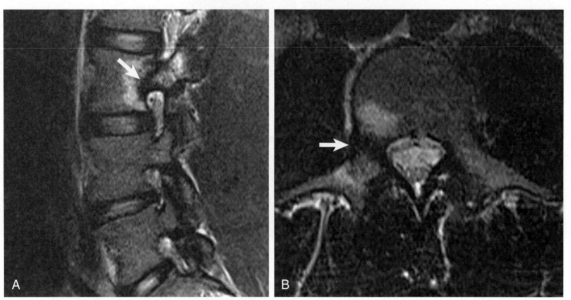

Fig. 30.5 Acute fracture of the right L3 pedicle in a 16-year-old. Sagittal (A) and axial (B) short-tau inversion recovery images show a linear hypointense fracture of the right L3 pedicle (*arrows*) with marrow edema of the adjacent vertebral body and superior articular process.

Initial imaging evaluation consists of plain radiographs. CT may be indicated to further evaluate disease or for preoperative planning. MR is useful in evaluating associated apophyseal ring fractures.

Treatment is mainly conservative, particularly for patients with remaining spinal growth and for those who respond well to physical therapy and bracing. Surgical treatment is reserved for patients with severe curvatures (>75–80 degrees) or skeletally mature patients with rigid curvatures.

Sacral Meningocele

An intrasacral meningocele consists of a cyst of fibrous tissue usually lined by arachnoid, located within an expanded sacral spinal canal that is attached to the caudal termination of the dural sac by a pedicle and allows flow of cerebrospinal fluid (CSF) from the tip of the subarachnoid space into the meningocele. Intrasacral meningoceles do not contain nerve roots, unlike perineural (Tarlov) cysts. Other terms used to refer to this entity

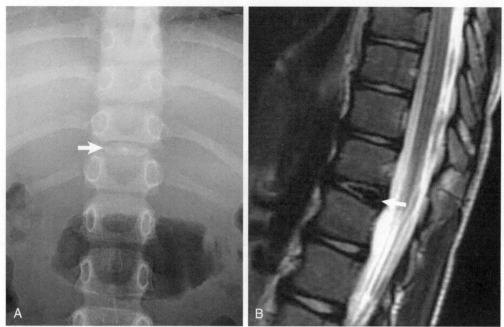

Fig. 30.6 Disk calcification in a 6-year-old boy. (A) Anteroposterior view of the thoracolumbar spine shows calcification of the T11/12 intervertebral disk (*arrow*). (B) Sagittal T2-weighted magnetic resonance image shows dark signal within the calcified T11/12 disk (*arrow*).

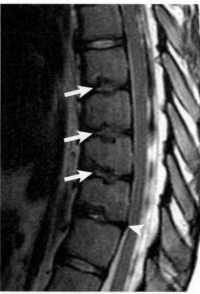

Fig. 30.7 Scheuermann disease in a 13-year-old boy. Sagittal T2-weighted image with fat saturation shows mild anterior wedge deformity of three consecutive thoracic vertebrae with irregular end plates and presence of Schmorl nodes (*arrows*). There is decreased height and T2 signal of the intervertebral disks and mildly increased kyphotic thoracic curvature. Notice posterior disk bulging of a lower thoracic disk with mass effect on the thecal sac but no cord compression (*arrowhead*).

include occult intrasacral meningocele, intrasacral cyst, intrasacral extradural arachnoid cyst, intraspinal meningocele, or giant sacral meningeal diverticula. Although these cysts can be discovered incidentally, the most common symptom is chronic, intermittent low back pain. Other symptoms such as urinary incontinence and constipation result from bowel and bladder dysfunction caused by local nerve root compression.

Of the various theories of pathogenesis proposed, the most accepted one is that it results from a primary mesenchymal defect involving the dura. Despite being considered a congenital abnormality, intrasacral meningoceles can expand over time because of hydrostatic pressure. There is an association with other intraspinal abnormalities, such as sacral vertebral anomalies, diastematomyelia, or tethered spinal cord.

MRI is the imaging modality of choice and provides fine anatomic detail for presurgical planning. Findings consist of an extradural, thin-walled cyst with smooth contours located within the sacral spinal canal adjacent to the distal thecal sac, without neural elements in the cyst and following CSF signal intensity on all sequences. Conventional MRI is usually sufficient for diagnosis and will demonstrate a hyperintense structure on T2WI and a hypointense structure on T1WI (Fig. 30.8). However, identifying the site of connection between the cyst and the thecal sac (isthmus or pedicle) can be difficult. Thin-section T2-weighted (steady-state acquisition) imaging can provide additional anatomic detail and can occasionally depict the connection between the cyst and the dura. Usually if the apex of the lesion is midline, it is more likely to be an intrasacral meningocele rather than a perineural cyst that is located eccentrically within an enlarged neural foramen, with dilatation of the nerve root meningeal sleeve. These cysts do not enhance with contrast material. Diffusion-weighted imaging can help differentiate an intrasacral meningocele from an epidermoid/dermoid cyst.

Myelography and CT myelography can depict the connection between the cyst and the thecal sac, depending on the size of the opening. However, these methods are invasive, time-consuming, painful, and associated with ionizing radiation, and therefore are rarely used in the pediatric population.

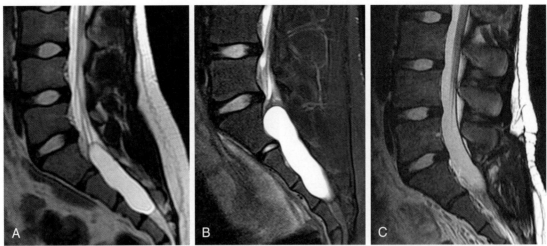

Fig. 30.8 *Sacral meningocele in a 9-year-old boy.* (A) Sagittal T2-weighted image of the lumbosacral spine shows a well-circumscribed cystic structure within the sacral canal with remodeling of the sacral vertebrae. (B) A 5-year follow-up study shows increased size of the intraspinal cystic lesion with further bone remodeling and mass effect on the cauda equina nerve roots. (C) Postoperative sagittal T2-weighted image shows complete removal of the cyst.

Plain radiographs can show remodeling of the sacral canal, or other bony abnormalities such as vertebral segmentation anomalies and spinal dysraphism. In infants younger than 3 to 4 months, ultrasound can effectively identify an intrasacral meningocele. Clinical indications for evaluation with ultrasound most often include sacral dimple and/or asymmetrical gluteal folds.

Differential diagnosis includes dorsal meningocele and dural ectasia. A dorsal meningocele consists of protrusion of the meninges through a dorsal dysraphism with extension into the paraspinal soft tissues. Dural ectasia consists of dilatation of the thecal sac with or without lateral components, and usually involves both the lumbar and sacral spine.

Surgical treatment, which consists of surgical ligation and obliteration of the cyst, is indicated in growing or symptomatic lesions.

Disk Degeneration and Herniation

Disk degeneration in children is detected with MRI in 50% of symptomatic patients, compared with 20% in asymptomatic patients, and requires no treatment. MR findings consist of loss of disk height and decreased signal intensity on T2WI.

Disk herniation in adults has a lifetime prevalence rate of 40%, whereas symptomatic disk herniation in adolescents and children is rare, with a prevalence rate of 0.2% to 3.2%. Traumatic and genetic factors are thought to play a role in the development of pediatric disk herniation. Approximately 30% to 45% of pediatric patients report history of trauma or sports-related injury preceding the onset of symptoms. Disk herniation is associated with activities such as weightlifting, falls, repetitive axial loading, and poor conditioning.

Disk herniation consists of injury to the annulus fibrosus that allows disk material to exit, causing irritation of the adjacent nerve roots. Disk herniations are classified into three types: (1) protrusion (bulging of the disk beyond the vertebral body border but contained within the annulus), (2) extrusion (extension through fibers of annulus, but connection preserved between the disk and extruded disk material), and (3) sequestration (no connection between the disk and the herniated material).

Clinical presentation in children and adolescents consists most often of nerve root tension and gait abnormalities, rather than lower-extremity numbness or weakness. In the acute posttraumatic setting, back pain is a common symptom, while radiating sciatic pain is less frequent. Pain is triggered by flexion and Valsalva maneuvers. Neurological symptoms, such as bowel and bladder dysfunction, can also be present.

In children, disk herniations tend be larger than in adults and can calcify. In addition, pediatric traumatic disk herniation is frequently accompanied by a fracture of the adjacent vertebral end plate (apophyseal ring fracture). Apophyseal ring fractures, also known as end plate avulsion fractures, occur more frequently in the lumbosacral spine. On CT, these present as an arc-shaped or rectangular bone fragment posterior to the dorsal end plate margin. MR will demonstrate bone marrow edema in the donor vertebral body with the disk extending into the defect. The disk between the fragment and the vertebral body is hyperintense on T2WI, whereas the bone fragment is hypointense. Disk desiccation occurs with time, appearing hypointense on T2WI.

Although in the adult population conservative versus surgical treatment has shown similar long-term outcomes, this is still unknown in children. In the absence of neurological symptoms, conservative treatment should always be attempted before considering surgery. Duration of conservative therapy varies between 6 weeks and 3 months and consists of a short period of rest (no more than 2 weeks) and NSAIDs, followed by physiotherapy. Although open micro-diskectomy remains the surgical standard of care for adults and children, there are reports of small series in children treated sucuessfully with minimally invasive lumbar microdiskectomy.

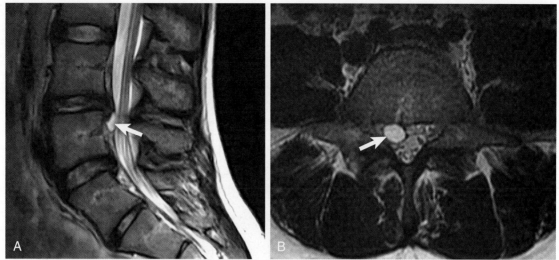

Fig. 30.9 Intervertebral disk cyst in a teenager. Sagittal (A) and axial (B) T2-weighted images show a well-circumscribed oval cystic lesion posterior and inferior to the L4/5 disk with mass effect on the ventral thecal sac (*arrows*). There is decreased height and signal of the disk, as well as herniation (protrusion and extrusion), as shown in (A).

Disk Cyst

Disk cysts are rare intraspinal extradural lesions that may present in the pediatric population with symptoms similar to acute lumbar disk herniation. These cysts are located along the ventral and lateral aspect of the thecal sac and appear to communicate with the disk. These are separate from the CSF space and contain connective fibrous tissue without synovial lining. Their natural history and pathogenesis remain unknown. The origin of these cysts is unclear but may be related to trauma or degenerative changes. Compared with disk herniation, these tend to occur at a younger age and can potentially grow. Clinical symptoms include low back pain, sciatica, and nerve root tension.

On MRI, disk cysts are well-circumscribed, round rim-enhancing, T2 hyperintense, T1 hypointense lesions (Fig. 30.9).

Although optimal management of this rare entity is still unclear, microsurgical diskectomy and cyst excision have been successful in treating radiculopathy caused by these cysts.

■ Infectious Disorders

Spinal infection may involve the vertebral body, intervertebral disk, paravertebral soft tissues, epidural space, leptomeninges, or the spinal cord. Infectious processes of the spine in children include vertebral osteomyelitis, sacroiliac pyarthrosis, diskitis, epidural abscess, meningitis, arachnoiditis, myelitis, and spinal cord abscess.

Spondylodiskitis

Spondylodiskitis refers to infection of the intervertebral disk and adjacent osseous structures (mostly the verte-

bral body). There is a bimodal distribution occurring in early childhood (6 months to 4 years of age) and adolescence (10–14 years of age). The pathophysiology is thought to be related to the presence of vascular channels in the cartilaginous portion of the disk that predispose the disk to infection and later disappear in life. Routes of infection include: (1) hematogenous spread, (2) direct implantation, and (3) contiguity. Isolated vertebral infection (osteomyelitis) is less frequent in children. Children are less susceptible to infection and infarction of the vertebral body from septic emboli than adults due to the presence of multiple intraosseous arterial anastomoses that promote clearance of microorganisms or entrapped emboli. In adults, infection occurs more often in the setting of significant bacteremia, while pyogenic spondylodiskitis in children is seen more often secondary to minor bacteremia caused by ear or upper respiratory system infections, or minor skin cuts and abrasions. History of trauma in children also has been associated with vertebral osteomyelitis and diskitis (Fig. 30.10).

The diagnosis may be delayed because of nonspecific clinical presentation, especially in the young child. Signs and symptoms may include fever, back pain, irritability, and refusal to walk or sit up. Gait abnormality is often reported by parents in children younger than 28 months. The L2-L3 and L3-L4 levels are most commonly affected. Mild leukocytosis and an elevated ESR and C-reactive protein level are usually present. Blood cultures can be negative in more than 50% of cases. Infection is most often bacterial; the most common organism is *Staphylococcus aureus*, followed by *Streptococcus pyogenes*, *Enterobacter* species, and *Haemophilus influenza*. Fungal and mycobacterial infections should be excluded when bacterial cultures are negative.

Radiographs are normal in the early stages but can be positive 12 days after onset of symptoms. Bone scintigraphy, however, can be positive as soon as 1 to 2 days

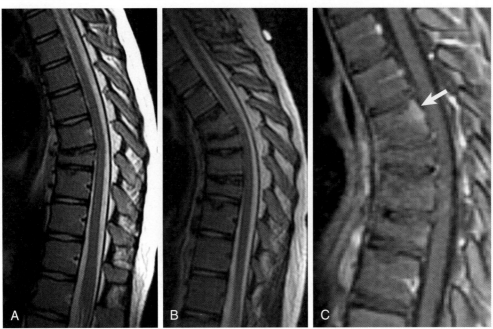

Fig. 30.10 *Compression fractures with superimposed osteomyelitis in a 10-year-old girl with history of fall from the monkey bars.* (A) Sagittal T2-weighted image shows a T9 subacute compression fracture with approximately 50% height loss and minimal anterior wedge deformity of T8 with mild focal kyphosis at T8/9. (B) One-month follow-up sagittal T2-weighted image shows multiple compression fractures from T6 to T9 and increased focal kyphosis. (C) Postcontrast sagittal T1-weighted image with fat saturation shows a focus of enhancement in the T8 vertebral body (*arrow*). Needle biopsy confirmed superimposed bacterial osteomyelitis.

after the onset of symptoms, showing increased radiotracer uptake in the intervertebral bodies on each side of the disk involved. MRI is the imaging modality of choice and should include T1WI and T2WI with fat saturation, or STIR, and postcontrast T1WI with fat saturation. Bone marrow edema, an early nonspecific finding, presents as low signal intensity on T1WI and high signal intensity on STIR or T2WIs with fat saturation. Findings include loss of the normal hyperintense signal intensity of the disk on T2WI, narrowing or complete absence of the disk, and abnormally increased T2-weighted signal intensity in the adjacent vertebral bodies, consistent with marrow edema. There is usually contrast enhancement of the disk and adjacent vertebral bodies. MRI can detect disk extrusion, as well as the presence of paraspinal or epidural abscesses, and spinal cord compression (Fig. 30.11).

Differential diagnosis includes leukemia/lymphoma or metastatic disease. However, these entities usually affect several noncontiguous vertebral bodies and do not involve the disk space; an associated paraspinal mass also can be present.

Treatment is nearly always nonsurgical, consisting of appropriate antibiotic treatment for the pathogen isolated and immobilization with a thoracolumbar orthotic brace. Antibiotics are initiated parenterally for 5 to 10 days, followed by oral antibiotics for 2 to 4 weeks. Duration of treatment depends on the presence of soft tissue involvement or osteomyelitis. Symptoms usually resolve within 3 weeks, and the disk may sometimes recover its height. Surgery is occasionally necessary when medical treatment fails, to decompress the spinal cord and nerve roots from an epidural abscess, or to obtain spinal stability when there is significant osseous destruction.

Epidural Abscess

Spinal epidural abscess is a rare condition in children that requires prompt diagnosis and treatment for optimal outcome. Risk factors for spinal epidural abscess include spinal trauma, previous skin infections, intravenous drug use, and immunodeficiency. The most common causative organism is *S. aureus*. However, an increased incidence of community-acquired methicillin-sensitive *S. aureus* (MRSA) infections is seen nowadays in children without risk factors.

Although clinical presentation has been traditionally described as a triad of back pain, fever, and neurological deficits, these are not always present. Patients can present with refusal to bear weight and pain with movement. Inflammatory markers (C-reactive protein and ESR) are increased, and ESR is specifically a good indicator of disease, even superior to leukocyte count.

MRI is the imaging modality of choice and will show an epidural fluid collection, hypointense on T1WI and hyperintense on T2WI, with possible proteinaceous content and decreased diffusivity due to purulent contents. Postcontrast images will show peripheral thick rim enhancement and adjacent dural thickening and enhancement (Fig. 30.12).

Treatment consists of surgical drainage or CT-guided percutaneous needle drainage with systemic antibiotics for 4 to 6 weeks.

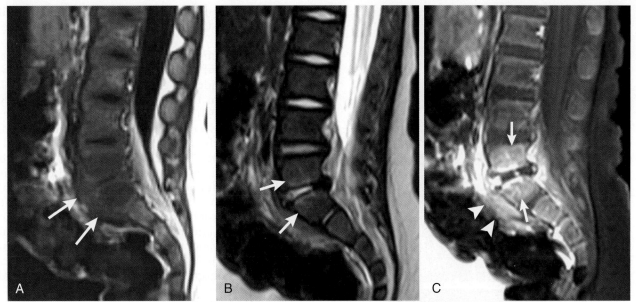

Fig. 30.11 Spondylodiskitis in a 1-year-old boy refusing to bear weight. (A) Sagittal T1-weight-ed image shows heterogeneous soft tissue mass in the prevertebral lumbosacral region (*arrows*) and de-creased T1 signal of the L5 and S1 vertebral bodies. (B) Sagittal T2-weighted image shows mild marrow edema of the L5 and S1 vertebral bodies (*arrows*), as well as paravertebral soft tissue edema. (C) Postcon-trast sagittal T1-weighted image with fat saturation shows diffuse abnormal enhancement of L5, sacral segments (*arrows*), and the anterior aspect of the L5/S1 disk, as well as heterogeneous enhancement of the paravertebral soft tissues (*arrowheads*).

Chronic Recurrent Multifocal Osteomyelitis/Chronic Noninfectious Osteomyelitis

Chronic recurrent multifocal osteomyelitis (CRMO), or chronic noninfectious osteomyelitis (CNO), is a dis-ease that was first described by Giedion et al. (1972) as "subacute and chronic symmetric osteomyelitis." CNO is considered an autoinflammatory skeletal dis-order presenting as severe chronic, nonbacterial osteo-myelitis. Etiology and pathogenesis remain unknown; however, genetic and autoinflammatory factors seem to be implicated. It mainly occurs in childhood and ado-lescence, with female predilection, and tends to resolve after puberty. Although any bone can be involved, the most frequent sites of involvement include the long bones (with metaphyseal predilection), clavicles, spine, and pelvis.

Clinical presentation is variable, and osseous lesions can be found incidentally or can manifest with pain and swelling. Spinal involvement has been reported in up to 39% of cases, with the thoracic spine most frequently affected, and manifests clinically with back pain, stiff-ness, scoliosis, or kyphosis.

Histopathology is nonspecific, consistent with sub-acute or chronic osteomyelitis, and ESR is usually elevated. Biomarkers are under investigation to differen-tiate CNO from other diseases and to monitor treatment response and remission.

Imaging findings play an important role in suggest-ing the diagnosis of CNO. Radiographs can be normal in more than 50% of cases. Radiographic signs include end plate irregularities, notched appearance of the end plates, vertebral body height loss, or vertebra plana. On CT, osseous lesions are mixed lytic and sclerotic. Marrow edema is the main finding on MRI and is best demonstrated on STIR (short-tau inversion recovery) pulse sequence, which uses fat suppression and is sen-sitive to inflammatory tissue processes. Marrow signal changes are most often confined to one or more verte-brae at multiple levels, usually without involvement of the adjacent disks or contiguous vertebrae, which can help to differentiate CNO from bacterial osteomyeli-tis. In the rare occurence that there is involvement of the disk and contiguous vertebra mimicking bacterial osteomyelitis, foci elsewhere in the body will aid in the diagnosis of CNO (Fig. 30.13). Vertebral collapse (vertebra plana) tends not to recover after treatment, and fatty marrow transformation is usually seen with healing. Whole-body MRI is now the imaging modal-ity of choice to identify further areas of disease, which may not be symptomatic on initial presentation, as well as for follow-up and evaluation of treatment response.

There is consensus among authors that when CNO is suspected based on clinical history (good general health), mild inflammatory syndrome with elevated ESR, and radiological findings, further evaluation with whole-body MRI is indicated. If MRI shows multifo-cality, a trial with antiinflammatory drugs should be started. Response to treatment will confirm the diag-nosis; consequently, there is no need for biopsy. If MRI findings are inconclusive, biopsy will differentiate CNO from other entities, such as Langerhans cell histiocytosis (LCH), bacterial osteomyelitis, and malignancy, such as leukemia. Isotope bone scans can also demonstrate the

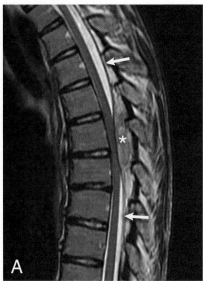

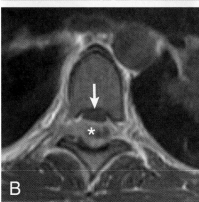

Fig. 30.12 Thoracic epidural abscess in a teenage girl. (A) Sagittal T2-weighted image demonstrates a heterogeneous low-intensity dorsal epidural mass (*asterisk*) with anterior displacement and compression of the thecal sac and spinal cord, which preserves normal signal intensity. Hypointense line (*arrows*) represents the dura. (B) Postcontrast axial T1-weighted image with fat saturation shows enhancement of the epidural abscess (*asterisk*) with anterior displacement and compression of the thecal sac and spinal cord (*arrow*).

multifocal lesions but are less commonly used because of exposure to radiation. Although long-term prognosis of CNO is favorable, usually resolving in the postpubertal period, approximately 25% of patients will continue to have active disease.

Complications from spinal involvement (vertebral body compression) can result in kyphosis and scoliosis; therefore, early detection is important and may require treatment with bisphosphonates.

■ Neoplastic Disorders

Spinal neoplasms can be classified depending on site of origin. Neoplasms of the spinal column include primary and secondary tumors of the vertebra. Primary tumors include aneurysmal bone cysts (ABC), osteoid osteoma, osteoblastoma, Ewing sarcoma, and rarely, osteosarcomas. Secondary tumors of the ver-

tebra include leukemia, lymphoma, Langerhans Cell Histiocystosis (LCH), neuroblastoma, and other metastases.

Intraspinal tumors can be intramedullary (originating from the cord) in 35% to 40% of cases or extramedullary (outside the cord) in approximately 60%. Astrocytomas are the most common intramedullary tumor (45%–60%), occuring more often in younger children with a decrease in frequency into adulthood. Ependymomas, the second most common intramedullary tumors (30%–35%), occur in the older child and are usually seen in association with neurofibromatosis type 2 (NF2). Extramedullary tumors can be extradural or intradural. These include meningiomas (from the meninges), neurofibromas and schwannomas (from the nerve roots and nerve root sheaths), extraspinal tumors that invade the epidural space (neuroblastoma–ganglioneuroblastoma–ganglioneuroma spectrum), or lymphomas or primitive neuroectodermal tumors.

Clinical presentation varies depending on tumor type and location and the patient's age. Pain, the most common symptom, is present in 25% to 30% of cases and can be diffuse or radicular, dull and aching, localized to the vertebral body adjacent to the tumor. Pain usually precedes the development of other symptoms, such as weakness, gait deterioration, torticollis, sensory disturbance, and sphincter dysfunction. Young children and infants can present with severe pain, motor regression, weakness, or frequent falls, whereas older children can present with clumsiness, progressive scoliosis, or gait disturbance. Malignant tumors tend to present with shorter duration of symptoms and show increased incidence of associated neurological deficits. Nocturnal pain that awakens the child from sleep can be associated with intramedullary tumors; this is thought to be secondary to venous congestion and dural distention in decubitus position.

■ Spinal Column Tumors

Langerhans Cell Histiocytosis

LCH refers to a group of disorders consisting of abnormal proliferation of histiocytes that can affect the bone, skin, and internal organs. Previously described eponyms associated with particular presentations of LCH, such as eosinophilic granuloma, Hand-Schüller-Christian, and Letterer-Siwe disease should be disregarded in clinical practice. LCH is now characterized as single systemic, which may be unifocal or multifocal, or multisystem, involving two or more organs and may or may not have risk organ involvement (spleen, liver, or bone marrow).

Spinal involvement of LCH usually presents with local back pain. The thoracic vertebrae are most commonly affected (54%), followed by the lumbar spine (35%) and cervical spine (11%). There may be associated leukocytosis and fever.

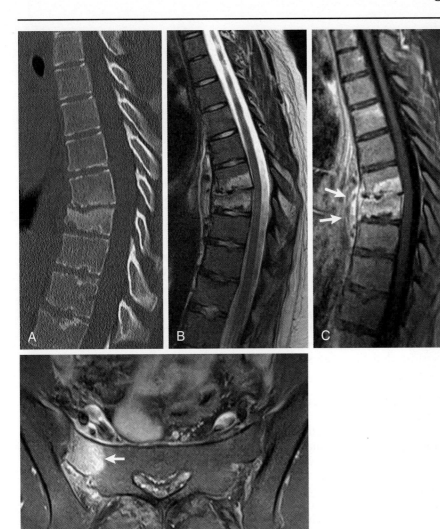

Fig. 30.13 Chronic noninfectious osteomyellitis (CRMO) in a 14-year-old with history of ulcerative colitis and chronic back pain. (A) Sagittal computed tomography image shows anterior wedge deformity of T9 with diffuse sclerosis and end plate irregularity. There is T8/9 disk height loss with a sclerotic and irregular T8 inferior end plate. Minimal retrolisthesis of T8 on T9 is noted with associated focal kyphosis. (B) Sagittal T2-weighted image with fat saturation shows marrow edema of T8 and T9 vertebral bodies with prevertbral soft tissue swelling. There is focal kyphosis with mild mass effect on the ventral thecal sac, without cord compression. (C) Postcontrast sagittal T1-weighted image with fat saturation shows enhancement of T8 and T9 vertebral bodies and prevertebral soft tissue enhancement and edema (*arrows*). (D) Postcontrast axial T1-weighted image with fat saturation of the sacroiliac joints shows a large area of abnormal enhancement in the right sacral wing (*arrow*) with surrounding soft tissue edema.

Radiographs may show a lytic, nonsclerotic destructive vertebral lesion or a collapsed vertebra (vertebra plana) with preservation of the adjacent disk spaces. The posterior elements are rarely involved. On CT, aside from the nonsclerotic destructive osseous lesion, a paraspinal enhancing soft tissue mass may be present with possible epidural extension (Fig. 30.14A–B). MRI is the imaging modality of choice to further assess extension of disease and to monitor treatment response. When only the vertebra is affected, it will manifest with marrow edema and contrast enhancement. Paraspinal disease with appear as homogeneously enhancing, T1 hypointense, T2 hyperintense soft tissue mass. In the presence of vertebra plana the typical appearance is apposition of two intervertebral disks without an intervening normal vertebral body (Fig. 30.14C–E). The differential diagnosis for vertebra plana includes LCH, neoplasms, infections such as tuberculosis, leukemia, lymphoma, trauma, Gaucher disease, and neurofibromatosis.

Treatment for LCH varies depending on severity of disease and may consist of conservative management with spontaneous resolution, curettage with allograft implantation, chemotherapy, steroids, and external beam radiation therapy.

Aneurysmal Bone Cyst

ABC is a benign osteolytic lesion that can affect any bone, but most often arises in the metaphyses of long bones. Spinal involvement is seen in 20% of cases, mostly affecting the posterior elements, but can also involve the vertebral body. ABCs may span two to three adjacent vertebrae. The World Health Organization (WHO) (2020) considers ABC a "benign cystic lesion of bone composed of blood-filled spaces separated by connective tissue septa containing fibroblasts, osteoclast-type giant cells and reactive woven bone." ABCs can be primary lesions (arising de novo) or secondary lesions arising from benign or malignant osseous lesions, such as giant cell tumor, chondroblastoma, or osteosarcoma. ABCs can present at any age but tend to affect the immature spine and have a slight female predilection.

Clinical presentation varies depending on size, location, and destructive behavior of the tumor. The most common symptom is back pain of insidious onset that is more severe at night. Acute pain may present with pathological fractures. Neurological symptoms from nerve root or spinal cord compression occur with large lesions. Scoliosis may be a presenting sign.

On plain radiographs, ABCs appear as radiolucent, expansile lesions that can be unilocular but are most often multiloculated with "soap-bubble" appearance. CT and MRI can show cortical thinning, internal thin septations, and blood-filled spaces with fluid–fluid levels, as well as extension of tumor with involvement of adjacent structures. Osseous changes are best demonstrated with CT, while fluid–fluid levels are typically more apparent on MRI (Fig. 30.15).

Given the aggressive nature of ABCs and high rates of recurrence with residual disease, gross total excision is the goal of surgery in most cases. Treatment options vary widely in the literature including a combination of intralesional curettage and bone grafting, piecemeal excision, en bloc resection, endovascular embolization, intralesional injection of ablating agents, and radiation.

Osteoid Osteoma

Osteoid osteoma is a benign osteoblastic lesion that consists of a nidus of osteoid matrix surrounded by a stroma of loose vascular connective tissue. The nidus may be calcified and surrounded by sclerotic reactive bone. Osteoid osteomas represent 10% to 12% of benign osseous tumors, with 10% of these localized in the spine. These lesions usually measure less than 15 mm and affect the posterior elements (mostly the lamina and pedicles), but they can also occur in the transverse and spinous processes. The etiology is still unknown. These tumors have a predilection for boys and are usually diagnosed at around age 10 to 12 years.

Clinical presentation consists of back pain that worsens at night and improves with NSAIDs. Scoliosis can develop secondarily, with the lesion located on the concave side of the spinal curvature.

Bony sclerosis of an osteoid osteoma of the posterior elements is usually not seen on plain radiographs. CT, in contrast, can accurately identify and localize the nidus and surrounding sclerosis, and thus considered the imaging modality of choice. However, the most sensitive technique for detection of suspected osteoid osteoma continues to be ^{99m}Tc bone scintigraphy, which shows marked uptake of bone tracer. Osteoid osteomas have a heterogeneous and variable appearance on MRI. The nidus is isointense on T1WI and hypointense on T2WI, with surrounding areas of enhancing marrow edema (Fig. 30.16). Paraspinal soft tissue edema may be present as well. MRI can also assess for spinal canal and spinal cord involvement.

Treatment options depend on the location of the lesion and include surgical excision or percutaneous ablation. CT-guided radiofrequency ablation is a minimally invasive and safe method that has proved to be an effective treatment. Lesions that cause nerve root compression usually require surgical resection.

Osteoblastoma

Osteoblastoma basically represents a giant osteoid osteoma, with a lytic nidus greater than 2 cm, and can measure up to 10 cm. This lesion is composed of fibrovascular stroma with osteoblasts, osteoid tissue, well-formed woven bone, and giant cells. Spinal osteoblastomas account for 40% of these tumors and affect the neural arch with potential extension to the vertebral body. A

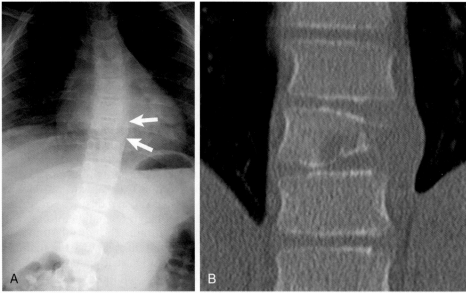

Fig. 30.14 Langerhans cell histiocytosis in a 10-year-old boy with history of painful thoracic levoscoliosis. Anteroposterior radiograph (A) and coronal computed tomography image (B) demonstrate decreased height of the left lateral aspect of the T9 vertebra with absent left pedicle and bony erosion. There is prominence of the left paraspinal soft tissues (*arrows*) and levoscoliosis. (C) Postcontrast sagittal T1-weighted image with fat saturation shows diffuse enhancement of T9. (D) Axial T1-weighted image with fat saturation shows enhancement of the vertebral body with associated left paraspinal enhancing soft tissue mass (*arrows*). There is extension of the mass into the spinal canal on the left with mild compression of the thecal sac (*small arrow*). (E) One-year follow-up. Sagittal short-tau inversion recovery image shows development of T9 vertebra plana. The adjacent intervertebral disks are preserved.

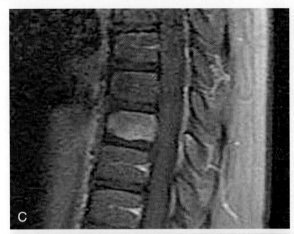

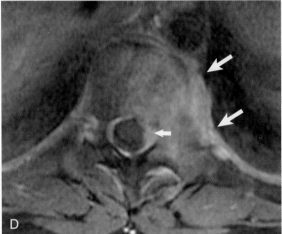

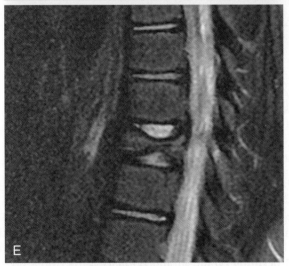

Fig. 30.14—cont'd

soft tissue mass may be present as well. These tumors have slow growth, cause bony destruction, and tend to recur. Clinical presentation often includes neurological deficits, as well as nocturnal back pain that is less severe than osteoid osteoma and does not respond to aspirin.

On imaging, osteoblastomas are lytic, expansile, geographic, destructive lesions, with multiple small internal calcifications and a thin sclerotic rim, with a lytic nidus measuring greater than 2 cm. This is best demonstrated with CT. On MRI, these lesions show variable signal intensity on T1WI and T2WI, and contrast enhancement can be lobular, marginal, or septal. Extension to the spinal canal and neuroforamina, as well as paraspinal soft tissue involvement, is best shown with MRI. Differential diagnosis includes osteosarcoma.

Treatment consists of curettage with bone graft or methylmethacrylate placement and preoperative embolization.

Ewing Sarcoma

Ewing sarcoma can present as a primary spinal tumor in 10% of cases, most often affecting the vertebral body, posterior elements, or sacrum. Occasionally, Ewing sarcoma presents as an extraosseous lesion in the epidural space.

Although local pain is the most common symptom, patients may report neurological deficits, such as muscle weakness, and sensory deficiencies at initial presentation. Bladder and bowel dysfunction tend to manifest later.

Ewing sarcoma presents as a permeative osteolytic lesion with a "moth-eaten" appearance on radiographs and CT. An associated soft tissue mass can be present in 50% of cases. MRI best shows soft tissue extension and invasion into the spinal canal. This tumor shows hypointense signal on T1WI and hyperintense signal on T2WI with moderate postcontrast enhancement. There is corresponding restricted diffusion due to its high nuclear/cytoplasmic ratio of tumor cells (Fig. 30.17). Differential diagnosis includes lymphoma and neuroblastoma. Metastatic disease can be seen in 25% of cases at presentation.

Treatment consists of neoadjuvant chemotherapy, as well as local control with radiation and/or surgery, and postoperative chemotherapy.

Lymphoma and Leukemia

Spinal involvement lymphoma is rare and may be the first form of presentation of disease, but most often it represents disseminated disease or relapse. Primary osseous lymphomas can be focal or diffuse appearing, and constitute 3% to 4% of all malignant bone tumors. Epidural mass presents in 4% of non-Hodgkin lymphomas (Fig. 30.18). Leukemia often presents with back pain together with constitutional symptoms, such as lethargy, fever, pallor, or unexplained bruising or bleeding. Children with acute myelogenous leukemia can present with an epidural solid spinal mass, known as granulocytic sarcoma (chloroma), which is a highly vascularized epidural mass. On MRI, these lesions are isointense to hyperintense on T1WI and isointense to hypointense on T2WI, and they show moderate-to-marked contrast enhancement. These tumors respond rapidly to chemotherapy.

Lymphoma and leukemia can also present as purely lytic or patchy sclerotic lesions, ivory vertebra, or vertebra plana (Fig. 30.19). The bone marrow in children with lymphoma and leukemia may show hypointense signal intensity on T1WI, unlike hyperintense T1 signal intensity seen in the bone marrow of healthy children. It

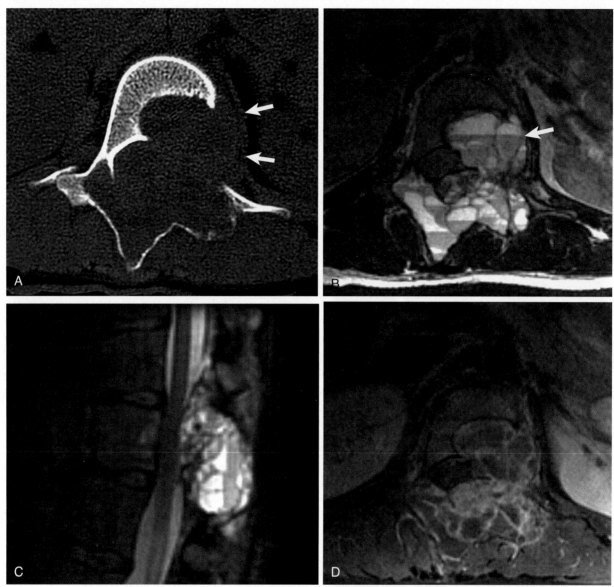

Fig. 30.15 Aneurysmal bone cyst in a teenager. (A) Axial computed tomography image of T12 demonstrates a large osteolytic mass lesion involving the body and posterior elements. There are extensive erosive changes of the vertebral body on the left side (*arrows*). (B) Axial T2-weighted image shows a large, multiloculated, cystic mass lesion involving the body and posterior elements of T12 with multiple fluid–fluid levels (*arrow*). (C) Sagittal T2-weighted image shows extension of the mass into the spinal canal, causing moderate compression of the spinal cord. (D) Postcontrast axial T1-weighted image with fat saturation shows septal enhancement of the multiloculated mass.

is unclear whether this is related to leukemic infiltration and/or increased bone marrow activity. This finding can be difficult to identify in children younger than 5 years because bone marrow may still have active hematopoiesis (red marrow), which typically exhibits low signal intensity on T1WI. Marrow contrast enhancement is also seen in patients with lymphoproliferative disease.

■ Intramedullary Tumors

Astrocytoma

Astrocytoma is the most common spinal cord tumor in children, accounting for 40% to 60% of intramedullary tumors. The most common histological types based on the WHO classification are low-grade astrocytomas: pilocytic astrocytoma (grade 1) and fibrillary astrocytoma (WHO grade 2), which occur in 80% to 90% of cases. High-grade neoplasms, anaplastic astrocytoma (grade 3) and glioblastoma (grade 4), are rare. Astrocytomas are slow-growing tumors that occur in the cervical and thoracic spinal cord and tend to be eccentrically located. Involvement of the entire cord, known as holocord tumor, also can occur.

Back pain is the most common symptom; however, motor deficits and scoliosis may be present as well.

Expansion and remodeling of the spinal canal can be well demonstrated with CT, MR, and occasionally with plain radiographs. On MRI, astrocytomas show cord expansion with cystic areas and necrosis and, rarely,

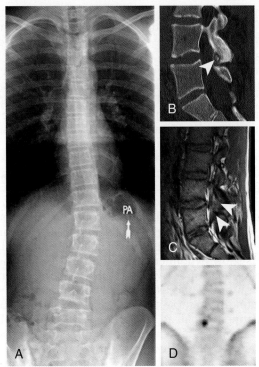

Fig. 30.16 Osteoid osteoma in a 13-year-old boy. (A) Anteroposterior radiograph of the entire spine shows focal levoscoliosis centered at T12/L1. Vertebral bodies are normal in height and shape with no osseous lesion identified. (B) Sagittal computed tomography (CT) image of the lower lumbar spine demonstrates a well-circumscribed low-attenuation lesion with a central hyperdensity within the right inferior L4 process with significant surrounding sclerosis and expansion (*arrowhead*). (C) Postcontrast sagittal T1-weighted image at the same level shows focal heterogeneous enhancement of the L4 inferior process (*arrowheads*). (D) Technetium-99m methylene diphosphonate single-photon emission CT coronal image shows corresponding increased radiotracer uptake of L4 on the right side.

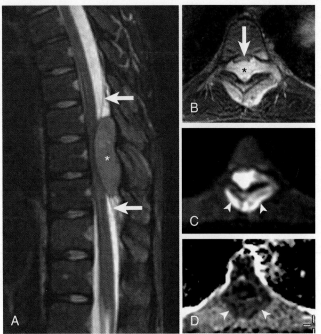

Fig. 30.17 Ewing sarcoma in a teenager. (A) Sagittal short-tau inversion recovery image of the midthoracic spine shows a well-circumscribed hypointense extradural mass within the posterior aspect of the spinal canal (*asterisk*) causing moderate anterior displacement and compression of the spinal cord. See hypointense dura (*arrows*). (B) Postcontrast axial T1-weighted image shows the enhancing mass within the spinal canal (*asterisk*) and surrounding the posterior elements. Again, significant anterior displacement and compression of the spinal cord (*arrow*) with intrinsic bright T2 signal are demonstrated. (C) Axial diffusion-weighted image shows decreased diffusivity (restricted diffusion) of this mass lesion (*arrowheads*) and corresponding hypointense signal on (D) apparent diffusion coefficient (ADC) map (*arrowheads*). These findings are consistent with a highly cellular malignant neoplasm.

hemorrhage involving several vertebral levels. These tumors show hypointense-to-isointense signal on T1WI and hyperintense signal on T2WI.

Edema or a syrinx may be seen above and below the level of the lesion. Intense contrast enhancement can be homogeneous or heterogeneous, partial, or diffuse (Fig. 30.20).

Differential diagnosis includes other intramedullary tumors, such as ependymoma, ganglioglioma, and hemangioblastoma; autoimmune or inflammatory myelitis; and rarely, vascular diseases, such as cord ischemia or infarction. Treatment mainly consists of gross total resection (GTR).

Ependymoma

Spinal ependymomas are rare tumors in children and can be seen in association with NF2. The WHO categorized ependymomas into three histological subtypes: grade I myxopapillary, grade II ependymoma, and grade III anaplastic ependymoma. Grade II ependymomas are slow-growing tumors that can affect any level of the spinal cord and present more frequently in adolescent boys. Ependymomas in patients with NF2 are usually low-grade gliomas that occur more often in the cervical

spinal cord, tend to have a more indolent course, and are often asymptomatic.

Ependymomas presumably originate from the ependymal cell remnants of the central canal and show circumferential and vertical growth along the central canal with expansion of the gray matter.

Associated osseous changes, such as spinal canal widening, posterior vertebral body scalloping, and widened interpediculate distance with thinning of the pedicles, can be identified on radiographs but are best evaluated with CT. Scoliosis can be seen occasionally. On MRI, ependymomas are well-circumscribed, expansile intramedullary lesions that show hypointense or isointense signal on T1WI and T2 hyperintense signal on T2WI. Hemorrhage and cysts can be present. Hemosiderin deposition may be seen in the cranial and caudal margins of the lesion, the so-called cap sign, in less than 20% of cases. The solid components of the lesion show intense contrast enhancement.

The treatment goal is gross total resection (GTR). However, recurrence may occur even after achieving GTR. The role of adjuvant radiation is still a matter of debate: some studies recommend postoperative radiation therapy in cases of subtotal resection, but not GTR, whereas others advocate for postoperative radiation therapy after GTR.

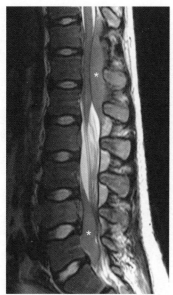

Fig. 30.18 Burkitt lymphoma in a 13-year-old boy. Sagittal T2-weighted image with fat saturation of the thoracolumbar spine shows two well-circumscribed intraspinal, extradural low T2-hypointense mass lesions (*asterisk*) with mild remodeling of the adjacent osseous structures. The more superior mass is centered at the T11-L1 level, causing moderate compression of the spinal cord. The lower mass lesion extends from L4 to S1 (*asterisk*), and causes mass effect on the distal cauda equina nerve roots. In addition, there is abnormally increased T2 signal of the L4 vertebral body.

Myxopapillary ependymoma, a WHO grade I tumor, may originate from the conus medullaris, terminal filum, or cauda equine, and it accounts for 13% of all spinal ependymomas. Although these tumors are considered benign, they tend to be more aggressive in children than in adults. Craniospinal dissemination may be seen at presentation. Tumor spread may occur via the subarachnoid space, invade locally, or metastasize outside the central nervous system. Mean age of presentation is 13 years with a male predominance. Back pain is a common symptom that can present with neurological deficits, such as motor, sensory, urinary, and gait abnormalities.

MRI findings of myxopapillary ependymoma include intradural extramedullary thoracolumbar mass spanning several vertebral levels in the lumbosacral canal and often with additional mass in the distal thecal sac. These tumors show hypointense signal on T1WI, show hyperintense signal on T2WI, and enhance homogeneously with contrast. Remodeling of the adjacent bone is a frequent finding in these slow-growing tumors (Fig. 30.21).

Treatment goal is GTR. However, myxopapillary ependymomas show a high rate of recurrence (50%) even after GTR. Adjuvant radiotherapy seems to play a key role in improving recurrence-free survival in patients with myxopapillary ependymoma in the first two decades of life.

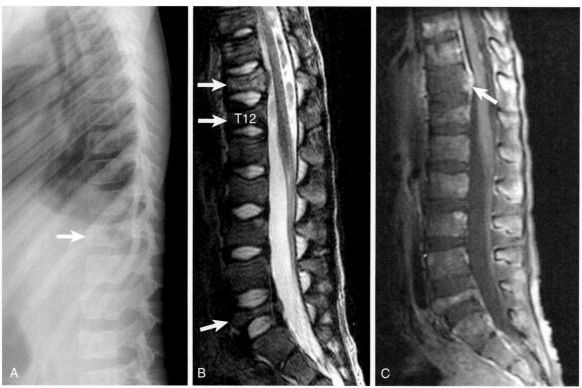

Fig. 30.19 Acute leukemia in 7-year-old boy. (A) Lateral radiograph of the thoracic spine shows moderate height loss of T12 with depression of its superior end plate (*arrow*). There is height loss of other vertebrae, including T5-T9, T11, and L3. (B) Sagittal short-tau inversion recovery image shows vertebral body height loss at multiple levels and L5 vertebra plana (*arrows*). (C) Postcontrast sagittal T1-weighted image with fat saturation shows dark signal of the T12 vertebral body with patchy enhancement posteriorly and along the adjacent dura (*arrow*).

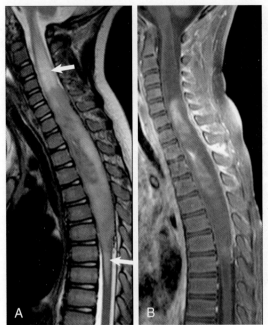

Fig. 30.20 Spinal astrocytoma in a 5-year-old boy. (A) Sagittal T2-weighted image of the cervical-thoracic spine shows a large intramedullary, expansile heterogeneous bright lesion from C5-T7. Above and below this level there is increased T2 signal of the cord, consistent with perilesional edema (*arrows*). There is expansion and remodeling of the spinal canal. (B) Postcontrast sagittal T1-weighted image with fat saturation shows heterogeneous patchy enhancement of the central portion of the intramedullary mass.

■ Extramedullary Intradural Tumors

Schwannoma

Spinal schwannomas are rare tumors in children that present as solitary tumors or may be multiple when associated with schwannomatosis or NF2. Schwannomatosis is the third major form of neurofibromatosis and is characterized by the development of multiple schwannomas in the spine or elsewhere in the body in the absence of bilateral vestibular schwannomas. The causative gene remains undetermined. It can be at times difficult to differentiate schwannomatosis from NF2 based on clinical manifestations. Spinal schwannomas of patients with NF2 appear to be more aggressive than those in patients with solitary schwannomas and schwannomatosis. Clinical presentation of schwannomas most often consists of pain and paresthesias; however, these can be asymptomatic as well. In schwannomatosis, chronic pain (68%) and recurrent headaches (28%) are the two most common presenting symptoms.

Solitary spinal schwannomas tend to occur in the high cervical and thoracolumbar levels, whereas tumors in schwannomatosis occur most often in the lumbar area.

Solitary schwannomas are well-circumscribed dumbbell-shaped masses within an enlarged neural foramen and are most often extramedullary intradural (75%). Bone remodeling with vertebral body scalloping can be seen as well. On MRI, this tumor is typically isointense on T1WI, is hyperintense on T2WI, and shows intense

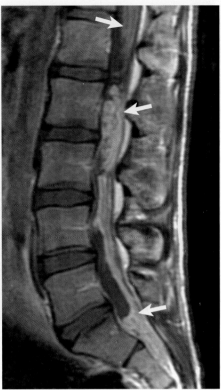

Fig. 30.21 Myxopapillary ependymoma in a 17-year-old boy. Postcontrast sagittal T1-weighted image of the lumbar spine shows an intradural, extramedullary enhancing mass lesion centered at L2 (*middle arrow*) and another mass at S1 and S2 (*bottom arrow*), consistent with neoplasm. Clumping and enhancement of the cauda equina nerve roots is seen between the mass lesions from L3 to L5. The distal spinal cord (conus medullaris) preserves normal caliber and signal intensity (*top arrow*).

contrast enhancement (Fig. 30.22). However, signal may be variable because of the two different cell types: Antoni A (compact) and Antoni B (less compact), with cystic degeneration. Rarely hemorrhage can be present as well.

In NF2 and schwannomatosis, these tumors present as multiple, well-circumscribed, subcentimeter diameter nodules that show isointense signal on T1WI and T2WI and enhance with contrast in the cervical and thoracic spinal canal and along the course of the cauda equina nerve roots. The differential diagnosis for nodules within the spinal canal and along the cauda equina nerve roots includes multiple schwannomas, neurofibromas, or metastatic disease.

Most tumors can be treated successfully with surgery. However, prognosis varies among spinal schwannomas of schwannomatosis, because some patients may need multiple operations as a result of newly developed schwannomas.

Meningioma

Spinal meningiomas are rare and account for about 4% of all spinal tumors, mostly affecting the cervical or thoracic spine. These are mainly intradural-extramedullary in location, although extradural tumors can occur

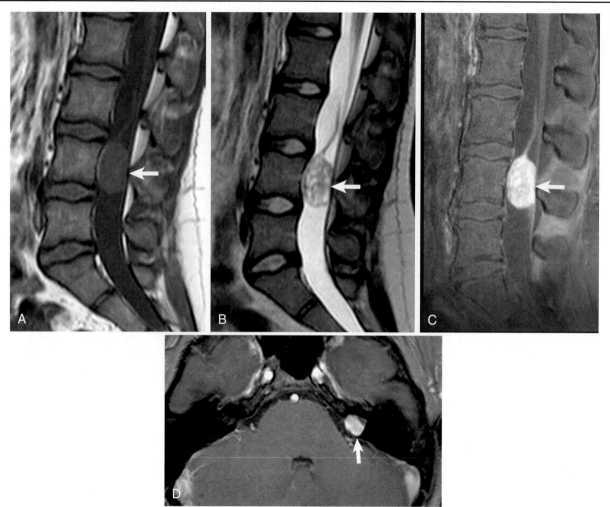

Fig. 30.22 Spinal schwannoma in a 13-year-old girl. (A) Sagittal T1-weighted image shows an oval, extramedullary mass centered at L4 (*arrow*) with mild remodeling of the posterior aspect of the vertebral body. (B) Sagittal T2-weighted image shows heterogeneous bright signal of the mass (*arrow*) and mass effect on the adjacent cauda equina nerve roots. (C) Postcontrast sagittal T1-weighted image shows diffuse, intense enhancement of the spinal mass (*arrow*). (D) Postcontrast axial T1-weighted image with fat saturation at the level of the internal auditory canals of the same patient shows an expansile, well-circumscribed, enhancing mass lesion within the left internal auditory canal consistent with acoustic schwannoma in this patient with neurofibromatosis type 2 (*arrow*).

as well. The most common histological subtypes are psammomatous and fibroblastic meningiomas. Spinal meningiomas in children are often associated with NF2 in which case they may present with multiple spinal lesions, and are frequently associated with vestibular schwannomas. There is a slight male predominance in children with NF2. Prognosis in children with NF2 is lower compared with patients with isolated meningioma, due to difficulty in resecting and treating multiple lesions, and their tendency to recur.

Back pain is the most frequent presenting symptom, and is usually followed by neurological deficits such as limb weakness, gait disturbance, and urinary incontinence. Occasionally patients may present with painful, progressive scoliosis.

On imaging these tumors are well-circumscribed masses which show isointense or hypointense signal on T1WI, and mild hyper intense or isointense signal on T2WI relative to the spinal cord. Contrast enhancement is diffuse and intense. These lesions cannot be differ-entiated from schwannomas by imaging characteristics (Fig. 30.23).

Treatment goal is total resection with dural clearance. Radiation treatment is controversial and mostly avoided in children. Tumor recurrence depends on the extent of resection and pathological subtype.

■ Summary

The prevalence of back pain in children has increased, especially among adolescents. Most pediatric back pain is mechanical and responds to conservative treatment without requiring imaging. Identification of clinical *red flags* will allow the clinician determine the need for evaluation with imaging studies. Evaluation typically begins with radiographs. Subsequent evaluation with advanced imaging (CT, MRI or bone scintigraphy) depends on the clinical presentation, suspected underlying pathology, child's age, and exposure to radiation. In addition to

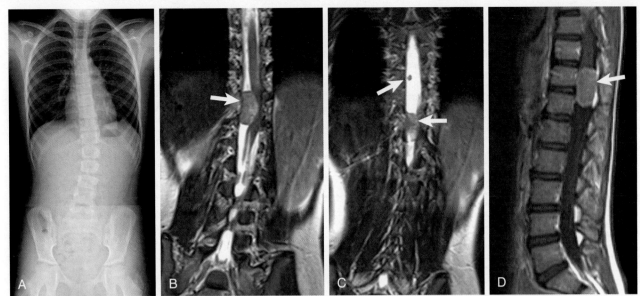

Fig. 30.23 Meningioma in a 9-year-old girl with a history of painful, progressive levoscoliosis. (A) Anteroposterior view of the entire spine shows atypical levoscoliosis centered at the thoracolumbar junction. (B) Coronal T2-weighted image shows an intradural extramedullary mass lesion centered at T11/12 level with hypointense T2 signal, causing compression of the distal spinal cord (*arrow*). (C) Coronal T2-weighted image demonstrates a smaller, round hypointense lesion at the T9 level consistent with a synchronous lesion (*top arrow*). (D) Postcontrast sagittal T1-weighted image shows increased enhancement of this mass with mild adjacent dural enhancement (*arrow*). Bilateral acoustic schwannomas were also present in this patient with neurofibromatosis type 2 (not shown).

common causes of pediatric back pain like spondylolysis, more serious conditions such as infectious, inflammatory, and neoplastic disorders may occur in children.

■ Acknowledgments

I acknowledge Brad Hoehne, Radiology Digital Imaging Specialist (Nationwide Children's Hospital), for preparation of figures.

Bibliography

Aartun, E., Degerfalk, A., Kentsdotter, L., & Hestbaek, L. (2014a). Screening of the spine in adolescents: Inter- and intra-rater reliability and measurement error of commonly used clinical tests. *BMC Musculoskeletal Disorders*, 10(15), 37.

Aartun, E., Hartvigsen, J., Wedderkopp, N., & Hestbaek, L. (2014b). Spinal pain in adolescents: Prevalence, incidence, and course: A school-based two-year prospective cohort study in 1,300 Danes aged 11-13. *BMC Musculoskeletal Disorders*, 29(15), 187.

Altaf, F., Heran, M. K., & Wilson, L. F. (2014). Back pain in children and adolescents. *Bone Joint J.*, 96-B(6), 717–723.

Ardern-Holmes, S., Fisher, G., & North, K. (2017). Neurofibromatosis type 2. *Journal of Child Neurology*, 32(1), 9–22.

Auerbach, J. D., Ahn, J., Zgonis, M. H., Reddy, S. C., Ecker, M. L., & Flynn, J. M. (2008). Streamlining the evaluation of low back pain in children. *Clinical Orthopaedics and Related Research*, 466(8), 1971–1977.

Beck, N. A., Miller, R., Baldwin, K., et al. (2013). Do oblique views add value in the diagnosis of spondylolysis in adolescents? *Journal of Bone and Joint Surgery American Volume*, 95(10), e65.

Booth, T. N., Iyer, R. S., Falcone, R. A., Jr., Hayes, L. L., Jones, J. Y., Kadom, N., et al. (2017). ACR appropriateness Criteria® back pain-child. *Expert Panel on Pediatric Imaging Am Coll Radiol*, 14(5S), S13–S24.

Boriani, S., Lo, S. F., Puvanesarajah, V., et al. (2014). Aneurysmal bone cysts of the spine: Treatment options and considerations. *Journal of Neuro-oncology*, 120(1), 171–178.

Burton, A. K., Clarke, R. D., McClune, T. D., & Tillotson, K. M. (1996). The natural history of low back pain in adolescents. *Spine*, 21(20), 2323–2328.

Davis, P. J., & Williams, H. J. (2008). The investigation and management of back pain in children. *Archives of Disease in Childhood - Education and Practice*, 93(3), 73–83.

Fadell, M. F., Gralla, J., Bercha, I., et al. (2015). CT outperforms radiographs at a comparable radiation dose in the assessment for spondylolysis. *Pediatric Radiology*, 45(7), 1026–1030.

Falip, C., Alison, M., Boutry, N., et al. (2013). Chronic recurrent multifocal osteomyelitis (CRMO): A longitudinal case series review. *Pediatric Radiology*, 43(3), 355–375.

Feldman, D. S., Straight, J. J., Badra, M. I., Mohaideen, A., & Madan, S. S. (2006). Evaluation of an algorithmic approach to pediatric back pain. *Journal of Pediatric Orthopedics*, 26(3), 353–357.

Giedion, A., Holthusen, W., Masel, L. F., & Vischer, D. (1972). Subacute and chronic "symmetrical" osteomyelitis. *Ann Radiol*, 15(3), 329–342.

Hawkins, M., Langendoerfer, M., von Kalle, T., Maier, J., & Bolton, M. (2013). Pediatric spinal epidural abscess: A 9-year institutional review and review of the literature. *Pediatrics*, 132(6), e1680–e1685.

Hospach, T. , & Langendoerfer, M. , von Kalle, T., Maier, J., & Dannecker, G. E. (2010). Spinal involvement in chronic recurrent multifocal osteomyelitis (CRMO) in childhood and effect of pamidronate. *European Journal of Pediatrics*, 169(9), 1105–1111.

James, S. L., & Davies, A. M. (2006). Imaging of infectious spinal disorders in children and adults. *European Journal of Radiology*, 58(1), 27–40.

Jones, G. T., & Macfarlane, G. J. (2005). Epidemiology of low back pain in children and adolescents. *Archives of Disease in Childhood*, 90(3), 312–316.

Khalatbari, M. R., Wedderkopp, N., Korsholm, L., & Moharamzad, Y. (2012). Discal cyst in pediatric patients: Case report and review of the literature. *Neuropediatrics*, 43(5), 289–292.

Kjaer, P., Wedderkopp, N., Korsholm, L. , & Leboeuf-Yde, C. (2011). Prevalence and tracking of back pain from childhood to adolescence. *BMC Musculoskeletal Disorders*, 12(4), 98–407.

Kukreja, S., Ambekar, S., Sin, A. H., & Nanda, A. (2014). Cumulative survival analysis of patients with spinal myxopapillary ependymomas in the first 2 decades of life. *Journal of Neurosurgery: Pediatrics*, 13(4), 400–407.

Kutluk, T., & Varan, A. , Kafali, C., et al. (2015). Pediatric intramedullary spinal cord tumors: A single center experience. *European Journal of Paediatric Neurology*, 19(1), 41–47.

Leboeuf-Yde, C., & Kyvik, K. O. (1998). At what age does low back pain become a common problem? A study of 29,424 individuals aged 12-41 years. *Spine*, 23(2), 228–234.

Ledonio, C. G., Burton, D. C., Crawford, C. H., 3rd., et al. (2017). Current evidence regarding diagnostic imaging methods for pediatric lumbar spondylolysis: A report from the scoliosis research society evidence-based medicine committee. *Spine Deform.*, 5(2), 97–101.

Lin, N., Schirmer, C. M., Lidov, H. G., Scott, R. M., & Proctor, M. R. (2011). Presentation and progression of a disc cyst in a pediatric patient. *Journal of Neurosurgery: Pediatrics*, 7(2), 209–212.

Lohani, S. , Rodriguez, D. P., Lidov, H. G., Scott, R. M., & Proctor, M. R. (2013). Intrasacral meningocele in the pediatric population. *Journal of Neurosurgery: Pediatrics, 11*(6), 615–622.

Luksik, A. S., Garzon-Muvdi, T. , Yang, W. , Huang, J., Flynn, J. M., & Jallo, G. I. (2017). Pediatric spinal cord astrocytomas: A retrospective study of 348 patients from the seer database. *Journal of Neurosurgery: Pediatrics, 19*(6), 711–719.

Miller, R., Beck, N. A., Sampson, N. R., Zhu, X., Flynn, J. M., & Drummond, D. (2013). Imaging modalities for low back pain in children: A review of spondyloysis and undiagnosed mechanical back pain. *Journal of Pediatric Orthopedics, 33*(3), 282–288.

Ramirez, N. , & Flynn, J. M., Hill, B. W., et al. (2015). Evaluation of a systematic approach to pediatric back pain: The utility of magnetic resonance imaging. *Journal of Pediatric Orthopedics, 35*(1), 28–32.

Rodriguez, D. P., & Poussaint, T. Y., Mase, Y. (2010). Imaging of back pain in children. *AJNR American Journal of Neuroradiology, 31*(5), 787–802.

Sairyo, K. , & Sakai, T., Mase, Y., et al. (2011). Painful lumbar spondylolysis among pediatric sports players: A pilot MRI study. *Archives of Orthopaedic and Trauma Surgery, 131*(11), 1485–1489.

Shah, S. A., Mitra, A., Cochrane, D., & Saller, J. (2016). Evaluation and diagnosis of back pain in children and adolescents. *Journal of the American Academy of Orthopaedic Surgeons, 24*(1), 37–45.

Singhal, A. , Mitra, A. , Cochrane, D. , & Steinbok, P. (2013). Ring apophysis fracture in pediatric lumbar disc herniation: A common entity. *Pediatric Neurosurgery, 49*(1), 16–20.

The World Health Organization (WHO). (2020). Classification of Soft Tissue and Bone Tumours, 5th Edition, Volume 3.

Thomas, A. K., Egelhoff, J. C., & Curran, J. G., & Thomas, B. (2016). Pediatric schwannomatosis, a rare but distinct form of neurofibromatosis. *Pediatric Radiology, 46*(3), 430–435.

Trout, A. T., Sharp, S. E., Anton, C. G., Gelfand, M. J., & Mehlman, C. T. (2015). Spondylolysis and beyond: Value of SPECT/CT in evaluation of low back pain in children and young adults. *RadioGraphics, 35*(3), 819–834.

Tsutsumi, S., Yasumoto, Y., Luo, C., Ai, F., & Ito, M. (2011). Idiopathic intervertebral disk calcification in childhood: A case report and review of literature. *Child's Nervous System, 27*(7), 1045–1051.

Wang, X. Q., Zeng, X. W., Zhang, B. Y., Jernigan, S., Hedequist, D., & Proctor, M. R., et al. (2012). Spinal meningioma in childhood: Clinical features and treatment. *Child's Nervous System, 28*(1), 129–136.

Yao, W., Mai, X., Luo, C., Ai, F., & Chen, Q. (2011). A cross-sectional survey of nonspecific low back pain among 2083 schoolchildren in China. *Spine, 36*(22), 1885–1890.

Zenonos, G., Jamil, O., Governale, L. S., Jernigan, S., Hedequist, D., & Proctor, M. R. (2012). Surgical treatment for primary spinal aneurysmal bone cysts: Experience from Children's Hospital Boston. *Journal of Neurosurgery: Pediatrics, 9*(3), 305–315.

INDEX

Note: Page numbers followed by "b" indicate boxes, those followed by "f" indicate figures, and those followed by "t" indicate tables.

A

AARS. *See* Atlantoaxial rotary subluxation (AARS)
ABC. *See* Aneurysmal bone cyst (ABC)
Abdomen. *See also* Fetal abdomen and pelvis.
  obstructed bowel, 390–391, 390f
  plain film pitfalls, 391–392
  postnatal imaging, 393–394
  radiograph, 392–393
Abdominal cyst
  choledochal cysts, 393, 393f
  duplication cysts, 392f, 393
  large ovarian cysts, 393
  lymphatic malformation, 393
  midline cyst, 393
Abdominal masses
  in children older than 1 year
    germ cell tumors, 142–144
    hepatic masses, 140–142
    lymphoma, 144–146
    neuroblastoma, 140
    renal masses, 136–140
    rhabdomyosarcoma, 144
    soft tissue sarcomas, 144
  computed tomography, 127–128
  differential diagnosis, 128
  gastrointestinal tract masses, 131–135
    bowel-related masses, 133–135
    hepatobiliary masses, 131–133
  infradiaphragmatic pulmonary sequestration, 135, 137f
  lymphatic malformations, 135
  magnetic resonance imaging (MRI), 127–128
  neonates/infants
    adrenal masses, 130, 130f
    cystic renal diseases, 128, 128f–129f
    ovarian and uterine masses, 130–131, 131f
    renal masses, 128–129
  palpable, 127
  sacrococcygeal teratoma, 135–136, 137f
  symptoms, 127
  ultrasound (US), 127–128
Abdominal pain
  age-based differential considerations
    infants, 101
    older children and teenagers, 103
    toddlers and school-age children, 101–103
  diagnostic etiologies
    appendicitis, 106–108, 108f
    colonic volvulus, 104, 105f
    constipation, 124–125, 125f
    gastroenteritis, 108–109
    hemolytic uremic syndrome (HUS), 118, 120f
    Henoch-Schönlein purpura (HSP), 116–118, 119f

Abdominal pain *(Continued)*
    inflammatory bowel disease (IBD), 118–120, 121f
    intussusception, 104–106
    malrotation/midgut volvulus, 103–104, 103f–104f
    Meckel diverticulum, 109–110
    mesenteric adenitis, 110, 112f
    pancreatitis, 113–116, 115f
    pneumonia, 112
    trauma, 121–124
    urinary tract infections (UTIs), 110–112
  etiology, 98–99, 99t
  gas pattern
    ileus, 100, 101f
    normal, 100, 100f–101f
    obstruction, 100
  history and physical examination, 98–99
  radiography, 98–99, 99t
Abdominal situs, 11f
Aberrant thymus, 36–37, 36f
Abusive head trauma (AHT)
  administering gadolinium, 409
  causes, 396–397
  child protection team (CPT), 397
  clinical outcomes, 398
  computed tomography (CT), 408, 407–408, 409f–410f
  definition, 396
  features, 396
  follow-up, 409–410
  healthcare professionals, 397
  imaging, 398, 398f–399f
  incidence, 396
  magnetic resonance imaging (MRI), 408
  mechanisms of injury, 397
  parenchymal brain injury, 404–405, 406f–407f
  radiologist's role, 397
  red flags, 396
  retinal hemorrhages, 406, 408f
  risk of, 397
  signs and symptoms, 396
  skull fractures, 399, 399f–400f
  subarachnoid and intraventricular hemorrhage, 404
  subdural and epidural hematomas
    appearance, 400–402, 401f–403f
    birth-related SDHs, 404
    causes, 400, 401f
    characteristics, 404
    convexity, 404
    enlarged low-density extraaxial spaces, 404
    hematohygromas, 402–403, 405f
    heterogeneous-appearing, 403–404
    injury dating, 404

Abusive head trauma (AHT) *(Continued)*
    membrane, 404
    retroclival subdural/epidural collections, 404
  suspected abuse, 397
  triggers, 397
  ultrasonography, 409
Abusive spine trauma
  clinical outcomes, 411
  clinical presentation, 410
  differential diagnosis, 413
  fracture-subluxations, 411–413, 411f–413f
  imaging, 411–414
  mechanisms of injury, 410
  prevalence, 410
  spinal cord and soft tissue injury, 413, 414f
  spinal fractures, 411–413, 411f–413f
  subdural and epidural hematomas, 413
Accidental caustic ingestion, 519
Achondroplasia, 240, 243f, 576, 576f
Acquired thymic cysts, 37
Acrocephalosyndactyly, 236, 237f
ACS. *See* Acute chest syndrome (ACS)
Acute arterial stroke, 496, 496f
Acute bilateral L2 spondylolysis, 595, 598f
Acute chest syndrome (ACS), 21–22
  chest CT, 22
  diagnostic criteria, 22
  pathophysiology, 22
  recurrent episodes, 22
  sickle cell disease, 21
Acute L5 spondylolysis, 595, 596f
Acute laryngotracheitis, 515
Acute pulmonary exacerbation, cystic fibrosis, 29f
Acute scrotum, ultrasound
  anatomy and appearance, 152, 153f
  diagnostic work-up, 152–154
  differential diagnosis, 155t
  nontwisted spermatic cord, 155–161
  normal spermatic cord, 153f
  technetium-99m scrotal scintigraphy, 151
  testicles, 151–152
Acute testicular torsion, 156f
Adenoids, 512–514, 514f
Adnexal torsion, 196–197
Adolescents
  aggressive
    osteosarcoma, 299
    primary lymphoma of bone, 301
  nonaggressive
    aneurysmal bone cyst (ABCs), 311–312
    chondroblastoma, 304–305
    chondromyxoid fibroma, 307–308

Adolescents *(Continued)*
    distal femoral avulsive irregularity, 308
    enchondromas, 305–306
    fibrous dysplasia, 302–304
    fibroxanthomas, 306–307
    osteoid osteoma/osteoblastoma, 308–310
    osteosarcoma, 301
    simple (unicameral) bone cyst, 310–311
Adrenal masses, 130, 130f
AEC. *See* Automatic exposure control (AEC)
Aggressive lesions, bone
    adolescents, 288b
    children, 288b
    infants and toddlers, 287b
AHL. *See* Anterior humeral line (AHL)
AHT. *See* Abusive head trauma (AHT)
Alar ligament, 555–556
Alveolar growth abnormalities, 380–381
Alveolar soft part sarcoma (ASPA), 333
Ameloblastoma, 538
Anal atresia, 460, 464f
Andersonian terminology, 55, 57f, 58
Aneurysmal bone cyst (ABC), 311–312, 312f, 605–606, 608f
Angiogenesis, 25–26
Angiographic classification, arteriovenous malformations (AVMs), 321t
Annular pancreas, 83, 85f
Anophthalmia/microphthalmia, 486, 486f
Anterior atlantooccipital (AAO) membranes, 556
Anterior humeral line (AHL), 269–270, 270f
Anterior neck masses
    branchial apparatus and remnants, 539
    branchial apparatus cysts, 539–540, 540f
    cyst near midline, 538–539, 539f
    cystic lesions, 538
    ear, 539
    ectopic thyroid tissue, 541, 541f
    foregut structure, 540, 541f
    lower neck, 540
    lymph node, 541–542, 543f
    "starry sky" appearance, 541, 542f
    thyroid carcinoma, 541
    thyroid gland, 540
Anterior pneumothorax, 382f
Anteroposterior renal pelvic diameter (APRPD), 172f–173f, 173–174
Anticongestive therapy, Shone complex, 73, 73f
Antrochoanal polyp, 518
Aorta, 58
Aortic arch anomalies, 47
    coarctation of the aorta (COA), 73–75
    interrupted aortic arch, 73–75
    vascular rings, 75–76
Aortic arch sidedness, 4–5
Apical ligament, 556
Apical lordotic technique, 369, 369f
Apophysis, 347
Appendicitis, 103
Appendicoliths, 108
Appendix epididymis, 156
Appendix testis, 160f
APRPD. *See* Anteroposterior renal pelvic diameter (APRPD)

Aqueductal stenosis, 475, 476f
Arachnoid cyst, 478, 479f
Arteriovenous fistula (AVF), 322f, 484–485
Arteriovenous malformations (AVMs), 316–317, 320f–321f, 343, 484–485
Aseptic synovitis, 229
ASPA. *See* Alveolar soft part sarcoma (ASPA)
Aspirated foreign body
    chest radiograph
        focal atelectasis, 20, 25f
        left mainstem bronchus, 20, 25f–26f
        linear radiopaque foreign body, 20, 24f
    incidence, 19
    large foreign bodies, 20
    nonorganic foreign bodies, 20
    smaller foreign bodies, 20
Asthma, 11–12
Astrocytoma, 608–609, 611f
Asymmetrical smaller lung, 382–385
Atlantoaxial rotary subluxation (AARS), 565–567
Atlantodental interval (ADI), 560, 561f
Atlantooccipital dislocation (AOD)/ craniocervical dissociation, 562, 563f–567f, 563b
Atrial arrangement/situs, 55, 56f–57f
Atrial septal defects (ASDs)
    cardiac magnetic resonance (CMR), 60–61, 61f
    clinical presentation, 60
    echocardiography, 60
    morphology, 60
    pathophysiology, 60
    primum, 60
    secundum, 60
    sinus venosus defects, 60
    treatment, 61–62
Atrioventricular connections, 58–59, 59f
Atrioventricular septal defect (AVSD), 58–59
    clinical presentation, 65
    complete, 64
    imaging, 65, 65f–66f
    incidence, 64
    incomplete, 64
    morphology and pathophysiology, 64–65
    transitional, 64
    treatment, 65
Atypical hemolytic uremic syndrome (HUS), 118
Autoimmune diseases, 519, 520f
Automatic exposure control (AEC), 434, 438, 438f
Autosomal dominant polycystic kidney disease, 128
Autosomal recessive polycystic kidney disease, 128, 129f, 462, 466f
AVF. *See* Arteriovenous fistula (AVF)
Avian spur, 279–280
AVMs. *See* Arteriovenous malformations (AVMs)
AVSD. *See* Atrioventricular septal defect (AVSD)

B
Back pain
    clinical evaluation, 593
    clinical history, 592
    epidemiology, 592, 593t

Back pain *(Continued)*
    extramedullary intradural tumors
        meningioma, 611–612, 613f
        schwannomas, 611, 612f
    imaging evaluation, 593
    infectious disorders
        chronic recurrent multifocal osteomyelitis/chronic noninfectious osteomyelitis, 603–604, 605f
        epidural abscess, 602, 604f
        spondylodiskitis, 601–602, 602f–603f
    intramedullary tumors
        astrocytoma, 608–609, 611f
        ependymomas, 609–610, 611f
    neoplastic disorders, 604
    radiographs
        computed tomography (CT), 594
        disk calcification, 595–596, 599f
        disk cysts, 601, 601f
        disk degeneration and herniation, 600
        magnetic resonance imaging (MRI), 594
        sacral meningocele, 598–600, 600f
        scheuermann disease/kyphosis, 596–598, 599f
        spondylolysis and spondylolisthesis, 594–595, 595f–598f
    spinal column tumors
        aneurysmal bone cyst (ABC), 605–606, 608f
        Ewing sarcoma, 607, 609f
        Langerhans cell histiocytosis (LCH), 604–605, 606f–607f
        leukemia and lymphoma, 607–608, 610f
        osteoblastoma, 606–607
        osteoid osteoma, 606, 609f
Bacterial pneumonia
    chest radiograph
        airspace opacity and consolidation, 14
        Chlamydia trachomatis pneumonia, 15, 19f
        community-acquired bacterial pneumonia (CAP), 15f
        empyema, 16
        intrapulmonary abscess, 23f–24f
        lobar bacterial pneumonia, 16f
        necrotizing pneumonia, 16–19, 22f
        round pneumonia, 14–15, 17f
        segmental bacterial pneumonia, 17f
        silhouette sign, 14, 16f
        sterile parapneumonic effusion, 15–16
    computed tomography, 22f
        early necrotizing pneumonia, 22f
        intrapulmonary abscess, 23f–24f
    tachypnea, 14
    ultrasound, 16
Bacterial tracheitis, 515–516, 517f
BAI. *See* Basion-axial interval (BAI)
Baker cyst, 328–329, 330f
Basal cell nevus syndrome, 503, 503f
Basion-axial interval (BAI), 563
Basion-dens interval (BDI), 563
BDI. *See* Basion-dens interval (BDI)
Benign enlargement of the subarachnoid space (BESS), 500, 500f
Bilateral intratesticular solid masses, 167

Bilious vomiting
  bedside upper gastrointestinal series, 90–91, 91f
  midgut malrotation, 82, 83f–84f
  newborn infant, 81–86
  obstruction, 82
Biparietal diameter (BPD), 474
Biventricular atrioventricular connections, 58–59, 59f
Bladder outlet obstructions
  congenital anomaly, 188
  full urinary bladder, 191f
  genitourinary anomalies, 189–191
  increased intravesical pressure, 186
  posterior urethral valves (PUV), 188
  Prune belly, 188–189, 193f
  reflux, 186
Blount disease, 246
Bone anatomy, 346–347, 347f
Bone lesions
  adolescents, 288, 288b
  benign/nonaggressive lesions, 286
  children, 287
  chronological age, 287–288, 287b
  computed tomography (CT), 287
  diagnostic challenge, 286
  diagnostic questions, 287b
  host bone
    axial plane, 289–290, 289b
    bone destruction patterns, 291
    calcaneal lesion, 288, 288b
    hemangioma, 288
    legion margins, 290
    longitudinal plane, 288–289, 289f
    matrix and mineralization, 292
    osteosarcoma, 288
    periosteal reaction, 290–292
    soft tissue component, 292
  infants and toddlers, 287
  magnetic resonance imaging (MRI), 287
  nuclear medicine bone scintigraphy, 287
  radiographs, 286
  single/multiple lesions
    adolescents, 299–312
    children, 298–299
    infants and toddlers, 292–298
  tumor-like, 286
Bone mineral density, 244–246, 252f
Bones evaluation
  congenital abnormalities, 4, 6f
  lung inflation, 4, 5f
  nonaccidental trauma, 4, 6f
  posteroanterior (PA) chest radiograph, 4
Bowel obstruction, 102
Bowel-related masses
  enteric duplication cysts, 133–135, 135f
  meconium pseudocysts, 135, 136f
BPD. See Biparietal diameter (BPD)
BPS. See Bronchopulmonary sequestration (BPS)
Branchial apparatus cysts, 539–540, 540f
Brodie abscess, 295
Bronchial artery hypertrophy, cystic fibrosis (CF), 30f
Bronchiectasis, 23
Bronchogenic cyst, 48–49, 452–453, 456f
Bronchomalacia, 372–373
Bronchopulmonary malformations (BPMs), 382
Bronchopulmonary sequestration (BPS)
  extralobar, 386, 387f
  intralobar, 388f

Bronchoscopy, 25–26
Buckle fracture, 347–348, 348f
Buckled appearance, thoracic trachea, 4f
Bunk-bed fractures, 224, 225f
Burkitt lymphoma, 146, 607, 610f

C
C1 vertebra fractures, 568–570, 569f
C2 vertebra fractures
  Hangman fracture, 569f, 570
  odontoid fractures, 573
  synchondrosal fractures, 570–573, 570f–571f
Café-au-lait lesions, 303–304
Calcaneal lesion, 288, 288b
Calcaneus positioning, 256
Campomelic dysplasia, 239, 241f
Capillary malformations (CMs), 313
Capitellum, radial head, internal (medial) epicondyle, trochlea, olecranon, external (lateral) epicondyle (CRITOE), 268–269, 268b–269b, 269f–270f
CAPTA. See Child Abuse Prevention and Treatment Act (CAPTA)
Carcinoma, thymus, 37–39
Cardiac magnetic resonance (CMR)
  atrial septal defects (ASD), 60–61, 61f
  coarctation of the aorta (COA), 75f
  double-outlet right ventricle, 70, 71f
  hypoplastic left heart syndrome, 72
  interrupted aortic arch, 75f
  Shone complex, 73, 73f
  tetralogy of fallot (TOF), 69, 69f
  transposition of the great arteries (TGA), 67
  vascular rings, 76f
  ventricular septal defects (VSDs), 63–64
Cardiac position, 54
Cardiac segments, morphological identification
  atrial identification
    atrial arrangement/situs, 55, 56f–57f
    great arterial arrangement, 58
    great arterial identification, 58, 58f
    inferior vena cava (IVC), 55
    left atrium (LA), 55, 55f
    right atrium, 55, 55f
    ventricular identification, 55–57, 57f
    ventricular topology/looping, 57, 58f
  atrioventricular connections, 58–59, 59f
  ventriculoarterial connections, 59
Cardiac transplantation, hypoplastic left heart syndrome, 72
Cardiopulmonary resuscitation (CPR), 423–424
Caudal regression syndrome, 489, 583
Cavum septum pellucidum, 478
CCI. See Condyle-C1 interval (CCI)
CDH. See Congenital diaphragmatic hernia (CDH)
Cecal volvulus, 104
Central cystic necrosis, 334
Central intramedullary lesion, bone, 289b
Central nervous system (CNS) MRI
  fetal brain, 473–475
  gestational age, 473
  head and neck

Central nervous system (CNS)
  MRI (Continued)
    anophthalmia/microphthalmia, 486, 486f
    flow voids, 488
    interocular/binocular distance abnormal, 486
    mandible, 487
    midline cystic scalp lesion, 485–486
    midline facial mass, 487, 487f
    solid and cystic components, 487f, 488
    upper lip/palate, 486–487
  indications, 473
  monochorionic twin pregnancy, 485
  posterior fossa
    brainstem "kinking", 484, 484f
    cerebellar hemispheres, 483
    cystic enlargement, 481–482
    torcular herophili, 482, 482f
    vermis normal, 482–483, 483f
  protocol, 473, 474t
  spine, 488–489, 488f
  vascular, 484–485
  ventriculomegaly
    causes of, 475, 475t
    cavum septum pellucidum, 478
    central gray matter, 476–478, 477f
    corpus callosum, 475–476, 476f–477f
    cortical irregularity, 479, 479f
    hemimegalencephaly, 479–480, 480f
    lobar cerebral brain parenchyma, 478–479, 478f–479f
    normal signal intensity, 480–481, 481f
    obstructive/nonobstructive, 475, 476f
    right and left cerebral hemispheres, 476–478, 477f
    solid and cystic intracranial mass, 481
    unilateral ventriculomegaly, 480, 480f
    value of, 475
    ventricle margins smooth, 480–481, 481f
Cerebral contusional tears, 405, 407f
Cerebral edema, 496–497, 497f, 497b
Cerebral vascular malformations, 501
Cervical spine (C-spine)
  atlantooccipital dislocation/craniocervical dissociation, 562, 563f–567f, 563b
  C1 vertebra fractures, 568–570, 569f
  C2 vertebra fractures
    Hangman fracture, 569f, 570
    odontoid fractures, 573
    synchondrosal fractures, 570–573, 570f–571f
  clearance of, 556–559, 559b
  clinical presentation, 559
  computed tomography (CT), 561–562
  craniocervical junction (CCJ) and ligaments, 555–556, 558f–559f
  developmental anatomy
    craniocervical junction and ligaments, 555–556, 558f–559f
    ossification patterns, 552–554, 555f–558f, 555b
    vertebral body shape, 552, 553f–554f
  epidemiology, 551–552
  ligamentous injury, 564–565, 568f

Cervical spine (C-spine) (Continued)
  magnetic resonance imaging (MRI), 562
  plain radiographs
    atlantodental interval (ADI), 560, 561f
    C1 spread/pseudospread, 560, 561f
    flexion and extension lateral views, 559–560
    interspinous distances, 560–561
    lateral radiograph, 560, 560f–561f
    modality, 559
    prevertebral soft tissues, 560
    pseudosubluxation, 560
  predisposing conditions
    achondroplasia, 576, 576f
    Down syndrome, 573f, 574–575
    Klippel-Feil syndrome (KFS), 575–576, 575f
    Os odontoideum, 574f, 575
    subaxial C3-C7 fractures, 573
Cervical teratoma, 450, 453f, 544
CF. See Cystic fibrosis (CF)
CHAOS. See Congenital high airway obstruction syndrome (CHAOS)
CHD. See Congenital heart disease (CHD)
Chest radiograph. See also Thorax.
  airway evaluation, 3, 4f
  bacterial pneumonia. See Bacterial pneumonia
  bones evaluation, 3–4
  cardiomediastinal silhouette evaluation
    aortic arch sidedness, 4–5
    cardiac structures, 4, 8f
    left and right aortic arch, 4–5, 8f
    size and age, 4
    thymus, 5, 9f
  diaphragm, 5–6, 9f
  gastric sidedness, 7, 11f
  hilum, 7–8, 11f
  lung fields, 6–7, 10f
  oblique fissure, 376, 377f
  pleural effusion, 6, 9f
  pulmonary vascularity, 377–389
  retrosternal triangular density, 376–377
  suprasternal fossa, 377, 377f
  term infant
    humeral ossification centers, 372, 373f
    mesenchymal hamartoma, 373f
    normal radiograph, 371f
    spurious pneumothorax, 372f
    sternal ossification center, 371f
Chest X-ray (CXR)
  coarctation of the aorta (COA), 74
  double-outlet right ventricle, 70
  hypoplastic left heart syndrome, 72
  interrupted aortic arch (IAA), 74
  tetralogy of fallot (TOF), 68
  vascular rings, 76
ChILD. See Childhood interstitial lung disease (ChILD)
Child abuse, 222b
  American College of Radiology Criteria, 421, 422f
  CAPTA, 416
  CPS, 416
  differential diagnosis, skeletal injuries
    accidental injuries, 422, 422f
    birth trauma, 422–423, 423f
    copper deficiency, 425

Child abuse (Continued)
    CPR, 423–424
    infections, 426f
    normal variants, 422, 423f
    osteogenesis imperfecta, 424, 426f
    rickets, 424, 424f–425f
    scurvy, 424–425, 426f
  fracture dating, 416–418, 417f–418f, 417t
  history, 416
  periostitis, 425–427, 427f–428f
  physical abuse, 416
  soft tissue injuries, 418–421, 419f–420f
Child Abuse Prevention and Treatment Act (CAPTA), 416
Child protection team (CPT), 397
Childhood interstitial lung disease (ChILD), 378, 380–381
Chlamydia trachomatis pneumonia, 15, 19f, 380
Chocolate cyst, 205
Choledochal cyst, 133, 134f, 393, 393f, 458
Chondroblastoma, 288, 304–305
Chondrodysplasia punctata, 240, 244f
Chondromyxoid fibroma, 307–308
Chronic bilateral L5 spondylolysis, 595, 597f
Chronic lung disease (CLD), 358, 360f
Chronic noninfectious osteomyelitis, 603–604, 605f
Chronic recurrent multifocal osteomyelitis (CRMO), 232b, 603–604, 605f
Chronic regional pain syndrome, 232b
Cisterna magna (CM), 474, 474f
Classic metaphyseal lesion (CML), 416–417, 422
Clavicle abnormalities, 372, 374f
CLD. See Chronic lung disease (CLD)
Clear cell sarcoma, 140
Cleidocranial dysostosis, 236–237, 238f, 372
CLO. See Congenital lobar overinflation (CLO)
Clubfoot, 258, 260f, 469, 470f
CM. See Cisterna magna (CM)
CML. See Classic metaphyseal lesion (CML)
CMR. See Cardiac magnetic resonance (CMR)
CMs. See Capillary malformations (CMs)
COA. See Coarctation of the aorta (COA)
Coarctation of the aorta (COA)
  aortic arch development, 74
  clinical presentation, 74
  imaging, 74
  incidence, 73–74
  pathophysiology, 74
Cockayne syndrome, 504, 504f
Cohen cross-trigonal ureteral reimplantation, 187f
Colon cutoff sign, pancreatitis, 113–115
Colonic atresia, 84, 87f
Colonic volvulus, 104, 105f
Community-acquired bacterial pneumonia (CAP), 15f
Community-acquired pneumonia, 20–21
Complete fracture, 348

Computed tomography (CT)
  abusive head trauma (AHT), 408, 407–408, 409f–410f
  abusive spine trauma, 413–414, 415f
  appendicitis, 108
  back pain, 594
  Burkitt lymphoma, 146, 146f
  cervical spine (C-spine), 561–562, 566
  chondroblastoma, 305
  congenital pulmonary airway malformation (CPAM), 385f
  dose optimization
    CT Dose Index, 431–432, 432f
    dose length product (DLP), 432
    effective dose, 433
    image quality targets, 433, 434f
    protocol design, 434–436, 435t, 436f
    radiation dose, 431
    size-specific dose estimate (SSDE), 432–433
  double-outlet right ventricle, 70
  Ewing sarcoma (ES), 299
  limping child, 218
  musculoskeletal (MSK) trauma, 346
  osteoid osteoma, 310
  pancreatitis, 116f–117f
  pediatric head
    cerebral edema, 496–497, 497f, 497b
    cerebrospinal fluid and extraaxial spaces normal, 499–501, 500f–501f
    CT angiography, 494
    foreign bodies, 505
    hydrocephalus, 498, 499f
    intracranial calcifications, 502–505, 503f–505f
    intraparenchymal hemorrhage, 501–502, 501f
    mass effect/midline shift or herniation, 497–498, 497b, 498f
    midline structures, 502, 502f
    radiation awareness, 493–494, 494t
    skull/soft tissues, 505–506
    vascular structures hyperdense
      acute arterial stroke, 496, 496f
      sinovenous thrombosis, 494–496, 495f
  periostitis, 425–426
  risk management
    benefits, 439
    challenging, 439–440
    dose, 439–440
    graphical representation, 440, 440f
  Shone complex, 73, 73f
  tetralogy of fallot (TOF), 69
  tracheal stenosis, 374, 375f
  transposition of the great arteries (TGA), 67
  urinary tract dilation (UTD), 179
  Wilms tumors, 140
Computed tomography angiography (CTA)
  bronchopulmonary sequestration (BPS)
    extralobar, 386, 387f
    intralobar, 386, 388f
  infradiaphragmatic pulmonary sequestration, 135, 137f
  vascular rings, 76, 76f

Condylar gap method, 563, 564f–567f
Condyle-C1 interval (CCI), 563, 564f–567f
Congenital and posttraumatic deformities
  congenital proximal radioulnar synostosis, 278–279, 280f
  fishtail deformity, 280, 281f
  supracondylar process, 279–280, 281f
Congenital caudal tumor, 584–585, 586f
Congenital cytomegalovirus, 503, 503f
Congenital diaphragmatic hernia (CDH), 387–388, 389f
  checklist, 457b
  fetal lung volumes, 456–457, 457f
  gastrointestinal and genitourinary anomalies, 457
  hernia sac, 454
  liver, 454
Congenital heart disease (CHD)
  aortic arch anomalies
    coarctation of the aorta (COA), 73–75
    interrupted aortic arch, 73–75
    vascular rings, 75–76
  cardiac segments identification
    atrial identification, 55–58
    atrioventricular connections, 58–59, 59f
    ventriculoarterial connections, 59
  left heart lesions
    hypoplastic left heart syndrome (HLHS), 71–72
    Shone complex, 72–73
  outflow tract anomalies
    double-outlet right ventricle, 69–71
    tetralogy of fallot (TOF), 68–69
    transposition of the great arteries (TGA), 65–68
  segmental approach, 54, 54f
  septal defects
    atrial septal defects and interatrial communications, 60–62
    atrioventricular septal defects (AVSDs), 64–65
    ventricular septal defects, 62–64
Congenital hemangioma, 450, 453f
Congenital high airway obstruction syndrome (CHAOS), 451–452
Congenital lesions, 517–518
Congenital limb overgrowth syndromes, 326t
Congenital lipomatous overgrowth, vascular malformations, epidermal nevi, scoliosis/spine (CLOVES) anomalies, 325f
Congenital lobar overinflation (CLO), 382, 383f, 452, 456f
Congenital proximal radioulnar synostosis, 278–279, 280f
Congenital pseudoarthrosis, 372
Congenital pulmonary adenomatoid malformation (CPAM), 452, 455f
Congenital pulmonary airway malformation (CPAM), 385–386
Congenital talipes equinovarus, 258, 260f
Congenital thymic cysts, 37
Congenital toxoplasmosis, 503, 503f
Congenital vertical talus, 262, 263f–264f
Constipation, 124–125, 125f
Contralateral lung, 383–384
Contrast enema, 93, 93f
Copper deficiency, 425

Coronary artery anatomy, 67
Corpus callosum, 475–476, 476f–477f, 502, 502f
Cortical dysplasia, 479, 479f
Cortical scintigraphy, urinary tract dilation (UTD), 177
Cortically based lesions, bone, 289–290, 290b
Cotwin demise, 470
CPR. See Cardiopulmonary resuscitation (CPR)
CPT. See Child protection team (CPT)
Crackles/rales, 12t
Craniocervical junction (CCJ) ligaments, 555–556, 558f–559f
Craniocervical/cervical spinal injuries, 590
Craniopharyngiomas, 504, 505f
Craniosynostosis, 236
CRMO. See Chronic recurrent multifocal osteomyelitis (CRMO)
Crohn disease, 121f
Croup, 515, 516f
Crouzon syndrome, 236
CT. See Computed tomography (CT)
CT Dose Index (CTDI), 431–432, 432f
Cyst
  abdomen, 393–394
  ovarian, 467, 468f
  thymus, 37
Cystic dysplasia, testes, 166
Cystic enlargement, 481–482
Cystic fibrosis (CF)
  acute pulmonary exacerbation, 29f
  advanced, 29f
  bronchial artery hypertrophy, 30f
  CFTR gene mutation, 23
  chest CT, 23–24, 29f
  diagnosis, 23
  mucous secretions, 23
  radiographic findings, 23–24, 28f
Cystic hygroma, 314
Cystic renal diseases, 128, 128f–129f

D
Dacryocystocele, 526, 527f
Dandy-Walker malformation, 482, 482f, 500, 501f
Deep neck masses, 542–545, 543f, 545f–546f
Dental disease, 536–537, 537f
Dentigerous cysts, 538
Dermoid and epidermoid inclusion cysts, 525–526, 526f
Dextrocardia, 54
Diametaphysis, bone lesions, 289b
Diaphragm
  hemidiaphragm, 5–6
  paralysis, 9f
Diaphysis, 289b, 347
Diastematomyelia, 586
Diffuse cerebral edema, 497f, 497b
Diffuse neurofibromas, 336
Discitis, 228
Disk cysts, 601, 601f
Disk degeneration, 600
Disk herniation, 600
Distal femoral avulsive irregularity, 308
Distal obstruction, 84–86, 86f
DLP. See Dose length product (DLP)
Dorsal dermal sinuses, 581–583
Dose length product (DLP), 432

Dose optimization
  automatic exposure control (AEC), 438, 438f
  component, 429
  computed tomography (CT) dosimetry
    CT Dose Index, 431–432, 432f
    dose length product (DLP), 432
    effective dose, 433
    radiation dose, 431
    size-specific dose estimate (SSDE), 432–433
  computed tomography protocol design, 434–436, 435t, 436f
  filtered backprojection, 438
  image quality targets, 433, 434f
  ionizing radiation
    carcinogenic effects, 430–431
    damage cell, 430
    DNA, 430
    iterative reconstruction, 438, 439f
    kilovolt peak, 436–437, 437f
    kilovoltage ranges, 437
    long-term studies, 429–430
    pitch, 437–438, 438f
    tube current (mA) and rotation time (mS), 436, 436f
Double aortic arch, 48
Double-outlet right ventricle
  clinical presentation, 70
  diagnosis, 70
  imaging, 70
  incidence, 69–70
  morphology, 70
  subtypes, 69–70
  treatment, 70–71
Down syndrome, 573f, 574–575
Duodenal atresia, 391f, 458, 462f
Duodenal hematoma, 124f
Duodenal web, 82–83, 85f
Duodenal-jejunal junction (DJJ), 82f
Duplex kidneys, 183–184, 188f–189f
Duplication cysts, 392f, 393
Dyggve-Melchior-Clausen (DMC) syndrome, 242, 246f
Dysplasia epiphysealis hemimelica, 302

E
Eccentric intramedullary lesion, bone, 289, 289b
Echocardiography
  atrial septal defects (ASD), 60
  coarctation of the aorta (COA), 74
  double-outlet right ventricle, 70
  hypoplastic left heart syndrome, 72, 72f
  Shone complex, 73
  tetralogy of fallot (TOF), 68–69
  transposition of the great arteries (TGA), 67
  ventricular septal defects (VSDs), 63
Ectopic pregnancy, pelvic pain, 204–205
Ectopic thymus, 36–37
Ectopic thyroid tissue, 541, 541f
EDHs. See Epidural hematomas (EDHs)
Effective dose, 433
Eisenmenger syndrome, 60, 63
Elbow, pediatric
  chronic elbow injuries
    juvenile osteochondritis dissecans, 283–284, 284f
    Little League elbow, 280–283, 281b, 282f

Elbow, pediatric (Continued)
  congenital and posttraumatic
      deformities worth mentioning
    congenital proximal radioulnar
        synostosis, 278–279, 280f
    fishtail deformity, 280, 281f
    supracondylar process, 279–280,
        281f
  dislocation
    posterior dislocation, 277, 278f, 278b
    radial head dislocations, 277, 279f,
        279b
    raise suspicion, 277
  FOOL checklist, 267b, 285b
    anterior humeral line (AHL),
        269–270, 270f
    fat pads, 267–268, 268f
    ossification centers, 268–269,
        268b–269b, 269f
    overt findings and outlines, 268
    radiocapitellar line (RCL), 270, 271f
  imaging modalities, 267
  oblique views, 267
  pediatric elbow fractures, 272b
    lateral condylar fracture, 272–274,
        273f–274f, 274b
    medial epicondyle fracture, 274–
        275, 275f, 275b–276b
    olecranon fractures, 276
    radial head fractures, 276
    radial neck fractures, 275, 276f, 277b
    supracondylar fracture, 272,
        272f–273f, 273b
    transphyseal distal humeral fractures,
        275–276, 277f–278f
  radial head subluxation, 270–271,
      271b
  radiographic views, 267, 268f
Ellis von Creveld syndrome, 241–242, 245f
Empyema, 16
Encephalocele, 531, 531f
Enchondroma, 305–306
Enchondromatosis, 306
Endometriosis, pelvic pain, 205
Enlarged bifrontal extraaxial spaces, 404
Enteric duplication cysts, 133–135, 135f
Ependymomas, 609–610, 611f
Epididymal cysts, 164–165, 167f
Epididymitis, 156–159
Epididymo-orchitis, 158b, 161
Epidural abscess, 602, 604f
Epidural hematomas (EDHs)
  abusive head trauma (AHT)
    appearance, 400–402, 401f–403f
    birth-related SDHs, 404
    causes, 400, 401f
    characteristics, 404
    convexity, 404
    enlarged low-density extraaxial
        spaces, 404
    hematohygromas, 402–403, 405f
    heterogeneous-appearing, 403–404
    injury dating, 404
    membrane, 404
    retroclival subdural/epidural
        collections, 404
  abusive spine trauma, 413
Epiglottis, 512
Epiglottitis, 514–515, 515f–516f
Epiphysis, 288b, 346
Epithelial tumors, thymus, 37–39,
    38f–39f

Equinus positioning, 256, 257f
ES. See Ewing sarcoma (ES)
Esophageal atresia (EA), 388–389, 390f,
    457–458, 459f
Esophageal duplication cysts, 49
Esthesioneuroblastoma, 533
Ewing sarcoma (ES), 337–338, 607,
    609f
  cortical bone destruction, 298
  CT evaluation, 299
  flat bones, 298
  Frank periosteal disruption, 298
  metastases, 298
  MRI, 298–299
  permeative lesion, 298, 298f
Expiratory chest radiograph, spurious
    findings, 370, 371t
Extralobar sequestrations, 458
Extramedullary hematopoiesis, 52
Extramedullary intradural tumors
  meningioma, 611–612, 613f
  schwannomas, 611, 612f
Extranasal glial heterotopia, 531–532,
    532f
Extraocular masses
  cystic and unilocular, 525–526, 526f
  eroding adjacent bone
    aggressive periosteal reaction, 529,
        530f
    expansile, ground-glass appearance
        to, 529–530, 530f
    leukemia, 529
    superior orbit, 528–529
    superolateral orbit, 529, 529f
  medial canthus, 526, 526f
  multicystic lesion, 527, 528f
  solid and hypervascular, 527, 528f
  unilocular cystic lesion, 526–527

F
18F sodium fluoride (18F-NaF), 218, 220f
Face and neck
  cleft lip and palate, 449, 450f
  micrognathia, 450, 451f
  neoplasms and masslike
      malformations, 450, 452f–454f
  normal appearance, 448–449, 449f
Fairbank disease, 240, 244f
Fall on an outstretched hand (FOOSH),
    272
Familial hypocalciuric hypercalcemia,
    424, 425f
Fascicular sign, schwannoma, 336, 337f
Fat necrosis, 338
FCDs. See Fibrous cortical defects
    (FCDs)
Fecal impaction, 125f
Fetal abdomen and pelvis
  abdominal wall defects, 460–462,
      464f–466f
  cystic mass, 465–467, 468f
  distal bowel obstruction, 460,
      463f–464f
  gastrointestinal system structures, 458,
      460f–461f
  genitourinary system structures, 458,
      460f–461f
  hydronephrosis, 463–465, 466f–467f,
      467b
  large kidneys, 462, 466f
  presacral mass, 467–468, 468f
  suprarenal mass, 458, 461b, 462f

Fetal abdomen and pelvis (Continued)
  upper abdominal cystic mass, 458,
      462f–463f
  visceral abdominopelvic neoplasms,
      468–469, 469f
Fetal hydrops, 585
Fetal musculoskeletal system, 469–470,
    469f–470f
Fetal situs, 448, 448t, 449f
18F-FDG PET/CT
  malignant peripheral nerve sheath
      tumor (MPNST), 337
  osteosarcoma, 300–301
Fibroids, 447, 447f
Fibromatosis colli, 333, 542, 543f
Fibrous cortical defects (FCDs), 306
Fibrous dysplasia (FD), 529–530, 530f
  CT evaluation, 304
  intramedullary lesions, 304
  McCune-Albright syndrome (MAS),
      303–304
  medullary expansion, 304, 304f
  nuclear medicine bone scan, 304
  polyostotic and syndromic
      cases, 303
Fibroxanthoma, 306–307
Fishtail deformity, 280, 281f
Flatfoot, 261, 262f
Focal atelectasis, 20, 25f
Focal cerebral edema, 497b
Focal scoliosis/hyperkyphosis, 588–589,
    589f
Follicular cysts, 538
FOOL checklist, pediatric elbow, 267b,
    285b
  anterior humeral line (AHL), 269–270,
      270f
  fat pads, 267–268, 268f
  ossification centers, 268–269,
      268b–269b, 269f
  overt findings and outlines, 268
  radiocapitellar line (RCL),
      270, 271f
Foot, pediatric
  anatomy, 254
  lines and positions, 254–255,
      255f–256f
  pathologies and radiographic findings
    clubfoot, 258, 260f
    congenital vertical talus, 262,
        263f–264f
    flatfoot, 261, 262f
    metatarsus adductus, 258–259,
        261f
    skewfoot, 259–261, 261f
    tarsal coalition, 262, 265f
  technique, 254
  terminology
    forefoot, 256–258, 257t, 260f
    heel, 256, 257f, 257t
    hindfoot, 256, 257t, 258f–259f
    plantar arch, 256, 257t, 259f
Forefoot eversion, 258
Forefoot inversion, 257–258
Forefoot terminology, 256–258, 257t,
    260f
Foregut anomalies, 48–49, 48f
Foregut duplication cysts, 540, 541f
Foreign body aspiration
  focal atelectasis, 25f
  left mainstem bronchus, 25f–26f
  linear radiopaque foreign body, 24f

Fractures
  buckle fracture, 347–348, 348f
  complete fracture, 348
  limping child, 232, 232f–233f
  physeal fractures, 348–349, 349f
  plastic deformation, 347, 347f
  skull, 399, 399f–400f
  testicular, 162
Fracture-subluxations, 411–413, 411f–413f
Functional cyst, 195–196
Functional immaturity of the colon, 84–85, 88f

G
Galen fistulas, 485
Ganglioneuroblastoma, 49, 51f
Ganglioneuromas, 49
Garré sclerosing osteomyelitis, 296
Gartland fractures
  type 1, 272, 272f
  type 2, 272, 273f
Gastroenteritis, 108–109
Gastroesophageal reflux, 88–89, 90f, 94
Gastroschisis, 460, 465f
GCTs. See Germ cell tumors (GCTs)
GCTTS. See Giant cell tumor of the tendon sheath (GCTTS)
Genitourinary system structures, 458, 460f–461f
Germ cell tumors (GCTs), 41–42, 43f, 166–167
  malignant, 144f
  nonseminomatous, 142–143
  nonteratomatous, 42
  retroperitoneal extragonadal, 142–143
  seminoma, 142–143
  teratoma, 42, 143
Germinal matrix, 480–481, 481f
Germinal matrix hemorrhage, 361–366
  bilateral grade III, 366f
  cystic change, 365–366
  grade I, 365f
  grading system, 361–363, 366b
  left grade II, 366f
  posthemorrhagic hydrocephalus, 365
  right grade IV, 366f
  white matter injury, 365–366
Giant cell tumor (GCT), 289
Giant cell tumor of the tendon sheath (GCTTS), 330
Glutaric aciduria, 500, 500f
Goiter, fetal, 450, 454f
Goldenhar syndrome, 238
Granulocytic sarcoma, 529
Great arterial identification, 58, 58f
Greenstick fracture, distal radial diaphysis, 348f
Group B Streptococcus pneumonia, 378

H
Haemophilus influenza, 514
Hamartoma, 339–340, 342f
Hand rule, 57, 58f
Hangman fracture, 569f, 570
Harris method, 563, 563b
Haustral folds, bowel obstruction, 390, 390f
Head and neck
  anophthalmia/microphthalmia, 486, 486f
  flow voids, 488
  interocular/binocular distance abnormal, 486

Head and neck (Continued)
  mandible, 487
  midline cystic scalp lesion, 485–486
  midline facial mass, 487, 487f
  solid and cystic components, 487f, 488
  upper lip/palate, 486–487
Head and neck masses
  anterior neck masses
    branchial apparatus and remnants, 539
    branchial apparatus cysts, 539–540, 540f
    cyst near midline, 538–539, 539f
    cystic lesions, 538
    ear, 539
    ectopic thyroid tissue, 541, 541f
    foregut structure, 540, 541f
    lower neck, 540
    lymph node, 541–542, 543f
    "starry sky" appearance, 541, 542f
    thyroid carcinoma, 541
    thyroid gland, 540
  deep neck masses, 542–545, 543f, 545f–546f
  extraocular masses. See Extraocular masses
  floor of mouth masses, 536–537, 536f–537f
  mandibular masses, 537–538, 537f
  ocular masses
    anatomy, 523f
    Coats disease, 524, 524f
    iris, 524
    optic nerve glioma, 525, 525f
    PHPV, 524, 524f
    retina with calcifications, 522–523, 523f
    retina without calcifications, 523–524
    retinal detachment, 524
  oral cavity masses, 535
  radiographs, 522
  sinonasal masses
    nasofrontal masses, 530–532, 531f–532f
    nasopharynx masses, 533–535, 534f–535f
    sinus masses, 532–533, 533f
Heel alignment, 254, 255f, 256, 257f, 257t
Hemangioma, 288
Hematocele, 162
Hematohygromas, 402–403, 405f
Hematoma, 338–339
Hemimegalencephaly, 479–480, 480f
Hemolytic uremic syndrome (HUS), 118, 120f
Hemorrhage, 25–26
Hemorrhagic cyst, ovary
  fishnet pattern, 196f
  internal clot, 196f–197f
Henoch-Schönlein purpura (HSP), 116–118, 119f, 160
Hepatic angiosarcoma, 142, 143f
Hepatic fibrosis, 462
Hepatobiliary masses
  choledochal cyst, 133, 134f
  hepatoblastoma, 132, 133f
  infantile hepatic hemangiomas (IHHs), 131–132, 132f
  mesenchymal hamartoma, 132–133, 134f

Hepatoblastoma, 132, 133f, 140
Hepatocellular carcinoma (HCC), 140
Hernia sac, 454
Herpes pneumonia, 380
Heterotaxy syndrome, 55
HII. See Hypoxic ischemic injury (HII)
Hilum, 7–8, 11f
Hindfoot alignment, 255–256, 255f–256f, 257t, 258f–259f
Hindfoot valgus deformity, 256, 258f
Hindfoot varus deformity, 256, 259f
Hirschsprung disease, 86, 89f, 125, 125f, 390f
HLHS. See Hypoplastic left heart syndrome (HLHS)
Hodgkin disease (HD), 144–146
Hodgkin lymphoma, 542
Holoprosencephaly, 476–478, 477f
HPS. See Hypertrophic pyloric stenosis (HPS)
HSP. See Henoch-Schönlein purpura (HSP)
Hunter syndrome, 500–501, 501f
Hydrocele, 160f, 163
Hydrocephalus, 498, 499f
Hydrometrocolpos, 131, 131f, 200–202
Hydronephrosis, 111, 128, 462–465, 466f–467f, 467b
  diuresis renography, 183f–184f
  prenatal, 183f–184f
  ultrasound, 183f–184f
Hydroureteronephrosis
  Cohen cross-trigonal ureteral reimplantation, 187f
  megaureter tapering, 182
  orthotopic distal ureter, 180
  periureteral diverticula, 182
  primary megaureter, 180
  primary reflux, 182, 186f
  vesicoureteral reflux, 182
  voiding cystourethrogram (VCUG), 182, 185f
Hynes-Anderson pyeloplasty, 184f
Hyperplastic thymic gland, 37
Hypertrophic pyloric stenosis (HPS), 86–87, 90f
  pylorospasm-simulating, 96f
  ultrasound, 94f–95f
Hypogenetic lung syndrome, 384–385
Hypoperfusion complex, 124f, 419, 420f
Hypophosphatasia, 246, 251f
Hypoplastic left heart syndrome (HLHS)
  clinical presentation, 71
  imaging, 72
  incidence, 71
  morphology, 71
  pathophysiology, 71
  treatment, 72
Hypoplastic lower extremities, 583–584, 584f–586f
Hypoxic ischemic injury (HII), 398, 398f, 401f, 405

I
IAA. See Interrupted aortic arch (IAA)
Iatrogenic respiratory distress, 519
Idiopathic bilious vomiting, 81
Idiopathic scrotal fat necrosis, 160
IFA. See Inferior facial angle (IFA)
IH. See Infantile hemangioma (IH)

IHHs. *See* Infantile hepatic hemangiomas (IHHs)
ILD. *See* Interstitial lung disease (ILD)
Ileal atresia, 84, 87f
Ileocolic intussusception, 105
Ileus pattern, 100, 101f
Imperforate hymen, 200–202
Indirect inguinal hernias, 163
Infantile fibrosarcoma
    congenital, 335
    MRI, 335, 336f
Infantile hemangioma (IH), 131–132, 340, 532, 544
Infantile hepatic hemangiomas (IHHs), 468, 469f
    contrast-enhanced MRI, 132, 132f
    infantile hemangiomas (IHs), 131–132
    sonographic appearance, 132
Infantile myofibroma
    MRI characteristics, 334, 335f
    multicentric myofibromatosis, 334
    natural history, 334
    nodules, 334
    solitary myofibroma, 334
    ultrasound, 334, 335f
Infants and toddlers
    bone lesions
        acute leukemia, 292, 293f
        infantile myofibromatosis, 296–297
        multifocal langerhans cell histiocytosis, 292–293, 294f
        neuroblastoma, 293–295, 295f
        osteofibrous dysplasia, 297–298, 297f
        osteomyelitis, 295–296, 296f
    preterm infant. *See* Preterm infant
Infectious disorders
    chronic recurrent multifocal osteomyelitis/chronic noninfectious osteomyelitis, 603–604, 605f
    epidural abscess, 602, 604f
    spondylodiskitis, 601–602, 602f–603f
Inferior facial angle (IFA), 450
Inflammatory bowel disease (IBD), 118–120, 121f
Infradiaphragmatic pulmonary sequestration (IPS), 130, 135, 137f
Infundibulum, 58
Inguinal hernia, 164f
Intermittent nonbilious vomiting, 88–89
Interocular/binocular distance (IOD/BOD), 486
Interrupted aortic arch (IAA)
    aortic arch development, 74
    clinical presentation, 74
    imaging, 74
    incidence, 73–74
    pathophysiology, 74
    types, 73–74
Interstitial lung disease (ILD), 380–381, 381f
Intramedullary lesion, bone lesions, 289, 289b
Intramedullary tumors
    astrocytoma, 608–609, 611f
    ependymomas, 609–610, 611f
Intraparenchymal hemorrhage, 501–502, 501f
Intrapulmonary abscess, 23f–24f
Intratesticular cysts, 166
Intratesticular solid lesions, 166–170

Intrathoracic foregut cysts, 48–49
Intrathoracic trachea, 3
Intraventricular hemorrhage, 404
Intussusception
    ileocolic, 104–106
    meniscus sign, 105–106, 106f
    symptoms, 105
    treatment, 106
    ultrasound, 106, 107f
IPS. *See* Infradiaphragmatic pulmonary sequestration (IPS)
Ipsilateral lung, 383–384
Ipsilateral renal anomalies, 166
IR. *See* Iterative reconstruction (IR)
Isolated fallopian tube torsion (IFTT), 199–200
Iterative reconstruction (IR), 438, 439f

J
Jaffe-Campanacci syndrome, 307
Jakob classification, 273
Jejunal atresia, 84, 86f, 460, 463f
Jeune syndrome, 241, 245f
Joubert syndrome, 483, 483f
Juvenile idiopathic arthritis (JIA), 230–231, 231b
Juvenile ossifying fibroma, 533, 533f
Juvenile osteochondritis dissecans, 283–284, 284f
Juxtacortical location, 290b

K
Kaposiform hemangioendothelioma (KHE), 327, 341–343, 344f
Kawasaki disease, 160
Keratocystic odontogenic tumor, 538
KFS. *See* Klippel-Feil syndrome (KFS)
Kilovolt peak (kVp), 436–437, 437f
Klippel-Feil syndrome (KFS), 575–576, 575f, 588
Kniest dysplasia, 242, 248f

L
Ladd bands, 82
Langerhans cell histiocytosis (LCH), 604–605, 606f–607f
    monostotic, 299
    multifocal
        classification, 292–293
        extensive, 292–293
        FDG-PET/CT, 293
        punched-out lesions, 293, 294f
        restricted, 292–293
        whole-body STIR MRI, 293
Laryngomalacia, 372–373
Lateral condylar fracture, 272–274, 273f–274f, 274b
Lateral neck radiograph
    accidental and iatrogenic causes, 519, 519f
    anatomy, 511–512, 512f
    approaches, 511
    autoimmune diseases, 519, 520f
    bacterial tracheitis, 515–516, 517f
    congenital lesions, 517–518
    croup, 515, 516f
    "edge of film" findings, 513
    epiglottis, 512
    epiglottitis, 514–515, 515f–516f
    foreign bodies, 516–517, 517f–518f
    neoplasms, 518, 519f

Lateral neck radiograph *(Continued)*
    prevertebral soft tissues, 513
    retropharyngeal abscess, 514, 515f
    subglottic airway, 512–513, 513f
    technique, 511, 512f
    tonsils and adenoids, 512–514, 514f
LCH. *See* Langerhans cell histiocytosis (LCH)
Left ventricle (LV), 57
Legg-Calvé-Perthes (LCP), 213, 229–230, 230b
Leg-length discrepancy, 222b
Leukemia, 167, 169f, 529, 607–608, 610f
    infants and toddlers, 292, 293f
    limping child, 220–221, 221b
Levocardia, 448
Limping child
    bone scans, 218, 219f–220f
    causes, 213
    clinical history, 213
    computed tomography, 218
    infection
        clinical and laboratory evidence, 225
        discitis, 228
        Lyme arthritis, 229
        Lyme disease, 228–229
        MRI, 225–226
        osteomyelitis, 226
        primary psoas abscesses, 228
        scintigraphic bone scan, 226–227
        septic arthritis, 226b
    juvenile idiopathic arthritis (JIA), 230–231, 231b
    Legg-Calvé-Perthes (LCP), 229–230, 230b
    magnetic resonance imaging
        drawbacks, 219–220
        leukemia, 220–221, 221b
        osteoid osteoma, 221b
        osteomyelitis, 220
    pain, 231–232
    pathological fractures, 232, 232f–233f
    patient's age, 221
    plain radiographs, 213–214
        anteroposterior radiograph, 215f
        hip pathologies, 214, 216f
        lateral radiograph, 214, 214f
    septic arthritis, 229
    slipped capital femoral epiphysis (SCFE), 230, 230b
    sonography, 215–217, 217b, 218f
    subacute/chronic limp, 231
    synovitis, 229
    trauma
        newly ambulating child, 222–223
        radiographs, 221–222
        young children, 224
    trendelenburg gait, 213
Lingular pneumonia, 17f
Lipoblastoma, 339, 341f
Lipoma, 339, 340f
Liposarcoma, 339
Little League elbow, 280–283, 281b, 282f
Liver injury, 418–419
Liver Injury Scale, 123t
LMs. *See* Lymphatic malformations (LMs)
Lobar bacterial pneumonia, 16f
Lobular simplification, 380–381
Localized neurofibroma, 336
Long bones anatomy, 346
Looping/topology, heart, 58f
Lower airway structural abnormality, 10

Lung abscesses, 16–19
Lung inflation, 4, 5f
Lyme arthritis, 229
Lyme disease, 228–229
Lymph node, anterior neck masses, 541–542, 543f
Lymphangiectasia, 379
Lymphangioma, 314
Lymphatic malformations (LMs), 314–315, 344, 450, 452f
  macrocystic, 314–315
  mediastinum, 44–47
  microcystic, 314–315
  treatment, 315
Lymphoma, 607–608, 610f
  Burkitt lymphoma, 146
  F-18 FDG PET, 146
  mediastinum
    chest pain, 44, 46f
    chest radiograph, 42, 45f
    FDG-PET/CT, 42, 45f
    Hodgkin disease (HD), 42
    non-Hodgkin lymphoma (NHL), 42
    staging, 42
    T cell lymphoblastic lymphoma, 44f
  splenic involvement, 144–146
  US, 144

M
Macrocystic lymphatic malformations (LMs), 314–315
Macrocystic malformations, 344
Maffucci syndrome, 306
Magnetic resonance enterography (MRE)
  Crohn disease, 121f
  inflammatory bowel disease (IBD), 119–120
Magnetic resonance imaging (MRI)
  abdomen and pelvis. See Fetal abdomen and pelvis
  abdomen, neonate
    choledochal cyst, 393f
  abusive head trauma (AHT), 408
  abusive spine trauma, 413–414, 415f
  aneurysmal bone cyst (ABCs), 312f
  appendicitis, 108, 109f
  back pain, 594
  central nervous system. See Central nervous system (CNS) MRI
  cervical spine (C-spine), 562, 567
  chondroblastoma, 305
  chondromyxoid fibroma, 307–308, 308f
  enchondroma, 306
  endometriosis, 205
  Ewing sarcoma (ES), 298–299
  face and neck
    cleft lip and palate, 449, 450f
    micrognathia, 450, 451f
    neoplasms and masslike malformations, 450, 452f–454f
    normal appearance, 448–449, 449f
  fetal musculoskeletal system, 469–470, 469f–470f
  fetal situs, 448, 448t, 449f
  fibroxanthoma, 307
  hepatic angiosarcoma, 142, 143f
  hepatoblastoma, 132, 133f
  indications, 446, 446t
  intravenous contrast, 447
  limping child
    drawbacks, 219–220

Magnetic resonance imaging (MRI) (Continued)
    leukemia, 220–221, 221b
    osteoid osteoma, 221b
    osteomyelitis, 220
  lymphatic malformations, 135
  maternal structures, 447–448, 447f–448f
  mesenchymal hamartoma, 132–133, 134f
  multifetal gestations, 470, 470f
  musculoskeletal (MSK) trauma, 346
  nephroblastomatosis, 139f
  neuroblastoma, 130, 130f
  osteofibrous dysplasia (OFD), 297–298
  osteoid osteoma, 310
  overview, 445–446
  patient preparation, 446
  pediatric elbow, 267
  periostitis, 425–426
  protocol, 446–447
  renal cell carcinoma, 141f
  rhabdomyosarcoma, 144, 145f
  sacrococcygeal teratoma (SCTs), 136, 137f
  soft tissue masses, 328
    alveolar soft part sarcoma (ASPA), 333
    fat necrosis, 339f
    ganglion cyst, 328, 329f
    hamartoma, 342f
    infantile hemangioma (IH), 340, 343f
    Kaposiform hemangioendothelioma (KHE), 341–343, 344f
    lipoblastoma, 339, 341f
    lipoma, 339, 340f
    lymphatic malformation, 344, 345f
    meniscal cysts, 329
    rhabdomyosarcoma, 336, 337f
    schwannoma, 336, 337f
    synovial sarcoma, 330–331, 332f
    torticollis, 333, 334f
    venous malformations, 333
  thorax
    cardiac position, 457
    congenital diaphragmatic hernia, 454–457, 457f, 457b
    determination, 457
    diffuse T2 hyperintensity, 451–452, 454t, 455f
    esophageal atresia, 457–458, 459f
    focal signal abnormalities, 452–453, 455f–456f
    mesenchymal hamartoma, 372, 373f
    normal fetal thorax, 451, 454f
    pleural effusions, 453–454
  unicameral bone cyst (UBCs), 311
  vascular malformations
    arteriovenous fistulas (AVFs), 322f
    arteriovenous malformations (AVMs), 322f
    CLOVES syndrome, 325f
    Klippel-Trenaunay syndrome (KTS), 324f
    lymphatic malformations (LMs), 315f
    venous malformations (VMs), 319f
  Wilms tumors, 138f
Magnetic resonance urography (MRU), urinary tract dilation (UTD), 177–178, 179f

Malignant peripheral nerve sheath tumor (MPNST), 49–52, 337
Malrotation/midgut volvulus, 103–104, 103f–104f
Mandibular masses, 537–538, 537f
Maternal hydronephrosis, 447, 447f
MCA. See Middle cerebral artery (MCA)
McCune-Albright syndrome (MAS), 303–304
MCDK. See Multicystic dysplastic kidney (MCDK)
MDAs. See Müllerian duct anomalies (MDAs)
Meckel diverticulum, 109–110
Meconium, 458
  cyst, 85
  ileus, 85, 88f
  periorchitis, 165–166, 167f
  peritonitis, 392f
  plugs, 84–85, 88f
  pseudocysts, 135, 136f
Meconium aspiration syndrome, 380
Medial epicondyle fracture, 274–275, 275f, 275b–276b
Medial epicondylitis/apophysitis, 281–283, 282f
Medial malleolar secondary ossification center, 351f
Mediastinal masses
  anterior, 34–47, 34t
    ectopic thymus, 36–37
    germ cell tumors, 41–42, 43f
    lymphatic malformations (LM), 44–47
    lymphoma, 42–44
    normal thymus, 34–35, 35f–36f
    thymic abscess, 39–40
    thymic cysts, 37
    thymic epithelial tumors, 37–39, 38f–39f
    thymic hyperplasia, 37, 37f
    thymolipoma, 41
  differential diagnosis, 33, 34t
  middle, 34t
    foregut anomalies, 48–49, 48f
    vascular rings and slings, 47–48, 47f
  posterior, 34t
    ages, 49
    extramedullary hematopoiesis, 52
    ganglioneuroblastoma, 49
    ganglioneuromas, 49
    nerve sheath tumors, 49–52
    neurogenic masses, 49
    thoracic neuroblastoma, 49, 50f
  vs. pulmonary parenchymal masses, 33
Mediastinal shift, 382–383
Mediastinum, 5, 9f, 33, 34f
  abscess, 39–40, 41f
  anterior, 34–47
  Langerhans cell histiocytosis, 41, 41f
Medulloepithelioma, 524
Megacystis megaureter association, 182
Megacystis-microcolon-intestinal hypoperistalsis syndrome, 464
Meniscal cyst, 329
Mercaptoacetyltriglycine (MAG3) study, urinary tract dilation (UTD), 174f, 177f–178f
Mesenchymal hamartoma, 132–133, 134f, 373f
Mesenteric adenitis, 110, 112f
Mesoblastic nephroma, 129, 129f

Metadiaphysis, 347
Metaphysis, 347
    bone lesions, 289b
Metatarsus adductus, 258–259, 261f
Metatropic dysplasia, 242, 247f
Microcystic lymphatic malformations
    (LMs), 314–315
Microcystic malformations, 344
Micrognathia, 450, 451f
Middle cerebral artery (MCA), 496, 496f
Midgut malrotation
    duodenal–jejunal junction, 82f
    imaging techniques, 94
    Ladd bands, 82
    with partial proximal obstruction, 83f
    with volvulus, 83f–84f
    without volvulus, 83f
Milch classification, 273
Mitral valve (MV), 57
MO. See Myositis ossificans (MO)
Monochorionic twin pregnancy, 485
Monteggia fracture dislocation, 279f,
    279b
Morquio syndrome, 244
Moth-eaten bone destruction, 291
MPNST. See Malignant peripheral nerve
    sheath tumor (MPNST)
MRI. See Magnetic resonance imaging
    (MRI)
Mucoid-filled cysts, 166
Mucopolysaccharidoses, 242–244,
    249f–250f
Müllerian duct anomalies (MDAs), 202,
    208f
Multicystic dysplastic kidney (MCDK),
    128, 128f, 463, 466f
Multicystic lesion, 527, 528f
Multifetal gestations, 470, 470f
Multiple epiphyseal dysplasia, 240, 244f
Muscular ventricular septal defects, 62–63
Musculoskeletal trauma
    abusive fractures, 349
    computed tomography (CT), 346
    fractures, 347–349
    magnetic resonance imaging (MRI),
        346
    plain radiographs, 346
    ultrasound, 346
Myasthenia gravis, thymoma, 37–38, 40f
Mycoplasma pneumonia, 20–21
Myofibroma, 297
Myofibromatosis, 296–297
Myositis ossificans (MO)
    components, 331
    MRI, 331
    peripheral ossification, 333
    serpiginous calcification, 331, 332f
Myxopapillary ependymoma, 610, 611f

N
Nasal glioma, 531
Nasofrontal masses, 530–532,
    531f–532f
Nasopharyngeal carcinoma, 535
Nasopharynx masses, 533–535,
    534f–535f
Necrotizing enterocolitis (NEC)
    clinical signs and symptoms, 360
    etiology, 359–360
    perforation, 360
    radiographic findings, 360–361, 360b,
        361f–363f

Necrotizing pneumonia, 16–19, 22f
NEHI. See Neuroendocrine cell
    hyperplasia of infancy (NEHI)
Neonate imaging study
    abdomen
        obstructed bowel, 390–391, 390f
        plain film pitfalls, 391–392
        postnatal imaging, 393–394
        radiograph, 392–393
    thorax, neonates. See Thorax
Neoplasms, renal, 129, 129f
Nephroblastomatosis, 137–140, 139f
Nerve sheath tumors
    malignant peripheral, 49–52
    malignant peripheral nerve sheath
        tumor (MPNST), 337
    neurofibroma, 336
    primitive neuroectodermal tumors,
        337–338
    scapular mass, 338, 338f
    schwannoma, 49, 336, 337f
Neurenteric cysts, 49
Neuroblastoma, 49, 130, 130f, 140, 166f
    infants and toddlers, 293–295, 295f
    orbital metastasis, 529, 530f
Neuroendocrine cell hyperplasia of
    infancy (NEHI), 381, 381f
Neurofibroma, 336
Neurofibromatosis type 1 (NF1), 52f,
    240, 242f, 525
Nodular fasciitis, 334–335
    imaging appearances, 334–335
    manifestations, 334
Nonaccidental spinal injury, 590, 591f
Nonaccidental trauma, 4, 6f, 416–417,
    417t
Nonaggressive lesions, bone, 288b
Nonbilious vomiting
    hypertrophic pyloric stenosis (HPS),
        86–87, 90f
    intermittent, 88–89
    upper gastrointestinal series, 91–93,
        92f
Noncommitted ventricular septal defects-
    type double-outlet right ventricle, 70
Nongerm cell tumors, 166–167
Non-Hodgkin lymphoma (NHL),
    144–146, 542
Nonorganic foreign bodies, 20
Nonseminomatous germ cell tumors,
    142–143
Nontwisted spermatic cord
    decreased vascularity, 162–163
    increased vascularity
        epididymo-orchitis, 161
        orchitis, 162
        torsion-detorsion sequence, 162
    normal testicular vascularity
        acute idiopathic scrotal edema, 160
        blue dot sign, 156
        epididymitis, 156–159
        fountain sign, 160
        Henoch-Schönlein purpura (HSP),
            160
        hydrocele and appendix testis, 156,
            160f
        idiopathic scrotal fat necrosis, 160
        Kawasaki disease, 160
        testicular appendage torsion, 156
        torsion-detorsion sequence, 160
Normally related great arteries (NRGAs),
    58

Nuclear medicine bone scan
    fibrous dysplasia (FD), 304
    osteomyelitis, 295–296
Nursemaid's elbow, 270–271, 271b

O
Obstructed bowel, 390–391, 390f
    haustral folds, 390
    high bowel obstruction, 391–392
    low obstruction, 390–391
    proximal point, 391
Obstruction, gas pattern, 100
Obstructive/nonobstructive process, 475,
    476f
Occipital osteodiastasis, 589–590
Occipitofrontal diameter (OFD), 474
OCD. See Osteochondritis dissecans (OCD)
Ocular masses
    anatomy, 523f
    Coats disease, 524, 524f
    iris, 524
    optic nerve glioma, 525, 525f
    PHPV, 524, 524f
    retina with calcifications, 522–523, 523f
    retina without calcifications, 523–524
    retinal detachment, 524
Odontoid fractures, 573
OFD. See Occipitofrontal diameter
    (OFD); Osteofibrous dysplasia
    (OFD)
OI. See Osteogenesis imperfecta (OI)
Olecranon fractures, 276
Oligohydramnios, 467
Ollier disease, 306
Omphalocele, cloacal exstrophy,
    imperforate anus, and spinal
    dysraphism (OEIS), 461–462, 464f,
    466f
Optic nerve glioma, 525, 525f
Oral cavity masses, 535
Orchitis, 162
Os odontoideum, 574, 575
Ossification patterns
    C1 (atlas), 552–553, 555f–556f, 555b
    C2 (axis), 553, 556f–557f
    C3-C7 vertebrae, 554, 557f–558f
Osteoblastoma, 309–310, 309f, 537–538,
    606–607
Osteochondritis dissecans (OCD),
    283–284, 284f
Osteofibrous dysplasia (OFD), 289
    adamantinoma, 298
    bubbly lesion, 297f
    MRI, 297–298
Osteogenesis imperfecta (OI), 242–246,
    250f–251f, 424, 426f
Osteoid osteoma, 221b, 308–310, 309f,
    606, 609f
Osteomyelitis, 289, 425, 426f
    infants and toddlers
        Brodie abscess, 295
        chronic osteomyelitis, 296
        hematogenous bacterial seeding, 295
        juxtacortical and/or periarticular soft
            tissue edema, 295
        nuclear medicine bone scan,
            295–296
        osseous infection site, 295
        osteolysis and periosteal reaction, 295
        septic arthritis, 295
        subperiosteal purulent debris, 296
    limping child, 220, 226b

Osteopetrosis, 246, 252f
Osteosarcoma, 537
  bone metaphysis, 289
    adventitial bursa formation, 302
    dysplasia epiphysealis hemimelica, 302
    monostotic, 302
    osteochondromas, 302
    pedunculated osteochondroma, 302, 303f
    pseudoaneurysm formation, 302
    sites of occurrence, 302
    vascular compression, 302
Outflow tract anomalies
  double-outlet right ventricle
    clinical presentation, 70
    diagnosis, 70
    imaging, 70
    incidence, 69–70
    morphology, 70
    subtypes, 69–70
    treatment, 70–71
  tetralogy of fallot (TOF)
    clinical presentation, 68
    imaging, 68–69
    incidence, 68
    morphology, 68
    pathophysiology, 68
    prevalence, 68
    treatment, 69
  transposition of the great arteries (TGA), 65–68
    cardiac magnetic resonance, 66f–67f
    clinical manifestations, 67
    imaging, 67
    incidence, 65–67
    morphology and pathophysiology, 67
    treatment, 68
Ovarian cyst, 467, 468f
  functional cyst, 195–196
  hemorrhagic cyst, 195–196, 196f–197f
  simple cyst, 196
  treatment, 196
Ovarian masses, 130
Ovarian torsion
  adnexal torsion, 196–197
  calcification, 197–198, 200f–201f
  clinical presentation, 196–197
  echogenicities and mural nodule, 201f
  enlarged ovary, 198–199, 203f
  enlarged ovary with peripheral follicles, 199, 206f
  extraadnexal position, 198–199, 204f
  hemorrhagic cyst, 197, 199f
  hemorrhagic ovarian cyst, 205f
  ligaments, 197
  polycystic ovary syndrome (PCOS), 198–199, 204f
  teratoma, 197–198, 200f, 202f
Overexposure, digital radiography, 371

P
Painless scrotal swelling, 163b
Pancreas divisum, 116, 117f
Pancreatitis
  abdominal radiographs, 113–115, 116f
  acute-on-chronic, 117f
  chronic, 115
  clinical symptoms, 113
  computed tomography, 115, 116f
  etiologies, 113

Pancreatitis (Continued)
  MRCP, 116
  MRI findings, 115
  ultrasound, 115
Panner disease, 283–284, 284f
Papillary muscles, 55–57
Paraadnexal cyst
  fimbrial cyst, 199–200
  hydrosalpinx and mesosalpinx, 200
  isolated tubal torsion, 200, 207f
  paraovarian cysts, 199–200
  torsed cyst, 199–200
Paraovarian cysts, 199–200
Parapneumonic effusion, 19f–20f
Paratesticular rhabdomyosarcoma, 165, 166f
Parenchymal brain injury, 404–405, 406f–407f
Parenchymal contusions, 405, 406f
Pars interarticularis fracture, 569f, 570
Partial testicular torsion, 154, 157f
Patent ductus arteriosus, 359, 360f
Patlak number, 178
Pedunculated osteochondroma, 303f
Pelvic congestion syndrome, 208, 209b
Pelvic inflammatory disease, pelvic pain, 203–204, 209b
Pelvic involvement, skeletal dysplasias, 242, 246f
Pelvic pain
  chronic, 205
  ectopic pregnancy, 204–205
  endometriosis, 205
  gynecological causes, 196b
  imperforate hymen, 200–202
  müllerian duct anomalies (MDAs), 202, 208f
  obstructed hemivagina, 203
  ovarian cyst
    functional cyst, 195–196
    hemorrhagic cyst, 195–196, 196f–197f
    simple cyst, 196
    treatment, 196
  ovarian torsion
    adnexal torsion, 196–197
    calcification, 197–198, 200f–201f
    clinical presentation, 196–197
    echogenicities and mural nodule, 201f
    enlarged ovary, 198–199, 203f
    enlarged ovary with peripheral follicles, 199, 206f
    extraadnexal position, 198–199, 204f
    hemorrhagic cyst, 197, 199f
    hemorrhagic ovarian cyst, 205f
    ligaments, 197
    polycystic ovary syndrome (PCOS), 198–199, 204f
    teratoma, 197–198, 200f, 202f
  paraadnexal cyst
    fimbrial cyst, 199–200
    hydrosalpinx and mesosalpinx, 200
    isolated tubal torsion, 200, 207f
    paraovarian cysts, 199–200
    torsed cyst, 199–200
  pelvic congestion syndrome, 208, 209b
  pelvic inflammatory disease, 203–204, 209b
  renal agenesis, 203
  ultrasound, 195

Penumbra sign, 295
Perimembranous ventricular septal defects (VSDs), 62
Periosteal chondromas, 310
Periosteal reaction, bone lesions
  aggressive forms, 290, 291f
  nonaggressive forms, 290, 290f
Periostitis, 425–427, 427f–428f
Peritoneal calcification, 392–393, 392f
Periureteral diverticula, 182
Periventricular leukoencephalopathy, 365–366
Permeative bone destruction, 291
Persistent hyperplastic primary vitreous (PHPV), 524
Pes cavus deformity, 256, 259f
Pes planus deformity, 256, 259f
Pfeiffer syndrome, 236
Phlebectasia, 325f
Phleboliths, 333, 333f
Physeal fractures, 222b, 348–349, 349f
Physis, 347
Pierre Robin sequence, 238–239
Pigmented villonodular synovitis (PVNS), 330
Pitch, 437–438, 438f
Placenta previa, 447–448, 448f
Plain radiographs
  appendicitis, 106–107
  Cervical spine. See Cervical spine (C-spine)
  gastroenteritis, 108–109
  limping child, 213–214
  limping child osteomyelitis, 226
  Meckel diverticulum, 109
  musculoskeletal (MSK) trauma, 346
Planovalgus deformity, 261, 262f
Plantar arch alignment, 256, 257t, 259f
Plastic bending fractures, 224
PLB. See Primary lymphoma of bone (PLB)
Pleural effusions, 6, 9f, 453–454
Pleuropulmonary blastoma, 452
Plexiform neurofibroma, 336, 544, 545f
Pneumatosis, 360b
Pneumococcal pneumonia, 14–15
Pneumomediastinum, 357–358, 359f, 381–382, 382f
Pneumonia, 16, 21f
  alba, 380
  neonatal, 379–380
Pneumoperitoneum, 360b
Pneumothorax, 357–358, 359f
  management, 27
  physical examination, 27
  spontaneous, 26–27
  supine radiographs, 10f
  tension, 27, 32f
  unilateral, 27
Poland syndrome, 382
Popliteal cysts, 328–329, 330f
Porencephalic cysts, 478, 478f
Portal venous gas, 360b
Posterior atlantooccipital (PAO) membrane, 556
Posterior fossa, 405
  brainstem "kinking", 484, 484f
  cerebellar hemispheres, 483
  cystic enlargement, 481–482
  torcular herophili, 482, 482f
  vermis normal, 482–483, 483f
Posterior urethral valves (PUV), 188
Posthemorrhagic hydrocephalus, 365

Postintubation subglottic narrowing, 519
Powers ratio, 563, 563f
Preterm infant
    brain
        magnetic resonance imaging (MRI), 361
        ultrasound technique, 361–366
    gastrointestinal, 359–361
    lung opacities
        neonatal chronic lung disease (CLD), 358
        patent ductus arteriosus, 359
        respiratory distress syndrome (RDS), 357
        umbilical arterial catheters (UACs), 355–356
        umbilical venous catheters (UVCs), 355
Prevertebral soft tissues, 513
Primary lymphangiectasia, 452, 455f
Primary lymphoma of bone (PLB), 301
    cortical disruption, 301
    CT, 301
    MRI, 301, 301f
    osseous lesions, 301
    sclerotic reactive bone, 301
    soft tissue extension, 301
Prominent diaphyseal involvement, 239–240, 239f–241f
Prominent epiphyseal involvement, 240, 244f
Prominent metaphyseal involvement, 240, 243f
Prune belly syndrome, 188–189, 193f, 463–464
Pseudocysts, pancreatitis, 115–116
Pseudosubluxation, 560
Pulmonary agenesis, 383
Pulmonary aplasia, 383
Pulmonary artery abnormality, 383–384
Pulmonary fissures, 10f
Pulmonary hemorrhage, surfactant administration, 358f
Pulmonary hypoplasia, 380–381, 383
Pulmonary interstitial emphysema (PIE), 357–358, 359f
Pulmonary interstitial glycogenosis, 381
Pulmonary parenchymal masses, 33
Pulmonary sequestration, 452, 456f
Pulmonary sling, 382
Pulmonary vascularity
    asymmetrical smaller lung, 382–385
    bronchopulmonary sequestration (BPS), 386–387, 387f–388f
    cardiac catheterization, 377–378
    congenital diaphragmatic hernia (CDH), 387–388, 389f
    congenital pulmonary airway malformation, 385–386
    congenitally hyperlucent lung, 381–382
    diffuse granular hazy appearance, 378
    esophageal atresia, 388–389, 390f
    pulmonary artery abnormality, 383–384
    pulmonary venous abnormality, 384–385
    reticular pattern
        altered fluid dynamics, 378–379
        infection, 379–380
        interstitial lung disease (ILD), 380–381, 381f
        meconium aspiration syndrome, 380, 382f
    vascular resistance, 378

Pulmonary venous abnormality, 384–385
Pulmonary vessels and bronchi, 7–8
Purulent pericarditis, 41f
PVNS. See Pigmented villonodular synovitis (PVNS)
Pyknodysostosis, 237
Pylorospasm-simulating hypertrophic pyloric stenosis, 96f
Pyogenic granuloma, 340
Pyogenic thymic abscess, 39–40

Q
Qualified Medical Physicist (QMP), 431

R
Radial head dislocations, 277, 279f, 279b
Radial head fractures, 276
Radial head subluxation, 270–271, 271b
Radial neck fractures, 275, 276f, 277b
Radiation therapy brain effects, 504, 504f
Radiocapitellar line (RCL), 270, 271f
Radiographs. See also Plain radiographs; Chest radiographs
    abdominal pain. See Abdominal pain
    back pain
        computed tomography (CT), 594
        disk calcification, 595–596, 599f
        disk cysts, 601, 601f
        disk degeneration and herniation, 600
        magnetic resonance imaging (MRI), 594
        sacral meningocele, 598–600, 600f
        scheuermann disease/kyphosis, 596–598, 599f
        spondylolysis and spondylolisthesis, 594–595, 595f–598f
Ranulas, 536, 536f
RCL. See Radiocapitellar line (RCL)
RDS. See Respiratory distress syndrome (RDS)
Reactive airways disease, 11–12
Redundant duodenum, 91, 92f
Reflux, 179
Relapsing polychondritis, 519
Renal cell carcinoma, MRI, 140, 141f
Renal masses, 128–129
    children older than 1 year
        nephroblastomatosis, 137–140, 139f
        renal tumors, 140
        Wilms tumors, 136–137
    neonates/infants
        hydronephrosis, 128
        neoplasms, 129, 129f
Renal medullary carcinoma, 140
Respiratory distress
    clinical characteristics, 3
    older child and adolescent
        acute chest syndrome (ACS), 21–22
        community-acquired pneumonia, 20–21
        cystic fibrosis (CF), 23–26
        spontaneous pneumothorax, 26–27
    toddler and young child, 8–20
        airways, 10
        infections, 12–13, 13t
        reactive airways disease/asthma, 11–12
Respiratory distress syndrome (RDS), 357, 357f–358f
    air leak complications, 357–358
    treatment, 357

Respiratory infections
    age group, 13t
    aspirated foreign body, 19–20
    bacterial pneumonia, 14–19
    viral bronchiolitis, 14, 14f
Retinal hemorrhages (RHs), 406, 408f
Retinoblastoma, 522–523, 523f
Retinoschisis, 408f
Retroclival subdural/epidural collections, 404
Retroperitoneal extragonadal germ cell tumors, 142–143
Retropharyngeal abscess, 514, 515f, 545, 546f
Rhabdoid tumor, 142f
Rhabdomyosarcoma, 144, 336, 337f
Rhombencephalosynapsis, 483f
RHs. See Retinal hemorrhages (RHs)
Rib lesions, 288b
Rickets, 424, 424f–425f
Risk management
    benefits, 439
    challenging, 439–440
    dose, 439–440
    graphical representation, 440, 440f
Rocker-bottom deformity, 256, 259f
Round pneumonia, 14–15, 17f

S
Sacral meningocele, 598–600, 600f
Sacrococcygeal teratoma (SCTs), 135–136, 137f
Sad sausages, obstruction, 102f
Salter-Harris classification of fracture
    distal femur, 350f–351f
    distal tibia, 350f
    proximal tibia, 350f
Scheuermann disease/kyphosis, 596–598, 599f
Schizencephaly, 502, 503f
Schwannoma, 49
Scimitar syndrome, 384–385, 384f
Scintigraphy
    limping child infection, 226–227
    neuroblastoma, 294–295
SCIWORA. See Spinal cord injury without radiographic abnormality (SCIWORA)
Scrotal trauma, 162
Scrotal ultrasound
    acute scrotum, 154
        anatomy and appearance, 153f
        diagnostic work-up, 152–154
        differential diagnosis, 155t
        nontwisted spermatic cord. See Nontwisted spermatic cord
        normal spermatic cord, 153f
        technetium-99m scrotal scintigraphy, 151
        testicles, 151–152
    scrotal pain and swelling
        extratesticular cystic lesions, 163–165
        extratesticular solid lesions, 165–166
        intratesticular cystic lesions, 166
        intratesticular solid lesions, 166–170
    twisted spermatic cord, 154–155
SCTs. See Sacrococcygeal teratoma (SCTs)
Scurvy, 424–425, 426f
SDH. See Subdural hematoma (SDH)
Segmental bacterial pneumonia, 17f

Septal defects
    atrial septal defects (ASDs)
        cardiac magnetic resonance (CMR), 60–61, 61f
        clinical presentation, 60
        echocardiography, 60
        morphology, 60
        pathophysiology, 60
        primum, 60
        secundum, 60
        sinus venosus defects, 60
        treatment, 61–62
    atrioventricular septal defects (AVSDs)
        clinical presentation, 65
        complete, 64
        imaging, 65, 65f–66f
        incidence, 64
        incomplete, 64
        morphology and pathophysiology, 64–65
        transitional, 64
        treatment, 65
    interatrial communications, 60
    ventricular septal defects (VSDs)
        incidence, 62
        morphology and pathophysiology, 62–63
Septic arthritis, 225, 226b, 229
Septo-optic dysplasia, 502, 503f
Septophobic mitral valve (MV), 57
Sequential segmental approach, congenital heart disease (CHD), 54, 54f
Serpiginous calcification, myositis ossificans, 331, 332f
Shock syndrome, 419, 420f
Shone complex
    clinical presentation, 73
    complete form, 72–73
    imaging, 73
    incomplete form, 72–73
    morphology, 73
    pathophysiology, 73
    treatment, 73
Shouldering, subglottic trachea, 3, 4f
Sigmoid volvulus, 104, 105f
Simple ureteroceles, 185
Sinonasal masses
    nasofrontal masses
        brain tissue, 531–532, 532f
        encephalocele, 531, 531f
        fonticulus frontalis, 531
        hypervascular, 532
        sinus tract/inclusion cyst, 532
    nasopharynx masses, 533–535, 534f–535f
    sinus masses, 532–533, 533f
Sinonasal polyp, 532, 533f
Sinovenous thrombosis, 494–496, 495f
Sinus masses, 532–533, 533f
Sinus pericranii, 506, 506f
Sinus tract/inclusion cyst, 532
Size-specific dose estimate (SSDE), 432–433
Skeletal dysplasias
    bone mineral density, 236, 244–246, 252f
    classification systems, 235
    clinical information, 236
    clinical suspicion, 235
    differential diagnosis, 235
    extraosseous organ involvement, 242–244, 249f–251f

Skeletal dysplasias (Continued)
    extremities
        prominent diaphyseal involvement, 239–240, 239f–241f
        prominent epiphyseal involvement, 240, 244f
        prominent metaphyseal involvement, 240, 243f
    head, 235
    length, 235–236
    mimickers, 246, 253f
    pelvic involvement, 236, 242, 246f
    predominant skull involvement, 236–239, 237f–238f
    spine involvement, 236, 242, 247f
    thoracic involvement, 241–242, 245f
Skewfoot, 259–261, 261f
Skin and subcutaneous fat
    hamartoma, 339–340
    lipoblastoma, 339, 341f
    lipoma, 339, 340f
    liposarcoma, 339
    trauma
        hematoma, 338–339
        subcutaneous fat necrosis, 338
Skin-covered dysraphias, 579–581
Skull fractures, 398–399, 399f–400f
Slipped capital femoral epiphysis (SCFE), 213, 230, 230b
Soft tissue injuries, 413, 414f, 418–421, 419f–420f
Soft tissue masses
    anesthesia and surgical procedures, 327
    articular/periarticular mass
        appearance, 328
        Baker cyst, 328–329
        gadolinium contrast agent, 330–331
        ganglion cysts, 328
        giant cell tumor of the tendon sheath (GCTTS), 330
        meniscal cyst, 329
        pigmented villonodular synovitis (PVNS), 330
        synovial cysts, 328–329
        synovial sarcoma, 330–331
        synovial venous malformations, 329–330
    calcification
        alveolar soft part sarcoma (ASPA), 333
        myositis ossificans (MO), 331
        venous malformations, 333, 333f
    central cystic necrosis, 334
    imaging, 327
    infantile fibrosarcoma, 335
    infantile myofibroma, 334
    magnetic resonance imaging (MRI), 328
    nerve sheath tumors, 336–338
    nodular fasciitis, 334–335
    pathology, 327
    radiographs, 327
    rhabdomyosarcoma, 336, 337f
    skin and subcutaneous fat
        hamartoma, 339–340
        hematoma, 338–339
        lipoblastoma, 339, 341f
        lipoma, 339, 340f
        liposarcoma, 339
    subcutaneous fat necrosistorticollis, 333, 334f, 338
    ultrasound (US), 327–328
    vascular lesions, high-flow, 340–343

Solitary arterial trunk, 58
Solitary myofibroma, 334
Spermatoceles, 164–165
Spinal column tumors
    aneurysmal bone cyst (ABC), 605–606, 608f
    Ewing sarcoma, 607, 609f
    Langerhans cell histiocytosis (LCH), 604–605, 606f–607f
    leukemia and lymphoma, 607–608, 610f
    osteoblastoma, 606–607
    osteoid osteoma, 606, 609f
Spinal cord, 413, 414f
Spinal cord injury without radiographic abnormality (SCIWORA), 552
Spinal fractures, 411–413, 411f–413f
Spinal meningiomas, 611–612, 613f
Spinal schwannomas, 611, 612f
Spine, fetal
    abruptly, 489
    fluid-filled sac anterior, 489
    segment, 489
Spine lesions, 288b
Splenic Injury Scale, 124t
Split-fat sign, schwannoma, 336, 337f
Spondylodiskitis, 601–602, 602f–603f
Spondyloepiphyseal dysplasia, 242, 247f
Spondylolisthesis, 594–595, 595f–598f
Spondylolysis, 594–595, 595f–598f
Spontaneous pneumothorax, 26–27, 31f–32f
Spurious pneumothorax, 372f
SSDE. See Size-specific dose estimate (SSDE)
Staphylococcal pneumonia, 14–15
Stepladder configuration, obstruction, 102f
Sterile parapneumonic effusion, 15–16
Sternal ossification centers, 371f
Sternocleidomastoid muscle, 542
Stertor, 10, 12t
Stridor, 10, 12t
Sturge-Weber syndrome, 505, 505f
Subarachnoid hemorrhage, 404
Subaxial C3-C7 fractures, 573
Subdural hematoma (SDH), 398, 398f
    abusive head trauma (AHT)
        appearance, 400–402, 401f–403f
        birth-related SDHs, 404
        causes, 400, 401f
        characteristics, 404
        convexity, 404
        enlarged low-density extraaxial spaces, 404
        hematohygromas, 402–403, 405f
        heterogeneous-appearing, 403–404
        injury dating, 404
        membrane, 404
        retroclival subdural/epidural collections, 404
    abusive spine trauma, 413
Subfalcine herniation, 497–498, 498f
Subglottic airway, 512–513, 513f
Subperiosteal purulent debris, 296
Supracondylar fracture, 272, 272f–273f, 273b
Supracondylar process, 279–280, 281f
Suprasternal fossa, 377, 377f
Surfactant deficiency syndrome, 357, 357f–358f

Swiss cheese defect, 63–64
Swyer-James syndrome, 382–383
Synchondrosal fractures, 570–573, 570f–571f
Synovial sarcoma
    clinical manifestation, 330
    juxtaarticular location, 330–331
    magnetic resonance imaging (MRI), 331
    ultrasound, 332f
Synovial venous malformations, 329–330
Synovitis, 229
Syphilitic pneumonia, 380

T

T cell lymphoblastic lymphoma, 44f
Tachypnea, 14
Talipes equinovarus, 469, 470f
Target sign sign, schwannoma, 336, 337f
Tarsal coalition, 262, 265f
TCD. See Transverse cerebellar dimension (TCD)
Tectorial membrane, 556
Tension pneumothorax, 27, 32f
Teratoma, 143, 168f, 487, 487f
Testicular torsion, 154, 156f
    acute, 156f
    intermittent, 155, 155b
    partial, 157f
Testicular tumors, 166–170
Testis
    adrenal rests, 169f, 170
    fracture, 162
    hematomas, 162
    rupture, 162–163
Tet spells, 69
Tetralogy of fallot (TOF)
    clinical presentation, 68
    imaging
        CT and CMR, 69, 69f
        CXR, 68
        echocardiography, 68–69
    incidence, 68
    morphology, 68
    pathophysiology, 68
    prevalence, 68
    treatment, 69
Tetralogy-type double-outlet right ventricle, 70
TGA. See Transposition of the great arteries (TGA)
Thanatophoric dysplasia, 239, 240f, 469, 469f
The Battered-Child Syndrome, 416
Thoracic involvement, 241–242, 245f
Thoracic neuroblastoma, 50f
Thoracic vertebral body compression fractures, 411, 411f
Thoracoabdominal visceral arrangement, 55, 56f–57f
Thoracolumbar injury, 590
Thorax
    airway narrowing
        fluoroscopic finding, 372–373
        multidetector computed tomography (CT), 373–374
        tracheal stenosis, 374, 375f
        tracheomalacia, 374
    cardiac position, 457
    clavicle abnormalities, 372, 374f
    congenital diaphragmatic hernia, 454–457, 457f, 457b

Thorax (Continued)
    determination, 457
    diffuse T2 hyperintensity, 451–452, 454t, 455f
    esophageal atresia, 457–458, 459f
    focal signal abnormalities, 452–453, 455f–456f
    imaging pitfalls
        oblique fissure, 376, 377f
        retrosternal triangular density, 376–377
        suprasternal fossa, 377, 377f
    normal fetal thorax, 451, 454f
    pleural effusions, 453–454
    pulmonary vascularity, 377–389
    radiograph
        collimation, 369
        exposure factors, 371
        humeral ossification centers, 372, 373f
        lordotic projection, 370t
        mesenchymal hamartoma, 373f
        patient positioning, 369, 370f
        projection/angulation, 369, 369f
        respiration, 369–370, 371f
    thymus
        ductus bump, 375
        inferior margin, 375
        MRI, 375
        tethered cord, 376f
        ultrasound, 375
    tracheal buckling, 372
Thymic cysts, 540
Thymic rebound, 5
Thymolipoma, 41
Thymoma
    invasive, 38
    myasthenia, 37–38, 40f
    noninvasive type A, 38
Thymus, 5, 9f
    aberrant, 36–37, 36f
    abscess, 39–40
    carcinoma, 39
    cysts, 37
    ectopic, 36–37
    epithelial tumors, 37–39, 38f–39f
    hyperplasia, 37, 37f
    Langerhans cell histiocytosis, 41
    lipoma, 41
    normal
        computed tomography (CT), 35f
        magnetic resonance imaging, 36f
        radiographs, 35f
        ultrasound, 35f
Thyroglossal duct cyst, 539, 539f
Toddler fracture, 222–223, 224b
TOF. See Tetralogy of fallot (TOF)
Tonsillar herniation, 498, 498f
Tonsillar/peritonsillar abscesses, 544–545
Tonsils, 512–514, 514f
TORCH infections, pneumonia, 380
Torcular herophili, 482, 482f
Torsion-detorsion sequence
    nontwisted spermatic cord, 162
    testicular torsion, 155, 155b, 159f
Torticollis
    fibromatosis colli, 333
    MRI, 333
    ultrasound, 333, 334f
Toulouse-Lautrec syndrome, 237
Toxic synovitis, 229
Toxocara endophthalmitis, 523–524
Trachea evaluation, 3, 4f

Tracheal buckling, 372
Tracheal disease, 519
Tracheal stenosis, 374
    long-segment, 374
    short-segment, 374
Tracheobronchomalacia, 10
Tracheomalacia, 372–374
Transient synovitis, 229
Transient tachypnea of the newborn (TTN), 378–379
Transphyseal distal humeral fractures, 275–276, 277f–278f
Transposition of the great arteries (TGA), 65–68
    cardiac magnetic resonance, 66f–67f
    clinical manifestations, 67
    imaging, 67
    incidence, 65–67
    management, 68
    morphology and pathophysiology, 67
    treatment, 68
Transposition-type double-outlet right ventricle, 70
Transverse cerebellar dimension (TCD), 474, 474f
Transverse ligament, 555, 559f
Trauma
    abdominal pain, 121–124
    limping child, 221–224
    scrotal, 162
    skin and subcutaneous fat, 338–339
Traumatic spondylolysis, 412, 413f
Trendelenburg gait, 213
Trevor- Fairbank disease, 302
Tricuspid valve (TV), 55–57
Truncal vascular malformations, 318
Truncus arteriosus, 58
TS. See Tuberous sclerosis (TS)
Tuberous sclerosis (TS), 481, 481f
Twin-twin transfusion syndrome, 470
Twisted spermatic cord, 154–155
Typical hemolytic uremic syndrome (HUS), 118

U

UACs. See Umbilical arterial catheters (UACs)
UBCs. See Unicameral bone cyst (UBCs)
Ultrasound (US)
    abusive head trauma (AHT), 409
    appendicitis, 107–108, 108f
    hamartoma, 339–340, 342f
    Henoch-Schönlein purpura (HSP), 118, 119f
    infantile hemangioma (IH), 340, 342f
    intussusception, 106, 107f
    limping child, 215–217, 217b, 218f
    lipoma, 339
    lymphatic malformation, 344
    lymphoma, 144
    Meckel diverticulum, 109, 111f
    musculoskeletal (MSK) trauma, 346
    neonatal spine
        congenital caudal tumor, 584–585, 586f
        development, 578
        "duplicated"/widened spinal canal, 586–587, 586f–588f
        focal scoliosis/hyperkyphosis, 588–589, 589f
        hypoplastic lower extremities, 583–584, 584f–586f

Ultrasound (US) (Continued)
  midline fluid-discharging skin pit, 581–583, 583f
  nonaccidental spinal injury, 590, 591f
  non-skin-covered bump/lesion, 578–579, 579f–581f
  sacral dimple, 578
  skin-covered bump/lesion, 579–581, 582f
  spinal abnormalities, 589
  spinal injury, 589–590, 590f
  nephroblastomatosis, 139f
  osteosarcoma, 300
  pancreatitis, 115
  pediatric elbow, 267
  pyelonephritis, 113f
  rhabdoid tumor, 142f
  rhabdomyosarcoma, 145f
  soft tissue masses, 327–328
    rhabdomyosarcoma, 336, 337f
    synovial sarcoma, 332f
    torticollis, 333, 334f
    venous malformation, 333, 333f–334f
  urinary tract dilation (UTD). See Urinary tract dilation (UTD)
  vascular malformations
    arteriovenous fistulas (AVFs), 322f
    arteriovenous malformations (AVMs), 321f, 321t
    macrocystic lymphatic malformations (LMs), 316f
    venous malformations (VMs), 318f
Umbilical arterial catheters (UACs)
  chronic lung disease (CLD), 358
  course, 355–356
  patent ductus arteriosus, 359
  respiratory distress syndrome (RDS), 357, 357f–358f
Umbilical venous catheters (UVCs)
  appropriate positioning, 356f
  malposition, 356f–357f
Unicameral bone cyst (UBCs), 310–311
Unilateral pneumothorax, 27
Unilateral ventriculomegaly, 480, 480f
UPJO. See Ureteropelvic junction obstruction (UPJO)
Upper airway obstruction, 10
Ureteral duplication, 185
Ureterocele, 185, 190f
Ureteropelvic junction obstruction (UPJO)
  diuretic renography, 180
  Hynes-Anderson pyeloplasty, 184f
Urinary tract dilation (UTD)
  bladder outlet obstructions, 186–191
  causes, 171
  classification system, 171, 172f–173f
  computed tomography (CT), 179
  differential diagnosis, 179–191
  duplex kidneys, 183–184, 188f–189f
  dynamic renal scintigraphy, 174f, 177f–178f
  ectopic ureters, 183–184
  hydronephrosis, 180
  hydroureteronephrosis, 180–182
  magnetic resonance urography, 177–178, 179f
  ultrasound
    central and peripheral calyces, 173–174, 174f

hypoechoic pyramid versus dilated calyx, 173f
    kidneys, 173f–174f
    normal ureteral jets, 174
    normal-appearing bladder, 176f
    oliguria, 171
    prenatal hydronephrosis, 171
    renal parenchyma, 173
    trabeculated bladder, 176f
    vesicoureteral reflux (VUR), 173–174, 175f
  ureteral duplication, 185
  ureterocele, 185, 190f
  vesicoureteral reflux, 178–179
  wall chart, 172f–173f
Urinary tract infections (UTIs)
  bladder wall thickening, 111
  CT/MRI findings, 111
  pyelonephritis, 111, 113f
  scintigraphy, 112
  uncomplicated cystitis, 111
  urinalysis, 110
US Child Protective Services (CPS), 416
UTD. See Urinary tract dilation (UTD)
Uterine masses, 131
UVCs. See Umbilical venous catheters (UVCs)

V
Vallecular cyst, 515
Varicoceles, 165, 165f
Vascular lesions
  high-flow
    arteriovenous malformations (AVMs), 343
    infantile hemangioma (IH), 340
    kaposiform hemangioendothelioma (KHE), 341–343, 344f
    malformations, 340
    rapidly involuting congenital hemangioma (RICH), 340–341, 344f
  slow-flow, 343–344
Vascular malformations
  channel-type, 318
  combined, 318, 323t
  computed tomographic angiography (CTA), 313
  magnetic resonance imaging (MRI), 313, 314t
  major named vessels, 323f
  overgrowth vascular anomaly syndromes, 318
  simple
    arteriovenous fistulas (AVFs), 318
    arteriovenous malformations (AVMs), 316–317, 320f–321f
    capillary malformations (CMs), 313
    lymphatic malformations, 314–315
    venous malformations (VMs), 315–316, 317f–319f
  ultrasound, 313, 314t
  vascular anomalies, 318
Vascular nidus, 484–485
Vascular rings
  clinical presentation, 76
  imaging, 76, 76f
  morphology and pathophysiology, 76
  and slings, 12f, 47–48, 47f
  treatment, 76
Vein of Galen malformation (VOGM), 484–485, 485f

Venolymphatic malformation, 487, 487f
Venous malformations (VMs), 333, 333f, 343–344
  dilated venous varicosities, 317f
  infantile hemangioma, 316
  low-flow malformations, 315–316
  MRI, 333
  natural history, 316
  physical examination, 316
  sonographic findings, 333, 334f
  thrombophlebitis and coagulopathy, 316
Ventricular identification, 55–57, 57f
Ventricular septal defects (VSDs)
  clinical presentation, 63
  doubly committed, 63
  imaging
    CT and CMR, 63–64
    echocardiography, 63
  incidence, 62
  inlet, 62–63
  malalignment, 62–63
  morphology and pathophysiology, 62–63
  muscular, 62–63
  perimembranous, 62–63
  size, 63
  treatment, 64
Ventricular septal defects-type double-outlet right ventricle, 70
Ventricular topology/looping, 57, 58f
Ventriculoarterial connections, 59
Ventriculomegaly
  causes of, 475, 475t
  cavum septum pellucidum, 478
  central gray matter, 476–478, 477f
  corpus callosum, 475–476, 476f–477f
  cortical irregularity, 479, 479f
  hemimegalencephaly, 479–480, 480f
  lobar cerebral brain parenchyma, 478–479, 478f–479f
  normal signal intensity, 480–481, 481f
  obstructive/nonobstructive, 475, 476f
  right and left cerebral hemispheres, 476–478, 477f
  solid and cystic intracranial mass, 481
  unilateral ventriculomegaly, 480, 480f
  value of, 475
  ventricle margins smooth, 480–481, 481f
Vesicoureteral reflux (VUR), 173–174, 175f, 178–179
  contrast-enhanced voiding urosonography, 180f–182f
  hydroureteronephrosis, 182
  International Reflux Study grading system, 182f
  radionuclide cystogram (RNC), 180f–182f
  voiding cystourethrogram (VCUG), 180f–182f
Viral bronchiolitis, 14, 14f
Visceral pleura, 7
Visceroatrial arrangement/situs, 55, 56f–57f
Vitamin C deficiency, 246
Vitamin D deficiency, 246
VMs. See Venous malformations (VMs)
VOGM. See Vein of Galen malformation (VOGM)

Vomiting infant
    annular pancreas, 83, 85f
    bilious vomiting
        bedside upper gastrointestinal series,
            90–91, 91f
        midgut malrotation, 82, 83f–84f
        newborn infant, 81–86
        obstruction, 82
    causes, 97t
    colonic atresia, 84, 87f
    distal obstruction, 84–86, 86f
    duodenal stenosis and atresia, 82–83,
        84f
    duodenal web, 82–83, 85f
    functional immaturity of the colon,
        84–85, 88f
    Hirschsprung disease, 86, 89f
    ileal atresia, 84, 87f
    imaging evaluation, 81

Vomiting infant (Continued)
    imaging techniques
        abdominal radiograph, 89–90, 90f
        abdominal ultrasound, 93–94
        contrast enema, 93, 93f
        gastroesophageal reflux, 94
        midgut malrotation, 94
        pyloric stenosis, 93f–96f, 94–96
        upper gastrointestinal series,
            90–93
    jejunal atresia, 84, 86f
    meconium ileus, 85, 88f
    nonbilious vomiting
        hypertrophic pyloric stenosis (HPS),
            86–87, 90f
        intermittent, 88–89
        upper gastrointestinal series, 91–93,
            92f
    preduodenal location, portal vein, 83

Von Recklinghausen disease, 240
VSDs. *See* Ventricular septal defects
    (VSDs)
VUR. *See* Vesicoureteral reflux (VUR)

W
Wackenheim line, 563, 564f
Walker-Warburg syndrome, 484, 484f
Wegener granulomatosis, 519
Wheezing, 12t
Whirlpool sign, testicular torsion, 154
Widened spinal canal, 586–587,
    586f–588f
Wilms tumors, 129, 136–137

Y
Yolk sac tumor, 167, 167f